TABLE OF CONTENTS

Reviewers vii

Foreword xi

Introduction xiii

Studying for the ACE Personal Trainer Exam xvii

PART I – Introduction

Chapter 1 – Role and Scope of Practice for the Personal Trainer *Todd Galati* 3

PART II – Leadership and Implementation

Chapter 2 – Principles of Adherence and Motivation *Tracie Rogers* 25

Chapter 3 – Communication and Teaching Techniques *Barbara A. Brehm* 39

Chapter 4 – Basics of Behavior Change and Health Psychology *Tracie Rogers* 63

PART III – The ACE Integrated Fitness Training™ Model

Chapter 5 – Introduction to the ACE Integrated Fitness Training Model *Todd Galati* 81

Chapter 6 – Building Rapport and the Initial Investigation Stage *Kelly Spivey* 99

Chapter 7 – Functional Assessments: Posture, Movement, Core, Balance, and Flexibility *Fabio Comana* 135

Chapter 8 – Physiological Assessments *Kelly Spivey* 173

Chapter 9 – Functional Programming for Stability-Mobility and Movement *Fabio Comana* . . 245

Chapter 10 – Resistance Training: Programming and Progressions *Wayne Westcott* 311

Chapter 11 – Cardiorespiratory Training: Programming and Progressions *Carl Foster & John P. Porcari* 369

Chapter 12 – The ACE Integrated Fitness Training Model in Practice *Pete McCall* 411

PART IV – Special Exercise Programming Topics

Chapter 13 – Mind-body Exercise *Ralph La Forge* 451

Chapter 14 – Exercise and Special Populations *Brad A. Roy* 479

PART V – Injury Prevention and First Aid

Chapter 15 – Common Musculoskeletal Injuries and Implications for Exercise *Scott Cheatham* 533

Chapter 16 – Emergency Procedures *Julia Valentour* 559

PART VI – Professional and Legal Responsibilities and Business Strategies

Chapter 17 – Legal Guidelines and Professional Responsibilities *Mark S. Nagel* 593

Chapter 18 – Personal-training Business Fundamentals *Pete McCall* 625

Appendix A – ACE Code of Ethics 659

Appendix B – Exam Content Outline 667

Appendix C – ACE Position Statement on Nutritional Supplements 687

Glossary 689

Index 717

ACE Personal Trainer Manual

The Ultimate Resource for Fitness Professionals

Fourth Edition

American Council on Exercise®

Editors

Cedric X. Bryant, Ph.D., FACSM

Daniel J. Green

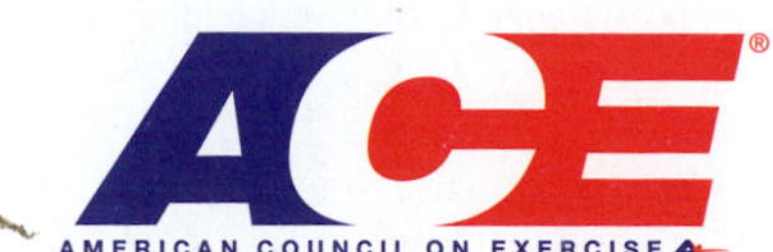

Library of Congress Catalog Card Number: 2009911158

ISBN 9781890720292

Copyright © 2010 American Council on Exercise® (ACE®)

Printed in the United States of America

All rights reserved. Except for use in a review, the reproduction or utilization of this work in any form or by any electronic, mechanical, or other means, now know or hereafter invented, including xerography, photocopying, and recording, and in any information retrieval system, is forbidden without the written permission of the American Council on Exercise.

C D E F G

Distributed by:
American Council on Exercise
4851 Paramount Drive
San Diego, CA 92123
(858) 576-6500
(858) 576-6564 FAX
www.acefitness.org

Project Editor: Daniel J. Green

Technical Editor: Cedric X. Bryant, Ph.D., FACSM

Cover Design & Art Direction: Karen McGuire

Associate Editor: Marion Webb

Special Contributor & Proofreader: Sabrena Merrill, M.S.

Production: Nancy Garcia

Photography: Dennis Dal Covey

Anatomical Illustrations: James Staunton

Index: Kathi Unger

Chapter Models: Doug Balzarini, Fabio Comana, Keith Crockett, Patricia A. Davis, Todd Galati, Jessica Matthews, Alexandra Morrison, Leslie R. Thomas, Julia Valentour, Matthew Zuniga, Randy Zuniga

Acknowledgments:
Thanks to the entire American Council on Exercise staff for their support and guidance through the process of creating this manual.

NOTICE

The fitness industry is ever-changing. As new research and clinical experience broaden our knowledge, changes in programming and standards are required. The authors and the publisher of this work have checked with sources believed to be reliable in their efforts to provide information that is complete and generally in accord with the standards accepted at the time of publication. However, in view of the possibility of human error or changes in industry standards, neither the authors nor the publisher nor any other party who has been involved in the preparation or publication of this work warrants that the information contained herein is in every respect accurate or complete, and they are not responsible for any errors or omissions or the results obtained from the use of such information. Readers are encouraged to confirm the information contained herein with other sources.

P11-015

REVIEWERS

Scott Cheatham, DPT, OCS, ATC, CSCS, PES, is owner of Bodymechanix Sports Medicine & PT. He previously taught at Chapman University and is currently a national presenter. He has authored various manuscripts and has served on the exam committee for the National PT Board Exam and the National Athletic Training Certification Exam. Dr. Cheatham is currently a reviewer for the *Journal of Athletic Training* and *NSCA Strength & Conditioning Journal,* and is on the editorial board for NSCA's *Performance Training Journal.*

Daniel Cipriani, P.T., Ph.D., is a licensed physical therapist and an associate professor in the School of Exercise and Nutritional Sciences at San Diego State University. His areas of teaching and research include applied biomechanics, rehabilitation sciences, and measurement. Prior to his appointment at SDSU, Dr. Cipriani served on the Physical Therapy faculty at the University of Toledo, with a focus on orthopaedic rehabilitation. Dr. Cipriani serves on the editorial boards of the *Journal of Physical Therapy* and the *Journal of Orthopaedic and Sports Physical Therapy.*

Fabio Comana, M.A., M.S., is an exercise physiologist and spokesperson for the American Council on Exercise and faculty at San Diego State University (SDSU) and the University of California San Diego (UCSD), teaching courses in exercise science and nutrition. He holds two master's degrees, one in exercise physiology and one in nutrition, as well as certifications through ACE, ACSM, NSCA, and ISSN. Prior to joining ACE, he was a college head coach and a strength and conditioning coach at SDSU. Comana also managed health clubs for Club One. He lectures, conducts workshops, and writes on many topics related to exercise, fitness, and nutrition both nationally and internationally. As an ACE spokesperson and presenter, he is frequently featured in numerous media outlets, including television, radio, Internet, and more than 100 nationwide newspaper and print publications. Comana has authored chapters in various textbooks.

Todd Galati, M.A., is the certification and exam development manager for the American Council on Exercise and serves on volunteer committees with the Institute for Credentialing Excellence, formerly the National Organization for Competency Assurance. He holds a bachelor's degree in athletic training and a master's degree in kinesiology and four ACE certifications (Personal Trainer, Advanced Health & Fitness Specialist, Lifestyle & Weight Management Coach, and Group Fitness Instructor). Prior to joining ACE, Galati was a program director with the University of California, San Diego School of Medicine, where he spent 14 years designing and researching the effectiveness of youth fitness programs in reducing risk factors for cardiovascular disease, obesity, and type 2 diabetes. Galati's experience includes teaching classes in biomechanics and applied kinesiology as an adjunct professor at Cal State San Marcos, conducting human performance studies as a research physiologist with the U.S. Navy, working as a personal trainer in medical fitness facilities, and coaching endurance athletes to state and national championships.

Carolyn Kaelin, M.D., M.P.H., FACS, is founding director of the Comprehensive Breast Health Center at Brigham and Women's Hospital, a major teaching hospital of Harvard Medical School. She is a surgical oncologist at Dana Farber Cancer Institute, a leading researcher in quality of life after breast cancer, and author of the award-winning book *Living Through Breast Cancer.*

Len Kravitz, Ph.D., is the program coordinator of exercise science and researcher at the University of New Mexico, where he won the "Outstanding Teacher of the Year" award. Dr. Kravitz was honored with the 2009 Canadian Fitness Professional "Specialty Presenter of the Year" award and was chosen as the American Council on Exercise "Fitness Educator of the Year" in 2006. He has also received the prestigious Canadian Fitness Professional "Lifetime Achievement Award."

John R. Martínez, P.T., M.P.T., is the sole principle and president of Executive Operations Management, which provides executive-level business consulting to companies in and around New York City. Additionally, he is the owner and clinical director of Physical Therapy Experts, P.L.L.C., and the Australian Physiotherapy Centers in Manhattan. Martinez has a B.A. in psychology from Swarthmore College, a B.S. in health sciences and an M.S. in physical therapy from the University of the Sciences in Philadelphia, and is a doctoral candidate in physical therapy at Temple University. He also brings his knowledge and skills to the classroom, teaching neurology and anatomy and physiology to local undergraduate students.

Pete McCall, M.S., is an exercise physiologist with the American Council on Exercise (ACE), where he creates and delivers fitness education programs to uphold ACE's mission of enriching quality of life through safe and effective exercise and physical activity. Prior to working with ACE, McCall was a full-time personal trainer and group fitness instructor in Washington, D.C. He has a master's of science degree in exercise science and health promotion from California University of Pennsylvania and is an ACE-certified Personal Trainer.

Sabrena Merrill, M.S., is a former full-time faculty member in the Kinesiology and Physical Education Department at California State University, Long Beach. She has a bachelor's degree in exercise science as well as a master's degree in physical education/biomechanics from the University of Kansas, and has numerous fitness certifications. Merrill, an ACE-certified Personal Trainer and Group Fitness Instructor and ACE Faculty Member, educates other fitness professionals about current industry topics through speaking engagements at local establishments and national conferences, as well as through educational videos. She is a spokesperson for ACE and is involved in curriculum development for ACE continuing education programs.

David Ohton has been the director of strength and conditioning at San Diego State University since 1985. After graduating from Arizona State University (ASU), he signed a free agent contract with the Kansas City Chiefs and attended graduate school at ASU with an emphasis in sports psychology and biomechanics while serving as a member of the strength and conditioning staff. Ohton is a long-time member of the National Strength and Conditioning Association and has published several articles in their periodical journal.

Justin Price, M.A., is the owner of The BioMechanics, a private training facility located in San Diego, Calif., that specializes in providing exercise alternatives for sufferers of chronic pain. He is the creator of The BioMechanics Method, a method for pain reduction that combines structural assessment, movement analysis, corrective exercise, and life coaching and teaches trainers how to help clients alleviate chronic pain and improve their function. He is also an IDEA Personal Trainer of the Year and an educator for the American Council on Exercise, PTontheNet, PTA Global, and the National Strength and Conditioning Association.

David K. Stotlar, Ed.D., serves as the director of the School of Sport & Exercise Science at the University of Northern Colorado and teaches on the faculty in the areas of sport management and sport marketing. He has had more than 70 articles published in professional journals and has written more than 40 textbooks and book chapters on sport marketing and management. During his career, Dr. Stotlar has given more than 200 presentations and workshops at national and international professional conferences.

Kimberly Summers, M.S., is an ACE-certified Personal Trainer and Group Fitness Instructor. She has a bachelor's degree in exercise science and a master's degree in kinesiology. Summers, former ACE Resource Center Coordinator and Academy staff member, has also been active in the fitness industry as a stroller fitness franchise owner, group fitness instructor, personal trainer, and an ACE Exam Development Committee member.

FOREWORD

Like the American Council on Exercise itself, the *ACE Personal Trainer Manual* has long stood as the standard of excellence in the fitness industry. And like previous editions of this manual, this Fourth Edition of the *ACE Personal Trainer Manual* was written based on feedback from individuals who are active in the fitness world—practicing personal trainers, university professors, and industry experts—who worked together to create the Exam Content Outline (see Appendix B). This document presents the skills and knowledge that a personal trainer needs to have a successful career and should serve as a guide as you prepare for the ACE exam.

That said, this textbook also marks a shift in the way that ACE is presenting this content to aspiring and practicing fitness professionals. Gone are the days when a personal trainer could study resistance training, cardiorespiratory training, and flexibility training as isolated components of physical fitness. Modern fitness consumers demand comprehensive programs that are truly individualized based on their physical-activity levels, current health status, and needs and desires. And, though clients may not even know it, the programs must also take into account each individual's psychological readiness for change. The core challenge for any fitness professional is to somehow translate all of the feedback he or she receives from health-history forms, physical assessments, and conversations with the client into a successful program. The all-new ACE Integrated Fitness Training™ Model (ACE IFT™ Model) meets this challenge head on.

The ACE IFT Model addresses some of the most common concerns and questions offered by personal trainers. What is the best way to take advantage of that initial contact with a prospective client? What should be accomplished during a client's first handful of sessions? When is the best time to perform the seemingly endless array of available assessments, and how does the trainer know which ones are appropriate for a specific client? How does the personal trainer use the results of those assessments to design an exercise program for a client? And, finally, how does the trainer keep clients motivated and progressing over the long haul?

Answering that final question is really the key to becoming a successful personal trainer and having a long, rewarding career. Passing the ACE Certification Exam is only the first step. By joining the more than 50,000 current ACE-certified Fitness Professionals, you will be earning a distinguished mark of excellence. It is then up to you to become a leader in your community as we work together to make the world a more active and healthy place.

Make good use of this textbook and all else that ACE has to offer—and don't hesitate to contact us if you need any additional guidance. In closing, good luck and congratulations on taking this important first step.

Scott Goudeseune
President and CEO

INTRODUCTION

The American Council on Exercise is proud to introduce the Fourth Edition of its *ACE Personal Trainer Manual.* This all-new textbook, which was written by a group of 14 industry experts, is designed to fill an important need in the fitness industry. In the past, many newcomers to personal training would read a textbook presenting fitness assessments, detailing resistance-, flexibility-, and cardiorespiratory-training programs, and providing motivational tools, and ask the same question—"Okay, so now what?" In other words, how does the reader assimilate all of this seemingly disparate information into a safe and effective training program for each of his or her clients?

The ACE Integrated Fitness Training™ (ACE IFT™) Model, which is a central feature of this new manual and is presented in **Part III: The ACE Integrated Fitness Training Model** (Chapters 5–12), should serve as a blueprint when meeting, assessing, and training clients, from recently sedentary adults who are just getting started and seek improved overall health to elite-level athletes working to enhance a specific aspect of their athletic performance. After introducing the various components of the ACE IFT Model, detailing the various assessments that personal trainers have at their disposal, and covering functional, resistance, and cardiorespiratory training, this part of the textbook closes with **Chapter 12: The ACE Integrated Fitness Training Model in Practice**. This chapter offers six case studies that are representative of the types of clientele that personal trainers can expect to see over the course of their careers. Each case study presents the health history of the client, along with his or her goals, and then follows the client over the course of the program, offering progression templates, discussing obstacles, and offering solutions along the way. This chapter is designed to help the reader synthesize the material presented in the previous seven chapters in a very practical sense. By combining the ACE IFT Model with appropriate leadership and implementation strategies as presented in **Part II: Leadership and Implementation** (Chapters 2–4), personal trainers can provide a truly individualized, integrated approach to achieving optimal health, fitness, and performance.

Of course, to be successful as a personal trainer, there is other foundational information that individuals need to understand and be able to utilize. **Chapter 1: Role and Scope of Practice for the Personal Trainer** defines the personal trainer's role within the healthcare continuum and details the scope of practice. In addition, this chapter discusses various avenues of career development for personal trainers.

Chapter 13: Mind-body Exercise explains how mind-body fitness, which includes everything from classical forms of yoga and tai chi to more contemporary options like the Alexander Technique and Nia, fits into the modern fitness industry. **Chapter 14: Training Special Populations** presents essential information for working with individuals with various diseases and disorders once they have been cleared to exercise by their physicians. These two chapters comprise **Part IV: Special Exercise Programming Topics.**

Part V: Injury Prevention and First Aid is also composed of two chapters. **Chapter 15: Common Musculoskeletal Injuries and Implications for Exercise** begins by explaining common tissue injuries before presenting guidelines for managing these common injuries, including rotator cuff injuries, carpal tunnel syndrome, ankle sprains, and plantar fasciitis. **Chapter 16: Emergency Procedures** discusses emergency policies and procedures for fitness facilities. Common emergencies are also discussed, ranging from choking and asthma to stroke and neck injuries.

The final two chapters combine to form **Part VI: Professional and Legal Responsibilities and Business Strategies. Chapter 17: Legal Guidelines and Professional Responsibilities** addresses many of the standard legal and business concerns that personal trainers may have regarding business structure, employment status, contracts, insurance, and risk management. **Chapter 18: Personal-training Business Fundamentals** presents a topic new to ACE textbooks: how to thrive on the business side of your personal-training career. This chapter covers creating a brand, financial planning, choosing a business structure, and effective marketing practices.

Our goal when putting together this textbook was to meet the needs of personal trainers at every stage of their careers, from deciding whether to work as an employee or independent contractor to owning one's own fitness facility, from training people who walk in off the street to specializing in a niche clientele that allows you to increase your income and become a recognized expert in your community. We wish you good luck in your efforts and sincerely hope that this manual serves you well as you prepare to become an ACE-certified Personal Trainer and remains a trusted resource throughout your career.

Cedric X. Bryant, Ph.D., FACSM
Chief Science Officer

Daniel J. Green
Project Editor

Studying for the ACE Personal Trainer Exam

ACE has put together a comprehensive package of study tools that should serve as your core materials while preparing for the ACE Certification Exam. Using the following study tips will optimize your chances of success.

Begin by studying *ACE's Essentials of Exercise Science for Fitness Professionals.* This book covers the foundational knowledge that you will need to take full advantage of the training-specific information presented in the *ACE Personal Trainer Manual,* Fourth Edition. The authors of the *Personal Trainer Manual* wrote with the assumption that readers had already mastered the content presented in the *Essentials* book. For example, **Chapter 10: Resistance Training: Programming and Progressions** assumes an understanding of human anatomy and the physiology of training, both of which are presented in the *Essentials* book. If at any point in your reading you come across a topic that you are not entirely confident with, revisit the *Essentials* book to sharpen your understanding.

Each chapter of *ACE's Essentials of Exercise Science for Fitness Professionals* includes a Study Guide that will help you identify areas that require additional study time and more focused attention. In addition, multiple-choice questions are included that mirror the style and types of questions that are included on the ACE certification exams.

Review the Exam Content Outline, which is presented in Appendix B of this book. This document was created by active members of the fitness industry and is the basis from which the ACE Personal Trainer Exam is written. Using this document to target your studies and identify areas of weakness will be a powerful study tool.

Use the *Master the Manual* to focus your studies as you work your way through the *ACE Personal Trainer Manual.* The *Master the Manual* uses the same format as the Study Guides in the *Essentials* book, with the addition of chapter summaries that point out key topics, and will be an invaluable tool as you prepare for the ACE Exam.

Other ACE study materials include the following:

- *Flashcards:* ACE's flashcards focus on foundational anatomy and physiology topics and feature detailed illustrations that will help strengthen your understanding of these essential topics.
- *Companion DVD for the ACE Personal Trainer Manual:* This DVD, which is included in the back of this book, presents many of the exercises and drills discussed in the textbook in a user-friendly, practical format. This will be a valuable tool whether you are teaching basic exercises to beginner clients or more advanced movement exercises for your more fit and experienced clients.
- *Glossary and Index:* Keep an eye out for boldface terms as you read. Each of these important terms is included in the book's glossary as a quick reference whenever a new concept is introduced. If you need more in-depth information on the topic, check the indexes of both the *Personal Trainer Manual* and the *Essentials* book.
- *www.acefitness.org:* The ACE website offers everything from calculators using equations commonly utilized in the fitness setting to online continuing education courses—which means that it will remain a valuable resource for tools and information throughout your fitness career.
- *ACE Resource Center:* ACE's Resource Center specialists are available to answer your questions as you prepare for the exam. The Resource Center can be reached at (800) 825-3636, ext. 715.

PART I
Introduction

Chapter 1

Role and Scope of Practice for the Personal Trainer

IN THIS CHAPTER:

The Allied Healthcare Continuum

The ACE Personal Trainer Certification

- Defining "Scope of Practice"
- Scope of Practice for ACE-certified Personal Trainers
- Knowledge, Skills, and Abilities of the ACE-certified Personal Trainer
- Professional Responsibilities and Ethics

Accreditation of Allied Healthcare Credentials Through the NCCA

- Recognition From the Fitness and Health Industry
- Recognition From the Education Community
- Recognition From the Department of Labor

Career Development

- Continuing Education
- Degrees
- Additional Fitness Certifications
- New Areas of Expertise Within Allied Healthcare

Summary

TODD GALATI, M.A., *is the certification and exam development manager for the American Council on Exercise and serves on volunteer committees with the Institute for Credentialing Excellence, formerly the National Organization for Competency Assurance. He holds a bachelor's degree in athletic training and a master's degree in kinesiology and four ACE certifications (Personal Trainer, Advanced Health & Fitness Specialist, Lifestyle & Weight Management Coach, and Group Fitness Instructor). Prior to joining ACE, Galati was a program director with the University of California, San Diego School of Medicine, where he spent 14 years designing and researching the effectiveness of youth fitness programs in reducing risk factors for cardiovascular disease, obesity, and type 2 diabetes. Galati's experience includes teaching classes in biomechanics and applied kinesiology as an adjunct professor at Cal State San Marcos, conducting human performance studies as a research physiologist with the U.S. Navy, working as a personal trainer in medical fitness facilities, and coaching endurance athletes to state and national championships.*

CHAPTER 1

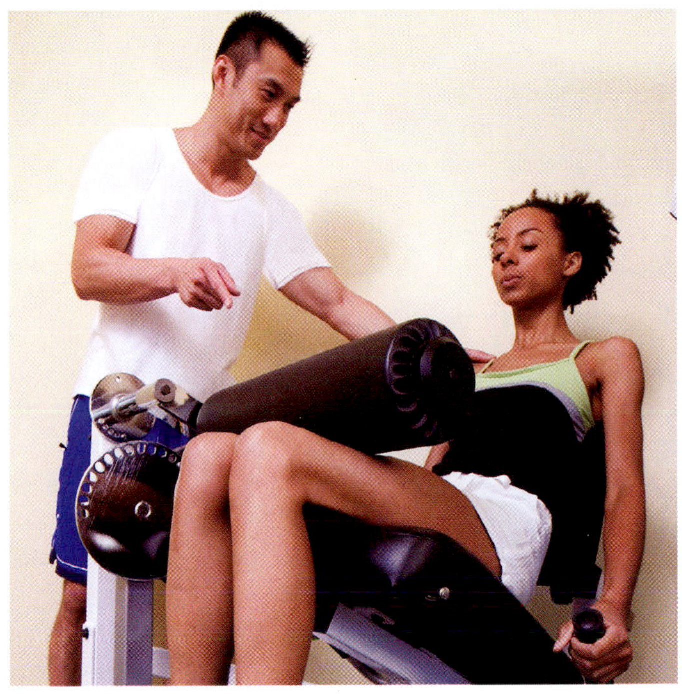

Role and Scope of Practice for the Personal Trainer

Todd Galati

The benefits resulting from regular physical activity are well documented (Table 1-1). After a comprehensive review of the research linking physical activity to health, the U.S. Department of Health & Human Services released the *2008 Physical Activity Guidelines for Americans,* the first comprehensive guidelines on physical activity to be issued by the U.S. government. These guidelines list the following major research findings regarding physical activity and its associated health benefits:

- Regular physical activity reduces the risk of many adverse health outcomes.
- Some physical activity is better than none.
- For most health outcomes, additional benefits occur as the amount of physical activity increases through higher intensity, greater frequency, and/or longer duration.

Table 1-1

Health Benefits Associated With Regular Physical Activity

Children and Adolescents

Strong evidence
- Improved cardiorespiratory and muscular fitness
- Improved bone health
- Improved cardiovascular and metabolic health biomarkers
- Favorable body composition

Moderate evidence
- Reduced symptoms of depression

Adults and Older Adults

Strong evidence
- Lower risk of early death
- Lower risk of coronary heart disease
- Lower risk of stroke
- Lower risk of high blood pressure
- Lower risk of adverse blood lipid profile
- Lower risk of type 2 diabetes
- Lower risk of metabolic syndrome
- Lower risk of colon cancer
- Lower risk of breast cancer
- Prevention of weight gain
- Weight loss, particularly when combined with reduced calorie intake
- Improved cardiorespiratory and muscular fitness
- Prevention of falls
- Reduced symptoms of depression
- Better cognitive function (for older adults)

Moderate to strong evidence
- Better functional health (for older adults)
- Reduced abdominal obesity

Moderate evidence
- Lower risk of hip fracture
- Lower risk of lung cancer
- Lower risk of endometrial cancer
- Weight maintenance after weight loss
- Increased bone density
- Improved sleep quality

U.S. Department of Health & Human Services (2008). *2008 Physical Activity Guidelines for Americans: Be Active, Healthy and Happy.* www.health.gov/paguidelines/pdf/paguide.pdf

Note: The Advisory Committee rated the evidence of health benefits of physical activity as strong, moderate, or weak. To do so, the Committee considered the type, number, and quality of studies available, as well as consistency of findings across studies that addressed each outcome. The Committee also considered evidence for causality and dose response in assigning the strength-of-evidence rating.

- Most health benefits occur with at least 150 minutes a week of moderate-intensity physical activity, such as brisk walking. Additional benefits occur with more physical activity.
- Both aerobic (endurance) and muscle-strengthening (resistance) physical activity are beneficial.
- Health benefits occur for children and adolescents, young and middle-aged adults, older adults, and those in every studied racial and ethnic group.
- The health benefits of physical activity occur for people with disabilities.
- The benefits of physical activity far outweigh the possibility of adverse outcomes.

These findings reinforce what fitness professionals have known for years; the human body was meant to move and, when it does so with regularity, it responds to the stress of physical movement with improved fitness and health. Guidelines with similar goals and recommendations have been published in the past by the American College of Sports Medicine (ACSM) and American Heart Association (AHA) (2007), U.S. Department of Health & Human Services and U.S.Department of Agriculture (USDA) (2005), International Association for the Study of Obesity (Saris et al., 2003), Institute of Medicine (2002), and the U.S. Department of Health & Human Services (1996). But, the 2008 guidelines mark the first time the U.S. government has confirmed that fitness is an important part of medicine and that fitness professionals are important members of the allied healthcare continuum.

Even with well-established guidelines for physical activity, the majority of healthcare professionals have little or no formal education or practical experience in designing and leading exercise programs. Physicians often give patients recommendations to exercise, but they generally do not provide specific instructions for *how* to exercise. ACE-certified Personal Trainers, therefore, play a vital role in allied healthcare by providing services that help clients participate in effective exercise programs that result in positive health and fitness improvements.

In the past, personal trainers have primarily worked with fitness enthusiasts in traditional fitness facilities. This role is changing due to the increasing number of adults and children who are **overweight** or obese and have related health issues. Personal trainers must now be prepared to work with clients ranging in age from youth to older adults, and ranging in health and fitness status from overweight and **sedentary** to athletic. The need for personal trainers to help combat the rising **obesity** epidemic has led to a positive outlook for personal training as a profession.

The Allied Healthcare Continuum

The allied healthcare continuum is composed of health professionals who are credentialed through certifications, registrations, and/or licensure and provide services to identify, prevent, and treat diseases and disorders. Physicians are at the top of the allied healthcare pyramid, evaluating patients to diagnose ailments and implement treatment plans that can include medication, surgery, rehabilitation, or other actions. Physicians are assisted in their efforts by nurses, physician's assistants, and a number of other credentialed technicians. When ailments or treatment plans fall outside their areas of expertise, physicians refer patients to specialists for specific medical evaluations, physical or occupational therapy, psychological counseling, dietary planning, and/or exercise programming.

Physicians and nurses teach patients the importance of implementing their treatment plans. **Physical therapists** and **occupational therapists** lead patients through therapeutic exercise and teach them to perform additional exercises at home to facilitate rehabilitation.

The Future of Personal Training

The U.S. Department of Labor (DOL), Bureau of Labor Statistics (2009), refers to the professionals in the fitness industry as Fitness Workers, with Personal Trainers classified as the primary profession within the industry. The DOL defines the nature of the job of personal trainers as working "one-on-one with clients either in a gym or in the client's home. They help clients assess their level of physical fitness and set and reach fitness goals. Trainers also demonstrate various exercises and help clients improve their exercise techniques. They may keep records of their clients' exercise sessions to monitor clients' progress toward physical fitness. They may also advise their clients on how to modify their lifestyles outside of the gym to improve their fitness."

Expected Growth in Personal-training Jobs

According to the DOL, employment of fitness workers is projected to increase by 27% between 2006 and 2016. This expected increase is much faster than the average for all occupations, and is attributed to a number of factors, including the following:

- Increasing numbers of baby boomers who want to stay healthy, physically fit, and independent
- Reduction in the number of physical-education programs in schools
- Growing concerns about childhood obesity
- Increasing club memberships among young adults concerned about physical fitness
- An aging population seeking relief from arthritis and other ailments through individualized exercise, yoga, and Pilates
- A need to replace workers who leave fitness occupations each year

Personal-trainer Qualifications

See "Recognition From the Department of Labor" on page 17 for the DOL's statement regarding the importance of obtaining a quality personal-training certification.

Athletic trainers teach athletes exercises to prevent injury and take them through therapeutic exercises following injury. **Registered dietitians** teach clients proper nutrition through recipes, meal plans, food-preparation methods, and implementation of specialized diets. While these professionals might also give patients or clients guidelines for general exercise (e.g., "try to walk up to 30 minutes per day, most days of the week"), few of them actually teach clients *how* to exercise effectively. This is where personal trainers hold a unique position in the allied healthcare continuum.

The majority of personal trainers will work with apparently healthy clients, helping them improve fitness and health. Experienced personal trainers with advanced education and training will generally have the skills necessary to work with clients who have special needs for exercise programming following medical treatment for an injury or disease. An advanced fitness professional providing post-rehabilitative exercise programs will need to have a solid position within the local healthcare community. In more clinical settings, the advanced fitness professional may work under the direction of a physician, physical therapist, or other rehabilitation professional, while in a club setting he or she may be more autonomous. In all situations, it is crucial for the fitness professional to stay within the boundaries of his or her education, certification, and legal **scope of practice**, and to work closely with each client's referring physician and other healthcare providers to ensure that the exercise program is complementary to their treatments. Refer to Chapter 18 for tips on how to utilize these relationships to expand a personal-training business.

It is important that every personal trainer understands the role of fitness professionals in relation to the other members of the healthcare team (Figure 1-1). Each client will generally have a primary care physician

Figure 1-1
Specialty areas within allied healthcare

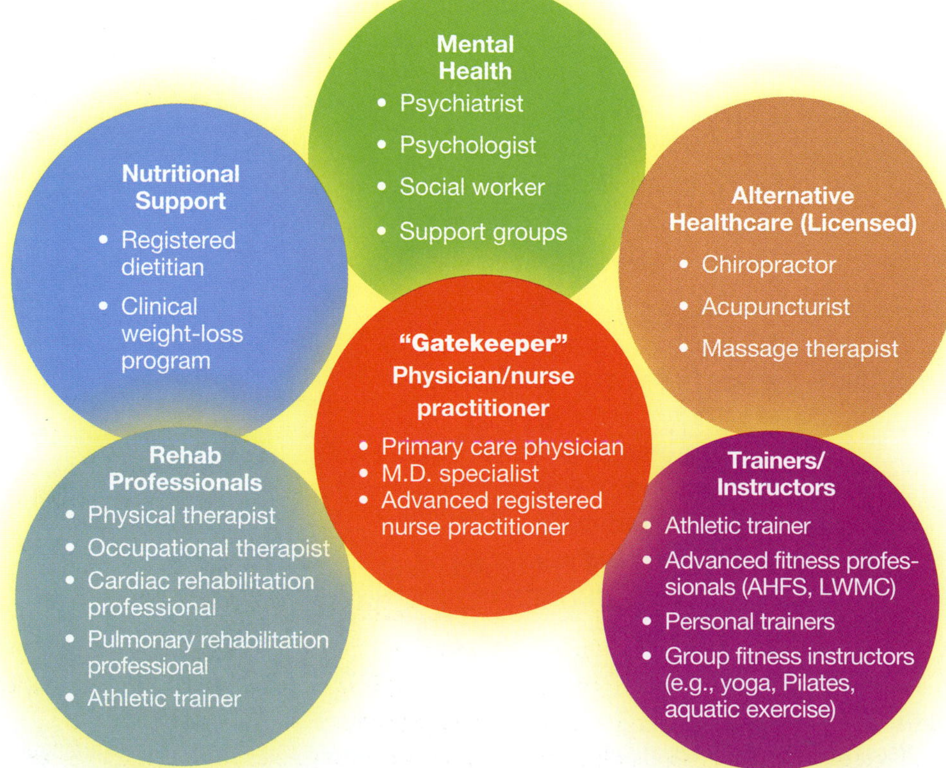

Note: AHFS = Advanced Health & Fitness Specialist; LWMC = Lifestyle & Weight Management Coach

who is responsible for his or her general medical care. If the client is referred by his or her physician, the personal trainer should obtain written permission from the client to communicate with the referring physician to provide regular reports regarding the client's progress with the exercise program. Even when clients do not have a physician's referral, it is important for the personal trainer to maintain confidential records that include the client's program, progress, and health-history information.

The ACE Personal Trainer Certification

The decision to pursue certification as a personal trainer is an important step in being recognized as a competent professional. The ACE Personal Trainer Certification Program was developed to assess candidate competency in making safe and effective exercise program decisions for apparently healthy clients. Candidates who achieve a passing score on the ACE Personal Trainer Certification Exam meet or exceed the level of competency required to work as a professional personal trainer with minimum supervision. In the credentialing world, this threshold of professional competence is referred to as the "minimum competency" required for a person to work in the profession. The primary purpose of a certification is always to protect the public from harm by assessing if the professional meets established levels of competence in the knowledge, skills, and abilities necessary to perform the job in a safe and effective manner. For the professional, a certification can separate him or her from others who have not proven themselves to be at the same level of competence.

Fitness professionals who earn the ACE Personal Trainer Certification are competent to work as professional personal trainers for apparently healthy individuals and small groups with minimal supervision. This does not mean that an ACE-certified Personal Trainer knows everything there is to know about personal training, just as successfully passing one's medical board exams does not mean that the individual knows everything there is to know about medicine. Instead, by earning an ACE Personal Trainer Certification, the professional has proven his or her competence in applying knowledge to make safe and effective exercise-programming decisions in a variety of practical situations, while minimizing client risk and exposure to harm (e.g., physical, emotional, psychological, financial, or other harm).

Defining "Scope of Practice"

A scope of practice defines the legal range of services that professionals in a given field can provide, the settings in which those services can be provided, and the guidelines or parameters that must be followed. Many factors go into defining a scope of practice, including the education, training, and certifications or licenses required to work in a given field, the laws and organizations governing the specific profession, and the laws and organizations governing complementary professions within the same field. Most laws defining a profession are determined and regulated by state regulatory agencies, including licensure. As a result, the scope of practice for licensed practitioners can vary from state to state in a given profession. In addition, most professions have organizations that serve as governing bodies within the profession that set eligibility requirements to enter educational programs or sit for certification exams, and establish codes for professional conduct and disciplinary procedures for professionals who break these codes.

The laws, rules, and regulations that govern a profession are established for the protection of the public. The laws governing a personal trainer's scope of practice and the ramifications faced by trainers who provide services that fall outside the defined scope are detailed in Chapter 17. The eligibility and certification requirements to work within this legal scope of practice are defined by the professional organizations that offer personal-trainer certifications. These organizations also establish codes of ethical conduct and mandate that they are upheld by certified professionals and applicants in all actions related to personal training. It is crucial for practitioners in every industry to be aware of the scope of practice for their given profession, to ensure that they practice within the realm of the specific education, experience, and demonstrated competency of their credential.

Scope of Practice for ACE-certified Personal Trainers

Fitness professionals as a collective group have a general scope of practice (Table 1-2). While this table provides general guidance, each professional must know what is within the specific scope of practice for his or her credential. The ACE-certified Personal Trainer scope of practice is presented in Figure 1-2. ACE-certified Personal Trainers must work within this defined scope of practice to provide effective services to their clients, gain and maintain support from the healthcare community, and avoid the legal ramifications of providing services outside their professional scope.

Personal trainers should never provide services that are outside their defined scope of practice. For example, a personal trainer may be asked nutrition questions by clients wanting to reduce weight and/or **body fat.** Personal

Table 1-2

IDEA Personal Fitness Trainers' Scope of Practice

Fitness Professionals DO NOT:	Fitness Professionals DO:
Diagnose	• Receive exercise, health, or nutrition guidelines from a physician, physical therapist, registered dietitian, etc. • Follow national consensus guidelines for exercise programming for medical disorders • Screen for exercise limitations • Identify potential risk factors through screening • Refer clients to an appropriate allied health professional or medical practitioner
Prescribe	• Design exercise programs • Refer clients to an appropriate allied health professional or medical practitioner for an exercise prescription
Prescribe diets or recommend specific supplements	• Provide general information on healthy eating, according to the MyPyramid Food Guidance System • Refer clients to a dietitian or nutritionist for a specific diet plan
Treat injury or disease	• Refer clients to an appropriate allied health professional or medical practitioner for treatment • Use exercise to help improve overall health • Help clients follow physician or therapist advice
Monitor progress for medically referred clients	• Document progress • Report progress to an appropriate allied health professional or medical practitioner • Follow physician, therapist, or dietitian recommendations
Rehabilitate	• Design an exercise program once a client has been released from rehabilitation
Counsel	• Coach • Provide general information • Refer clients to a qualified counselor or therapist
Work with patients	• Work with clients

IDEA Health & Fitness Association's Opinion Statement: Benefits of a working relationship between medical and allied health practitioners and personal fitness trainers. *IDEA Health and Fitness Source,* September 2001. www.ideafit.com. Reprinted with permission.

Figure 1-2
The ACE-certified Personal Trainer Scope of Practice

ACE-certified Personal Trainer Scope of Practice

The ACE-certified Personal Trainer is a fitness professional who has met all requirements of the American Council on Exercise to develop and implement fitness programs for individuals who have no apparent physical limitations or special medical needs. The ACE-certified Personal Trainer realizes that personal training is a service industry focused on helping people enhance fitness and modify risk factors for disease to improve health. As members of the allied healthcare continuum with a primary focus on prevention, ACE-certified Personal Trainers have a scope of practice that includes:

- Developing and implementing exercise programs that are safe, effective, and appropriate for individuals who are apparently healthy or have medical clearance to exercise
- Conducting health-history interviews and stratifying risk for cardiovascular disease with clients in order to determine the need for referral and identify contraindications for exercise
- Administering appropriate fitness assessments based on the client's health history, current fitness, lifestyle factors, and goals utilizing research-proven and published protocols
- Assisting clients in setting and achieving realistic fitness goals
- Teaching correct exercise methods and progressions through demonstration, explanation, and proper cueing and spotting techniques
- Empowering individuals to begin and adhere to their exercise programs using guidance, support, motivation, lapse-prevention strategies, and effective feedback
- Designing structured exercise programs for one-on-one and small-group personal training
- Educating clients about fitness- and health-related topics to help them in adopting healthful behaviors that facilitate exercise program success
- Protecting client confidentiality according to the Health Insurance Portability and Accountability Act (HIPAA) and related regional and national laws
- Always acting with professionalism, respect, and integrity
- Recognizing what is within the scope of practice and always referring clients to other healthcare professionals when appropriate
- Being prepared for emergency situations and responding appropriately when they occur

trainers can help clients with their weight-loss goals by designing effective exercise programs that bring about positive **body composition** changes and helping them to adopt more healthful behaviors. This can include showing clients how to utilize the tools available at www.MyPyramid.gov or educating them about the recommendations in the *Dietary Guidelines* to help them gain a better understanding of healthful foods and make better choices (U.S. Department of Health & Human Services and U.S. Department of Agriculture, 2005). Clients who are looking for more detailed nutritional programming, such as specific meal plans, recipes, or recommendations for nutritional supplements should be referred to a registered dietitian, as these services are beyond the scope of practice of personal trainers and are in the legal domain of services provided by registered dietitians in most states.

There is overlap among professions within the healthcare field that must be understood if fitness professionals are going to stay within the realm of their professional qualifications and training. For example, the same registered dietitian who can create specific meal plans for clients can also provide general guidelines about exercise to help them understand the important role that physical activity plays in improving health and creating a negative energy balance. However, if a client working with a registered dietitian wants a thorough exercise plan, he or she should be referred to a qualified personal trainer.

A personal trainer should *not* make recommendations that contradict those of the client's healthcare team. For example, if a client's physician's release has specific guidelines for exercise intensities, modalities, or exercises, the trainer must follow these guidelines when designing the client's exercise program. While the physician generally will not have the same knowledge about specific exercises as a personal trainer, the physician's guidelines will be based on the knowledge of the client's health, medications, ailments, injuries, and diseases, and *must* be followed for the health and safety of the client. Each state, province, and country has specific laws about the responsibilities of different healthcare professions. It is the responsibility of the personal trainer to learn and adhere to the laws in his or her geographical area, as well as adhere to the ACE-certified Personal Trainer scope of practice (see Figure 1-2).

Knowledge, Skills, and Abilities of the ACE-certified Personal Trainer

The ACE Personal Trainer Certification is designed for fitness professionals wanting to provide one-on-one and small-group exercise instruction to apparently healthy individuals. The certification program is continually evaluated to ensure that it is up to date with the most current research and industry standards. In addition, every five years a group of industry experts analyzes the specific job requirements for personal trainers to update the outline of tasks, knowledge, and skills required to perform the job of personal training effectively. After being validated by several thousand ACE-certified Personal Trainers, this outline is published as the ACE Personal Trainer Exam Content Outline (Appendix B), which serves as the blueprint for the ACE Personal Trainer Certification Exam and provides a template for candidates preparing for the exam. It is also a written job description of the knowledge, skills, and abilities required to be an effective ACE-certified Personal Trainer.

Education and Experience

There is no single course of study for individuals looking to enter the profession of personal training. To become an ACE-certified Personal Trainer, a candidate must show that he or she is able to apply the knowledge required to be a safe and effective personal trainer by passing the ACE Personal Trainer Certification Exam. There are many paths to reaching this goal, including self-study using preparatory materials from ACE or other sources that cover the ACE Personal Trainer Certification Exam Content Outline, preparatory courses or workshops delivered live or online, educational internships, professional experience, and college courses. Each candidate must select his or her own path based on time, financial resources, learning styles, and personal factors. As a general rule, ACE recommends that candidates allow three to six months of study time to adequately prepare for the ACE Personal Trainer Certification Exam.

The growth in personal training has led numerous colleges and universities to offer programs to help students prepare to become qualified fitness professionals. These programs help students prepare for certification exams by offering courses that teach the specific knowledge and skills required to become personal trainers or group fitness instructors, or to work with clients who have special needs. ACE has an Educational Partnership Program that provides colleges, universities, and technical/professional schools with curricula, instructor materials, and discounts to students preparing for ACE certification programs. These programs are not required to earn an ACE certification, but they provide students with helpful instruction from people with advanced degrees and experience in the field.

Preparation and Testing

The knowledge, skills, and abilities tested include developing and enhancing **rapport** with clients, collecting adequate health-history information and determining the appropriateness of referral, conducting appropriate assessments, designing and modifying exercise programs to help clients progress toward their goals, motivating clients to exercise and adhere to their programs, and always acting in a professional manner within the personal trainer's scope of practice.

Fitness professionals interested in sitting for the ACE Personal Trainer Certification Exam should download the *ACE Certification Candidate Handbook* from the ACE website (www.acefitness.org/getcertified/pdfs/Certification-Exam-Candidate-Handbook.pdf). This complimentary handbook explains how ACE certification exams are developed, what the candidate should expect, and the procedures for earning and maintaining an ACE certification. The handbook also includes explanations about the multiple-choice and client-scenario questions found on the ACE certification exams, along with sample questions to help candidates understand the difference between questions that assess *recall* knowledge and those that assess *applied* knowledge. In addition, the handbook provides candidates with test-taking strategies and a list of available study resources.

Professional Responsibilities and Ethics

The primary purpose of professional certification programs is to protect the public from harm (e.g., physical, emotional, psychological, financial). Professionals who earn an ACE Personal Trainer Certification validate their capabilities and enhance their value to employers, clients, and other healthcare providers. This does not happen simply because the individual has a new title. This recognition is given because the ACE credential itself upholds rigorous standards established for assessing an individual's competence in making safe and effective exercise-programming decisions. ACE has established a professional ethical code of conduct and disciplinary procedures, and ACE certifications have all received third-party accreditation from the National Commission for Certifying Agencies (NCCA).

To help ACE-certified Professionals understand the conduct expected from them as healthcare professionals in protecting the public from harm, ACE has developed the ACE Code of Ethics (Appendix A). This code of conduct serves as a guide for ethical and professional practices for all ACE-certified Professionals. This code is enforced through the ACE Professional Practices and Disciplinary Procedures (www.acefitness.org/getcertified/certified-code.aspx). All ACE-certified Professionals and candidates for ACE certification must be familiar with, and comply with, the ACE Code of Ethics and ACE Professional Practices and Disciplinary Procedures.

ACE Code of Ethics

The ACE Code of Ethics governs the ethical and professional conduct of ACE-certified Professionals when working with clients, the public, or other health and fitness professionals. Every individual who registers for an ACE certification exam *must* agree to uphold the ACE Code of Ethics throughout the exam process and as a professional, should he or she earn an ACE certification. Exam candidates and ACE-certified Personal Trainers must have a comprehensive understanding of the code and the consequences and public harm that can come from violating each of its principles.

ACE Professional Practices and Disciplinary Procedures

The ACE Professional Practices and Disciplinary Procedures are intended to assist and inform ACE-certified Professionals, candidates for ACE certification, and the public about the ACE application and certification standards relative to professional conduct and disciplinary procedures. ACE may revoke or otherwise take action with regard to the application or certification of an individual in the case of:

- Ineligibility for certification
- Irregularity in connection with any certification examination
- Unauthorized possession, use, access, or distribution of certification examinations, score reports, trademarks, logos, written materials, answer sheets, certificates, certificant or applicant files, or other confidential or proprietary ACE documents or materials (registered or otherwise)

- Material misrepresentation or fraud in any statement to ACE or to the public, including but not limited to statements made to assist the applicant, certificant, or another to apply for, obtain, or retain certification
- Any physical, mental, or emotional condition of either temporary or permanent nature, including, but not limited to, substance abuse, which impairs or has the potential to impair competent and objective professional performance
- Negligent and/or intentional misconduct in professional work, including, but not limited to, physical or emotional abuse, disregard for safety, or the unauthorized release of confidential information
- The timely conviction, plea of guilty, or plea of nolo contendere ("no contest") in connection with a felony or misdemeanor that is directly related to public health and/or fitness instruction or education, and that impairs competent and objective professional performance. These include, but are not limited to, rape, sexual abuse of a client, actual or threatened use of a weapon of violence, or the prohibited sale, distribution, or possession with intent to distribute of a controlled substance.
- Failure to meet the requirements for certification or recertification

ACE has developed a three-tiered disciplinary process of review, hearing, and appeals to ensure fair and unbiased examination of alleged violation(s) of the Application and Certification Standards in order to (1) determine the merit of allegations and (2) impose appropriate sanctions as necessary to protect the public and the integrity of the certification process.

Certification Period and Renewal

ACE certifications are valid for two years from the date earned, expiring on the last day of the month. To renew certification for a new two-year cycle, ACE-certified Professionals must complete a minimum of 20 hours of continuing education credits (2.0 CECs) and maintain a current certificate in **cardiopulmonary resuscitation (CPR)** and, if living in North America, **automated external defibrillation (AED).**

Continuing education is a standard requirement in healthcare to help ensure that professionals stay up-to-date with the latest research in their respective fields for the protection of the public. Given the dynamic nature of the fitness industry and the rapidly advancing research in exercise science, it is imperative for fitness professionals to complete continuing education on a regular basis. By completing continuing education, ACE-certified Professionals can stay current with the latest findings in exercise science and keep their services in line with the most recent guidelines for fitness and healthcare.

ACE encourages its certified professionals to complete additional continuing education as necessary to help advance their careers and enhance the services they provide. Each year, the ACE Academy approves thousands of continuing education courses, providing ACE-certified Professionals with many options for maintaining their credentials and advancing their careers. ACE-certified Professionals holding more than one ACE certification can apply the CECs they earn to each of their current certifications.

ACE-certified Professionals are encouraged to renew their certifications before they expire. ACE offers a six-month extension of the renewal period for professionals who go beyond the deadline, but it is merely a grace period for certification renewal, not an extension of the actual certification. During this grace period, the certification is expired and will only become current again once renewed. The ramifications for ACE-certified Professionals that allow their certifications to expire can include not being able to advertise the fact that they hold the ACE certification until it is renewed, discontinued professional liability insurance, and loss of employment.

Client Privacy

Beginning with the initial health-history interview, clients will share confidential information with the personal trainer.

Although the client–trainer relationship does not currently have the same legal requirements for confidentiality as client–physician or client–psychologist relationships, personal trainers should maintain that same level of security for each client's personal information. Failure to do so could prove detrimental for the client and the client–trainer relationship, and may violate the ACE Code of Ethics and state or federal privacy laws.

To help prevent violations of client privacy, ACE-certified Professionals should become familiar with, and adhere to, the **Health Insurance Portability and Accountability Act (HIPAA),** which addresses the use and disclosure of individuals' protected health information. By following HIPAA regulations, personal trainers can maintain the confidentiality of each client's protected health information according to the same rules that govern most healthcare professions. More details about client privacy and keeping clients' protected health information secure can be found in Chapter 17 and Appendix A.

Referral

It is important for healthcare professionals, including personal trainers, to understand their professional qualifications and boundaries, and to always refer clients who require services outside their scope of practice to the appropriate qualified healthcare professionals. Doing so ensures that clients are provided with appropriate care from qualified providers and prevents healthcare professionals from offering services that they do not have the education, training, credentials, and/or legal right to offer.

Sometimes a personal trainer will need to investigate a bit further to determine if referral is warranted. For example, if a client wants to lose more weight than would be advisable based on his or her current body composition, the trainer can first explain healthy body-fat ranges, point out that the client's body composition is within the normal range, and work with him or her to determine a safe and achievable weight-loss goal. If the client is comfortable with this new goal, the personal trainer can design a program to help the client achieve it. However, if the client feels that he or she still wants to aim for the original weight-loss goal, the personal trainer should refer him or her to a registered dietitian who has experience with body image and related issues.

Referrals can also come to the personal trainer from other health professionals. For example, a physician may provide a patient with exercise guidelines and then refer him or her to an ACE-certified Personal Trainer. In a situation like this, the trainer should provide the physician with regular updates on the client's progress and program direction. It is always important for clients to be referred to the appropriate healthcare professional and for all health professionals involved to correspond regularly regarding each client's progress, provided they have the client's written permission to do so.

Developing a Referral Network

It is important for a personal trainer to develop a network of referral sources to meet the varying needs of his or her clientele. Trainers should identify allied health professionals who are reputable and aspire to the same professional standards as an ACE-certified Personal Trainer. Potential referral sources include the following:

- Mind/body instructors (e.g., yoga, tai chi, qigong)
- Smoking cessation programs
- Aquatic exercise programs
- Support groups (e.g., cardiac rehabilitation, cancer survivors, Overeaters Anonymous)
- Massage therapist

As the personal trainer develops a referral network, it is important to research instructors, programs, or organizations before recommending any programs or services to a client. Do they have the proper licensure or certification? Can they provide a list of references? How many years of experience do they have? The personal trainer does not want to jeopardize his or her reputation by referring clients to substandard health and fitness "professionals." With proper networking, the personal trainer may also gain referrals from the other health and fitness professionals within the network.

Safety

All fitness professionals should do what they can to minimize risk for everyone in the fitness facility. This includes having equipment that is properly spaced and in good working order; having racks, shelves, hooks, or other storage spots for portable equipment, including stability balls and dumbbells; and ensuring that floors and equipment are cleaned, maintained, and free from clutter and moisture. Trainers should also pay attention to the cleanliness of the facility, including the availability of wipes or other sterilizers for cleaning equipment following usage. An emergency plan, AED, and appropriate first-aid supplies are essential in case an injury or incident occurs.

A personal trainer has additional client-specific risk-management responsibilities, beginning with the first meeting, when the trainer should conduct a health-history assessment to determine whether the client requires a physician's referral prior to exercise or has limitations or **contraindications** for certain exercises. The trainer also needs to determine appropriate levels of intensity for initial exercise program design. Then, by helping clients perform exercises in a safe and effective manner with proper progressions, the personal trainer can minimize the risk of injury and enhance the quality of service provided. Even with the best risk-management program, injuries and incidents can still occur. As such, ACE recommends that all ACE-certified Professionals carry professional liability insurance for protection in the event a client is injured during training (see Chapter 17).

Supplements

Supplements are not regulated by the U.S. Food and Drug Administration (FDA), so their strength, purity, safety, and effects are not guaranteed. Some supplements can cause adverse interactions and complications with other prescribed medications or congenital problems. Still, the supplement market constitutes a multimillion-dollar industry. The lure of this profitable revenue stream, coupled with consumer interest for a quick fix, leads some fitness facilities to sell nutritional supplements as a profit center. It is not illegal for fitness facilities to sell commercial nutritional supplements, but it is irresponsible for them to provide supplement recommendations without staff that have the expertise and legal qualifications required to give such advice (e.g., registered dietitians, medical doctors). Facilities selling dietary supplements are assuming a huge liability risk in the event that a member has a negative reaction to a supplement recommended by a staff member who is not qualified (see Chapter 17).

Some personal trainers amass substantial knowledge about dietary supplements. However, they are no more qualified to recommend these supplements to clients than they are to recommend or prescribe medications. Unless a personal trainer is also a registered dietitian or a physician, he or she does not have the expertise or legal qualifications necessary to recommend supplements. The ACE Position Statement on Nutritional Supplements can be found in Appendix C.

Personal trainers should, however, educate themselves about supplements. Clients often ask personal trainers about supplements, thinking that supplements are necessary to achieve fitness, weight loss, or other goals. The personal trainer can help the client understand that fitness goals can be reached without supplements and that supplements can have negative and potentially harmful side effects. If a client insists on using dietary supplements, the personal trainer should refer the client to a qualified physician or registered dietitian for guidance.

Ramifications of Offering Services Outside the Scope of Practice

To achieve their fitness goals, clients must adopt healthful behaviors that can include a regular exercise program, eating a more healthful diet, and initiating lifestyle changes to decrease stress. An ACE-certified Personal Trainer is qualified to help clients with comprehensive exercise programming needs, but the level of assistance the trainer can provide when it comes to nutrition, lifestyle, or post-rehabilitation programming can be confusing, especially to the newly certified trainer. The client scenarios in Table 1-3 are designed to provide personal trainers with a better understanding of services that are within and outside their scope of practice.

ACE-certified Professionals offering services that are within the legal realm of another healthcare profession are in violation of the ACE Code of Ethics and are at risk for potential legal prosecution. For example, if a client tells a trainer that he or she experiences muscle soreness following long training runs, the trainer can provide education about the benefits of massage, but cannot perform hands-on massage therapy for the client, as this would constitute the practice of massage without a license. All responses listed in Table 1-3 as "Inappropriate for an ACE-certified Personal Trainer" are examples of services that could result in an ACE-certified Personal Trainer facing legal ramifications, with possible prosecution for practicing other forms of medicine or healthcare without appropriate credentials.

Accreditation of Allied Healthcare Credentials Through the NCCA

Healthcare professionals recognize the important role that physical activity plays in improving and maintaining good health. Unfortunately, the lack of professional credentials held by some individuals working in fitness has slowed the acceptance of fitness professionals as legitimate members of the allied healthcare team by some healthcare providers. As a result, ACE and other top professional fitness organizations

Table 1-3
Appropriate Scope of Practice

Client Scenario	Inappropriate for an ACE-certified Personal Trainer	Appropriate for an ACE-certified Personal Trainer
Client stands with a lordosis posture	Diagnosing the cause of the client's lordosis	Implementing a core conditioning program to improve strength and flexibility imbalances in muscles acting on the hips and spine
Client wants to lose weight by trying the latest commercial diet	Helping the client to understand and implement the diet	Helping the client to make more healthful choices using the *Dietary Guidelines* and tools on www.MyPyramid.gov
Client is cleared for exercise following physical therapy for rotator cuff impingement	Continuing the PNF shoulder mobilization exercises used during physical therapy	Implementing exercises to improve shoulder stability and building on the work done in physical therapy
Client has tight iliotibial (IT) bands	Providing deep tissue massage to relieve tightness in the IT bands	Teaching the client self–myofascial release techniques for the IT bands using a foam roller
Client has soreness following a weekend tennis tournament	Recommending use of over-the-counter anti-inflammatory medications	Discussing proper techniques for icing
Client tells you she is depressed due to problems with her spouse	Listening to the client and providing her with recommendations for improving the situation	Listening to the client with empathy and maintaining her confidentiality

Note: PNF = Proprioceptive neuromuscular facilitation

have earned third-party accreditation from the NCCA for their fitness certification programs. For a complete list of NCCA-accredited fitness certifications organizations, visit www.credentialingexcellence.org.

The NCCA is the accreditation body of the Institute for Credentialing Excellence (ICE) [formerly known as the National Organization for Competency Assurance (NOCA)] a non-profit, 501(c)(3) organization. Formed in 1977, ICE originated as the National Commission for Health Certifying Agencies (NCHCA). Originally funded through the U.S. Department of Health & Human Services, the NCHCA had a mission to develop standards for quality certification in allied health fields and to accredit organizations that met those standards. The NCHCA evolved into NOCA (in 1987) and then ICE (in 2009) to expand accreditation globally to certification programs outside healthcare that met the rigorous standards of the NCCA.

The NCCA has reviewed and accredited the certification programs for most professions within allied healthcare. This includes the credentials for registered dietitians, occupational therapists, athletic trainers, podiatrists, nurses, nurse practitioners, massage therapists, personal trainers, group fitness instructors, and advanced fitness professionals. By earning NCCA accreditation for all four of its certification programs, the American Council on Exercise has taken the professional and responsible steps necessary for ACE-certified Professionals to be accepted as legitimate members of the allied healthcare continuum.

Recognition From the Fitness and Health Industry

In the fitness industry, NCCA accreditation has become recognized as the third-party standard for accreditation of certifications for personal trainers and other fitness professionals, as seen in the following professional standards, guidelines, and recommendations:

- The Medical Fitness Association (MFA), the professional membership organization for medically integrated health and fitness facilities, has made it a standard that medical fitness facilities hire only fitness professionals who hold NCCA-accredited certifications.
- *ACSM's Health/Fitness Facility Standards and Guidelines* (ACSM, 2007) recommends that clubs hire only fitness directors, group exercise directors, fitness instructors (including personal trainers), and group exercise instructors who hold a "certification from a nationally recognized and accredited certifying organization" [American College of Sports Medicine (ACSM), 2007]. It then states that "In this instance, the term accredited refers to certification programs that have received third-party approval of its certification procedures and practices from an appropriate agency, such as the National Commission for Certifying Agencies (NCCA)."
- The International Health, Racquet, and Sportsclub Association (IHRSA) recommends that club owners only hire personal trainers with certifications from agencies accredited by the NCCA or an equivalent accrediting organization.

There are other professional organizations currently in the process of developing voluntary fitness facility standards that will include requirements for hiring fitness professionals that recognize the NCCA accreditation. In reference to the ACSM and IHRSA recommendations, the only other organization for possible consideration as a credible accreditation organization for certifying agencies is the American National Standards Institute (ANSI), which focuses primarily on third-party accreditation of industrial and workplace safety and quality standards.

Recognition From the Education Community

The ACE Educational Partnership Program offers four separate college curricula that instructors can use to teach courses in personal training, group exercise, exercise for weight management, and exercise for special populations, and to help students prepare for the corresponding ACE certification exam. The ACE Personal Trainer curriculum is the most widely utilized of the four, with more than 150 ACE Educational Partners using this curriculum in their regular course offerings. The ACE Personal Trainer curriculum helps instructors with course design, provides discounts for students, and helps exercise science departments meet one of the primary outcome assessments stated in the *Standards and Guidelines for the Accreditation of Educational Programs for Personal Fitness Training* from the Commission on Accreditation of Allied Health Education Programs (CAAHEP, 2007).

The CAAHEP is the largest programmatic accreditor in the health sciences field. The Committee on the Accreditation for the Exercise Sciences (CoAES) was formed under the guidance and sponsorship of CAAHEP to establish standards that academic programs in kinesiology, physical education, and exercise science must meet to become accredited by CAAHEP (2007).

One of the primary outcomes assessed by the CAAHEP *Standards and Guidelines for the Accreditation of Educational Programs for Personal Fitness Training* is the students' performance on a national credentialing examination accredited by the National Commission for Certifying Agencies. This recognition of NCCA-accredited personal-trainer certifications as the standard for this outcome assessment is an important endorsement of the NCCA accreditation by the educational community. The ACE Personal Trainer Certification Program, with its NCCA accreditation, helps universities and colleges meet this outcome assessment standard for exercise science departments to earn accreditation from CAAHEP.

Recognition From the Department of Labor

The Department of Labor (DOL) reports that most personal trainers *must* obtain certification in the fitness field to gain employment, explaining that there are many fitness organizations that offer certifications and that "becoming certified by one of the top certification organizations is increasingly important, especially for personal trainers." The DOL then goes on to state that, "One way to ensure that a certifying organization is reputable is to see that it is accredited by the National Commission for Certifying Agencies." The American Council on Exercise is one of the few organizations specifically identified by the DOL as offering quality certifications for personal trainers.

Other professions listed as fitness workers by the DOL include group exercise instructors, fitness directors, and those teaching specializations such as yoga and Pilates.

Career Development

It is important for every personal trainer to have a general idea of the career path that he or she wants to follow. Career paths can include becoming a fitness director or general manager of a larger club, opening a personal-training studio, opening a home-based personal-training business, or simply working part-time as a personal trainer. Career goals are personal. They are based on the specific needs of the professional to meet his or her career objectives and are balanced with his or her other commitments.

Career paths should be viewed as guidelines to help the professional reach certain career goals, with the flexibility to be modified as needed based on new clientele, changes in family, industry recessions, and other important events. A career plan can help a professional determine if a new opportunity or continuing education offering is in line with his or her goals. After setting a career plan that spans one, three, five, or more years, a personal trainer can use this plan as a template for researching and selecting continuing education to work toward his or her goals.

Continuing Education

ACE-certified Professionals are encouraged to select continuing education based on areas of interest, client needs, and desired career path. By completing continuing education in one or more areas of focus, a personal trainer can advance his or her career by becoming a specialist in areas such as weight management, youth fitness, sports conditioning, or older adult fitness. This can help the trainer become recognized as an expert in a given field, attracting specific clientele and advancing his or her career. Factors that should be considered when selecting continuing education courses include checking if the course will be at the appropriate level, seeing if the instructor has the appropriate qualifications to teach the course, learning if the course is ACE-approved or will have to be petitioned for CECs, and determining if the education provided is within the scope of practice.

Advanced Knowledge

ACE-certified Professionals should select continuing education that will help advance their current knowledge, skills, and abilities, without being too advanced. The continuing education needs for a newly certified trainer and a trainer with 10 years of experience will be different. If these two professionals attend the same conference together, it would be beneficial for them to independently select sessions that meet their individual career paths and needs, rather than going to the same sessions and having the new trainer be overwhelmed by the advanced subject matter, or the veteran bored by information that he or she already knows.

Continuing education should help the personal trainer work toward one or more career goals. For a management-focused personal trainer, this could include taking management courses, while a trainer who works with older adults and is looking for new programming ideas would have a different course of study entirely. It is also important for ACE-certified Professionals to stay current, as standards and guidelines are released based on new findings in exercise science and related healthcare research. A personal trainer can do this through continuing education courses or through his or her own research of the published scientific literature.

Specialization

Specialization is a great way for a personal trainer to become recognized as an "expert" for a particular type of training or client population. By gaining advanced knowledge and skills in a specialized area, a personal trainer can enhance the training services provided to clients with special needs—and hopefully attract more clients seeking these specialty services. For example, a personal trainer who is interested in working with athletes might go on to do extensive continuing education in sports performance, possibly earning a specialty certificate in sports conditioning. Once the trainer is a recognized sports conditioning specialist, he or she should more readily attract athletic clients, and should be able to earn more per session when providing these advanced sessions.

Areas of specialization should be selected by the personal trainer based on his or her desired career path, interests, and client base. The area of specialization should also fall within the scope of practice, or provide the trainer with knowledge that is complementary to what he or she does within the scope of practice. For example, a course teaching techniques for manual manipulations of the shoulder would be educational, but would provide the trainer with techniques that he or she could not use within the defined scope of practice.

Degrees

Having a degree in exercise science or a related field is not a requirement to earn an ACE Personal Trainer Certification or most other NCCA-accredited personal-training certifications, but it can be helpful to the professional as he or she prepares for a certification exam. More than 70% of ACE-certified Professionals have four-year degrees, with many holding degrees in exercise science. Whether earned before or after becoming an ACE-certified Professional, a degree can prove helpful as trainers try to advance their careers into management or advanced positions within medical fitness or even teaching. For this reason, some personal trainers will decide years into their careers to earn a degree in exercise science, nutrition, business, or other subject areas. Upon earning the degree, the trainer can advance his or her career, fulfill a personal goal, and earn ACE continuing education credits for courses that provide education related to fitness and health.

Additional Fitness Certifications

Another way for a personal trainer to earn continuing education and advance his or her career is to earn additional certifications. ACE encourages professionals to earn certifications that provide them with new areas of expertise. ACE offers four certifications, each providing a different area of expertise for fitness professionals. For a personal trainer looking to become a better leader or motivator, or simply to pick up some group exercise classes to supplement his or her personal-training income, ACE offers its Group Fitness Instructor (GFI) certification. To meet the needs of the growing number of individuals who are trying to change behaviors and lose weight, ACE offers an advanced credential titled the ACE Lifestyle & Weight Management Coach (LWMC) certification. And, for advanced fitness professionals who want to work with clients who have special needs or are post-rehabilitation for cardiovascular, respiratory, metabolic, or musculoskeletal diseases and disorders, ACE offers the Advanced Health & Fitness Specialist (AHFS) certification.

New Areas of Expertise Within Allied Healthcare

A personal trainer who wants to expand the services that he or she provides into another area of allied healthcare must earn the appropriate credentials to ethically and legally provide those services. This could include becoming a licensed massage therapist, earning a nutrition degree and becoming a registered dietitian, earning a doctorate in physical therapy and becoming a licensed physical therapist, or going to medical school and becoming a medical doctor. In all of these situations, the trainer earning the new credential will advance his or her career and the services that he or she can provide, becoming an advocate for exercise and personal training in his or her new professional arena.

Summary

It is important for people interested in becoming personal trainers to realize that it is a service profession. The U.S. Department of Labor, Bureau of Labor Statistics (2009), reports that people planning fitness careers should be:

- Outgoing
- Excellent communicators
- Good at motivating people
- Sensitive to the needs of others
- In excellent health and physical fitness, due to the physical nature of the job
- Good at sales if they want to work as personal trainers, particularly in large commercial fitness centers
- Personable and motivating to attract and retain clients

Understanding the ACE-certified Personal Trainer's scope of practice can be empowering, as it defines a unique profession dedicated to helping people improve their fitness, health, and quality of life through physical activity. Many of the professions in healthcare are devoted to *treating* disease, while a personal trainer primarily helps people *avoid* disease. In a society where almost two-thirds of the adult population is overweight and physically inactive, and youth are projected to possibly live shorter lives than their parents, the role that ACE-certified Personal Trainers play in the healthcare continuum has never been more important.

References

American College of Sports Medicine (2007). *ACSM's Health/Fitness Facility Standards and Guidelines* (3rd ed.). Champaign, Ill.: Human Kinetics.

American College of Sports Medicine & American Heart Association (2007). *Physical Activity and Public Health Guidelines.* www.americanheart.org/presenter.jhtml?identifier=3049282

Commission on Accreditation of Allied Health Education Programs (2007). *Standards and Guidelines for the Accreditation of Educational Programs for Personal Fitness Training*. www.caahep.org/documents/Personal%20Fitness%20Standards%20January%202007.pdf

IDEA Health & Fitness Association (2001). IDEA Opinion Statement: Benefits of a working relationship between medical and allied health practitioners and personal fitness trainers. *IDEA Personal Trainer*, 13, 6, 26–31.

Institute of Medicine (2002). *Dietary reference intake for energy, carbohydrate, fiber, fat, fatty acids, cholesterol, protein and amino acids*. Washington, D.C.: National Academy Press.

Saris, W.H. et al. (2003). How much physical activity is enough to prevent unhealthy weight gain? Outcome of the International Association for the Study of Obesity 1st Stock Conference and consensus statement. *Obesity Reviews*, 4, 2, 101–114.

U.S. Department of Health & Human Services (2008). *2008 Physical Activity Guidelines for Americans: Be Active, Healthy and Happy.* www.health.gov/paguidelines/pdf/paguide.pdf

U.S. Department of Health & Human Services (1996). *Physical Activity and Health: A Report of the Surgeon General.* Atlanta, Georgia: U.S. Department of Health & Human Services, Public Health Service, CDC, National Center for Chronic Disease Prevention and Health Promotion.

U.S. Department of Health & Human Services and U.S. Department of Agriculture (2005). *Dietary Guidelines for Americans 2005.* www.healthierus.gov/dietaryguidelines

U.S. Department of Labor, Bureau of Labor Statistics (2009). *Occupational Outlook Handbook 2008–09 ed. Fitness Workers*. www.bls.gov/oco/ocos296.htm. Retrieved April 22, 2009.

Suggested Reading

American College of Sports Medicine (2010). *ACSM's Guidelines for Exercise Testing and Prescription* (8th ed.). Philadelphia: Wolters Kluwer/Lippincott Williams & Wilkins.

American Council on Exercise (2009). *ACE Advanced Health & Fitness Specialist Manual*. San Diego, Calif.: American Council on Exercise.

American Dietetic Association, Dietitians of Canada & American College of Sports Medicine (2007). *Joint Position Statement: Nutrition and Athletic Performance*. www.ms-se.com/pt/pt-core/template-journal/msse/media/0309nutrition.pdf

Eickhoff-Shemek, J.M., Herbert, D.L., & Connaughton, D.P. (2009). *Risk Management for Health/Fitness Professionals: Legal Issues and Strategies.* Philadelphia: Lippincott Williams & Wilkins.

Janot, J. (2004). Do you know your scope of practice? *IDEA Fitness Journal*, 1, 1, 44–45.

Riley, S. (2005). Respecting your boundaries. *IDEA Trainer Success*, 2, 4, 12–13.

U.S. Department of Health & Human Services (2003). *Summary of the HIPAA Privacy Rule*. www.hhs.gov/ocr/privacy/hipaa/understanding/summary/privacysummary.pdf

Additional Resources

Ethics Resource Center: www.ethics.org

Institute for Credentialing Excellence (ICE): www.credentialingexcellence.org

International Health, Racquet, and Sportsclub Association: www.cms.ihrsa.org/

Medical Fitness Association: www.medicalfitness.org

Medline Plus Reference on Drugs and Supplements (A service of the National Library of Medicine and National Institutes of Health): www.medlineplus.gov

1 B

2 D

3 B

4 C

---

5 A

6 B

7 A

8 D

---

9 B

10 B

11 D

12 B

---

13 B

14 A

15 D

16 C

---

17 D

18 C

19 D

20 A

PART II

Leadership and Implementation

Chapter 2
Principles of Adherence and Motivation

Chapter 3
Communication and Teaching Techniques

Chapter 4
Basics of Behavior Change and Health Psychology

IN THIS CHAPTER:

Factors Influencing Exercise Participation and Adherence
- Personal Attributes
- Environmental Factors
- Physical-activity Factors

Understanding Motivation
- Intrinsic and Extrinsic Motivation
- Self-efficacy

Feedback

Leadership Qualities

The Personal Trainer's Role in Building Adherence
- Program Design
- Role Clarity
- Goal Setting
- Contracts/Agreements

Strategies to Maintain Client Motivation
- Relapse Prevention

Summary

TRACIE ROGERS, Ph.D., *is a sport and exercise psychology specialist and an assistant professor in the Human Movement program at the Arizona School of Health Sciences at A.T. Still University. She is also the owner of the BAR Fitness Studio in Phoenix, Arizona. Dr. Rogers teaches, speaks, and writes on psychological constructs related to behavior change and physical-activity participation and adherence.*

CHAPTER 2

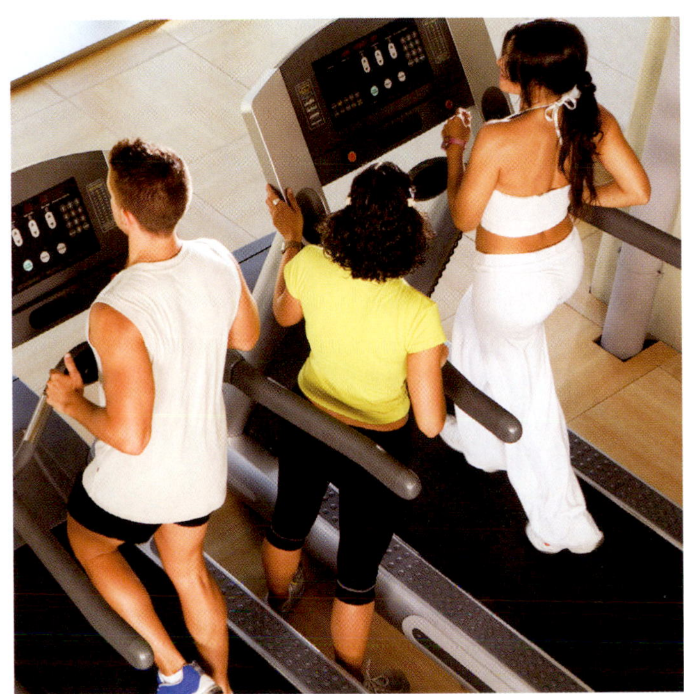

Principles of Adherence and Motivation

Tracie Rogers

With only about 45% of American adults engaging in physical activity at the minimum recommended levels [Centers for Disease Control and Prevention (CDC), 2005a], and with some reports indicating that levels of leisure time physical activity have actually declined since 1994 (CDC, 2005b), it is clear that fitness professionals have a significant challenge in getting people motivated to start—and then stick with—an exercise program. From a fitness perspective, these are really two separate issues. There is a great difference between motivating someone to start a new program and motivating someone to stick with a program once he or she has begun. For the purpose of this chapter, and to best address the issues that personal trainers face on a daily basis related to **adherence,** the focus will be on increasing the likelihood that people will adhere to a program once they have started. In other words, personal trainers must learn to maximize the experiences of their current clients.

The issue of exercise adoption has received more research attention than exercise adherence and is based mainly around the concept of behavior change. Adopting any lifestyle-modification program, including exercise, requires an individual to break old habits and develop new ones. The motivation to start a new program can come from any source, such as concern over health, an upcoming event, wanting to look better, and peer pressure. The most important factor, however, in starting an exercise program is the individual. A person cannot be coerced into starting to work out, but he or she must be somewhat ready to make a change. This poses an ongoing challenge to all health professionals who spend their careers trying to get people to change. Understanding the **transtheoretical model of behavioral change** (see Chapter 4) and using interventions specific to an individual's stage of change will help increase the success of any health professional who is trying to help others adopt a new behavior.

It is important to note, however, that factors that may motivate an individual to start exercising are not the same factors that will keep them participating in an exercise program over the long haul. While getting people to start a new program can be challenging and frustrating, it is a mistake to think that this is the only battle that fitness professionals will face. The true challenge for the health and fitness industry is creating programming and exercise environments that maximize the likelihood that a person will stick with the program and adopt an active lifestyle.

Motivation is a complex construct that refers to the psychological drive that gives behavior direction and purpose. There is no simple answer or magic pill to create motivation, which requires the personal trainer to practice awareness, communication, and consistency. Once trainers become proficient at helping to motivate others, they will understand the impact they have in changing lives and promoting life-long physical activity.

For the purposes of a fitness professional, exercise adherence refers to voluntary and active involvement in an exercise program. For the majority of clients, a moderate-intensity exercise program is appropriate, and according to the United States Department of Health & Human Services (2008), adults should engage in at least 2.5 hours of moderate-intensity aerobic physical activity each week. These guidelines are based on the substantial health benefits received from this amount of activity, but they also recognize that any activity is better than none. Additionally, it is recommended that adults engage in muscle-strengthening activities that are moderate or high intensity and involve all major muscle groups on two or more days a week, as these activities provide additional health benefits. For people who are physically active, reaching these recommended levels is typically not a problem, but they may seem intimidating for a new exerciser. Therefore, it is the fitness professional's responsibility to break these guidelines down into a manageable and achievable program. Researchers have also suggested that following such guidelines too closely can prevent a trainer from creating an individualized program. Recommended activity guidelines should only guide a trainer in creating a program that meets the needs and preferences of each individual client. Taking a "one size fits all" approach to program design is detrimental to long-term adherence. Instead, trainers should be mindful of general guidelines while personalizing exercise programs that people actually enjoy (Morgan, 2001).

Most people know that being physically active has many health benefits and have even started an exercise program at some time in their lives. Yet, a well-known statistic states that more than 50% of people who start a new program will drop out within the first six months (Dishman, 1988), which demonstrates that existing programming models may not be effective for getting the majority of people to stick with a program. Unfortunately, the solution is not simple. There are many factors related to exercise that influence adherence and dropout (e.g., environment, support, leadership, knowledge), and despite all of the knowledge and research about safe and effective exercise programming, not nearly enough is known about the specifics related to maintaining a regular exercise program (Dishman & Buckworth, 1997). In fact, much of the research has examined the people who quit, when it really may be much more relevant to understand the reasons why certain people stick with a program. Because there is no exact formula for helping people continue with a program, it is up to personal trainers to combine all of their interpersonal, communication, and program-design skills to create well-rounded exercise programs that not only get people fit and healthy, but that also create an exercise experience that is positive and worthwhile.

Factors Influencing Exercise Participation and Adherence

Much research has examined the factors related to physical-activity participation, creating a solid knowledge base for understanding the potential determinants for physical activity. In this context, determinants can be described as the factors that influence a person's decision to engage in exercise behavior. The potential determinants for physical activity can be broken down into three categories (Dishman & Buckworth, 1997):

- Personal attributes
- Environmental factors
- Physical-activity factors

Having a general understanding of these factors can help prepare personal trainers for the various challenges that clients may face during the course of participation in an exercise program.

Personal Attributes

Demographic Variables

Adherence to physical-activity programs has proven to be consistently related to education, income, age, and gender (CDC, 2005b; Morgan et al., 2003). Specifically, lower levels of activity are seen with increasing age, fewer years of education, and low income. Age, however, has been shown to be unrelated to adherence levels when examined in supervised exercise settings. Since personal trainers are directly involved with supervised fitness programs, this is particularly relevant (Oldridge, 1982). Regarding gender, men demonstrate higher and more consistent activity adherence rates than women (CDC, 2005b, 2003; Dishman & Buckworth, 1997). Demographic variables always occur concurrently, so it can be difficult to understand the specific effects of one demographic variable versus another. Nevertheless, the general trends are apparent and consistent.

Biomedical Status

Biomedical status refers to health conditions, including obesity and cardiovascular disease, and is typically a weak predictor of exercise behavior. In general, research has shown that obese individuals are typically less active than normal-weight individuals, and are less likely to adhere to supervised exercise programs. Unfortunately, these relationships have not remained consistent in more recent research, leaving experts a bit unsure about the exact relationship between obesity and physical-activity program adherence (Dishman & Buckworth, 1997). No consistent relationship between cardiovascular disease and activity adherence has been seen. It is likely that the relationship between these biomedical variables and behavior change is significantly related to the characteristics of the exercise program and the fitness industry itself.

Activity History

Activity history is arguably the most important and influential personal attribute variable. In supervised exercise programs, past program participation is the most reliable predictor of current participation. This relationship between past participation and current participation is consistent across gender, obesity, and coronary heart disease status (Dishman & Buckworth, 1997). Therefore, it is important that personal trainers gather activity history information from their clients. This information can help in the development of the current program, as client preferences should be considered, and it will also give the personal trainer a good idea of the challenges that the client may face in adhering to the current program.

Psychological Traits

Psychological traits refer to general tendencies that people have in their personality or psychological makeup. Psychological traits account for individual differences among people and are often difficult to define and measure. However, the trait of self-motivation, which is reflective of one's ability to set goals, monitor progress, and self-reinforce, has been shown to have a positive relationship with physical-activity adherence (Dishman, 1982).

Knowledge, Attitudes, and Beliefs

Individuals have a wide variety of knowledge, attitudes, and beliefs about starting and sticking with an exercise program. Modifying the way an individual thinks and feels about exercise has been shown to influence his or her intentions regarding being active. Health perception, which is a knowledge, attitude, and belief variable, has been linked to adherence, such that those who perceive their health to be poor are unlikely to start or adhere to an activity program. Furthermore, if they do participate, it will likely be at an extremely low intensity and frequency (Dishman & Buckworth, 1997). **Locus of control** is another variable in this category, as a belief in personal control over health outcomes is a consistent predictor of unsupervised exercise activity among healthy adults. Finally, the variable of perceived barriers, such as lack of time, consistently demonstrates a negative relationship with physical-activity program adherence.

Environmental Factors

Access to Facilities

Access to facilities most frequently refers to facility location. When fitness facilities are conveniently located near a person's home or work, he or she is more likely to adhere to the program. Specifically, when facility access is measured objectively (i.e., true access and availability of a facility), it is a consistent predictor of physical-activity behavior, such that people with greater access are more likely to be physically active than people with less access (Dishman, 1994). Personal trainers should ask their clients about access issues and understand how convenient or inconvenient it is for each client to reach the facility.

Time

A lack of time is the most common excuse for not exercising and for dropping out of an exercise program, as people perceive that they simply do not have time to be physically active (Oldridge, 1982). The perception of not having enough time to exercise is likely a reflection of not being interested in or enjoying the activity, or not being committed to the activity program. Personal trainers must teach their clients to change their perception of time availability through the use of goal setting, time management, and prioritizing. If an individual considers health and physical activity top priorities, he or she will find—or make—the time to be active.

Social Support

Social support from family and friends is an important predictor of physical-activity behavior (Duncan & McAuley, 1993). It is difficult for an individual to maintain an exercise program if he or she does not have support at home. When support is broken down into specific types, support from a spouse is shown to be an important and reliable predictor of program adherence. Social support is also a critical topic for personal trainers and clients to discuss. If a client is lacking support from family and friends, personal trainers must be proactive in creating and establishing a support network for the client.

Physical-activity Factors

Intensity

The drop-out rate in vigorous-intensity exercise programs is almost twice as high as in moderate-intensity activity programs. Additionally, when people are able to choose the type of activity they engage in, six times as many women and more than twice as many men choose to start moderate-intensity programs than vigorous-intensity programs. These results are true regardless of whether intensity is measured physiologically, such as by percentage of **heart-rate reserve,** or psychologically, such as by **ratings of perceived exertion (RPE)** (Sallis et al., 1986).

Injury

There is a reliable relationship between physical activity and injury, and it is estimated that as many as half of all people who engage in high-intensity activities (such as running) are injured each year (Macera et al., 1989). The red flag with this statistic is that injuries that occur as a result of program participation are directly related to program dropout. Research has also shown that injured exercisers are able to participate in modified exercise programs and often report engaging in significantly more walking than non-injured exercisers (Hofstetter et al., 1991).

Understanding Motivation

What is motivation and how does a person get it? The answer to this question is complex and multifaceted. It would be much easier to "build" motivation if it came from a single source and worked the same for all people. The reality is that motivation can be a lot of different things. It can come from within a person and is sometimes described as a personality trait. It can also come from other people's encouragement, guidance, and support. Motivation can even come from things, ideas, and events. Regardless of the source of motivation, even if it is external, the individual always plays an important role. Most fitness professionals will attest to the fact that it is nearly impossible to motivate someone who does not want to be motivated. The individual must buy into the process and into the motivators, whatever they may be. Because of the complexity of motivation, it is often a difficult topic for personal trainers to handle. Some clients are self-motivated, eager to be in the gym, and ready to get to work, while others make excuses, are inconsistent, and constantly complain. The natural tendency is for personal trainers to describe an eager, hard-working client as motivated and a difficult client as unmotivated, and this is likely an accurate assessment. However, it is more important to evaluate how trainers deal with each type of client: Is it true that the eager client will never need any motivational support from the trainer? Is the difficult client a lost cause? The truth is that while the individual plays a critical role, his or her attitude toward exercise is not the only factor influencing motivation. Both of these clients will need guidance and help in maintaining and building motivation for continued exercise participation (Duda & Treasure, 2005).

Because of the importance and complexity of motivation, numerous theoretical constructs have been proposed to explain motivation and its relationship with performance and achievement. Two commonly discussed approaches for evaluating motivation are **intrinsic** and **extrinsic motivation** and **self-efficacy.**

Intrinsic and Extrinsic Motivation

To be intrinsically motivated, in the exercise context, means that a person is engaged in exercise activity for the inherent pleasure and experience that comes from the engagement itself. For true intrinsic motivation to be in effect, no other factors (e.g., people or things) are instigating the client's participation (Vallerand & Losier, 1999). People who are intrinsically motivated report being physically active because they truly enjoy it. Such involvement in an activity is associated with positive attitudes and emotions (e.g., happiness, freedom, and relaxation), maximal effort, and persistence when faced with barriers. Consider an individual who is offered a "magic pill" that will make him or her lose weight, be healthy and fit, and look great without having to work out. An intrinsically motivated exerciser would still want to continue with the exercise program, regardless of the potential of the pill (Vallerand, 2001). While many people truly enjoy being physically active, very few (if any) adults are completely intrinsically motivated. The goal of personal trainers should be to maximize enjoyment and engagement, but not expect that their clients will always demonstrate intrinsic motivation.

The reality is that most adults depend on some amount of extrinsic motivation. This type of motivation involves the engagement in exercise for any benefit other than for the joy of participation. People who are extrinsically motivated report being physically active because of some external factor (e.g., to lose weight, to be healthy, to make my spouse happy, to look good, to meet new people) and are likely to experience feelings of tension, guilt, or pressure related to their participation. Very few people are entirely intrinsically or extrinsically motivated. Instead, most everyone falls somewhere on the continuum between the two.

Instead of feeling like they need to make their clients more intrinsically motivated, personal trainers should strive to enhance the feelings of enjoyment and accomplishment that come with program participation. This can be done through creating mastery, providing consistent and clear **feedback,** including the client in aspects of program design, and creating a workout environment that is aesthetically pleasing. These things will help increase the state of motivation during the actual workout. This is called situational motivation and refers to motivation as people are actually exercising. The second task of a personal trainer is to foster the development of motivation at the contextual level, which means how the client generally views exercise and physical activity. The most important thing a personal trainer can do to help build this type of motivation is to empower the client with the perception of control of his or her own participation and to actually give the client control. In general, personal trainers must teach, not control. Trying to control or manipulate a client to act in a certain way will actually diminish intrinsic motivation. Instead, by encouraging client ownership and involvement in the program and by teaching self-sufficiency and autonomy, personal trainers can help facilitate the development of intrinsic motivation. Many personal trainers are afraid to teach their clients to be independent because they fear that their services will no longer be needed. In reality, failing to build client independence is related to less-motivated clients who will ultimately be more likely to drop out. On the other hand, people who enjoy the experience are likely to continue working with a personal trainer and remain involved in an exercise program.

Self-efficacy

Self-efficacy is an important motivational concept for personal trainers to clearly understand because it deals with positive thinking, which is an important precursor to motivation. Self-efficacy is particularly relevant in challenging situations in which people are trying to achieve a goal, as is the case with exercise adherence. In the exercise context, self-efficacy is defined as the belief in one's own capabilities to successfully engage in a physical-activity program. Self-efficacy beliefs influence thought patterns, emotional responses, and behavior (Bandura, 1986). Self-efficacy is positively related to motivation, because when people believe that they can effectively engage in exercise behavior, they do so with a positive attitude and more effort and persistence.

It is important that personal trainers use communication and ongoing awareness to understand the self-efficacy levels of their clients. These levels can change quickly, so personal trainers should be in touch with these thought patterns of their clients. Personal trainers can use the sources of self-efficacy (see Chapter 4) to help influence efficacy levels. This can be as simple as creating short-term success by designing a workout that the client will master and that will demonstrate growth and achievement. In fact, this should be the case for the program in general, as each workout should build on previous accomplishments.

Different clients will require different amounts of verbal encouragement and statements of belief. Being aware of how much feedback a client needs and then providing that verbal support is an important motivational tool. Also, it is important to help clients re-evaluate appraisals of their physiological states to create more positive interpretations. By teaching clients to appropriately identify muscle fatigue, soreness, and tiredness, as well as the implications of these states, trainers can help clients view the "feelings" of working out in a more positive light. In general, by being aware of self-efficacy levels, personal trainers will be better able to consistently motivate their clients and help them create positive self-belief.

Feedback

Providing clients with information about their progress and performance in an exercise program is one of the most important roles of a personal trainer. This information is called feedback. Learning is non-existent without feedback, because if clients do not know how they are doing, they do not have a reason to make adjustments and change their behaviors.

Feedback can be either intrinsic or extrinsic, and both are important for enhancing learning and building motivation. Extrinsic feedback is the reinforcement, error correction, and encouragement that personal trainers give to their clients. Intrinsic feedback is information that the clients provide themselves based on their own sensory systems (i.e., what they feel, see, or hear). While extrinsic feedback is always important in the exercise environment, long-term program adherence is dependent on the client's ability to provide his or her own feedback. It is important for personal trainers to not give too much feedback. As client motivation, efficacy, and ability develop, personal trainers should allow their clients more opportunity to provide themselves feedback by tapering off the amount of external feedback provided.

Feedback serves an important role in motivation because it provides a guide to clients of how they are doing. The type of feedback that provides information on progress can be referred to as **knowledge of results** and without it, persistence suffers and people give up. General motivation comments during a training session can keep clients on track. Feedback also helps in the goal-setting process. Both intrinsic and extrinsic feedback can contribute to knowledge of results and provide information about progress toward goal attainment. Whether a client is achieving goals and experiencing success or is falling short of desired performance levels, it is up to the personal trainer to help the client use the feedback information to adjust and reestablish goals for continued motivation and program participation (Coker, Fischman, & Oxendine, 2005).

Leadership Qualities

The individual qualities of the personal trainer play a substantial role in a client's likelihood for long-term adherence. An effective personal trainer will become a leader who successfully influences the way his or her clients think, feel, and behave. Much has been written about the qualities of influential leaders, and personal trainers should learn from this information and not discount their leadership role. Leadership is both an art and a science and must be practiced and perfected. It may be helpful for some trainers to view their role as that of a coach who is working together with the client to achieve common goals. This analogy makes the importance of the role of the personal trainer clearer and demonstrates that the trainer is truly part of the process, not just a person who designs a workout.

Some of the components of being an effective leader are simple and straightforward. The first component is professionalism. The personal trainer's appearance should be clean, neat, and non-threatening. A personal trainer should look like someone who is at work and available to help others. Personal trainers should never look like they are ready for a workout or like they just finished a workout. At the same time, personal trainers should practice what they preach and exemplify what it means to live an active and healthy life. This initial credibility will help build client trust and help clients justify the time and financial commitment that they are making. Other requirements that define professionalism include being punctual and prepared. A client should never perceive that a trainer is "making it up as he or she goes along."

The trust in a client–trainer relationship should never be broken. A great deal of confidential information is shared with personal trainers. If a client perceives that personal information has been shared or mocked, the credibility of the trainer is compromised, trust is lost, and the client will likely withdraw from program participation with a negative perception of the fitness industry. This is a common occurrence and clients are often left feeling that they have nowhere to turn for help.

Personal trainers should take every opportunity to demonstrate to their clients that they listen. This can be accomplished effectively in the customization of the program based on client preferences and apprehensions. Clients will appreciate and value the fact that their trainer took the time to make their experience unique and personalized.

Clients will also appreciate personal trainers who demonstrate excitement for their craft. They want to work with trainers who are innovative and educated. By bringing new things to the table, a personal trainer not only builds motivation and adherence, but also enhances his or her credibility and the client's level of trust.

Continuing to show clients that they care and are interested in their progress is an ongoing part of the personal-training profession. By using systematic goal setting and by teaching relapse-prevention techniques, trainers are telling their clients that they care about them for more than the one-hour session. People like to be thought of and appreciated, and when clients perceive that their trainer is thinking of their overall well-being, the client–trainer relationship is further enhanced and the client becomes more vested in the program. Additionally, an effective personal trainer will include the client in all aspects of the program. After all, it is the client's program and he or she should be given the respect to be part of the planning and decision-making process. Personal trainers are the experts; however, by including the client in the process, the trainer has succeeded in getting the client to buy into the program, which will maximize long-term adherence.

Personal trainers should take time to think about their clients' experiences through the clients' eyes. What type of overall experience is the trainer providing? How clear are the communication and the plan for success? How stable is the support? How professional is the environment and interaction? These are all critical questions that personal trainers should be able to answer about their own services.

The Personal Trainer's Role in Building Adherence

Program Design

A significant and time-consuming part of a personal trainer's job is exercise program design. The trainer must have the ability to design a safe and effective physical-activity program. In the real world, however, clients are individuals and place unique demands on the trainer that he or she must be able to meet. Not all people have the time or money to participate in the "ideal" program. A personal trainer must be able to design a program with regard to each client's preferences, schedule, experience, apprehensions, and constraints (money, access, time, etc.). If a trainer is unable to create customized programs, he or she will be unable to build a stable business that is based on promoting long-term adherence to physical activity. A great deal of patience, listening skills, and creativity are required to successfully customize a program, but once a trainer takes the time and energy to hear and meet the needs of a client, the trainer will understand what it means to truly make a difference.

Role Clarity

In every relationship, there are formal and informal roles that people play. The client–trainer relationship is no different. A common cause of disagreements and conflict in a relationship is the lack of role clarity. In other words, if expectations are not clearly defined, there is room for misinterpretations and assumptions, which may lead to problems. From the beginning of the relationship with each client, a personal trainer should clarify his or her role, as well as that of the client, as part of the written agreement. What are the responsibilities and expectations of both parties? What does each person need to do to hold up his or her end of the deal? This information should be written down and agreed upon. If there are any issues or questions about the expectations, they should be discussed and modified from the start. This task is not difficult or time-consuming, but it is something that will help the client be vested in the program and feel supported, as well as maximize the client's experience and likelihood for adherence.

Goal Setting

Goal setting is an important process for initial and continued behavior change. It is an integral part of all fitness programs. The best thing about goal setting is that it is relatively simple to employ and extremely effective when done properly. Goal setting must be used systematically and should be an active part of the program to maximize adherence. As discussed in Chapter 3, goals should follow the SMART guidelines (i.e., specific, measurable, attainable, relevant, and time-bound) and personal trainers should take the time to teach their clients about setting proper goals. This education will be beneficial to clients as they progress through their programs and take more control over their experiences. The following are a few issues to keep in mind during the goal-setting process:

- *Avoid setting too many goals:* Keep the number of goals manageable and attainable so that the client is not overwhelmed with all that he or she needs to accomplish.
- *Avoid setting negative goals:* If the client wants to set a goal of not missing any workouts, the trainer should help the client reword this goal in a positive way: "I will attend every scheduled workout session." Setting negative goals puts the focus on the behavior that should be avoided, not the behavior to be achieved. It is important that the client is thinking about achievement, not avoidance.
- *Set short- and long-term goals, as well as outcome and performance goals:* Clients should be achieving short-term successes in each workout.
- *Revisit the goals on a regular basis:* This is the most important thing that a trainer can do to maximize the effectiveness of the goal-setting process. Goals need regular adjusting and should be consistently used as a tool to help direct attention and effort, and to promote persistence.

Contracts/Agreements

As previously mentioned, creating clarity within a program related to expectations and goals can be the difference between success and failure. An effective way to create clarity is through the use of behavioral contracts and written agreements. When used effectively, these documents can give the entire training process clarity by defining what the client should expect, what the program entails, and the rationale for the program design. This process enhances the communication between the client and the personal trainer and should give the client an accurate perception of the program. More information on contracts and agreements can be found in Chapter 4.

Strategies to Maintain Client Motivation

Relapse Prevention

It is important for any individual who participates regularly in a physical-activity program to implement strategies to prevent the occurrence of a **relapse** to an inactive state. Relapse from regular physical-activity participation is common and should be expected. From unexpected events and schedule changes to vacations and illnesses, there are countless things that can trigger such a relapse. The most important tool in dealing with a relapse is planning ahead and being prepared. Personal trainers should educate their clients about the potential occurrence of a relapse and prepare them in advance, so that they are able to get back on track with their activity programs soon after experiencing a relapse. The vast majority of people face one or more barriers, such as time, finances, prioritizing, scheduling, support issues, or dislike or dissatisfaction with the program, so it is important to develop strategies before adherence problems arise. Remember, the program and the overall experience ultimately have to be valued by the client for long-term adherence to occur.

Social Support

An important coping strategy for relapse prevention is to develop and maintain a social-support network for exercise. Personal trainers must be creative in increasing their clients' support systems at home, as it is important to get family members and/or friends involved to some degree in the program. In fact, adherence to an exercise program has shown to be increased when an exerciser has support from his or her spouse, either by joint participation or by demonstration of a positive attitude toward participation (Raglin, 2001). In general, individuals in a support network must understand the commitment the client has made to being physically active. Something easier for a personal trainer to do is create a support system within the exercise environment. Trainers should maximize opportunities for group involvement and social interaction, making their clients feel as though they belong in the program and are part of a team of people who have common interests and goals.

Assertiveness

Another strategy that personal trainers can use to help prevent program relapse is to teach their clients to be assertive. Assertiveness is an important characteristic for achieving success and is defined as the honest and straightforward expression of one's thoughts, feelings, and beliefs. Typically, when an individual is not assertive, it is because he or she lacks self-confidence or feels vulnerable. The more assertive clients are with regard to their progress, concerns, accomplishments, and struggles, the more likely they are to achieve long-term success.

Self-regulation

Personal trainers should strive to teach their clients to become effective self-regulators of their own behaviors, schedules, time, and priorities. The more control a client has over these things, the more likely he or she will be to adhere to the program. Personal trainers and other fitness professionals have a tendency to want to regulate clients' behavior for them. Instead, clients must be taught to self-monitor and to make behavior changes that will maximize their success. Once clients perceive control over their behavioral outcomes, they are more able to deal with barriers and challenges as they arise.

High-risk Situations

Clients and trainers who identify high-risk situations will be more prepared to deal with program barriers and relapses. By being prepared for common relapse-inducing events before they occur and by understanding the challenges of dealing with such changes, trainers and clients can come up with a plan to remain active through such times. It is also important for personal trainers to identify those clients who appear to be most at risk for program relapse. Individuals who have poor time-management skills, a lack of social support, or busy schedules are most likely to relapse. By providing extra education, support, and guidance for these clients as they participate in their programs, trainers can help them be better prepared to deal with the barriers they will face in terms of adherence. Personal trainers must be constantly aware and watch for signs that clients are overwhelmed, frustrated, or worn out. If these signs are present, personal trainers must take the time to teach these individuals additional coping skills, including time management and prioritizing. By working with clients on developing a plan for adherence, and by being supportive, understanding, and empathetic, personal trainers will be better able to help clients continue participating in their exercise programs.

Summary

Motivating clients every day can be among the most challenging and frustrating tasks for personal trainers. Because there is no single right way to create and enhance motivation and adherence, trainers must be aware, creative, and compassionate with their interactions and programming. Successful personal trainers understand and implement interpersonal and motivational skills during each workout. Motivation and adherence are perfect examples of why personal training is about so much more than exercise science and exercise program design. Effective personal trainers take the time to enhance their communication and relationship-building skills and work on a daily basis to effectively use these skills with their clients. The end result will be motivated and consistent clients who not only receive great workouts, but who are also having experiences that will keep them coming back for more.

References

Bandura, A. (1986). *Social Foundations of Thought and Action: A Social Cognitive Theory*. Englewood Cliffs, N.J.: Prentice-Hall.

Centers for Disease Control and Prevention (2005a). Adult participation in recommended levels of physical activity: United States, 2001 and 2003. *Morbidity and Mortality Weekly Report,* 54, 47, 1208–1212.

Centers for Disease Control and Prevention (2005b). Trends in leisure-time physical inactivity by age, sex, and race/ethnicity: United States, 1994–2004. *Morbidity and Mortality Weekly Report,* 54, 39, 991–994.

Centers for Disease Control and Prevention (2003). Physical activity among adults: United States, 2000. *Advance Data,* 333.

Coker, C.A., Fischman, M.G., & Oxendine, J.B. (2005). Motor skill learning for effective coaching and performance. In: Williams, J.M. (Ed.) *Applied Sport Psychology: Personal Growth to Peak Performance.* New York, NY: McGraw-Hill.

Dishman, R.K. (1994). *Advances in Exercise Adherence*. Champaign, Ill.: Human Kinetics.

Dishman, R.K. (Ed.). (1988). *Exercise Adherence: Its Impact On Public Health.* Champaign, Ill.: Human Kinetics.

Dishman, R.K. (1982). Compliance/adherence in health-related exercise. *Health Psychology,* 1, 237–267.

Dishman, R.K. & Buckworth, J. (1997). Adherence to physical activity. In: Morgan, W.P. (Ed.) *Physical Activity & Mental Health* (pp. 63–80). Washington, D.C.: Taylor & Francis.

Duda, J.L. & Treasure, D.C. (2005). Toward optimal motivation in sport: Fostering athletes' competence and sense of control. In: Williams, J.M. (Ed.) *Applied Sport Psychology: Personal Growth to Peak Performance.* New York: McGraw-Hill.

Duncan, T. E. & McAuley, E. (1993). Social support and efficacy cognitions in exercise adherence: A latent growth curve analysis. *Journal of Behavioral Medicine,* 16, 199–218.

Hofstetter, D.R. et al. (1991). Illness, injury, and correlates of aerobic exercise and walking: A community study. *Research Quarterly for Exercise and Sport,* 62, 1–9.

Macera, C.A. et al. (1989). Predicting lower-extremity injuries among habitual runners. *Archives of Internal Medicine,* 149, 2565–2568.

Morgan, C.F. et al. (2003). Personal, social, and environmental correlates of physical activity in a bi-ethnic sample of adolescents. *Pediatric Exercise Science*, 15, 288–301.

Morgan, W.P. (2001). Prescription of physical activity: A paradigm shift. *Quest,* 53, 336–382.

Oldridge, N.G. (1982).Compliance and exercise in primary and secondary prevention of coronary heart disease: A review. *Preventive Medicine*, 11, 56–70.

Raglin, J.S. (2001). Factors in exercise adherence: Influence of spouse participation. *Quest,* 52, 356-361.

Sallis, J.F. et al. (1986). Predictors of adoption and maintenance of physical activity in a community sample. *Preventive Medicine,* 15, 331–341.

U.S. Department of Health & Human Services (2008). *2008 Physical Activity Guidelines for Americans: Be Active, Healthy and Happy.* www.health.gov/paguidelines/pdf/paguide.pdf

Vallerand, R.J. (2001). A hierarchical model of intrinsic and extrinsic motivation in sport and exercise. In: Roberts, G. (Ed.) *Advances in Motivation in Sport and Exercise*. Champaign, Ill.: Human Kinetics.

Vallerand, R.J. & Losier, G.F. (1999). An integrative analysis of intrinsic and extrinsic motivation in sport. *Journal of Applied Sport Psychology,* 11, 142–169.

Suggested Reading

Bandura, A. (2001). Social cognitive theory: An agentive perspective. *Annual Review of Psychology,* 52, 1–26.

Bandura, A. (1997). *Self-efficacy: The Exercise of Control.* New York: Freeman.

Dishman, R.K. & Sallis, J. (1990). Determinants and interventions for physical activity and exercise. In: Bouchard, C. et al. (Eds.) *Exercise, Fitness, and Health*. Champaign, Ill.: Human Kinetics.

McAuley, E., Pena, M.M., & Jerome, G.J. (2001). Self-efficacy as a determinant and an outcome of exercise. In: Roberts, G.C. (Ed.) *Advances in Motivation in Sport and Exercise.* Champaign, Ill.: Human Kinetics.

Sallis, J.F. & Hovell, M.F. (1990). Determinants of exercise behavior. In: *Exercise and Sports Sciences Reviews*, 18. Baltimore: Williams & Wilkins, 307–330.

U.S. Department of Health & Human Services (1996). *Physical Activity and Health: A Report of the Surgeon General*. Atlanta, Georgia: U.S. Department of Health & Human Services, Public Health Service, CDC, National Center for Chronic Disease Prevention and Health Promotion.

IN THIS CHAPTER:

Stages of the Client–Trainer Relationship

Rapport Stage

Investigation Stage

Planning Stage

Action Stage

Strategies for Effective Communication

Cultural Competence Increases Empathy and Rapport

Difficult Clients May Require More Effort

Empathy and Rapport Enhance Adherence

Professional Boundaries Enhance the Effectiveness of Personal Trainers

Stages of Learning and Their Application to the Client–Trainer Relationship

How to Incorporate Effective Communication and Teaching Techniques Into Daily Interactions With Clients

Summary

BARBARA A. BREHM, ED.D., *is a professor of exercise and sport studies at Smith College, Northampton, Mass., where she teaches courses in stress management, nutrition, and health. She is also the director of the Smith Fitness Program for Faculty and Staff. Dr. Brehm writes extensively for fitness professionals and has received widespread recognition for the regular columns she writes as a contributing editor for* Fitness Management *magazine. She is the co-author of* Applied Sports Medicine for Coaches, *and author of several other books, including* Successful Fitness Motivation Strategies.

CHAPTER 3

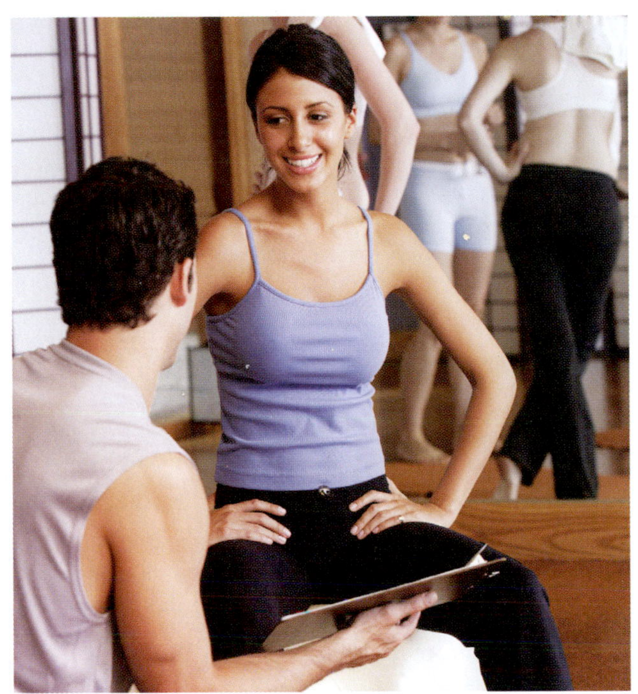

Communication and Teaching Techniques

Barbara A. Brehm

Successful personal trainers consistently demonstrate excellent communication and teaching techniques while working closely with their clients to understand their concerns, formulate health and fitness goals, design effective fitness programs, and teach exercise skills. Fitness professionals who excel in exercise science and understand the intricacies of training principles will still lack effectiveness if they cannot establish positive and productive working relationships with their clients. These relationships are based on good communication and teaching techniques.

Stages of the Client–Trainer Relationship

The early days of the client–trainer relationship can be thought of as consisting of four stages, each requiring somewhat different communication skills on the part of the personal trainer (Figure 3-1). When personal trainers meet new clients for the first time, they begin by breaking the ice and building **rapport,** which refers to a relationship marked by mutual understanding and trust. The rapport stage begins with first impressions, so it is extremely important that personal trainers present themselves in an approachable, professional manner from day one, using both verbal and nonverbal communication skills. Rapport continues to build over time, and the longer personal trainers and clients work together, the more they come to understand one another. An early foundation of trust and respect increases the likelihood that clients seeking a long-term personal-training relationship will stay with a given personal trainer.

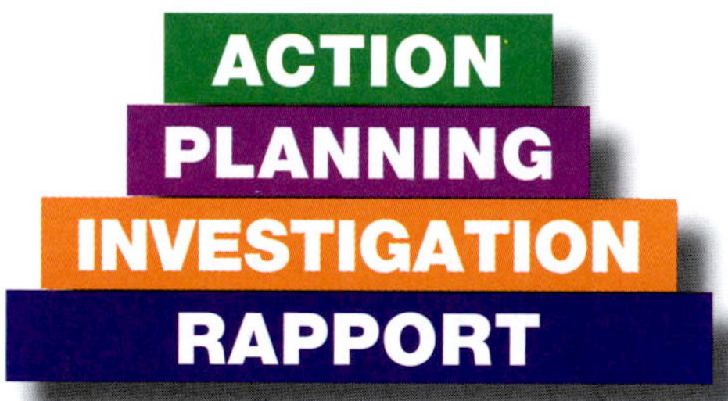

Figure 3-1
Stages of the client–trainer relationship

Client–trainer relationships quickly enter the investigation stage. Personal trainers and clients review clients' health and fitness data, any available test results, medical clearance information, and clients' goals and exercise history. During the investigation stage, good listening skills help the personal trainer understand the client and elicit as much helpful information as possible.

When all of this information has been gathered and discussed, the client–trainer relationship progresses to the planning stage, during which the personal trainer designs an exercise program in partnership with the client, using both good listening and teaching skills. At this point, clients are ready to begin working out, signaling the beginning of the action stage of the client–trainer relationship. The ability to effectively teach new motor skills is essential at this point.

It is important to remember that while these stages describe the traditional progression of the client–trainer relationship, they often overlap and recur. For example, rapport building continues throughout the first several weeks or months of a new client–trainer relationship. Similarly, personal trainers frequently reinvestigate client data as they review workout records and new fitness test results, and then update the exercise plan and teach new skills. Personal trainers who complete only a single session with clients may go through all of the stages during that session. Excellent communication skills and teaching techniques are essential during all of these stages.

Rapport Stage

During the rapport stage, the personal trainer sets the scene for establishing understanding and trust. Obviously, it takes time for trust and understanding to fully develop, but most people have a "gut response" or first impression when meeting another person. Many factors influence clients' first impressions of a personal trainer, including the personal trainer's physical appearance, facial expression, attire, and self-confidence. Rapport continues to develop through the use of good verbal and nonverbal communication, as personal trainers work to create a climate of respect and trust.

First Impressions

One way to think about the importance of the first impression a personal trainer makes is to consider the factors that generally contribute to a positive client–provider relationship in the health and fitness industry. When people are asked to recall both negative and positive experiences with healthcare providers, allied health professionals, and/or health and fitness professionals, many common themes emerge (Brehm, 2004).

Negative experiences are marked by rudeness, indifference, ineptitude, neglect, and even malpractice. When describing negative experiences, people often report being left waiting a long time in environments that are dirty, disorganized, or dull. Personal trainers are described as appearing bored, uninterested in the client, uncaring, or distracted. Communications with personal trainers are perceived as unclear, with clients saying they did not understand the information or the reasons for the recommendations. Questions are not encouraged or answered clearly.

On the other hand, positive experiences with personal trainers are characterized by a sense of caring, respect, clear communication, and professionalism on the part of the personal trainer. Clients perceive that their concerns are taken seriously and that the personal trainer is highly qualified, knowledgeable, and helpful. Questions are carefully considered and clearly answered. The environment is usually clean and organized. Characteristics of positive client–trainer experiences are listed in Table 3-1.

Positive first impressions provide a great start for the rapport-building process. Clients' first impressions are based on many controllable factors, as listed in Table 3-1. Because first impressions are so important, personal trainers should always conduct themselves appropriately, even when not planning to be in the public eye, since opportunities to meet future clients may unexpectedly arise. During the first meeting with clients, personal trainers should be sure that clients know about their education, training, certifications, qualifications, and work experience. In emerging professions, such as personal training, where credentialing is not always required or well-understood by the public, it is especially important to establish one's professional credibility (George, 2008).

Table 3-1

Characteristics of Positive Client–Trainer Experiences

Environment
• The facility is neat and clean. • Offices and staff have a well-organized appearance.
Appearance of the Personal Trainer
• The personal trainer wears professional attire. • The personal trainer's appearance is fit, neat, and clean. • The personal trainer is friendly and interested in the client. • The personal trainer shows a warm, positive attitude. • The personal trainer makes a positive first impression.
Interactions With the Personal Trainer
• Clients have confidence in the trainer's qualifications, training, experience, and skills. • Clients have enough time to express their concerns. • The personal trainer listens carefully and tries to understand the client's concerns. • Clients believe that the personal trainer is genuinely interested in what clients have to say. • Clients perceive an unconditional positive regard from the personal trainer. • Clients believe that the personal trainer respects them and their opinions. • Clients trust that the personal trainer will maintain their confidentiality and has their best interests at heart. • Instructions are clearly explained and clients' questions are answered.

Reprinted, with permission, from B.A. Brehm (2004). *Successful Fitness Motivation Strategies,* Champaign, Ill.: Human Kinetics.

Verbal and Nonverbal Communication

People's verbal communication is only a small part of the messages they send. People pay attention to much more than words in their effort to decipher messages and understand social situations. While people hear each other's words, they seek to verify verbal content by evaluating the speaker's appearance, facial expressions, body language, and tone of voice. If someone's words ("I am glad to meet you") and body language (lack of eye contact, disinterested facial expression, body turned away, low energy) do not match, people generally trust body language over verbal content (Ambady & Gray, 2002).

When speaking with clients, the personal trainer should speak clearly and use language that is easily understood by clients, without talking down to them. It is certainly appropriate to use exercise science vocabulary, but the personal trainer should be sure to define terms that may be unfamiliar to clients. Verbal content can be enhanced with visual information that illustrates concepts (e.g., pictures, diagrams, charts). Exercise demonstrations may accompany verbal explanations.

Nonverbal communication has many components, including the following:

- *Voice quality:* A weak, hesitant, or soft voice does not inspire client confidence. On the other hand, a loud, tense voice tends to make people nervous. Personal trainers should try to develop a voice that is firm and confident to communicate professionalism. Some people end their sentences with a higher pitch, as though asking a question. This communicates indecisiveness and can detract from the confident impression that the personal trainer should always be trying to make.
- *Eye contact:* Direct, friendly eye contact shows clients they are the center of the personal trainer's attention, whether the personal trainer is listening or talking. When a listener looks away while a person is speaking, the speaker feels as though he or she is not being heard. Similarly, when a speaker looks away, the listener does not feel important; the speaker does not seem to care about the listener's reaction.
- *Facial expression:* Facial expressions convey emotion, but work best when the emotion is sincere. Most clients can sense an artificial smile, so personal trainers must always portray a genuine display of positive regard for clients. As personal trainers work with clients, their faces should display the concern, thoughtfulness, and/or enjoyment they are feeling.
- *Hand gestures:* Use of hand gestures varies from culture to culture. In general, people are most comfortable when a speaker uses relaxed, fluid hand gestures while explaining something. When listening, a personal trainer's hands should be quiet. Fidgeting hands, clenched fists, abrupt gestures, and finger pointing are distracting to many clients.
- *Body position:* An open, well-balanced, erect body position communicates confidence. Good posture is especially important for personal trainers, whose bodies serve as symbols of their professional expertise (Maguire, 2008). A body posture that is leaning or stooped suggests fatigue and boredom (not to mention poor physical fitness), while a rigid, hands-on-hips stance may be interpreted as aggressive. When the personal trainer and client are seated together in discussion, the personal trainer should look attentive by leaning slightly forward and keeping the arms uncrossed. The personal trainer should eliminate distracting nervous activity such as foot or finger tapping, or constantly shifting position.

In addition to body language, many other behaviors serve as forms of communication. For example, when the personal trainer is late for an appointment, this communicates a lack of respect to the client. A lack of involvement is communicated when the personal trainer interrupts an appointment to make a phone call or perform other tasks.

Personality Styles

Successful personal trainers adapt their communication and teaching techniques to the personality style of the clients with whom they work. Personality style can be defined as an individual's characteristics, thoughts, feelings, attitudes, behaviors, and coping mechanisms. It is the distinctive pattern of an individual's psychological functioning—the way a person thinks, feels, and behaves.

Psychologists have devised many interesting theories of personality as well as scales for analyzing and categorizing personality styles. One of the most applicable is that of Daves and Holland (1981), who categorize people based on two important scales. The "dominance scale" measures how strongly a person is driven to influence the thinking and actions of others. The "sociability scale" is a measure of a person's tendency to express feelings openly, and to be extroverted and outgoing with others. People can be classified based on whether they score low or high on these two scales. Figure 3-2 illustrates the four personality styles that are described in this model. Table 3-2 describes the general traits associated with each personality style.

Personal trainers can benefit from assessing their own personality styles using Figure 3-3. The most helpful approach is for personal trainers to complete the survey describing

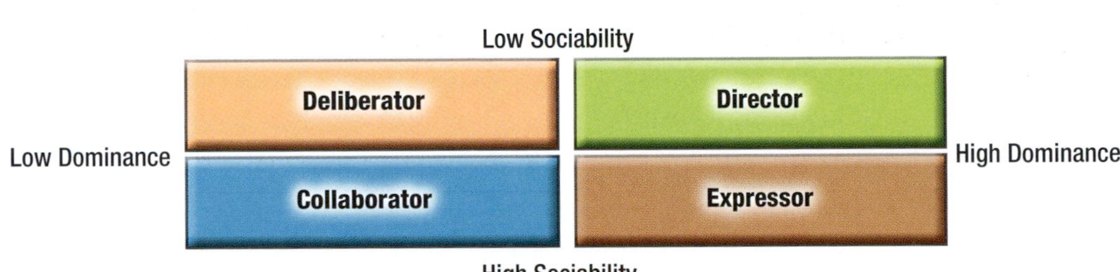

Figure 3-2
Personality styles

Table 3-2
General Personality Style Traits

Personality Style	General Traits
Deliberators Low sociability Low dominance	• More cognitive (thinking), less affective (emotion) • Ask-oriented (collect information before making decisions) • Methodical, favoring logic, objectivity, analysis, and accuracy • Problem-solvers, working alone or in small groups • Careful planners, interested in reducing the risk of the unknown • Appear rigid, formal, and cautious • Highly creative, but thorough and detail-oriented • Emotionally reserved initially, opening up once strong relationships are forged • Appear distant (less trusting) and uninterested in social interaction
Directors Low sociability High dominance	• More cognitive (thinking), less affective (emotion) • Action-oriented, competitive, take-charge, dominant personalities • Resourceful and tell-oriented, favoring teamwork where they can define problems, identify solutions, formulate plans and goals, and delegate to others to achieve results • Appear insensitive, impatient, direct, and unafraid to voice opinions • Poor listeners, as they proactively think ahead to problem solving • Appear unapproachable, unyielding, inflexible, and blunt • Emotionally reserved, valuing time over relationships
Collaborators High sociability Low dominance	• More affective (emotion), less cognitive (thinking) • Emotionally open, relationship-oriented, favor relationships over results • Amiable, warm, trusting and honest, sociable, easy-going, supportive, and non-dominant • Avoid unnecessary risks, slow to decide, non-confrontational, and sometimes exploited • Team- and ask-oriented, gather information to reach consensus over conflict
Expressors High sociability High dominance	• More affective (emotion), less cognitive (thinking) • Strong communicators, highly motivational and persuasive, but impatient • Overly ambitious, more risk-driven, favor incentives and rewards • Impulsive and lack discipline in completing projects • Dominant, tell-orientated visionaries who thrive on excitement, challenge, and creativity

themselves, have three close friends or colleagues complete the survey describing the personal trainer, and then compare these results.

Personal trainers may also find it helpful to use the scales to categorize the personality styles of their clients. As personal trainers spend time with clients and observe clients answering questions, interacting, and exercising, personality styles begin to emerge. Identifying personality styles can help personal trainers understand how their clients communicate, behave, and want to be treated. A personal trainer should never assume that people should all be treated the same, or that what works with one client always works for everyone. Table 3-3 provides guidelines for adapting rapport-building strategies to a client's personality style.

Figure 3-3
Identifying personality styles

1. Complete the surveys assessing dominance and sociability by circling an appropriate score for each word that best reflects the person's personality.

2. A score of 1 is "not descriptive of the person" while a score of 7 is "very descriptive of the person."

3. Sum the scored numbers to reach a total for each dimension.

Dominance Scale							
Aggressive	1	2	3	4	5	6	7
Challenging and confronting	1	2	3	4	5	6	7
Forceful	1	2	3	4	5	6	7
Outspoken	1	2	3	4	5	6	7
Takes charge	1	2	3	4	5	6	7
Assertive	1	2	3	4	5	6	7
Competitive	1	2	3	4	5	6	7
Straightforward	1	2	3	4	5	6	7
Frank	1	2	3	4	5	6	7
Blunt	1	2	3	4	5	6	7
						Total Score:	

Sociability Scale							
Accepting and supporting	1	2	3	4	5	6	7
Easy to know	1	2	3	4	5	6	7
Friendly and outgoing	1	2	3	4	5	6	7
People-orientated	1	2	3	4	5	6	7
Sociable	1	2	3	4	5	6	7
Agreeable	1	2	3	4	5	6	7
Cares how others feel	1	2	3	4	5	6	7
Flexible	1	2	3	4	5	6	7
Warm	1	2	3	4	5	6	7
Fun-loving	1	2	3	4	5	6	7
						Total Score:	

4. Score the dimensions of dominance and sociability scale according to the table presented below.

DOMINANCE SCALE			SOCIABILITY SCALE	
51–70	High		53–70	High
10–50	Low		10–52	Low

Table 3-3

Guidelines for Working With Different Personality Styles

Deliberators	Directors
• Supply information to support their need for detail • Appeal to their need to be right, believing that actions were clearly planned in detail • Establish credibility with research and supporting facts • Help secure clients' decisions by illustrating successful outcomes • Provide consistent, accurate follow-ups • Be well-prepared, detail-oriented, and organized • Avoid being too casual or informal, being vague or too general, and relying on intuition	• Minimize social aspects and desire to foster relationships • Appeal to clients' need for action and problem-solving • When planning, focus on facts, exploring solutions and possible outcomes • Be clear, concise, and business-like, and results- and goal-oriented • Avoid being overly personal or casual, vague or too general, and careless with facts • Avoid being too directive or forceful, as clients might become argumentative
Collaborators	**Expressors**
• Build trust and confidence through personal support and concern • Move carefully into the planning and action stages, informing clients that all possible options have been explored and risks minimized • Be candid, open and patient, personally interested and supportive, and goal-directed • Avoid being impatient, forceful and pressing for rapid decisions, aloof or too formal, or disengaged	• Offer incentives and rewards • Share clients' visions and enthusiasm and show support for their goals by stressing the exciting facets of their visions • Be stimulating and positive and provide adequate information; support ideas without overwhelming these clients with details, as they are not detail-oriented • Try to appear supportive of clients' ideas • Stimulate clients' thoughts and provoke ideas • Demonstrate commitment • Avoid being directive, unyielding, inflexible or too structured, too restrained or conservative, and indecisive or wavering

Investigation Stage

Rapport continues to build during the investigation stage, as personal trainers gather information from their clients. Much of this information is very personal in nature, including medical concerns, fitness assessment results, body weight, and exercise history. Clients may be somewhat embarrassed and uneasy discussing this information with someone they have just met. Clients who sense that the personal trainer is a professional who has their best interests at heart are likely to be more honest and comfortable in this investigation stage.

Gathering Information

Many personal trainers ask clients to complete forms such as health-history and lifestyle questionnaires. Taking time to review these forms with clients can help the personal trainer clarify questions and elicit more information. Personal trainers should use the investigation stage not only to learn about a client's current health and fitness, but also to understand a client's exercise likes and dislikes. Personal trainers should ask clients about their previous experiences with physical activity to uncover factors that furthered or disrupted exercise **adherence.** A personal trainer who listens carefully to clients' descriptions of past experiences can learn a great deal about clients' personal preferences, such as whether they like to exercise alone or with a friend, in the morning or at the end of the day, or at moderate or vigorous intensities. What has worked (or not worked) in previous exercise programs may work (or not work) again. Careful attention can help personal trainers read between the lines of fitness forms, while good listening skills help their understanding of the emotions behind the stories that clients tell.

Demonstrating Effective Listening

Some personal trainers tend to believe that because they get paid to give advice, the more they say, the better. They love to talk about exercise and health, and equate information delivery with performance and clients getting their money's worth. Unfortunately, this focus on talking can interfere with good communication if the personal trainer always dominates discussions with clients and interrupts clients before they are finished speaking.

Effective listening means listening closely and carefully to both the words and the emotions behind the speaker's words. Anyone who works with people needs to be able to listen effectively. During the investigation stage, careful listening is critical so that the personal trainer can understand the new client. Effective listening can help the personal trainer gather information that will enhance exercise program design as well as the personal trainer's working relationship with that client.

Effective listening takes a great deal of attention and energy, so people do not tend to listen carefully to each other most of the time. People sometimes pretend to listen, but do not pay careful attention. They may pretend to listen so as not to appear rude, but may only hear part of what the speaker says, tuning out parts they find uninteresting, offensive, or hard to understand. Instead of listening carefully, the listener is often busy formulating arguments, forming judgments about the speaker, or thinking about what to say next. Sometimes the listener is simply daydreaming and thinking about other things. Listeners are often preoccupied with themselves and their own thoughts, perhaps distracted by their own problems.

Even when listeners try to listen, they miss much of what the speaker is trying to say. Listeners often reconstruct messages in accordance with their own beliefs or needs. The listener may have prejudices about the speaker and look for confirmation of these feelings in the speaker's words. Listeners may project their own feelings onto the speaker, or only hear what they expect to hear.

Effective listening occurs when the personal trainer listens to a client carefully, empathetically, and with an open mind, trying to put him- or herself in the client's shoes. When trying to listen effectively, personal trainers should give clients their full attention. Close communication occurs most easily in quiet, private spaces that limit distraction.

Personal trainers should direct the conversation during the investigation stage by asking clients questions. As clients answer, personal trainers should show that they are listening by maintaining appropriate eye contact, using proper body language, and taking notes as necessary. Personal trainers can also demonstrate good listening skills by responding to clients' answers in several ways, including the following:

- *Encouraging:* The personal trainer may use short words or phrases such as "I see," "Yes," and "I know what you mean," that encourage the client to continue speaking when there is a natural pause in the client's speech. These phrases let the client know the personal trainer is listening carefully and following what is being said. Nodding and smiling can also indicate that a person is listening and encourage speakers to continue.
- *Paraphrasing:* The personal trainer can demonstrate understanding by restating in a clear and concise way the essence of what the client has been saying. Paraphrasing may also extend the meaning of the client's answers. For example, a client may tell a story about how he or she maintained a lighter weight for several years. The personal trainer might paraphrase, "So that feels like a realistic weight for you." If the paraphrase is not

accurate, the speaker then has a chance to correct an erroneous impression.

- *Questioning:* Open-ended questions demonstrate good listening and encourage the client to share relevant information. The personal trainer might follow up a client's story with a comment such as, "You said you quit exercising last year. What made you stop?" Personal trainers should ask questions at appropriate times to clarify points they do not understand or to move the conversation in a more productive direction.
- *Reflecting:* The personal trainer can demonstrate understanding or seek clarification by trying to restate the main points and feelings in the client's communication. For example, "It sounds like you have been most successful exercising in the past when you have a friend to exercise with." The listener can correct this conclusion if it is wrong, or explore this reflection in more depth if it is correct. Reflections should help to move the conversation in productive directions as well as indicate effective listening.
- *Summarizing:* At appropriate points in the conversation, the personal trainer should try to summarize key points that have a bearing on exercise program design. The personal trainer should allow clients to comment on the summary to confirm its accuracy. Summarizing not only demonstrates effective listening, but gives the personal trainer an opportunity to direct a conversation that is wandering too far off topic or keep an appointment on track in terms of time.

Personal trainers can also use a limited amount of self-disclosure to demonstrate understanding and forge bonds with clients. Personal trainers may choose to reveal similar personal experiences to indicate that they understand a client's position. These self-disclosures should be limited to one or two sentences, keeping the focus on the client. For example, a personal trainer might say, "I think I know what you mean. When I moved to a new city last year, I didn't exercise for several weeks either. What did you do then?"

Responding to Difficult Disclosures

Personal trainers are sometimes unsure of how to respond when clients share information that is very sad, such as a disclosure of a client's serious illness, or the illness or death of someone close to the client. Often, a short response is all that is required, such as "I'm so sorry," "That must have been very hard," or "I can't even imagine how difficult that must have been for you and your family." The personal trainer should follow the client's lead as to whether he or she wants to say anything more on a topic or not. If the situation affects exercise program design in any way, the personal trainer can turn the conversation back to the practical details. For example, "Now that your mother has moved in with you and your family, what is the best time for you to get to the fitness center?" If clients reveal new medical information that causes concern, they should be referred back to their healthcare providers for medical clearance. If a new medical condition places a client outside of the personal trainer's **scope of practice** and expertise, the client should be referred to someone with the necessary training and experience.

Sometimes personal trainers hear information that worries or even alarms them. For example, a personal trainer may suspect a client is suffering from **depression,** an **eating disorder,** or another serious health problem. In such cases, personal trainers should follow referral procedures that encourage the client to seek professional help. Personal trainers may also wish to share their concerns (while ensuring the confidentiality of the client) with their supervisors or a colleague to confirm their referral plan.

Planning Stage

The planning stage of the client–trainer relationship should be viewed as a give-and-take opportunity in terms of communication. While personal trainers move into a more active role during this stage, they must continue to listen to clients' responses to their ideas and suggestions. Client adherence is usually better when clients help take responsibility for exercise program design. The planning stage generally moves through the following steps:

- Setting goals
- Generating and discussing alternatives
- Formulating a plan
- Evaluating the exercise program

Setting Goals

Clients often express fairly general personal-training goals, such as wanting to "tone muscles" or "lose some weight." The personal trainer should help clients define goals in more specific and measurable terms so that progress can be evaluated. Effective goals are commonly said to be **SMART goals,** which means they are:

- *Specific:* Goals must be clear and unambiguous, stating specifically what should be accomplished.
- *Measurable:* Goals must be measurable so that clients can see whether they are making progress. Examples of measurable goals include performing a given strength-training workout two times a week or losing 5 pounds (2.3 kg).
- *Attainable:* Goals should be realistically attainable by the individual client. The achievement of attaining a goal reinforces commitment to the program and encourages the client to continue exercising. Attaining goals is also a testimony to the personal trainer's effectiveness.
- *Relevant:* Goals must be relevant to the particular interest, needs, and abilities of the individual client.
- *Time-bound:* Goals must contain estimated timelines for completion. Clients should be evaluated regularly to monitor progress toward goals.

The personal trainer should err on the conservative side of goal setting in terms of what might be realistically achieved by the client. Lofty goals feel good and sound inspirational, but clients are soon disappointed when progress is slow (Sears & Stanton, 2001). Fitness indicators that may demonstrate change include those listed in Table 3-4. These indicators may be incorporated into SMART goals, depending upon a client's specific interests.

The personal trainer should be sure to include **process goals** as well as **product goals.** A process goal is something a client does, such as walk 2 miles a certain number of times. A product goal is something achieved, like weight loss or a resistance lifted on a strength-training machine. Clients often achieve process goals before noticeable changes occur in weight or fitness test results. More suggestions for setting goals are presented in Table 3-5.

Generating and Discussing Alternatives

Once goals have been clarified, the personal trainer and client are ready to generate and discuss alternative ways of achieving these goals. The personal trainer should remember that, although it may not have been formally stated, the ultimate goal for every client is adherence to the exercise program. Similarly, the personal trainer hopes that the client will find the exercise program achievable and rewarding, so that the client continues working with the personal trainer.

A number of variables influence client adherence, as described in Chapter 2, and these should be taken into consideration as the personal trainer suggests alternatives. For example, one of the most common causes of exercise dropout is that clients perceive the exercise program as too time-consuming. If a client has dropped out of programs for this reason in the past, it makes sense for the personal trainer to encourage a fairly modest exercise program that may necessitate some goal adjustment, but will be preferable to an ambitious program that is never performed.

When clients are only going to be working with a personal trainer for one session or a few sessions, the exercise program design must be simple enough that a client can perform the program on his or her own. When a long-term client–trainer relationship is anticipated, the program can be more complex, since the personal trainer will be providing guidance. As the trainer and client work together to evaluate alternatives, the personal trainer

Table 3-4
Fitness Indicators for SMART Goal Setting
• *Emotional health indicators:* Clients may have measurable improvements in mood, energy level, and sleep quality, and fewer feelings of stress and irritability following exercise.
• *Resting heart rate:* Many personal trainers have their clients measure resting heart rate, either first thing in the morning or before falling asleep at night. Clients new to exercise often experience a decrease in resting heart rate after a few months of exercise.
• *Heart rate during a given submaximal workload:* Clients performing aerobic exercise are also likely to experience a decrease in exercise heart rate during exercise performed at a standard workload on a piece of equipment that reproduces the type of exercise training the client is performing. The submaximal load or loads must be identical each time the client is tested.
• *Muscular strength and endurance:* Gains in muscular strength and endurance occur fairly quickly during the first few months of an exercise program. A client's gains in terms of the amount of resistance used or the number of repetitions performed are easily measured.
• *Walking test:* Measuring fitness improvement with some sort of timed walking test usually yields positive results if clients have been walking as part of their exercise programs for several weeks.
• *Flexibility:* Flexibility is very slow to improve and should only be included in the assessment if the exercise program includes regular stretching.
• *Balance:* Balance measures show the most improvement for adults participating in some sort of balance-training program, which are becoming increasingly popular, especially among older adults.
• *Skill level:* Clients participating in an activity that requires skill (e.g., rock climbing, tennis, golf) will be pleased to see improvements in their motor-skill levels. Skill improvement may be measured via motor-skill tests or game performance.
• *Medical indicators, such as resting blood pressure, blood lipid levels, or blood sugar levels:* If any of these are the focus of clients' exercise programs, clients should have these measures taken at regular intervals as established by their healthcare providers. These variables may be affected by many other factors, including diet or changes in body weight, and these factors should be taken into consideration when evaluating exercise results.
• *Body weight:* Body weight is easily measured, but is a poor indicator of body-composition changes. Body weight may remain unchanged even though changes in body composition are occurring, or it may change by several pounds or kilograms due to changes in hydration. Nevertheless, clients on a weight-reduction program who are more than a few pounds or kilograms overweight will probably see a decrease in weight. Clients should work for slow and consistent weight loss, which is more likely to yield long-term weight loss.
• *Body size:* Clients who are only slightly overweight may not see much change in scale weight. Body-composition changes (fat loss with an increase in muscle mass) may still lead to a change in body size. Lean tissue, because of its greater density, takes up less space than fat tissue. Many people are happy when a waistband on a skirt or pair of pants fits more loosely. Many personal trainers encourage clients to watch for changes in the way their clothes fit.
• *Body composition:* If body composition is measured, the same test should be used consistently. Some personal trainers record circumferences or skinfolds without predicting body composition. Changes in these measures may be indicative of fat loss or increases in muscle size.

Table 3-5
How to Set Health and Fitness Goals That Motivate Clients for Long-term Adherence

- Listen carefully to understand what clients hope to accomplish with an exercise program.
- Help them define specific, measurable goals.
- Suggest additional goals that clients may not have thought of, such as feeling more energetic and less stressed.
- Break large goals (reachable in six months or more) into small goals (reachable in about eight to 10 weeks) and even weekly goals (such as completing a certain number of exercise sessions).
- Include many process goals, such as the completion of exercise sessions. In other words, simply completing workouts accomplishes a goal.
- Record goals and set up a record-keeping system to record workouts and track progress toward goals.
- Be sure clients understand what types of exercise will help them reach their health and fitness goals.
- Reevaluate and revise goals and exercise recommendations periodically to prevent discouragement if large goals are not being met.

Reprinted, with permission, from B.A. Brehm (2004). *Successful Fitness Motivation Strategies,* (Champaign, Ill.: Human Kinetics), 11.

should encourage the client to take the lead in what seems realistic, especially in terms of time commitment and scheduling.

Formulating a Plan

Personal trainers should incorporate material on effective exercise program design as they consider clients' goals and discuss alternatives (see Chapters 5 through 12). Once a plan is decided upon, it should be written down and given to the client. The plan should include all the information that the client needs to get started.

The personal trainer should also take this opportunity to help the client feel prepared to begin an exercise program. Many clients appreciate advice on what to wear, where to go, and any other tips on facility etiquette and customs that might help them feel more at home. Personal trainers often fail to realize how intimidating a fitness facility can be to a newcomer. Some guidance on "fitting in" is especially important if a client will be exercising on his or her own.

Evaluating the Exercise Program

Exercise program evaluation occurs regularly, as the personal trainer and client review exercise records at their sessions together and discuss what is working and what needs to change. Clients should also be reassessed periodically to measure progress toward goals. The exercise program should be evaluated both in terms of exercise challenge and adherence. Programs can be modified as necessary to provide a more realistic or challenging stimulus. If adherence is faltering, the personal trainer and client should discuss what is causing problems and revise the exercise program design as necessary.

Using Motivational Interviewing Techniques

Occasionally, personal trainers may find themselves working with clients who are not ready to commit to an exercise program. They may have been pushed into trying a personal-training session by a friend or family member, or they may know they should exercise but be unwilling to exert the effort required to become more active. While it is tempting to forge ahead and tell these clients what they should be doing, the personal trainer's advice may be wasted on clients who have not yet made a commitment to exercise. Unless a client has made a decision to change, his or her exercise attempts are likely to fail. Refer to Chapter 4 for more information on determining a client's readiness to change. A more beneficial approach is to discuss why clients feel unable to become more active. **Motivational interviewing** may help clients feel the need to become more active and make a decision to start exercising. Motivational interviewing refers to a method of speaking with people in a way that motivates them to make a decision to change their behavior. Motivational interviewing, which was originally designed for therapists working in addiction-counseling programs, is designed to show supportive concern while challenging a client's current behavior (Goldstein, DePue, & Kazura, 2008; Miller & Rollnick, 2002), but it can also be used by personal trainers discussing physical activity with their clients.

The personal trainer's goal in motivational interviewing is to create awareness in clients that a sedentary lifestyle will likely cause health problems. Using direct questions, the personal trainer can make clients realize that good health is important, and that a **sedentary** lifestyle is actually dangerous to their health and well-being. Personal trainers who use motivational interviewing will be most successful if they do the following (Brehm, 2004):

- *Ask probing questions:* The personal trainer may begin the motivational discussion by asking clients open-ended questions about their daily activity levels, health concerns, and physical-activity history. The personal trainer should move to questions that will hopefully help the client conclude that good health is important and that physical activity is essential for good health. For example, if clients have a family history of heart disease, the personal trainer could follow up by asking "Did you know that regular physical activity helps to prevent heart disease?"
- *Listen effectively:* The personal trainer should listen carefully to the client's answers. Listening effectively will help the personal trainer understand why a client feels unable to exercise or does not feel the need to exercise. By listening carefully, the personal trainer can uncover valuable information and show clients that they are respected, even when the trainer and client do not see eye to eye.
- *Provide educational information:* The personal trainer can explain the dangers of a sedentary lifestyle and the health benefits of regular physical activity. Attractive, readable handouts may help clients understand these issues.
- *Keep the conversation friendly:* While personal trainers may challenge statements made by clients ("I don't have a weight problem, so I don't need to exercise."), they should avoid heated arguments, since negative feelings may make clients defensive. If a client starts to seem angry, the personal trainer should switch to a more neutral, information-gathering question. The personal trainer may also express **empathy** and respect for the difficulties that clients face.
- *Build self-confidence:* The personal trainer can help clients identify areas of success, no matter how small. For example, the personal trainer might praise a client who currently walks the dog twice a day for five minutes, and then suggest that perhaps the client would consider increasing the walk time by a minute or two each week.
- *Encourage clients to generate ideas:* If clients seem willing to make even small changes, the personal trainer should let them take the lead in making suggestions that might work for them.

A personal trainer should monitor clients' responses to motivational interviewing attempts. If the personal trainer senses that the client has stopped listening, it is time to stop talking. Instead, the personal trainer can ask clients what they are thinking about or if they have any questions. A motivational interview can feel somewhat uncomfortable for personal trainers who tend to avoid conflict, but mild discomfort may help clients feel the need to change. The personal trainer's job in a motivational interview is to be supportive of the client (he or she is okay), but to challenge sedentary behavior (the behavior is not okay, and could be harmful to his or her health).

Action Stage

Once the exercise program design is complete, the client is ready to begin exercising. In many cases, the program is a combination of exercise completed by clients on their own (for example, taking a walk twice a week at home) and exercise performed with the personal trainer instructing and supervising. The personal trainer can enhance client success in many ways during the action stage.

Setting Up Self-monitoring Systems

In addition to a specific written exercise plan, the personal trainer should give the client—or better yet, design with the client's input—a system for recording exercise sessions, including any relevant data the personal trainer and client wish to track. An example is a flashcard or electronic system that is used at the fitness center that records the station, resistance, repetitions, and sets of a workout, and/or the time, intensity, heart rate, and so forth for cardiovascular exercise. If clients will also be exercising outside of the fitness center, the self-monitoring system should include a way to record these sessions as well.

Research has shown that self-monitoring is one of the most effective ways to support behavior change, including exercise program adherence (Berkel et al., 2005). Self-monitoring systems help in two ways. First, they increase client self-awareness. A log with nothing recorded for several days testifies to the fact that clients are neglecting their exercise programs. Self-monitoring acts as a mirror to give clients a more objective view of their behaviors. Second, self-monitoring systems enhance client–trainer communication. Clients come to expect careful surveillance of their records, which they present to the personal trainer at each session. Knowing that someone will be checking on their adherence may prod clients into action. As the personal trainer reviews the workout record, questions about what is working and what is not working will arise, leading to productive discussions between trainers and their clients.

Individualizing Teaching Techniques

Personal trainers often find themselves in the role of teacher. Personal trainers teach motor skills such as correct lifting techniques for strength training, how to use exercise machines, and how to perform **flexibility** exercises. Depending upon their training and expertise, personal trainers may coach sports drills, teach yoga postures, or explain rehabilitation exercises. Personal trainers may also teach clients about information in the **cognitive domain,** such as explaining health problems, how physical activity affects physiological variables, and how to prevent injury. Understanding how people learn most effectively can help personal trainers provide sound instruction to diverse groups of clients.

Clients learn in many different ways. People gather information through their senses (primarily visual, auditory, and kinesthetic), and process the information in their muscles and nervous systems, including the many areas of the brain. People usually have a preference for gathering information with one pathway over others, although most people use a combination of pathways. The personal trainer can identify which pathway a client prefers by observing actions during learning situations and by listening for clues in language (Table 3-6). Using a combination of visual, auditory, and kinesthetic approaches gives a client more information to enhance learning and understanding. All three techniques may be used to introduce a new skill, but once a trainer learns what works best for each client, he or she should emphasize the preferred learning style.

Clients who prefer auditory learning may like a lot of explanation and ask many questions. Visual learners learn by watching and appreciate longer demonstrations with less talking, while kinesthetic learners learn by doing, needing to feel the movement before catching on. Once the personal trainer has been working with a particular client for a period of time, his or her preferred learning style should become apparent.

Teaching pace should also be modified for each client. Clients should feel successful in their mastery of new exercises. Success improves **self-efficacy**, which means that clients will continue to exert the effort required to meet new challenges. While some clients catch on to new skills quickly, others do so more slowly and require a great deal of patience on the part of the personal trainer.

Table 3-6

Preferred Learning Style Indicators

	Visual	Auditory	Kinesthetic
Client actions	Watches intently Prefers reading	Listens carefully Prefers hearing	Touches or holds Prefers to be spotted
Client statement	"Oh, I see" "Let me see that again"	"Yeah, I hear you" "Say that one more time"	"I feel that" "This does not feel right"
Strategy	Demonstrations	Question and answer	Hands-on supervision

"Tell, Show, Do"

> Tell me and I'll forget
> Show me and I may remember
> Involve me and I'll understand
> —Chinese Proverb

This proverb should be understood by all personal trainers as they teach exercises to clients. **Motor learning** is the process of acquiring and improving motor skills. Many adult clients are quite self-conscious in the motor-skill domain, especially if they have had little experience with sports and physical activity. Personal trainers with a strong background in physical education and sport are often surprised at the lack of motor ability they see in many adult clients. Motor skills will be taught most effectively if the following points are kept in mind:

- *Remind beginners that it takes time and practice to improve motor skills:* Physical education specialists have noted that many people tend to believe that good coordination and athletic ability are something a person is born with (Rink, 2004). While ability in the motor-skills domain certainly varies from person to person, motor skills are more strongly related to practice and experience than to natural ability alone. It is important for people new to physical activity to understand that motor-skill improvement takes a great deal of practice—and that the people they see in the fitness center have often been performing similar movement patterns and choreography for years. The same holds true for athletes in every sport.

  Many clients new to exercise feel self-conscious participating in a personal-training session. They may feel out of place, awkward, and clumsy. The personal trainer must help new clients feel at home in the exercise environment, and reassure clients learning new skills that it is okay to be a beginner, and that with practice they will eventually look like fitness center regulars.
- *Introduce new skills slowly and clearly:* "Tell, show, do," illustrates a good way to introduce a new skill. The personal trainer should begin with a very short explanation of what he or she is going to do and why. Explanations should be short and clear. Safety information should be emphasized, along with guidelines for preventing injury. Skills should be explained in terms of what the skill is accomplishing or why it is important.

  A personal trainer may often combine the telling and showing phases of skill introduction, demonstrating while explaining the skill. When describing certain movements, the personal trainer should focus on explaining the goal of the movement rather than giving distracting details about limb position (Marchant, Clough, & Cramshaw, 2005). For example, a personal trainer would not teach someone how to use an elliptical trainer by describing when to bend and straighten the knees. Instead, the personal trainer would emphasize moving the pedals around in a smooth, steady motion. The personal trainer should demonstrate the skill accurately and allow clients time to watch.

Teaching strength-training exercises or exercise positions does require some explanation of limb position for safety and efficacy. For example, when teaching squats, the personal trainer might ask the client to focus on bending the knees only to 90 degrees and not moving the knees beyond the toes. These descriptions should be brief and simple.

- *Allow clients the opportunity for focused practice:* Once the personal trainer has "told and shown," the client is ready to "do," or perform the motor skill. People learn more quickly when they focus on performing the motor skill without being distracted by talking or listening. The personal trainer should observe the client's practice and prepare to give helpful **feedback.**

Providing Feedback

Once a client has tried the skill, the personal trainer should respond by giving helpful feedback. The feedback should do three things:

- Provide reinforcement for what was done well
- Correct errors
- Motivate clients to continue practicing and improving

The correcting of errors, which may be seen as the more "negative" point, should be sandwiched between reinforcement and motivation (Coker, Fischman, & Oxendine, 2006). For example, "Your breathing and timing were just right on the first four lifts. Remember to keep breathing, even as the exercise starts to feel harder. You'll find the work easier now that you are learning how to breathe correctly."

The personal trainer should limit feedback to a few simple points and avoid overloading the client with information. The personal trainer should decide which errors are the most important to correct first, which typically include those that involve safety, occur earliest in the movement sequence, or are fundamental in some other way. Feedback should be phrased positively, pointing out what the clients should do. For example, a personal trainer might say "Remember to breathe," rather than "Don't hold your breath."

Sometimes personal trainers can provide helpful feedback by touching clients to indicate where they are supposed to feel the movement, or to help them achieve the correct body position. Some clients are uncomfortable being touched or may misinterpret physical contact. Personal trainers should discuss their training methods early in the client–trainer relationship, explain the purpose of any physical contact, and ask clients for permission for this contact.

Using Effective Modeling

It is important for personal trainers to model the healthful lifestyle advice they are giving to their clients (Kamwendo et al., 2000). First, it is good for business, since it enhances a personal trainer's credibility (Maguire, 2008). Personal trainers must promote the notion that physical fitness and regular exercise are important and deliver benefits that are worth the cost—the financial cost of personal training and the cost of the time and energy the client must put into the exercise program. If personal trainers are not personally passionate about physical activity, they will lack persuasive power. Similarly, personal trainers should model other healthful lifestyle attributes, such as not smoking and following a generally healthful diet.

Second, when personal trainers model a healthful lifestyle, clients see that it can be done and it gives them confidence that they can do it, too. Cultivating a healthful lifestyle is not easy in a culture that has engineered physical activity out of daily living. If a personal trainer cannot achieve a physically active lifestyle, who can?

In addition to serving as role models themselves, personal trainers can increase clients' motivation to exercise and self-confidence in their ability to stick to a regular exercise program by exposing clients to role models similar to the clients themselves. For example, a client who is older and coping with the joint pain of **arthritis** may not see the personal trainer as a realistic model if the personal trainer is young and healthy. But if the personal trainer can arrange for a friend, client, or colleague who is more similar to the client to attend a session or simply work out while the client is nearby, this can provide a more suitable model for the client. People who see people like themselves exercising will develop more confidence in their own exercise abilities (Kerstin, Gabriele, & Richard, 2006).

Personal trainers should model not only healthful behaviors, but good attitudes as well. Especially important is the modeling of exercise for positive reasons, as opposed to negative reasons that might promote negative body image or disordered eating and exercise behavior (DiBartolo et al., 2007). Research suggests that exercise adherence is better in people who exercise for positive reasons. For example, personal trainers should promote the attitude that physical activity can feel good, reduce stress, and lead to wonderful health and fitness improvements. Underlying this attitude is the idea that the client is "good," and exercise can make his or her life even better.

Negative reasons for exercise include exercising primarily to lose weight or improve appearance. Underlying these negative reasons is the idea that clients are not good enough the way they are, and that they must lose weight and improve their appearance to be acceptable. But is it not true that many clients sign up for personal training to lose weight and improve appearance? Of course, but personal trainers can still emphasize exercise as a means for improving health rather than as punishment for eating too much at lunchtime. The personal trainer can model self-acceptance along with self-discipline, and the idea that while they exercise to look good, they also exercise to feel good. People are more likely to adopt an exercise habit if personal trainers model the idea that exercise improves quality of life, rather than the idea that exercise is just something painful one must do to lose weight and look better to conform to some unrealistic societal standard.

Personal trainers should be especially careful to model a healthful attitude when working with young people, since young people are more likely than adults to have fragile self-esteem. Careless remarks about physical features may be taken to heart by a young exerciser who may have a tendency to develop problems with body image, self-esteem, and eating behavior.

Behavior Contracts

Some personal trainers use behavior contracts with their clients to help them make a commitment to behavior change. Contracts typically spell out the behavior the client is expected to perform and a reward that will be given to the client upon successful achievement. Contracts work best when the behavioral goal is realistic and when clients feel motivated to earn the reward (Hayes et al., 2000).

Behavior-change contracts may be motivational for some clients, especially if they feel the reward is worth their effort. But contracts can also be problematic. Some personal trainers have found that contracts that set behavioral expectations too high may instill a sense of frustration in clients, especially when high expectations are not achieved and the reward is not obtained. Some fitness professionals have tried contracts in which the personal support of others close to the client is enlisted. For example, a friend or family member might contract with the client to offer a reward if the behavior is achieved. This type of contract is problematic because people (the clients) do not like to be nagged or told what to do, and tension can arise between contract members. **Social support** is better offered in an accepting, affirming manner rather than via contract. A friend who exercises with the client is more helpful than one who monitors the client's behavior and distributes (or does not distribute) rewards.

Behavior-change contracts offer **extrinsic motivation** for exercise, which may be helpful for getting clients started. People who exercise to achieve an external reward, such as a free personal-training session or movie passes, are said to be extrinsically motivated. People who exercise because they enjoy competition or because exercise feels good are said to have **intrinsic motivation.** Most people exercise for both intrinsic and extrinsic reasons. Research shows that people who exercise regularly for extended periods of time often do so because of intrinsic motivation (Duda & Treasure, 2006).

Nevertheless, people seem to do just about anything for a free T-shirt, so offering rewards can help move people in the right direction. A contract between the personal trainer and the client is fine. Process goals (complete 50 miles of walking) work better than product goals (lose 50 pounds), since they are more predictable and controllable. For example, a personal trainer might offer a free training session for every nine sessions the client completes. Hopefully, as clients get further into their programs, they will develop intrinsic motivation to continue.

Strategies for Effective Communication

Personal trainers must continually work to practice and improve their communication and teaching techniques. Effective communication involves more than superficial words and behaviors, and grows out of personal trainers' knowledge and understanding of, and attitudes toward, their clients.

Cultural Competence Increases Empathy and Rapport

Personal trainers who have had little difficulty developing rapport with clients similar to themselves may find it takes a little more effort to build trust with people who differ from themselves in terms of age, gender, ethnicity, size, socioeconomic status, educational background, ability, and fitness level. Personal trainers can improve their rapport-building ability by learning as much as possible about each client, and by trying to understand clients different from themselves. Personal trainers who work with people from different backgrounds can develop **cultural competence** by taking time to learn about clients' beliefs, attitudes, and lifestyles. Cultural competence can be defined as the ability to communicate and work effectively with people from different cultures.

Training programs for cultural competence for healthcare providers typically focus on communication skills. Culturally competent workers have the ability to recognize social and cultural differences that may exist between providers and clients and adapt their communication styles accordingly (Teal & Street, 2008). Providers are encouraged to elicit and understand clients' perspectives and individualize recommendations based on client input. Many medical schools have incorporated training programs in cultural competence and patient-centered care into their classes.

Ethnicity and race have been the most studied factors in terms of cultural competence training. While little research exists on racial and ethnic discrimination in the fitness industry, one can assume that this service sector would be vulnerable to America's national ethos. Research in healthcare suggests that ethnic minorities, who often work with providers of different ethnic backgrounds, rate the quality of healthcare more negatively than whites (Johnson et al., 2004).

Personal trainers can increase their own cultural competence in several ways. Personal trainers should begin by acknowledging their own biases regarding people of other backgrounds, including ethnic background, gender, sexual orientation, age, socioeconomic level, size, and physical ability. For example, some people may hold the idea that older adults are frail, overweight people are lazy, or that men are less communicative. People who are not fluent in English may be perceived as less smart than native speakers. Uncoordinated people who learn motor skills slowly may be perceived as inferior to athletes.

Personal trainers who are working with clients from an unfamiliar demographic can learn about clients' beliefs, attitudes, and lifestyles by talking to others who work with similar groups and reading any information they can find about that group. It is important to know, for example, that some older people and some cultural groups may believe that asking questions is rude and indicates that the speaker has been unclear. Many people pretend they agree with and understand a health professional, when in fact they may not agree or understand at all (Wright, Frey, & Sopory, 2007). Sometimes people say they have been performing their exercise programs when in fact they have not been doing so, simply to appear in a good light.

Once personal trainers have thought about their own biases and learned more about other groups, they should then be careful not to form new stereotypes. Personal trainers should work to understand each individual client using effective listening skills and by treating each client with dignity and respect.

Difficult Clients May Require More Effort

Building rapport can take more effort when clients are reluctant to begin exercising, are afraid of getting injured, or are depressed and anxious about their health. Some clients may have had bad experiences that led them to develop prejudices against athletes and physical educators, and therefore may initially be critical of information coming from a personal trainer. Some individuals may have less trust in young people, old people, women, people who appear to be overweight, or people of a different ethnicity. Nevertheless, personal trainers who behave professionally and try to understand their clients often win the hearts and trust of even the most reluctant clients.

Personal trainers who encounter resistance from their clients may be able to ask questions that expose problems and promote productive discussion. For example, a personal trainer who senses distrust from a client might explain his background working with clients with similar injuries, health problems, or whatever a particular client's worry might be. Personal trainers should display their certifications and other credentials and mention the various training programs and other continuing education opportunities they pursue or have completed.

Empathy and Rapport Enhance Adherence

Empathy and good rapport evolve over time from good communication between the personal trainer and client. Research suggests that the time spent establishing a good working relationship enhances adherence to behavior-change programs (Aikens, Bingham, & Piette, 2005; Larson & Yao, 2005).

Personal trainers develop empathy with a client when they put themselves in the client's position. While one person may never truly understand what it is like to be another person, the client usually appreciates the personal trainer's willingness to try to understand. Personal trainers' attempts to understand are conveyed through effective listening with an open, nonjudgmental mind as they ask questions and try to paraphrase, reflect, and summarize what they are hearing.

Professional Boundaries Enhance the Effectiveness of Personal Trainers

Empathy can develop into a double-edged sword if personal trainers fail to maintain professional distance from their clients. When personal trainers and clients work together for an extended period of time, it is normal for each to experience a feeling of friendliness toward the other. However, the professional effectiveness of personal trainers is undermined when they become too personally involved with their clients.

What is the difference between empathy and personal involvement? Empathy occurs when the trainer demonstrates understanding and acceptance toward the client. Empathy can be demonstrated without leaving one's role as a professional helping a client. Personal involvement occurs when the trainer becomes friends with the client or enters into a sexual relationship. It is difficult to maintain a client–trainer relationship once this has occurred. In fact, the client–trainer relationship should cease immediately if a sexual relationship has developed. What is appropriate professional behavior for one trainer may not feel right to another. For example, should a personal trainer attend a party given by a client? Most personal trainers could participate professionally in such a situation, while others might feel uncomfortable, or at least unable to really enjoy the party. Over time, personal trainers develop certain boundaries that allow them to behave professionally and express empathy without becoming best friends with clients.

In general, personal trainers should express empathy for situations and information pertaining to the client–trainer relationship. When clients start chatting about intimate issues, trainers can keep their distance and not feel compelled to show understanding or even a strong interest, especially if a client is particularly talkative.

Stages of Learning and Their Application to the Client–Trainer Relationship

Many researchers have developed models to describe the stages of motor learning. One model popular in the personal-training literature divides motor learning into three stages: cognitive, associative, and autonomous (Fitts & Posner, 1967). This model works well for the types of motor skills that personal trainers tend to teach, since clients are usually building onto motor skills they already know (e.g., walking, cycling, lifting). In such cases, explaining the upcoming skill is helpful. As clients try to understand the new skill, they are said to be in the **cognitive stage of learning.** Neuroscientists have demonstrated that different brain activity occurs when new motor skills are first being learned, as compared to the brain activity demonstrated once the motor skill has become more established (Floyer-Lea & Matthews, 2005; Rosenkranz, Kacar, & Rothwell, 2007). Personal trainers introducing a new motor skill can almost "see" clients thinking about what to do. Movements in this stage are often uncoordinated and jerky. In this stage of learning, personal trainers should use the "tell, show, do" teaching technique and provide ample opportunity for practice. This stage of learning occurs most frequently in the early stages of the client–trainer relationship. The personal trainer should be careful at this stage to not overwhelm clients by teaching them too many new motor skills.

In the **associative stage of learning,** clients begin to master the basics and are ready for more specific feedback that will help them refine the motor skill. At this learning stage, personal trainers must balance giving appropriate feedback, so that clients do not learn the skill incorrectly, with giving too much feedback.

In the **autonomous stage of learning**, clients are performing motor skills effectively and naturally, and the personal trainer is doing less teaching and more monitoring. Once some skills are learned, the personal trainer may decide to introduce new exercises or routines, and the process begins all over again.

Personal trainers working with athletes and clients trying to master complex motor skills, such as skiing and other sports skills, may find the Fitts and Posner model (1967) less helpful. Some research suggests that too much explanation and cognitive work may actually interfere with client learning of complex motor skills (Hodges & Franks, 2002). Personal trainers working with such skills should study with professional coaches in these sports to understand how best to help clients learn complex skills.

How to Incorporate Effective Communication and Teaching Techniques Into Daily Interactions With Clients

Personal trainers must continue to build productive relationships with clients throughout all of their daily interactions by using the following techniques.

- Personal trainers should periodically reinforce their credentials. Personal trainers should let clients know when they are away for conferences and other continuing education opportunities. This helps clients perceive personal trainers as educated and competent.

- Personal trainers should prepare for each personal-training session by cultivating a mindful focus. Instead of rushing into a new session preoccupied with other matters, personal trainers should take a minute to review the materials on upcoming clients, set goals for the upcoming session, and prepare to focus mindfully on the next client. A mindful focus means keeping one's awareness in the present moment with an open, nonjudgmental attitude. This allows personal trainers to listen effectively and put fresh energy into each personal-training session.
- Personal trainers should ask clients for feedback on their own performance. Client feedback may be obtained from a feedback form that is either returned directly to the personal trainer or to the personal trainer's supervisor. Client feedback can be helpful as personal trainers evaluate their communication and teaching skills.
- Personal trainers should use electronic communication channels with discretion. Both clients and personal trainers should give clear direction on how they prefer to be contacted. Many clients do not wish to receive email every day reminding them to exercise, although they may not mind a reminder of an upcoming personal-training session. Personal trainers may wish to let clients contact them at a work telephone number, but not on their mobile or home telephone numbers. In addition, personal trainers who allow clients access to their Internet pages, such as Facebook or Myspace, should be sure to maintain such pages in a professional manner.
- Personal trainers should try to make training fun. While certain stages of the client–trainer relationship tend to be more focused and serious, personal trainers should do what they can to make sessions fun and enjoyable. Some clients are more open to joking around than others, though playfulness should never detract from the personal-training activities. But appropriately funny stories that help pass the time are often appreciated.

Summary

Successful personal trainers consistently demonstrate excellent communication and teaching techniques throughout the various stages of the client–trainer relationship. During the rapport stage, personal trainers begin to establish trust and understanding with their clients. In the investigation stage, personal trainers use good listening skills to gather information from clients. In the planning stage, personal trainers use both good listening and teaching skills to design an exercise program in partnership with the client. During the action stage, personal trainers use effective, individualized teaching techniques to help clients learn motor skills and increase self-confidence.

Personal trainers who work with clients who differ from themselves can benefit from developing cultural competence and learning about their clients' beliefs, attitudes, and lifestyles. Trainers must become adept at developing an empathetic understanding of their clients while maintaining professional boundaries. Personal trainers must learn to provide helpful direction to clients through all the stages of learning and incorporate effective communication and teaching techniques into their daily interactions with clients.

References

Aikens, J.E., Bingham, R., & Piette, J.D. (2005). Patient-provider communication and self-care behavior among type 2 diabetes patients. *The Diabetes Educator*, 31, 5, 681–690.

Ambady, N. & Gray, H.M. (2002). On being sad and mistaken: Mood effects on the accuracy of thin-slice judgments. *Journal of Personality and Social Psychology,* 83, 4, 947–961.

Berkel, L.A. et al. (2005). Behavioral interventions for obesity. *Journal of the American Dietetic Association,* 105, 5 (Suppl 1), 35–43.

Brehm, B.A. (2004). *Successful Fitness Motivation Strategies.* Champaign, Ill.: Human Kinetics.

Coker, C.A., Fischman, M.G., & Oxendine, J.B. (2006). Motor skill learning for coaching and performance. In: Williams, J.M. (Ed.) *Applied Sport Psychology.* New York: McGraw-Hill.

Daves, W.F. & Holland, C.L. (1981). Interpersonal style: Reliability and validity. Research and development of the interpersonal style profile. In: Dodd, J. & Corbett, J. *Managing Relationships for Productivity*. Atlanta, Ga.: International Learning, Inc.

DiBartolo, P.M. et al. (2007). Are there "healthy" and "unhealthy" reasons for exercise? Examining individual differences in exercise motivations using the Function of Exercise Scale. *Journal of Clinical Sport Psychology*, 1, 2, 93–120.

Duda, J.L. & Treasure, D.C. (2006). Motivational processes and the facilitation of performance, persistence, and well-being in sport. In: Williams, J.M. (Ed.) *Applied Sport Psychology.* New York: McGraw-Hill.

Fitts, P.M. & Posner, M.I. (1967). *Human Performance.* Belmont, Calif.: Brooks/Cole.

Floyer-Lea, A. & Matthews, P.M. (2005). Distinguishable brain activation networks for short- and long-term motor skill learning. *Journal of Neurophysiology*, 94, 2, 512–518.

George, M. (2008). Interactions in expert service work: Demonstrating professionalism in personal training. *Journal of Contemporary Ethnography*, 37, 1, 108–131.

Goldstein, M.G., DePue, J., & Kazura, N.A. (2008). Models for provider-patient interaction and shared decision making. In: Shumaker, S.A., Ockene, J.A., & Riekert, K.A. (Eds.) *The Handbook of Health Behavior Change* (3rd ed.). New York: Springer.

Hayes, R.A. et al. (2000). The effects of behavioural contracting and preferred reinforcement on appointment keeping. *Behaviour Change,* 17, 2, 90–96.

Hodges, N.J. & Franks, I.M. (2002). Modeling coaching practice: The role of instruction and demonstration. *Journal of Sports Sciences,* 20, 10, 793–812.

Johnson, R.L. et al. (2004). Racial and ethnic differences in patient perceptions of bias and cultural competence in health care. *Journal of General Internal Medicine,* 19, 2, 101–110.

Kamwendo, K. et al. (2000). Adherence to healthy lifestyles: A comparison of nursing and physiotherapy students. *Advances in Physiotherapy,* 2, 2, 63–74.

Kerstin, W., Gabriele, B., & Richard, L. (2006). What promotes physical activity after a spinal cord injury? An interview study from a patient perspective. *Disability and Rehabilitation*, 28, 8, 481–488.

Larson, E.B. & Yao, X. (2005). Clinical empathy as emotional labor in the patient-physician relationship. *Journal of the American Medical Association,* 293, 9, 1100–1106.

Maguire, J.S. (2008). The personal is professional: Personal trainers as a case study of cultural intermediaries. *International Journal of Cultural Studies* 11, 2, 211–229.

Marchant, D., Clough, P., & Cramshaw, M. (2005). Influence of attentional focusing strategies during practice and performance of a motor skill. *Journal of Sports Sciences,* 23, 11–12, 1258–1259.

Miller, W.R. & Rollnick, S. (2002). *Motivational Interviewing: Preparing People to Change Addictive Behavior* (2nd ed.). New York: Guilford.

Rink, J.E. (2004). It's okay to be a beginner: Teach a motor skill, and the skill may be learned. *Journal of Physical Education, Recreation, and Dance,* 75, 6, 31–35.

Rosenkranz, K., Kacar, A., & Rothwell, J.C. (2007). Differential modulation of motor cortical plasticity and excitability in early and late phases of human motor learning. *Journal of Neuroscience,* 27, 44, 12058–12066.

Sears, S.R. & Stanton, A.L. (2001). Expectancy-value constructs and expectancy violation as predictors of exercise adherence in previously sedentary women. *Health Psychology,* 20, 5, 326–333.

Teal, C.R. & Street, R.L. (2009). Critical elements of culturally competent communication in the medical encounter: A review and model. *Social Science & Medicine,* 68, 3, 533–543.

Wright, K.B., Frey, L., & Sopory, P. (2007). Willingness to communicate about health as an underlying trait of patient self-advocacy: The development of the willingness to communicate about health (WTCH) measure. *Communication Studies,* 58, 1, 35–52.

Suggested Reading

Brehm, B.A. (2004). *Successful Fitness Motivation Strategies.* Champaign, Ill.: Human Kinetics.

George, M. (2008). Interactions in expert service work: Demonstrating professionalism in personal training. *Journal of Contemporary Ethnography,* 37, 1, 108–131.

McKay, M., David, M., & Fanning, P. (1995). *Messages: The Communication Skills Book.* Oakland, Calif.: New Harbinger Publications.

IN THIS CHAPTER:

Behavioral Theory Models

Health Belief Model

Self-efficacy

Transtheoretical Model of Behavioral Change

Principles of Behavior Change

Operant Conditioning

Shaping

Observational Learning

Cognitions and Behavior

Behavior-change Strategies

Stimulus Control

Written Agreements and Behavioral Contracting

Cognitive Behavioral Techniques

Implementing Basic Behavior-change and Health-psychology Strategies

Behavioral Interventions

Summary

TRACIE ROGERS, Ph.D., *is a sport and exercise psychology specialist and an assistant professor in the Human Movement program at the Arizona School of Health Sciences at A.T. Still University. She is also the owner of the BAR Fitness Studio in Phoenix, Arizona. Dr. Rogers teaches, speaks, and writes on psychological constructs related to behavior change and physical-activity participation and adherence.*

CHAPTER 4

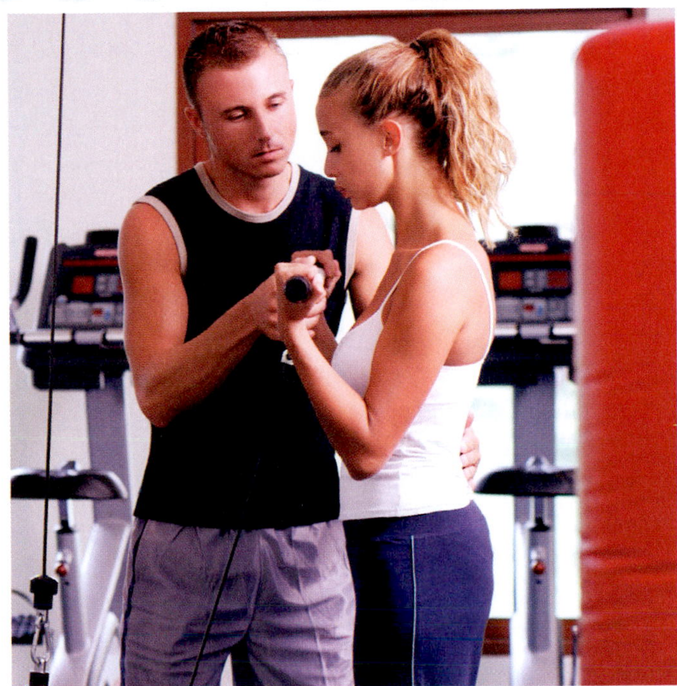

Basics of Behavior Change and Health Psychology

Tracie Rogers

Whether an individual is studying to become a personal trainer or is already working in that capacity, much focus is placed on learning and understanding program development and implementation with regard to exercise science. Personal trainers spend a great deal of time designing exercise programs and coming up with new and creative ways to target different muscle groups. Understanding the components of an exercise program is critical for all fitness professionals. However, if this is a trainer's sole focus, he or she will have a difficult time establishing a solid client base and helping clients achieve optimal success. In other words, the ultimate success of a trainer is based on how well he or she understands each individual client. Client **adherence** is crucial for a personal trainer to achieve long-term success in the fitness industry. A personal trainer cannot expand a business with constant client turnover, but this type of turnover is inevitable if a trainer treats all clients the same and does not take the time to understand the individual differences that each client brings to the client–trainer relationship.

For years, the health and medical communities focused primarily on the physiological components of disease, which led to great advances in knowledge and technology. However, as healthcare costs continue to rise, along with the occurrence of lifestyle diseases, the importance of understanding the psychological factors related to behavior and disease has become increasingly relevant. In the 1970s, **health psychology** emerged as a field that examines the causes of illnesses and studies ways to promote and maintain health, prevent and treat illness, and improve the healthcare system (Sarafino, 2008). Health psychology took the traditional biomedical model and added the individual to the equation, resulting in a broader picture of the correlates of health and illness (Engel, 1977). This biopsychosocial approach to health has provided a framework for studying health behaviors and behavior change. As awareness has increased about the role of physical activity in disease prevention, the United States government has become progressively more involved in increasing the physical-activity levels of Americans and in the promotion of the health benefits of physical activity. In 2008, the U.S. Department of Health & Human Services released physical-activity guidelines stating that adults gain substantial health benefits from engaging in 150 minutes a week of moderate-intensity aerobic physical activity, or 75 minutes of vigorous physical activity. More extensive health benefits can be achieved by increasing aerobic activity levels to five hours a week of moderate-intensity exercise or 150 minutes a week of vigorous-intensity aerobic physical activity. Additionally, it was recommended that adults incorporate muscle-strengthening activities at least two days a week.

Personal trainers are truly in a unique position to help people adopt significant lifestyle changes that will decrease their risk for numerous diseases and increase the overall quality of their lives. It is critical that personal trainers understand the psychological and social components of behavior change and use them in their practices to help each client adopt and maintain an active lifestyle.

Behavioral Theory Models

There is no simple formula to predict why some people adopt healthy behaviors and others do not. Understanding health behaviors is challenging in general, but the behavior of exercise is uniquely complicated, as it is perceived to take more time and effort than other health behaviors (Turk, Rudy, & Salovey, 1984). Despite this complexity, personal trainers must be able to deal with real people and the unique challenges that come with each individual. A personal trainer's goal should go beyond designing a great workout. Instead, the goal should be to help teach and inspire each individual client to adopt a life-long activity program. There is no doubt that adopting an active lifestyle is complex and trying to make someone change can sometimes seem like an impossible task. Over the years, in an effort to create clarity in guiding behavior change, numerous explanations have been developed regarding the factors affecting health behaviors. These explanations include examinations of people's beliefs about their health, their beliefs about their ability to change, and their readiness to make a change. Each of the following models has relevance for personal trainers.

Health Belief Model

The most accepted theory focusing on health beliefs is the **health belief model** (Becker, 1974). The health belief model predicts that people will engage in a health behavior (e.g., exercise) based on the perceived threat they feel regarding a health problem and the pros and cons of adopting the behavior. Perceived threat is defined as the degree to which a person feels threatened or worried about the prospect of a particular health problem and is influenced by several factors:

- *Perceived seriousness* of the health problem refers to the feelings one has about the seriousness of contracting an illness or leaving an illness untreated. This judgment is based on the severity of the potential consequences of the problem. The more serious the consequences are perceived to be, the more likely people are to engage in a health behavior.

- *Perceived susceptibility* to the health problem is based on a person's subjective appraisal of the likelihood of developing the problem. People have a higher perceived threat and an increased likelihood to engage in a health behavior when they believe they are vulnerable to a particular health problem.
- *Cues to action* are events, either bodily (e.g., physical symptoms) or environmental (e.g., health promotion information), that motivate people to make a change. The more people are reminded about a potential health problem, the more likely they are to take action and engage in a health behavior.

The pros and cons of engaging in a health behavior are examined by the health belief model in terms of perceived benefits and perceived barriers of the health behavior. In other words, the client will assess the benefits (getting healthier and feeling and looking better) along with the barriers (financial cost, effort, and time) of making a lifestyle modification. According to the health belief model, if an individual perceives more or stronger barriers than benefits regarding a health behavior, he or she will be unlikely to make a behavior change. However, if the perceived benefits outweigh the perceived barriers and the perceived threat of illness is high, people are likely to take preventative action, thus engaging in exercise and healthy nutrition behaviors. It is important for personal trainers to understand the perceptions that clients have regarding illness and a healthy lifestyle, including the perceived benefits and barriers to program participation and success. If an individual perceives very little threat of developing an illness related to his or her lifestyle, success of the modification program is unlikely. The trainer would need to make the seriousness of the illness more apparent and make the individual feel more susceptible to developing the condition. Personal trainers need to learn to implement appropriate cues to action by introducing health information along with educating and focusing attention on physical symptoms.

The following case study is an example of how the health belief model explains behavior. A personal trainer is approached by a 39-year-old **sedentary** male who is nearly 100 pounds (45 kg) overweight. His father recently died at age 65 of complications related to **chronic obstructive pulmonary disease (COPD)** (a disease with a significant lifestyle component). This individual is very busy with his family and job, but knows that if he does not take action, he will likely develop a disease similar to the one that took his father's life. As the personal trainer talks to this person, it becomes clear that even though he knows he needs to exercise, making a change has not yet become a priority in his life and he is not prepared to make a commitment to an exercise program. He gives numerous excuses for his lack of activity and for his current dietary habits. In fact, it seems he has an explanation for everything.

According to the health belief model, there are numerous reasons why this individual is not ready to start an exercise program. Despite his high perception of the seriousness of developing a lifestyle-related disease, and his high susceptibility to developing a lifestyle-related disease, he does not have any noticeable symptoms of a disease state. In fact, he says he feels fine, only complaining of a lack of energy to make it through a typical day. This should signal to the personal trainer that this individual may need a cue to action to help him get started. It is likely that this individual has not had a recent physical exam, and this may be a good place to start. He could receive information during a physical that would serve as motivation to get started on making a change. His numerous comments about his busy life and his feelings of being overwhelmed by how much weight he has gained should serve as instant cues that he perceives many barriers to succeeding at an exercise program. It is important for the personal trainer in this example to create a program that is flexible and easy to stick with. If the trainer presents program options that require a huge time commitment and schedule reorganization, this individual will be immediately turned off. Instead, the trainer needs to set him up to succeed, giving him something to build on (i.e., start with small, achievable steps).

Self-efficacy

While numerous questionnaires have been developed to measure **self-efficacy** in research, personal trainers can best gain an understanding of a client's self-efficacy level through consistent communication and rapport-building strategies. Because self-efficacy is a subjective perception of one's own ability to succeed, it is difficult to quantify and is interpreted, for practical purposes, through interpersonal communication. To develop an understanding of a client's self-efficacy regarding exercise participation, a trainer should ask clients questions about the sources of self-efficacy information. Specifically, through conversation, a trainer should gain knowledge about a client's previous experience with exercise, feelings and emotions associated with starting a new program, expectations and apprehensions related to program involvement (i.e., physiological, psychological, adherence), and potential barriers for program adherence. The assessment of self-efficacy is an ongoing part of the client–trainer relationship and should not be thought of as a one-time measurement. Client self-efficacy will continually change and trainers should take advantage of increases in self-efficacy and make program modifications when self-efficacy levels drop.

Self-efficacy is an important concept to understand when working with clients. In the exercise-behavior context, self-efficacy can be defined as the belief in one's own capabilities to successfully be physically active (Bandura, 1986). Self-efficacy beliefs are important because they are thought to influence thought patterns, emotional responses, and behavior. Self-efficacy is also positively related to motivation (i.e., higher levels of self-efficacy are linked to increases in motivation) (Bandura, 1994). Personal trainers should be aware of each client's self-efficacy for exercise behavior. Does the client believe he or she has the ability to be active and fit and to adhere to a fitness program? If personal trainers ignore self-efficacy information, they are likely creating a barrier to long-term success for their clients and for their own business development. Due to the importance of having high levels of self-efficacy, it is worth understanding how self-efficacy is developed. Specifically, there are six sources of self-efficacy information.

- *Past performance experience* is the most influential source of self-efficacy information. Personal trainers should ask clients about their previous experiences with exercise, fitness facilities, and personal trainers. These previous experiences will strongly influence their current self-efficacy levels.
- *Vicarious experience* is important for a client who is starting a brand new exercise program and who has little previous experience with a supervised program. The observation or knowledge of someone else who is successfully participating in a similar program—or has done so in the past—can increase one's self-efficacy. This is particularly true if the person being observed is perceived by the client to be similar to him- or herself.
- *Verbal persuasion* typically occurs in the form of **feedback** from teaching or encouragement. Statements from others are most likely to influence self-efficacy if they come from a credible, respected, and knowledgeable source.
- *Physiological state appraisals* related to exercise participation are important because a client may perceive arousal, pain, or fatigue. It is important to be aware of the types of appraisals clients are making about their physiological states because these beliefs may lead to judgments about their ability to participate successfully.
- *Emotional state and mood appraisals* of program participation can also influence self-efficacy. Negative mood states and emotional beliefs associated with exercise, such as fear, anxiety, anger, and frustration, are related to reduced levels of self-efficacy and lower levels of participation. On the other hand, positive mood states and

emotional beliefs, including mastery, are related to higher levels of self-efficacy.

- *Imaginal experiences* refer to the imagined experiences (positive or negative) of exercise participation. It is important to understand a client's preconceived notion of what exercise will be like, as this information will influence actual self-efficacy levels.

Personal trainers should always take the time to gain an understanding of the self-efficacy levels of their clients. This is most effectively done through conversation and by taking the time to understand what an individual believes about his or her ability to succeed. With this information, the personal trainer will be better able to design a program that sets up the client for success. In an exercise program, self-efficacy levels will influence the types of tasks an individual wants to engage in, how hard they will try, and if they will persist. Specifically, people with high self-efficacy will choose challenging tasks, set goals, and display a commitment to master those tasks. They will display maximum effort to reach their goals and will even increase their effort when challenges arise. These people will work to overcome obstacles and challenges and will recover from setbacks. In general, individuals with high self-efficacy are much more likely to adhere to a program (Bandura, 1994).

On the other hand, people with low self-efficacy will be more likely to choose non-challenging tasks that are non-threatening and easy to accomplish. They will display minimal effort to protect themselves in the face of a challenge—since failing when not working hard will be a lesser blow to their self-efficacy than failing when doing their best—and, if faced with too many setbacks, they are likely to lose faith, give up, and drop out of the program (Bandura, 1994).

Transtheoretical Model of Behavioral Change

An important factor in the successful adoption of any exercise program is the client's readiness to make a change. This individual readiness for change is the focus of a well-accepted theory examining health behaviors called the **transtheoretical model of behavioral change (TTM)** (Prochaska & DiClemente, 1984). More commonly called the **stages-of-change model,** the TTM is important for personal trainers to understand when promoting the adoption of exercise programs. Not everyone is necessarily ready to start a regular exercise program, and personal trainers must stop using the "one-size-fits-all" approach to exercise program design and implementation (Marcus et al., 2000; Morgan, 2001). Succeeding at making a behavioral change is not a simple task. To better delineate the process of starting and maintaining a behavioral change, the TTM is separated into four components:

- Stages of change
- Processes of change
- Self-efficacy
- Decisional balance

Stages of Change

The first component of the TTM is made up of the five stages of behavior change. These stages can be related to any health behavior, but in the exercise context the stages are as follows:

- The first stage is the **precontemplation** stage, during which people are sedentary and are not even considering an activity program. These people do not see activity as relevant in their lives, and may even discount the importance or practicality of being physically active.
- The next stage is the **contemplation** stage. People in the contemplation stage are still sedentary. However, they are starting to consider activity as important and have begun to identify the implications of being inactive. Nevertheless, they are still not ready to commit to making a change.
- The **preparation** stage is marked by some physical activity, as individuals are mentally and physically preparing to adopt an activity program. Activity during the preparation stage may be a sporadic walk, or even a periodic visit to the gym, but it is inconsistent. People in the preparation stage are ready to adopt and live an active lifestyle.

- Next is the **action** stage. During this stage, people engage in regular physical activity, but have been doing so for less than six months.
- The final stage is the **maintenance** stage. This stage is marked by regular physical-activity participation for longer than six months.

Processes of Change

The second component of the TTM is likely the most important for personal trainers to understand, as it entails the processes of change that people use to get from one stage to the next. Each stage transition has a unique set of processes and is based on specific individual decisions and mental states, including individual readiness and motivation. The most effective change strategies are stage-specific interventions that target the natural processes people use as they move from one stage to the next. The first step for a personal trainer is to identify the current stage of the client. If someone is actively seeking information about fitness programs, it is highly unlikely that this individual is a precontemplator. The personal trainer needs to listen to the types of questions an individual is asking and to the types of hesitations he or she has in an effort to identify the current stage of change and choose an appropriate program option. Trainers also must remember that the general goal of any intervention should be to advance the individual to the next stage of change (Table 4-1).

Self-efficacy

The third component of the TTM is self-efficacy. As previously mentioned, self-efficacy in the exercise context is the belief in one's own capabilities to successfully engage in an exercise program (Bandura, 1986). Self-efficacy is an important component of exercise behavior change because it is strongly related to program adoption and maintenance. There is a circular relationship between self-efficacy and behavior change, such that a person's self-efficacy is related to whether he or she will participate in an activity, and a person's participation in activity influences his or her self-efficacy level. Therefore, self-efficacy acts as both a determinant and an outcome of behavior change. Additionally, there is a reliable relationship between self-efficacy for activity and stage of behavior change, such that precontemplators and contemplators have significantly lower levels of self-efficacy than people in the action and maintenance stages. This is a logical relationship, as those in the precontemplation and contemplation stages are not exercising at all or are doing so very infrequently, which may be reflective of the belief that they do not have the ability or knowledge required to be active, while those in the action and maintenance stages are engaged in regular activity programs, thus demonstrating a belief in the ability to be active.

So how does a person develop self-efficacy? The most important and powerful predictor of self-efficacy is past performance experience. This means that an individual who has had past success in adopting and maintaining a physical-activity program will have higher self-efficacy regarding his or her ability to be active in the future. It also means that those individuals with no exercise experience will have much lower self-efficacy regarding their abilities to engage in an exercise program. Therefore, it should be the trainer's primary goal to get these non-exercisers some sort of positive exercise experience. The self-efficacy has to come from somewhere, so those initial encounters with exercise are extremely critical for promoting and triggering change.

The relationship between stage of change and self-efficacy implies that by influencing self-efficacy, a person may progress through the stages more efficiently. This is critical for people in the contemplation and preparation stages, as they are thinking about or wanting to be active and working toward the point where they can be regularly active, but still have some doubts about achieving that goal. By specifically trying to increase these individuals' levels of self-efficacy, a personal trainer may be able to help them progress to the action stage more quickly.

Table 4-1

Transtheoretical Model of Behavioral Change—Processes of Change

Stage of Change	Goal	Interventions
Precontemplation	To make inactivity a relevant issue and to start thinking about being active	• Provide information about the risks of being inactive and the benefits of being active. • Provide information from multiple sources (e.g., news, posters, pamphlets, general health-promotion material). Information is more effective from multimedia sources than from family and friends. • Make inactivity a relevant issue.
Contemplation	To get involved in some type of activity	• Provide opportunities to ask a lot of questions and to express apprehensions. • Provide information about exercise in general. • Provide information about different types of activity options, fitness facilities, programs, and classes. • Provide cues for actions, such as passes to nearby facilities and invitations to facility open houses, tours, or information sessions.
Preparation	Regular physical-activity participation	• Provide the opportunity to be active. • Provide a lot of support, feedback, and reinforcement. • Provide clients the opportunity to express their concerns and triumphs. • Introduce different types of exercise activities to find something they enjoy. • Help create support groups of similar people who are also adopting exercise programs.
Action	Maintain regular physical activity	• Provide continued support and feedback. • Identify things and events that are potential barriers to adherence. • Identify high-risk individuals and situations. • Educate clients about the likelihood of relapse and things that may trigger relapse. • Teach physical and psychological skills to deal with potential barriers. • Provide continuous opportunities to be active and a plan to maintain activity in the changing seasons, during vacations, and through schedule changes.
Maintenance	Prevent relapse and maintain continued activity	• Maintain social support from family and friends and from within the exercise environment. • Provide continued education about barrier identification. • Keep the exercise environment enjoyable and switch it up to fight boredom. • Create reward systems for continued adherence. • Identify early signs of staleness to prevent burnout.

Decisional Balance

The final of the four components of the TTM is **decisional balance,** which refers to the number of pros and cons perceived about adopting and/or maintaining an activity program. Precontemplators and contemplators perceive more cons (e.g., sweating, sore muscles, time, cost, unwanted physical changes, and boredom) related to being regularly active than pros. The perceived cons do not have to be logical or realistic to prevent an individual from being active. As people progress through the stages of change, the balance of pros and cons shifts, such that people in the action and maintenance stages perceive more pros about being active than cons. The active behavior of people in these later stages reflects this change in decisional balance. The decisional balance worksheet presented in Figure 4-1 can be used to help clients weigh the perceived benefits against the potential losses involved with making a change. While this worksheet is a valuable tool to help trainers and clients work together to clarify potential barriers or psychological roadblocks, it is important that trainers do not become overly reliant on worksheets. The most effective approach is for trainers to use worksheets in conjunction with continued communication and observation to build a complete understanding of client needs and to develop appropriate programming.

The natural change in decisional balance that occurs as people progress through the stages of change suggests that influencing their perceptions about being active may help encourage them to start an activity program. When working on shifting decisional balance, it is important to remember the processes of change related to moving from one stage to the next. For example, when working with a precontemplator or contemplator, it is important to emphasize a wide variety of benefits of being physically active and avoid arguing about the cons they perceive about exercise. Often, the cons that non-exercisers perceive about physical activity are a result of misinformation and a lack of experience. Additionally, it is important that the discussed benefits are both short- and long-term. For example, emphasizing only the long-term weight-loss benefits of an activity program can be overwhelming and may make those benefits seem unattainable. Focusing on the short-term benefits, such as increased energy and mastery of the exercise itself, will give the client something to look forward to immediately.

Relapse can occur at any stage of the TTM, including during the maintenance stage. Any change that may occur in an individual's life, such as moving, starting school, family changes, or suffering an injury, can trigger a relapse into irregular activity or even to no activity. The commitment of long-term exercisers should not be taken for granted, as this behavior can change, and relapse can occur on any given day.

Figure 4-1
Decisional balance worksheet

Instructions:

- Work with the client to document the gains and potential losses that he or she might experience when making a lifestyle change.
- Identify and list the recommended implementation strategies needed to achieve the gains and list coping strategies that can be used to deal with the potential losses or obstacles associated with the change.

DECISIONAL BALANCE WORKSHEET

Perceived gains associated with adopting desired behaviors	Perceived losses associated with adopting desired behaviors
1. ______	1. ______
2. ______	2. ______
3. ______	3. ______
4. ______	4. ______
Strategies to maximize potential for achieving gains	**Strategies to minimize potential of perceived losses**
1. ______	1. ______
2. ______	2. ______
3. ______	3. ______
4. ______	4. ______

Examples of the Processes of Change in the TTM

Precontemplation: A personal trainer is having a discussion with his uncle, who is questioning how anyone can make a living by helping people exercise. The uncle is sedentary and thinks that exercise is for women who take aerobics or for bodybuilder types who are looking to bulk up. He views exercise as completely irrelevant to his life. The trainer's initial thought is to argue with his uncle and to tell him that he is completely misinformed, but this would be counterproductive. The trainer needs to educate his uncle without lecturing or arguing with him. The trainer decides to pull up his website, which contains videos of some of his workouts. He shows his uncle how exercise has transformed over the years and the diversity of his clientele. Additionally, he shares some of the successes of his clients, including weight loss and changes in blood pressure and cholesterol. The trainer presents and shares this information in a very general context that is not specific to, or directed at, his uncle. As the discussion continues, he answers his uncle's questions and even invites him into the gym to meet a couple of his clients and to watch him go through a few workouts.

Contemplation: A personal trainer receives a phone call at the gym from a woman who saw an advertisement for a free trial week. She says that she does not currently work out and that she has never exercised in a gym before. She seems very apprehensive and nervous on the phone and says that she is not sure if it is for her, but that she knows she needs to be more active. She asks if there is any programming for beginners and if someone will be available to help her if she comes in, since she does not know what she is doing. The trainer talks to the woman for a few minutes and then invites her into the gym for a tour and a meeting, during which they can talk and he can answer any questions she may have. They set an appointment for the next day. During the meeting, the trainer serves as a sounding board for her questions and concerns. He introduces her to the staff members at the gym that they encounter and describes the various options for activity. He even talks about what people typically wear when they work out. The woman has a lot of doubt about starting a program and the trainer emphasizes the benefits of being active. To help her learn more about the different options, he invites her to a beginner-level group fitness class and introduces her to the instructor of that class. He then gives her a pass for an introductory training session that will teach her the basics of strength training and how she could start a program. Before she leaves, he invites her to the facility's health fair, which is taking place the following weekend. He explains that it will be a good opportunity to meet more people and get additional information about exercise options.

Preparation: A personal trainer is approached by a member at the gym who comes in a few times a month and goes through a basic workout. He tells the trainer that he wants to be more consistent and lose weight, but that he is having a difficult time finding the motivation. He says that he is not really sure what he needs to be doing and that he needs help. The personal trainer talks with the member and ensures him that he is off to a great start. He emphasizes that he just needs a little more direction and accountability in his workouts. The trainer asks if he would like some help setting new goals. As they talk, the trainer casually introduces the member to a couple of the staff people at the gym whom he has never met. The trainer offers to show him a couple of new exercises and goes over the different programming options at the club. The member comments that he had no idea there were so many activities. The trainer then tells him about a group of men he trains two days a week who are also trying to lose weight. He invites the member to join them for their next workout.

Action: A personal trainer has a female client who has been consistently training three days a week for a couple of months. She is seeing great results and loves her workouts. She is always happy to come in and never misses an appointment. The client has two children and with the school year coming to an end knows her schedule will change. She really wants to continue to train. The trainer encourages the client by telling her how great she has done, reminding her how much she has accomplished. They then talk about the challenges she will face trying to stick to her workouts when her children are out of school. He tells her that she will likely be less consistent with her workouts and proposes developing a plan to help her stay with the program. The trainer teaches her the importance of flexibility in her program and offers a couple of exercise options she can do outside of the gym with her children. They also look at changing the times of her workouts to accommodate her new schedule. The trainer tells the client that he knows she can do it and to not hesitate to ask for help if she is having challenges with her schedule.

Maintenance: A long-time client of a personal trainer has lost more than 60 pounds (27 kg) and feels great. He has reached his goals and loves being physically active. He has even started taking his family for hikes on the weekends. He rarely misses an appointment and is one of the trainer's easiest clients to deal with. The trainer understands, however, that this state of consistency may not last forever, so she plans a sit-down session with the client to evaluate the program and set new goals. The trainer tells her client that she wants to switch up his program a bit and introduce some more functional training. She also recommends switching to a group-training session for one of his sessions each week. The trainer explains that she thinks he would really enjoy the group activity, which will give him an opportunity to meet more people in the gym. They also talk about the client's upcoming schedule, work activities, and travel plans, and discuss strategies to help him stay active during any inconsistencies in his schedule. The trainer also emphasizes to the client that he should keep her posted if he starts to get bored or lose motivation. Finally, the trainer praises the client for his continued success and dedication to the program.

Principles of Behavior Change

One of the biggest mistakes a fitness professional can make is to assume that starting and sticking with an activity program is easy or simple. This may seem like a basic point, but most fitness professionals are active themselves and sometimes have difficulty relating to the challenge of getting started from a sedentary state. This is part of the reason why it is important for personal trainers to understand and apply theoretical constructs (e.g., TTM and self-efficacy) in their work with clients. The main benefit of using such models is that they properly address exercise as a behavior. The adoption of physical activity is a complicated process that requires replacing sedentary behaviors with healthy, active behaviors. It is the personal trainer's job to provide guidance and support to help change client behaviors by influencing their attitudes, motives, emotions, and performance. This process of behavior change is a gradual progression that requires effort, dedication, and commitment. As previously discussed, for a personal trainer to be successful in building a client base and a business, he or she must understand the factors that control behavior and be able to teach clients new ways of doing things.

Operant Conditioning

Operant conditioning is an effective and widely used approach to understanding human behavior. Operant conditioning is the process by which behaviors are influenced by their **consequences.** More specifically, it examines the relationship between **antecedents,** behaviors, and consequences (Martin & Pear, 2007). Operant conditioning examines the **behavior chains** that lead to the engagement of certain behaviors and the avoidance of others, taking into account the consequences associated with each behavior.

Antecedents

Part of the learning experience is realizing the consequences of specific behaviors under certain conditions. Antecedents help in this process, as they are stimuli that precede a behavior and often signal the likely consequences of the behavior. Antecedents help guide behavior so that it will most likely lead to positive or desirable consequences. An example of an antecedent is a man looking at the clock and realizing he is late for his workout. This would lead to the behavior of rushing out the door and speeding to the gym, where he is able to complete only part of his scheduled training appointment.

Antecedents can be manipulated in the environment to maximize the likelihood of desirable behaviors. This type of influence by antecedents on behavior is called **stimulus control.** Stimulus control is a valuable tool in behavior modification. For example, a client who frequently leaves the office late and is therefore late for his workout is getting only half of his scheduled workout time. To help with this problem, he sets an alarm on his computer for the days of his workouts to remind him five minutes before it is time to leave. This reminder triggers him to prepare to leave his office and head to the gym—resulting in a full workout session.

Consequences

The most important component of operant conditioning is what happens after a behavior is executed. The consequence following a behavior will influence the future occurrence of that behavior. Consequences fall under the categories of presentation, non-occurrence, or removal of a positive or aversive stimulus. **Positive reinforcement** is the presentation of a positive stimulus that increases the likelihood that the behavior will reoccur in the future. **Negative reinforcement,** which consists of the removal or avoidance of aversive stimuli following undesirable behavior, also increases the likelihood that the behavior will reoccur. For example, if a client is late to a training session and the trainer does not say anything about the time and just extends the workout in accordance with the number of minutes that the client was late, this client will likely be late again because there was not an aversive consequence to his tardiness. **Extinction** occurs when a positive stimulus that once followed a behavior is removed and the likelihood that the behavior will reoccur is decreased. **Punishment** also decreases the likelihood of the behavior reoccurring, and consists of an aversive stimulus following an undesirable behavior. If a tardy client was told that his appointment was cancelled due to his tardiness and that he must be on time to work out, he will likely not be late again. However, despite the fact that punishment is effective at decreasing an unwanted behavior, it also increases fear and decreases enjoyment, so it must be used sparingly and only when appropriate (never for poor performance, only for lack of effort).

Personal trainers are in a unique position to provide feedback and encouragement to their clients. It is important that trainers learn to provide appropriate feedback and consequences to clients' behaviors. Actions that are done well should be positively reinforced and actions that need improvement should not be ignored. Target behaviors should be clear and concise, and consistent consequences should be established for specific behaviors (Smith, 2005).

Shaping

Shaping refers to the process of using reinforcements to gradually achieve a target behavior. This process begins with the performance of a basic skill that the client is currently capable of doing. The skill demands are then gradually raised and reinforcement is given as more is accomplished. This process of continually increasing the demands at an appropriate rate, accompanied by positive reinforcement, leads to the execution of the desired behavior and is a powerful behavior-control and teaching technique. Part of the reason that shaping is so effective is that it starts with having the client execute a task at an appropriate skill level (Smith, 2005). This not only helps in the learning of new behaviors, but it is also critical for building self-efficacy. The many benefits that come from shaping make it an important tool for all personal trainers. For shaping to be maximally effective, each client must have his or her own starting point. The effectiveness of the program will be based on the trainer's ability to successfully identify the appropriate starting level. If the starting point is too easy, the client will likely get bored, and if the starting point is too difficult, the client will likely feel discouraged, inadequate, and overwhelmed. Either situation will lead to increased dropout from program participation.

Observational Learning

A personal trainer can never underestimate the role that a client's environment plays in his or her ability to make behavioral changes. All people are influenced to some degree by the behaviors of people around them at home, at work, and in social environments. It is important for trainers to be aware of the exercise behaviors of the people closest to their clients, as these behaviors may impact the likelihood of client success. Once a person starts an exercise program, trainers should encourage interactions with other people who are also physically active.

Cognitions and Behavior

As reflected in the health belief model and in the TTM, a person's exercise behavior is influenced by how he or she thinks about exercise and about succeeding in an exercise program. Not only should personal trainers understand what their clients think about exercise participation, but they should also be aware of the types of thoughts that their clients have about lapses in program participation. Thoughts, or **cognitions,** can serve as great motivational tools, but they can also handicap an individual from achieving success if they are negative or discouraging in nature.

Behavior-change Strategies

Helping clients successfully adopt and adhere to exercise programs is an integral part of a personal trainer's job. Therefore, personal trainers must be able to teach their clients behavior-change strategies. These strategies are the actual tools that a fitness professional will use to enhance the likelihood that clients will successfully adopt and maintain a physical-activity program. Behavior-change strategies, as related to exercise, are important for beginners as well as for those who have been regularly participating for a long time. Being physically active, or not being active, is a habit. Similar to other habits, like a person brushing his or her teeth after getting out of bed or sitting on the couch when getting home from work, it is possible to learn to be more "automatically" active throughout the day. By helping a client find time for regular exercise, a personal trainer will often identify undesirable, time-wasting behaviors that can, over time, be replaced by healthy, productive, active habits.

Behavior-change programs have been proven effective in increasing physical activity in research settings. By using principles of operant and classical conditioning to change behavior, people learn to be more physically active (Dishman, 1991). Additionally, research has shown that adoption of an exercise program may potentially be triggered by emphasizing the benefits of exercise, such as changes to physical appearance. However, the motives for sustaining a program are likely much different and include increased well-being and enjoyment of activity participation (Ingledew & Markland, 2008).

Stimulus Control

One effective behavior-change strategy is stimulus control. As previously discussed, stimulus control refers to making adjustments to the environment to increase the likelihood of healthy behaviors. Simple and effective stimulus-control strategies may include choosing a gym that is in the direct route between home and work; keeping a gym bag in the car that contains all the required items for a workout; having workout clothes, socks, and shoes laid out for early morning workouts; and writing down workout times as part of a weekly schedule. A less obvious, but very important stimulus-control technique is for personal trainers to encourage their clients to surround themselves with other people who have similar health and fitness goals. By associating with people who are also interested in being active, clients will naturally develop support systems for behavior change. The overall goal of stimulus control is to make being physically active as convenient as possible. Personal trainers should listen continuously for cues from their clients that are reflective of difficulty with adherence, and should be prepared to provide tips and strategies to help reduce the effort required to stick with the program.

Written Agreements and Behavioral Contracting

Written agreements and behavioral contracting are effective behavior-change tools that can be used together or on their own to help people stick with their exercise programs. Written agreements should be developed first and can be between the personal trainer and the client or just by the client on his or her own terms. Each agreement should outline the expectations of the client and the trainer. This is an effective tool, as it decreases ambiguity and clarifies the roles of all people involved. Agreements should be so specific that behaviors, attitudes, and commitments are clearly outlined. A personal trainer cannot create an agreement for a client, as this tool will only be effective if the client has an active role in its development. Each agreement should be signed by the personal trainer, the client, and anyone else who plays an integral role in the agreement (e.g., the client's spouse). It is important that this document is reviewed and adjusted at all program-modification points.

Once a written agreement has been established, an effective behavior contract should be created by the personal trainer and client and should outline a system of rewards for maintaining the program and maximizing adherence. It is important that the rewards are outlined by, and meaningful to, the client. Otherwise, they will not be worth working toward. As with written agreements, this process must be revised and updated as goals are met and programs are modified.

Cognitive Behavioral Techniques

Cognitive behavioral techniques are effective tools that influence behavior change by targeting how people think and feel about being physically active. The first step in using cognitive techniques is to identify problematic beliefs that are barriers to change. The next step is to change the obstructive thoughts. As with all behavior-change techniques, cognitive behavioral techniques are effective when used alone and when used together with other behavior-change strategies (Dishman, 1991). Effective techniques include goal setting, feedback, decision making, and self-monitoring.

Goal Setting

Goal setting is one of the most widely used and straightforward cognitive behavioral techniques. However, it is often used ineffectively. People tend to set some goals and then get started on the program, quickly forgetting about the goals. This type of goal setting does not help trigger or stabilize behavior change. Goal setting, to be maximally effective, must be included as a regular part of the exercise program. Clients should always be aware of what they are working toward and what it will take to get there. Additionally, the goals should be written following the **SMART goal** guidelines (specific, measurable, attainable, relevant, and time-bound) (see Chapter 3). Personal trainers should be able to clearly guide clients through the goal-setting process and help them understand how to set effective and appropriate goals.

Feedback

Feedback can be intrinsic or extrinsic. The most common type of feedback is extrinsic feedback, which includes the reinforcement and encouragement that personal trainers give to their clients. However, long-term program adherence is dependent on a client's ability to provide internal feedback. It is important for personal trainers to not give too much feedback. Instead, as efficacy and ability builds, trainers should taper off the amount of external feedback they provide, encouraging the clients to start providing feedback for themselves. Clients must learn to reinforce their own behaviors by providing internal encouragement, error correction, and even punishment.

Decision Making

Decision making is reflective of a client's ability to control a situation and choose appropriately among alternative courses of action. Personal trainers can teach effective decision-making skills by giving clients control over their own program participation. It is important that trainers do not make every decision and micromanage their clients' programs. Trainers must provide their clients the information needed to determine the outcome of their programs. Trainers should continuously educate their clients on everything from the principles of behavior change to exercise techniques to give the clients the knowledge they need to be successful on their own.

Self-monitoring

Self-monitoring helps a client keep track of program participation and progress, or lack thereof. This is an information-gathering process that will help clients and trainers identify potential barriers to success (e.g., people, events). Only committed clients will be able to successfully self-monitor, as it requires honesty and self-reflection. Self-monitoring is most effectively done in the form of keeping a journal that records thoughts, experiences, and emotions that are related to program participation. The gathered information is extremely helpful in developing an effective plan for long term adherence.

Implementing Basic Behavior-change and Health-psychology Strategies

Effective and successful personal trainers will not only understand the theoretical constructs of behavior change, but will also be able to apply that information when working with clients. It is this application of knowledge that will generate adherence and long-term success for the trainer and the client.

No assessment tool is available that personal trainers can give to their clients that will provide all the information they need about self-efficacy, health beliefs, and readiness to change. It is up to the trainer to be able to use effective and consistent communication to gain a better understanding about each client. All information that is gathered through effective communication and observation should be used in program design and implementation. Personal trainers cannot create programs based solely on physical skill level and ability; they must also use the psychological information. The gathering of information about the client's attitudes, thoughts, and beliefs is a continuous process that is part of each training session. Minor adjustments and modifications should be made to training programs on an ongoing basis because the psychological variables will change and shift as a client progresses in a program. Old barriers will be overcome and new challenges will arise, so personal trainers must use systems of feedback and communication to be aware of the changes occurring with the client and make appropriate program adjustments that maximize adherence.

Behavioral Interventions

There are several pieces of information that trainers need to obtain when working with a new client. The first one is past activity experience and the client's feelings and perceptions about that experience. In other words, what issues from past experiences will influence the current experience? In this discussion, the personal trainer should be able to identify client apprehensions, comfort zones, and abilities and should be able to get a pretty good idea of the client's current exercise-specific self-efficacy level.

A trainer should also seek information about the client's social-support network. If the client does not have a support network that embraces and encourages an active lifestyle, he or she will face many more obstacles to making a successful lifestyle change. Everything from family and friend activity levels to work environment is relevant and important in building an appropriate program. Some of this information will be easily gathered in initial meetings, and some of it will surface over time as the client–trainer relationship is better established.

Personal trainers should also identify clients' attitudes, opinions, and beliefs about physical activity and then make an effort to manipulate client decisional balance and self-efficacy. Almost all new exercisers have misconceptions about being physically active. It is up to the personal trainer to teach the truths about living an active lifestyle. This is best done through a continual process of education, experience, and trust development that provides logical information to dispute irrational beliefs and fosters the creation of a rational and realistic assessment of fitness. In other words, each training session is an opportunity for the trainer to teach the client about making lasting changes. It is critical that initial program experiences build mastery and positive emotional states. Clients must believe early on that they can do it. If doubt lingers for an extended period of time, the client will drop out. Personal trainers must treat each client as an individual and address the unique goals, needs, attitudes, and beliefs of each person.

Lastly, all personal trainers need to establish an effective goal-setting program from the very beginning. This requires the trainer to teach goal-setting techniques and self-monitoring strategies. Personal trainers should empower their clients to take their physical-activity experiences into their own hands.

Summary

Helping others make changes in their exercise behaviors is a challenging and ongoing process. It requires a personal trainer to excel at communication, rapport building, and program design. A firm understanding of the theoretical behavior models will provide personal trainers with the knowledge required to help their clients make lasting behavior changes. The psychological component of exercise programming is also an ongoing process. Psychological states change and require unique strategies to help foster positive behavior modification. It is critical that personal trainers are respectful of how difficult it is to adopt and maintain an exercise program, as the success of both the client and trainer is based on how well the processes of change are implemented and used on a regular basis.

References

Bandura, A. (1994). Self-efficacy. In: Ramachaudran, V.S. (Ed.) *Encyclopedia of Human Behavior* (Vol. 4; pp. 71–81). New York: Academic Press.

Bandura, A. (1986). *Social Foundations of Thought and Action: A Social Cognitive Theory*. Englewood Cliffs, N.J.: Prentice-Hall.

Becker, M.H. (1974). The health belief model and personal health behavior. *Health Education Monographs,* 2, 324–473.

Dishman, R.K. (1991). Increasing and maintaining exercise and physical activity. *Behavior Therapy,* 22, 345–378.

Engel, G.L. (1977). The need for a new medical model: A challenge for biomedicine. *Science*, 196, 129–136.

Ingledew, D.K. & Markland, D. (2008). The role of motives in exercise participation. *Psychology and Health,* 23, 807–828.

Marcus, B.H. et al. (2000). Physical activity behavior change: Issues in adoption and maintenance. *Health Psychology*, 19, 32–41.

Martin, G. & Pear, J. (2007). *Behavior Modification: What It Is and How to Do It* (8th ed.). Englewood Cliffs, N.J.: Prentice-Hall.

Morgan, W.P. (2001). Prescription of physical activity: A paradigm shift. *Quest,* 53, 336–382.

Prochaska, J.O. & DiClemente, C.C. (1984). *The Transtheoretical Approach: Crossing Traditional Boundaries of Therapy.* Homewood, Ill.: Dow Jones/Irwin.

Sarafino, E.P. (2008). *Health Psychology: Biopsychosocial Interactions* (6th ed.). New York: John Wiley & Sons.

Smith, R.E. (2005). Positive reinforcement, performance feedback, and performance enhancement. In: Williams, J.M. (Ed.) *Applied Sport Psychology: Personal Growth to Peak Performance* (5th ed.). Mountain View, Calif.: Mayfield Publishing Company.

Turk, D.C., Rudy, T.E., & Salovey, P. (1984). Health protection: Attitudes and behaviors of LPNs, teachers, and college students. *Health Psychology*, 3, 189–210.

U.S. Department of Health & Human Services (2008). *2008 Physical Activity Guidelines for Americans: Be Active, Healthy and Happy.* www.health.gov/paguidelines/pdf/paguide.pdf

Suggested Reading

Bandura, A. (2001). Social cognitive theory: An agentive perspective. *Annual Review of Psychology,* 52, 1–26.

Bandura, A. (1997). *Self-efficacy: The Exercise of Control.* New York: Freeman.

Centers for Disease Control and Prevention (2005). Adult participation in recommended levels of physical activity: United States, 2001 and 2003. *Morbidity and Mortality Weekly Report,* 54, 47, 1208–1212.

Centers for Disease Control and Prevention (2005). Trends in leisure-time physical inactivity by age, sex, and race/ethnicity: United States, 1994-2004. *Morbidity and Mortality Weekly Report,* 54, 39, 991–994.

Centers for Disease Control and Prevention (2003). Physical activity among adults: United States, 2000. *Advance Data,* 333.

Dishman, R. K. (1990). Determinants of participation in physical activity. In: Bouchard, C. et al. (Eds.) *Exercise, Fitness, and Health* (pp. 75–102). Champaign, Ill.: Human Kinetics.

Dishman, R.K. & Buckworth, J. (1996). Increasing physical activity: A quantitative synthesis. *Medicine & Science in Sports & Exercise,* 28, 706–719.

Dunn, A.L. & Blair, S.N. (1997). Exercise prescription. In: Morgan, W.P. (Ed.) *Physical Activity & Mental Health* (pp. 49–62). Washington, D.C.: Taylor & Francis.

Kirschenbaum, D.S. (1997). Prevention of sedentary lifestyles: Rationale and methods. In: Morgan, W.P. (Ed.) *Physical Activity & Mental Health* (pp. 33–48). Washington, D.C.: Taylor & Francis.

Masui, R. et al. (2002). The relationship between health beliefs and behaviors and dietary intake in early adolescence. *Journal of the American Dietetics Association*, 102, 421–424.

McAuley, E., Pena, M.M., & Jerome, G.J. (2001). Self-efficacy as a determinant and an outcome of exercise. In: Roberts, G.C. (Ed.) *Advances in Motivation in Sport and Exercise.* Champaign, Ill.: Human Kinetics.

Orleans, C.T. (2000). Promoting the maintenance of health behavior change: Recommendations for the next generation of research and practice. *Health Psychology,* 19, 76-83.

Sallis, J.F. & Hovell, M.F. (1990). Determinants of exercise behavior. In: *Exercise and Sports Sciences Reviews*, 18. Baltimore, Md.: Williams and Wilkins, 307–330.

U.S. Department of Health & Human Services (1996). *Physical Activity and Health: A Report of the Surgeon General*. Atlanta, Georgia: U.S. Department of Health & Human Services, Public Health Service, CDC, National Center for Chronic Disease Prevention and Health Promotion.

PART III

The ACE Integrated Fitness Training™ Model

ACE would like to acknowledge the contributions of Fabio Comana, M.A., M.S., Todd Galati, M.A., and Pete McCall, M.S., who helped develop the ACE Integrated Fitness Training Model and served as section reviewers for Part III: Chapters 5 through 12.

Chapter 5
Introduction to the ACE Integrated Fitness Training™ Model

Chapter 6
Building Rapport and the Initial Investigation Stage

Chapter 7
Functional Assessments: Posture, Movement, Core, Balance, and Flexibility

Chapter 8
Physiological Assessments

Chapter 9
Functional Programming for Stability-Mobility and Movement

Chapter 10
Resistance Training: Programming and Progressions

Chapter 11
Cardiorespiratory Training: Programming and Progressions

Chapter 12
The ACE Integrated Fitness Training™ Model in Practice

IN THIS CHAPTER:

Health—Fitness—Performance Continuum

Introduction to the ACE Integrated Fitness Training™ Model

Rapport and Behavioral Strategies

Training Components and Phases

Functional Movement and Resistance Training

Cardiorespiratory Training

Special Population Clientele

Summary

TODD GALATI, M.A., *is the certification and exam development manager for the American Council on Exercise and serves on volunteer committees with the Institute for Credentialing Excellence, formerly the National Organization for Competency Assurance. He holds a bachelor's degree in athletic training and a master's degree in kinesiology and four ACE certifications (Personal Trainer, Advanced Health & Fitness Specialist, Lifestyle & Weight Management Coach, and Group Fitness Instructor). Prior to joining ACE, Galati was a program director with the University of California, San Diego School of Medicine, where he spent 14 years designing and researching the effectiveness of youth fitness programs in reducing risk factors for cardiovascular disease, obesity, and type 2 diabetes. Galati's experience includes teaching classes in biomechanics and applied kinesiology as an adjunct professor at Cal State San Marcos, conducting human performance studies as a research physiologist with the U.S. Navy, working as a personal trainer in medical fitness facilities, and coaching endurance athletes to state and national championships.*

CHAPTER 5

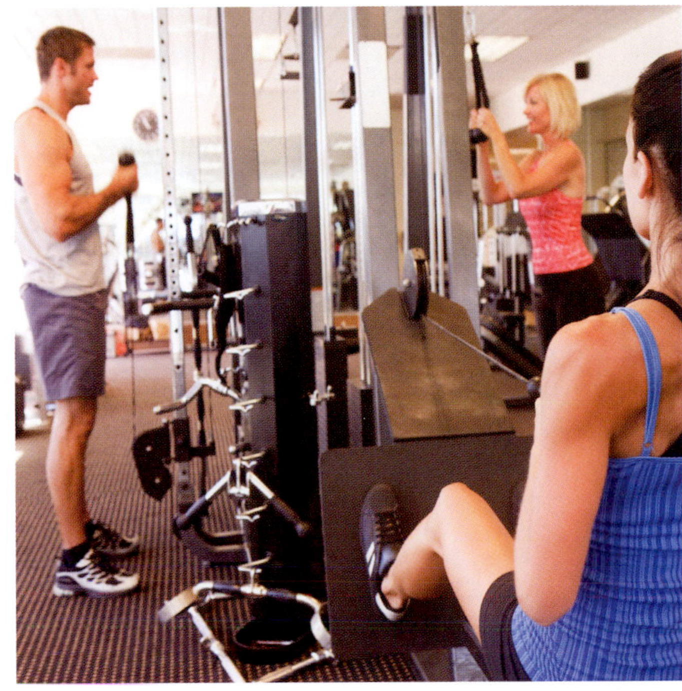

Introduction to the ACE Integrated Fitness Training™ (ACE IFT™) Model

Todd Galati

Personal training is a fairly new profession compared to other fields in allied healthcare. Originally a relatively straightforward profession, it has evolved to meet the mounting challenges of an aging and increasingly **overweight** population and an overburdened healthcare system that is often unable to meet the need for preventative care. Personal trainers are seeing an influx of clientele with an increasingly long list of special needs. Fortunately, there has been concurrent growth in the body of knowledge in exercise science, which has led to advances in technology, equipment, and programming solutions to meet the expanding needs of a growing diversity of personal-training clients.

This shift in programming toward specialized needs and interests has led to some confusion among personal trainers when it comes to designing exercise programs. What was once a relatively simplistic approach to programming for health-related fitness has become a seemingly complicated process that includes a myriad of training modalities, equipment, and differing schools of thought.

The process of learning these new exercise-programming methods and the science behind them seems relatively easy when each is considered individually. It is when determining which training method, or methods, would be most appropriate for each client that the full weight of these rapid advances is felt, often leaving the personal trainer confused about where to begin and how to progress the client's program (Table 5-1).

Table 5-1

Traditional Physiological Training Parameters versus New Physiological Training Parameters

Traditional Training Parameters	New Training Parameters
Cardiorespiratory (aerobic) fitness Muscular endurance Muscular strength Flexibility	Postural (kinetic chain) stability Kinetic chain mobility Movement efficiency Core conditioning Balance Cardiorespiratory (aerobic) fitness Muscular endurance Muscular strength Flexibility Metabolic markers (ventilatory thresholds) Agility, coordination, and reactivity Speed and power

Both novice and veteran personal trainers are well aware of the positive benefits exercise can yield in improving health, fitness, mood, weight management, stress management, and other health-related parameters. The *2008 Physical Activity Guidelines for Americans* reinforce these positive benefits by acknowledging that regular exercise is a critical component of good health and that individuals can reduce their risk of developing **chronic disease** by staying physically active and participating in structured exercise on a regular basis (U.S. Department of Health & Human Services, 2008). The guidelines specifically state that regular exercise will help *prevent* many common diseases, such as **type 2 diabetes, coronary artery disease,** high blood pressure, and the health risks associated with **obesity.** Michael Leavitt, the former Secretary of Health & Human Services, stated "There is strong evidence that physically active people have better health-related physical fitness and are at lower risk of developing many disabling medical conditions than inactive people." The *2008 Physical Activity Guidelines for Americans* suggest that adults should participate in structured physical activity at a moderate intensity for at least 150 minutes per week or a vigorous intensity for at least 75 minutes per week to experience the health benefits of exercise. While this document endorses exercise as a means to achieve good health, it does not provide specific instructions for *how* to exercise.

A summary of general exercise programming guidelines for apparently healthy adults can be found in Table 5-2. These guidelines are based on sound research for providing safe and effective exercise for apparently healthy adults, but they are so broad that trainers require additional information on how to appropriately implement them for each individual client.

In addition, there are exercise guidelines for many specific groups, including youth, older adults, pre- and postnatal women, and people who have obesity, **hypertension, hyperlipidemia, osteoporosis,** and a variety of other special needs (see Chapter 14). These guidelines are based on medical and scientific research, are published by the governing body of practitioners for each respective special-needs group, and provide specific exercise guidelines to help these individuals improve their health and quality of life. So how does a personal trainer pull it all together? How does a novice or even an experienced personal trainer know which assessments to perform, when to perform them, which guidelines are most important, when to address foundational imbalances in **posture** or movement, and how to progress or modify a program based on observed and reported feedback? To address these questions and more, the American Council on Exercise developed the ACE Integrated Fitness Training (ACE IFT™) Model to provide personal trainers with a systematic and comprehensive approach to exercise programming that integrates assessments and programming to facilitate behavior change, while also improving posture,

Table 5-2
General Exercise Recommendations for Healthy Adults

Training Component	Frequency (days per week)	Intensity	Time (Duration) or Repetitions	Type (Activity)
Cardiorespiratory	>5 or >3 or 3–5	Moderate (40% to <60% $\dot{V}O_2$R/HRR) Vigorous (≥60% $\dot{V}O_2$R/HRR) Combination of moderate and vigorous (40% to <60% $\dot{V}O_2$R/HRR; or ≥60% $\dot{V}O_2$R/HRR)	>30 minutes* 20–25 minutes* 20–30 minutes*	Aerobic (cardiovascular endurance) activities and weightbearing exercise
Resistance	2–3	60–80% of 1 RM or RPE = 5 to 6 (0–10 scale) for older adults	2–4 sets of 8–25 repetitions (e.g., 8–12, 10–15, 15–25; depending upon goal)	8–10 exercises that include all major muscle groups (full body or split routine); Muscular strength and endurance, calisthenics, balance, and agility exercise
Flexibility	>2–3	Stretch to the limits of discomfort within the ROM, to the point of mild tightness without discomfort	>4 repetitions per muscle group Static: 15–60 seconds; PNF: hold 6 seconds, then a 10–30 second assisted stretch	All major muscle tendon groups Static, PNF, or dynamic (ballistic may be fine for individuals who participate in ballistic activities)

*Continuous exercise or intermittent exercise in bouts of at least 10 minutes in duration to accumulate the minimum recommendation for the given intensity

Note: $\dot{V}O_2$R = $\dot{V}O_2$ reserve; HRR = Heart-rate reserve; 1 RM = One-repetition maximum; RPE = Ratings of perceived exertion; ROM = Range of motion; PNF = Proprioceptive neuromuscular facilitation

Source: American College of Sports Medicine (2010). *ACMS's Guidelines for Exercise Testing and Prescription* (8th ed.). Philadelphia: Wolters Kluwer/Lippincott Williams & Wilkins.

movement, **flexibility, balance,** core function, **cardiorespiratory fitness, muscular endurance,** and **muscular strength.**

Health—Fitness—Performance Continuum

The health—fitness—performance continuum is based on the premise that exercise programs should follow a progression that first improves health, then develops and advances fitness, and finally enhances performance (Figure 5-1). Each client will have different needs based on his or her personal health, fitness, and goals. Therefore, each client will start his or her exercise program at a unique point along the continuum. The first component of this model is exercise for improved health, which serves as the foundation of every exercise program, even if the client's ultimate goal is to achieve optimum athletic performance for a specific competition. For a client who has been **sedentary,** improved health should be a primary program goal. For clients who have progressed into the fitness or performance domains, their comprehensive training programs should still feature components that maintain or help improve health as well as address their specific fitness or athletic goals.

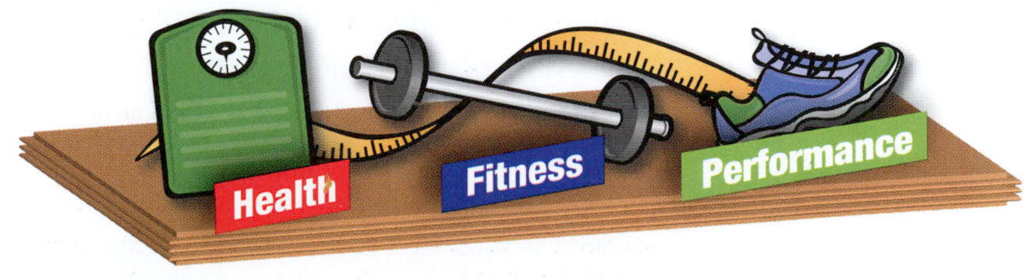

Figure 5-1
The health—fitness—performance continuum

Throughout this continuum, programs should progress at a rate that is safe and effective, while taking into account the client's schedule or time availability, capacity for recovery, and outside stressors such as work, family, and travel. Clients who have been sedentary for many years will generally need to adhere to a regular exercise program focused on improved health for at least the initial conditioning stage—approximately four to six weeks—before focusing on exercise program variables such as frequency, intensity, and duration that move them into the fitness domain. This should seem fairly straightforward for a sedentary client, but what about the client who has focused primarily on resistance training for many years, or the long-time runner who runs at least five days per week but does not do any resistance training? Should a client fitting one of these profiles automatically train all components of fitness at intensity levels that fall into the fitness or performance domains? The answer to this question is different for each client based on his or her unique strengths, weaknesses, imbalances, and goals. Meeting each client's individualized needs can be a welcome challenge for an experienced personal trainer—and a confusing and frustrating venture for a newly certified professional. While the health—fitness—performance continuum provides a suggested sequence for training clients from sedentary to performance, it does not address the individual components of fitness and how they fit together.

Introduction to the ACE Integrated Fitness Training Model

The foundation of the ACE IFT Model is built upon **rapport.** Successful personal trainers consistently demonstrate excellent communication skills and teaching techniques, while understanding the psychological, emotional, and physiological needs and concerns of their clients. Building rapport is a critical component of successful client–trainer relationships, as this process promotes open communication, develops trust, and fosters the client's desire to participate in an exercise program. Rapport should be developed early through open communication and initial positive experiences with exercise, and then enhanced through behavioral strategies that help build long-term **adherence.** The components of, and techniques for, open communication, rapport development, and the facilitation of program adherence are presented in Chapters 2 through 4, while effective strategies for implementing these techniques as the foundation for the ACE IFT Model are presented in Chapter 6.

After establishing initial rapport, the trainer should collect health-history information to determine if the client has any contraindications or requires a physician's evaluation prior to exercise. The collection of health-history information and other pre-exercise paperwork is covered in Chapter 6, along with health-related physiological measurements such as **resting heart rate** and **blood pressure.** This is a critical process not only to ensure the safety of the client, but also to provide an opportunity for the personal trainer to establish trust and create an open source of communication. The ACE IFT Model includes functional and physiological assessments that can be performed at specific phases to provide key information for exercise programming in that phase. Some assessments, such as those that focus on functional movement, balance, and **range of motion,** may be conducted within the first few sessions with a new client, while other assessments might not be conducted until the client has progressed from one phase to another. Ideally, the trainer should utilize a sequential approach to conducting client assessments that begins with reviewing the client's health history; discussing desires, preferences, and general goals; completing a needs assessment; and then determining which assessments are relevant and the timelines in which to conduct them (Figure 5-2). The various assessment protocols included in the ACE IFT Model are covered in Chapters 7 and 8, while the parameters for when to use many of these assessments and how to program based on the data collected are presented in Chapters 9 through 11.

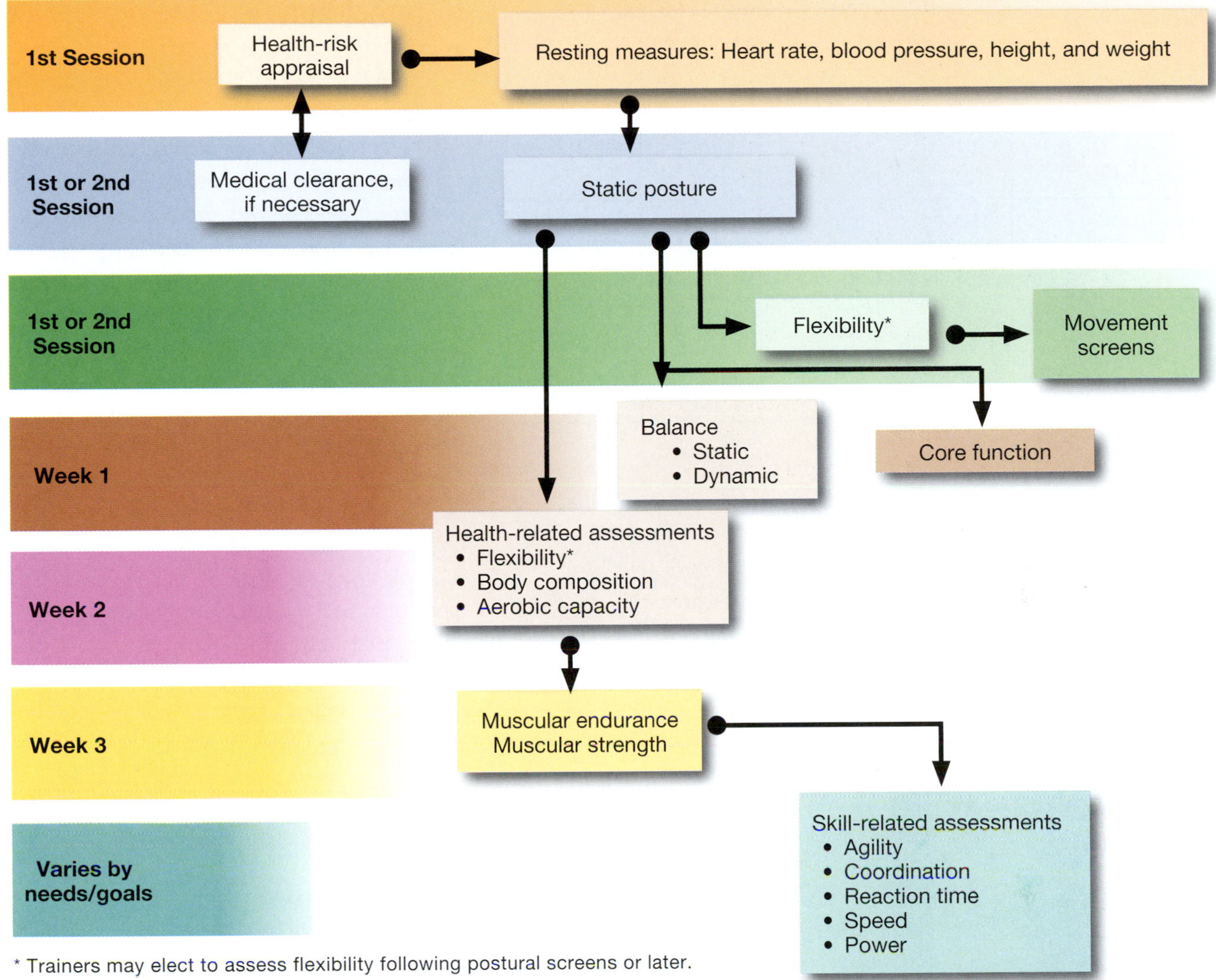

Figure 5-2
Sample assessment sequencing for the general client

The ACE IFT Model is a comprehensive system for exercise programming that pulls together the multifaceted training parameters required to be a successful personal trainer. It organizes the latest exercise science research into a logical system that helps trainers determine appropriate assessments, exercises, and progressions for clients based on their unique health, fitness, needs, and goals. The ACE IFT Model has two principal training components:

- Functional movement and resistance training
- Cardiorespiratory training

Each of these components is composed of four phases that provide trainers with strategies to determine and implement the most appropriate assessments and exercise programs for clients at all levels of fitness.

The training components are broken down into four phases, each with a title that is descriptive of the principal training focus during that specific phase (Table 5-3). Rapport is the foundation for success during all phases, whether a trainer is working with a highly motivated fitness enthusiast or a sedentary adult looking to adopt more healthful habits.

The four training phases run parallel to the health—fitness—performance training continuum that was presented in Figure 5-1 (Figure 5-3). In phase 1, the primary focus is on improving health by correcting imbalances through training to improve joint stability and mobility prior to training movement patterns

Table 5-3
ACE Integrated Fitness Training Model—Training Components and Phases

Training Component	Phase 1	Phase 2	Phase 3	Phase 4
Functional Movement & Resistance Training	Stability and Mobility Training	Movement Training	Load Training	Performance Training
Cardiorespiratory Training	Aerobic-base Training	Aerobic-efficiency Training	Anaerobic-endurance Training	Anaerobic-power Training

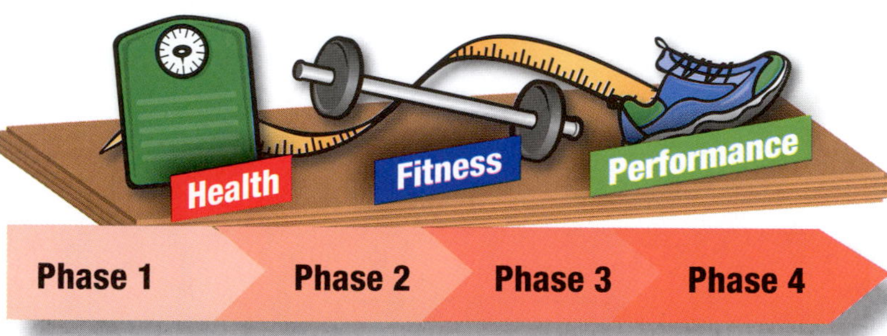

Figure 5-3
ACE IFT Model phases and the health—fitness—performance continuum

and building an **aerobic** base to improve parameters of cardiorespiratory health. The primary focus of phase 2 is to progress clients toward improved fitness by introducing aerobic intervals to improve aerobic efficiency and training movement patterns prior to loading the movements. In phase 3, clients progress to higher levels of fitness through load training and the development of **anaerobic** endurance, with programming at the advanced stages of phase 3 moving into the performance area of the health—fitness—performance continuum. Phase 4 is focused entirely on improving performance through training for power, speed, agility, reactivity, and anaerobic power. Each client will progress from one phase to the next according to his or her unique needs, goals, and available time to commit to training. Many clients will be at different phases of the two training components based on their current health and fitness, and only clients with performance-oriented goals will reach phase 4.

Rapport and Behavioral Strategies

The greatest impact a personal trainer can have on a client's life is to help that person change his or her habits and establish a positive relationship with exercise. For this reason, rapport is the foundation of the ACE IFT Model. Exercise programming has traditionally had a primary focus on helping clients make physiological changes, placing early emphasis on fitness assessments for program design and tracking progress. However, to the out-of-shape client, a complete battery of initial assessments can be detrimental to early program success by reinforcing his or her negative self-image and beliefs that he or she is hopelessly out of shape or overweight. The most important initial adaptations come from helping a client modify behavior to establish a habit of regular exercise. A personal trainer can have an immediate impact on a client's health by first creating a positive exercise experience that can lead to exercise adherence, and then gradually progressing the training plan by applying program-design strategies that produce results.

Successful personal trainers provide integrated training solutions to clients by helping them have positive experiences with exercise. Applying strategies for fitness-related behavior change and exercise adherence, along with implementing comprehensive exercise programs that help clients reach their unique fitness and wellness goals are two primary functions of personal trainers who want to help clients achieve meaningful results. Some of the key steps that facilitate fitness-related behavior change include:

- Implementing strategies for developing and enhancing rapport
- Identifying each client's readiness to change behavior and stage of behavioral change (see Chapter 4)
- Fostering exercise adherence by creating positive exercise experiences and building self-efficacy
- Appropriately selecting and timing assessments and reassessments

- Designing programs, supervising workouts, and implementing progressions that match each client's current health and fitness status, needs, and goals
- Fostering a sense of self-reliance to enable clients to take ownership of their lifestyle changes
- Implementing lapse-prevention strategies
- Helping clients transition from **extrinsic** to **intrinsic motivation**
- Using tools for identifying, and strategies for working with, a client's personality style
- Establishing realistic short- and long-term goals to prevent burnout and promote adherence
- Helping clients transition to the **action** and then **maintenance** stages of behavior change
- Providing extrinsic motivation and introducing visualization techniques during performance training
- Factoring a client's external stresses into total fatigue to avoid training plateaus and prevent overtraining
- Empowering clients by helping them gain the self-efficacy and knowledge to train on their own
- Helping clients make exercise a long-term habit

The first time that a trainer and client meet, it is important for the trainer to encourage the client and create an environment where he or she can feel successful. It is also important for the trainer to be mindful that many adults who are inactive might have been inactive since childhood. After two to four weeks of regular physical activity, clients will generally experience more stable positive moods due to:

- Changes in **hormone** and **neurotransmitter** levels (e.g., **endorphins, serotonin,** and **norepinephrine**)
- Increased self-efficacy with task and possibly short-term goal accomplishment
- Improved performance due to the positive neuromuscular adaptations to exercise that follow the initial **delayed onset muscle soreness (DOMS)** and accompanying temporary decreases in strength

These positive factors will enhance adherence behaviors, but the client must make it through two to four weeks of regular exercise to reap these benefits. To help a client transition to the action stage of behavior change, the trainer should make exercise fun and emphasize regular adherence to a program *first* before switching the primary focus toward any other specific goals such as weight loss or changes in **body composition.** By providing regular positive experiences with exercise, personal trainers can help clients have continued success. Chapter 6 provides the tools and techniques for putting these behavioral strategies into action.

Training Components and Phases

The ACE IFT Model provides a comprehensive training model for health, fitness, and performance that can be implemented with all apparently healthy clients. To effectively utilize the ACE IFT Model with a variety of clients, personal trainers must understand how to assess which stage a client is in for *each* training component, how to design exercise programs in each component, and how to integrate and progress each component to provide clients with comprehensive training solutions. Some clients will be at the same phase for cardiorespiratory training and functional movement and resistance training, while others will be at distinctly different phases for these two training components. Many clients, regardless of their current exercise frequency and fitness level, will have muscle imbalances, postural issues, and improper movement mechanics that should be addressed through early programming in the stability and mobility training phase (phase 1) before they progress to the movement-training phase (phase 2). It is important for personal trainers to understand the different phases and training components of the ACE IFT Model, in order to assess each client individually and determine which phase of training to apply to his or her specific training goals. By doing this, personal trainers will be able to design individualized programs that apply the appropriate training stimulus.

The phase descriptions that follow provide an overview of the objectives, assessments, and exercise programming and progressions within each training phase, and provide a guideline for how clients should progress from one phase to the next within each training component. Initial emphasis is placed on behavioral strategies as the foundation for the ACE IFT Model. Chapters 6 through 11 provide detailed descriptions of the tools and strategies necessary for trainers to determine which phase a client is in for each training component, which assessments are appropriate to conduct with the client, what to include in the client's initial exercise program, and appropriate progressions to help the client reach his or her goals. Chapter 12 will then help trainers synthesize all of this information by presenting case studies that take clients through programs that meet their unique needs.

Functional Movement and Resistance Training

Functional movement and resistance training are often treated as two separate and unrelated types of training. However, at the core of human movement is posture. Individuals who have weak core muscles, muscle imbalances, and/or postural deviations are in poor postural health and at increased risk for injury when external loads are applied to movements. For that reason, the functional movement and resistance training component begins in phase 1 with assessments and training for postural and joint stability and mobility. Once a client gains or restores good postural integrity, he or she is ready to move on to phase 2, where assessments and exercise selection are focused on training the basic movement patterns of single-leg actions, squatting or bending, pushing, pulling, and rotating. Before the client can move on to phase 3, where these movement patterns will be loaded with external resistance, he or she needs to demonstrate proficiency with:

- Performing bodyweight movement sequences with proper form
- Core stabilization
- Control of the **center of gravity (COG)**
- Control of the velocity of movement

Once movement training has been successfully completed, it is time to progress to phase 3, where the focus is on applying external resistances, or loads, to these functional movement patterns. Phase 3 applies the traditional resistance-training methodology for endurance, hypertrophy (or strength-endurance), and strength to the client's particular goals. Finally, those clients who have performance-oriented goals and have successfully progressed to advanced levels of training in phase 3 of resistance training can move on to training for performance in phase 4.

The four phases of the functional movement and resistance training component—stability and mobility, movement, load, and performance—are based on the principles of **specificity, overload,** and progression. For an exercise program to be successful, the selection of exercises needs to be specific to the client's individual needs and goals while providing the appropriate overload so that he or she can progressively improve his or her fitness level. Recognizing that all movement begins and ends from a position of posture, the focus of the first level of the functional movement and resistance training component is to apply the variables of exercise-program design to help clients improve posture.

Phase 1: Stability and Mobility Training

The training focus during phase 1 is on the introduction of low-intensity exercise programs to improve muscle balance, muscular endurance, core function, flexibility, and static and dynamic balance to improve the client's posture. Teaching a client how to find and hold a relatively neutral posture will create the foundation for the movement skills that will be introduced in the phases that follow. It is important to note that this neutral position will be unique for each client, so the personal trainer will want to assist each client in learning and practicing this position. Exercise selection in this phase will focus on core and balance exercises that improve the strength and function of the tonic muscles responsible for stabilizing the spine and COG during movement. Exercises will use primarily bodyweight or body-segment weight as resistance. No assessments of muscular strength or endurance are required prior to designing and implementing an exercise program during this phase. Assessments that should be conducted early in this phase include basic assessments of:

- Posture
- Balance
- Movement
- Range of motion of the ankle, hip, shoulder complex, and thoracic and lumbar spine

Based on the results of these assessments, the personal trainer should implement an exercise program that addresses the client's weaknesses and imbalances. Two to three weeks into this phase, personal trainers can consider assessing muscular endurance of the torso muscles based on the client's current level of postural stability and core muscle activation. Assessment protocols for posture, balance, movement screens, range of motion, and torso muscular endurance are covered in detail in Chapter 7.

The principal goal of this phase of the training program will be to develop postural stability throughout the kinetic chain without compromising mobility at any point in the chain. Exercises should emphasize supported surfaces that offer stability against gravity (e.g., floor, backrests) and focus on restorative flexibility, **isometric** contractions, limited-ROM strengthening, static balance, core activation, spinal stabilization, and muscular endurance to promote stability. Exercise-programming tools and strategies for stability and mobility training are presented in Chapter 9.

Phase 2: Movement Training

The primary focus during phase 2 of the functional movement and resistance training component of the ACE IFT Model is on training movement patterns. Through programming that builds on the training completed during phase 1, trainers can help clients develop mobility within the kinetic chain without compromising stability. Movement training focuses on the five primary movements of exercise:

- *Bend-and-lift movements (e.g., squatting):* Squatting movements are performed many times throughout the day as a person sits or stands from a chair or squats down to lift an object off of the floor.
- *Single-leg movements (e.g., lunging):* Single-leg balance and movements are a critical part of walking. In addition, lunging movements are performed when a person steps forward to reach down with one hand to pick something small up off the floor.
- *Pushing movements:* Pushing movements occur in four directions: forward (e.g., during a push-up exercise or when pushing open a door), overhead (e.g., during a shoulder press or when putting an item on a tall shelf), lateral (e.g., pushing open double sliding doors or lifting one's torso when getting up from a side-lying position), and downward (e.g., during dips or when lifting oneself up from a chair or out of the side of a swimming pool).
- *Pulling movements:* Pulling movements occur during an exercise such as a bent-over row or pull-up, or during a movement like pulling open a car door.
- *Rotational (spiral) movements:* Rotation occurs during many common movements, such as the rotation of the thoracic spine during gait or when reaching across the body to pick up an object on the left side and placing it on the right side.

Most pushing, pulling, and squatting motions can be performed either unilaterally or bilaterally, while lunges require alternating unilateral movements of the legs. Most everyday pushing, pulling, and squatting movements also have a rotational component that requires either rotational mobility or stability to prevent motion in the **transverse plane.** Assessments that are recommended during this phase are covered in Chapter 7.

Exercise programs during this phase should emphasize the proper sequencing of movements and control of the body's COG throughout normal ROM during body-segment and full-body movements to develop efficient neural patterns. Exercises that promote **dynamic balance** and active flexibility should be introduced as part of a dynamic warm-up, or as part of the principal exercise program to facilitate proper movement patterns. Any resistance training performed during this phase should include exercises that build muscular endurance and promote mobility, with an emphasis on controlled motion and deceleration performed via controlled **eccentric** muscle actions.

Whole-body movement patterns that utilize gravity as the source of external resistance should be emphasized until proper movement patterns are established. Once a client can perform the movement patterns effectively while maintaining stable neutral posture, COG, and movement speed, he or she can then progress to load training in phase 3. The general timeframe for movement training is two to eight weeks, depending on the level of movement corrections required. Personal trainers should keep in mind that every client is unique and will progress at his or her own rate based on ability and adherence to training. Detailed tools and strategies for training movement patterns can be found in Chapter 9.

Phase 3: Load Training

Training in phases 1 and 2 focuses on addressing postural imbalances and muscle motor control to help clients develop the prerequisite postural stability and proper movement sequences to allow for external loads to be added during full-body movements. In phase 3, load training, the exercise program is advanced with the addition of an external force, placing emphasis on muscle force production where the variables of training can be manipulated to address a variety of exercise goals. These goals may include positive changes in body composition, muscular strength, muscle **hypertrophy,** or muscular endurance, or simply looking more "toned." It is during load training that personal trainers will apply the body of knowledge of exercise science related to resistance training to design and progress exercise programs to meet the diverse goals of their clients.

Traditional resistance-training programs for muscle hypertrophy, strength, or endurance all require external loads to facilitate increased muscular force production. Therefore, during load training, exercise program design variables are applied in a manner consistent with the standard FITT model (frequency, intensity, time, and type) for increasing muscular hypertrophy, enhancing muscular endurance, or improving muscular strength. Exercise selection is consistent with traditional resistance-training exercises and is dictated by the client's specific goals and needs. Resistance, or loading, can be applied through a number of different options, including selectorized equipment, plate-loaded machines, barbells, dumbbells, kettlebells, medicine balls, elastic tubing, or even non-traditional strength-training equipment such as tires or water-filled containers. Regardless of the exercise selected or the type of load used, the focus during load training is on increasing the ability of muscles to generate force.

Personal trainers can play a crucial role in helping clients stay motivated by designing and modifying programs to introduce variety and work toward goal attainment. This can be accomplished through programs utilizing **linear** or **undulating periodization** models to progress the total training volume (see Chapter 10). Exercise selection may initially focus on isolated or single-joint movements, but should transition to integration of body segments and full-body movements. Programs can range from exercises for all major muscle groups performed two to three times per week, to circuit training or split routines, depending on the client's goals, available time for training, and motivation. Stability and mobility– and movement-training exercises should be maintained during phase 3 as part of a dynamic warm-up and to maintain flexibility during the cool-down. During phase 3, assessments of muscular strength and endurance are introduced to facilitate program design and quantify progress. Protocols for assessing muscular strength and endurance are detailed in Chapter 8, while exercise programming strategies for load training (phase 3) are presented in Chapter 10.

Each client's specific training goals will dictate the unique focus of his or her program within phase 3. Since phase 3 is focused on resistance training, many clients will stay in this phase for many years, especially those clients who have no interest in training for performance. If the client has a significant lapse during this phase of training, the personal trainer should assess the client's stability, mobility, and movement patterns before reintroducing load training to determine if the client has developed or reestablished postural deviations, muscle imbalances, or movement errors. Before progressing to phase 4 (performance training), clients should develop the prerequisite strength necessary to move into training for power, speed, agility, and quickness. If the client moves on to phase 4 before this base is developed, he or she will be at risk for injuries.

Phase 4: Performance Training

Phase 4 of the functional movement and resistance training component emphasizes specific training to improve speed, agility, quickness, reactivity, and power. Many clients will not progress to this stage of training, as they will not have athletic or performance-oriented goals. All clients who progress to the performance phase of training should continue to maintain good postural stability and proper movement patterns. Personal trainers can facilitate this progress by incorporating the techniques of mobility and stability training (phase 1) and movement training (phase 2) as dynamic warm-ups.

Strength training performed during load training increases muscular force production, but it does not specifically address speed of force production. Power training enhances the velocity of force production by improving the ability of muscles to generate a large amount of force in a short period of time. Power is needed in all sports and activities that require repeated acceleration and deceleration. Power can be defined as both the velocity of force production and the rate of performing work.

Power Equations

Power = Force x Velocity

or

Power = Work/Time

Where:

Force = Mass x Acceleration

Velocity = Distance/Time

Work = Force x Distance

These equations are provided to illustrate that power can be defined as the rate at which force is produced over a given distance. Personal trainers can use these equations to manipulate training to help clients increase their ability to produce power. During load training, clients will have actually created some increase in their power by increasing strength and the ability to produce muscular force. To advance power, clients must also work on the rate at which they produce force. By manipulating the time of force production through different loading techniques that involve quick accelerations and decelerations, clients can improve power. Speed, agility, quickness, and reactivity are the skill-related parameters that will directly benefit from enhanced power.

Exercise selection during performance training can include a variety of techniques, including **plyometric** jump training, medicine ball throws, kettlebell lifts, and traditional Olympic-style lifts. The FITT components used during this phase are applied in a manner consistent with program design for power training and emphasize intensity and technique over repetitions. During load training (phase 3), the focus is on strength training to improve muscle **motor unit** recruitment, while the goal of power training is to increase **rate coding,** or the speed at which the motor units stimulate the muscles to contract and produce force. The emphasis is on maximizing the **stretch reflex** by minimizing the transition time between the eccentric and **concentric** phases of muscle action. The faster a muscle can convert from the lengthening to shortening phases (i.e., eccentric to concentric muscle actions), the greater the amount of force generated by the muscle during the concentric, or shortening, phase where the desired movement (e.g., vertical jump) is performed.

In most sports, power originates at the body's point of contact with a stable surface, which is generally the ground or court surface, as seen in running, jumping, throwing, and striking/hitting skills. The power originates from the legs and torso first loading eccentrically as the body gets closer to the ground and rotates. As the muscles transition from eccentric loading to concentric force production, the body recoils as the force transfers from the feet, through the legs and torso, and, in the case of throwing and striking, through the shoulders, arms, and hands. For this reason, power training is applied with integrated full-body exercises to improve power in the legs, hips, core, shoulder complex, and arms. Failure to involve the full body when training for power puts the client at an increased risk for injuries. Protocols for assessments for measuring power (e.g., Margaria-Kalamen) and speed, agility, and quickness (e.g., pro agility) are provided in Chapter 8. In addition, detailed descriptions for designing and progressing exercise programs for phase 4 can be found in Chapter 10.

Power-based training can also be an effective strategy to help clients improve their body-composition levels, since this can be one of the most efficient methods of expending energy during a training session. Clients will have to develop the prerequisite stability, mobility, strength, and skills during the previous three phases prior to beginning phase 4 training methods. An additional benefit of training for power is the development of lean muscle, since **type II muscle fibers** are responsible for high-force, short-duration contractions, and the enhancement of muscle size and definition.

Cardiorespiratory Training

Cardiorespiratory-training programs have traditionally focused on **steady state** training to improve cardiorespiratory fitness, with progressions based on increased duration and intensity. Intervals have been loosely categorized and have primarily been focused on reducing boredom through higher- and lower-intensity segments, or training intervals at or near the **lactate threshold** to improve speed during endurance events. While these methods are effective, they have often been looked at as very different training programs for individuals trying to improve health, fitness, or performance. The ACE IFT Model provides a systematic approach to cardiorespiratory training that can take a client all the way from being sedentary to training for a personal record in a half-marathon. While this will not be the training goal of most sedentary individuals, having an organized system of training that can allow for a long-term progression is empowering for the personal trainer because it provides strategies for implementing cardiorespiratory programs for the entire spectrum of apparently healthy individuals—from the sedentary person to the competitive athlete. During each phase of the cardiorespiratory training component, the exercise mode should accommodate the level of exertion required during that phase, while also being appropriate for the client based on his or her preferences, health and fitness status, and contraindications. Recommended cardiorespiratory fitness assessment protocols are presented in Chapter 8, along with guidelines for which assessments to conduct during each phase. Exercise programming guidelines for each phase are presented in Chapter 11.

Phase 1: Aerobic-base Training

Phase 1 of the cardiorespiratory training component of the ACE IFT Model is focused on developing an initial aerobic base in clients who have been sedentary or near-sedentary. This should not be confused with the "aerobic-base training" that is performed by endurance athletes as the endurance-performance foundation for them to be able to complete their events, often lasting two or more hours in length. Instead, aerobic-base training during phase 1 of the cardiorespiratory training component is focused on establishing baseline aerobic fitness to improve health and to serve as a foundation for training for cardiorespiratory fitness in phase 2.

The intent of this phase is to develop a stable aerobic base upon which the client can build improvements in health, endurance, energy, mood, and caloric expenditure.

How quickly a client progresses through phase 1 will depend on the client's goals, training volume, and initial fitness level. A client who has been fairly fit in the past and is in relatively good health will likely progress through this phase more quickly than a client who has led a mostly sedentary life and is currently obese. Exercise during this phase should be performed at steady-state intensities in the low-to-moderate range, which is in line with the lower portion of the range of the guidelines for cardiorespiratory exercise [American College of Sports Medicine (ACSM), 2010]. The easiest method for monitoring intensity with clients in this aerobic-base phase is to use the **talk test.** If the client can perform the exercise and talk comfortably in sentences that are more than a few words in length, he or she is likely below the **first ventilatory threshold (VT1).** By exercising below or up to the talk-test threshold, clients should be exercising at **ratings of perceived exertion (RPE)** of 3 to 4 (0 to 10 scale).

The cardiorespiratory exercise performed by the client should initially be of an appropriate duration that the client can tolerate. For the sedentary client who is starting his or her cardiorespiratory exercise in this aerobic base phase, this duration could be as short as five minutes and up to 10 to 20 minutes. Regardless of the initial duration, the goal for all clients in this phase is to progress cardiorespiratory training by gradually increasing the duration and frequency until the client is performing cardiorespiratory exercise three to five days per week for a duration of 20 to 30 minutes at an RPE of 3 to 4. Clients who progress to this level of exercise will see improvements in health, endurance, and energy expenditure, and should notice decreased stress and improved function during **activities of daily living (ADL).** As the primary focus during this phase is to establish an initial aerobic base for clients who have little to no base at the time of their first personal-training session, steady-state exercise is recommended. No assessments are recommended during the aerobic-base phase, since many of the clients who start in this phase will be unfit and may have difficulty completing an assessment of this nature.

Phase 2: Aerobic-efficiency Training

This second phase of cardiorespiratory training is dedicated to enhancing the client's aerobic efficiency by progressing the program through increased duration of sessions, increased frequency of sessions when possible, and the introduction of aerobic intervals. Aerobic intervals are introduced at a level that is at or just above VT1, or an RPE of 5 ("strong") on the 0 to 10 scale. The goal of these intervals will be to improve aerobic endurance by raising the intensity of exercise performed at VT1, and to improve the client's ability to utilize fat as a fuel source The addition of these aerobic intervals will also allow the personal trainer to add variety to the client's cardiorespiratory exercise program by introducing sets of intervals that differ in number and length of work and rest intervals, as well as intervals that utilize different methods for increasing intensity, such as increased speed, incline, and resistance.

To enhance exercise program design, trainers can conduct the submaximal talk test to determine heart rate at VT1. A protocol for this assessment can be found in Chapter 8. The talk test can also be used to help clients gain a better understanding of RPE, as VT1 has been found to be approximately between an RPE of 4 and 5 ("somewhat strong" to "strong") (Foster, 1998). This assessment tool requires little equipment and is easy to administer, providing a simple method for determining VT1 that can be used for exercise programming during phases 2 through 4 of cardiorespiratory training. The use of aerobic intervals will allow the personal trainer to introduce a more intense training stimulus to elicit the desired adaptations.

The training goals for clients during this phase will vary greatly. Because there are aerobic intervals included in this phase, the training stimulus will be adequate for some clients to perform cardiorespiratory exercise in phase 2 for many years if they have no goals of improving speed or fitness beyond that gained in phase 2 training.

Phase 3: Anaerobic-endurance Training

During phase 3 of cardiorespiratory training, the primary focus is on designing training programs that help improve performance in endurance events or to train fitness enthusiasts for higher levels of cardiorespiratory fitness. This is accomplished through the introduction of higher-intensity intervals that load the cardiorespiratory system enough to develop anaerobic endurance, and balancing training time spent below VT1, between VT1 and the **second ventilatory threshold (VT2),** and at or above VT2. This type of training is sometimes referred to as lactate threshold or tolerance training and is designed to increase the amount of sustained work that an individual can perform at or near VT2. In addition to improving cardiorespiratory capacity at or near VT2, this type of work will also help to increase the ability of the working muscles to produce force for an extended period. A protocol for determining heart rate at VT2 is presented in Chapter 8. This protocol provides a useful field test for determining estimated VT2 that can be performed with minimal equipment.

Depending on the individual, his or her available training time, and the dates of the client's goal event(s), a client may train three to seven days per week with sessions that are 20 minutes to multiple hours in length. Exercise at or near VT2 cannot be sustained for extended periods during multiple training sessions per week. For clients looking to improve speed and performance, research has shown that world-class endurance athletes in multiple sports spend approximately 70 to 80% of their training time at or below VT1 (RPE of 3 to 4), only brief periods (less than 10% of training time) between VT1 and VT2 (RPE of 5 to 6), and the remaining approximately 10 to 20% of their training time at or above VT2 (RPE ≥7) (Esteve-Lanao et al., 2007). The ACE IFT Model utilizes a three-zone model for cardiorespiratory training. The full cardiorespiratory exercise program should be composed of:

- Zone 1 (at or below VT1): 70–80% of training time—Focus on developing a solid base of exercise below the talk-test threshold or VT1 (RPE = 3 to 4) on several days per week: recovery workouts, warm-up, cool-down, and long-distance workouts
- Zone 2 (between VT1 and VT2): <10% of training time—Aerobic intervals at or just above VT1 (RPE of 5) during one or two cardiorespiratory sessions per week: aerobic efficiency
- Zone 3 (at or above VT2): 10–20% of training time—Anaerobic intervals at or above VT2 (RPE = 6 to 7) during one or two cardiorespiratory sessions per week: anaerobic endurance (Foster, 1998)

This will add great variety to the client's cardiorespiratory program, but will also increase fatigue due to the increased interval intensity. Having the client perform a warm-up, cool-down, and active rest intervals at an intensity that falls below the talk-test level will allow him or her to better prepare for, and recover from, the intervals performed at or above VT2. This can be valuable information for a personal trainer who is trying to explain the importance of active recovery and rest to a client who believes that if a few intervals are good, more must be better. Exercise programming strategies for phase 3 cardiorespiratory exercise are presented in Chapter 11.

If the client begins showing signs of overtraining (e.g., increased resting heart rate, disturbed sleep, or decreased hunger on multiple days), the personal trainer should decrease the frequency and/or intensity of the client's intervals and focus more time on recovery. Also, if during an interval workout the client cannot reach the desired intensity during a training interval, or is unable to reach the desired recovery intensity or heart rate during a recovery interval, the session should be stopped and the client should recover with low-to-moderate cardiorespiratory exercise (an RPE of 3, and no more than 4) to prevent overtraining. Personal trainers should take time to explain to clients the crucial role that recovery plays in improving fitness and performance, and that it is more important to perform, and fully recover from, a few intervals than it is to do all intervals and take the body to a point of fatigue where recovery before the next workout is less likely to occur. While situations of this nature may seem more common during the next phase (phase 4) of the cardiorespiratory training component, the intervals introduced in this phase, coupled with additional life stresses, can be enough to induce overtraining in some clients.

Phase 4: Anaerobic-power Training

Many clients will never reach this phase of cardiorespiratory training, as the challenges introduced during the anaerobic-endurance training phase (phase 3) will be at the highest level of work they will want or need to perform based on their goals and motivation. This is fine, as the primary focus in this phase is on building on the training done in the previous three phases, while also introducing new intervals that are designed to enhance anaerobic power. These new intervals are designed to develop peak power and aerobic capacity with intervals performed well above VT2, or an RPE of ≥9 ("very, very strong"). These intervals will overload the **fast glycolytic system** and challenge the **phosphagen system,** enhancing the client's ability to perform work for extended periods above the lactate threshold. These intervals are short-duration, high-intensity intervals that are very taxing; therefore, they require a great deal of intrinsic motivation to meet the physical and mental challenges of completing them.

Clients working in this phase of cardiorespiratory training will be training for competition and have specific goals that relate to short-duration, high-intensity efforts during longer endurance events, such as speeding up to stay with a pack in road cycling, or paddling vigorously for several minutes to navigate some difficult rapids while kayaking. Depending on the individual, his or her available training time, and the dates of the client's goal event(s), clients will train three to seven days per week with sessions that are 20 minutes to several hours in length. The same principles of work intervals, recovery, and avoiding overtraining described in the anaerobic-endurance training phase (phase 3) apply to the anaerobic-power training phase as well. In addition, it is important for the personal trainer to keep in mind that most of the client's time spent performing cardiorespiratory exercise should be at or below VT1 (RPE of 3 to 4), especially during the warm-up, cool-down, rest intervals, recovery workouts, and on days when the client is working on increasing maximum training time during his or her longest weekly workout sessions. Exercise-programming strategies for cardiorespiratory training phase 4 are presented in Chapter 11.

Special Population Clientele

Personal trainers in most settings will work with clients who have a variety of special needs. Once these clients have been cleared for exercise by their physicians, they can begin an exercise program based on specific guidelines provided by their physicians and the guidelines for their conditions as provided by the appropriate governing bodies. Specific guidelines for a variety of special populations are provided in Chapter 14. Personal trainers working with special-population clients should still utilize the integrated training process provided in the ACE IFT Model, being sure to adjust exercise selection, intensity, sets, repetitions, and duration to fit the special needs of each client. Many of these clients may never progress beyond the aerobic-efficiency phase of cardiorespiratory training (phase 2), and many of them will never progress beyond the loading phase of functional movement and resistance training (phase 3). The most important goal with all clients is to provide them with initial positive experiences that promote adherence through easily achieved initial successes. Transitioning a special-population client into the action stage and then on to the maintenance stage of change will have a significant impact on that client's health and overall quality of life, and may even have a positive impact on the client's state of physical and mental fitness.

Summary

The ACE IFT Model offers personal trainers a systematic approach to providing integrated assessment and programming solutions for clients at various ages and levels of fitness. The phases of the model provide appropriate levels of programming to improve health, basic fitness, advanced fitness, and performance, while the training components—functional movement and resistance training, and cardiorespiratory training—allow the personal trainer to provide comprehensive training solutions that are appropriate for each client's current health, fitness, and goals in each area of training. The central focus of creating positive experiences that develop and enhance program adherence is crucial to success for all clients and will set a personal trainer apart from peers who are more focused on sets and repetitions. The many tools of personal training have been delivered though a variety of books, courses, and workshops, requiring a personal trainer to spend years learning new material and figuring out how to convert that knowledge into practical programs. The ACE IFT Model provides personal trainers with a comprehensive solution that synthesizes all of these assessments and training components for easy use.

References

American College of Sports Medicine (2010). *ACSM's Guidelines for Exercise Testing and Prescription* (8th ed.). Philadelphia: Wolters Kluwer/ Lippincott Williams & Wilkins.

Esteve-Lanao, J. et al. (2007). Impact of training intensity distribution on performance in endurance athletes. *Journal of Strength and Conditioning Research,* 21, 943–949.

Foster, C. (1998). Monitoring training in athletes with reference to overtraining syndrome. *Medicine & Science in Sports & Exercise,* 30, 1164–1168.

U.S. Department of Health & Human Services (2008). *2008 Physical Activity Guidelines for Americans: Be Active, Healthy and Happy.* www.health.gov/paguidelines/pdf/paguide.pdf

Suggested Reading

American Council on Exercise (2010). *ACE's Essentials of Exercise Science for Fitness Professionals*. San Diego, Calif.: American Council on Exercise.

American Council on Exercise (2009). *ACE Advanced Health & Fitness Specialist Manual.* San Diego, Calif.: American Council on Exercise.

IN THIS CHAPTER:

Facilitating Change and Motivational Interviewing

The Health-risk Appraisal

Evaluation Forms

Health Conditions That Affect Physical Activity

- Cardiovascular
- Respiratory
- Musculoskeletal
- Metabolic
- Other Conditions

Medications

- Antihypertensives
- Bronchodilators
- Cold Medications

Sequencing Assessments

Choosing the Right Assessments

- Goals of the Assessment
- Physical Limitations of the Participant
- Testing Environment
- Availability of Equipment
- Age of the Participant

Tools to Get Started

Conducting Essential Cardiovascular Assessments

- Heart Rate
- Blood Pressure

Ratings of Perceived Exertion

The Exercise-induced Feeling Inventory

Summary

KELLY SPIVEY, N.D., *is a continuing education provider for health and fitness professionals and maintains her own personal-training business. As a member of the American Alternative Medical Society, Dr. Spivey's primary focus is on disease prevention and complementary medicine. She is an adjunct professor in the Exercise Science Department at the University of Tampa. Dr. Spivey has been working as an exam development subject-matter expert with ACE since 2006.*

CHAPTER 6

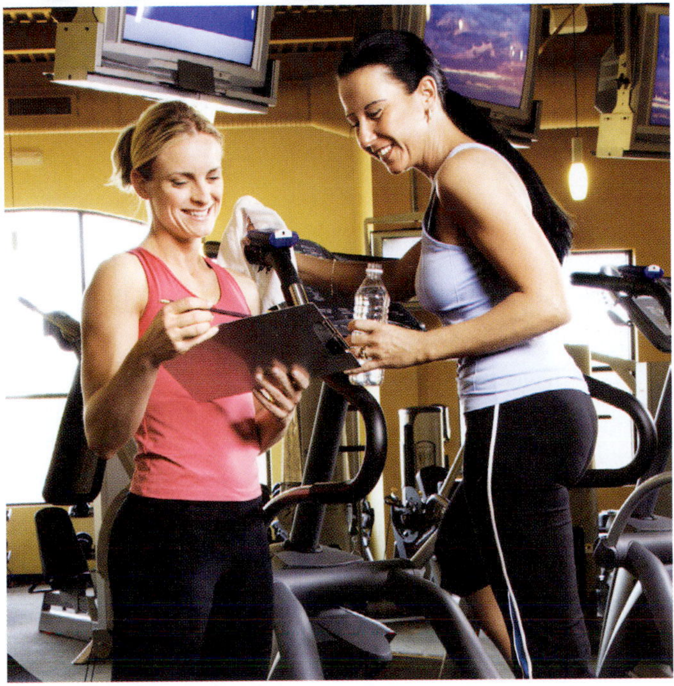

Building Rapport and the Initial Investigation Stage

Kelly Spivey

Certified personal trainers have a lot of useful information to share with prospective clients, but until trust and respect have been earned, that information will go unheard. Before designing any programs, explaining any exercises, or discussing nutritional habits, the trainer must take full advantage of lessons learned from behavioral scientists and begin to cultivate a strong client–trainer relationship.

The first impression a personal trainer makes on a prospective client is perhaps the most critical, as it may influence the individual's hiring decision, regardless of the trainer's qualifications or reputation. Trainers must be aware that this first impression may be made in person through a casual meeting or introduction, over the phone, or even through an email. It is therefore imperative to make a strong, convincing, and positive first impression. Assuming the trainer makes a good first impression, a targeted approach to building **rapport** is essential to developing a solid level of trust and a foundation for a solid client–trainer relationship.

As discussed in Chapter 3, rapport implies a relationship of mutual trust, harmony, or emotional affinity. It is essentially the development of a professional/personal relationship with mutual respect and understanding. Three attributes are essential to successful relationships:

- *Empathy:* The ability to experience another person's world as if it were one's own
- *Warmth:* An unconditional positive regard, or respect, for another person regardless of his or her individuality and uniqueness. This quality will convey a climate that communicates safety and acceptance to the client.
- *Genuineness:* Authenticity, or the ability to be honest and open

Rapport-building is considered one of the four essential stages of a successful client–trainer relationship. Unlike the three latter stages, which have somewhat clearly defined timelines, rapport is ongoing, in that it continues to develop throughout the relationship (Figure 6-1).

- *Rapport:* Involves the personal interaction a trainer establishes and maintains with a client, as well as the ability to communicate effectively with clients. This stage includes:
  - ✓Impressions of professionalism, developing trust, demonstrating warmth and genuineness, and exhibiting **empathy**
- *Investigation:* Involves the collection of all relevant information to identify the comprehensive needs of clients. This stage includes:
  - ✓Identifying readiness to change behavior; identifying the client's stage of behavioral change and personality style; collecting health and safety information; learning about lifestyle preferences, interests, and attitudes; understanding previous experiences; and conducting assessments
- *Planning:* Involves collaborative goal setting with the client after the investigation is complete to design an effective and comprehensive program. This stage includes:
  - ✓Goal setting, programming considerations, and designing **motivation** and **adherence** strategies
- *Action:* Involves the successful implementation of all programming components and providing the appropriate instruction, **feedback**, and progression as needed. This stage includes:
  - ✓Instruction, demonstration, and execution of programs; implementing strategies to improve motivation and promote long-term adherence; providing feedback and evaluation; making necessary adjustments to programs; and monitoring the overall exercise experience and progression toward goals

If a client finds the trainer trustworthy and genuinely concerned about his or her needs, desires, and goals, it helps promote open, effective communication channels in which the client is willing to share challenges and obstacles with the trainer. This in turn will allow the trainer to problem-solve and strategize solutions with the client, which not only improves the client's willingness to participate in the training program, but will also enhance long-term compliance in his or her health and fitness program.

It is important to remember that the first objective when meeting a prospective client is to first build a foundation for a personal relationship with the individual; gathering information on the client's goals and objectives is secondary. This entails taking an appropriate

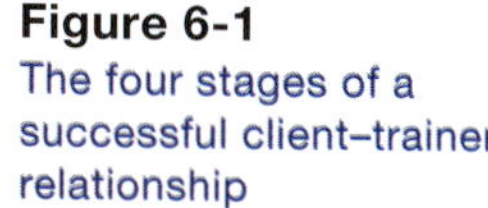
Figure 6-1
The four stages of a successful client–trainer relationship

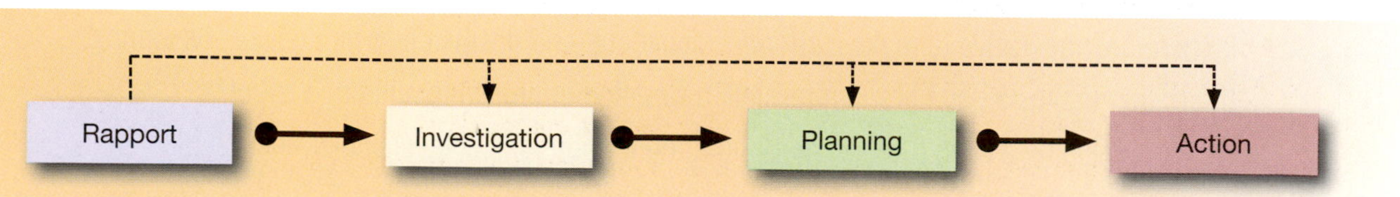

amount of time to get to know the client and discover his or her individual characteristics. Trainers frequently make the mistake of immediately collecting information pertinent to personal training and neglect the need to develop rapport. However, while rapport is critical, a trainer must also be attentive to the personality style of the person with whom he or she is interacting. For example, a "director" who scores low on the sociability scale and high on the dominance scale cares little for casual conversation initially, while a "collaborator" who scores high on the sociability scale and low on the dominance scale favors an extended exchange of ideas and a friendly manner.

A successful trainer can quickly identify the basic personality style of the individual and then adapt a communication style to treat the individual the way he or she needs to be treated (i.e., allowing the client to remain in his or her comfort zone). A trainer should avoid treating each client in the same manner. One critical skill to successful personal training is the ability to be versatile and adapt one's personality style to meet that of new clients. A thorough review of the personality traits (i.e., director, deliberator, collaborator, and expressor) and how to work effectively with each individual style is presented in Chapter 3 and will certainly improve a trainer's rapport-building skills.

Trainers should also be attentive to general communications skills and factors (e.g., active listening, verbal and nonverbal communication, environment). Many of these skills are discussed in Chapter 3, but key strategies are highlighted here as well.

Environment:

- A trainer must attend to the environment where he or she meets prospective/current clients.
  - ✓ Create a nurturing, yet professional environment by meeting in a quiet, comfortable area.
  - ✓ Avoid high-traffic areas and member distractions, and do not attempt to establish rapport with a simple facility tour or orientation.
  - ✓ Do not sit behind a desk, but rather sit facing the client to create a level of comfort.
- Be attentive to personal appearance (e.g., clothing, grooming, jewelry, scent, breath).

Effective communication:

- Verbal communication translates only part of the messages people send. While people hear each other's words, they often seek to verify the verbal content by evaluating the speaker's nonverbal messages, including posture, facial expressions, gestures, and eye contact. Success with nonverbal communication is influenced by attending behavior, which involves the nonverbal things people do to communicate:
  - ✓ *Distance and orientation (body positioning):* Trainers should face the client squarely and maintain appropriate distances to demonstrate respect for personal space [1½ to 4 feet (0.5 to 1.2 m) is considered ideal, and in many cultures, less than 1½ feet (0.5 m) is considered intimate space].
  - ✓ *Posture and position:* Trainers should adopt an open, well-balanced, erect, but relaxed posture with a slight forward lean toward the client to show confidence and interest in the conversation.
    - ○ Leaning on a desk or wall or stooping suggests boredom and fatigue.
    - ○ Rigid hands placed upon the hips can be interpreted as aggressive behavior.
    - ○ Crossing the arms or legs conveys a defensive stance.
  - ✓ *Mirroring and gestures:* Trainers can sensitively mimic a client's posture, gestures, and voice tone and tempo to help place the individual at ease and facilitate open communication. People generally feel more comfortable when others use relaxed, fluid gestures to convey messages.
    - ○ Reduce distracting movements that may disrupt the client's communication (e.g., tapping one's feet, clicking a pen).

- Avoid making postural changes while listening. Postural changes are effective when preparing to speak or while speaking.
- Avoid pointing or other intimidating gestures

✓ *Eye contact:* Trainers should maintain a relaxed look to help instill comfort, but avoid fixed stares.

- Looking away while a person speaks is inattentive behavior and conveys disinterest, while suggesting that what the client is saying is only moderately important.

✓ *Facial expressions:* These convey emotion and work to the trainer's benefit best when the emotion is sincere.

- Try to wear a genuine smile to demonstrate positive regard for the client.
- Eye expressions also portray a lot about a person's intentions.

• Voice quality (tonality and articulation) is an important determinant of successful communication. A weak, hesitant voice does not inspire confidence, whereas a loud, overbearing voice can make others nervous. Trainers should develop a voice that is firm, confident, and professional, yet conveys warmth and compassion. It is important to avoid too many voice fluctuations, which often prove distracting.

• Listening effectively is the *primary* nonverbal communication skill. Being an effective communicator involves listening perhaps more than speaking. While humans can speak 125 to 250 words per minute, they are capable of listening to up to 500 words per minute.

✓ Effective listening implies listening to both the content and emotions behind the speaker's words.

✓ Listening occurs at different levels:

- *Indifferent listening:* A person is not really listening and is tuned out.
- *Selective listening:* A person listens only to key words.
- *Passive listening:* A person gives the impression of listening by using minimal noncommittal agreements (e.g., head nods, "uh huhs").
- *Active listening:* A person shows empathy and listens as if he or she is in the speaker's shoes. This is the key to effective listening.

Empathy:

• Trainers must be attentive and empathetic, regardless of personal opinion.

✓ Separate meaningful content from superfluous information and do not get caught on trigger words (hot buttons) that distract from listening to, and understanding, the entire message.

✓ Be aware of how the client's emotional patterns change based on the nature of the content being discussed (e.g., how a client may become defensive when discussing weight challenges).

✓ Be conscious of how cultural and ethnic differences affect communication (e.g., averting one's eyes from a person while speaking).

• Trainers must distinguish between verbal messages that reflect apparent (cognitive) and underlying (affective) content of the communication.

✓ Cognitive messages are more factual.

✓ Affective messages are composed of feelings, emotions, and behaviors and are often expressed via both verbal and nonverbal communication.

Interviewing techniques:

• It is important to use a variety of interviewing techniques to clearly understand the content of a client's message. Avoid questions that simply require a "yes" or "no" answer.

✓ *Minimal encouragers:* Brief words or phrases that encourage the client to share additional information (e.g., "*Please explain* what you mean by occasional knee pain")

✓ *Paraphrasing:* Responding to the client's communication by restating the essence of the content of his or her communication

✓ *Probing:* Asking additional questions in an attempt to gather more information

(e.g., "Please tell me more about the medications you are taking")

- ✓ *Reflecting:* Restating the feelings and/or content of what the speaker conveys, but with different words. This verifies information and displays empathy and understanding. This is different than paraphrasing in that feelings or attitudes may be included (e.g., "I hear you say you've been unsuccessful at losing weight, but it appears that it makes you uncomfortable to discuss your previous attempts at weight loss").
- ✓ *Clarifying:* Verifying an understanding of the content of the client's communication. Trainers must be careful not to interpret or analyze based on their own opinions or experiences.
- ✓ *Informing:* Expanding upon shared information. If a client is concerned about having an **asthma** attack while working out, the trainer can share factual information on strategies to avoid an asthma attack.
- ✓ *Confronting:* Using mild to strong feedback with a client. This can encourage accountability when clients display lethargy or a lack of motivation toward their workout sessions. This technique should be used with caution because the trainer's perceptions may not be based on factual data.
- ✓ *Questioning:* Directing both open and closed questions to a client
- ✓ *Deflecting:* Changing the focus of one individual onto other, usually to devalue and diminish the content of the communication. Use of this style is ill-advised unless the trainer is intentionally attempting to be empathetic by sharing appropriate experiences.

Trainers must always be aware that a client's emotional patterns may change based on the nature of the content being discussed. General psychological states and personality traits, as well as relevant cultural and ethnic factors, should all be considered when communicating with a client.

Just as an appropriate interview technique is important in establishing rapport, trainers should select a communication style that matches the client's needs and personality style, and the situation.

- A preaching style is judgmental and delivers information in a lecture-type format by describing what the client should do. This minimizes the chances for establishing rapport.
- An educating style is informational, providing relevant information in a concise manner, and allows the client to make a more informed decision.
- A counseling style is supportive, utilizing a collaborative effort to problem-solve and help the client make an informed decision. This is the most effective style and is recommended when implementing a plan and/or modifying a program design.
- A directing style is more instructive, in that the trainer provides instructions and direction. This style is most effective when safety and proper form and technique are essential.

Facilitating Change and Motivational Interviewing

Once a trainer has developed a foundation of rapport through effective communication and appropriate interviewing techniques, he or she should identify the client's readiness to change behavior and his or her stage in the behavioral change process. Success in personal training also requires skill in understanding behavioral change and how to facilitate lifestyle changes. Adopting healthy behavior is a complex process, and several theories have been developed to explain factors affecting lifestyle change. One such model is the **transtheoretical model of behavioral change (TTM)**—also called the **stages-of-change model**—which is detailed in Chapter 4. This model begins with identifying a client's readiness to change. This readiness provides a good indication of when an individual is ready to adopt healthy behavior. Trainers should never make the assumption that because someone purchases personal-training sessions, he or she is actually committed and ready to change his or her behavior. The person may simply be appeasing a significant other, using gifted sessions before they expire, or have been pressured into starting an exercise program after a doctor's stern recommendation.

As many trainers stake their reputation on facilitating successful behavioral change, it would be prudent for the trainer to determine each client's or prospective client's (1) readiness to change behavior; and (2) stage of behavioral change, before attempting to design and implement a program. Employing strategies to change behavior that are inappropriate for the individual's current stage of change may result in failure on the part of the individual to adopt the strategies and successfully change the behavior.

Figure 6-2 presents a simple eight-item questionnaire that trainers can administer to clients verbally during the lifestyle and health-history portion of the investigation stage (interview) or distribute to them to complete on their own. Keep in mind that individuals may not always be completely honest when completing self-administered surveys and questionnaires. The more "yes" responses indicated on the questionnaire, the more likely the person is to commit to changing key behaviors.

Motivational interviewing can be used by the trainer to facilitate behavioral change, as it helps the client feel as if he or she has control (see Chapter 3 for more information on how to incorporate motivational interviewing into your interactions with clients). Motivational interviewing, as defined by Miller and Rollnick (2002), is a client-centered, directive method for enhancing **intrinsic motivation** to change by exploring and resolving ambivalence. In other words, it is an interviewing technique to get clients "off the fence" about exercise. Motivational interviewing is not about questioning; it involves careful listening and strategic questioning.

To promote behavioral change, it is important for the client to buy into the process. If he or she is not willing, any behavioral change that does take place is not likely to remain. Motivational interviewing is an interview process that helps the personal trainer determine the client's level of readiness, or current stage of change. This technique also helps the client learn more about the reasons for change, and then participate in the behavioral change process.

There is more to personal training than sets and repetitions, which is why there are a number of chapters in this book devoted to the behavioral components associated with personal training. This information is important when fostering behavioral change and providing the motivation needed to achieve personal goals. The trainer should become very familiar with the psychological aspects of the profession. The behavioral tactics described should be incorporated into the personal-training program, starting with the initial interview. The following section of this chapter focuses on the next integral aspect of the personal-training experience: The initial interview and the pre-exercise screening.

Figure 6-2
Readiness to change questionnaire

	YES	NO
Are you looking to change a specific behavior?	❑	❑
Are you willing to make this behavioral change a top priority?	❑	❑
Have you tried to change this behavior before?	❑	❑
Do you believe there are inherent risks/dangers associated with not making this behavioral change?	❑	❑
Are you committed to making this change, even though it may prove challenging?	❑	❑
Do you have support for making this change from friends, family, and loved ones?	❑	❑
Besides health reasons, do you have other reasons for wanting to change this behavior?	❑	❑
Are you prepared to be patient with yourself if you encounter obstacles, barriers, and/or setbacks?	❑	❑

The Health-risk Appraisal

Research demonstrates the positive impact that exercise and physical activity have on reducing a person's risk for developing cardiovascular, pulmonary, and metabolic diseases, as well as cancer, **anxiety, depression,** and premature death (Haskell et al., 2007; U.S. Department of Health & Human Services, 2008). While exercise and physical activity promote numerous physiological, psychological, and emotional benefits, there are some inherent risks. In general, moderate levels of exercise and physical activity do not provoke any dangerous cardiovascular or musculoskeletal events in healthy individuals, but there is an increased risk for harm in individuals who are unhealthy, or who present with existing disease or are at *risk* for disease [American College of Sports Medicine (ACSM), 2010]. A systematic screening will address signs and/or symptoms of disease, **risk factors,** and family history. The purposes of the pre-participation screening include the following (ACSM, 2010):

- Identifying the presence or absence of known cardiovascular, pulmonary, and/or metabolic disease, or signs or symptoms suggestive of cardiovascular, pulmonary, and/or metabolic disease
- Identifying individuals with medical **contraindications** (health conditions and risk factors) who should be excluded from exercise or physical activity until those conditions have been corrected or are under control
- Detecting at-risk individuals who should first undergo medical evaluation and clinical exercise testing before initiating an exercise program
- Identifying those individuals with medical conditions who should participate in medically supervised programs

Further consideration should be given when assessing an individual's risk as to whether the exercise program is self-directed or being conducted under the consultation and supervision of a qualified fitness professional. With self-directed exercise, a standard questionnaire is completed by the individual with little to no feedback from the fitness professional. These questionnaires are designed to provide information regarding existing risks for participation in activity and the need for medical clearance beforehand. A pre-participation screening *must* be performed on all new participants, regardless of age, upon entering a facility that offers exercise equipment or services. The screening procedure should be valid, simple, cost- and time-efficient, and appropriate for the target population. Additionally, there should be a written policy on referral procedures for at-risk individuals.

Individuals participating in self-guided activity should at least complete a general health-risk appraisal. The **Physical Activity Readiness Questionnaire (PAR-Q)** has been used successfully when a short, simple medical/health questionnaire is needed (Figure 6-3). Experts recognize the PAR-Q as a *minimal,* yet safe, pre-exercise screening measure for low-to-moderate, but not vigorous, exercise training:

- It serves as a minimal health-risk appraisal prerequisite.
- It is quick, easy, and non-invasive to administer.
- It is, however, limited by its lack of detail and may overlook important health conditions, medications, and past injuries.

If someone is identified by the PAR-Q as having multiple health risks, it is recommended that a more detailed health risk-appraisal that gathers more in-depth information relative to cardiovascular disease and other disorders and dysfunctions be used.

The process of conducting a health-risk appraisal involves detailed information gathering and a thorough review of the client's health information, medical history, and lifestyle habits, which will enable the trainer to determine risk stratification or the need for medical examination, as well as develop recommendations for lifestyle modifications and strategies for exercise testing and programming. In 1998, ACSM and the American Heart Association published a screening tool that is more comprehensive than the PAR-Q

Physical Activity Readiness
Questionnaire - PAR-Q
(revised 2002)

PAR-Q & YOU

(A Questionnaire for People Aged 15 to 69)

Regular physical activity is fun and healthy, and increasingly more people are starting to become more active every day. Being more active is very safe for most people. However, some people should check with their doctor before they start becoming much more physically active.

If you are planning to become much more physically active than you are now, start by answering the seven questions in the box below. If you are between the ages of 15 and 69, the PAR-Q will tell you if you should check with your doctor before you start. If you are over 69 years of age, and you are not used to being very active, check with your doctor.

Common sense is your best guide when you answer these questions. Please read the questions carefully and answer each one honestly: check YES or NO.

YES	NO		
☐	☐	1.	**Has your doctor ever said that you have a heart condition and that you should only do physical activity recommended by a doctor?**
☐	☐	2.	**Do you feel pain in your chest when you do physical activity?**
☐	☐	3.	**In the past month, have you had chest pain when you were not doing physical activity?**
☐	☐	4.	**Do you lose your balance because of dizziness or do you ever lose consciousness?**
☐	☐	5.	**Do you have a bone or joint problem (for example, back, knee or hip) that could be made worse by a change in your physical activity?**
☐	☐	6.	**Is your doctor currently prescribing drugs (for example, water pills) for your blood pressure or heart condition?**
☐	☐	7.	**Do you know of any other reason why you should not do physical activity?**

If you answered

YES to one or more questions

Talk with your doctor by phone or in person BEFORE you start becoming much more physically active or BEFORE you have a fitness appraisal. Tell your doctor about the PAR-Q and which questions you answered YES.

- You may be able to do any activity you want — as long as you start slowly and build up gradually. Or, you may need to restrict your activities to those which are safe for you. Talk with your doctor about the kinds of activities you wish to participate in and follow his/her advice.
- Find out which community programs are safe and helpful for you.

NO to all questions

If you answered NO honestly to all PAR-Q questions, you can be reasonably sure that you can:

- start becoming much more physically active – begin slowly and build up gradually. This is the safest and easiest way to go.
- take part in a fitness appraisal – this is an excellent way to determine your basic fitness so that you can plan the best way for you to live actively. It is also highly recommended that you have your blood pressure evaluated. If your reading is over 144/94, talk with your doctor before you start becoming much more physically active.

DELAY BECOMING MUCH MORE ACTIVE:

- if you are not feeling well because of a temporary illness such as a cold or a fever – wait until you feel better; or
- if you are or may be pregnant – talk to your doctor before you start becoming more active.

PLEASE NOTE: If your health changes so that you then answer YES to any of the above questions, tell your fitness or health professional. Ask whether you should change your physical activity plan.

Informed Use of the PAR-Q: The Canadian Society for Exercise Physiology, Health Canada, and their agents assume no liability for persons who undertake physical activity, and if in doubt after completing this questionnaire, consult your doctor prior to physical activity.

No changes permitted. You are encouraged to photocopy the PAR-Q but only if you use the entire form.

NOTE: If the PAR-Q is being given to a person before he or she participates in a physical activity program or a fitness appraisal, this section may be used for legal or administrative purposes.

"I have read, understood and completed this questionnaire. Any questions I had were answered to my full satisfaction."

NAME ______________________

SIGNATURE ______________________ DATE ______________________

SIGNATURE OF PARENT ______________________ WITNESS ______________________
or GUARDIAN (for participants under the age of majority)

Note: This physical activity clearance is valid for a maximum of 12 months from the date it is completed and becomes invalid if your condition changes so that you would answer YES to any of the seven questions.

CSEP SCPE © Canadian Society for Exercise Physiology   Supported by: Health Canada Santé Canada

Figure 6-3
The Physical Activity Readiness Questionnaire

©2000 Used with permission from the Canadian Society for Exercise Physiology. www.csep.ca

and has undergone several revisions since its conception (ACSM, 2010). The basis for performing a risk stratification prior to engaging in a physical-activity program is to determine the following (ACSM, 2010):

- The presence or absence of known cardiovascular, pulmonary, and/or metabolic disease
- The presence or absence of cardiovascular risk factors
- The presence or absence of signs or symptoms suggestive of cardiovascular, pulmonary, and/or metabolic disease

Risk stratification is important because someone with only one positive risk factor will be treated differently than someone with several positive risk factors. Recommendations for physical activity/exercise, medical examinations or exercise testing, and medically supervised exercise are based on the number of associated risks; risk stratification is categorized as low, moderate, or high.

This process involves three basic steps that should be followed chronologically:

- Identifying **coronary artery disease (CAD)** risk factors
- Performing a risk stratification based on CAD risk factors
- Determining the need for a medical exam/clearance and medical supervision

The worksheet presented in Table 6-1 presents clinically relevant CAD health risks that should be used to identify the total number of positive risk factors an individual possesses. Each positive risk factor category equals one point. There is also a *negative* risk factor for a high level of **high-density lipoprotein (HDL),** as a point is subtracted if the individual has an HDL cholesterol score that is equal to, or exceeds, 60 mg/dL. It is the total number of risk factors and the presence or absence of signs or symptoms that ultimately categorizes an individual's CAD risk during exercise and/or physical activity (ACSM, 2010). The trainer should add up the total number of risk factors for a client, subtracting one point for higher HDL cholesterol if appropriate, and use this score to stratify the client's risk (Figure 6-4).

Signs or symptoms are also included in risk stratification, but given the need for specialized training to make a diagnosis, and respecting the **scope of practice** of personal trainers, these signs and symptoms must *only* be interpreted by a qualified licensed professional within the clinical context in which they appear. These signs and symptoms include the following (ACSM, 2010):

- Pain (tightness) or discomfort (or other **angina** equivalent) in the chest, neck, jaw, arms, or other areas that may result from **ischemia**
- Shortness of breath or difficulty breathing at rest or with mild exertion (**dyspnea**)
- **Orthopnea** (dyspnea in a reclined position) or paroxysmal nocturnal dyspnea (onset is usually two to five hours after the beginning of sleep)
- Ankle **edema**
- **Palpitations** or **tachycardia**
- Intermittent **claudication** (pain sensations or cramping in the lower extremities associated with inadequate blood supply)
- Known heart murmur
- Unusual fatigue or difficulty breathing with usual activities
- Dizziness or **syncope**, most commonly caused by reduced **perfusion** to the brain

Trainers should be familiar with each of these conditions and document them in a client's file if (1) the client has a history of any of these symptoms; or (2) develops these signs of symptoms while under the trainer's supervision. While personal trainers cannot diagnose signs or symptoms, it is helpful to know that:

- These symptoms are more likely to be apparent in individuals with a greater number of positive risk factors
- The stratification between low-, moderate-, and high-risk individuals only requires differentiation between zero, one, and two risk factors, and the medical diagnosis of diseases. The flow chart shown in Figure 6-4 is an easy reference tool for the personal trainer to use in determining an appropriate plan of care.

Table 6-1

Atherosclerotic Cardiovascular Disease Risk Factor Thresholds for Use With ACSM Risk Stratification

Positive Risk Factors	Defining Criteria	Points
Age	Men ≥45 years Women ≥55 years	+1
Family history	Myocardial infarction, coronary revascularization, or sudden death before 55 years of age in father or other first-degree male relative, or before 65 years of age in mother or other first-degree female relative	+1
Cigarette smoking	Current cigarette smoker or those who quit within the previous six months, or exposure to environmental tobacco smoke (i.e., secondhand smoke)	+1
Sedentary lifestyle	Not participating in at least 30 minutes of moderate-intensity physical activity (40–60% $\dot{V}O_2R$) on at least three days/week for at least three months	+1
Obesity*	Body mass index ≥30 kg/m^2 or waist girth >102 cm (40 inches) for men and >88 cm (35 inches) for women	+1
Hypertension	Systolic blood pressure ≥140 mmHg and/or diastolic blood pressure ≥90 mmHg, confirmed by measurements on at least two separate occasions or currently on antihypertensive medications	+1
Dyslipidemia	Low-density lipoprotein (LDL) cholesterol ≥130 mg/dL (3.37 mmol/L) or high-density lipoprotein (HDL) cholesterol <40 mg/dL (1.04 mmol/L) or currently on lipid-lowering medication; If total serum cholesterol is all that is available, use serum cholesterol >200 mg/dL (5.18 mmol/L)	+1
Prediabetes	Fasting plasma glucose ≥100 mg/dL (5.50 mmol/L), but <126 mg/dL (6.93 mmol/L) or impaired glucose tolerance (IGT) where a two-hour oral glucose tolerance test (OGTT) value is ≥140 mg/dL (7.70 mmol/L), but <200 mg/dL (11.00 mmol/L), confirmed by measurements on at least two separate occasions	+1
Negative Risk Factor	**Defining Criteria**	**Points**
High serum HDL cholesterol	≥60 mg/dL (1.55 mmol/L)	–1
	Total Score:	

*Professional opinions vary regarding the most appropriate markers and thresholds for obesity; therefore, allied health professionals should use clinical judgment when evaluating this risk factor.

Note: $\dot{V}O_2R = \dot{V}O_2reserve$

Note: It is common to sum risk factors in making clinical judgments. If HDL is high, subtract one risk factor from the sum of positive risk factors, because high HDL decreases cardiovascular disease risk.

American College of Sports Medicine (2010). *ACSM's Guidelines for Exercise Testing and Prescription* (8th ed.). Philadelphia: Wolters Kluwer/Lippincott Williams & Wilkins.

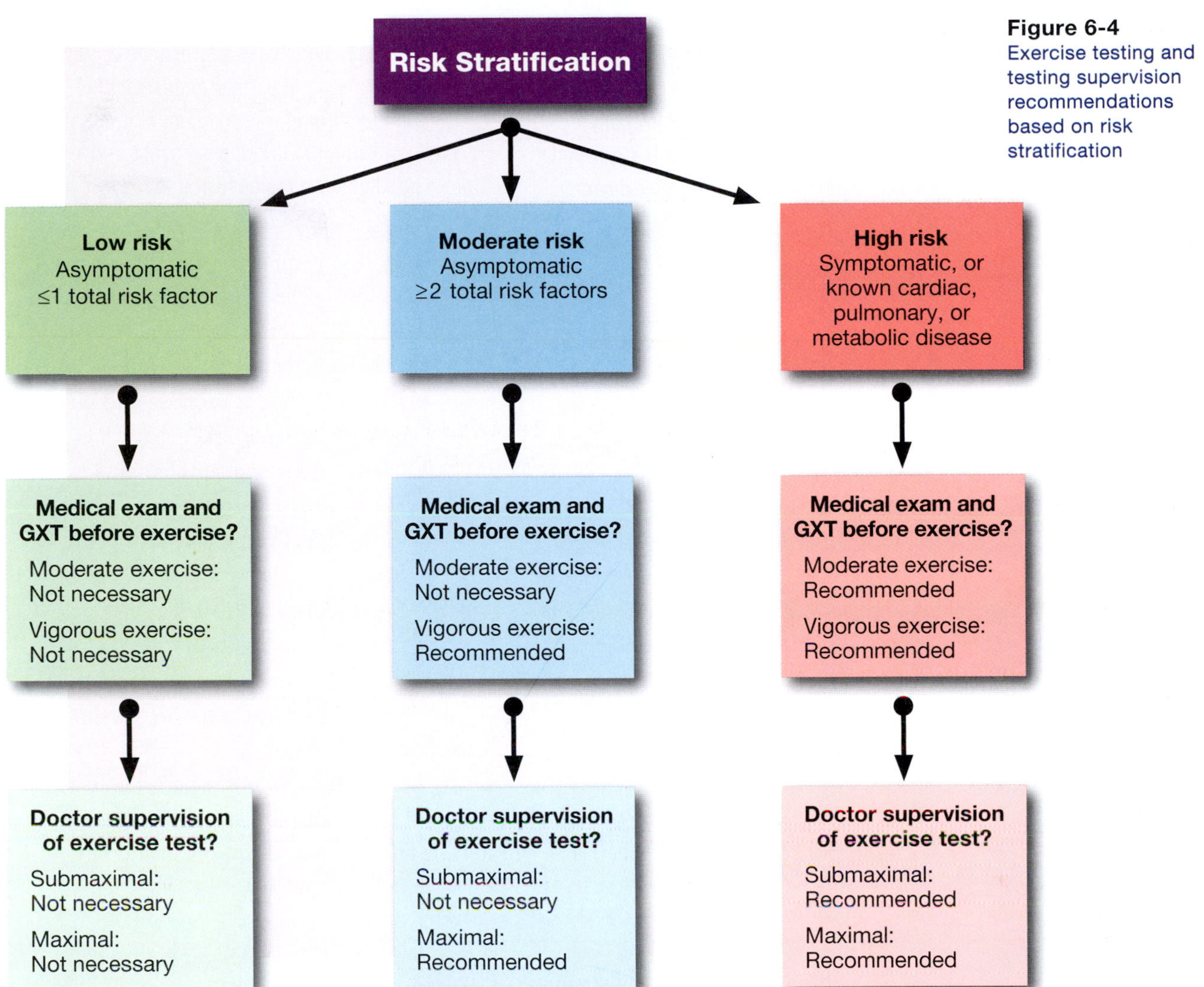

Figure 6-4
Exercise testing and testing supervision recommendations based on risk stratification

Moderate exercise:*	Moderate intensity equivalent to 40–60% $\dot{V}O_2$max, 3–6 METs, or an intensity well within an individual's capacity that can be comfortably sustained for ~45 minutes
Vigorous exercise:†	Vigorous intensity equivalent to >60% $\dot{V}O_2$max, >6 METs, or a level of intensity sufficient enough to represent a substantial cardiorespiratory challenge
Not necessary:	Reflects the notion that a medical examination, exercise test, and physician supervision of testing would not be essential in the pre-participation screening. However, this does not mean that it cannot be considered.
Recommended:	Reflects the notion that a medical examination is strongly encouraged. Exercise testing with physician supervision indicates that a physician should be in close proximity and readily available should there be a need.

*<VT1 (zone 1) in ACE IFT™ Model

†≥VT1 (zones 2 and 3) in ACE IFT Model

Note: GXT = Graded exercise test; METs = Metabolic equivalents; Cardiovascular disease = Cardiac, peripheral artery, or cerebrovascular disease; Pulmonary disease = Chronic obstructive pulmonary disease (COPD), cystic fibrosis, interstitial lung disease, or asthma; Metabolic disease = Diabetes mellitus (type 1 or 2), thyroid disorders, and renal or liver disease

American College of Sports Medicine (2010). *ACSM's Guidelines for Exercise Testing and Prescription* (8th ed.). Philadelphia: Wolters Kluwer/Lippincott Williams & Wilkins.

> It is imperative that the client's personal physician be made aware of any signs or symptoms suggestive of CAD that may have been discovered as a result of this pre-screening session or during an ongoing exercise program.

> It is recommended that personal trainers consult a legal professional familiar with local and regional laws prior to utilizing the informed consent and agreement and release of liability forms.

Evaluation Forms

Once the client's risk for exercise has been assessed, the need for outside referral has been determined (yes or no), and the client is clear for exercise, an appropriate health and fitness plan can then be developed. Beyond the initial PAR-Q or CAD health-risk assessment, there are several important forms that personal trainers should review, keep accessible, and utilize as needed with their clients. These forms include the following:

Informed consent, or "assumption of risk," form (see Figure 17-3, page 608)

- When a client signs an informed consent form, he or she is acknowledging having been specifically informed about the risks associated with activity.
- This form is also used prior to assessments and provides evidence of disclosure of the purposes, procedures, risks, and benefits associated with the assessments.
- Limitations:
  - ✓Not a liability waiver, and therefore does not provide legal immunity
  - ✓Intended to communicate the dangers of the exercise program or test procedures; it is recommended that the trainer also *verbally* review the content to promote understanding.

Agreement and release of liability waiver (see Figure 17-1, page 603)

- This document is used to release a personal trainer from **liability** for injuries resulting from a supervised exercise program.
- It represents a client's voluntary abandonment of the right to file suit.
- Limitations include the fact that it does not necessarily protect the personal trainer from being sued for **negligence.**

Health-history questionnaire (Figure 6-5)

- This form collects more detailed medical and health information beyond the CAD risk-factor screen, including the following:
  - ✓Past and present exercise and physical-activity information
  - ✓Medications and supplements
  - ✓Recent or current illnesses or injuries, including **chronic** or **acute** pain
  - ✓Surgery and injury history
  - ✓Family medical history
  - ✓Lifestyle information (related to nutrition, stress, work, sleep, etc.)

Exercise history and attitude questionnaire (Figure 6-6)

- This form provides the personal trainer with a detailed background of the client's previous exercise history, including behavioral and adherence experience.
- This information is important when developing goals, designing programs incorporating the client's preferences and attitudes toward exercise, and implementing strategies for improving motivation and adherence.

Medical release (Figure 6-7)

- This form provides the personal trainer with the client's medical information, and explains physical-activity limitations and/or guidelines as outlined by his or her physician. *Deviation from these guidelines must be approved by the personal physician.*

Testing forms (see Chapters 7 and 8)

- These forms are used for recording testing and measurement data during the fitness assessment.
- Testing instructions and normative tables are used to determine client rankings for each fitness test. These forms can be assembled in a notebook or be accessible via a computer, PDA, or website.

Case Study Example

Joe is a 49-year-old male who stands 5'11" (1.8 m) and weighs 240 pounds (109 kg). He currently smokes one pack of cigarettes a day and indicates no history of regular physical activity over the past 10 years. He also has a **sedentary** occupation and travels frequently for work. His latest physical examination revealed the following information:

- **Blood pressure** (repeated twice): 136/88 mmHg
- Total **cholesterol:** 208 mg/dL; HDL cholesterol: 41 mg/dL; **low-density lipoprotein (LDL)** cholesterol: 134 mg/dL
- No medications
- Fasting blood glucose (last medical exam): 98 mg/dL
- Family history:
  Father diagnosed with CAD at age 62
  Mother diagnosed with **type 2 diabetes** at age 50

Questions:

- What are his positive risk factors for heart disease?
- What is his risk stratification according to the ACSM's guidelines?
- What testing and programming guidelines should a personal trainer follow prior to working with Joe?

Positive Risk Factor	Defining Criteria/Comments		Score
Age	49	≥45-year-old threshold for men	1
Family history	Male	None (father diagnosed with CAD at age 62)	0
	Female	None	0
Cigarette smoking	Current	1 pack a day	1
	Quit in past 6 months		0
Physical activity	Sedentary		1
Hypertension	SBP	136 mmHg	0
	DBP	88 mmHg	0
	Medications	None reported	N/A
Dyslipidemia	Cholesterol	Do not use, as LDL and HDL scores are available	
	HDL	41 mg/dL	0
	LDL	134 mg/dL	1
	Medications	None reported	N/A
Impaired fasting glucose	Blood glucose	98 mg/dL	0
Obesity	BMI	33.6	1
	Circumference	No measurement at this time	N/A
	Body fat	No measurement at this time	N/A
Negative Risk Factor	**Comments**		**Score**
HDL	Score <60 mg/dL		0
		Total Score:	5

Note: CAD = Coronary artery disease; SBP = Systolic blood pressure; DBP = Diastolic blood pressure; LDL = Low-density lipoprotein; HDL = High-density lipoprotein; BMI = Body mass index

- *What are his positive risk factors for CAD?* Age, current smoker, high LDL, high BMI, and sedentary lifestyle
- *What is his risk stratification according to the ACSM's guidelines?* Moderate, as he has no known diagnosis, although he has five positive risk factors
- *What testing and programming guidelines should a personal trainer follow prior to working with Joe?* Theoretically, he could participate in moderate-intensity activity and submaximal testing without a medical exam. However, given his number of risk factors, Joe should consider getting a medical exam before starting an exercise program.

Sample Health-History Form

Name ______________________________ Date______________

Age__________ Sex ☐ M ☐ F

Physician's Name ______________________________

Physician's Phone (________) ______________________

Person to contact in case of emergency:

Name ______________________________ Phone ______________

Are you taking any medications, supplements, or drugs? If so, please list medication, dose, and reason.

____

____

____

Does your physician know you are participating in this exercise program?

____

Describe any physical activity you do somewhat regularly.

____

____

Do you now, or have you had in the past:	Yes	No
1. History of heart problems, chest pain, or stroke	☐	☐
2. Elevated blood pressure	☐	☐
3. Any chronic illness or condition	☐	☐
4. Difficulty with physical exercise	☐	☐
5. Advice from physician not to exercise	☐	☐
6. Recent surgery (last 12 months)	☐	☐
7. Pregnancy (now or within last 3 months)	☐	☐
8. History of breathing or lung problems	☐	☐
9. Muscle, joint, or back disorder, or any previous injury still affecting you	☐	☐
10. Diabetes or thyroid condition	☐	☐
11. Cigarette smoking habit	☐	☐
12. Obesity (BMI $\geq$30 kg/m^2)	☐	☐
13. Elevated blood cholesterol	☐	☐
14. History of heart problems in immediate family	☐	☐
15. Hernia, or any condition that may be aggravated by lifting weights or other physical activity	☐	☐

Figure 6-5
Sample health-history form

Exercise History and Attitude Questionnaire

Name ______________________________ Date ______________

General Instructions: Please fill out this form as completely as possible. If you have any questions, DO NOT GUESS; ask your trainer for assistance.

1. Please rate your exercise level on a scale of 1 to 5 (5 indicating very strenuous) for each age range through your present age:
   15–20 _____ 21–30 _____ 31–40 _____ 41–50 _____ 51+_____

2. Were you a high school and/or college athlete?
   ☐ Yes ☐ No If yes, please specify ______________________________

3. Do you have any negative feelings toward, or have you had any bad experience with, physical-activity programs?
   ☐ Yes ☐ No If yes, please explain ______________________________

4. Do you have any negative feelings toward, or have you had any bad experience with, fitness testing and evaluation?
   ☐ Yes ☐ No If yes, please explain ______________________________

5. Rate yourself on a scale of 1 to 5 (1 indicating the lowest value and 5 the highest). Circle the number that best applies.

   Characterize your present athletic ability.
   1 2 3 4 5

   When you exercise, how important is competition?
   1 2 3 4 5

   Characterize your present cardiovascular capacity.
   1 2 3 4 5

   Characterize your present muscular capacity.
   1 2 3 4 5

   Characterize your present flexibility capacity.
   1 2 3 4 5

6. Do you start exercise programs but then find yourself unable to stick with them?
   ☐ Yes ☐ No

7. How much time are you willing to devote to an exercise program?
   ________ minutes/day ________ days/week

8. Are you currently involved in regular endurance (cardiovascular) exercise?
   ☐ Yes ☐ No If yes, specify the type of exercise(s) ____________________
   ________ minutes/day ________ days/week

   Rate your perception of the exertion of your exercise program (circle the number):
   (1) Light (2) Fairly light (3) Somewhat hard (4) Hard

Figure 6-6 Sample exercise history and attitude questionnaire

Figure 6-6
continued

9. How long have you been exercising regularly?
   ________ months ________ years

10. What other exercise, sport, or recreational activities have you participated in?
    In the past 6 months? ________________________
    In the past 5 years? ________________________

11. Can you exercise during your work day?
    ☐ Yes ☐ No

12. Would an exercise program interfere with your job?
    ☐ Yes ☐ No

13. Would an exercise program benefit your job?
    ☐ Yes ☐ No

14. What types of exercise interest you?

☐ Walking	☐ Jogging	☐ Strength training
☐ Cycling	☐ Traditional aerobics	☐ Racquet sports
☐ Stationary biking	☐ Elliptical striding	☐ Yoga/Pilates
☐ Stair climbing	☐ Swimming	☐ Other activities

15. Rank your goals in undertaking exercise:
    What do you want exercise to do for you? ________________________
    ____
    ____

    Use the following scale to rate each goal separately:

Not at all important				Somewhat important					Extremely important
1	2	3	4	5	6	7	8	9	10

    a. Improve cardiovascular fitness _____
    b. Lose weight/body fat _____
    c. Reshape or tone my body _____
    d. Improve performance for a specific sport _____
    e. Improve moods and ability to cope with stress _____
    f. Improve flexibility _____
    g. Increase strength _____
    h. Increase energy level _____
    i. Feel better _____
    j. Enjoyment _____
    k. Social interaction _____
    l. Other _____

16. By how much would you like to change your current weight?
    (+) ________ lbs (-) ________ lbs

Sample Medical Release Form

Date ____________________

Dear Doctor:

Your patient, ____, wishes to start a personalized training program. The activity will involve the following:

(type, frequency, duration, and intensity of activities)

If your patient is taking medications that will affect his or her exercise capacity or heart-rate response to exercise, please indicate the manner of the effect (raises, lowers, or has no effect on exercise capacity or heart-rate response):

Type of medication(s) ____

Effect(s) ____

Please identify any recommendations or restrictions that are appropriate for your patient in this exercise program:

____

____

____

Thank you.
Sincerely,

Fred Fitness
Personalized Gym
Address
Phone

____ has my approval to begin an exercise program with the recommendations or restrictions stated above.

Signed____ Date__________ Phone____________________

Figure 6-7
Sample medical release form

Health Conditions That Affect Physical Activity

The benefits of regular physical activity are well established, but there also are risks inherent in physical activity. Identifying these risks is the first step in preventing them. Regular physical activity increases the risk of both musculoskeletal injury and cardiovascular problems, such as cardiac arrest. While clients need to be informed of these risks (see Chapter 17 for more information on informed consent), they also should know that the overall absolute risk in the general population is low, especially when weighed against the health benefits of regular exercise (ACSM, 2010). Injuries related to physical activity usually come from:

- Aggravating an existing condition (either known or unknown by the client), or
- Precipitating a new condition

The primary systems of the body that experience stress during physical activity are the cardiovascular, respiratory, and musculoskeletal systems. Certain metabolic and other medical conditions also will be affected by regular physical activity. A complete health history provides the trainer with essential information in these areas that will ensure that each client gets the most benefit from an exercise program with the lowest degree of risk. The following material covers health conditions that may affect a client's benefit-to-risk ratio and should be considered when developing a physical-activity program.

Cardiovascular

Atherosclerosis is a process in which fatty deposits of cholesterol and calcium accumulate on the walls of the arteries, causing them to harden, thicken, and lose elasticity. When this process affects the arteries that supply the heart, it is called CAD. As with other muscles, the heart contracts during exercise. The increased contraction of the heart muscle requires an increased supply of oxygen-rich blood that provides necessary nutrients. The greater the exercise intensity, the larger the demand for blood and oxygen to the heart muscle. If the vessels that supply this blood to the heart are narrowed from atherosclerosis, the blood supply is limited, and the increased oxygen demand by the heart cannot be met. This can result in angina and possibly a **myocardial infarction,** or heart attack.

Angina is usually described as a pressure or tightness in the chest, but can also be experienced in the arm, shoulder, or jaw. This pain may be accompanied by shortness of breath, sweating, nausea, and palpitations (pounding or racing of the heart). Although regular exercise may be an important part of the treatment and rehabilitation for CAD, limitations may be necessary.

Anyone with a history of CAD or chest pain should have a physician's release, along with a description of any specific limitations, before beginning an exercise program.

Risk Factors

Unfortunately, many people with CAD have no known symptoms and are unaware of their potential risk for a heart attack. Long-term studies have helped researchers identify several factors that correlate with an increased risk for CAD (see Table 6-1).

Hypertension

Hypertension, or high blood pressure, is more prevalent among the elderly and African-American individuals, but is becoming more common in the general population. An individual's risk of CAD, **stroke,** and kidney disease increases progressively with higher levels of **systolic blood pressure (SBP)** and **diastolic blood pressure (DBP)** (Chobanian et al., 2003). This is important information for personal trainers because blood pressure increases with exercise, especially in activities involving heavy resistance, such as weight lifting, or isometric exercises. If a person's resting blood pressure is already high, it may elevate to dangerous levels during exercise, increasing the likelihood of a stroke.

Respiratory

The lungs (major component of the respiratory system) extract oxygen from inhaled air and deliver it to the body's tissues via the cardiovascular system. Oxygen is essential to all body tissues for survival. A problem in the respiratory system will interfere with the body's ability to provide enough oxygen for the increasing demand that occurs during aerobic exercise. Bronchitis, asthma, and **chronic obstructive pulmonary disease (COPD)** are some of the more common respiratory problems. Each of these conditions may result in dyspnea (difficult or labored breathing), making exercise difficult. Regular exercise may aggravate the condition for some people, and may improve it for others. Anyone with a disorder of the respiratory system should have a physician's clearance and recommendations before beginning or continuing an exercise program. More information on respiratory conditions and programming concerns can be found in Chapter 14.

Musculoskeletal

The musculoskeletal system consists of the muscles, bones, **tendons,** and **ligaments** that support and move the body. This is the system most commonly injured during exercise. Aside from the pain and discouragement of an injury, there are other factors to contend with. Client motivation and the trainer's scope of practice create concerns when working with a client with previous or current musculoskeletal injuries. Changes or modifications in the exercise program are necessary to accommodate the injury. For these reasons, it is important to be cognizant of potentially hazardous situations before they occur. Most minor **sprains** and **strains** are easily managed, but a persistent problem or a more serious injury requires physician referral for appropriate treatment.

The health screening evaluation is crucial to identifying both old injuries and risk factors for potential new injuries. Asking the client about current conditions, previous injuries, and pain that comes and goes is critical in detecting potential problems. The most common type of injury sustained by persons participating in physical activity is the **overuse injury.** These injuries are usually the result of poor training techniques, poor body mechanics, or both. Examples of overuse injuries include runner's knee, swimmer's shoulder, tennis elbow **(lateral epicondylitis), shin splints** (pain in the anterior lower leg), and **iliotibial band syndrome (ITBS)** (pain along the outside of the thigh and knee). To avoid aggravating an existing injury, and to allow for healing to occur, trainers should modify the client's exercise program using a **cross-training** strategy (see Chapter 15).

Other common conditions to screen for in the health-history interview are sprains (ligament) or strains (muscle or its tendon), **herniated discs, bursitis, tendinitis,** and **arthritis.** Information on arthritis and low-back disorders can be found in Chapter 14. These conditions must be recognized before implementing an exercise program to avoid worsening the condition. Guidelines for recognizing and preventing injuries can be found in Chapter 15. Any musculoskeletal disorder that a trainer is not qualified to deal with should be referred to an appropriate healthcare professional, and a client with an injury more severe than a simple sprain or strain must have a physician's approval before beginning an exercise program. If significant muscle weakness or joint laxity exists, medical referral is recommended, and appropriate accommodations to the program are necessary.

A client who has recently undergone orthopedic surgery may not be ready for a standard exercise program. Depending on the type of surgery performed, it may take up to one year (in the case of knee reconstruction, for example) for the tissues to heal completely. Also, disuse **atrophy** of the muscles surrounding an injury may begin after just two days of inactivity. Properly rehabilitating the weakened area requires knowledge of the type of surgery as well as the indicated rehabilitation program. This information can be obtained from the client's surgeon and physical therapist. Beginning an exercise program before complete rehabilitation may lead to biomechanical imbalances that could predispose the client to other injuries. Communication with the physician is paramount, particularly for clients who have had surgery within the last year.

Metabolic

There are many metabolic diseases that may interfere with metabolism, or the utilization of energy. Two of the more common types are **diabetes** and thyroid disorders. A client with either condition requires physician approval before initiating an exercise program. Exercise, both as a means to regulate blood glucose and to facilitate fat loss, is an important component of the lifestyle of an individual with diabetes. Clients with diabetes should discuss their situations and exercise programs with their physicians before working with a personal trainer. Physician referral is especially important if a client is receiving **insulin.** Diabetes types and exercise programming concerns are discussed further in Chapter 14.

The thyroid is a small gland in the neck that secretes hormones (thyroxine and triiodothyronine) that increase oxygen consumption and heat production and affect many metabolic functions. Hyperthyroid individuals have an increased level of these hormones and a higher metabolic rate, while individuals suffering from hypothyroidism have a reduced level of these hormones and require thyroid medication to regulate their metabolism to normal levels. Because physical-activity status also influences the metabolism, it is important for trainers to know if a client suffers from thyroid disease.

Other Conditions

Hernia

Another condition that needs consideration, especially when incorporating weight lifting into a program, is a history of an inguinal or abdominal **hernia.** This is a protrusion of the abdominal contents into the groin or through the abdominal wall, respectively. Pain is usually present, but may not be in some cases. During an activity involving increased abdominal pressure, such as the **Valsalva maneuver,** the hernia may be further aggravated. A hernia is a **relative contraindication** for weight lifting unless cleared by a physician. If there is a history of a hernia, it is very important for the trainer to instruct and educate the client on proper breathing and lifting techniques.

Pregnancy

Optimum fitness levels during pregnancy are beneficial to the health of both the mother and the unborn infant. This is not a good time to pursue maximum fitness goals, but rather to focus on maintaining a good fitness level. A client should have a physician's approval for exercise during pregnancy and until three months after delivery. Please refer to Chapter 14 for more information on modifying an exercise program during pregnancy.

Illness or Infection

A recent history of illness or infection may impair a client's ability to exercise. Moderate exercise may be acceptable during a mild illness such as a cold. A more serious condition, however, requires more of the body's energy reserves, and exercise would be contraindicated until the client improves. The human body has a given amount of available energy that must be balanced between its physiological requirements, which include fighting infections, and the energy used during exercise. This balance varies from person to person, but it is generally not advisable to start a new exercise program during an illness. To distinguish between a minor and a major illness, the trainer may need to consult with the client's physician.

Medications

Medication or drug use is another important topic to cover when taking a health history. These substances alter the biochemistry of the body and may affect a client's ability to perform or respond to exercise. The properties of these drugs must be understood by the trainer and discussed with the client. When designing and supervising an exercise program, it is important to realize that many over-the-counter medications and prescription or illicit drugs affect the heart's response to exercise. There are hundreds of thousands of different drugs on the market and each may be referred to by the manufacturer's brand name (e.g., Inderal®) or by the scientific generic name (e.g., propranolol). Table 6-2 lists many medication categories that may affect a person's response to exercise. To use the table, consult the client, the client's physician, or a medical reference to find the correct category for the medication. Then refer to the general category under which each drug is grouped, such as **beta blockers,** antihistamines, or **bronchodilators.** The drugs in each group are thought to have a similar effect on most people, although individual responses will vary.

A particular response is usually dose dependent; the larger the dose, the greater the response. An important factor to consider in this dose-related response is the time when the medication is taken. As medications are metabolized, their effects diminish. If a trainer has any questions concerning a client's medications, it is essential that the trainer discuss them with the client and his or her physician.

Any client taking a prescription medication that could potentially have an effect on exercise should have a physician's clearance for physical activity. The following are some of the most common categories of medications of which personal trainers should be aware.

Antihypertensives

High blood pressure, or hypertension, is common in modern society, and there are many medications used for its treatment. Most antihypertensives primarily affect one of four different sites: the heart, to reduce its force of contraction; the peripheral blood vessels, to open or dilate them to allow more room for the blood; the brain, to reduce the sympathetic nerve outflow; or the kidneys, to deplete body water and decrease blood volume. The site that the medication acts on helps to determine its effect on the individual as well as any potential side effects. The following are common antihypertensives.

Beta Blockers

Beta-adrenergic blocking agents, or beta blockers, are commonly prescribed for a variety of cardiovascular and other disorders. These medications block beta-adrenergic receptors and limit **sympathetic nervous system** stimulation. In other words, they block the effects of **catecholamines** (**epinephrine** and **norepinephrine**) throughout the body, and reduce resting, exercise, and maximal heart rates. This reduction in heart rate requires modifying the method used for determining exercise intensity. Using RPE, for example, would be appropriate for a safe and effective aerobic exercise program for someone on beta blockers.

Calcium Channel Blockers

Calcium channel blockers prevent calcium-dependent contraction of the smooth muscles in the arteries, causing them to dilate, which lowers blood pressure. These agents also are used for angina and heart dysrhythmias (rapid or irregular heart rate). There are several types of calcium channel blockers on the market, and their effect on blood pressure and heart rate depends on the specific agent. Notice in Table 6-2 that calcium channel-blocking drugs may increase, decrease, or have no effect on the heart rate. Therefore, while it is important to know the general effects of a category of medication, remember that individual responses can vary.

Angiotensin-converting Enzyme (ACE) Inhibitors

ACE inhibitors block an enzyme secreted by the kidneys, preventing the formation of a potent hormone that constricts blood vessels. If this enzyme is blocked, the vessels dilate, and blood pressure decreases. ACE inhibitors should not have an effect on heart rate, but will cause a decrease in blood pressure at rest and during exercise.

Angiotensin-II Receptor Antagonists

Angiotensin-II receptor antagonists (or blockers) are a newer class of antihypertensive agents. These drugs are selective for angiotensin II (type 1 receptor). Angiotensin-II receptor antagonists are well tolerated, and do not adversely affect blood lipid profiles or cause "rebound hypertension" after discontinuation. Clinical trials indicate that angiotensin-II receptor antagonists are effective and safe in the treatment of hypertension.

Table 6-2
Effects of Medication on Heart-rate (HR) Response

Medications	Resting HR	Exercising HR	Maximal Exercising HR	Comments
Beta-adrenergic blocking agents	↓	↓	↓	Dose-related response
Diuretics	←→	←→	←→	
Other antihypertensives	↑, ←→, or ↓	↑, ←→, or ↓	Usually ←→	Many antihypertensive medications are used. Some may decrease, a few may increase, and others do not affect heart rates. Some exhibit dose-related response
Calcium channel blockers	↑, ←→, or ↓	↑, ←→, or ↓	Usually ←→	Variable and dose-related responses
Antihistamines	←→	←→	←→	
Cold medications:				
without sympathomimetic activity (SA)	←→	←→	←→	
with SA	←→ or ↑	←→ or ↑	←→	
Tranquilizers	←→, or if anxiety reducing may ↓	←→	←→	
Antidepressants and some antipsychotic medications	←→ or ↑	←→	←→	
Alcohol	←→ or ↑	←→ or ↑	←→	Exercise prohibited while under the influence; effects of alcohol on coordination increase possibility of injuries
Diet Pills:				Discourage as a poor approach to weight loss; acceptable only with physician's written approval
with SA	↑ or ←→	↑ or ←→	←→	
containing amphetamines	↑	↑	←→	
without SA or amphetamine	←→	←→	←→	
Caffeine	←→ or ↑	←→ or ↑	←→	
Nicotine	←→ or ↑	←→ or ↑	←→	Discourage smoking; suggest lower target heart rate and exercise intensity for smokers

↑ = increase ←→ = no significant change ↓ = decrease

Note: Many medications are prescribed for conditions that do not require clearance. Do not forget other indicators of exercise intensity (e.g., client's appearance, ratings of perceived exertion).

Diuretics

Diuretics are medications that increase the excretion of water and **electrolytes** through the kidneys. They are usually prescribed for high blood pressure, or when a person is accumulating too much fluid, as occurs with congestive heart failure. They have no primary effect on the heart rate, but they can cause water and electrolyte imbalances, which may lead to dangerous cardiac **arrhythmias.** Since diuretics can decrease blood volume, they may predispose an exerciser to **dehydration.** A client taking diuretics needs to maintain adequate fluid intake before, during, and after exercise, especially in a warm, humid environment. Diuretics are sometimes used by athletes to try to lose weight for sport. This is a dangerous practice that should not be condoned by a responsible trainer.

Bronchodilators

Asthma medications, also known as bronchodilators, relax or open the air passages in the lungs, allowing better air exchange. There are many different types, but the primary action of each is to stimulate the sympathetic nervous system. Bronchodilators increase exercise capacity in persons limited by bronchospasm.

Cold Medications

Decongestants act directly on the smooth muscles of the blood vessels to stimulate **vasoconstriction.** In the upper airways, this constriction reduces the volume of the swollen tissues and results in more air space. Vasoconstriction in the peripheral vessels may raise blood pressure and increase heart rate both at rest and possibly during exercise.

Antihistamines block the histamine receptor, which is involved with the mast cells and the allergic response. These medications do not have a direct effect on the heart rate or blood pressure, but they do produce a drying effect in the upper airways and may cause drowsiness.

Most cold medications are a combination of decongestants and antihistamines and may have combined effects. However, they are normally taken in low doses and have minimal effect on exercise.

Sequencing Assessments

It has been standard practice to conduct physiological assessments at the beginning of a personal trainer's professional relationship with a client. Traditionally, these baseline assessments are conducted in an effort to do the following:

- Identify areas of health/injury risk for potential referral to the appropriate health professional(s)
- Collect baseline data that can be used to develop a personalized fitness program and allow for comparison of subsequent evaluations
- Educate a client about his or her present physical condition and health risks by comparing his or her results to normative data for age and gender
- Motivate a client by helping him or her establish realistic goals

There is much debate over the timing and specific testing modalities that are chosen during an initial assessment. The justification behind conducting assessments in this initial session is based on the long-standing notion that some, if not all, assessments need to be conducted at the beginning of the client–trainer relationship to collect baseline information from which personalized programming can be developed. Trainers need to be aware that not all clients need or desire a *complete* fitness assessment from the start. In fact, assessments may demotivate some individuals, as they may feel uncomfortable, intimidated, overwhelmed, or embarrassed by their current physical condition, their inadequacies in performing the test protocols, or even by the fear of the results. Proper test selection can minimize these aspects. Chapters 7 and 8 detail a variety of physiological tests that can be performed, as well as the likely populations that would benefit from such testing. Regardless of the assessments selected and how the assessment timelines are structured, trainers should remember that a health-risk appraisal *must* be included as a preparticipation screen.

Savvy trainers must have a good understanding of the client's needs, determine the appropriate testing battery, and then create a suitable timeline. It is important to understand each client's needs and goals, and be empathic when evaluating the relevance and timing of assessments.

The physiological assessments that merit consideration generally include the following:

- Resting vital signs (**heart rate,** blood pressure, height, weight)
- Static posture and movement screens
- Joint flexibility and muscle length
- Balance and core function
- Cardiorespiratory fitness
- **Body composition**
- Muscular endurance and strength
- Skill-related parameters (agility, coordination, power, reactivity, and speed)

Refer to Figure 5-2 on page 85 for a suggested template that trainers can follow when sequencing assessments relevant to clients' needs and desires. However, only after a trainer has identified a client's personality style (during rapport-building), readiness to change behavior, and stage of behavioral change, should he or she perform assessments (refer to Chapters 3 and 4).

The balance of this chapter covers tools and protocols for measuring heart rate and blood pressure. There is also a discussion on **ratings of perceived exertion (RPE)** and the exercise-induced feeling inventory. Chapter 7 presents protocols for assessing static posture, basic movement screens, joint flexibility (muscle length), balance, and core function, while Chapter 8 covers physiological assessment protocols.

Physiological influences on an assessment must be considered when establishing the testing sequence and timeline for a client. For example, resting BP and HR should be measured before any exertion to avoid falsely elevated scores; skinfold measures for body composition should be taken before activity to avoid either underestimation of fat stores from dehydration, or overestimation of fat stores due to **vasodilation** in surface vessels associated with **thermoregulation**; cardiovascular testing following resistance exercise may elevate HR responses and invalidate the results (ACSM, 2010; Wilmore, Costill, & Kenney, 2008). Additionally, testing for muscular strength and endurance is not suggested for many novice clients within the first few weeks, given the initial neurological adaptations and motor-skill changes that occur during the first one to four weeks of a resistance-training program.

It is important to note that the physiological demands of exercise can uncover underlying disease or dysfunction that may not be revealed while a person is sedentary. During the administration of any exercise test involving exertion (e.g., a cardiorespiratory fitness test), trainers must always be aware of signs or symptoms they can identify that merit immediate test termination and referral to a more qualified healthcare professional. These symptoms include:

- Onset of **angina pectoris** or angina-like symptoms that center around the chest
- Significant drop (>10 mmHg) in SBP despite an increase in exercise intensity
- Excessive rise in blood pressure: SBP >250 mmHg or DBP >115 mmHg
- Fatigue, shortness of breath, difficult or labored breathing, or wheezing (does not include heavy breathing due to intense exercise)
- Signs of poor perfusion: lightheadedness, pallor (pale skin), **cyanosis**, nausea, or cold and clammy skin
- Increased nervous system symptoms (e.g., **ataxia,** dizziness, confusion, syncope)
- Leg cramping or claudication
- Physical or verbal manifestations of severe fatigue

The test should also be terminated if the client requests to stop or the testing equipment fails.

Professionalism as a personal trainer includes management of the testing environment and gaining the proper experience. Trainers must embody the highest level of professionalism by being fully prepared when conducting assessments and integrating the following (ACSM, 2010):

- Distribution of instructions in advance of testing that clearly outline the client's responsibilities (e.g., clothing, eating, and hydration recommendations, abstaining from certain products like stimulants)
- Obtaining a signed informed consent from the client, a document required from both ethical and legal standpoints. This document must ensure that the client knows and understands the purposes and risks associated with testing and exercise. The trainer must allow the client the opportunity to ask questions pertaining to the protocol(s) and grant him or her the right to test participation, inclusion, and termination.
- Organization of all necessary documentation forms, data sheets, assessment tables, etc.
- Communication and demonstration skills, clearly explaining the tests, sequence, and instructions in a calm, confident manner
- Calibration and working condition of all exercise equipment
- Environmental control, ensuring room temperature is ideally between 68 and 72° F (20 to 22° C) with a relative humidity below 60%. Additionally, the testing environment should be quiet and private to reduce test anxiety.

Choosing the Right Assessments

Goals of the Assessment

One of the primary factors to consider when choosing the appropriate assessments is the goals of each client. This entails conducting a thorough assessment to identify evaluation tools that are consistent with his or her needs, desires, and goals. For example, when conducting the needs assessment with a client interested in performance-related training, personal trainers should answer the following relevant questions:

- What are the needed performance-related skills and abilities to be successful in the client's chosen activity (recreational or otherwise)?
  - ✓To make this determination, trainers can talk to coaches and watch top-level athletes in the sport to identify what skills and fitness levels are needed.
- Which of these needed skills and abilities are currently lacking in this client?
  - ✓Which specific skills and fitness levels currently need improvement?
- What are the prevalent injuries and weaknesses associated with the activity in which the client wants to participate? For example, lateral ankle sprains are common in soccer, and if the client has high arches or supinated ankles, he or she might be more prone to this injury.
  - ✓Talk to medical staff working with participants in the activity to learn more about common injuries and how to condition the body to prevent these injuries.
- Which energy systems are required to be successful in this activity?
- Which integrated movement patterns and planes of movement will need to be trained to be successful in this activity?

Clearly, the fitness goals of a high school athlete trying to enhance his or her sports performance will be considerably different from those of a new mother who is trying to drop her "baby weight." Since the fitness and training goals are different, the components of the testing battery should be unique to each individual.

Physical Limitations of the Participant

It is important for a trainer to choose tests that will provide valid results without causing undue stress on the client. For example, if a client complains of chronic knee inflammation due to arthritis, a weightbearing walking test may prove to be painful and the results will likely be tainted because the effort was limited by pain, not by **cardiorespiratory endurance.**

Testing Environment

Environmental conditions such as extreme heat or cold, uneven surfaces, or a crowded track can limit a client's performance on a cardiorespiratory endurance test. Privacy issues and distractions can also have a negative impact on testing outcomes. Trainers should be aware of the following considerations for testing:

- Proper calibration and routine maintenance (documented) of all equipment
- The ability of equipment to accommodate a range of exercise intensities and the client's specific needs
- Adequately illuminated areas for testing
- Proper emergency response protocol and access to emergency supplies
- Appropriate temperature range between 68 and 72° F (20 to 22° C)

Trainers should also avoid outdoor testing on excessively hot and humid days.

Availability of Equipment

Some personal trainers will have access to state-of-the art computerized testing equipment, while others may be limited by what they can carry in their vehicles. In either case, it is important to choose the best test with whatever equipment is available. Laboratory testing requires an investment in precision equipment, but there are a variety of valid and reliable field tests that can also be useful to the personal trainer.

Age of the Participant

Aging can carry with it certain health risks. In most cases, an older, deconditioned client will not perform the same battery of tests as a younger client. A thorough screening will ensure that important health risks are uncovered prior to risking injury or the client's health status. For example, a maximal strength test is not appropriate to use with a senior exerciser with **hypertension.**

Tools to Get Started

In some cases, a fitness facility provides the personal trainer with access to a variety of fitness-assessment instruments and equipment. Other times, the trainer is working for him- or herself and must have a portable system for providing a comprehensive battery of fitness assessments. Table 6-3 lists common assessment tools, as well as an approximate cost for each.

There are a number of computer and PDA software programs available to aid in calculations, documentation, and reporting.

Table 6-3
Common Physiological Assessment Tools

Assessment Tool	Approximate Cost
Blood pressure cuff	$10–35
Large blood pressure cuff (33.3 cm to 51 cm)	$15–45
Stethoscope	$6–25
Automatic blood pressure machine	$40–80
Heart-rate monitor	$60–120
Skinfold calipers (manual)	$20–400
Skinfold calipers (automated calculations using Jackson-Pollock method)	$470
Tape measure, retractable, non-elastic	$7
Crunch strap	$5
Metronome	$10–$35
Stopwatch	$7–$25
Portable first-aid kit	$10–$25
Pocket mask with gloves	$10–$20
Miscellaneous: calculator, floor mat, beach towel, masking tape	

The American Council on Exercise also provides valuable calculation tools and assessment support materials through its website (www.acefitness.org/calculators).

Conducting Essential Cardiovascular Assessments

Heart Rate

The pulse rate (which in most people is identical to the heart rate) can be measured at any point on the body where an artery's pulsation is close to the surface. The following are some commonly palpated sites:

- *Radial artery:* The ventral aspect of the wrist on the side of the thumb, and less commonly, the ulnar artery on the pinky side, which is deeper and harder to palpate
- *Carotid artery:* Located in the neck, lateral to the trachea. More easily palpated when the neck is slightly extended. Never palpate both carotid arteries at the same time and always press lightly to prevent decreased blood flow to the brain.

Though the radial and carotid arteries are the most common locations for detecting a pulse, the following sites will also provide a pulse location: brachial artery, femoral artery, posterior tibial artery, popliteal artery, and the abdominal aorta. It is also possible to auscultate the actual beat of the heart using a stethoscope placed over the chest. If when palpating the client's pulse, the trainer feels any irregularity in the rate or rhythm of the pulse, it is recommended that the client contact his or her personal physician.

Measurement of heart rate is a valid indicator of work intensity or stress on the body, both at rest and during exercise. Lower resting and submaximal heart rates may indicate higher fitness levels, since cardiovascular adaptations to exercise increase **stroke volume (SV),** thereby reducing heart rate. Conversely, higher resting and submaximal heart rates are often indicative of poor physical fitness. **Resting heart rate (RHR)** is influenced by fitness status, fatigue, body composition, drugs and medication, alcohol, caffeine, and stress, among other things. A traditional classification system exists to categorize RHRs:

- Sinus bradycardia, or slow HR: RHR <60 bpm
- Normal sinus rhythm: RHR 60 to 100 bpm
- Sinus tachycardia, or fast HR: RHR >100 bpm

Average RHR is approximately 70 to 72 bpm, averaging 60 to 70 bpm in males and 72 to 80 bpm in females. The higher values found in the female RHR is attributed in part to:

- Smaller heart chamber size
- Lower blood volume circulating less oxygen throughout the body
- Lower hemoglobin levels in women

The following are some key notes about heart rate:

- Knowing a client's heart rate provides insight into the overtraining syndrome, as any elevation in RHR >5 bpm over the client's normal RHR that remains over a period of days is good reason to offload or taper training intensities.
- Certain drugs, medications, and supplements can directly affect RHR. Individuals should abstain from consuming non-prescription stimulants or depressants for a minimum of 12 hours prior to measuring RHR.
- Body position affects RHR. Standing or sitting positions elevate HR more so than supine or prone positions due to the involvement of postural muscles and the effects of gravity.
- **Digestion** increases RHR, as the processes of **absorption** and digestion require energy, necessitating the delivery of nutrients and oxygen to the gastrointestinal tract.
- Environmental factors can affect RHR, as it is believed that noise, temperature, and sharing of personal information can place additional stress on the body, increasing heart rate as the body attempts to tolerate the stressors.

During exercise, heart rate reflects exercise intensity. Since the heart plays a pivotal role in supplying oxygen and nutrients and removing waste products, heart rate is a valid indicator of the demands placed upon the body. Several methods are used to measure heart rate, both at rest and during exercise:

- 12-lead **electrocardiogram (ECG** or **EKG)**
- **Telemetry** (often two-lead, including commercial heart-rate monitors)
- **Palpation**
- **Auscultation** with stethoscope

Palpation and auscultation are each accurate within 95% of a heart-rate monitor.

Procedure for Measuring Resting Heart Rate

Keep in mind that true RHR is measured just before the client gets out of bed in the morning. Therefore, in most personal-training environments, the trainer's assessment of RHR will not be entirely accurate. The pulsation heard through auscultation is generated by the expansion of the arteries as blood is pushed through after contraction of the left ventricle. This beat can be quite prominent in leaner individuals.

- The client should be resting comfortably for several minutes prior to obtaining RHR.
- The RHR may be measured indirectly by placing the fingertips on a pulse site (palpation), or directly by listening through a stethoscope (auscultation).
- Place the tips of the index and middle fingers (not the thumb, which has a pulse of its own) over the artery (typically, radial is used) and lightly apply pressure.
- To determine the RHR, count the number of beats for 30 or 60 seconds and then correct that score to beats/minute, if necessary.
  - ✓It is important to remember that a trainer is counting cardiac cycles. Therefore, the first pulse measured should commence with "zero."
- When measuring by auscultation, place the bell of the stethoscope to the left of the client's sternum just above or below the nipple line. (It is important to be respectful of the client's personal space).
- The client may also measure his or her own resting HR before rising from bed in the morning and report back.

Procedure for Measuring Exercise Heart Rate

- Measuring for 30 to 60 seconds is generally difficult. Therefore, exercise heart rates are normally measured for shorter periods that are then corrected to equal 60 seconds.
- Generally a 10- to 15-second count is recommended over a six-second count given the larger potential for error with the shorter count.
- Count the first pulse beat as "zero" at the start of the time interval, then multiply the counted score by either six (for a 10-second count) or four (for a 15-second count).

Blood Pressure

Blood pressure is defined as the outward force exerted by the blood on the vessel walls. It is generally recorded as two numbers. The higher number, the SBP, represents the pressure created by the heart as it pumps blood into circulation via ventricular contraction. This represents the greatest pressure during one cardiac cycle. The lower number, the DBP, represents the pressure that is exerted on the artery walls as blood remains in the arteries during the filling phase of the cardiac cycle, or between beats when the heart relaxes. It is the minimum pressure that exists within one cardiac cycle.

Blood pressure is measured within the arterial system. The standard site of measurement is the brachial artery, given its easy accessibility and the ability to hold it level to the heart position. Blood pressure is measured indirectly by listening to the **Korotkoff sounds,** which are sounds made from vibrations as blood moves along the walls of the vessel. These sounds are only present when some degree of wall deformation exists. If the vessel has unimpeded blood flow, no vibrations are

pressure cuff, vessel deformity facilitates hearing these sounds. This deformity is created as the air bladder within the cuff is inflated, restricting the flow of blood.

When inflated to pressures greater than the highest pressure that exists within a cardiac cycle, the brachial artery collapses, preventing blood flow. As the air is slowly released from the bladder, blood begins to flow past the compressed area, creating turbulent flow and vibration along the vascular wall. The first BP phase, signified by the onset of tapping Korotkoff sounds, corresponds with SBP. DBP is indicated by the fourth (significant muffling of sound) and fifth (disappearance of sound) phases (Figure 6-8). As the cuff is continuously released, blood pressure within the vessel increases and eventually will exceed the pressure within the cuff. At this point, the blood pressure completely distends the vessel wall back to its original shape and the Korotkoff sounds will fade (fourth phase) and then disappear (fifth phase). Typically, in adults with normal blood pressure, the fifth phase is recorded as DBP. However, in children and adults with a fifth phase below 40 mmHg, yet who appear healthy, the fourth phase may be used.

Equipment:

- Sphygmomanometer (BP cuff)
- Stethoscope
- Chair

Procedure:

- Have the client sit with both feet flat on the floor for two full minutes.
- Cuff placement:
  - ✓ While the right arm is considered standard, many individuals favor placing the cuff on the left arm due to the increased proximity to the heart, which amplifies the heart sounds.
  - ✓ Smoothly and firmly wrap the blood pressure cuff around the arm with its lower margin about 1 inch (2 cm) above the antecubital space (i.e., the front of the elbow).
    - ○ The tubes should cross the antecubital space.
    - ○ Since BP cuffs come in a variety of sizes, it is important to ensure the correct size is used, as obese or muscular clients may have falsely elevated BP readings, while thin, small-framed individuals may have falsely low BP readings with a standard-sized cuff.
  - ✓ The client's arm should be supported either on an armchair or by the trainer at an angle of 0 to 45 degrees.

Measuring procedure:

- Turn the bulb knob to close the cuff valve (turning it all the way to the right, no more than finger tight) and rapidly inflate the cuff to 160 mmHg, or 20 to

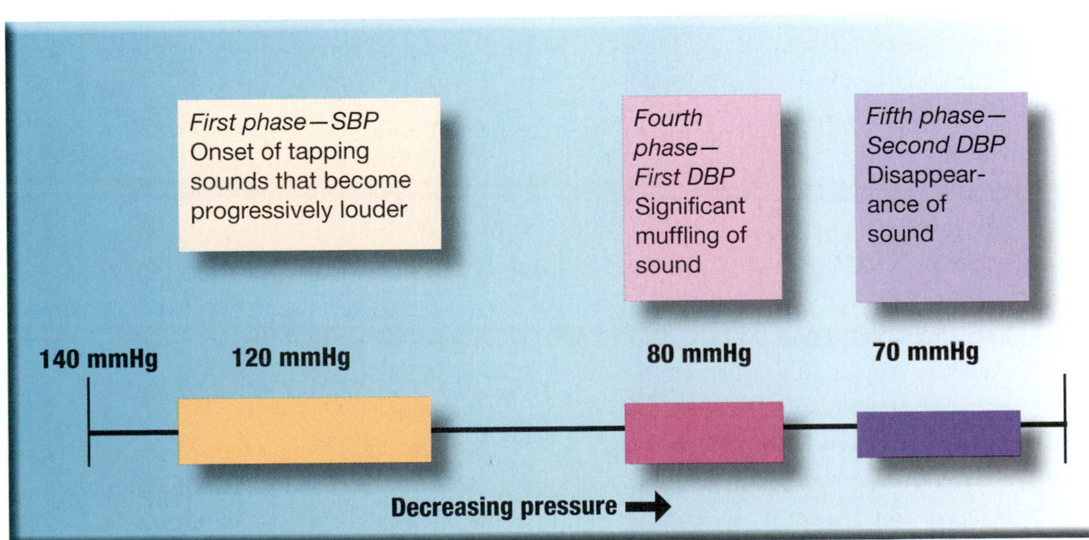

Figure 6-8
Korotkoff sounds and blood-pressure phases

Note: SBP = Systolic blood pressure; DBP = Diastolic blood pressure

30 mmHg above the point where the pulse can no longer be felt at the wrist.

- Place the stethoscope over the brachial artery using minimal pressure (do not distort the artery).
  - ✓The stethoscope should lie flat against the skin and should not touch the cuff or the tubing.
  - ✓The client's arm should be relaxed and straight at the elbow.
- Release the pressure by slowly turning the knob to the left at a rate of about 2 mmHg per second, listening for the Korotkoff sounds.
  - ✓SBP is determined by reading the dial at the first perception of sound (a faint tapping sound).
- DBP is determined by reading the dial when the sounds cease to be heard or when they become muffled.
- If a BP reading needs to be repeated on the same arm, allow at least 60 seconds between trials so that normal circulation can return to the area.
- Share measurements with the client as well as the classification of values.

Note: If abnormal readings result, repeat the measurement on the opposite arm. If there is a significant discrepancy between readings from arm to arm, it could represent a circulatory problem, and the client should be referred to his or her physician for a medical evaluation.

Common causes for mistakes in measuring blood pressure include:

- Cuff deflation that is too rapid
- Inexperience of the test administrator or inability of the test administrator to read pressure correctly
- Improper stethoscope placement and pressure
- Improper cuff size or an inaccurate/uncalibrated sphygmomanometer
- Auditory acuity of the test administrator or excessive background noise

The classification of blood pressure for adults is presented in Table 6-4.

During exercise:

- Blood pressure is very difficult to obtain during exercise due to the excessive amount of movement and noise, unless the person is riding a stationary bicycle.
- Traditionally, when exercise blood pressure measurements are justified, they are usually measured before and following exercise (to monitor against excessive **hypotension**).
- A sphygmomanometer with a stand and a hand-held gauge are better choices for measuring BP during exercise.
- If SBP drops during exercise, it should immediately be remeasured prior to terminating the session, just to ensure accuracy in measurement. If the client was anxious prior to the cardiorespiratory assessment, it is likely that the initial exercise SBP reading will drop.

Application:

The relationship between elevated blood pressure and cardiovascular events [e.g., myocardial infarction or **cerebrovascular accident (CVA)**] is unmistakable. For individuals 40 to 70 years old, each 20 mmHg

Table 6-4

Classification of Blood Pressure for Adults Age 18 and Older*

Category	Systolic (mmHg)		Diastolic (mmHg)
Normal†	<120	and	<80
Prehypertension	120–139	or	80–89
Hypertension‡			
Stage 1	140–159	or	90–99
Stage 2	≥160	or	≥100

* Not taking antihypertensive drugs and not acutely ill. When systolic and diastolic blood pressures fall into different categories, the higher category should be selected to classify the individual's blood pressure status. For example, 140/82 mmHg should be classified as stage 1 hypertension, and 154/102 mmHg should be classified as stage 2 hypertension. In addition to classifying stages of hypertension on the basis of average blood pressure levels, clinicians should specify presence or absence of target organ disease and additional risk factors. This specificity is important for risk classification and treatment.

† Normal blood pressure with respect to cardiovascular risk is below 120/80 mmHg. However, unusually low readings should be evaluated for clinical significance.

‡ Based on the average of two or more readings taken at each of two or more visits after an initial screening.

Chobanian, A.V. et al. (2003). *JNC 7 Express: The Seventh Report of the Joint National Committee on Prevention, Detection, Evaluation, and Treatment of High Blood Pressure.* NIH Publication No. 03-5233. Washington, D.C.: National Institutes of Health & National Heart, Lung, and Blood Institute.

increase in resting SBP or each 10 mmHg increase in resting DBP above normal *doubles* the risk of cardiovascular disease (ACSM, 2010). If the trainer discovers an abnormal BP reading, either at rest or during exercise, it is prudent to recommend that the client visit his or her personal physician.

Blood pressure can be reduced with medication or certain behavior modifications (i.e., exercise, weight loss, sodium restriction, smoking cessation, and stress management). For those with **prehypertension**, BP can realistically be reduced with lifestyle interventions; for those with true clinical hypertension (see Table 6-4), it is likely that their personal physicians will want to treat the hypertension with medication *and* lifestyle interventions (see Chapter 14). The personal trainer can provide guidance and motivation on appropriate lifestyle-modification practices.

Ratings of Perceived Exertion

RPE is used to subjectively quantify a participant's overall feelings and sensations during the stress of physical activity. Subjective measures of exertion are useful since they can be compared and have been validated against the physiological measure of heart rate. They can be used to complement or replace heart rates (when the client is taking certain drugs that may blunt the heart-rate response to exercise such as beta blockers) in providing feedback on exercise intensity. Two standardized ratings exist: the Borg 15-point scale (6 to 20 scale) and a modified 0 to 10 category ratio scale, which is a revision of the original Borg scale (Table 6-5). On the original 6-20 Borg scale, each value corresponds to a heart rate. For example:

- Borg score: 6 = corresponding heart rate of 60 bpm
- Borg score: 12 = corresponding heart rate of 120 bpm
- Borg score: 20 = corresponding heart rate of 200 bpm

Common trends:

- Men tend to underestimate exertion, while women tend to overestimate exertion.

Table 6-5

Ratings of Perceived Exertion (RPE)

RPE	Category Ratio Scale
6	0 Nothing at all
7 Very, very light	0.5 Very, very weak
8	1 Very weak
9 Very light	2 Weak
10	3 Moderate
11 Fairly light	4 Somewhat strong
12	5 Strong
13 Somewhat hard	6
14	7 Very strong
15 Hard	8
16	9
17 Very hard	10 Very, very strong
18	* Maximal
19 Very, very hard	
20	

Source: Adapted, with permission, from American College of Sports Medicine (2010). *ACSM's Guidelines for Exercise Testing and Prescription* (8th ed.). Philadelphia: Wolters Kluwer/Lippincott Williams & Wilkins

- The use of RPE has a significant learning curve that demonstrates deviation toward the mean as the client becomes more familiar with the scale.
- Initially, very sedentary individuals may find it difficult to use RPE charts, as they often find any level of exercise fairly hard.
- Conditioned individuals may under-rate their exercise intensity if they focus on the muscular tension requirement of the exercise rather than cardiorespiratory effort.

Recommendations for usage:

- The 6 to 20 scale is difficult to use and should only be utilized if HR equivalents are needed and the actual exercise HR is not a reliable indicator of exertion (e.g., when a client is taking medications that affect HR responses, such as beta blockers).
- The 0 to 10 scale should always be used to gauge intensity when the trainer does not need to measure HR via the RPE.

The Exercise-induced Feeling Inventory

The overall exercise experience strongly influences exercise adherence given how the decisions people make (e.g., "Should I exercise today?") are driven by the way they feel and think. Trainers should aim to leverage any positive emotional experiences associated with the exercise program to long-term adherence. Strategic use of a client's association of exercise with pleasant feelings will only serve to promote the client's willingness to continue exercising. The exercise-induced feeling inventory (EFI) quantifies a client's emotions and feelings following an exercise session (Figure 6-9).

The EFI should be administered during the initial interview, with the trainer asking the client to rate previous exercise experience. This will establish a baseline from which to compare future assessments. The EFI is then administered shortly after a client completes a workout to help trainers identify whether the recommended programming is a positive experience.

Instructions:

- Administer the survey verbally or give it to the client to self-complete. However, it is important to remember that clients are not always completely honest with self-administered surveys, so trainers should consider varying the delivery format.
- Administer the survey more frequently initially (e.g., every session or every other session for the first two weeks), then gradually diminish the frequency of admission to avoid a desensitization effect.
- The survey can also be readministered each time a change is made in the client's program.
- Instruct the client to score each of the 12 words using a 0 to 4 scale, checking the appropriate box that describes how he or she feels at this time.

Scoring the EFI:

- The survey consists of four distinct subscales, each defining a particular emotional state.
- As people define adjectives differently, the idea of using three adjectives to define the same emotional state (a subscale) tends to minimize deviations in how people define words.
- The four subscales are:
  - ✓ *Positive engagement:* Items 4, 7, and 12
  - ✓ *Revitalization:* Items 1, 6, and 9
  - ✓ *Tranquility:* Items 2, 5, and 10
  - ✓ *Physical exhaustion:* Items 3, 8, and 11
- Each adjective can earn a total of 4 points, creating a total for each subscale that ranges between 0 and 12.
- Track subscale scores over a period of four to six weeks and plot the results as illustrated in Figure 6-10 to determine aggregated trends.

Figure 6-9
Exercise-induced feeling inventory (EFI) survey

Instructions: Please use the following scale to indicate the extent to which each word describes how you feel at this moment in time. Record your responses by checking the appropriate box next to each word.

0 = Do not feel
1 = Feel slightly
2 = Feel moderately
3 = Feel strongly
4 = Feel very strongly

	0	1	2	3	4
1. Refreshed	❑	❑	❑	❑	❑
2. Calm	❑	❑	❑	❑	❑
3. Fatigued	❑	❑	❑	❑	❑
4. Enthusiastic	❑	❑	❑	❑	❑
5. Relaxed	❑	❑	❑	❑	❑
6. Energetic	❑	❑	❑	❑	❑
7. Happy	❑	❑	❑	❑	❑
8. Tired	❑	❑	❑	❑	❑
9. Revived	❑	❑	❑	❑	❑
10. Peaceful	❑	❑	❑	❑	❑
11. Worn out	❑	❑	❑	❑	❑
12. Upbeat	❑	❑	❑	❑	❑

Reprinted with permission from Gauvin, L. & Rejeski, W.J. (1993). The exercise-induced feeling inventory: Development and initial validation. *Journal of Sport & Exercise Psychology,* 15, 4, 409.

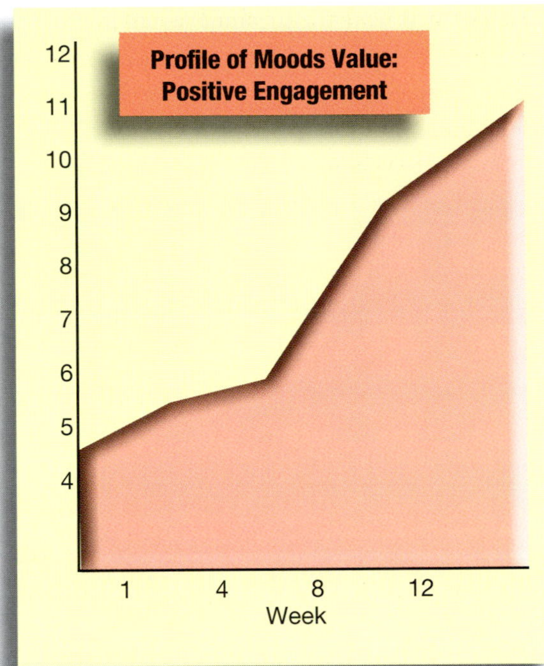

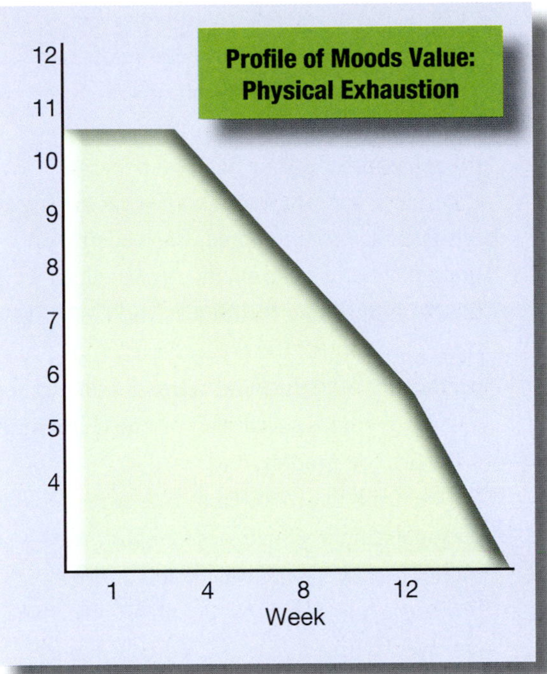

Figure 6-10 Examples of aggregated data for subscales of positive engagement and physical exhaustion over 12 weeks

- ✓ The objective is to build a positive emotional change with exercise over time by influencing the subscales accordingly.
- ✓ Plot the total scores of all four subscales against time to demonstrate each client's progress.

In trying to improve the overall experience of the exerciser, the trainer can determine the variables that promote or discourage exercise and use this information to manipulate these variables to increase the likelihood of continuing with his or her exercise program. For example, if the client repeatedly "feels strongly" that the exercise session makes him or her feel "worn out" or "fatigued," it would be appropriate to reduce the intensity of the exercise session, even if the exercise HR is within an acceptable range. If the client is not enjoying the exercise sessions, he or she is more likely to find excuses for skipping exercise sessions.

There is a reason why less than 35% of Americans exercise on a regular basis (U.S. Department of Health & Human Services, 2006). Many people do *not* enjoy exercise. Many are still haunted by the "no pain, no gain" signs hung around the school gymnasiums. The good news is that even a low-intensity workout will have a positive impact on overall health and well-being, without the "pain."

Summary

A personal trainer's role is to facilitate change and help his or her clients throughout the stages of establishing and building rapport with them, gathering vital information, developing fitness goals, and implementing a plan to accomplish them. As a facilitator of change, a trainer creates conditions and uses techniques that will help bring about the desired outcomes for each client. Merely possessing a fit body, technical skills, and a wide-based knowledge of health and fitness does not ensure a trainer's success. Perhaps the most crucial factor for determining a positive climate for the working relationship is the trainer's repertoire of communication skills. These skills include both verbal and nonverbal behaviors, such as attending, perceiving nonverbal messages, and verbal responding. These interpersonal communication skills can be learned, practiced, and mastered, and are important not only in the first stage of establishing rapport, but throughout the entire process.

Personal training is about behavioral change, which is the true measure of a successful client–trainer relationship. Every personal trainer is unique and brings into the relationship his or her own personal experience and opinions about what leads to lifestyle changes in people. Each client also is unique. Therefore, trainers must be flexible in matching teaching techniques and changing strategies to meet the goals, needs, and personality of each client, remembering that a technique that is successful for one client may not work for another.

The flexibility required to be a successful personal trainer sometimes demands the trainer use a personal touch, and at other times asks the trainer to remain an objective observer. Being able to move freely along the full range of interpersonal skills and teaching techniques will permit the trainer to respond appropriately at various stages of the relationship. The process of sizing up and assisting a client as he or she seeks a healthy lifestyle may be naturally intuitive, but it also needs to be a deliberate, rational process.

Prior to initiating any formal exercise program, it is up to the trainer to first get to know the client and determine his or her individual needs and wants. Through the effective use of appropriate communication and interviewing techniques, the trainer will establish rapport with the client and gain his or her trust. Second, it is important to conduct a thorough health assessment utilizing appropriate health-risk appraisals and risk stratifications. This will help ensure that the client is physically and mentally ready to embark on a structured fitness program. Measuring resting heart rate and blood pressure will further clarify the health status of the client. Finally, it is up to the trainer to be perceptive to the thoughts and feelings of his or her client, especially as it relates to the exercise experience, and tailor a balanced fitness program that will meet the specific wants and needs of each individual client.

References

American College of Sports Medicine (2010). *ACSM's Guidelines for Exercise Testing and Prescription* (8th ed.). Philadelphia: Wolters Kluwer/Lippincott Williams & Wilkins.

Chobanian, A.V. et al. (2003). *JNC 7 Express: The Seventh Report of the Joint National Committee on Prevention, Detection, Evaluation, and Treatment of High Blood Pressure.* NIH Publication No. 03-5233. Washington, D.C.: National Institutes of Health & National Heart, Lung, and Blood Institute.

Gauvin, L. & Rejeski, W.J. (1993). The exercise-induced feeling inventory: Development and initial validation. *Journal of Sport & Exercise Physiology,* 15, 4, 409.

Haskell, W.L. et al. (2007) Physical activity and public health: Updated recommendation for adults from the American College of Sports Medicine and the American Heart Association. *Circulation,* 116, 9, 1081.

Miller, W.R. & Rollnick, S. (2002). *Motivational Interviewing: Preparing People to Change Addictive Behavior* (2nd ed.). New York: Guilford.

U.S. Department of Health & Human Services (2008). 2008 Physical Activity Guidelines for Americans: Be Active, Healthy and Happy. www.health.gov/paguidelines/pdf/paguide.pdf

U.S. Department of Health & Human Services (2006). *Summary of Health Statistics for U.S. Adults: National Health Interview Survey.* Atlanta: U.S. Department of Health & Human Services.

Wilmore, J.H., Costill, D.L., & Kenney, W.L. (2008). *Physiology of Sport and Exercise* (4th ed.). Champaign, Ill.: Human Kinetics.

Suggested Reading

American College of Sports Medicine (2009). *ACSM's Exercise Management for Persons with Chronic Disease and Disabilities* (3rd ed.). Champaign, Ill.: Human Kinetics.

Burbank, P. & Riebe, D. (2002). *Promoting Exercise and Behavior Change in Older Adults: Interventions With the Transtheoretical Model.* New York: Springer Publishing Company.

Dubin, D. (2000). *Rapid Interpretation of EKGs* (6th ed.). Tampa, Fla.: COVER Inc.

Merrill, D. & Reid, R. (1981) *Personal Styles and Effective Performance*. Boca Raton, Fla.: CRC Press.

Peirce, A. (1999). *The American Pharmaceutical Association Practical Guide to Natural Medicines.* New York: Stonesong Press.

Pressman, A. & Shelley, D. (2000). *Integrative Medicine.* New York: St. Martin's Press.

Marcora, S.M., Staiano, W., & Manning, V. (2009). Mental fatigue impairs physical performance in humans. *Journal of Applied Physiology*, 106, 857–864.

U.S. Preventive Services Task Force (2002). *Guide to Clinical Preventive Services* (3rd ed.). Baltimore: International Medical Publishing.

IN THIS CHAPTER:

Static Postural Assessment

- Plumb Line Instructions
- Plumb Line Positions
- Deviation 1: Ankle Pronation/Supination and the Effect on Tibial and Femoral Rotation
- Deviation 2: Hip Adduction
- Deviation 3: Hip Tilting (Anterior or Posterior)
- Deviation 4: Shoulder Position and the Thoracic Spine
- Deviation 5: Head Position
- Postural Assessment Checklist and Worksheets

Movement Screens

- Clearing Tests
- Bend and Lift Screen
- Hurdle Step Screen
- Shoulder Push Stabilization Screen
- Shoulder Pull Stabilization Screen
- Thoracic Spine Mobility Screen

Flexibility and Muscle-length Testing

- Thomas Test for Hip Flexion/Quadriceps Length
- Passive Straight-leg (PSL) Raise

Shoulder Mobility

- Shoulder Flexion and Extension
- Internal and External Rotation of the Humerus at the Shoulder
- Apley's Scratch Test for Shoulder Mobility

Balance and the Core

- Sharpened Romberg Test
- Stork-stand Balance Test
- Core Function: Blood Pressure Cuff Test

Summary

***FABIO COMANA, M.A., M.S.**, is an exercise physiologist and spokesperson for the American Council on Exercise and faculty at San Diego State University (SDSU) and the University of California San Diego (UCSD), teaching courses in exercise science and nutrition. He holds two master's degrees, one in exercise physiology and one in nutrition, as well as certifications through ACE, ACSM, NSCA, and ISSN. Prior to joining ACE, he was a college head coach and a strength and conditioning coach at SDSU. Comana also managed health clubs for Club One. He lectures, conducts workshops, and writes on many topics related to exercise, fitness, and nutrition both nationally and internationally. As an ACE spokesperson and presenter, he is frequently featured in numerous media outlets, including television, radio, Internet, and more than 100 nationwide newspaper and print publications. Comana has authored chapters in various textbooks.*

CHAPTER 7

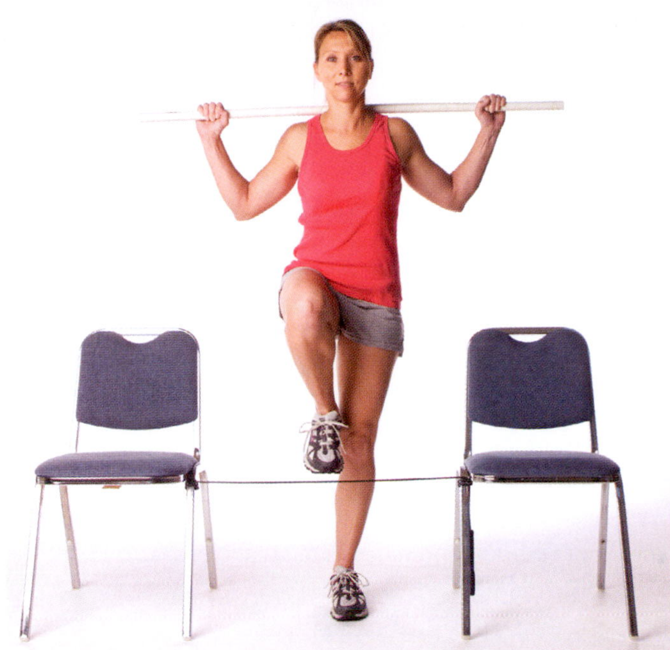

Functional Assessments: Posture, Movement, Core, Balance, and Flexibility

Fabio Comana

Sequencing a client's assessments involves consideration of both protocol selection and timing of the assessments. While trainers must always conduct the health-risk appraisal or assessment discussed in Chapter 6, the physiological assessments selected must be consistent with the client's goals and desires, and with the discoveries made during the needs assessment conducted during the initial interview. While clients often express a desire to lose weight, tone or shape their bodies, or improve their overall fitness levels, one primary objective of all training programs should be to improve functionality, which means that they should help clients enhance their ability to perform their **activities of daily living (ADL).** One key facet of functionality involves movement efficiency, or the ability of an individual to generate appropriate levels of force and movement at desired joints, while controlling or stabilizing the entire kinetic chain against **reactive** and **gravity-based forces**.

While movement is integral to human survival, it operates from a static base or alignment of the body segments, which is commonly referred to as **posture.** Since movement originates from this base, a postural assessment should be conducted to evaluate body-segment alignment in addition to movement screens that evaluate how posture, both good and bad, impacts the ability to move.

Static Postural Assessment

Static posture represents the alignment of the body's segments, or how the person holds him- or herself "statically" or "isometrically" in space. Holding a proper postural position involves the actions of multiple postural muscles, which are generally the deeper muscles that contain greater concentrations of **type I muscle fibers** and function to hold static positions or low-grade **isometric** contractions for extended periods. Good posture or structural integrity is defined as that state of musculoskeletal alignment and balance that allows muscles, joints, and nerves to function efficiently (Kendall et al., 2005; Soderberg, 1997). However, if a client exhibits deviations in his or her static position from good posture, this may reflect muscle-endurance issues in the postural muscles and/or potential imbalance at the joints. Movement begins from a position of static posture. Therefore, the presence of poor posture is a good indicator that movement may be dysfunctional. Although movement screens offer valuable information related to **neuromuscular efficiency,** a static postural assessment is considered very useful and serves as a starting point from which a personal trainer can identify muscle imbalances and potential movement compensations associated with poor posture (Kendall et al., 2005; Sahrmann, 2002). A static posture assessment may offer valuable insight into:

- Muscle imbalance at a joint and the working relationships of muscles around a joint
  - ✓ Muscle imbalance often contributes to dysfunctional movement.
- Altered neural action of the muscles moving and controlling the joint
  - ✓ For example, tight or shortened muscles are often overactive and dominate movement at the joint, potentially disrupting healthy joint mechanics (the concept of neural **hypertonicity** is covered in Chapter 9).

Muscle imbalance and postural deviations can be attributed to many factors that are both correctible and non-correctible, including the following:

- Correctible factors:
  - ✓ Repetitive movements (muscular pattern overload)
  - ✓ Awkward positions and movements (habitually poor posture)
  - ✓ Side dominance
  - ✓ Lack of joint **stability**
  - ✓ Lack of joint **mobility**
  - ✓ Imbalanced strength-training programs
- Non-correctible factors:
  - ✓ Congenital conditions (e.g., **scoliosis**)
  - ✓ Some pathologies (e.g., **rheumatoid arthritis**)
  - ✓ Structural deviations (e.g., tibial or femoral **torsion,** femoral **anteversion**)
  - ✓ Certain types of trauma (e.g., surgery, injury, amputations)

Proper postural alignment promotes optimal neural activity of the muscles controlling and moving the joint. When joints are correctly aligned, the length-tension relationships and force-coupling relationships function efficiently. This facilitates proper joint mechanics, allowing the body to generate and accept forces throughout the kinetic chain, and promotes joint stability and mobility and movement efficiency (refer to Chapter 9 for more information on the concept of mobility, stability, and movement efficiency). Figure 7-1 illustrates the importance of muscle balance and its contribution to movement efficiency. Given how an individual's static posture reflects

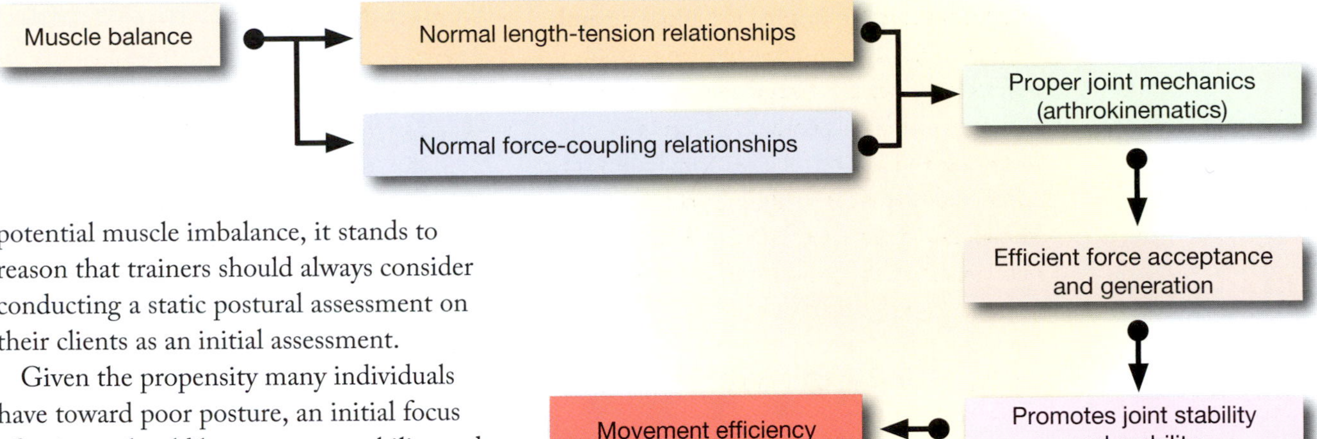

Figure 7-1
Movement efficiency pattern

potential muscle imbalance, it stands to reason that trainers should always consider conducting a static postural assessment on their clients as an initial assessment.

Given the propensity many individuals have toward poor posture, an initial focus of trainers should be to restore stability and mobility within the body and attempt to "straighten the body before strengthening it." The trainer should therefore start by looking at a client's static posture following the right-angle rule of the body (Kendall et al., 2005). This model demonstrates how the human body represents itself in vertical alignment across the major joints—the ankle (and subtalar joint), knee, hip, and shoulder, as well as the head. This model allows the observer to look at the individual in all three planes to note specific "static" asymmetries at the joints (e.g., front to back, left to right). As illustrated in Figure 7-2, the right-angle model implies a state in the **frontal plane** wherein the two hemispheres are equally divided, and in the **sagittal plane** wherein the anterior and posterior surfaces appear in balance. The body is in good postural position when the body parts are symmetrically balanced around the body's **line of gravity,** which is the intersection of the mid-frontal and mid-sagittal planes and is represented by a plumb line hanging from a fixed point overhead.

While this model helps trainers identify postural compensations and potential muscle imbalances, it is important to recognize that limitations exist in using this model.

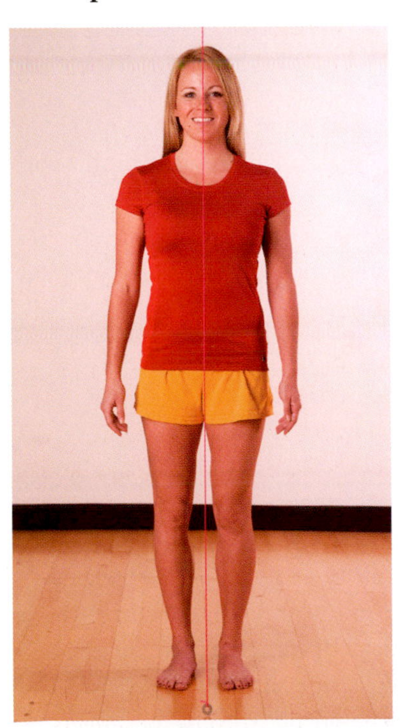
a.

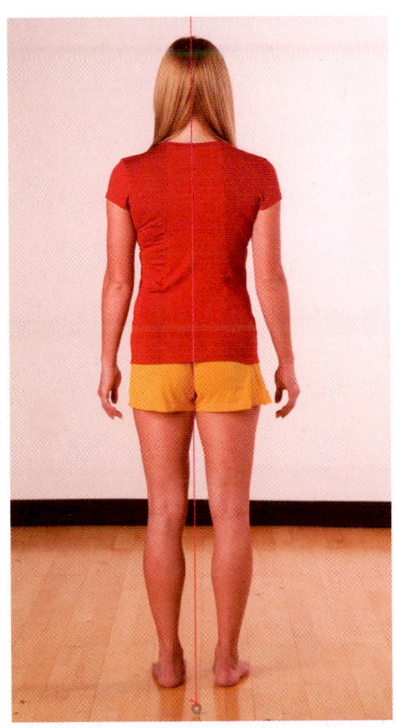
b.

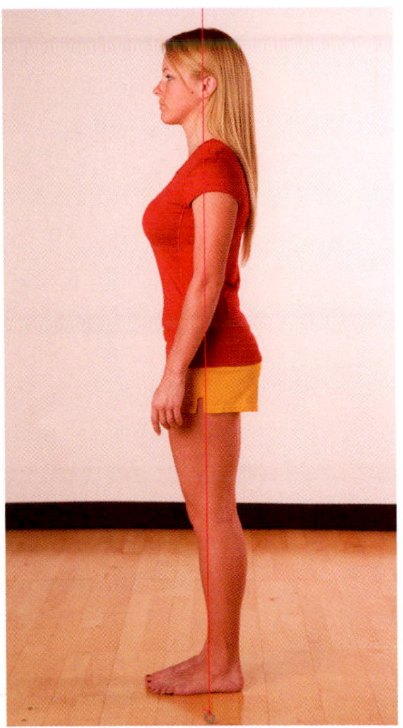
c.

Figure 7-2
The right-angle rule (frontal and sagittal views)

Plumb Line Instructions

Using a length of string and an inexpensive weight (e.g., a washer), trainers can create a plumb line that suspends from a ceiling or fixed point to a height 0.5 to 1 inch (1.3 to 2.5 cm) above the floor. It is important to select a location that offers a solid, plain backdrop or a grid pattern with vertical and horizontal lines that offer contrast against the client. When conducting these assessments, the trainer should instruct the client to wear form-fitting athletic-style clothing to expose as many joints and bony landmarks as possible, and have the client remove his or her shoes. The use of adhesive dots placed upon the bony landmarks may assist trainers in identifying postural deviations.

The objective of this assessment is to observe the client's symmetry against the plumb line and the right angles that the weightbearing joints make relative to the line of gravity. Individuals will consciously or subconsciously attempt to correct posture when they are aware they are being observed. Personal trainers should encourage clients to assume a normal, relaxed position, and utilize distractions such as casual conversation to encourage this relaxed position. It is important to remember that while postural assessments provide valuable information, they are only one piece to the movement efficiency puzzle, and thus should not be overemphasized. Personal trainers should focus on the obvious, gross imbalances and avoid getting caught up in minor postural asymmetries. Trainers should bear in mind that the body is rarely perfectly symmetrical and that overanalyzing asymmetries is time-consuming, potentially intimidating to clients, and may induce muscle fatigue in the client that can alter his or her posture even further. Therefore, when looking for gross deviations, the trainer should select an acceptable margin of asymmetry that he or she will allow and focus on larger, more obvious discrepancies. For example, start by focusing on gross deviations that differ by a quarter-inch (0.6 cm) or more between the compartments of the body. While postural assessments can be performed in great detail, this section addresses five key postural deviations that occur frequently in individuals.

Plumb Line Positions

Anterior and Posterior Views

Source: Kendall et al., 2005

- For the anterior view, position the client between the plumb line and a wall, facing the plumb line with the feet equidistant from the suspended line (using the inside of the heels or medial malleoli as a reference) (see Figure 7-2a).
- With good posture, the plumb line will pass equidistant between the feet and ankles, and intersect the pubis, umbilicus, sternum, manubrium, mandible (chin), maxilla (face), and frontal bone (forehead).
- For the posterior view, position the individual between the plumb line and a wall, facing away from the plumb line with the insides of the heels equidistant from the suspended line (see Figure 7-2b).
- With good posture, the plumb line should ideally intersect the sacrum [equidistant between the posterior superior iliac spines (PSIS)] and overlap the spinous processes of the spine.

Sagittal View

Source: Kendall et al., 2005

- Position the individual between the plumb line and the wall, facing sideways with the plumb line aligned immediately anterior to the lateral malleolus (anklebone) (see Figure 7-2c).
- With good posture, the plumb line should ideally pass through the anterior third of the knee, the greater trochanter of the femur, and the acromioclavicular (A-C) joint, and slightly anterior to the mastoid process of the temporal bone of the skull (in line with, or just behind, the ear lobe).

Transverse View

Source: Kendall et al., 2005

All transverse views of the limbs and torso are performed from frontal- and sagittal-plane positions.

Trainers must respect **scope of practice** when performing a postural assessment on clients, particularly in the presence of pain or injury. They must understand the need for referral to more qualified healthcare professionals when pain or underlying pathologies are present (e.g., scoliosis).

When conducting assessments of posture and movement, the following components are included following the outline provided in Figure 7-3.

- Client history—written and verbal
  - ✓ Collect information on musculoskeletal issues, congenital issues (e.g., scoliosis), trauma, injuries, pain and discomfort, the site of pain or discomfort, and what aggravates and relieves pain or discomfort (e.g., with discomfort in the upper back, the client may feel temporary relief by hunching forward and rounding the shoulders).
  - ✓ Collect lifestyle information, including occupation, side-dominance, and habitual patterns (information regarding these patterns may take time to gather).
- Visual and manual observation
  - ✓ Identify observable postural deviations.
  - ✓ Verify muscle imbalance as determined by muscle-length testing.
  - ✓ Determine the impact on movement ability or efficiency by performing movement screens.
  - ✓ Facilitate movement to distinguish correctible from non-correctible compensations.

Deviation 1: Ankle Pronation/Supination and the Effect on Tibial and Femoral Rotation

Both feet should face forward in parallel or with slight (8 to 10 degrees) **external rotation** (toes pointing outward from the midline, as the ankle joint lies in an oblique plane with the medial malleolus slightly anterior to the lateral malleolus). The toes should be aligned in the same direction as the feet and any excessive **pronation** (arch flattening) or **supination** (high arches) at the subtalar joint should be noted. To evaluate this, personal trainers can perform the following screen (Price, 2007) (Figure 7-4):

- The personal trainer places the palm of the left hand against the inside of the client's left ankle, resting the hand upon the medial malleolus.
- The client collapses the ankle inward without lifting the toes off the floor. The personal trainer marks this end-range position with the left hand.
- Next, the trainer places the palm of the right hand against the outside of the client's right ankle, resting the hand upon the lateral malleolus.
- The client rolls the ankle outward without lifting the big toe off the floor. The trainer marks this end-range position with the right hand.

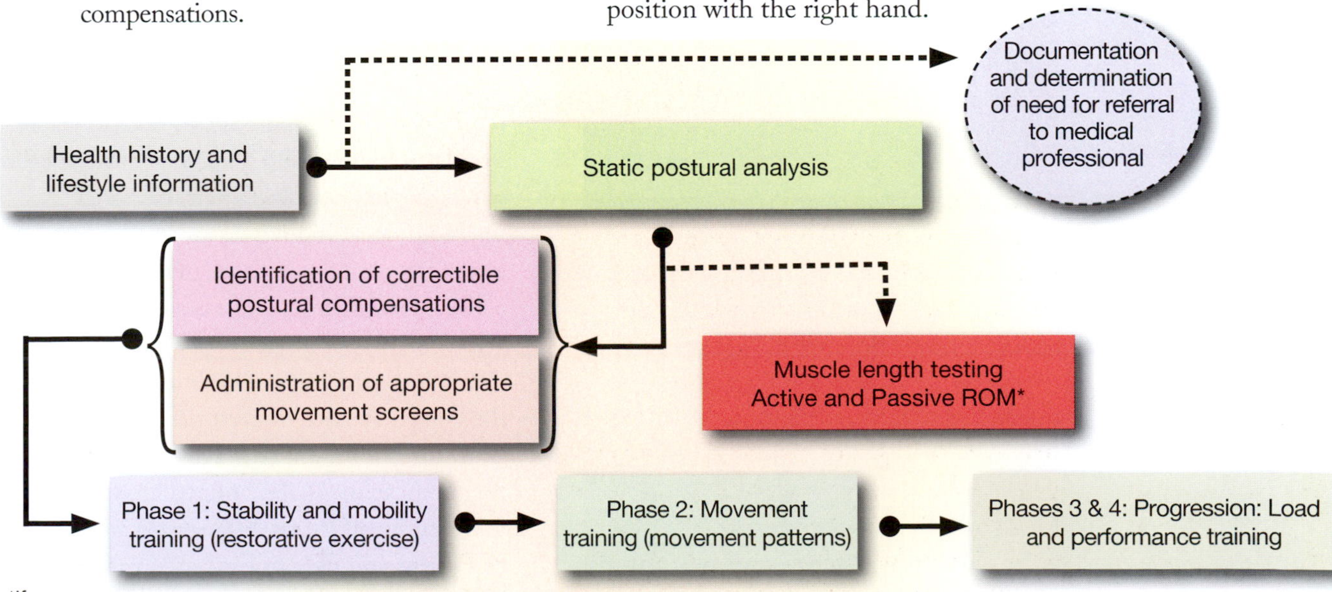

Figure 7-3
A chronological plan for conducting postural assessments and movement screens

- The trainer should slowly coach the client to move the ankle joint until it is positioned midway between both palms.
- On the trainer's command, the client relaxes the foot.
  - ✓ If the foot collapses inward, it indicates that this client may stand in a more pronated position, which is more common.
  - ✓ If the foot rolls outward, it indicates that the client stands in a more supinated position, which is less common.
- This procedure is then repeated with the opposite foot.

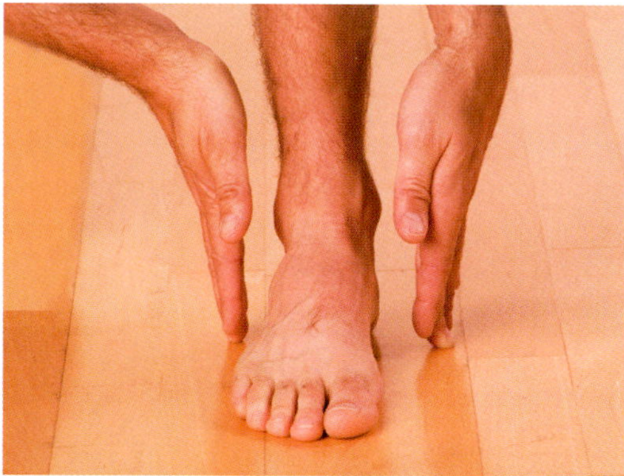
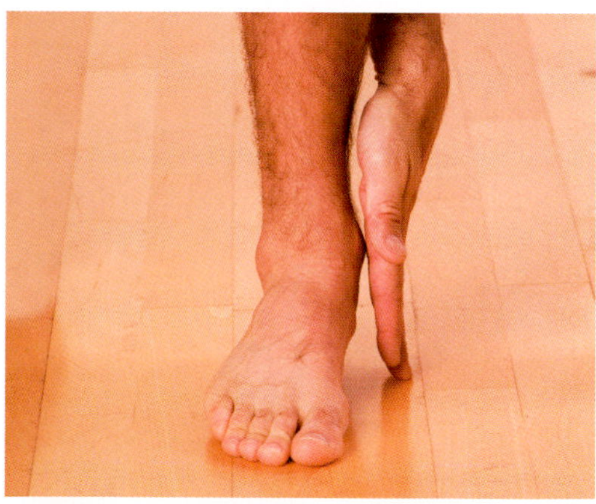
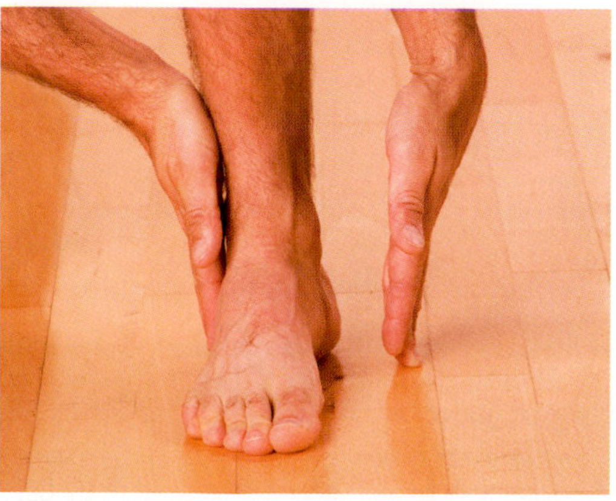

Figure 7-4
Evaluation of ankle pronation/supination

Because the body is one continuous kinetic chain, the position of the ankle will impact the position of the tibia and femur. Barring structural differences in the skeletal system (e.g., tibial torsion, femoral anteversion), a pronated ankle position typically forces internal rotation of the tibia and slightly less internal rotation of the femur (Figure 7-5 and Table 7-1). To demonstrate this point, stand with shoes off and place the hands firmly on the fronts of the thighs. Notice what happens to the orientation of the knees and thighs when moving between pronation and supination. Additionally, notice how the calcaneus everts as the ankle is pronated.

Ankle pronation forces rotation at the knee and places additional stresses on some knee ligaments and the integrity of the joint itself (Houglum, 2005). Additionally, as pronation tends to move the calcaneus into **eversion,** this may actually lift the outside of the heel slightly off the ground (moving the ankle into **plantarflexion**). In turn, this may tighten the calf muscles and potentially limit ankle **dorsiflexion,** but trainers should keep in mind that the opposite is also true: A tight gastrocnemius and soleus complex (triceps surae) may force calcaneal eversion in an otherwise neutral subtalar joint position (Gray & Tiberio, 2006). To illustrate this point, stand barefoot facing a wall with the feet 36 inches (0.9 m) away. Extend both arms in front of the body, placing the hands on the wall for support. Slowly lean forward, flexing the elbows and dorsiflexing the ankles while keeping both heels firmly pressed into the floor. Observe for any movement in the feet (e.g., appearance of the arch collapsing with calcaneal eversion). As a tight gastrocnemius and soleus complex (triceps surae) reach the limit of their extensibility, the body may need to evert the calcaneus to allow further movement. This scenario may occur repeatedly in gait immediately prior to the push-off phase if the gastrocnemius and soleus complex (triceps surae) are tight, forcing calcaneal eversion and pronation.

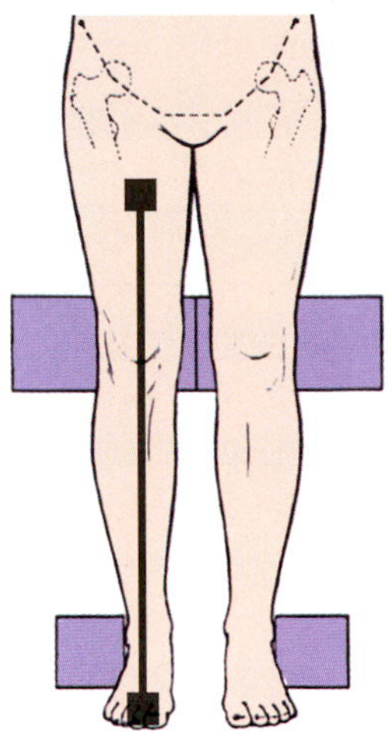
Neutral subtalar position with neutral knee alignment

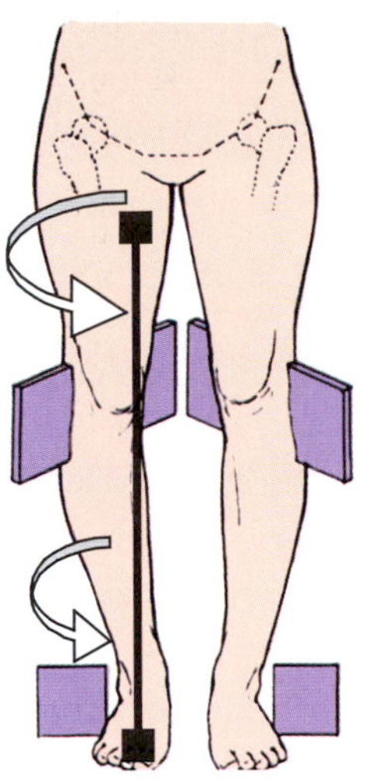
Pronation with internal rotation of the knee

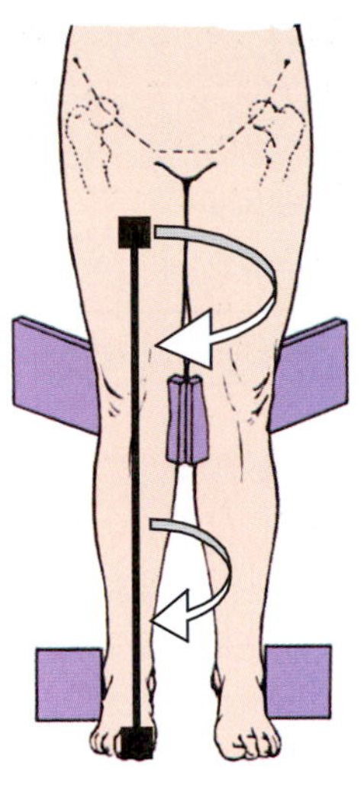
Supination with external rotation of the knee

Figure 7-5
Ankle pronation and supination and the effects up the kinetic chain

Source: LifeART image copyright 2008 Wolters Kluwer Health, Inc., Lippincott Williams & Wilkins. All rights reserved.

Table 7-1
Ankle Pronation/Supination and the Effect on the Feet, Tibia, and Femur

Ankle Movement	Foot Movement	Tibial (Knee) Movement	Femoral Movement	Plane of View
Ankle pronation	Eversion	Internal rotation	Internal rotation	View from front
Ankle supination	Inversion	External rotation	External rotation	View from front

Deviation 2: Hip Adduction

Hip **adduction** defines a lateral tilt of the pelvis that elevates one hip higher than the other, which may be evident in individuals who have a limb-length discrepancy (Sahrmann, 2002). If a person raises the right hip as illustrated in Figure 7-6, the line of gravity following the spine tilts over toward the left, moving the right thigh closer to this line of gravity. Consequently, the right hip is identified as moving into adduction. This position progressively lengthens and weakens the right hip abductors, which are unable to hold the hip level. Sleeping on one's side can produce a similar effect, as the hip abductors of the upper hip fail to hold the hip level.

To evaluate the presence of hip adduction with a client, a personal trainer must identify the alignment of the pelvis relative to the plumb line (Table 7-2). As mentioned previously, the plumb line should pass through the pubis with the anterior view and the middle of the sacrum with the posterior view (see Figure 7-2). By using a dowel or lightly weighted bar positioned across the iliac crests, the trainer can determine whether the iliac crests are parallel with the floor (Figure 7-7).

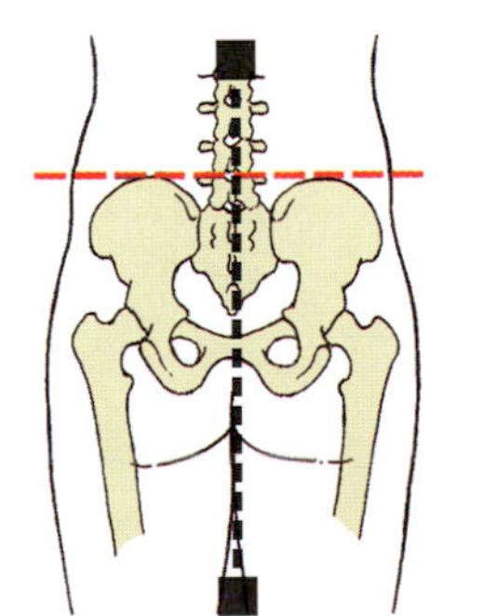
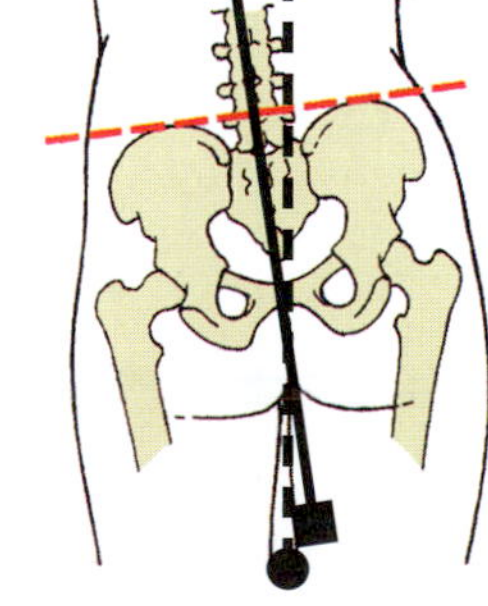

Figure 7-6
Normal hip position versus right hip adduction

Source: LifeART image copyright 2008 Wolters Kluwer Health, Inc., Lippincott Williams & Wilkins. All rights reserved.

Figure 7-7
Dowel placement to determine level pelvis

Table 7-2

Hip Adduction

Observation	Position	Plumb Line Alignment	Plane of View
Right hip adduction	Elevated (vs. left side)	Hips usually shifted right	View from front
Left hip adduction	Elevated (vs. right side)	Hips usually shifted left	View from front

Deviation 3: Hip Tilting (Anterior or Posterior)

Anterior tilting of the pelvis frequently occurs in individuals with tight hip flexors, which is generally associated with sedentary lifestyles where individuals spend countless hours in seated (i.e., shortened hip flexor) positions (Kendall et al., 2005). With standing, this shortened hip flexor pulls the pelvis into an anterior tilt (i.e., the superior, anterior portion of the pelvis rotates downward and forward). As illustrated in Figure 7-8, an anterior pelvic tilt rotates the superior, anterior portion of the pelvis forward and downward, spilling water out of the front of the bucket, whereas a posterior tilt rotates the superior, posterior portion of the pelvis backward and downward, spilling water out of the back of the bucket. An anterior pelvic tilt will increase **lordosis** in the lumbar spine, whereas a posterior pelvic tilt will reduce the amount of lordosis in the lumbar spine. To demonstrate this point, a personal trainer can stand with hands placed on the hips and gently tilt his or her pelvis anteriorly, noticing the change in position and increase in muscle tension in the lumbar region. Likewise, the trainer can tilt the pelvis posteriorly and notice how the lumbar spine flattens and reduces tension in the lumbar extensors.

Tight or overdominant hip flexors are generally coupled with tight erector spinae muscles, producing an anterior pelvic tilt, while tight or overdominant rectus abdominis muscles are generally coupled with tight hamstrings, producing a posterior pelvic tilt (Table 7-3). This coupling relationship between tight hip flexors and erector spinae is defined by Vladimir Janda as lower-cross syndrome

Figure 7-8
Anterior and posterior tilting of the pelvis—sagittal (side) view

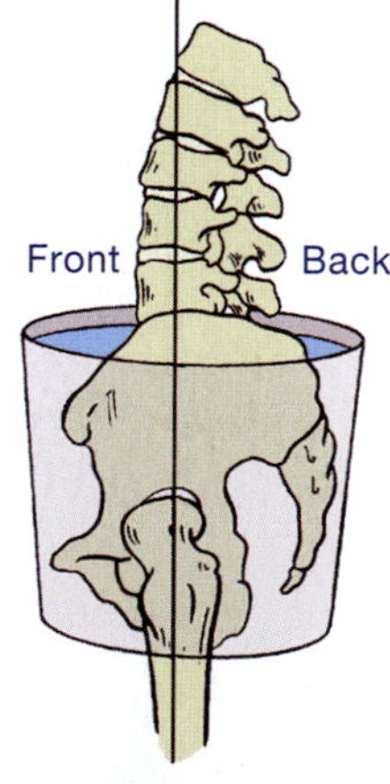

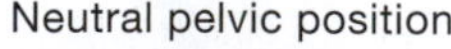
Neutral pelvic position

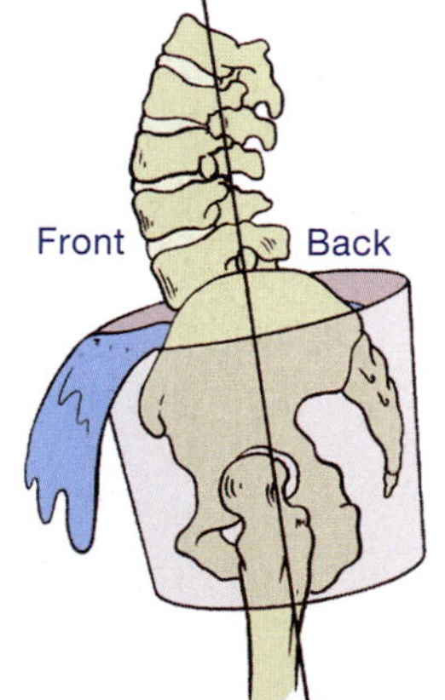

Anterior pelvic tilt

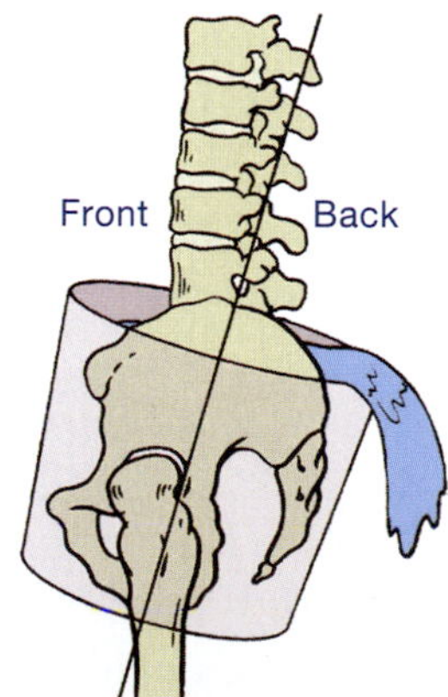

Posterior pelvic tilt

Table 7-3

Pelvic Rotation

Observation	Rotation	Muscles Suspected to Be Tight	Plane of View
Anterior tilt	ASIS tilts downward and forward	Hip flexors, erector spinae	Sagittal
Posterior tilt	ASIS tilts upward and backward	Rectus abdominis, hamstrings	Sagittal

Note: ASIS = Anterior superior iliac spine

(Morris et al., 2006). With ankle pronation and accompanying internal femoral rotation, the pelvis may tilt anteriorly to better accommodate the head of the femur, demonstrating the point of an integrated kinetic chain whereby ankle pronation can increase lumbar lordosis due to an anterior pelvic tilt (Sahrmann, 2002).

To evaluate the presence of a pelvic tilt, some trainers simply observe the natural line of a client's pants along the waistline. Trainers should use caution when using this technique, as the potential for error is high given the various preferences for how people wear pants and pant styles. Several more accurate evaluations can be performed, but because each has specific limitations and no technique is considered superior to the others, the trainer can consider using the consensus of what the four techniques listed reveal to determine the presence of a pelvic tilt.

- Relationship of two bony landmarks on the pelvis: the anterior superior iliac spine (ASIS) and the PSIS (Kendall et al., 2005)
  - ✓ Generally, the ASIS lies lower than the PSIS with the ASIS–PSIS angle deviating approximately 10 to 15 degrees from horizontal in men and between 5 and 10 degrees in women due to differences in pelvic structure. However, this cannot be viewed as an absolute valid marker given structural variations in the pelvic anatomy between individuals.
  - ✓ Additionally, the PSIS may prove very difficult to locate, especially in obese individuals.
- Appearance of lordosis in the lumbar spine
  - ✓ The client steps away from the plumb line and stands with his or her back against a wall with the heels touching the wall. The trainer then slides one hand between the wall and the small of the client's back, reaching all the way through or until the knuckles touch the client's back [a 2.0- to 2.5-inch (5.0 to 6.4 cm) space].
  - ✓ This technique may be invalid if an individual exhibits well-developed gluteal muscles, which will create a larger space and create a perception of increased lordosis.
- The alignment of the pubic bone to the ASIS as illustrated in Figure 7-9 (Sahrmann, 2002)
  - ✓ As illustrated in Figure 7-9, the ASIS and pubic bone lie in line vertically when the pelvis is in a neutral position. Have the client palpate his or her ASIS and pubic bone, pushing his or her fingers firmly against each bone to determine their relative orientation.

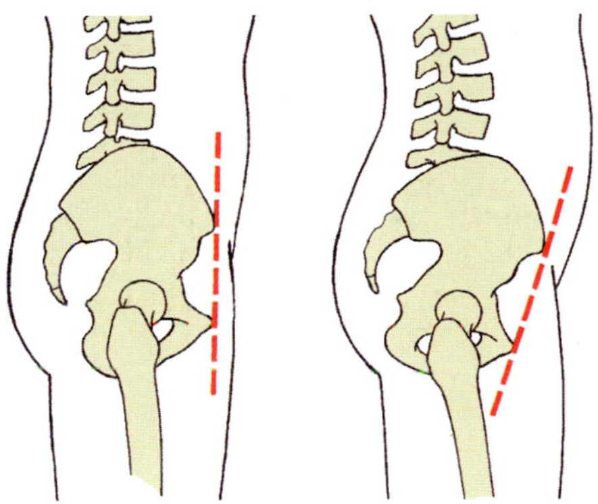
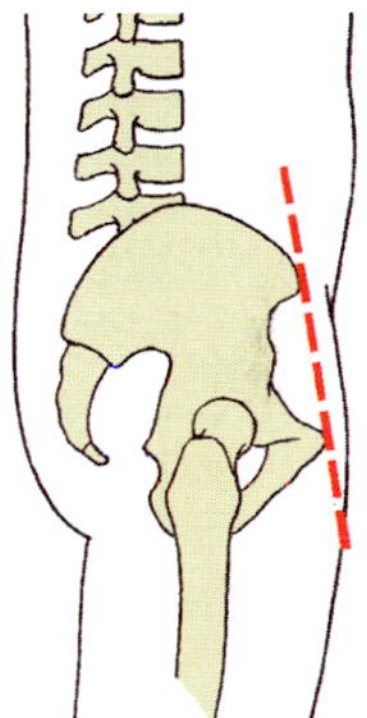

Figure 7-9
Alignment of the ASIS and pubic bone

Source: LifeART image copyright 2008 Wolters Kluwer Health, Inc., Lippincott Williams & Wilkins. All rights reserved.

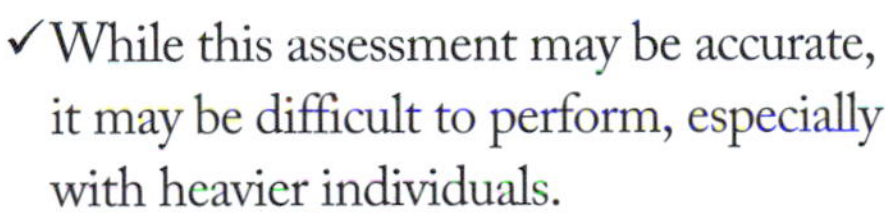

  - ✓ While this assessment may be accurate, it may be difficult to perform, especially with heavier individuals.
- The degree of **flexion** or **hyperextension** in the knees
  - ✓ Generally, as the pelvis tilts anteriorly, the knees exhibit a greater degree of hyperextension.
  - ✓ Generally, as the pelvis tilts posteriorly, the knees exhibit a greater degree of flexion.
  - ✓ To demonstrate this point, a trainer can place the hands on his or her own hips and observe the knee position while rotating the pelvis anteriorly and posteriorly.

Deviation 4: Shoulder Position and the Thoracic Spine

Limitations and compensations to movement at the shoulder occur frequently due to the complex nature of the shoulder girdle design and the varied movements performed at the shoulder. In Chapter 9, basic shoulder movements are discussed that outline the collaborative function of the scapulothoracic region (the scapulae and associated muscles attaching them to the thorax) and glenohumeral joint to produce shoulder movements. While the glenohumeral joint is highly mobile and perhaps a less stable joint, the scapulothoracic joint is designed to offer greater stability with less mobility. However, it is important to remember that it still contributes approximately 60 degrees of movement in raising the arms overhead, with the glenohumeral joint contributing the remaining 120 degrees (see Figure 9-60, page 299). Collectively, however, they allow for a diverse range of movements in the shoulder complex. Observation of the position of the scapulae in all three planes provides good insight into the quality of movement that a client has at the shoulders.

Figure 7-10 illustrates the "resting" position of the scapulae, which can vary considerably from person to person. The vertebral (medial) border of the scapula is typically positioned between the second and seventh ribs and vertically about 3 inches (7.6 cm) from the spinous processes (Kendall et al., 2005; Houglum, 2005). While the glenoid fossa is tilted upward 5 degrees and anteriorly 30 degrees to optimally articulate with the head of the humerus, the scapulae usually lie flat against the ribcage (Kendall et al., 2005). While the scapulae should appear flat against the ribcage, their orientation depends on the size and shape of the person and the ribcage.

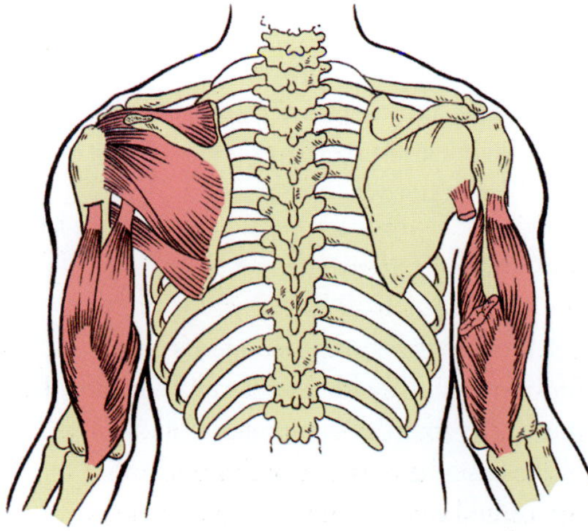

Figure 7-10
The normal position of the scapulae

To evaluate shoulder position, personal trainers can perform the following steps:

- Determine whether the shoulders are level. Place a level (dowel, broomstick, or lightly weighted bar) across either the spine of the scapulae or resting on each acromion process as illustrated in Figure 7-11.

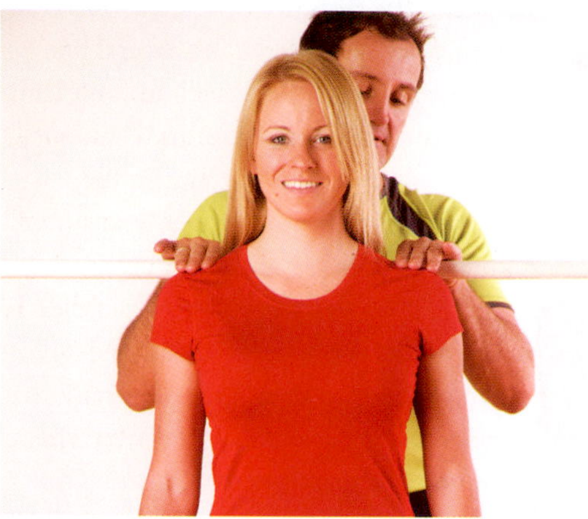

Figure 7-11
Dowel placement to determine level shoulders

  - ✓ If the shoulders are not level, trainers need to identify potential reasons. Remember that the presence of any congenital, traumatic, or skeletal (i.e., non-correctible) condition may be causing this asymmetry. Therefore, this imbalance is probably not correctible.
- Determine whether the torso and shoulders are symmetrical relative to the line of gravity [i.e., alignment of the plumb line through the sternum (anterior view) and spine (posterior view)].
  - ✓ A torso lean would shift the alignment of the sternum (anterior) and spine (posterior) away from the plumb line and create tightness on the flexed side of the trunk. This could explain why the shoulders are not level. Additionally, this may create uneven spacing between the arms and torso.
  - ✓ However, if the hips are level with the floor and the spine is aligned with the plumb line, but the shoulders are not level with the floor, this may represent muscle imbalance within the shoulder complex itself.
    - ○ An elevated shoulder may present

with an overdeveloped or tight upper trapezius muscle.
    - A depressed shoulder may present with more forward rounding of the scapula.
    - The shoulder on a person's dominant side may hang lower than the non-dominant side due to continual use that collectively loosens the shoulder ligaments.
- Determine whether the scapulae and/or arms are internally rotated.
  - ✓ From a posterior view, if the vertebral (medial) and/or inferior angle of the scapulae protrude outward, it indicates an inability of the scapulae stabilizers (primarily the rhomboids and serratus anterior) to hold the scapulae in place.
    - Noticeable protrusion of the vertebral (medial) border outward is termed "scapular protraction" (Figure 7-12a).
    - Noticeable protrusion of the inferior angle and vertebral (medial) border outward is termed "winged scapulae" (Figure 7-12b).
  - ✓ From an anterior view, if the knuckles or the backs of the client's hands are visible when the hands are positioned at the sides, this generally indicates internal (medial) rotation of the humerus or scapular protraction (Figure 7-13). This can also be viewed by looking at the orientation of the client's elbows while in the posterior position. The elbows will point outward instead of backward.
- Determine whether the spine exhibits normal **kyphosis** or whether there is insufficient (flat- or sunken-back) or excessive kyphosis (which is more common).
  - ✓ With the client's consent, the trainer can run one hand gently up the thoracic spine between the scapulae. The spine should exhibit a smooth, small, outward curve.

Table 7-4 lists key deviations of the thoracic spine and shoulders in various planes of view.

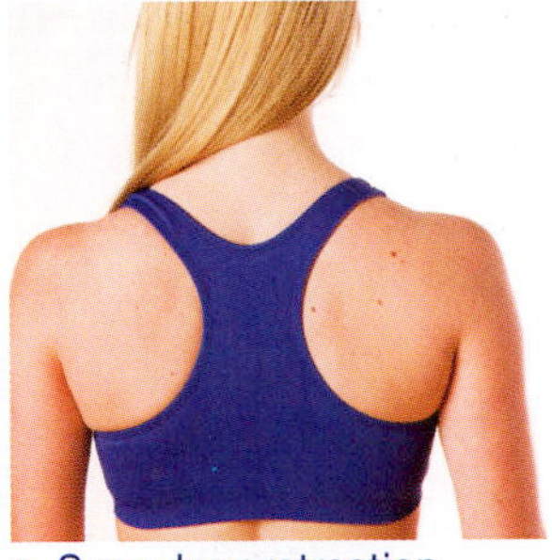
a. Scapular protraction

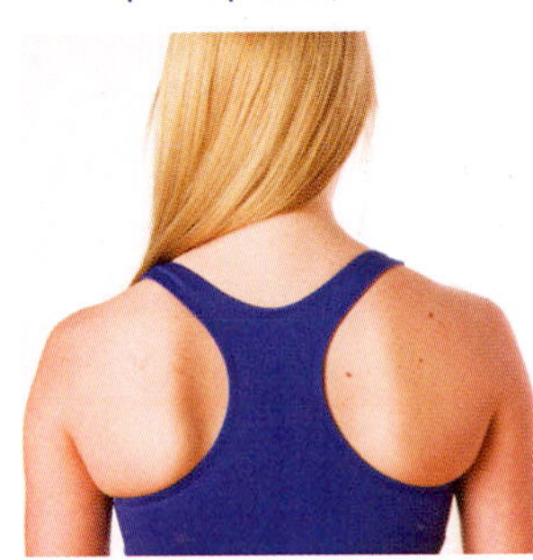
b. Scapular winging

Figure 7-12
Scapular protraction and winging: Posterior view

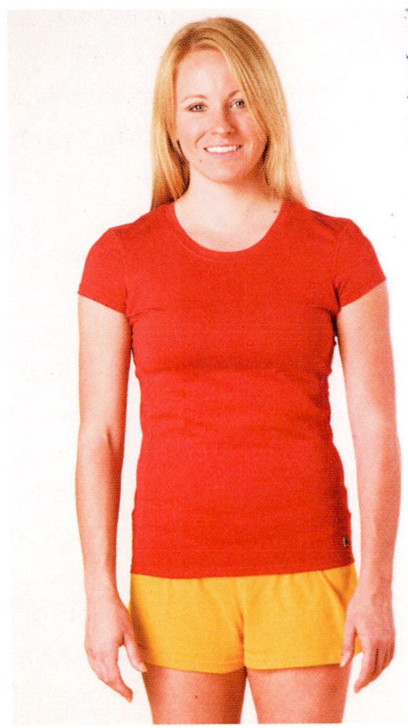

Figure 7-13
Scapular protraction: Anterior view

Table 7-4
Shoulder Position

Observation	Muscles Suspected to Be Tight	Plane of View
Shoulders not level	Upper trapezius, levator scapula, rhomboids	Frontal
Asymmetry to midline	Lateral trunk flexors (flexed side)	Frontal
Protracted (forward, rounded)	Serratus anterior*, anterior scapulo-humeral muscles, upper trapezius	Sagittal
Medially rotated humerus	Pectoralis major, latissimus dorsi, subscapularis	Frontal
Kyphosis and depressed chest	Shoulder adductors, pectoralis minor, rectus abdominis, internal oblique	Sagittal

*Serratus anterior is usually tight with scapular protraction and is usually weak with scapular winging.

Deviation 5: Head Position

With good posture, the earlobe should align approximately over the acromion process, but given the many awkward postures and repetitive motions of daily life, a forward-head position is very common (Table 7-5) (Kendall et al., 2005). This altered position does not tilt the head downward, but simply shifts it forward so that the earlobe appears significantly forward of the acromioclavicular (AC) joint. To observe the presence of this imbalance, use the sagittal view, aligning the plumb line with the AC joint, and observe its position relative to the ear (Figure 7-14). A forward-head position represents tightness in the cervical extensors and lengthening of the cervical flexors. To demonstrate this point, a trainer can place one thumb on his or her manubrium (top of the sternum) and the index finger of the same hand on the chin. Slowly slide the head forward and observe how the spacing between the fingers increases, representing the change in muscle length. An alternative option for observing forward-head position is via the alignment of the cheek bone and the collarbone. With good posture, they should almost be in vertical alignment with each other. To demonstrate this point, have a client place one finger on his or her collar bone (aligned under the cheek) and place another finger on the cheek bone (aligned under the eye) as illustrated in Figure 7-15. From the sagittal plane, the trainer can observe the vertical alignment of the two fingers.

Table 7-5
Head Position

Observation	Muscles Suspected to Be Tight	Plane of View
Forward-head position	Cervical spine extensors, upper trapezius, levator scapulae	Sagittal

Figure 7-14
Alignment of the acromioclavicular joint with the ear

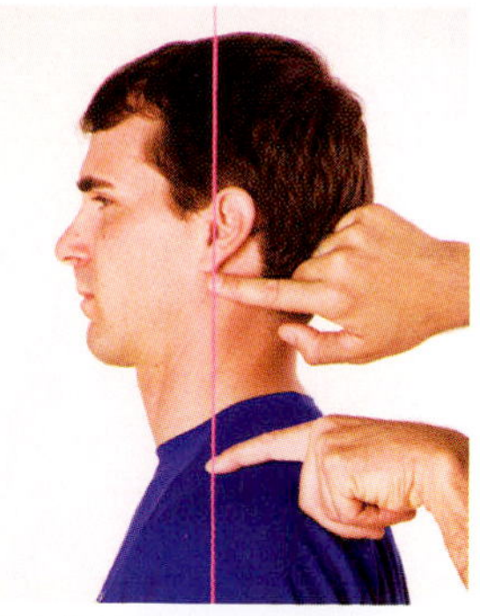
Good posture

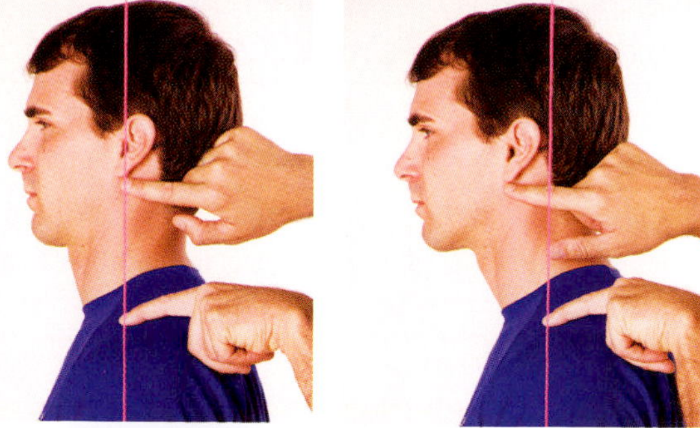
Forward-head position

Figure 7-15
Alignment of the collar bone and cheek bone

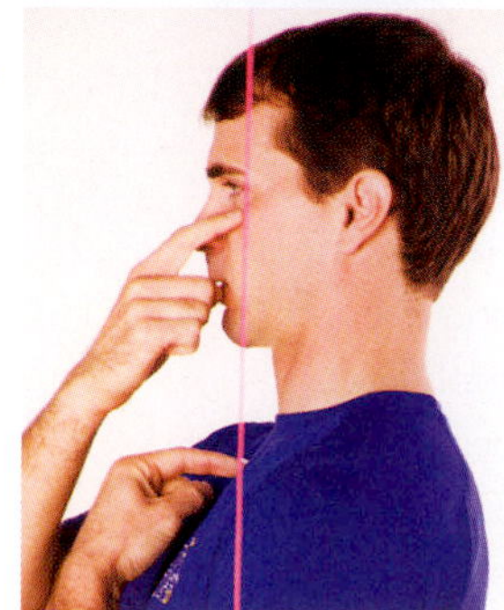
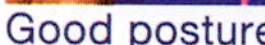
Good posture

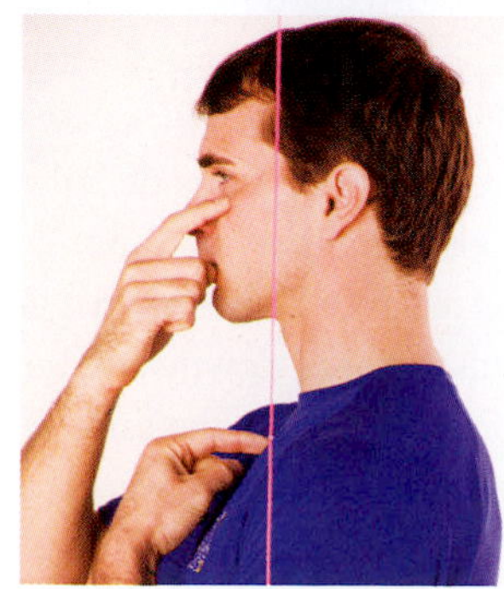
Forward-head position

The preceding information and techniques for assessing static posture have been adapted from The BioMechanics Method, an educational program created by ACE subject matter expert Justin Price, M.A. More in-depth information regarding postural assessments and corrective exercise can be obtained at www.TheBioMechanicsMethod.com.

Postural Assessment Checklist and Worksheets

When performing basic postural assessments, trainers can use the checklist provided in Figure 7-16 to guide themselves through their observations, and complete the worksheets provided in Figures 7-17 and 7-18 to mark any postural compensations they identify.

Movement Screens

Observing active movement is an effective method to determine the contribution that muscle imbalances and poor posture have on neural control, and also helps identify movement compensations (Whiting & Rugg, 2006; Sahrmann, 2002). When compensations occur during movement, it is usually indicative of some form of altered neural action, commonly referred to as "faulty neural control," which normally manifests due to muscle tightness or an imbalance between muscles acting at the joint.

Movement can essentially be broken down and described by five primary movements that people perform during many daily activities (Cook, 2003):

- Bending/raising and lifting/lowering movements (e.g., squatting)
- Single-leg movements
- Pushing movements (in vertical/horizontal planes) and resultant movement
- Pulling movements (in vertical/horizontal planes) and resultant movement
- Rotational movements

ADL are essentially the integration of one or more of these primary movements. For example, the action of picking up a child and turning to place the child in a car seat involves

Figure 7-16
Postural assessment checklist

Frontal View	
☐	Overall body symmetry: symmetrical alignment of the left and right hemispheres
☐	Ankle position: observe for pronation and supination
☐	Foot position: observe for inversion and eversion
☐	Knees: rotation and height discrepancies
☐	Hip adduction and shifting: observe for shifting to a side as witnessed by the position of the pubis in relation to the plumb line
☐	Alignment of the iliac crests
☐	Alignment of the torso: position of the umbilicus and sternum in relation to the plumb line
☐	Alignment of the shoulders
☐	Arm spacing: observe the space to the sides of the torso
☐	Hand position: observe the position relative to the torso
☐	Head position: alignment of the ears, nose, eyes, and chin
Posterior View	
☐	Overall body symmetry: symmetrical alignment of the left and right hemispheres
☐	Alignment of the spine: vertical alignment of the spinous processes (may require forward bending)
☐	Alignment of the scapulae: inferior angle of scapulae and presence of winged scapulae
☐	Alignment of the shoulders
☐	Head: alignment of the ears
Sagittal View	
☐	Overall body symmetry: symmetrical alignment of load-bearing joint landmarks with the plumb line
☐	Knees: flexion or extension
☐	Pelvic alignment for tilting: relationship of ASIS to PSIS
☐	Spinal curves: observe for thoracic kyphosis, lumbar lordosis, or flat-back position
☐	Shoulder position: forward rounding (protraction) of the scapulae
☐	Head position: neutral cervical curvature (versus forward position) and level (position above the clavicle)

Note: ASIS = Anterior superior iliac spine; PSIS = Posterior superior iliac spine

Figure 7-17
Anterior/posterior worksheet

Anterior View:			**Posterior View:**		
L	**R**	**Deviation**	**L**	**R**	**Deviation**
☐	☐	1. ______	☐	☐	1. ______
☐	☐	2. ______	☐	☐	2. ______
☐	☐	3. ______	☐	☐	3. ______
☐	☐	4. ______	☐	☐	4. ______
☐	☐	5. ______	☐	☐	5. ______
☐	☐	6. ______	☐	☐	6. ______
☐	☐	7. ______	☐	☐	7. ______

Circle or mark observed deviations

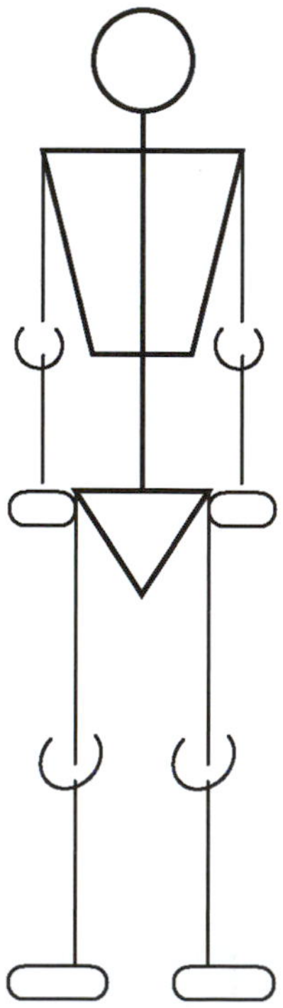

Circle or mark observed deviations

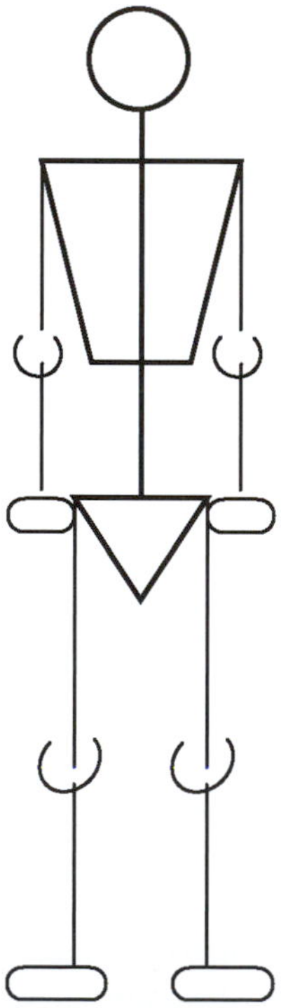

Figure 7-18
Sagittal worksheet

Sagittal: Left Side	Sagittal: Right Side
L **Deviation**	**R** **Deviation**
☐ 1. ______	☐ 1. ______
☐ 2. ______	☐ 2. ______
☐ 3. ______	☐ 3. ______
☐ 4. ______	☐ 4. ______
☐ 5. ______	☐ 5. ______
☐ 6. ______	☐ 6. ______
☐ 7. ______	☐ 7. ______
Circle or mark observed deviations	Circle or mark observed deviations

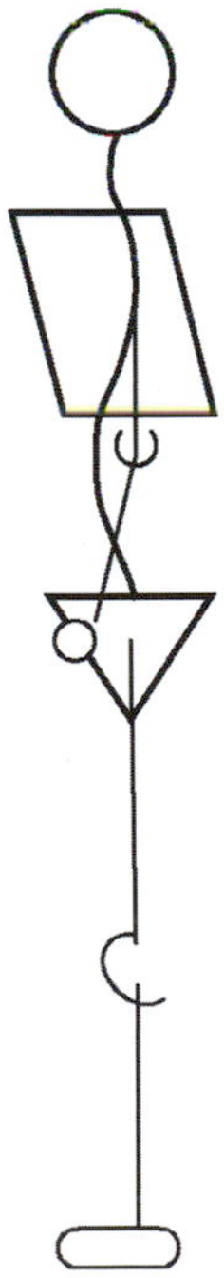

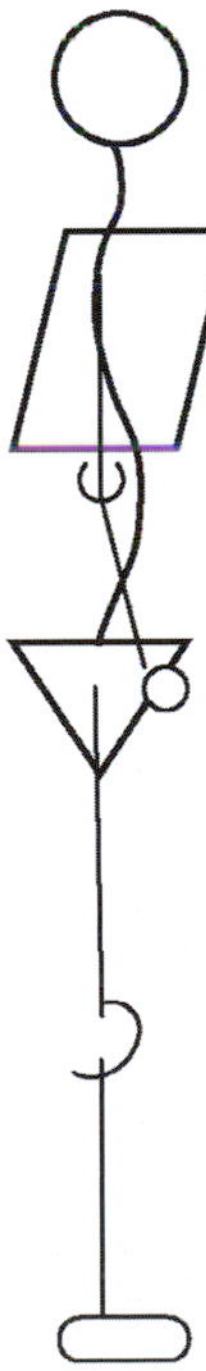

a squatting movement, a rotational movement, a possible single-leg movement if stepping is involved, a pushing movement, and finally a pulling movement to resist the effects of gravity as the child is lowered into the seat.

Movement screens help trainers observe the ability and efficiency with which a client performs many ADL. The movement screens, however, must be skill- and conditioning-level appropriate, and be specific to the client's needs. It is important to remember that almost any screen can evaluate functional capacity, as long as it is relevant to client needs and challenges, and provides useful feedback on movement efficiency (Sahrmann, 2002). Screens generally challenge clients with no recognized pathologies to perform basic movements and evaluate their ability to demonstrate appropriate levels of stability and mobility throughout the entire kinetic chain—namely, at the feet, knees, lumbo-pelvic-hip complex, shoulders, and head.

Clearing Tests

Prior to administering any movement screens, trainers should screen their clients for any potential contraindications associated with pain by using basic clearing tests. These tests may uncover issues that the individual did not know existed. Trainers should select clearing tests according to the movements that require evaluation. Remember, the objective when conducting clearing tests is *not* to uncover underlying pain that merits referral, but to ensure that pain is not exacerbated by movement. Any client who exhibits pain during a clearing test should be referred to his or her physician and should not perform additional assessments for that part of the body.

Cervical spine:

- From a seated position with the back resting against a backrest, the client performs the following movements while the personal trainer monitors for any indication of pain:
  - ✓ Move the chin to touch the chest (i.e., cervical flexion).
  - ✓ Tilt the head back until the face lies approximately parallel or near parallel to the floor (i.e., cervical **extension** without lumbar extension).
  - ✓ Drop the chin left and right to rest on, or within 1 inch (2.5 cm) of, the shoulder or collarbone.

Shoulder impingement:

- From a seated position with the back resting against a backrest, the client performs the following movement while the personal trainer monitors for any indication of pain:
  - ✓ Reach one arm across the chest to rest upon the opposite shoulder and slowly elevate the elbow as high as possible.

Low back:

- Starting from a prone position on a mat, the client performs the following movements while the personal trainer monitors for any indication of pain:
  - ✓ Slowly move into a "cobra pose" or trunk-extension position (body supported on the arms), producing lumbar extension, and compression in the vertebrae and shoulder joint (Figure 7-19).
  - ✓ Move into a quadruped (all-fours) position and slowly sit back on the heels with outstretched arms, producing lumbar and hip flexion (Figure 7-20).

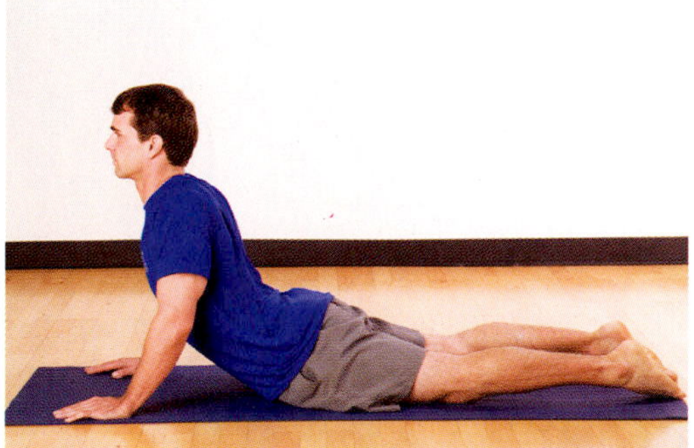

Figure 7-19
Low-back movement: Lumbar extension and compression in the vertebrae and shoulder joint

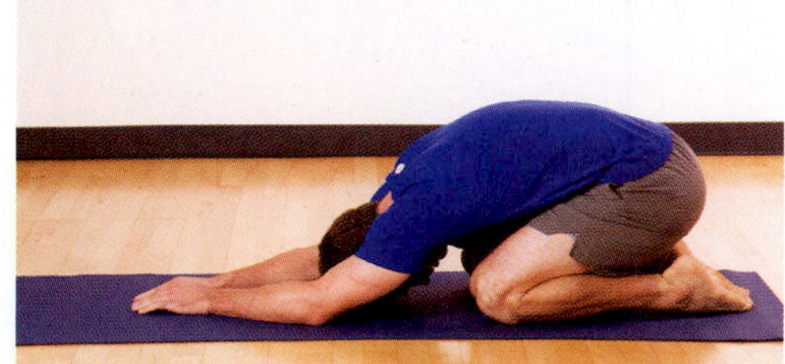

Figure 7-20
Low-back movement: Lumbar and hip flexion

Bend and Lift Screen

Objective: To examine symmetrical lower-extremity mobility and stability, and upper-extremity stability during a bend-and-lift movement

Equipment needed:

- Two 2- to 4-foot (0.6- to 1.2-m) dowels or broomsticks

Instructions:

- Briefly discuss the protocol so the client understands what is required.
- Ask the client to stand with the feet shoulder-width apart with the arms hanging freely to the sides.
- Place the two dowels on the floor adjacent to the outside of each foot.
- Ask the client to perform a series of basic bend-and-lift movements (i.e., a squatting movement) to grasp the dowels and lift them off the floor, holding the lowered position for one to two seconds to allow the trainer to make some brief observations before returning to the starting position. The number of repetitions performed is determined by the number needed to make the necessary evaluations.
  - ✓ Ask the client to pretend the dowels are 25-pound weights.
  - ✓ It is important to remember *not* to cue the client to use good technique, but instead observe his or her natural movement.

Observations (Table 7-6):

- Frontal view (Figure 7-21):
  - ✓ First repetition: Observe the stability of the foot (i.e., evidence of pronation, supination, eversion, **inversion**).
  - ✓ Second repetition: Observe the alignment of the knees over the second toe.
  - ✓ Third repetition: Observe the overall symmetry of the entire body over the base of support (i.e., evidence of a lateral shift or rotation).
- Sagittal view (Figure 7-22):
  - ✓ First repetition: Observe whether the heel remains in contact with the floor throughout the movement.
  - ✓ Second repetition: Determine whether the client exhibits "glute" or "knee" dominance (i.e., does he or she initiate the downward phase by driving the knees forward or pushing the hips backward?).
  - ✓ Third repetition: Observe whether the client achieves a parallel position between the tibia and torso in the lowered position (sometimes referred to as the "figure-4" position), while also observing whether he or she controls the descent to avoid resting the hamstrings against the calves.
  - ✓ Fourth repetition: Observe the degree of lordosis in the lumbar/thoracic spine during the lowering movement and while the client is in the lowered position (i.e., flat-to-neutral or demonstrated increased lordosis) and watch for excessive thoracic extension in the lowered position.
  - ✓ Fifth repetition: Observe any changes in head position during the lowering phase.

General interpretations:

- Identify origin(s) of movement limitation or compensation.
- Evaluate the impact on the entire kinetic chain.

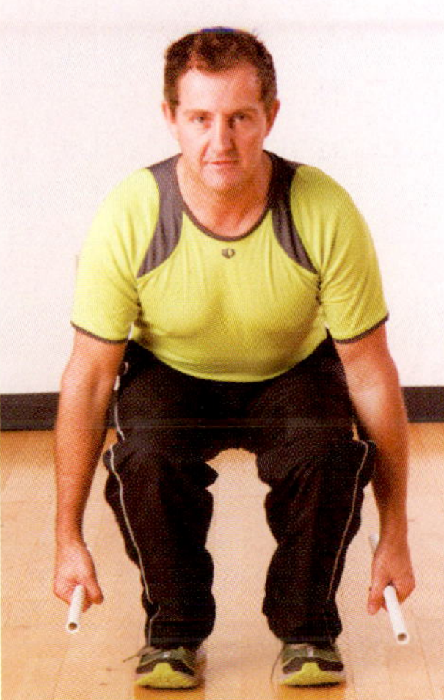

Figure 7-21
Bend and lift screen: Frontal view

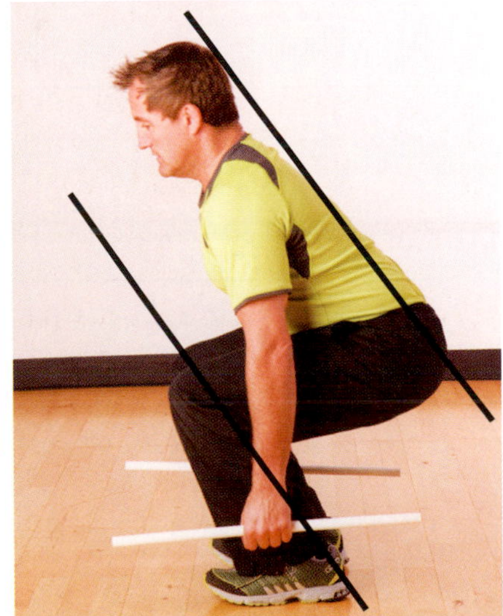

Figure 7-22
Bend and lift screen: Sagittal view

Table 7-6

Bend and Lift Screen

	View	Joint Location	Compensation	Key Suspected Compensations: Overactive (Tight)	Key Suspected Compensations: Underactive (Weak)
☐	Anterior	Feet	Lack of foot stability: Ankles collapse inward/ feet turn outward	Soleus, lateral gastrocnemius, peroneals	Medial gastrocnemius, gracilis, sartorius, tibialis group
☐	Anterior	Knees	Move inward	Hip adductors, tensor fascia latae	Gluteus medius and maximus
☐	Anterior	Torso	Lateral shift to a side	Side dominance and muscle imbalance due to potential lack of stability in the lower extremity during joint loading	
☐	Sagittal	Feet	Unable to keep heels in contact with the floor	Plantarflexors	None
☐	Sagittal	Hip and knee	Initiation of movement	Movement initiated at knees may indicate quadriceps and hip flexor dominance, as well as insufficient activation of the gluteus group	
☐	Sagittal	Tibia and torso relationship	Unable to achieve parallel between tibia and torso	Poor mechanics, lack of dorsiflexion due to tight plantarflexors (which normally allow the tibia to move forward)	
		Contact behind knee	Hamstrings contact back of calves	Muscle weakness and poor mechanics, resulting in an inability to stabilize and control the lowering phase	
☐	Sagittal	Lumbar and thoracic spine	Back excessively arches	Hip flexors, back extensors, latissimus dorsi	Core, rectus abdominis, gluteal group, hamstrings
			Back rounds forward	Latissimus dorsi, teres major, pectoralis major and minor	Upper back extensors
☐	Sagittal	Head	Downward	Increased hip and trunk flexion	
			Upward	Compression and tightness in the cervical extensor region	

Sources: Abelbeck, K.G. (2002). Biomechanical model and evaluation of a linear motion squat type exercise. *Journal of Strength and Conditioning Research,* 16, 516–524; Cook, G. (2003). *Athletic Body in Balance.* Champaign, Ill.: Human Kinetics; Donnelly, D.V. et al. (2006). The effect of directional gaze on kinematics during the squat exercise. *Journal of Strength and Conditioning Research,* 20, 145–150; Fry, A.C., Smith J.C., & Schilling, B.K. (2003). Effect of knee position on hip and knees torques during the barbell squat.*Journal of Strength and Conditioning Research,* 17, 629–633; Kendall, F.P. et al. (2005). *Muscles Testing and Function with Posture and Pain* (5th ed.). Baltimore, Md.: Lippincott Williams & Wilkins; Sahrmann, S.A. (2002). *Diagnosis and Treatment of Movement Impairment Syndromes.* St. Louis, Mo.: Mosby.

Hurdle Step Screen

Objective: To examine simultaneous mobility of one limb and stability of the **contralateral** limb while maintaining both hip and torso stabilization under a balance challenge of standing on one leg

Equipment needed:

- Two uprights to anchor string (chair or table legs)
- 36-inch (0.9-m) piece of string
- 48-inch (1.2-m) wooden or plastic dowel

Instructions:

- Briefly discuss the protocol so the client understands what is required.
- Fasten a piece of string spanning two points at a height even with the underside of the foot positioned parallel with the floor, when it is raised to a height that flexes the hip to 70 degrees (approximately just above halfway up the tibia).
- Have the client stand with both feet together and the front edge of the toes aligned directly beneath the string.
  - ✓Ultimately, this test should be performed with the feet positioned at gait-width [i.e., 2.8 to 3.5 inches (7 to 9 cm) apart] to simulate single-leg support during walking.
- Place the dowel across the client's shoulders, holding it parallel to the floor (similar to the placement of the bar during the traditional barbell squat).
- Instruct the client to load onto one leg and slowly lift the opposite leg over the string, flexing the hip to clear the string and then gently touching the heel of the raised leg to the floor in front of the string before returning to the starting position.
  - ✓The foot only needs to clear the string and does not need to be lifted as high as possible.
  - ✓It is important to remember *not* to cue the client to use good technique, instead observing the natural movement.
  - ✓Repetitions need to be performed slowly and with control.
- Have the client repeat the movement with the opposite leg, completing a series of repetitions with each leg so that the trainer can make the necessary evaluations.
- Allow sufficient practice trials to accommodate learning before administrating the test screens.

Observations (Table 7-7):

- Frontal view (Figure 7-23):
  - ✓First repetition: Observe the stability of the foot (i.e., evidence of pronation, supination, eversion, or inversion).
  - ✓Second repetition: Observe the alignment of the stance-leg knee over the foot (i.e., evidence of knee movement in any plane).
  - ✓Third repetition: Watch for excessive hip adduction greater than 2 inches (5.1 cm) as measured by excessive stance-leg adduction or downward hip-tilting toward the opposite side (Figure 7-24).
  - ✓Fourth repetition: Observe the stability of the torso (i.e., evidence of torso movement in any plane as demonstrated by movement of the dowel) (see Figure 7-24).
  - ✓Fifth repetition: Observe the alignment of the moving leg (i.e., lack of dorsiflexion at the ankle, deviation from the sagittal plane at the knee or ankle, or hiking of the moving hip) (see Figure 7-24).
- Sagittal view (Figure 7-25):
  - ✓First repetition: Observe the stability of the torso and stance leg.
  - ✓Second repetition: Observe the mobility of the hip (i.e., allowing 70 degrees of hip flexion without compensation—anterior tilting).

> Hip adduction involves weight transference over the stance leg while preserving hip, knee, and foot alignment. This weight transference requires a 1- to 2-inch (2.5- to 5-cm) lateral shift over the stance-leg, with a small hike in the stance-hip of 4 to 5 degrees or less.

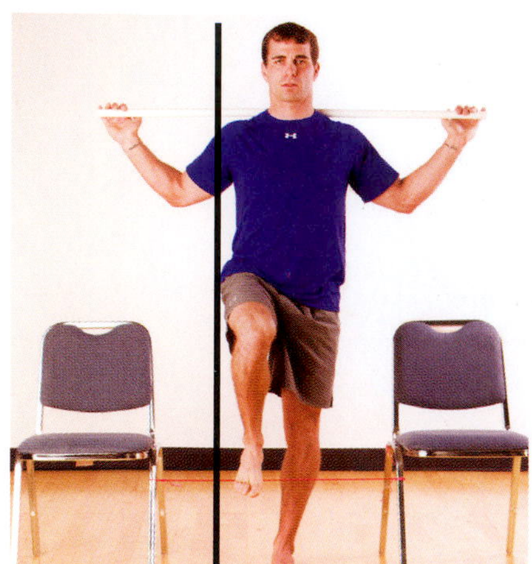
Figure 7-23
Hurdle step screen: Anterior view

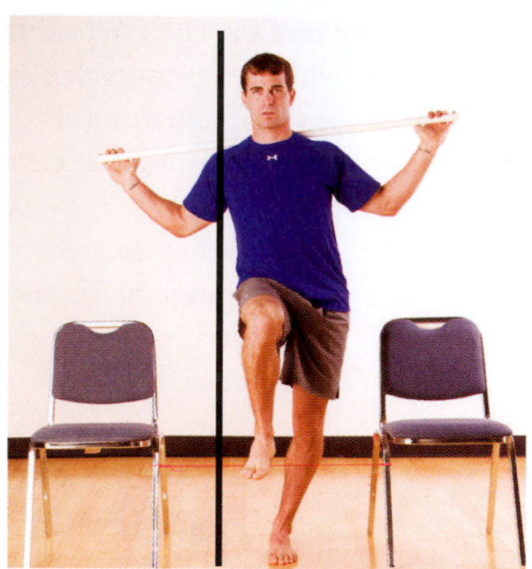
Figure 7-24
Hurdle step screen: Anterior view with compensations

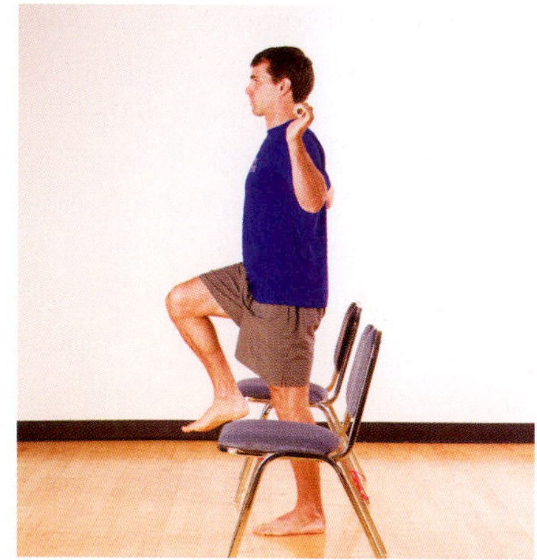
Figure 7-25
Hurdle step screen: Sagittal view

Table 7-7
Hurdle Step Screen

View		Joint Location	Compensation	Key Suspected Compensations: Overactive (Tight)	Key Suspected Compensations: Underactive (Weak)
☐	Anterior	Feet	Lack of foot stability: Ankles collapse inward/ feet turn outward	Soleus, lateral gastrocnemius, peroneals	Medial gastrocnemius, gracilis, sartorius, tibialis group, gluteus medius and maximus—inability to control internal rotation
☐	Anterior	Knees	Move inward	Hip adductors, tensor fascia latae	Gluteus medius and maximus
☐	Anterior	Hips	Hip adduction >2 inches (5.1 cm) Stance-leg hip rotation (inward)	Hip adductors, tensor fascia latae Stance-leg or raised-leg internal rotators	Gluteus medius and maximus Stance-leg or raised-leg external rotators
☐	Anterior	Torso	Lateral tilt, forward lean, rotation	Lack of core stability	
☐	Anterior	Raised-leg	Lack of ankle dorsiflexion Limb deviates from sagittal plane Hiking the raised hip	Ankle plantarflexors Raised-leg hip extensors Stance-leg hip flexors—limiting posterior hip rotation during raise	Ankle dorsiflexors Raised-leg hip flexors
☐	Sagittal	Pelvis and low back	Anterior tilt with forward torso lean Posterior tilt with hunched-over torso	Stance-leg hip flexors Rectus abdominis and hip extensors	Rectus abdominis and hip extensors Stance-leg hip flexors

Sources: Cook, G. (2003). *Athletic Body in Balance.* Champaign, Ill.: Human Kinetics; Kendall, F.P. et al. (2005). *Muscles Testing and Function with Posture and Pain* (5th ed.). Baltimore, Md.: Lippincott Williams & Wilkins; Sahrmann, S.A. (2002). *Diagnosis and Treatment of Movement Impairment Syndromes.* St. Louis, Mo.: Mosby.

General interpretations:

- Identify the origin(s) of movement limitation or compensation.
- Evaluate the impact on the entire kinetic chain.

Shoulder Push Stabilization Screen

Objective: To examine stabilization of the scapulothoracic joint during closed-kinetic-chain pushing movements

Instructions:

- Briefly discuss the protocol so the client understands what is required.
  - ✓The client presses his or her body off the ground as the trainer evaluates the ability to stabilize the scapulae against the thorax (ribcage) during pushing-type movements (Figure 7-26).
- Instruct the client to lie prone on the floor with arms abducted in the push-up position or bent-knee push-up position.
- Ask the client to perform several push-ups to full arm extension.
  - ✓Subjects should perform full push-ups; modify to bent-knee push-ups if necessary.
  - ✓It is important to remember *not* to cue the client to use good technique, but instead observe his or her natural movement.
  - ✓Repetitions need to be performed slowly and with control.

Observations (Table 7-8):

- Observe any notable changes in the position of the scapulae relative to the ribcage at both end-ranges of motion (i.e., the appearance of scapular "winging") (Figure 7-27).
- Observe for lumbar hyperextension in the press position.

General interpretations:

- Identify the origin(s) of movement limitation or compensation.
- Evaluate the impact on the entire kinetic chain.

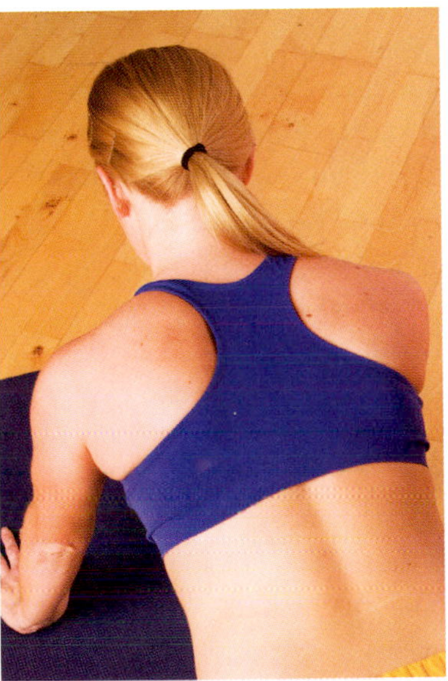

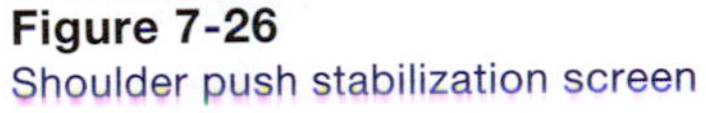

Figure 7-26
Shoulder push stabilization screen

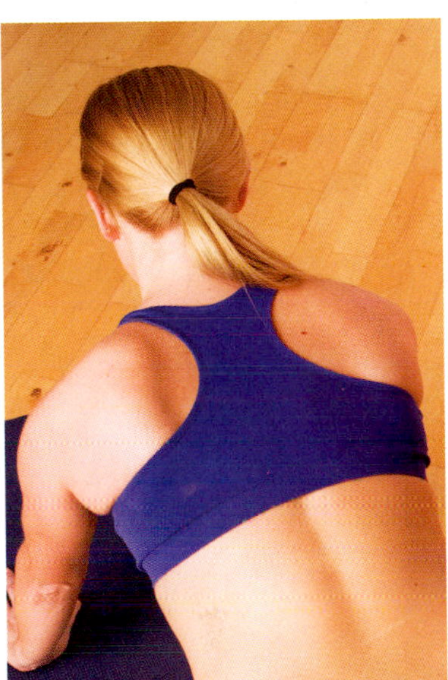

Figure 7-27
Shoulder push stabilization screen with scapular winging

Table 7-8
Shoulder Push Stabilization Screen

View		Joint Location	Compensation	Key Suspected Compensations
☐	Sagittal	Scapulothoracic	Exhibits "winging" during the push-up movement	Inability of the parascapular muscles (i.e., serratus anterior, trapezius, levator scapula, rhomboids) to stabilize the scapulae against the ribcage. Can also be due to a flat thoracic spine.
☐	Sagittal	Trunk	Hyperextension or "collapsing" of the low back	Lack of core, abdominal, and low-back strength, resulting in instability

Sources: Sahrmann, S.A. (2002). *Diagnosis and Treatment of Movement Impairment Syndromes.* St. Louis, Mo.: Mosby; Kendall, F.P. et al. (2005). *Muscles Testing and Function with Posture and Pain* (5th ed.). Baltimore, Md.: Lippincott Williams & Wilkins.

Shoulder Pull Stabilization Screen

Objective: To examine the client's ability to stabilize the scapulothoracic joint during closed-kinetic-chain pulling movements

Equipment needed:

- Yoga mat

Instructions:

- Briefly discuss the protocol so the client understands what is required.
  - ✓The objective is for the client to allow the shoulders to be lifted a few inches off the ground as the trainer evaluates the ability to stabilize the scapulae against the thorax (ribcage) during pulling-type movements.
- Instruct the client to lie supine on a mat with bent knees, flexing one shoulder with an extended elbow until the arm points vertically toward the ceiling.
- The client and trainer grasp each other's forearm to secure a tight grip (Figure 7-28).
  - ✓Ask the client to lock the elbow and maintain this position throughout the screen.
  - ✓Instruct the client to press the scapula toward the floor and try to maintain this position throughout the screen.
  - ✓Ask the client to stiffen the core, so that when he or she is lifted, the spine and shoulders will both lift together while he or she hinges at the hips. Instruct the client not to use the feet to push upward during the screen.
- The trainer assumes a split-stance position with a quarter-squat and, using the legs, gently and slowly lifts the client upward (raising the shoulders) until he or she is approximately 3 to 6 inches (8 to 15 cm) off the floor (Figure 7-29).
  - ✓It is important to remember *not* to cue the client to use good technique, but instead observe his or her natural movement.
  - ✓Observe the client's ability to maintain his or her scapula fixed against the rib cage and not let it protract during the lift.
  - ✓Perform one or two repetitions per arm, slowly and with control.
- Repeat the screen on the opposite side.

Observations (Table 7-9):

- Observe any bilateral discrepancies between the pulls on each arm.

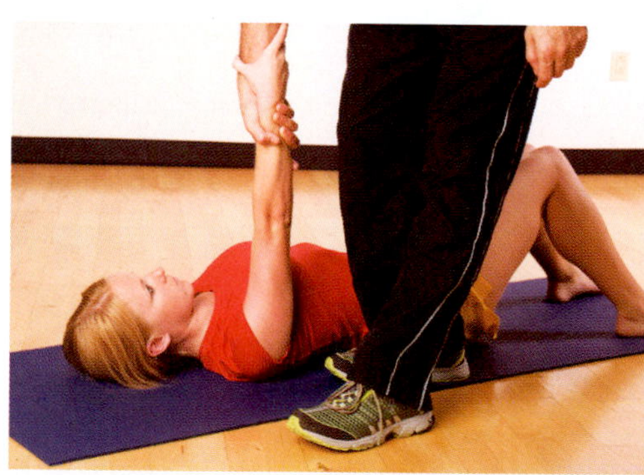

Figure 7-28
Shoulder pull stabilization screen: Starting position

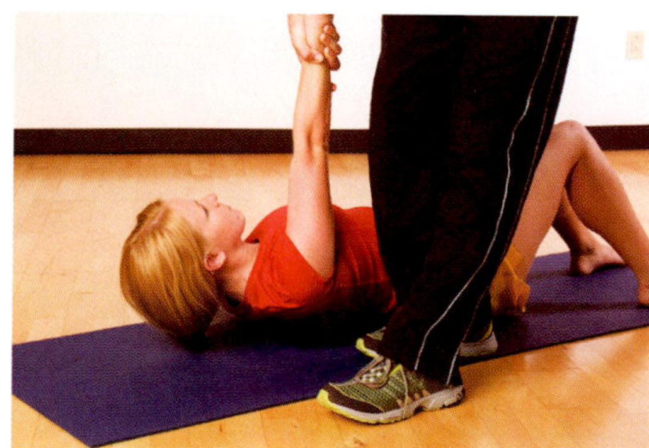

Figure 7-29
Shoulder pull stabilization screen: Test position

Table 7-9
Shoulder Pull Stabilization Screen

View		Joint Location	Compensation	Key Suspected Compensations
☐	Sagittal	Scapulothoracic	Scapula moves into protraction during the pull	Inability of the parascapular muscles (i.e., serratus anterior, trapezius, levator scapula, rhomboids) to stabilize the scapulae against the ribcage
☐	Transverse	Trunk	Rotation during the pull	Lack of core stability

Source: Cook, G. (2003). *Athletic Body in Balance.* Champaign, Ill.: Human Kinetics.

- Observe the ability to stabilize the trunk during the pull movement (i.e., the ability of the core to stiffen and lift the hips with the shoulders and resist trunk rotation during the lift).

General interpretations:

- Identify the origin(s) of movement limitation or compensation.
- Evaluate the impact on the entire kinetic chain.

Thoracic Spine Mobility Screen

Objective: To examine bilateral mobility of the thoracic spine. Lumbar spine rotation is considered insignificant, as it only offers approximately 15 degrees of rotation.

Equipment:

- Chair
- Squeezable ball or block
- 48-inch (1.2-m) dowel

Instructions:

- Briefly discuss the protocol so the client understands what is required.
- Instruct the client to sit upright toward the front edge of the seat with the feet together and firmly placed on the floor. The client's back should not touch the backrest.
- Place a squeezable ball or block between the knees and a dowel across the front of the shoulders, instructing the client to hold the bar in the hands (i.e., front barbell squat grip) (Figure 7-30).
- While maintaining an upright and straight posture, the client squeezes the ball to immobilize the hips and gently rotates left and right to an end-range of motion without any bouncing (Figure 7-31).
  - ✓ It is important to remember *not* to cue the client to use good technique, but instead observe his or her natural movement.
  - ✓ Ask the client to perform a few repetitions in each direction, slowly and with control.

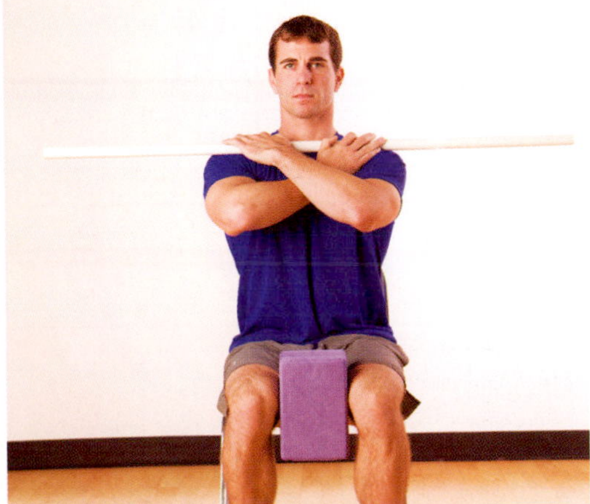

Figure 7-30
Thoracic spine mobility screen: Starting position

Observation (Table 7-10):

- Observe any bilateral discrepancies between the rotations in each direction.

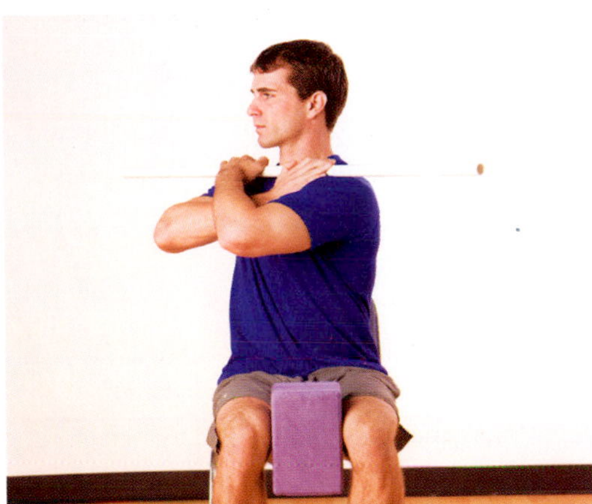

Figure 7-31
Thoracic spine mobility screen: End position

Table 7-10
Thoracic Spine Mobility Screen

View		Joint Location	Compensation	Possible Biomechanical Problems
☐	Transverse	Trunk	None if trunk rotation achieves 45 degrees in each direction	
☐	Transverse	Trunk	Bilateral discrepancy (Assuming no existing congenital issues in the spine)	Side-dominance Differences in paraspinal development Torso rotation, perhaps associated with some hip rotation *Note:* Lack of thoracic mobility will negatively impact glenohumeral mobility

Source: Sahrmann, S.A. (2002). *Diagnosis and Treatment of Movement Impairment Syndromes.* St. Louis, Mo.: Mosby.

General interpretations:

- Identify the origin(s) of movement limitation or compensation. As an individual rotates, the facet joints of each vertebra experience shearing forces against each other. One way to reduce this force and promote greater movement is to laterally flex the trunk during the movement or at the end-range of movement. This screen evaluates trunk rotation in the transverse plane. Therefore, any lateral flexion of the trunk (dowel tilting up or down) must be avoided.
- Evaluate the impact on the entire kinetic chain. Remember that the lumbar spine generally exhibits limited rotation of approximately 15 degrees (Sahrmann, 2002), with the balance of trunk rotation occurring through the thoracic spine. If thoracic spine mobility is limited, the body strives to gain movement in alternative planes within the lumbar spine (e.g., increase in lordosis to promote greater rotation).

Flexibility and Muscle-length Testing

During the initial assessments of posture and movement, a personal trainer may opt to assess the **flexibility** of specific muscle groups that he or she suspects demonstrate tightness or limitations to movement. While Table 7-11 provides

Table 7-11

Average Range of Motion for Healthy Adults

Joint and Movement	ROM (°)	Joint and Movement	ROM (°)
Shoulder/Scapulae		*Thoraco-lumbar Spine*	
Flexion	150–180	Lumbar flexion	40–45
Extension	50–60	Thoracic flexion	30–40
Abduction	180	Lumbar extension	30–40
Internal/medial rotation	70–80	Thoracic extension	20–30
External/lateral rotation	90	Lumbar rotation	10–15
Shoulder horizontal adduction	90*	Thoracic rotation	35
Shoulder horizontal abduction	30–40*	Lumbar lateral flexion	20
		Thoracic lateral flexion	20–25
Elbow		*Hip*	
Flexion	145	Flexion	100–120
Extension	0	Extension	10–30
Radio-ulnar		Abduction	40–45
Pronation	90	Adduction	20–30
Supination	90	Internal/medial rotation	35–45
		External/lateral rotation	45–60
Wrist		*Knee*	
Flexion	80	Flexion	125–145
Extension	70	Extension	0–10
Radial deviation	20	*Ankle*	
Ulnar deviation	45	Dorsiflexion	20
		Plantarflexion	45–50
Cervical Spine		*Subtalar*	
Flexion	45–50	Inversion	30–35
Extension	45–75	Eversion	15–20
Lateral flexion	45		
Rotation	65–75		

*Zero point (0 degrees) is with the arms positioned in frontal-plane abduction at shoulder height.

Source: Adapted from Kendall, F.P. et al. (2005). *Muscles Testing and Function with Posture and Pain* (5th ed.). Baltimore, Md.: Lippincott Williams & Wilkins.

normal ranges of motion for healthy adults at each joint, specific muscle groups that frequently demonstrate tightness or limitations to movement are discussed in this section. Figure 7-32 can be used to keep records when conducting the flexibility assessments presented in this section.

Figure 7-32
Worksheet for conducting flexibility assessments

Thomas Test

Left hip:	Normal ❑	Tight ❑	Right hip:	Normal ❑	Tight ❑
Additional notes:__________			Additional notes:__________		

Passive Straight-leg Raise

Left Hamstrings:	Normal ❑	Tight ❑	Right Hamstrings:	Normal ❑	Tight ❑
Additional notes:__________			Additional notes:__________		

Shoulder Flexion

Left shoulder:	Normal ❑	Tight ❑	Right shoulder:	Normal ❑	Tight ❑
Additional notes:__________			Additional notes:__________		

Shoulder Extension

Left shoulder:	Normal ❑	Tight ❑	Right shoulder:	Normal ❑	Tight ❑
Additional notes:__________			Additional notes:__________		

Internal Rotation

Left shoulder:	Normal ❑	Tight ❑	Right shoulder:	Normal ❑	Tight ❑
Additional notes:__________			Additional notes:__________		

External Rotation

Left shoulder:	Normal ❑	Tight ❑	Right shoulder:	Normal ❑	Tight ❑
Additional notes:__________			Additional notes:__________		

Apley's Scratch Test

Left reach-under:	Normal ❑	Tight ❑	Right reach-under:	Normal ❑	Tight ❑
Additional notes:__________			Additional notes:__________		
Left reach-over:	Normal ❑	Tight ❑	Right reach-over:	Normal ❑	Tight ❑
Additional notes:__________			Additional notes:__________		

Thomas Test for Hip Flexion/Quadriceps Length

Objective: To assess the length of the muscles involved in hip flexion. This test can actually assess the length of the primary hip flexors.

- Hip flexors or iliopsoas
- Rectus femoris (one of the four quadriceps muscles)

This test should not be conducted on clients suffering from low-back pain, unless cleared by their physician.

Equipment needed:

- Stable table

Instructions:

- Given the nature of the movement associated with this test, trainers may want to consider draping a towel over the client's groin area.
- Explain the objective of the test and allow a warm-up if necessary.
- Instruct the client to sit at the end of a table with the mid-thigh aligned with the table edge (Figure 7-33). Place one hand behind the client's back and the other under his or her thighs.
- While supporting the client, instruct him or her to gently flex both thighs toward the chest, and gradually assist as the client rolls back onto the table to touch the back and shoulders to the table top.

✓ Instruct the client to slowly pull one thigh (hip) toward the chest, reaching with both hands to grasp the thigh or the area behind the knee without raising or moving the torso.

✓ Ask the client to slowly relax the opposite leg, allowing the knee to slowly fall toward the table and the lower leg to hang freely off the table edge [a 1-inch (2.5 cm) spacing between the back of the knee and the table edge is adequate] (Figure 7-34).

Observations:

- Observe whether the back of the lowered thigh touches the table (hips positioned in 10 degrees of extension).
- Observe whether the knee of the lowered leg achieves 80 degrees of flexion.
- Observe whether the knee remains aligned straight or falls into internal or external rotation.

General interpretations:

- Use the information provided in Table 7-12 to determine the location and identity of the tight or limiting muscles.

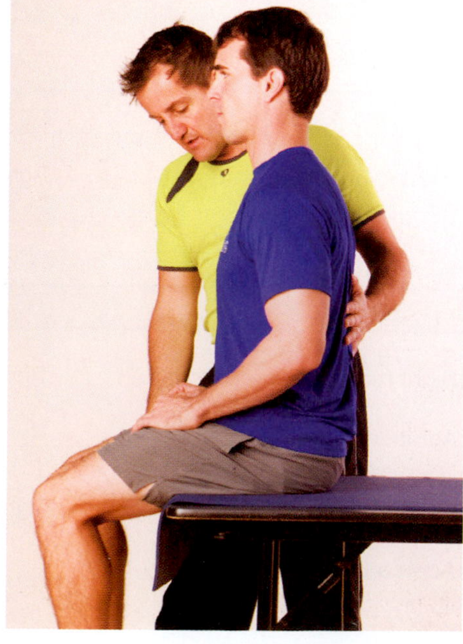

Figure 7-33
Thomas test: Starting position

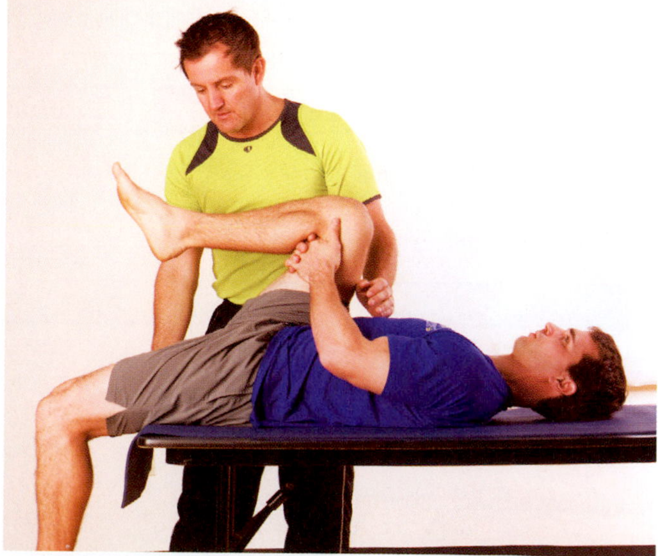

Figure 7-34
Thomas test: Test position

Table 7-12
Interpretation of the Thomas Test

Movement/Limitation	Suspected Muscle Tightness
With the back and sacrum flat, the back of the lowered thigh does not touch the table and the knee cannot flex to 80 degrees.	Primary hip flexor muscles
With the back and sacrum flat, the back of the lowered thigh does not touch the table, but the knee does flex to 80 degrees.	The iliopsoas, which is preventing the hip from rotating posteriorly (this would allow the back of the thigh to touch the table)
With the back and sacrum flat, the back of the lowered thigh does touch the table, but the knee does not flex to 80 degrees.	The rectus femoris, which does not allow the knee to bend

Source: Adapted from Kendall, F.P. et al. (2005). *Muscles Testing and Function with Posture and Pain* (5th ed.). Baltimore, Md.: Lippincott Williams & Wilkins.

Passive Straight-leg (PSL) Raise

Objective: To assess the length of the hamstrings

Equipment:

- Stable table or exercise mat

Instructions:

- Explain the objective of the test and allow a warm-up if necessary.
- Instruct the client to lie supine on a mat or table with the legs extended and the low back and sacrum flat against the surface.
- Place one hand under the calf of the leg that will be raised while instructing the client to keep the opposite leg extended on the mat or table. Restrain that leg from moving or rising during the test.
- Slide the other hand under the lumbar spine into the space between the client's back and the mat or table (Figure 7-35).
- Advise the client to gently plantarflex his or her ankles to point the toes away from the body. This position avoids a test limitation due to a tight gastrocnemius muscle (which would limit knee extension with the ankle in dorsiflexion). Additionally, a straight-leg raise with dorsiflexion may increase tension within the sciatic nerve and create some discomfort.
- Slowly raise the one leg, asking the client to keep that knee loosely extended throughout the movement.
  - ✓ Continue to raise the leg until firm pressure can be felt from the low back pressing down against the hand (Figure 7-36).
  - ✓ This indicates an end-range of motion of the hamstrings with movement now occurring as the pelvis rotates posteriorly.
- Throughout the movement, the client needs to maintain extension in the opposite leg and keep the sacrum and low back flat against the mat or table.
  - ✓ If the test is performed with the opposite hip in slight flexion, this allows the

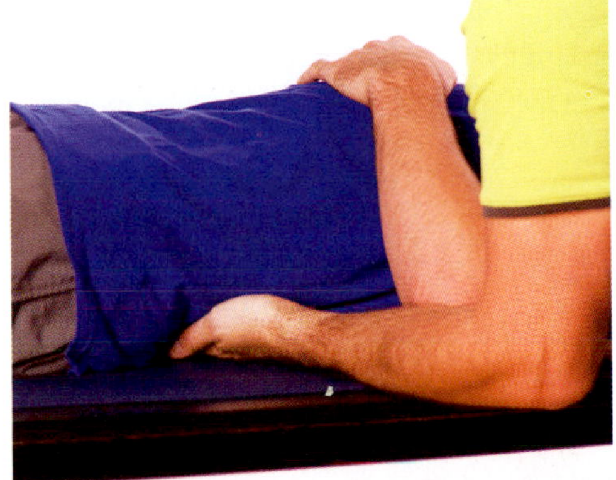

Figure 7-35
PSL raise: Trainer's hand position

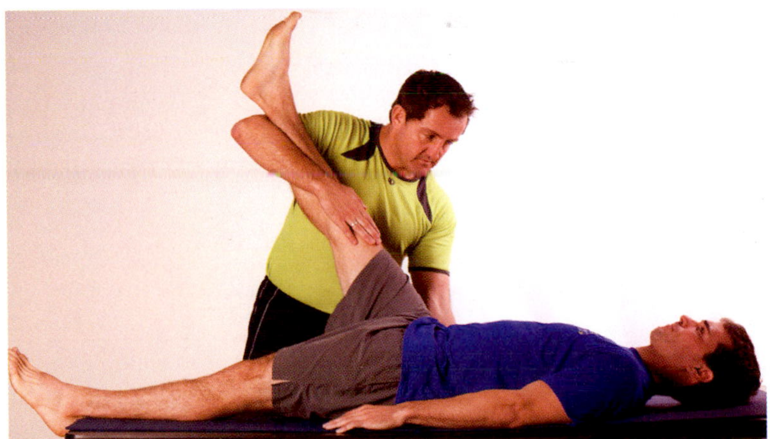

Figure 7-36
PSL raise: Test position

pelvis more freedom to move into a posterior tilt, allowing a greater range of motion and falsely increasing the length of the hamstrings.

Observation:

- Note the degree of movement attained from the table or mat that is achieved before the spine compresses the hand under the low back or the opposite leg begins to show visible signs of lifting off the table or mat.
  - ✓The mat or table represents 0 degrees.
  - ✓The leg perpendicular to the mat or table represents 90 degrees.

General interpretation:

- Use the information provided in Table 7-13 to determine the limitation(s).

Table 7-13

Interpretation of the Passive Straight-leg Raise

Movement/Limitation	Hamstrings Length
The raised leg achieves ≥80 degrees of movement before the pelvis rotates posteriorly.	Normal hamstrings length
The raised leg achieves <80 degrees of movement before the pelvis rotates posteriorly or there are any visible signs in the opposite leg lifting off the mat or table.	Tight hamstrings

Source: Kendall, F.P. et al. (2005). *Muscles Testing and Function with Posture and Pain* (5th ed.). Baltimore, Md.: Lippincott Williams & Wilkins.

Shoulder Mobility

Apley's scratch test involves multiple and simultaneous movements of the scapulothoracic and glenohumeral joints in all three planes. This represents a challenge in evaluating shoulder movement and identifying movement limitations. To identify the source of the limitation, trainers can first perform various isolated movements in single planes to locate potentially problematic movements. Consequently, the scratch test is completed in conjunction with:

- The shoulder flexion-extension test
- An internal-external rotation test of the humerus

Shoulder Flexion and Extension

Objective: To assess the degree of shoulder flexion and extension. This test should be performed in conjunction with Apley's scratch test (see page 165) to determine if the limitation occurs with shoulder flexion or extension.

Equipment needed:

- Exercise mat
- Pillow (optional)

Instructions:

- Explain the purpose of the test.
- Shoulder flexion:
  - ✓Instruct the client to lie supine on a mat, with the back flat and a bent-knee position (knees and second toe aligned with the ASIS), and with the arms at the sides.
  - ✓Have the client engage the abdominal muscles to hold a neutral spinet without raising the hips from the mat.
  - ✓Instruct the client to raise both arms simultaneously into shoulder flexion, moving them overhead, keeping them close to the sides of the head, and bringing them down to touch the floor or as close to the floor as possible (Figure 7-37).
    - The client must maintain extended elbows and neutral wrist position (the arms will naturally rotate internally during this movement).
    - Have the client avoid any arching in the low back during the movement.
    - Have the client avoid any depression of the ribcage, which may pull the shoulders off the mat.
- Shoulder extension:
  - ✓Instruct the client to lie prone, extending both legs, with arms at the sides, and resting the forehead gently on a pillow or the mat.
  - ✓Ask the client to slowly raise both arms simultaneously into extension, lifting them off the mat while keeping the arms close to the sides (Figure 7-38) (the arms will naturally rotate internally during this movement).

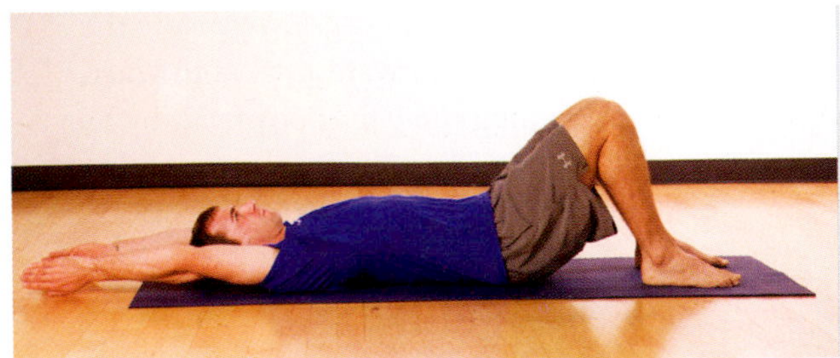

Figure 7-37
Shoulder flexion test

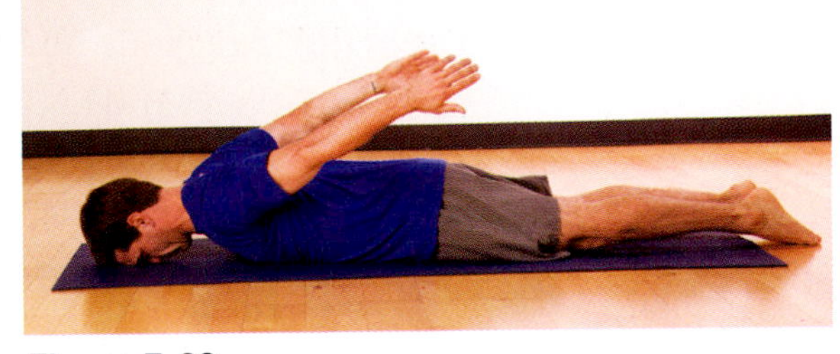

Figure 7-38
Shoulder extension test

- A small amount of extension in the thoracic spine is acceptable during the movement.
- The client should avoid any arching in the low back or any rotation of the torso during the movement.
- The client should avoid any attempts to lift the chest or head off the mat during the movement.

Observations:
- Measure the degree of movement in each direction.
- Note any bilateral differences between the left and right arms in performing both movements.

General interpretations:
- Use the information provided in Table 7-14 to determine the limitation(s) in this flexibility test.

Table 7-14
Interpretation of the Shoulder Flexion and Extension Test

Movement/Limitation—Flexion	Shoulder Mobility
Ability to flex the shoulders to 170–180 degrees (hands touching/nearly touching floor)	Good shoulder mobility
Inability to flex the shoulders to 170 degrees or discrepancies between the limbs	Potential tightness in the pectoralis major and minor, latissimus dorsi, teres major, rhomboids, and subscapularis Tightness in the latissimus dorsi will force the low back to arch. Tightness of the pectoralis minor may tilt the scapulae forward (anterior tilt) and prevent the arms from touching the floor. Tight abdominals may depress the ribcage, tilting the scapulae forward (anterior tilt), and prevent the arms from touching the floor. Thoracic kyphosis may round the thoracic spine and prevent the arms from touching the floor.
Movement/Limitation—Extension	**Shoulder Mobility**
Ability to extend the shoulders to 50–60 degrees off the floor	Good shoulder mobility
Inability to extend the shoulders to 50 degrees or discrepancies between the limbs	Potential tightness in pectoralis major, abdominals, subscapularis, certain shoulder flexors (anterior deltoid), coracobrachialis, and biceps brachii Tightness in the abdominals may prevent normal extension of the thoracic spine and ribcage. Tightness in the biceps brachii may prevent adequate shoulder extension with an extended elbow (but may permit extension with a bent elbow).

Sources: Kendall, F.P. et al. (2005). *Muscles Testing and Function with Posture and Pain* (5th ed.). Baltimore, Md.: Lippincott Williams & Wilkins; Houglum, P.A. (2005). *Therapeutic Exercise for Musculoskeletal Injuries* (2nd ed). Champaign, Ill.: Human Kinetics.

Internal and External Rotation of the Humerus at the Shoulder

Objective: To assess internal (medial) and external (lateral) rotation of the humerus at the shoulder joint. This test should be performed in conjunction with Apley's scratch test to determine if the limitation occurs with internal or external rotation of the humerus (see page 165).

Equipment needed:

- Mat

Instructions:

- Explain the purpose of the test.
- Instruct the client to lie supine, with his or her back flat on a mat in a bent-knee position (knees and second toe aligned with the ASIS) (see Figure 9-15, page 257).
- Ask the client to abduct the arms to 90 degrees, with a 90-degree bend at the elbows and the forearms perpendicular to the mat (i.e., pointing up toward the ceiling).
  - ✓The upper arms *must* remain aligned with the shoulders throughout the test.
  - ✓The backs of the upper arms should rest against the mat throughout the test.
- External (lateral) rotation to evaluate medial rotators
  - ✓Ask the client to slowly rotate his or her forearms backward toward the mat, aiming to rest the forearms and the backs of the hands on the mat adjacent to the head, while maintaining the 90-degree bend at the elbows (Figure 7-39).
    - ○ The client should engage the abdominals to avoid arching the low back, and avoid flexing the spine forward.
    - ○ The client should maintain a neutral wrist position throughout the movement.
- Internal (medial) rotation to evaluate lateral rotators
  - ✓Have the client return to the starting position (forearms perpendicular to the mat).
  - ✓Ask the client to slowly rotate the forearms forward toward the mat, turning the palms downward while maintaining the 90-degree bend at the elbows (Figure 7-40).
    - ○ The client should avoid raising the shoulders off the table or flexing the spine forward.
    - ○ The client must maintain a neutral wrist position throughout the movement.

Observations:

- Measure the degree of movement in each direction.
- Note any bilateral differences between the left and right arms in performing both movements.

General interpretation:

- Use the information provided in Table 7-15 to determine the limitation(s) in this flexibility test.

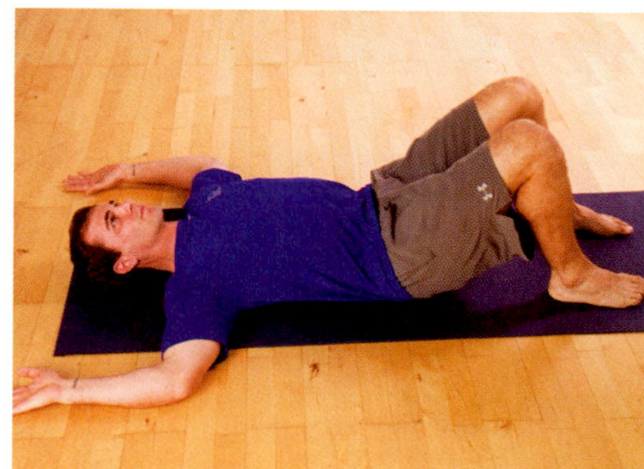

Figure 7-39
External (lateral) shoulder rotation

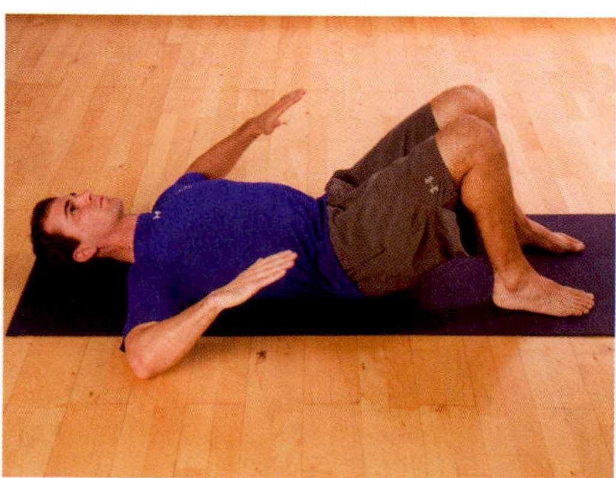

Figure 7-40
Internal (medial) shoulder rotation

Table 7-15

Interpretation of the External and Internal Rotation Test

Movement/Limitation—External/Lateral Rotation	Shoulder Mobility
Ability to externally rotate the forearms 90 degrees to touch the mat	Good mobility in the internal (medial) rotators, allowing the joint to move through the full range
Inability to reach the floor or discrepancies between the limbs	Potential tightness in the medial rotators of the arm (i.e., subscapularis) The joint capsule and ligaments may also be tight and limit rotation.
Movement/Limitation—Internal/Medial Rotation	**Shoulder Mobility**
Ability to internally rotate the forearms 70 degrees toward the mat (i.e., forearms are 20 degrees off the mat)	Good mobility in the external (lateral) rotators, allowing the joint to move through the full range
Inability to internally rotate the forearm 70 degrees, or discrepancies between the limbs	Potential tightness in the lateral rotators of the arm (i.e., infraspinatus and teres minor) The joint capsule and ligaments may also be tight and limit rotation.

Sources: Kendall, F.P. et al. (2005). *Muscles Testing and Function with Posture and Pain* (5th ed.). Baltimore, Md.: Lippincott Williams & Wilkins; Houglum, P.A. (2005). *Therapeutic Exercise for Musculoskeletal Injuries* (2nd ed). Champaign, Ill.: Human Kinetics.

Apley's Scratch Test for Shoulder Mobility

Objective: To assess simultaneous movements of the shoulder girdle (primarily the scapulothoracic and glenohumeral joints).

Movements include:

- Shoulder extension and flexion
- Internal and external rotation of the humerus at the shoulder
- Scapular **abduction** and adduction

Instructions:

- Explain the purpose of the test and allow a warm-up if necessary (e.g., forward and rearward arm circles).
- Shoulder flexion, external rotation, and scapular abduction
  - ✓From a sitting or standing position, the client raises one arm overhead, bending the elbow and rotating the arm outward while reaching behind the head with the palm facing inward to touch the medial border of the contralateral scapula or to reach down the spine (touching vertebrae) as far as possible (Figure 7-41).
  - ✓The client should avoid any excessive arching in the low back or rotation of the torso during the movement.
  - ✓Have the client repeat the test with the opposite arm.

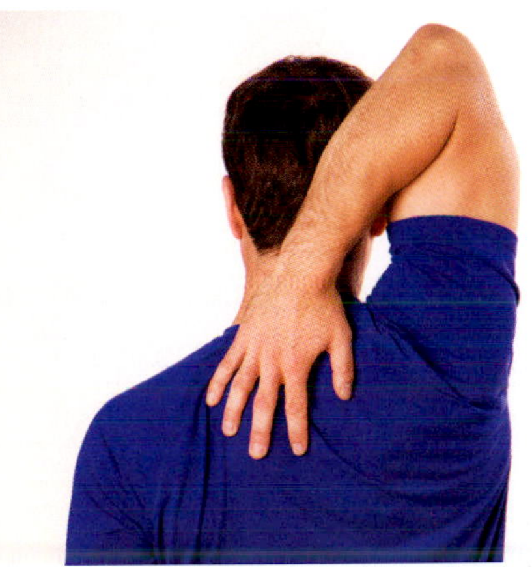

Figure 7-41
Apley's scratch test: Shoulder flexion, external rotation, and scapular abduction

- Shoulder extension, internal rotation, and scapular adduction
  - ✓From a sitting or standing position, the client reaches one arm behind the back, bending the elbow and rotating the arm inward with the palm facing outward to touch the inferior angle of the contralateral scapula or to reach up the spine (touching vertebrae) as far as possible (Figure 7-42).
  - ✓The client should avoid any excessive arching in the low back or rotation of the torso during the movement.
  - ✓Have the client repeat the test with the opposite arm.

Observations:

- Note the client's ability to touch the medial border of the contralateral scapula or how

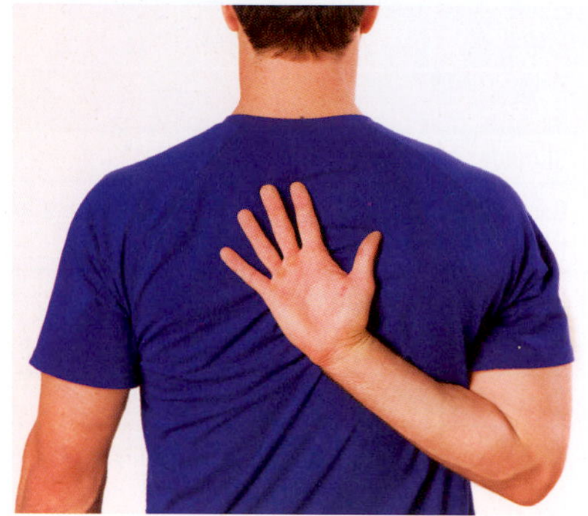

Figure 7-42
Apley's scratch test: Shoulder extension, internal rotation, and scapular adduction

far down the spine he or she can reach with shoulder flexion and external rotation.

- Note the client's ability to touch the opposite inferior angle of the scapula or how far up the spine he or she can reach with shoulder extension and internal rotation.
- Observe any bilateral differences between the left and right arms in performing both movements.

General interpretations:

- Use the information provided in Table 7-16 to determine the limitation(s) in this flexibility test.

Balance and the Core

Given the importance of balance and the condition of the core musculature to fitness and overall quality of life, these baseline assessments should be collected to evaluate the need for comprehensive balance training and core conditioning during the early stages of a conditioning program. While dynamic balance correlates more closely with people's daily activities, these tests are generally movement-specific and quite complex. Consequently, trainers should aim to first evaluate the basic level of static balance that a client exhibits by using the sharpened Romberg test or the stork-stand test. Table 7-17 can be used to record the client's performance on the balance and core assessments presented in this chapter.

Table 7-16
Interpretation of Apley's Scratch Test

Movement/Limitation	Shoulder Mobility*
Ability to touch specific landmarks	Good shoulder mobility
Inability to reach or touch the specific landmarks or discrepancies between the limbs	Requires further evaluation to determine the source of the limitation (i.e., which of the movements is problematic) • Shoulder flexion and extension • Internal and external rotation of the humerus • Scapula abduction and adduction

*Tightness of the joint capsules and ligaments may also contribute to limitations. It is common to see greater restriction on the dominant side due to increased muscle mass.

Source: Kendall, F.P. et al. (2005). *Muscles Testing and Function with Posture and Pain* (5th ed.). Baltimore, Md.: Lippincott Williams & Wilkins.

Sharpened Romberg Test

Sources: Black et al., 1982; Newton, 1989

Objective: To assess static balance by standing with a reduced base of support while removing visual sensory information

Equipment:

- Flat, non-slip surface
- Stopwatch

Instructions:

- Explain the purpose of the test.
- Instruct the client to remove his or her shoes and stand with one foot directly in front of the other (tandem or heel-to-toe position), with the eyes open.
- Ask the client to fold his or her arms across the chest, touching each hand to the opposite shoulder (Figure 7-43).

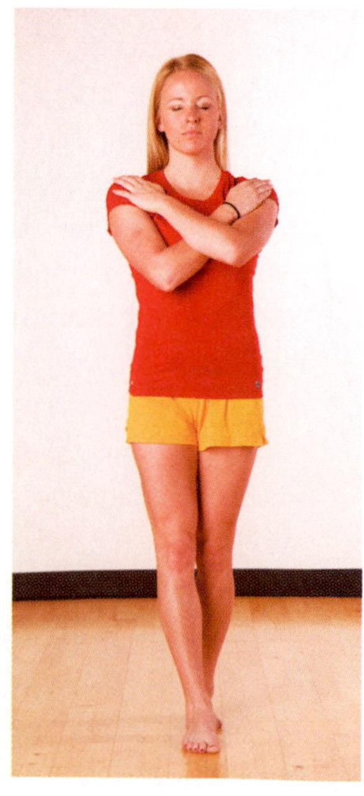

Figure 7-43
Sharpened Romberg test

Table 7-17
Balance and Core Worksheet

Balance	Right Leg			Left Leg	Difference	
Sharpened Romberg test	______ seconds			______ seconds	______ seconds	
Stork-stand balance test	______ seconds			______ seconds	______ seconds	
Core Function	**Change in Pressure**			**Score**	**Analysis**	
Blood pressure cuff test	Increase	No change	Decrease	+/– ______ mmHg	Need work	Maintain

- Allow sufficient practice trials. Once the client feels stable, instruct the client to close his or her eyes. Start the stopwatch to begin the test.
- Always stand in close proximity as a precaution to prevent falling.
- Continue the test for 60 seconds or until the client exhibits any test-termination cue, as listed in the Observations section.
- Allow up to two trials per leg position and record the best performance on each side.

Observations:

- Continue to time the client's performance until one of the following occurs:
  - ✓The client loses postural control and balance.
  - ✓The client's feet move on the floor.
  - ✓The client's eyes open.
  - ✓The client's arms move from the folded position.
  - ✓The client exceeds 60 seconds with good postural control.

General interpretations:

- The client needs to maintain his or her balance with good postural control (without excessive swaying) and not exhibit any of the test-termination criteria for 30 or more seconds.
- The inability to reach 30 seconds is indicative of inadequate static balance and postural control.

Stork-stand Balance Test

Source: Johnson & Nelson, 1986

Objective: To assess static balance by standing on one foot in a modified stork-stand position. This is a more challenging variation of the blind stork-stand test, where the stance foot remains flat on the floor, but the test is conducted with the eyes closed.

Equipment:

- Flat, non-slip surface
- Stopwatch

Instructions:

- Explain the purpose of the test.
- Ask the client to remove his or her shoes and stand with feet together, hands on the hips.
- Instruct the client to raise one foot off the ground and bring that foot to lightly touch the inside of the stance leg, just below the knee (Figure 7-44).
  - ✓The client must raise the heel of the stance foot off the floor and balance on the ball of the foot (Figure 7-45).

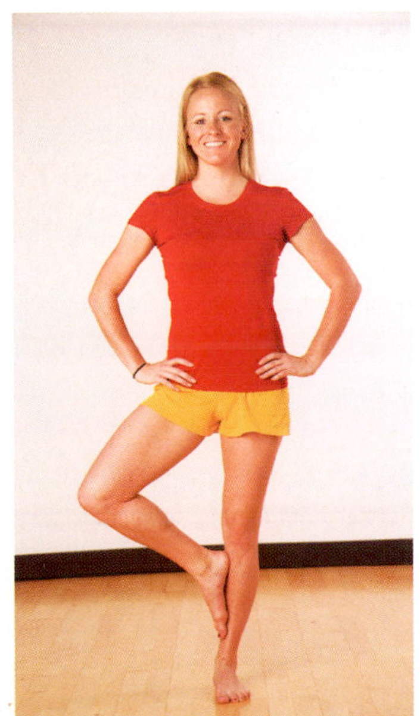

Figure 7-44
Stork-stand balance test: Starting position

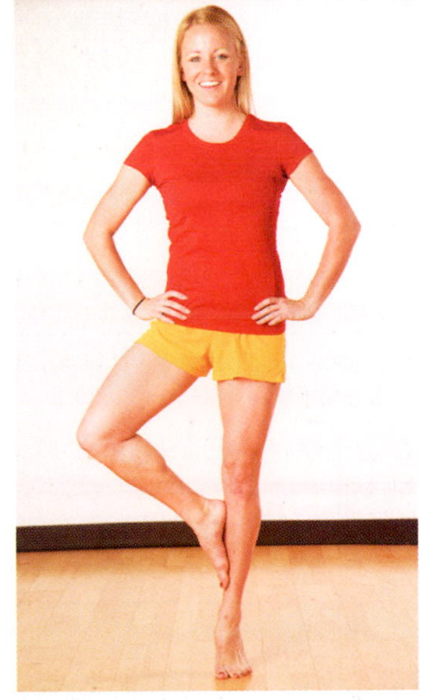

Figure 7-45
Stork-stand balance test: Test position

- ✓Stand behind the client for support if needed.
- ✓Allow 1 minute of practice trials.
- ✓After the practice trial, perform the test, starting the stopwatch as the heel lifts off the floor.
- ✓The test is performed with the eyes open.
- Repeat with the opposite leg.
- Allow up to three trials per leg position and record the best performance on each side.

Observations:

- Timing stops when any of the following occurs:
  - ✓The hand(s) come off the hips.
  - ✓The stance or supporting foot inverts, everts, or moves in any direction.
  - ✓Any part of the elevated foot loses contact with the stance leg.
  - ✓The heel of the stance leg touches the floor.
  - ✓The client loses balance.

General interpretation:

- Use the information provided in Table 7-18 to categorize the client's performance

Core Function: Blood Pressure Cuff Test

Source: Richardson et al., 1999

Objective: To assess core function, as demonstrated by the ability to draw the abdominal wall inward via the coordinated action of the transverse abdominis (TVA) and related core muscles without activation of the rectus abdominis. While the absolute validity of this test has been challenged, it does demonstrate the ability to activate the TVA independent of the rectus abdominis.

Equipment:

- Exercise mat
- Blood pressure cuff

Instructions:

- Explain the purpose of the test.
- Instruct the client to lie prone on an exercise mat while resting his or her forehead on a small padded surface or the mat.
- Ask the client to extend the legs, plantarflex the ankles, and abduct the arms out to the sides at shoulder height with the elbows extended and palms resting on the floor.
- Place the bladder of a blood pressure cuff directly under the client's umbilicus.
- Gently pump the bulb until the pressure gauge reads approximately 70 mmHg at end-tidal volume (between breaths, after an exhalation).
  - ✓If 70 mmHg proves to be uncomfortable, any number between 40 and 70 mmHg can be used.
  - ✓Small fluctuations in the pressure will be seen as the client continues to breathe in and out normally. This is attributed to movement of the diaphragm pressing downward against the abdomen.
  - ✓Continue to make slight adjustments to the cuff pressure until it fluctuates within the acceptable pressure range of 40 to 70 mmHg.
- Following a few normal breaths, the client slowly exhales. Before taking the next breath, the client slowly draws the umbilicus upward toward the spine, essentially trying to lift the stomach off the cuff and hold that contraction for a few seconds before relaxing (Figure 7-46).
  - ✓Allow a few practice trials before having the client complete three test trials.
  - ✓Record the direction and magnitude

Table 7-18

The Stork-stand Balance Test

Rating	Excellent	Good	Average	Fair	Poor
Males	>50 seconds	41–50 seconds	31–40 seconds	20–30 seconds	<20 seconds
Females	>30 seconds	25–30 seconds	16–24 seconds	10–15 seconds	<10 seconds

Source: Johnson B.L. & Nelson, J.K. (1986). *Practical Measurements for Evaluation in Physical Education* (4th ed.). Minneapolis, Minn.: Burgess.

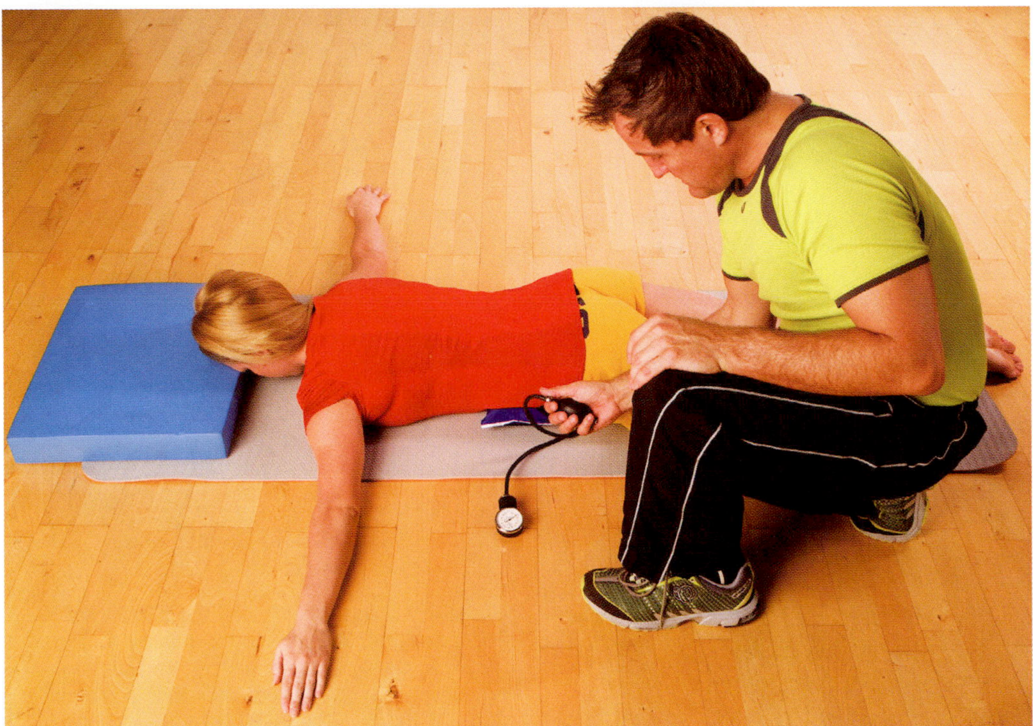

Figure 7-46
Blood pressure cuff test

of pressure changes in the blood pressure gauge.

Observations:

- While the client attempts the contraction, carefully monitor for any movement of the hips, ribcage, or shoulders (hip elevation or movement of the ribcage may indicate activation of the rectus abdominis and not the TVA).
- Clients must avoid any movement at the ankles (dorsiflexion) or pushing from the elbows that would be used as leverage to raise the torso.

General interpretation:

- A good indicator of TVA function is the ability to reduce the pressure in the cuff by 10 mmHg during the contraction.
- If a client lacks effective core function, he or she usually recruits the rectus abdominis muscle instead to achieve the desired movement.
  - ✓This will be evident by movement in the hips and/or ribcage (trunk flexion).
  - ✓This may also be evident by an increase in the blood pressure reading, as this muscle contraction actually pushes downward on the bladder of the blood-pressure cuff.
- No change or a change <10 mmHg does not necessarily represent a lack of core function. It represents control of muscle activation without being overly reliant on recruiting the rectus abdominis.

Summary

By adhering to the principle of "straightening the body before strengthening it" aided by the information provided by the assessments for stability and mobility in this chapter, trainers may witness improved efficacy in their programs and an increased likelihood of success in terms of their clients attaining their goals. Trainers should consider performing the assessments in this chapter in the sequence presented and utilizing them as prerequisites to the more traditional assessments of **body composition,** aerobic fitness, and muscular fitness.

References

Abelbeck, K.G. (2002). Biomechanical model and evaluation of a linear motion squat type exercise. *Journal of Strength and Conditioning Research,* 16, 516–524.

Black, F.O. et al. (1982). Normal subject postural sway during the Romberg test. *American Journal of Otolaryngology,* 3, 309–318

Cook, G. (2003). *Athletic Body in Balance*. Champaign, Ill.: Human Kinetics.

Donnelly, D.V. et al. (2006). The effect of directional gaze on kinematics during the squat exercise. *Journal of Strength and Conditioning Research*, 20, 145–150.

Fry, A.C., Smith J.C., & Schilling, B.K. (2003). Effect of knee position on hip and knees torques during the barbell squat. *Journal of Strength and Conditioning Research*, 17, 629–633.

Gray, G. & Tiberio, D. (2006). *Chain Reaction Function*. Adrian, Mich.: The Gray Institute.

Houglum, P.A. (2005). *Therapeutic Exercise for Musculoskeletal Injuries* (2nd ed). Champaign, Ill.: Human Kinetics.

Johnson B.L. & Nelson, J.K. (1986). *Practical Measurements for Evaluation in Physical Education* (4th ed.). Minneapolis, Minn.: Burgess.

Kendall, F.P. et al. (2005). *Muscles Testing and Function with Posture and Pain* (5th ed.). Baltimore, Md.: Lippincott Williams & Wilkins.

Morris, C.E. et al. (2006). Vladimir Janda: Tribute to a master of rehabilitation. *Spine,* 31, 9, 1060–1064.

Newton, R. (1989). Review of tests of standing balance abilities. *Brain Injury,* 3, 4, 335–343.

Price, J. (2007). *A Step-by-step Guide to the Fundamentals of Structural Assessment*. San Diego, Calif.: TheBiomechanics.com

Richardson, C. et al. (1999). Therapeutic exercise for spinal segmental stabilization. In: *Lower Back Pain: Scientific Basis and Clinical Approach.* London, England: Churchill Livingstone.

Sahrmann, S.A. (2002). *Diagnosis and Treatment of Movement Impairment Syndromes*. St. Louis, Mo.: Mosby.

Soderberg, G.L. (1997). *Kinesiology: Application to Pathological Motion* (2nd ed.) Baltimore, Md.: Lippincott Williams & Wilkins.

Whiting W.C. & Rugg, S. (2006). *Dynatomy: Dynamic Human Anatomy*. Champaign, Ill.: Human Kinetics.

Suggested Reading

American College of Sports Medicine (2010). *ACSM's Guidelines for Exercise Testing and Prescription* (8th ed.). Baltimore, Md.: Wolters Kluwer/Lippincott Williams & Wilkins.

Canadian Society for Exercise Physiology (2002). *Canada's Physical Activity Guide to Healthy Active Living*. Ottowa, Ontario: Health Canada.

Haskell, W.L. et al. (2007). Physical activity and public health: Updated recommendation for the American College of Sports Medicine and the American Heart Association. *Medicine & Science in Sports & Exercise,* 39, 8, 1423–1434.

Kendall, F.P. et al. (2005). *Muscles Testing and Function with Posture and Pain* (5th ed.). Baltimore, Md.: Lippincott Williams & Wilkins.

Morrow, J. et al. (2005). *Practical Measurements for Evaluation in Physical Education* (3rd ed.). Champaign, Ill.: Human Kinetics.

Shumway-Cook, A. & Woollacott, M.H. (1989). *Development of Posture and Gait: Across the Life Span.* Columbia, S.C.: University of South Carolina Press.

U.S. Department of Health & Human Services (1996). *Physical Activity and Health: A Report of the Surgeon General.* Atlanta, Ga.: U.S. Department of Health & Human Services, Centers for Disease Control and Prevention, National Center for Chronic Disease Prevention and Health Promotion.

Whiting W.C. & Rugg, S. (2006). *Dynatomy: Dynamic Human Anatomy*. Champaign, Ill.: Human Kinetics.

Wilmore, J.H., Costill, D.L., & Kenney, W.L. (2008). *Physiology of Sport and Exercise* (4th ed.). Champaign, Ill.: Human Kinetics.

IN THIS CHAPTER:

Testing and Measurement

Anthropometric Measurements and Body Composition

- Appropriate Use/Clientele
- Measurement of Lean and Fat Tissue
- Contraindications
- Hydrostatic Weighing
- Skinfold Measurements
- Body Composition Evaluation
- Programming Considerations
- Measurement of Body Size: Other Anthropometric Measures

Cardiorespiratory Fitness Testing

- Cardiorespiratory Assessments for the Lab or Fitness Center
- Treadmill Exercise Testing
- Cycle Ergometer Testing
- Ventilatory Threshold Testing
- Field Testing
- Step Tests

Muscular-fitness Testing

- Muscular-endurance Testing
- Muscular-strength Testing

Sport-skill Assessments

- Power Testing: Field Tests
- Speed, Agility, and Quickness Testing

Fitness Testing Accuracy

Summary

***KELLY SPIVEY, N.D.**, is a continuing education provider for health and fitness professionals and maintains her own personal-training business. As a member of the American Alternative Medical Society, Dr. Spivey's primary focus is on disease prevention and complementary medicine. She is an adjunct professor in the Exercise Science Department at the University of Tampa. Dr. Spivey has been working as an exam development subject-matter expert with ACE since 2006.*

CHAPTER 8

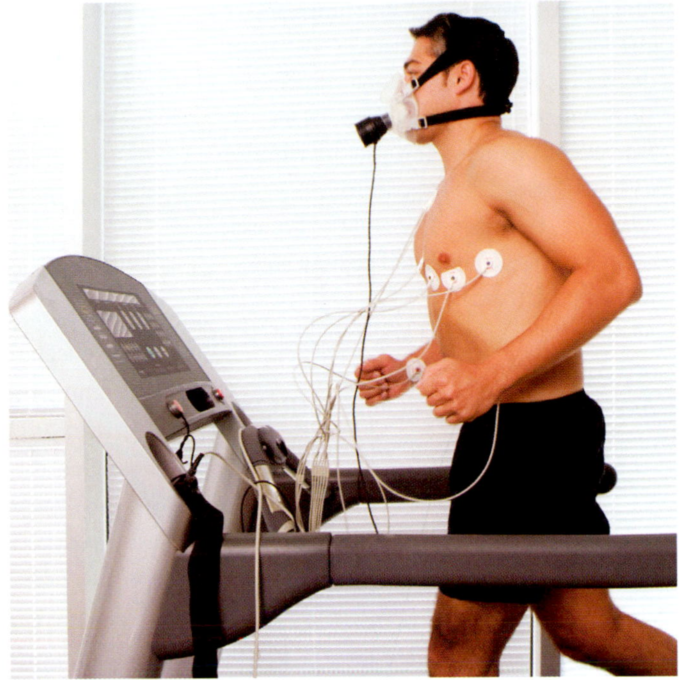

Physiological Assessments

Kelly Spivey

This chapter describes the various health- and fitness-related assessments that are commonly used by personal trainers. The selected modalities follow the sequence outlined in the ACE Integrated Fitness Training™ (ACE IFT™) Model (see Chapter 5). The personal trainer will select and administer tests according to each client's needs and desires using information obtained during the initial needs assessment. Testing methods are also determined by a number of other factors, including availability of equipment, time allotment, and the trainer's level of comfort with the assessment procedures.

Chapter 7 introduced important foundational assessments (posture, movement, flexibility, balance, and core function) that merit strong consideration given their contribution to movement. This chapter presents both health-related assessments and sports- or skill-related assessments that are often relevant to program development and ongoing evaluation. Client goals and lifestyles will often determine the appropriate test selection.

The health-related assessments focus on the following components:

- *Cardiorespiratory fitness:* Overall functioning of the heart and lungs and the efficiency of the cardiovascular system in delivering oxygen to working muscles
- *Body composition and anthropometry:* **Body composition** and the distribution of **body fat**
- *Muscular endurance:* The ability of muscle groups to sustain repeated activity and withstand fatigue
- *Muscular strength:* The ability of muscle to overcome external resistance
- *Flexibility:* The **range of motion (ROM)** of a given joint or group of joints or the level of tissue extensibility that a muscle group possesses

The skill-related assessments (excluding balance assessments, which are covered in Chapter 7) focus on the following components:

- *Anaerobic power:* The amount of work performed in a given unit of time; usually represents one single and explosive bout, event, or repetition performed at maximal efforts
- *Anaerobic capacity:* The ability to sustain high-intensity **anaerobic** activity
- *Speed:* The rate of motion or the rate of change of distance
- *Agility:* How accurately and rapidly a person can change direction; involves the stages of acceleration, stabilization, and deceleration
- *Reactivity:* The rate at which an individual responds to a stimulus
- *Coordination:* The ability of an individual to complete complex movements while providing accurate responses in both timing and intensity

Testing and Measurement

The list of fitness-assessment techniques presented in this section is by no means all-inclusive, as there are many assessments that can be used to measure physical-fitness status. Some of these assessments are very simple to perform, while others are more complicated and require practice. It is important for personal trainers to act professionally and be competent when evaluating a client's level of fitness. There are a number of resources for gaining hands-on training in fitness assessments, including the following:

- ACE-sponsored workshops
- Local colleges or universities with exercise science departments
- Experienced personal trainers, athletic trainers, or rehabilitation specialists
- Repeated practice, using friends, family members, or other trainers until comfortable and competent

During the administration of any exercise test involving exertion (e.g., cardiovascular or **muscular endurance** and/or strength test), trainers must always be aware of identifiable signs or symptoms that merit immediate test termination and possible referral to a qualified healthcare professional [American College of Sports Medicine (ACSM), 2010a]. These symptoms include:

- Onset of **angina,** chest pain, or angina-like symptoms
- Significant drop (>10 mmHg) in **systolic blood pressure (SBP)** despite an increase in exercise intensity
- Excessive rise in **blood pressure (BP)**: SBP >250 mmHg or **diastolic blood pressure (DBP)** >115 mmHg
- Excess fatigue, shortness of breath, or wheezing (does not include heavy breathing due to intense exercise)
- Signs of poor **perfusion**: lightheadedness, pallor (pale skin), **cyanosis** (bluish coloration, especially around the mouth), nausea, or cold and clammy skin
- Increased nervous system symptoms (e.g., **ataxia,** dizziness, confusion, **syncope**)
- Leg cramping or **claudication**
- Subject requests to stop
- Physical or verbal manifestations of severe fatigue
- Failure of testing equipment

Anthropometric Measurements and Body Composition

This section addresses key anthropometric measures of body shape and size, as well as the assessment of body composition. There are many methods for assessing body composition, though some prove to be impractical in a fitness setting given the expense and expertise needed to operate the equipment [e.g., **hydrostatic weighing, air displacement plethysmography** (e.g., Bod-Pod™), valid **bioelectrical impedance analysis, dual energy X-ray absorptiometry (DEXA)**]. Skinfold measurement determines body composition via the measurement of select subcutaneous **adipose tissue** sites (Wilmore, Costill, & Kenney, 2008). Given the ease of administration and low cost, skinfold measurements are still considered the most practical assessment tool for measuring body composition in the fitness setting. While some skinfold protocols demonstrate similar accuracy to the more expensive techniques, the margin of error increases when trainers are unfamiliar with identifying exact skinfold locations or lack experience or technique in correctly grasping the skinfold site. Considering how critical a body-composition score can be to a client's psyche and motivational levels, it is extremely important that trainers demonstrate strong skills and reliability when assessing body composition.

Anthropometric measures include measurements of height, weight, and/or circumference to assess body size or dimension. They are very easy to administer and require minimal equipment. Two examples of this approach are **body mass index (BMI)** and **waist-to-hip ratio (WHR).** While these measurements demonstrate strong correlations to health, **morbidity,** and **mortality,** they provide only *estimations* of body composition and fitness level. The personal trainer must consider his or her own skill level, protocol accuracy, and equipment availability, as well as the client's personal concerns, when determining the appropriate testing protocols to assess body composition and body shape/size. Trainers may also opt to use more than one protocol (e.g., skinfold, BMI, and waist circumference). Table 8-1 presents a list of various techniques and protocols available within health and fitness centers.

Table 8-1

Body Composition and Body Size Measurement Techniques

Body Composition	Body Size
Bioelectrical impedance	Body mass index
DEXA scans	Girth measurements, including waist-to-hip ratio
Hydrostatic weighing or underwater weighing	Height
Near-infrared interactance	Weight
Skinfold measurements	
Whole-body air displacement plethysmography	

Body composition refers to the proportion of lean tissue to body-fat tissue. Lean body mass is composed of muscles, **connective tissue,** bones, blood, nervous tissue, skin, and organs. For the most part, lean mass is metabolically active tissue that allows the body to perform work. A certain amount of body fat is necessary for insulation and **thermoregulation, hormone** production, cushioning of vital organs, and maintenance of certain body functions. For men, **essential body fat** is between 2 and 5%; for women it is between 10 and 13%. The remainder of body fat is stored throughout the body in adipose tissue, either subcutaneously or viscerally, acting as a readily available source of energy or to cushion and protect vital organs. Just as lean tissue contributes to athletic performance, an appropriate percentage of body fat can also be related to successful athletic performance. The calculation of desired body weight based on appropriate body composition is presented on page 184.

A certain amount of body fat is necessary for overall health and well-being, though too much body fat can be detrimental to health and increases the risk of many diseases, ranging from heart disease to **osteoarthritis.** A person's health can also be compromised if his or her body-fat percentage drops below recommended levels.

Appropriate Use/Clientele

Almost 70% of individuals who join a fitness center cite weight management as a top reason for their membership (ACE, 2007). Many clients are likely to be concerned with body composition and will have a desire to decrease their body fat in an effort to look fit and trim. When working with clients who are concerned with weight loss, it is important to focus primarily on fat loss, without sacrificing lean muscle tissue. The same holds true when working with clients who are interested in weight gain. Most desire to gain lean muscle tissue and not an excess amount of adipose tissue.

Others may wish to decrease their body fat for health reasons. Excess body fat has been linked to **coronary artery disease (CAD), metabolic syndrome, diabetes,** certain types of cancer (breast, colon, endometrial), osteoarthritis, low-back dysfunction, sleep **apnea,** and even premature death (Olshansky et al., 2005).

Measurement of Lean and Fat Tissue

It is important to differentiate between **overweight** and overfat. Overweight is defined as an upward deviation in body weight, based on the subject's height. Most normative data defines overweight as 20% or more above ideal weight. Since only height and weight are factored into the equation, excess body weight could be attributed to either fat mass or lean tissue. Overfat, a more accurate depiction of body composition, indicates an excess amount of body fat.

Assessment of body composition is often of great interest to a client. In fact, many clients are compelled to enroll in a personal-training program for the sole purpose of changing their body composition. To get a more detailed look at the actual lean and fat mass, it is necessary to perform tests that involve more than periphery measurements. The assessments presented in Table 8-2 are used to assess body composition. Due to the cost and limited availability of the equipment needed, not all are practical in a fitness setting.

The assessment of body composition can be quite invasive. It is important for personal trainers to conduct these assessments in a private area to put the client at ease. Clients should be instructed on appropriate attire to promote easy access to measurement sites. The trainer should act as a professional and be competent in the chosen method. Testing accuracy is improved by proper hydration, so it is important to instruct the client not to exercise prior to testing and to maintain adequate hydration throughout the day.

During subsequent reassessments, body composition will likely change due to a loss of body fat and an increase in lean tissue. Between measurements, a client may notice changes in the way his or her clothes fit. These subjective observations will be motivating to the client. Objective reassessments of body composition will be especially important for a client who has not noticed any significant change on the bathroom scale. Clients may need to be reminded that as lean mass increases and body fat decreases, the scale cannot differentiate between the two.

Contraindications

If a client is extremely obese, some of the body-composition techniques will not be accurate (see Table 8-2). In some cases, it may be more appropriate to utilize only BMI and girth measurements.

Hydrostatic Weighing

Hydrostatic weighing, which is also called underwater weighing, is considered the benchmark for computing body composition. When compared with cadaver assessments, there is only a 1.5 to 2.0% margin of error. Most of the other methods of computing body composition are based on formulas derived from underwater weighing research. The concept behind hydrostatic weighing is based on the Archimedes Principle, which provides the following equation:

$$\text{Density} = \text{Mass}/\text{Volume}$$

Table 8-2

Body-composition Assessments

Method	Description
Bioelectrical impedance analysis (BIA)* Whole-body BIA machines are found primarily in laboratory settings. Less-sophisticated BIA devices are found in fitness settings.	BIA measures electrical signals as they pass through fat, lean mass, and water in the body. In essence, this method assesses leanness, but calculations can be made based on this information. BIA accuracy is based primarily on the sophistication of the machine. Many fitness centers utilize BIA due to the simplicity of use. Optimal hydration is necessary for accurate results.
Air displacement plethysmography (ADP) Example: Bod Pod® (or Pea Pod® for children) Marketed for the fitness setting, but it is cost-prohibitive for most facilities	The Bod Pod is an egg-shaped chamber that measures the amount of air that is displaced when a person sits in the machine. Two values are needed to determine body fat: air displacement and body weight. ADP has a high accuracy rate but the equipment is expensive.
Dual energy x-ray absorptiometry (DEXA)* May be found in exercise physiology departments at colleges and universities	DEXA ranks among the most accurate and precise methods. DEXA is a whole-body scanning system that delivers a low-dose x-ray that reads bone and soft-tissue mass. DEXA has the ability to identify regional body-fat distribution.
Hydrostatic weighing (i.e., underwater weighing) The gold standard: Many later methods of body-fat assessment are based on calculations derived from hydrostatic weighing. May be found in exercise physiology departments at colleges and universities	This method measures the amount of water a person displaces when completely submerged, thereby indirectly measuring body fat. It is not practical in a fitness center setting due to the size of the apparatus and the complexity of the technique required for accurate measurements, which involves the individual going down to the bottom of a tank, exhaling all air from the lungs (expiratory quotient), and then holding the breath until the scale settles and records an accurate weight. The assessment must then be repeated to ensure accuracy.
Magnetic resonance imaging (MRI) Found in hospitals and diagnostic centers	MRI uses magnetic fields to assess how much fat a person has and where it is deposited. Since MRIs are located in clinical settings, using an MRI solely for calculation of body fat is not practical.
Near-infrared interactance (NIR)* Example: Futrex®	NIR uses a fiber optic probe connected to a digital analyzer that indirectly measures tissue composition (fat and water). Typically, the biceps are the assessment site. Calculations are then plugged into an equation that includes height, weight, frame size, and level of activity. This method is relatively inexpensive and fast, but not as accurate as most.
Skinfold measurement Very commonly used in fitness settings	Skinfold calipers are used to "pinch" a fold of skin and fat. Several sites on the body are typically measured. The measurements are plugged into an equation that calculates body-fat percentage.
Total body electrical conductivity (TOBEC) Found in clinical and research settings	TOBEC uses an electromagnetic force field to assess relative body fat. Much like the MRI, it is impractical and too expensive for the fitness setting.

*These body-composition assessment techniques are not accurate when used with obese clients.

This technique originally measured the amount of water displaced when a person was completely submerged and exhaled all available air from the lungs [leaving only the **residual volume (RV)** and a small volume of air in the **gastrointestinal tract**]. Fat tissue is less dense than lean tissue and displaces more water despite weighing less. The body is weighed on an underwater scale. As water buoyancy (i.e., the counterforce of water) reduces body weight significantly, and air and fat mass increase buoyancy, their respective contributions to underwater weight have to be determined. To minimize error with this protocol, the RV should be measured in water. This volume can be 100 to 200 mL lower underwater due to the non-compressible nature of water that helps compact the lungs. Given the costs, equipment, and expertise needed to accurately measure residual volume, mathematical calculations are often used to estimate RV, which may introduce a margin of error of 300 to 400 mL. For every 100 mL error in estimation of RV, the percent body fat error changes by 0.7%.

Hydrostatic weighing is not a practical approach for the standard fitness center. The apparatus is expensive and takes up a lot of room, testing takes a considerable amount of time and expertise, and many people feel uncomfortable remaining submerged under water after they have exhaled all available air from their lungs. This evaluation tool is often found in elite clinical settings and in many colleges and universities.

Skinfold Measurements

Subcutaneous body fat can be measured using a device called a skinfold caliper. In an average person, approximately 50% of body fat is distributed just below the skin. For this reason, body composition can be easily calculated using the right tools and formulas. Skinfold formulas are derived from calculations based on extensive research derived from hydrostatic weighing. In general, the skinfold caliper method produces a measurement that is ± 2.0 to 3.5% of that obtained in hydrostatic weighing. Further measurement error is likely if the trainer is inexperienced or uses poor technique, if the client is obese or extremely thin, or if the caliper is not properly calibrated (ACSM, 2010a). Before conducting skinfold measurements, trainers must familiarize themselves with the exact site locations and proper grasping technique.

Given the variability in fat distribution from site to site, it is recommended that multiple sites be analyzed (ACSM, 2010a). Most research supports using at least three sites when assessing body fat. The sites are also different between men and women. For men, the Jackson and Pollock three-site skinfold locations are as follows (Jackson & Pollock, 1985):

- *Chest (Figure 8-1):* A diagonal skinfold taken midway between the anterior axillary line (crease of the underarm) and the nipple
- *Thigh (Figure 8-2):* A vertical skinfold taken on the anterior midline of the thigh between the inguinal crease at the hip and the proximal border of the patella
- *Abdominal (Figure 8-3):* A vertical skinfold taken 2 cm (~1 inch) to the right of the umbilicus

For women, the Jackson and Pollock three-site skinfold locations are as follows (Jackson & Pollock, 1985):

- *Triceps (Figure 8-4):* A vertical fold on the posterior midline of the upper arm taken halfway between the acromion (shoulder) and olecranon (elbow) processes
- *Thigh (Figure 8-5)*: A vertical skinfold taken on the anterior midline of the thigh between the inguinal crease at the hip and the proximal border of the patella
- *Suprailium (Figure 8-6):* A diagonal fold following the natural line of the iliac crest taken immediately superior to the crest of the ilium and in line with the anterior axillary line

Body composition can be determined by adding the three skinfold measurements

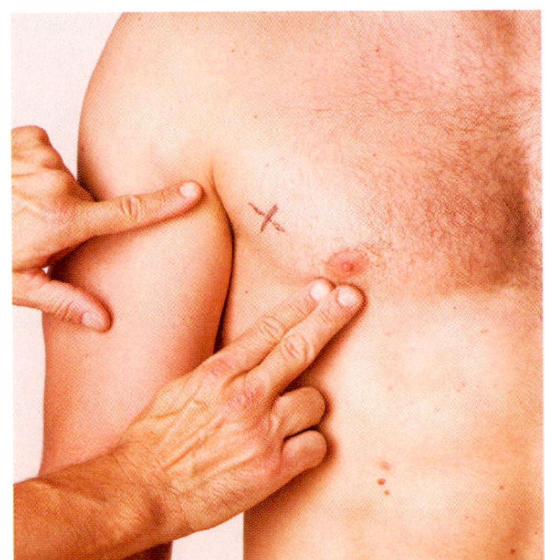

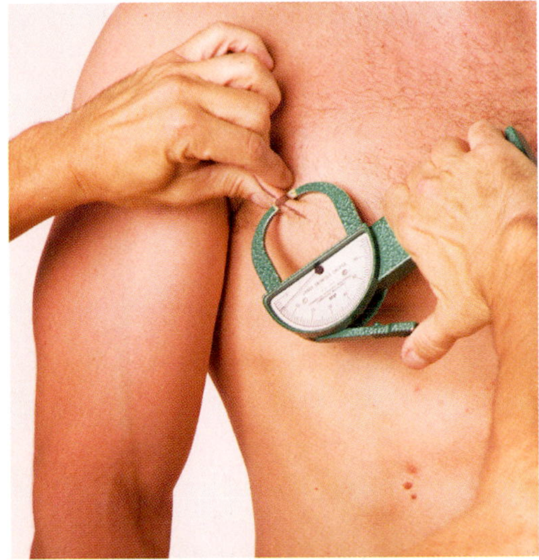

Figure 8-1
Chest skinfold measurement for men:

Locate the site midway between the anterior axillary line and the nipple.

Grasp a diagonal fold and pull it away from the muscle.

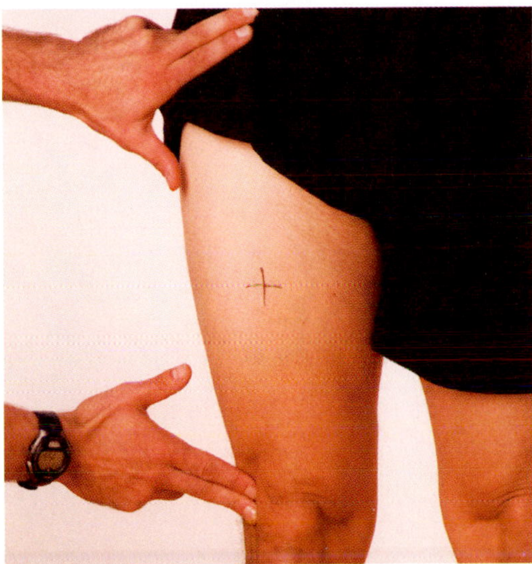

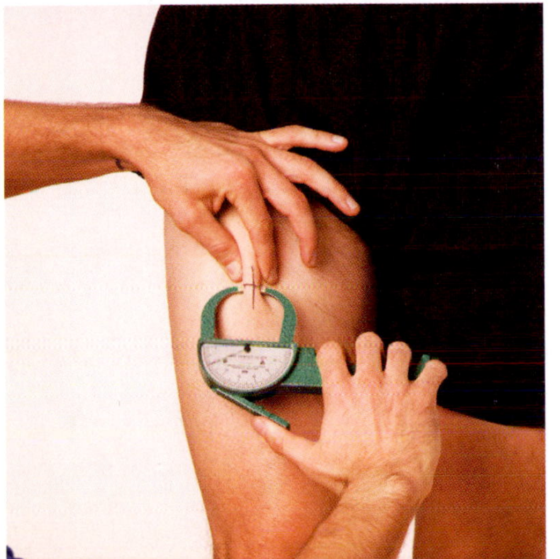

Figure 8-2
Thigh skinfold measurement for men:

Locate the hip and the knee joints and find the midpoint on the top of the thigh.

Grasp a vertical skinfold and pull it away from the muscle.

and plugging the values into the conversion tables (Tables 8-3 and 8-4) or by calculating body density, from which body composition can be computed (Jackson & Pollock, 1985).

Men (chest, thigh, and abdominal):
Body density = 1.10938 – 0.0008267 (sum of three skinfolds) + 0.0000016 (sum of three skinfolds)^2 – 0.0002574 (age)

Women (triceps, thigh, and suprailium):
Body density = 1.099421 – 0.0009929 (sum of three skinfolds) + 0.0000023 (sum of three skinfolds)^2 – 0.0001392 (age)

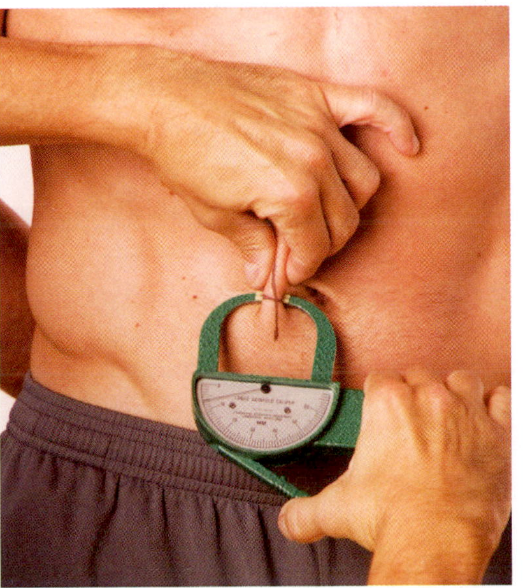

Figure 8-3
Abdominal skinfold measurement for men:

Grasp a vertical skinfold one inch to the right of the umbilicus.

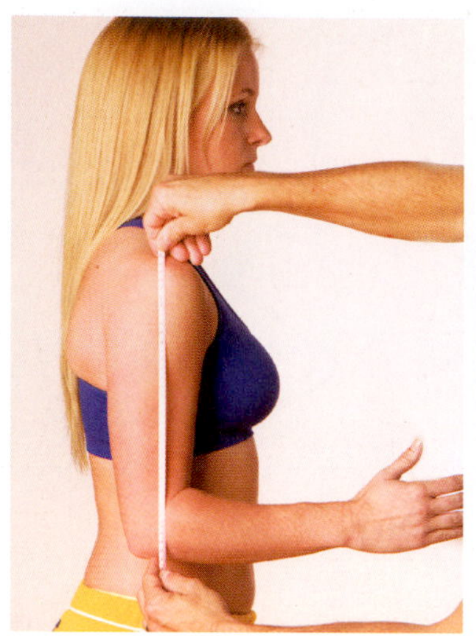
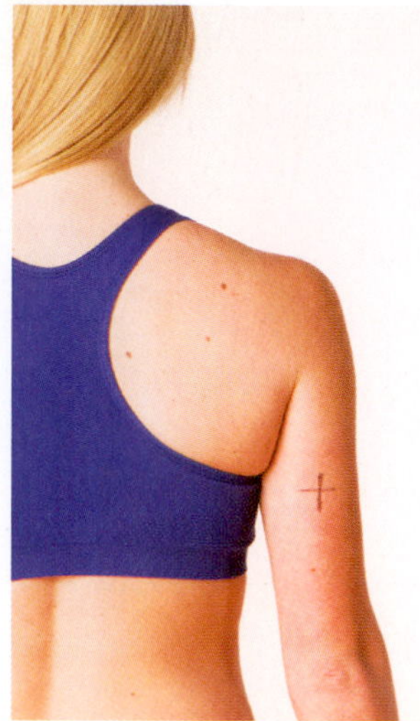
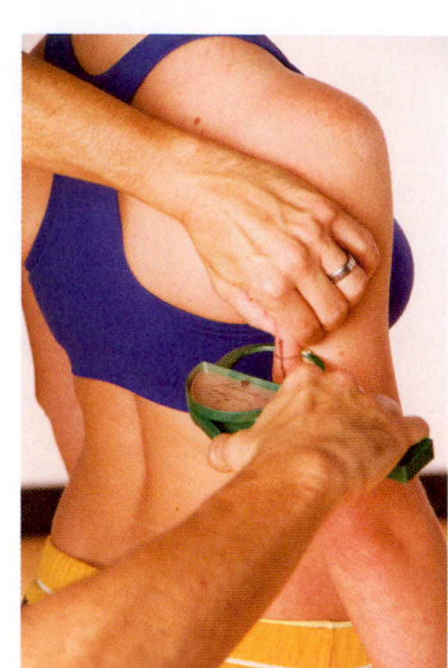

Figure 8-4
Triceps skinfold measurement for women:

Locate the site midway between the acromial (shoulder) and olecranon (elbow) processes.

Grasp a vertical fold on the posterior midline and pull it away from the muscle.

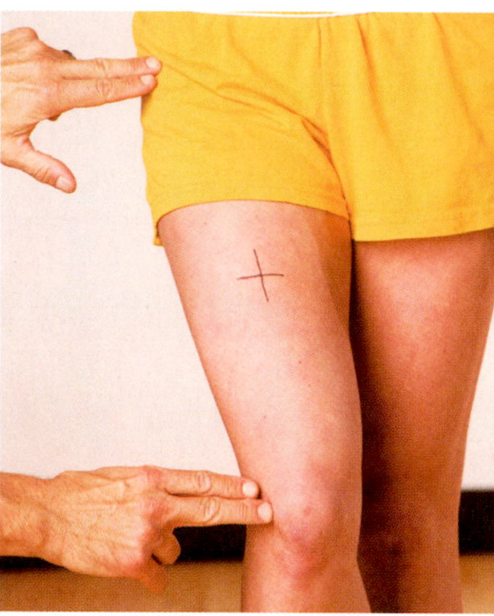
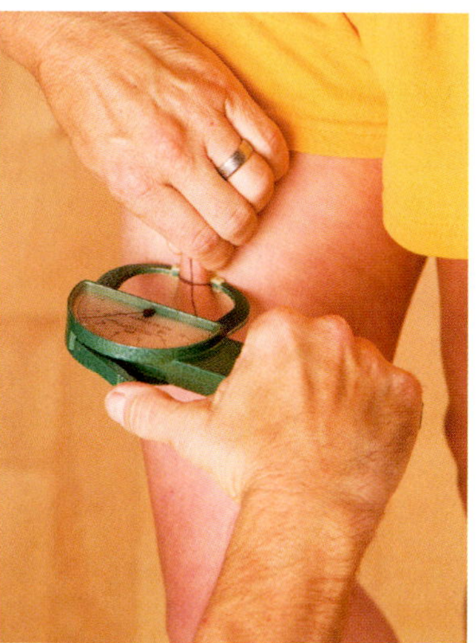

Figure 8-5
Thigh skinfold measurement for women:

Locate the hip and the knee joints and find the midpoint on the top of the thigh.

Grasp a vertical skinfold and pull it away from the muscle.

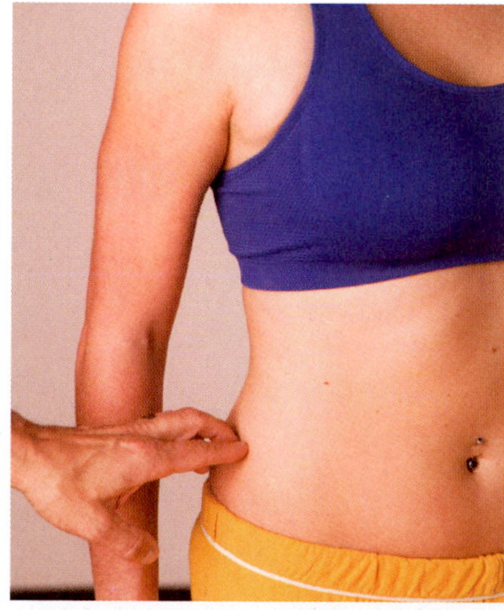
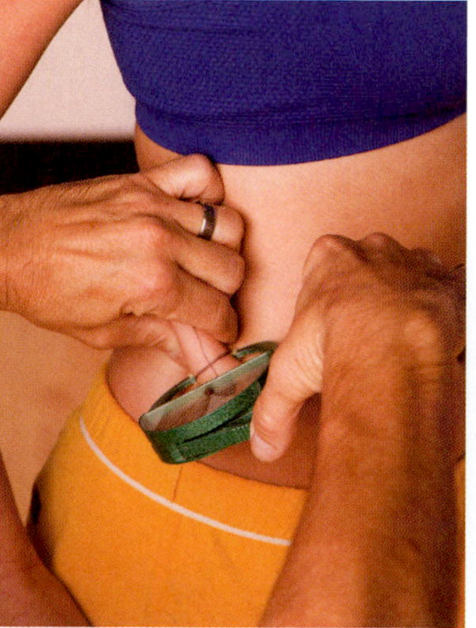

Figure 8-6
Suprailium skinfold measurement for women:

Grasp a diagonal skinfold just above, and slightly forward of, the crest of the ilium.

Table 8-3

Percent Body Fat Estimations for Men—Jackson and Pollock Formula

	Age Groups								
Sum of Skinfolds (mm)	**Under 22**	**23–27**	**28–32**	**33–37**	**38–42**	**43–47**	**48–52**	**53–57**	**Over 57**
8–10	1.3	1.8	2.3	2.9	3.4	3.9	4.5	5.0	5.5
11–13	2.2	2.8	3.3	3.9	4.4	4.9	5.5	6.0	6.5
14–16	3.2	3.8	4.3	4.8	5.4	5.9	6.4	7.0	7.5
17–19	4.2	4.7	5.3	5.8	6.3	6.9	7.4	8.0	8.5
20–22	5.1	5.7	6.2	6.8	7.3	7.9	8.4	8.9	9.5
23–25	6.1	6.6	7.2	7.7	8.3	8.8	9.4	9.9	10.5
26–28	7.0	7.6	8.1	8.7	9.2	9.8	10.3	10.9	11.4
29–31	8.0	8.5	9.1	9.6	10.2	10.7	11.3	11.8	12.4
32–34	8.9	9.4	10.0	10.5	11.1	11.6	12.2	12.8	13.3
35–37	9.8	10.4	10.9	11.5	12.0	12.6	13.1	13.7	14.3
38–40	10.7	11.3	11.8	12.4	12.9	13.5	14.1	14.6	15.2
41–43	11.6	12.2	12.7	13.3	13.8	14.4	15.0	15.5	16.1
44–46	12.5	13.1	13.6	14.2	14.7	15.3	15.9	16.4	17.0
47–49	13.4	13.9	14.5	15.1	15.6	16.2	16.8	17.3	17.9
50–52	14.3	14.8	15.4	15.9	16.5	17.1	17.6	18.2	18.8
53–55	15.1	15.7	16.2	16.8	17.4	17.9	18.5	19.1	19.7
56–58	16.0	16.5	17.1	17.7	18.2	18.8	19.4	20.0	20.5
59–61	16.9	17.4	17.9	18.5	19.1	19.7	20.2	20.8	21.4
62–64	17.6	18.2	18.8	19.4	19.9	20.5	21.1	21.7	22.2
65–67	18.5	19.0	19.6	20.2	20.8	21.3	21.9	22.5	23.1
68–70	19.3	19.9	20.4	21.0	21.6	22.2	22.7	23.3	23.9
71–73	20.1	20.7	21.2	21.8	22.4	23.0	23.6	24.1	24.7
74–76	20.9	21.5	22.0	22.6	23.2	23.8	24.4	25.0	25.5
77–79	21.7	22.2	22.8	23.4	24.0	24.6	25.2	25.8	26.3
80–82	22.4	23.0	23.6	24.2	24.8	25.4	25.9	26.5	27.1
83–85	23.2	23.8	24.4	25.0	25.5	26.1	26.7	27.3	27.9
86–88	24.0	24.5	25.1	25.7	26.3	26.9	27.5	28.1	28.7
89–91	24.7	25.3	25.9	26.5	27.1	27.6	28.2	28.8	29.4
92–94	25.4	26.0	26.6	27.2	27.8	28.4	29.0	29.6	30.2
95–97	26.1	26.7	27.3	27.9	28.5	29.1	29.7	30.3	30.9
98–100	26.9	27.4	28.0	28.6	29.2	29.8	30.4	31.0	31.6
101–103	27.5	28.1	28.7	29.3	29.9	30.5	31.1	31.7	32.3
104–106	28.2	28.8	29.4	30.0	30.6	31.2	31.8	32.4	33.0
107–109	28.9	29.5	30.1	30.7	31.3	31.9	32.5	33.1	33.7
110–112	29.6	30.2	30.8	31.4	32.0	32.6	33.2	33.8	34.4
113–115	30.2	30.8	31.4	32.0	32.6	33.2	33.8	34.5	35.1
116–118	30.9	31.5	32.1	32.7	33.3	33.9	34.5	35.1	35.7
119–121	31.5	32.1	32.7	33.3	33.9	34.5	35.1	35.7	36.4
122–124	32.1	32.7	33.3	33.9	34.5	35.1	35.8	36.4	37.0
125–127	32.7	33.3	33.9	34.5	35.1	35.8	36.4	37.0	37.6

Jackson, A.S. & Pollock, M.L. (1985). Practical assessment of body composition. *Physician & Sports Medicine,* 13, 76–90.

Table 8-4

Percent Body Fat Estimations for Women—Jackson and Pollock Formula

	Age Groups								
Sum of Skinfolds (mm)	**Under 22**	**23–27**	**28–32**	**33–37**	**38–42**	**43–47**	**48–52**	**53–57**	**Over 57**
23–25	9.7	9.9	10.2	10.4	10.7	10.9	11.2	11.4	11.7
26–28	11.0	11.2	11.5	11.7	12.0	12.3	12.5	12.7	13.0
29–31	12.3	12.5	12.8	13.0	13.3	13.5	13.8	14.0	14.3
32–34	13.6	13.8	14.0	14.3	14.5	14.8	15.0	15.3	15.5
35–37	14.8	15.0	15.3	15.5	15.8	16.0	16.3	16.5	16.8
38–40	16.0	16.3	16.5	16.7	17.0	17.2	17.5	17.7	18.0
41–43	17.2	17.4	17.7	17.9	18.2	18.4	18.7	18.9	19.2
44–46	18.3	18.6	18.8	19.1	19.3	19.6	19.8	20.1	20.3
47–49	19.5	19.7	20.0	20.2	20.5	20.7	21.0	21.2	21.5
50–52	20.6	20.8	21.1	21.3	21.6	21.8	22.1	22.3	22.6
53–55	21.7	21.9	22.1	22.4	22.6	22.9	23.1	23.4	23.6
56–58	22.7	23.0	23.2	23.4	23.7	23.9	24.2	24.4	24.7
59–61	23.7	24.0	24.2	24.5	24.7	25.0	25.2	25.5	25.7
62–64	24.7	25.0	25.2	25.5	25.7	26.0	26.7	26.4	26.7
65–67	25.7	25.9	26.2	26.4	26.7	26.9	27.2	27.4	27.7
68–70	26.6	26.9	27.1	27.4	27.6	27.9	28.1	28.4	28.6
71–73	27.5	27.8	28.0	28.3	28.5	28.8	29.0	29.3	29.5
74–76	28.4	28.7	28.9	29.2	29.4	29.7	29.9	30.2	30.4
77–79	29.3	29.5	29.8	30.0	30.3	30.5	30.8	31.0	31.3
80–82	30.1	30.4	30.6	30.9	31.1	31.4	31.6	31.9	32.1
83–85	30.9	31.2	31.4	31.7	31.9	32.2	32.4	32.7	32.9
86–88	31.7	32.0	32.2	32.5	32.7	32.9	33.2	33.4	33.7
89–91	32.5	32.7	33.0	33.2	33.5	33.7	33.9	34.2	34.4
92–94	33.2	33.4	33.7	33.9	34.2	34.4	34.7	34.9	35.2
95–97	33.9	34.1	34.4	34.6	34.9	35.1	35.4	35.6	35.9
98–100	34.6	34.8	35.1	35.3	35.5	35.8	36.0	36.3	36.5
101–103	35.3	35.4	35.7	35.9	36.2	36.4	36.7	36.9	37.2
104–106	35.8	36.1	36.3	36.6	36.8	37.1	37.3	37.5	37.8
107–109	36.4	36.7	36.9	37.1	37.4	37.6	37.9	38.1	38.4
110–112	37.0	37.2	37.5	37.7	38.0	38.2	38.5	38.7	38.9
113–115	37.5	37.8	38.0	38.2	38.5	38.7	39.0	39.2	39.5
116–118	38.0	38.3	38.5	38.8	39.0	39.3	39.5	39.7	40.0
119–121	38.5	38.7	39.0	39.2	39.5	39.7	40.0	40.2	40.5
122–124	39.0	39.2	39.4	39.7	39.9	40.2	40.4	40.7	40.9
125–127	39.4	39.6	39.9	40.1	40.4	40.6	40.9	41.1	41.4
128–130	39.8	40.0	40.3	40.5	40.8	41.0	41.3	41.5	41.8

Jackson, A.S. & Pollock, M.L. (1985). Practical assessment of body composition. *Physician & Sports Medicine,* 13, 76–90.

Body density of fat tissue equals 0.9 g/cc^3, while the density of fat-free tissue is approximately 1.1 g/cc^3, although these figures vary slightly by age, gender, and ethnicity. Once body density is determined, it needs to be converted to body composition. Two of the most commonly used prediction equations to estimate percent body fat are:

- Brozek et al. (1963):
  % Fat = (457/Body density) – 414
- Siri (1961):
  % Fat = (495/Body density) – 450

These calculations provide generalized measurements of subcutaneous fat for an average person based on the populations that were used to establish these coefficients. Tables 8-3 and 8-4 provide a quick reference for use with the three-site protocol for both men and women, based on the age of the individual.

Skinfold Measurement Protocol

Equipment:

- Skinfold caliper, properly calibrated (e.g., Slim Guide®, Lange®, Harpenden®)
- Marking pencil (optional)

Pre-test procedures:

To ensure testing accuracy, the client should be optimally hydrated and always be measured prior to exercise. Since this particular test can feel intrusive to a first-time client, the trainer should make sure the client is familiar and comfortable with the protocol. If a marking pencil is to be used, it should be washable; an eyeliner pencil works well.

Test protocol and administration:

To ensure accuracy in assessing body composition using the skinfold caliper method, it is important to measure each skinfold in the appropriate location and use standardized techniques:

- All measurements are taken on the right side of the body while the client is standing.
- Skinfold locations should be properly identified using anatomical landmarks and measurements. Use of a marking pencil will help ensure precise landmarks and consistency.
- Hold the calipers in the right hand, grasping the skinfold site with the left hand. (Left-handed calipers are available, which reverses the hand position.)
- The thumb and index finger of the left hand are opened to about 8 cm (~3 inches) and positioned 1 cm (~½ inch) above the measurement site. Grasp or pinch the skinfold site making a fold line (double fold of skin) that corresponds to the site instructions.
- To accurately assess subcutaneous fat, the skin and underlying fat are simultaneously pulled firmly away from the underlying muscle tissue.
- The pinch is maintained while the calipers are positioned perpendicular to the site and on the site location (1 cm below the thumb and index finger), midway between the top and the base of the fold.
- Slowly release the caliper trigger, reading the dial to the nearest 0.5 mm approximately two or three seconds after release.
- After taking the skinfold reading, gently squeeze the trigger to remove the caliper before releasing the skinfold pinch.
- Moving onto the next site, repeat the above steps. Each site should be measured a minimum of two times to ensure consistency between measurements. If subsequent readings produce a difference greater than 2 mm, a third measurement is necessary and the average of the two acceptable scores should be taken (i.e., within 2 mm of each other). It is recommended that the trainer wait 20 to 30 seconds between measurements to allow the skin and fat to redistribute.
- Record all measurements on a testing form.
- Evaluate and classify the client's body composition using normative data (Tables 8-5 and 8-6).

Body Composition Evaluation

Table 8-5 presents acceptable body-fat norms for both men and women. As previously mentioned, vanity is a fundamental

Table 8-5

General Body-fat Percentage Categories

Classification	Women (% fat)	Men (% fat)
Essential fat	10–13%	2–5%
Athletes	14–20%	6–13%
Fitness	21–24%	14–17%
Average	25–31%	18–24%
Obese	32% and higher	25% and higher

Table 8-6

Standard Values for Percentage Body Fat

	Age (years)				
Percentile (Men)	**20–29**	**30–39**	**40–49**	**50–59**	**60+**
90	7.1	11.3	13.6	15.3	15.2
80	9.4	13.9	16.3	17.9	18.4
70	11.8	15.9	18.1	19.8	20.3
60	14.1	17.5	19.6	21.3	22.0
50	15.9	19.0	21.2	22.7	23.5
40	17.4	20.5	22.5	24.1	25.0
30	19.5	22.3	24.1	25.7	26.7
20	22.4	24.2	26.1	27.5	28.5
10	25.9	27.3	28.9	20.3	31.2
Percentile (Women)	**20–29**	**30–39**	**40–49**	**50–59**	**60+**
90	14.5	15.5	18.5	21.6	21.1
80	17.1	18.0	21.3	25.0	25.1
70	19.0	20.0	23.5	26.6	27.5
60	20.6	21.6	24.9	28.5	29.3
50	22.1	23.1	26.4	30.1	30.9
40	23.7	24.9	28.1	31.6	32.5
30	25.4	27.0	30.1	33.5	34.3
20	27.7	29.3	32.1	35.6	36.6
10	32.1	32.8	35.0	37.9	39.3

Reprinted with permission from The Cooper Institute, Dallas, TX. For more information: www.cooperinstitute.org.

reason for lowering body fat; the trainer should also point out that personal health is negatively impacted when body fat stores are high.

There are no true recommendations for reassessment of body composition. Since time and significant energy expenditure are necessary to reduce body fat, assessments should not be conducted too frequently. Monthly or bimonthly assessments are appropriate.

Programming Considerations

Determination of body composition is essential for a personal trainer who is designing a personalized exercise program, especially if the primary goal is either weight loss or weight gain. Reducing excess adipose tissue is also important for any person trying to decrease his or her risk of major disease and dysfunction. To enhance the program's effectiveness, appropriate exercise should be used in conjunction with dietary recommendations. Body-composition values can also be used to determine a goal weight. This calculation is based on the assumption that throughout the fitness program, lean body weight or mass will not change. It should be noted that with any weight loss or gain, there is typically a change in the amount of both lean body mass and fat mass.

Desired body weight = [Lean body weight / (100% – Desired % fat)] x 100

Sample Goal Weight Calculation

To determine a goal weight based on body composition, a few simple calculations are necessary.

Starting information: Female client's current weight is 168 pounds, with 28% body fat

Initial goal: To achieve 24% body fat without losing lean tissue

- *Determine fat weight in pounds:*
  Body weight x body-fat percentage (BF%)
  168 lb x 28% = 47 lb of fat
- *Determine lean body weight (LBW):*
  Total weight – Fat weight
  168 lb – 47 lb = 121 lb of lean tissue
  (also called lean body mass)
- *Calculate goal weight:* Divide current LBW by 76% (100% – Goal BF%)
  121/0.76 = 159 lb

These and other formulas commonly used by personal trainers can be found at www.acefitness.org/calculators.

Measurement of Body Size: Other Anthropometric Measures

Though body-composition analysis provides a more three-dimensional look at the makeup of the human body, peripheral measurements can also be used to determine health and fitness status.

Anthropometry is the measurement of the size and proportions of the human body for the purposes of understanding human physical variation. The most frequently used anthropometric measures are height, weight, and circumference measures. For example, periodic height assessments are important, especially for women who may be at risk for **osteoporosis.** BMI is used extensively in healthcare settings to determine health risk and/or to establish target weight levels.

Body Mass Index

BMI provides an objective ratio describing the relationship between body weight and height. This peripheral measurement cannot determine actual body composition, which means that it can unfairly categorize some individuals. For example, individuals who are extremely muscular or have large frames can score high on the BMI charts, resulting in a label of "overweight" or even "obese," while older adults with decreased lean tissue and excess body fat may score "normal." BMI calculations are described below, though Table 8-7 can be used as a quick reference.

BMI Equations

BMI = Weight (kg)/Height^2 (m)

To convert pounds to kilograms, divide by 2.2

To convert inches to meters, multiply inches by 0.0254

or BMI = Weight (lb) x 703/Height (inches)/Height (inches)

For example, consider an individual who weighs 200 pounds and stands 5'10".

Weight = 200 pounds/2.2 = 90.9 kg

Height = 70 inches x 0.0254 = 1.778 m

BMI = 90.9/1.778^2 = 28.7

Using the standard formula: BMI = 200 lb x 703/70 inches/70 inches = 28.7

Table 8-7

Body Mass Index

	19	20	21	22	23	24	25	26	27	28	29	30	35	40
Height (inches)	**Weight (pounds)**													
58	91	95	100	105	110	115	119	124	129	134	138	143	167	191
59	94	99	104	109	114	119	124	128	133	138	143	148	173	198
60	97	102	107	112	118	123	128	133	138	143	148	153	179	204
61	100	106	111	116	121	127	132	137	143	148	153	158	185	211
62	104	109	115	120	125	131	136	142	147	153	158	164	191	218
63	107	113	118	124	130	135	141	146	152	158	163	169	197	225
64	110	116	122	128	134	140	145	151	157	163	169	174	203	233
65	114	120	126	132	138	144	150	156	162	168	174	180	210	240
66	117	124	130	136	142	148	155	161	167	173	179	185	216	247
67	121	127	134	140	147	153	159	166	172	178	185	191	223	255
68	125	131	138	144	151	158	164	171	177	184	190	197	230	263
69	128	135	142	149	155	162	169	176	182	189	196	203	237	270
70	132	139	146	153	160	167	174	181	188	195	202	209	243	278
71	136	143	150	157	165	172	179	186	193	200	207	215	250	286
72	140	147	155	162	169	177	184	191	199	206	213	221	258	294
73	144	151	159	166	174	182	189	197	204	212	219	227	265	303
74	148	155	163	171	179	187	194	202	210	218	225	233	272	311
75	152	160	168	176	184	192	200	208	216	224	232	240	279	319
76	156	164	172	180	189	197	205	213	221	230	238	246	287	328

Note: Find your client's height in the far left column and move across the row to the weight that is closest to the client's weight. His or her body mass index will be at the top of that column.

As BMI increases, so do health risks. It is estimated that 65% of Americans are overweight, and 28.1% of American men and 34.0% of American women are classified as obese. Even more shocking is the fact that 16% of American children and teens are in the obese category [Centers for Disease Control and Prevention (CDC), 2004]. A BMI greater than 25 increases a person's risk for **cardiovascular disease,** metabolic syndrome, **hypertension,** and **type 2 diabetes.** Table 8-8 is a BMI reference chart that can be used to discuss the health risks of being overweight or obese and to set long-term weight-loss goals for clients.

Calculating BMI is not only quick, but also inexpensive. BMI charts are used by many healthcare agencies to assess body mass and associated risks. If BMI charts are the *only* method of assessing body structure, the results could be misinterpreted and healthy individuals could be misclassified. A simple visual inspection should make the personal trainer question the label in these situations and proceed with a body-composition assessment to gain a more accurate indicator of health risk.

Table 8-8

BMI Reference Chart

Weight Range	BMI Category
Underweight	<18.5
Normal weight	18.5–24.9
Overweight	25.0–29.9
Grade I Obesity	30.0–34.9
Grade II Obesity	35.0–39.9
Grade III Obesity	>40

Table 8-9

Predicted Body-fat Percentage Based on Body Mass Index (BMI) for African-American and White Adults*

BMI (kg/m^2)	Health Risk	20–39 yr	40–59 yr	60–79 yr
Men				
<18.5	Elevated	<8%	<11%	<13%
18.6–24.9	Average	8–19%	11–21%	13–24%
25.0–29.9	Elevated	20–24%	22–27%	25–29%
>30	High	≥25%	≥28%	≥30%
Women				
<18.5	Elevated	<21%	<23%	<24%
18.6–24.9	Average	21–32%	23–33%	24–35%
25.0–29.9	Elevated	33–38%	34–39%	36–41%
>30	High	≥39%	≥40%	≥42%

*Standard error of estimate is +/–5% for predicting body fat from BMI (based on a four-compartment estimate of body-fat percentage).

Gallagher, D. et al. (2000). Healthy percentage body fat ranges: An approach for developing guidelines based on body mass index. *American Journal of Clinical Nutrition,* 72, 694–701.

Online BMI calculators are available where an individual can simply key in his or her height and weight and be given the BMI, including one on ACE's website (www.acefitness.org/calculators). The CDC website provides a BMI calculator specifically for children and teens (www.apps.nccd.cdc.gov/dnpabmi/Calculator.aspx). BMI can also be used to predict body-fat percentages, though the method is still in its initial stages of development (Table 8-9).

Girth Measurements

Girth measurements are not only good predictors of health problems (e.g., waist circumference as it correlates to heart disease), but an overall body assessment will also provide motivation as clients see changes in their body dimensions. In the case of excess fat mass, clients will be inspired by a decline in girth measurements, while individuals who are interested in muscular **hypertrophy** will likely be motivated by increases in girth.

When taking girth measurements, precision is necessary to validate the results. To ensure accuracy, the personal trainer must use exact anatomical landmarks for taking each measurement (Figures 8-7 through 8-9 and Table 8-10). In addition, procedures must be followed in accordance with established guidelines:

- When measuring body circumference, it is important to measure precisely and consistently.
- All measurements should be made with a non-elastic, yet flexible tape.
- The tape should be snug against the skin's surface without pressing into the subcutaneous layers. Individuals should wear thin, form-fitting materials that allow for accurate measurements.

- Trainers should rotate through the battery of sites, initially measuring each site only once.
- Duplicate measurements should be taken of each site. If recorded values are not within 5 mm, it is necessary to remeasure. Trainers should wait 20 to 30 seconds between measurements to allow the skin and subcutaneous tissue to return to its normal position.

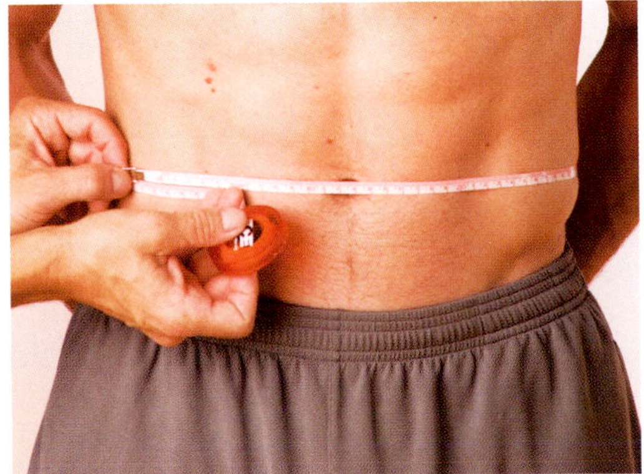

Figure 8-7
Abdominal circumference

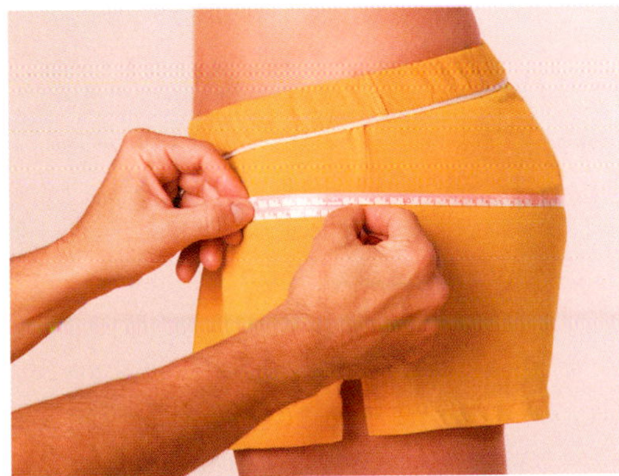

Figure 8-8
Hip circumference

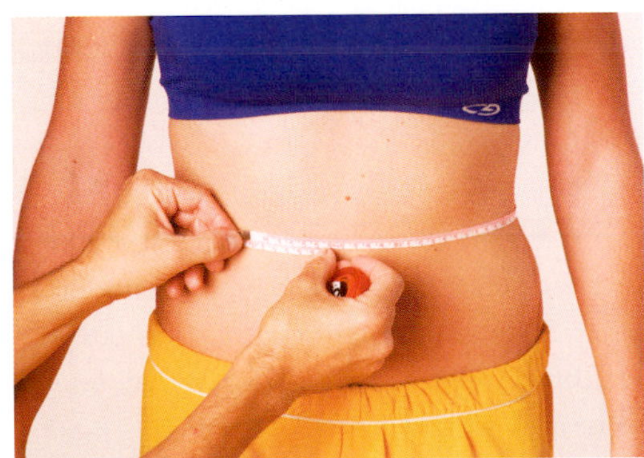

Figure 8-9
Waist circumference

Table 8-10

Standardized Description of Circumference Sites and Procedures

Site	Description
Abdomen	With the subject standing upright and relaxed, a horizontal measure is taken at the greatest anterior extension of the abdomen, usually at the level of the umbilicus (Figure 8-7).
Arm	With the subject standing erect and arms hanging freely at the sides with hands facing the thighs, a horizontal measure is taken midway between the acromion and olecranon processes.
Buttocks/hips	With the subject standing erect with the feet together, a horizontal measure is taken at the maximal circumference of the buttocks. This measure is used for the hip measure in a hip/waist measure (Figure 8-8).
Calf	With the subject standing erect [feet apart ~20 cm (8 inches)], a horizontal measure is taken at the level of the maximum circumference between the knee and the ankle, perpendicular to the long axis.
Forearm	With the subject standing, arms hanging downward but slightly away from the trunk, and palms facing anteriorly, a measure is taken perpendicular to the long axis at the maximal circumference.
Midthigh	With the subject standing with the and one foot on a bench so the knee is flexed at 90 degrees, a measure is taken midway between the inguinal crease and the proximal border of the patella, perpendicular to the long axis.
Upper thigh	With the subject standing, legs slightly apart [~10 cm (4 inches)] a horizontal measure is taken at the maximal circumference of the hip/upper thigh, just below the gluteal fold.
Waist	With the subject standing, arms at the sides, feet together, and abdomen relaxed, a horizontal measure is taken at the narrowest part of the torso (above the umbilicus and below the xiphoid process) (Figure 8-9). The National Obesity Task Force (NOTF) suggests obtaining a horizontal measure directly above the iliac crest as a method to enhance standardization. Unfortunately, current formulae are not predicated on the NOTF suggested site.

Procedures

- All measurements should be made with a flexible yet inelastic tape measure.
- The tape should be placed on the skin surface without compressing the subcutaneous adipose tissue.
- If a Gulick spring-loaded handle is used, the handle should be extended to the same marking with each trial.
- Take duplicate measures at each site, and retest if duplicate measurements are not within 5 mm.
- Rotate through measurement sites or allow time for skin to regain normal texture.

Adapted from American College of Sports Medicine (2010a). *ACSM's Guidelines for Exercise Testing and Prescription* (8th ed.). Philadelphia; Wolters Klumer/Lippincott Williams & Wilkins; Modified from Callaway, C.W. et al. (1988). Circumferences. In: Lohman, T.G., Roche, A.F., & Martorell, R. (Eds.). *Anthropometric Standardization Reference Manual.* Champaign, Ill.: Human Kinetics.

Waist-to-Hip Ratio

As mentioned previously, excess body fat poses significant health risks. The location of the fat deposits may even be a better indicator of disease risk (Chobanian et al., 2003). The WHR helps differentiate **android** (or apple-shaped) individuals from those who are **gynoid** (or pear-shaped). Those who are apple-shaped carry excess fat in the abdominal area, while pear-shaped individuals carry excess fat in the hips and thighs. Though any extra fat weight is detrimental to a person's health, those who are android and have a high WHR have a greater health risk. To determine a client's WHR, the waist measurement is divided by the hip measurement. Table 8-11 illustrates the relative risk ratings for waist-to-hip ratios.

Table 8-11

Waist-to-Hip Ratio (WHR) Norms

Gender	Excellent	Good	Average	At Risk
Males	<0.85	0.85–0.89	0.90–0.95	≥0.95
Females	<0.75	0.75–0.79	0.80–0.86	≥0.86

Bray, G.A. & Gray, D.S. (1988). Obesity: Part I: Pathogenesis. *Western Journal of Medicine,* 149, 429–441.

Waist Circumference

Visceral fat contributes to android fat distribution and is very damaging, not only because it encroaches on the vital organs of the body, but also because excess abdominal fat has been associated with **insulin resistance.** There is a strong correlation between excess abdominal fat and a number of health risks, including type 2 diabetes, hypertension, and **hypercholesterolemia.**

For every 1-inch (2.5-cm) increase in waist circumference in men, the following associated health risks are found (Janssen et al., 2004):

- Blood pressure increases by 10%
- Blood cholesterol level increases by 8%
- **High-density lipoprotein (HDL)** decreases by 15%
- **Triglycerides** increase by 18%
- Metabolic syndrome risk increases by 18%

Table 8-12 presents the risk categories associated with various waist circumferences for men and women.

Table 8-12

Criteria for Waist Circumference in Adults

	Waist Circumference	
Risk Category	Females	Males
Very low	<27.5 in (<70 cm)	<31.5 in (<80 cm)
Low	27.5–35.0 in (70–89 cm)	31.5–39.0 in (80–99 cm)
High	35.5–43.0 in (90–109 cm)	39.5–47.0 in (100–120 cm)
Very high	>43.5 in (>110 cm)	>47.0 in (>120 cm)

Bray, G.A. (2004). Don't throw the baby out with the bath water. *American Journal of Clinical Nutrition*, 70, 3, 347–349.

Many of the tests measuring body size and proportions can be used in conjunction with body-composition testing. Testing protocols are basically the same for all of the anthropometric tests:

- These tests should be performed prior to exercise.
- The trainer should explain the procedure for each test and ensure that the client is comfortable with the proposed measurement sites.
- Each measurement must be performed using the precise landmarks.
- The trainer should record values on the testing form and evaluate and classify the client's measurements using normative data.
- Trainers should discuss health and fitness concerns related to abnormal readings and educate clients on strategies to reduce personal risk and improve overall health.

Many people are often successful at losing weight or fat, but are unsuccessful at long-term weight management. It is important for the personal trainer to emphasize that exercise is a key component not only in effective weight loss, but also in maintaining a healthy weight:

- Exercise enhances daily caloric expenditure.

- Exercise, especially strength training, can minimize the loss of lean body weight.
- Exercise may suppress appetite and counteract the impact that diet may have on **resting metabolic rate (RMR).**
- Exercise makes the body more efficient at burning fat.

The previous sections in this chapter were devoted to resting measurements. Subsequent sections focus on physical-fitness assessments that are active and require submaximal to maximal effort. Not all tests are suitable for all populations. Test selection should be done with thoughtful consideration.

Cardiorespiratory Fitness Testing

Cardiorespiratory fitness (CRF) is defined by how well the body can perform dynamic activity using large muscle groups at a moderate to high intensity for extended periods of time. CRF depends on the efficiency and interrelationship of the cardiovascular, respiratory, and skeletal muscle systems.

CRF assessments are also valuable mechanisms in assessing the overall health of an individual. Exercise testing for cardiorespiratory fitness is useful to:

- Determine functional capacity, using predetermined formulas based on age, gender, and in some cases, body weight
- Determine a level of cardiorespiratory function [commonly defined as either **maximal oxygen uptake ($\dot{V}O_2$max)** or **metabolic equivalent (MET)** level] that serves as a starting point for developing goals for **aerobic** conditioning
- Determine any underlying cardiorespiratory abnormalities that signify progressive stages of cardiovascular disease
- Periodically reassess progress following a structured fitness program

The risk of heart attack and sudden cardiac death during exercise among fitness facility members is three times that of cardiac patients in a supervised rehabilitation program (Foster & Porcari, 2001). The risk can be reduced with appropriate pre-exercise screening and careful observation of clients during and following exercise.

$\dot{V}O_2$max, an excellent measure of cardiorespiratory efficiency, is an estimation of the body's ability to use oxygen for energy, and is closely related to the functional capacity of the heart. Measuring $\dot{V}O_2$max in a laboratory involves the collection and analysis of exhaled air during maximal exercise. Conducting a cardiorespiratory assessment at maximal effort is not always feasible and can actually be harmful to certain populations. Therefore, it is recommended that submaximal tests be used in the fitness setting.

Submaximal cardiorespiratory assessments will provide accurate values that can be extrapolated to determine expected maximal efforts. Repeated research demonstrates that as workload increases, so do **heart rate** and **oxygen uptake.** In fact, heart rate and oxygen uptake exhibit a fairly linear relationship to workload. This relationship allows the personal trainer to accurately estimate $\dot{V}O_2$max from the heart-rate response to exercise with fairly good accuracy. The lack of accuracy related to estimated maximum oxygen uptake is influenced by two key variables:

- Many estimation calculations are based on the calculation of 220 – age for estimating **maximum heart rate (MHR)** (Fox, Naughton, & Haskell, 1971). This formula is subject to a standard deviation of approximately ±12 beats per minute (bpm). This means that in a room of 100 40-year-old individuals (for whom this standard MHR calculation would yield an MHR of 180 bpm), the actual MHR for 68% of them would range between 168 and 192 bpm, while the remaining 32% would fall further outside that range.
- Maximal oxygen uptake is determined by estimating MHR at submaximal workloads. The charts and equations that are used to determine maximal oxygen uptake are based on the assumption that everyone expends exactly the same

amount of energy and uses the same amount of oxygen at any given work rate (remember, $\dot{V}O_2$max is calculated from equations devised after repeated tests that actually measured oxygen consumption). For this reason, a submaximal test is likely to *underestimate* the true maximum for an individual who is very deconditioned, and *overestimate* $\dot{V}O_2$max for a very fit individual. The true value of submaximal cardiorespiratory testing comes when the client can repeat the same test a few months later and then compare his or her individual test results.

There are a number of cardiorespiratory tests available to the personal trainer. The specific test used will depend on the availability of equipment, knowledge and experience of the trainer, fitness level of the client, and, in the case of field tests, the weather.

The following tests are described in this section:

- Treadmill tests:
  - ✓ Bruce submaximal treadmill exercise test
  - ✓ Balke & Ware treadmill exercise test
  - ✓ Ebbeling single-stage treadmill test
- Cycle ergometer tests:
  - ✓ YMCA bike test
  - ✓ Astrand-Ryhming cycle ergometer test
- Ventilatory threshold testing
  - ✓ Submaximal talk test for VT1
  - ✓ VT2 threshold test
- Field tests:
  - ✓ Rockport fitness walking test (1 mile)
  - ✓ 1.5-mile run test
- Step tests:
  - ✓ YMCA submaximal step test (12 inches)
  - ✓ McArdle step test (16 inches)

Maximum Heart Rate: How Useful Is The Prediction Equation?

Two methods exist for determining maximum heart rate (MHR). The most accurate way is to directly measure the MHR with an EKG monitoring device during a graded exercise test. The other way is to estimate MHR by using a simple prediction equation or formula. In 1971, the formula "220 – age" was introduced and was widely accepted by the health and fitness community (Fox, Naughton, & Haskell, 1971). However, the validity of the formula has come under attack for several reasons. The subjects used in the study to determine the formula were not representative of the general population. In addition, even if the prediction equation did represent a reasonable average, a significant percentage of individuals will not fit the average. In fact, standard deviations of plus or minus 10 to 20 beats per minute have been observed. Consequently, basing a client's exercise intensity (i.e., training heart rate) on a potentially flawed estimation of MHR is somewhat dubious. When the training heart rate is based on an estimated MHR, it should be used in combination with the ratings of perceived exertion scale (see Table 8-14 on page 192). Modify the intensity of the workout if a client reports a high level of perceived exertion, even if his or her training heart rate has not been achieved.

Cardiorespiratory Assessments for the Lab or Fitness Center

Cardiorespiratory testing in a laboratory or fitness center provides a controlled environment in which the setting is generally more private, the temperature is usually constant, and all the equipment is centrally located for easy test administration.

Graded exercise tests (GXT) conducted in laboratory and fitness settings typically use a treadmill, cycle ergometer, or arm ergometer to measure cardiorespiratory fitness. Some of the tests are administered in stages that incorporate gradual increases in exercise intensity, while others measure the heart-rate response to a single-stage bout of exercise. On a treadmill, the intensity is raised by increasing the speed and/or elevation; on the cycle or arm ergometer, the intensity is generally raised by increasing resistance, while the cadence, measured in revolutions per minute, is generally held constant.

Graded exercise tests are used extensively in both clinical and fitness settings. In the clinical setting, a GXT is typically performed to maximal exertion, which means that the test is terminated when the client can no longer tolerate the activity, when signs or symptoms arise that warrant test termination, or when the client has achieved a predetermined age-predicted MHR. There are certain risks associated with maximal GXTs, the most severe being cardiac arrest. For this reason, maximal exercise tests are not typically administered in fitness centers or other nonclinical settings.

Submaximal exercise testing is safer and, in many cases, provides a reliable indicator of maximal effort. The information obtained from a submaximal exercise test can be used to determine $\dot{V}O_2$max. Table 8-13 defines the norms for maximal oxygen uptake, or "aerobic fitness."

The workload can also be measured in METs. Workload is a reflection of oxygen consumption and, hence, energy use (i.e., 1 MET is the equivalent of oxygen consumption at rest, or approximately 3.5 mL/kg/min). For example, most **activities of daily living (ADL)** require a functional capacity of 5 METs.

In addition to measuring cardiorespiratory fitness, a GXT is also a valuable tool in identifying those who are at risk of a coronary event. The major indicators include the following (ACSM, 2010a; Miller, 2008):

- *A decrease—or a significant increase—in blood pressure with exercise:* SBP that is lower during exercise compared to SBP taken immediately prior to the test in the same posture as the test is being performed (i.e., baseline measurement); SBP that rises above 250 mmHg during exercise; or SBP that increases during immediate post-exercise recovery
- *An inadequate HR response to exercise:* An increase in HR of <80% of age-predicted value or <62% for clients on **beta blocker** medication during exercise
- *Exercise duration:* Stated simply, the longer the individual can tolerate the treadmill test, the less likely he or she is to die soon of CAD—or of any cause.
- *Heart-rate recovery:* An individual standing in an upright position should show a reduction of 12 bpm at one minute post-exercise, and an individual in a sitting position should show a reduction of 22 bpm two minutes post-exercise.

In addition to monitoring heart rate and blood pressure during the initial interview, it is essential to monitor the client before, during, and after any GXT. The following variables should be constantly assessed and recorded during an exercise test:

- *Heart rate:* Monitor continuously and record during the last 15 seconds of each minute
- *Blood pressure:* Measure and record during the last 45 seconds of each stage
- *Ratings of perceived exertion (RPE):* Record during the last five seconds of each minute (Table 8-14)
- *Signs and symptoms (S/S):* Monitor continuously and record both personal observations and subjective comments from the client

Table 8-13

Percentile Values for Maximal Oxygen Uptake (mL/kg/min)

	Age				
Percentile*	**20–29**	**30–39**	**40–49**	**50–59**	**60–69**
Men					
90	54.0	52.5	51.1	46.8	43.2
80	51.1	48.9	46.8	43.3	39.5
70	48.2	46.8	44.2	41.0	36.7
60	45.7	44.4	42.4	38.3	35.0
50	43.9	42.4	40.4	36.7	33.1
40	42.2	41.0	38.4	35.2	31.4
30	40.3	38.5	36.7	33.2	29.4
20	39.5	36.7	34.6	31.1	27.4
10	35.2	33.8	31.8	28.4	24.1
Women					
90	47.5	44.7	42.4	38.1	34.6
80	44.0	41.0	38.9	35.2	32.3
70	41.1	38.8	36.7	32.9	30.2
60	39.5	36.7	35.1	31.4	29.1
50	37.4	35.2	33.3	30.2	27.5
40	35.5	33.8	31.6	28.7	26.6
30	33.8	32.3	29.7	27.3	24.9
20	31.6	29.9	28.0	25.5	23.7
10	29.4	27.4	25.6	23.7	21.7

*To realize the health benefits of aerobic conditioning, personal-training clients should aim to achieve >30th percentile.

Note: $\dot{V}O_2$max below the 20th percentile is associated with an increased risk of death from all causes (Blair et al., 1995). Study population for the data set was predominately white and college educated. A modified Balke treadmill test was used with $\dot{V}O_2$max estimated from the last grade/speed achieved. The following may be used as descriptors for the percentile rankings: well above average (90), above average (70), average (50), below average (30), and well below average (10).

Reprinted with permission from The Cooper Institute, Dallas, Texas from *Physical Fitness Assessments And Norms For Adults And Law Enforcement*. Available online at www.cooperinstitute.org.

Table 8-14

Ratings of Perceived Exertion (RPE)

RPE	Category Ratio Scale
6	0 Nothing at all
7 Very, very light	0.5 Very, very weak
8	1 Very weak
9 Very light	2 Weak
10	3 Moderate
11 Fairly light	4 Somewhat strong
12	5 Strong
13 Somewhat hard	6
14	7 Very strong
15 Hard	8
16	9
17 Very hard	10 Very, very strong
18	* Maximal
19 Very, very hard	
20	

Source: Adapted, with permission, from American College of Sports Medicine (2010a). *ACSM's Guidelines for Exercise Testing and Prescription* (8th ed.). Philadelphia: Wolters Kluwer/Lippincott Williams & Wilkins.

There are a number of reasons to terminate an exercise test, ranging from chest pain to a drop in SBP. Additionally, a GXT *must* be terminated if the client requests to stop or fails to comply with testing protocol (i.e., cannot maintain proper cadence on the cycle ergometer). During the administration of any exercise test involving exertion (e.g., a cardiovascular test), trainers must always be aware of signs or symptoms they can identify that merit immediate termination and referral to a more-qualified professional (see page 174).

To better prepare the client and the tester, the personal trainer should clarify important information from the client's health-history form (see Figure 6-5, page 112) and review a few key procedural issues prior to any cardiorespiratory assessment:

- Medication/supplement usage. If the client is on a beta blocker (atenolol, metropolol, propranalol), the test will be invalid due to a blunted HR response. Use of stimulants may exaggerate the HR response.
- Recent musculoskeletal injury or limiting orthopedic problem(s)
- Any sickness or illness (cold, flu, infection)
- Time of last meal or snack (especially important to avoid **hypoglycemia**)
- It is the client's responsibility to perform the test as advised, as the validity of fitness testing is based on precise protocols being followed.
- Clients should provide RPE when requested, as well as information on personal signs and symptoms.
- The personal trainer will assess HR and BP at specific intervals throughout the test. The test may be terminated if there is an inappropriate HR or BP response to exercise, even without complaints from the client.
- The personal trainer should remind the client that the test will immediately cease if the client reports any significant discomfort at any point during the test. The client is free to stop the test at any time, for any reason.

Treadmill Exercise Testing

The type of test chosen to assess cardiorespiratory fitness should be individualized and based on the client's capabilities. Walking on a treadmill may make some clients uneasy. In such cases, a bicycle ergometer test or a field walking test could be used. Ideally, a submaximal *graded* fitness test should take between eight and 12 minutes (ACSM, 2010a), allowing ample time in each stage to allow the client's HR to reach **steady state (HRss).**

Treadmill tests are a simple and reliable means of assessing cardiorespiratory fitness. The type of treadmill test used will also depend on the client. Though the Bruce submaximal treadmill protocol is the most widely used, the incremental increases every three minutes are quite significant and may be overly taxing for deconditioned clients.

For this reason, the Bruce protocol is advised for younger and fitter individuals, whereas the Balke & Ware treadmill test is preferred for older and deconditioned clients, since the incremental increases are more modest.

Contraindications

Treadmill exercise testing should not be conducted when working with a client with:

- Visual or balance problems, or who cannot walk on a treadmill without using the handrails
- Orthopedic problems that create pain with prolonged walking. Low-back pain (LBP) can be aggravated at inclines exceeding 3 to 5%. As obese individuals may suffer from both balance and orthopedic issues, treadmill testing may not be an appropriate modality for them. They may be better suited to a bicycle test if cardiorespiratory testing is considered appropriate.
- Foot **neuropathy**

Bruce Submaximal Treadmill Exercise Test

The Bruce submaximal treadmill test is perhaps the most common test used to assess cardiorespiratory fitness, especially in clinical settings. The test is administered in three-minute stages until the client achieves 85% of his or her age-predicted MHR. In a clinical setting, the test is typically performed to maximal effort, to evaluate both fitness and cardiac function. Given the degree of difficulty with this test, it is generally not appropriate for deconditioned individuals or the elderly.

Equipment:

- Commercial treadmill
- Stopwatch
- Stethoscope and **sphygmomanometer** (with hand-held dial or with a stand)
- RPE scale
- HR monitor (optional)
- Medical tape

Pre-test procedure:

- Measure pre-exercise HR, sitting and standing, and record the values on a testing form or data sheet.
- Estimate the submaximal target exercise HR using the Tanaka, Monahan, and Seals (2001) formula for estimating MHR [(208 – (0.7 x Age) x 85%] (see Chapter 11 for more information on this formula). Record this value on a testing form (this is one of the test endpoints).
- Discuss RPE and remind the client that he or she will be asked for perceived exertion levels throughout the test.
- Describe the purpose of the treadmill test. Each of the stages is three minutes in length with a goal to achieve HRss at each workload. As long as HRss has been achieved, the speed and incline will increase at the end of each three-minute interval.
- Secure the BP cuff on the client's arm (tape the cuff in place with medical tape to avoid slippage). Check the accuracy of the HR monitor if one is being used.
- Allow the client to walk on the treadmill to warm up and get used to the apparatus (≤1.7 mph). He or she should avoid holding the handrails. If the client is too unstable without holding onto the rails, consider using another testing modality. The results will not be accurate if the client must hold on to the handrails the entire time.

Test protocol and administration:

- This treadmill tests begins at 1.7 mph and a 10% incline.
- Assess and record exercise HR and RPE at each minute; assess and record exercise BP at the 2:15 mark of each stage.
- The stages for the Bruce submaximal treadmill test progress are shown in Table 8-15.

Table 8-15

Bruce Submaximal Treadmill Exercise Test Protocol

Stage	Speed (mph)	Grade (%)	$\dot{V}O_2$ (mL/kg/min)
1	1.7	10	13.4
2	2.5	12	21.4
3	3.4	14	31.5
4	4.2	16	41.9

Note: Each stage is 3 minutes in duration.

- Each stage is three minutes in duration. If the difference in the client's exercise HR between the second and third minute is >6 bpm, the HR has not achieved steady state. In this case, the client should continue for an additional minute at the same speed and incline.
- The test should be performed until signs or symptoms develop that warrant test termination or until the subject's HR response exceeds 85% of MHR. To ensure test validity and accuracy, the client's HR responses should exceed 115 bpm for at least two stages.
- Upon completion of the test, the client should cool down on the treadmill, walking at a moderate speed until breathing returns to normal and HR drops below 100 bpm. Three to five minutes should be sufficient.
- Calculate $\dot{V}O_2$max and MET level using the following conversion formulas (Pollock et al., 1982; Foster et al., 1984).
  - ✓ Men: $\dot{V}O_2max = 14.8 - (1.379 \times time) + (0.451 \times time^2) - (0.012 \times time^3)$
  - ✓ Women: $\dot{V}O_2max = 4.38\ (time) - 3.90$
  - ✓ To calculate METs, divide the $\dot{V}$Omax by 3.5 mL/kg/min
- Record values on the testing form.
- Continue to observe the client after the test, as negative symptoms can arise immediately post-exercise.
- Evaluate the client's performance/maximum oxygen uptake and classify using the normative data found in Table 8-13.

Balke & Ware Treadmill Exercise Test

The Balke & Ware treadmill test is another common treadmill test used in both clinical and fitness settings to assess cardiorespiratory fitness. The test is administered in one- to three-minute stages until the desired HR is achieved or symptoms limit test completion. In a clinical setting, the test is typically performed to maximal effort, to evaluate cardiac function in addition to fitness. When performed in a fitness setting, this test should be terminated when the client achieves 85% of his or her age-predicted MHR. Since speed is held constant, this test is more appropriate for deconditioned individuals, the elderly, and those with a history of cardiovascular disease.

Equipment:

- Commercial treadmill
- Stopwatch
- Stethoscope and sphygmomanometer (with hand-held dial or with a stand)
- RPE scale
- HR monitor (optional)

Pre-test procedures:

- Measure pre-exercise HR, sitting and standing, and record the values on a testing form or data sheet.
- Estimate the submaximal target exercise HR using the Tanaka, Monahan, and Seals (2001) formula [(208 – (0.7 x Age) x 85%]. Record the value on the testing form.
- Discuss RPE and remind the client that he or she will be asked for perceived exertion levels throughout the test.
- Describe the purpose of the treadmill test. The protocols for men and women are different, as illustrated in Table 8-16:
  - ✓ For men, the treadmill speed is set at 3.3 mph, with the gradient starting at 0%. After one minute, the grade is raised to a 2% incline and increased by 1% each minute thereafter until any test termination criteria is achieved (i.e., signs, symptoms, or 85% of MHR).
  - ✓ For women, the treadmill speed is set at 3.0 mph, with the gradient starting at 0%. After three minutes, the grade is raised to a 2.5% incline and increased by 2.5% every three minutes thereafter until any test termination criteria is achieved (i.e., signs, symptoms, or 85% MHR).
- Secure the BP cuff on the client's arm (tape the cuff in place with medical tape to avoid slippage). Check the accuracy of the HR monitor if one is being used.
- Allow the client to walk on the treadmill to warm up and get used to the apparatus. He or she should avoid holding the handrails. If the client is too unstable without holding onto the rails, consider

Table 8-16

Balke & Ware Treadmill Exercise Test Protocol

Minute	Incline (Males)	Incline (Females)
1	0	0
2	2	
3	3	
4	4	2.5
5	5	
6	6	
7	7	5.0
8	8	
9	9	
10	10	7.5
11	11	
12	12	
13	13	10
14	14	
15	15	
16	16	12.5

Note: This test utilizes a constant speed of 3.3 mph for men and 3.0 mph for women.

using another testing modality, as test results will not be accurate.

Test administration:

- This treadmill test begins at 3.0 mph for a female client or 3.3 mph for a male client with a 0% grade.
- Assess and record exercise HR and RPE at each minute; assess and record exercise BP with 30 seconds to go in each stage. (Since men are only in each stage for 1 minute, BP assessment may be appropriate at every other stage.)
- The stages progress as shown in Table 8-16.
- The test should be performed until 85% maximal effort is achieved or until symptoms develop that warrant test termination.
- Upon completion of the test, allow the client to cool down on the treadmill by walking at a moderate speed until breathing returns to normal and HR drops below 100 bpm.
- Calculate $\dot{V}O_2$max and MET level using the following conversion formulas (Pollock et al., 1976; 1982).
  - ✓Men: $\dot{V}O_2$max = 1.444 (time) + 14.99
  - ✓Women: $\dot{V}O_2$max = 1.38 (time) + 5.22
  - ✓To calculate METs, divide the $\dot{V}O_2$max by 3.5 mL/kg/min
- Record all values on the testing form.
- Continue to observe the client as he or she cools down, as negative symptoms can arise immediately post-exercise.
- Using Table 8-13, rank the client's maximum oxygen uptake.

Ebbeling Single-stage Treadmill Test

The single-stage treadmill test developed by Ebbeling and colleagues (1991) is an optional treadmill test appropriate for low-risk, apparently healthy, non-athletic adults aged 20 to 59 years. This test estimates $\dot{V}O_2$max using a single-stage, four-minute submaximal treadmill walking protocol.

Equipment:

- Commercial treadmill
- Stopwatch
- RPE scale
- HR monitor (optional)

Pre-test procedure:

- Measure pre-exercise HR, sitting and standing, and record the values on a testing form or data sheet.
- Estimate the submaximal target exercise HR using the Tanaka, Monahan, and Seals (2001) formula [208 – (0.7 x Age) x 50% and 208 – (0.7 x Age) x 70%]. These values represent the warm-up range. Record these values on the testing form.
- Discuss RPE and remind the client that he or she will be asked for perceived exertion levels throughout the test.
- Describe the purpose of the treadmill test. This test consists of a four-minute warm-up stage and a single four-minute testing stage that should elicit HRss.
- Allow the client to walk on the treadmill to warm up and get used to the apparatus (≤1.7 mph). He or she should avoid holding the handrails. If the client is too unstable without holding onto the rails, consider using another testing modality. The results

will not be accurate if the client must hold on to the handrails the entire time.

Test administration:

- Warm-up stage:
  - ✓ The goal of the four-minute warm-up phase is to determine a comfortable speed between 2.0 and 4.5 mph at a 0% grade that elicits a heart rate response within 50 to 70% of age-predicted MHR.
  - ✓ For more deconditioned or elderly clients, target a warm-up intensity between 50 and 60% of MHR.
  - ✓ For apparently healthy individuals, target a warm-up intensity between 60 and 70% MHR.
    - If the HR response is not within that range at the end of the first minute, adjust the speed accordingly.
- Test:
  - ✓ The goal of the exercise phase is to complete a submaximal four-minute treadmill walk at the same speed determined during the warm-up phase, but at a 5% grade (Figure 8-10).
    - After the warm-up phase and an appropriate treadmill speed has been determined, elevate the treadmill to a 5% grade and continue into the workout stage without any stoppages.
    - Record HR in the last 15 seconds of the last two minutes of this workload to establish HRss.
    - If the HR varies by more than 5 bpm between the last two minutes, extend the workload by an additional minute and record the HRss from the new final two minutes.
    - Use the *average* of the two last heart rates as the final HR score.
- Record all values on a testing form.
- Continue to observe the client as he or she cools down, as negative symptoms can arise immediately post-exercise.
- After performing the following calculation, use Table 8-13 to rank the client's maximum oxygen uptake.

$\dot{V}O_2$max (mL/kg/min) Equation

$$\dot{V}O_2\text{max} = 15.1 + (21.8 \times \text{mph}) - (0.327 \times \text{HR}) - (0.263 \times \text{mph} \times \text{age}) + (0.00504 \times \text{HR} \times \text{age}) + (5.98 \times \text{sex*})$$

* Females = 0, males = 1, to account for gender differences (lean mass and oxygen-carrying capacity).

Example: A 30-year-old male walked at 4.0 mph (5% grade) with an HRss of 155 bpm.

✓ $\dot{V}O_2\text{max} = 15.1 + (21.8 \times 4) - (0.327 \times 155) - (0.263 \times 4 \times 30) + (0.00504 \times 155 \times 30) + (5.98 \times 1) = 15.1 + 87.2 - 50.685 - 31.56 + 23.436 + 5.98 = 49.47$ mL/kg/min

Cycle Ergometer Testing

Submaximal cycle ergometer tests, including the YMCA bike test and the Astrand-Ryhming cycle ergometer test, are useful assessment tools to estimate $\dot{V}O_2$max without maximal effort. As long as the heart rate has achieved a steady state at an appropriate workload, exercise HR can be used to predict $\dot{V}O_2$max. Calculations can be made using a simple chart (YMCA test) or a nomogram or formula (Astrand-Ryhming test).

Cycle ergometer testing has many advantages in assessing cardiorespiratory fitness. These tests are performed in a controlled environment, using stationary cycles, some of which are specifically designed for fitness

Figure 8-10
Ebbeling single-stage treadmill test

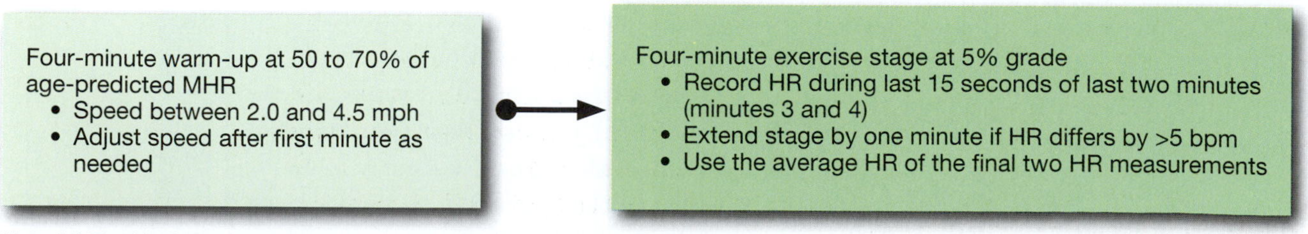

Four-minute warm-up at 50 to 70% of age-predicted MHR
- Speed between 2.0 and 4.5 mph
- Adjust speed after first minute as needed

→

Four-minute exercise stage at 5% grade
- Record HR during last 15 seconds of last two minutes (minutes 3 and 4)
- Extend stage by one minute if HR differs by >5 bpm
- Use the average HR of the final two HR measurements

Note: MHR = Maximum heart rate; HR = Heart rate; bpm = Beats per minute

testing.* These testing cycles are easy to maintain and very portable. Another advantage with this type of testing is the fact that it is easier to manually measure exercise HR and BP because the arms are relatively stationary as compared to treadmill testing. For those with balance problems or unfamiliarity with the treadmill, cycle ergometer testing is preferred.

There are disadvantages to cycle ergometer testing. Because many clients are not accustomed to cycling, the cycle ergometer test may underestimate the client's actual cardiorespiratory fitness, since he or she may prematurely experience leg fatigue (therefore underestimating $\dot{V}O_2$max). The exercise BP may also be higher than if the client was tested using a treadmill test. This is due to the prolonged muscular contractions, likely caused by the slow, controlled cadences of the test protocols themselves. And, as is the case with submaximal treadmill testing, the accuracy of these two tests is based on an initial MHR prediction calculated using the Tanaka, Monahan, and Seals (2001) formula [208 – (0.7 x Age)], which has approximately a ±7 bpm margin of error.

Contraindications

Cycle ergometer testing should be avoided when working with:

- Obese individuals who are not comfortable on the standard seats or are physically unable to pedal at the appropriate cadence
- Individuals with orthopedic problems that limit knee ROM to less than 110 degrees
- Individuals with neuromuscular problems who cannot maintain a cadence of 50 rotations per minute (rpm)

*Monarch™ and Bodyguard™ both make suitable cycle ergometers. These cycles are more expensive than standard stationary cycles and are often only utilized for the purpose of fitness testing. Because they lack many of the features of modern electronic cycles, they are typically not utilized on the fitness floor. Consequently, testing with these protocols using traditional health club bikes is difficult, as the workloads or levels are predetermined and may not match the intensities required for the test protocol.

YMCA Bike Test

This test measures HRss response to incremental (and predetermined) three-minute workloads that progressively elicit higher heart-rate responses. The HRss responses are then plotted on a graph against workloads performed. As exercise HR correlates to a $\dot{V}O_2$ score, the HR response line is extended to determine maximal effort (i.e., MHR) and estimate the individual's $\dot{V}O_2$max.

Equipment:

- Cycle ergometer
- Stopwatch
- HR monitor with chest strap
- Metronome (optional)
- Sphygmomanometer
- RPE chart

Pre-test procedures:

- Estimate the submaximal target exercise HR using the Tanaka, Monahan, and Seals (2001) formula [(208 – (0.7 x Age) x 85%]. Record this value on a testing form (this is one of the test endpoints). If an HR strap and monitor are unavailable, calculate a 15-second count for this value.
- Measure and record the client's weight in pounds and convert that value to kg by dividing the weight by 2.2.
- Measure and record seated, resting BP.
- Discuss RPE and remind the client that he or she will be asked for perceived exertion levels throughout the test.
- Adjust seat height and record the seat position for future tests to ensure consistency between tests:
  - ✓Position the pedal at the bottom of a revolution so that the crank arm is orientated vertically. Have the client place the heel of the foot on the pedal. The knee should be almost straight (5 to 10 degrees of **flexion**) in this position, with the ankle held in neutral (i.e., the toe should not be pointed in either direction). Test results may be inaccurately low if the seat is set too low.
  - ✓The seat and pedal position should be comfortable for the client.

- If a cadence meter is available on the bike, instruct the client to ride at 50 rpm. If the cadence meter is unavailable, use a metronome set to 100 bpm to coincide with each pedal stroke.
- Allow for a two- to three-minute warm-up period at a low intensity (3-out-of-10 effort) to allow the client to practice and familiarize him- or herself with the cadence. There should be no tension on the cycle during the warm-up.
- Let the client know that the test will be stopped once he or she has achieved a submaximal workload of 75 to 85%. The client can stop the test at any time and for any reason, but especially if he or she experiences chest pain, shortness of breath, dizziness, or nausea.

Test protocol and administration:

- Each stage is three minutes long. The first workload is set at 150 kilogram-meters per minute (kgm/min) or 0.5 kg (Figure 8-11).
- Continually coach the client to maintain the 50 rpm cadence. Measure and record HR and RPE at the end of each minute; measure and record BP at the start of the third minute. Before progressing to the next stage, the HR at the end of the third minute must be within 5 bpm of the HR at the end of second minute. If the subject has failed to achieve HRss between these two timeframes, have him or her perform another minute at the same workload. During the last 15 seconds of stage 1, measure the client's HR. This HR will determine which workload follows in stage 2. For example, if the client's HRss is 94 bpm at the end of stage 1, he or she will proceed to 450 kgm/min or 1.5 kg during stage 2; if the client's HRss is 88 bpm, he or she will proceed to 600 kgm/min or 2.0 kg during stage 2 (see Figure 8-11). Once a column is selected for stage 2, the next two workloads must remain consistent

Figure 8-11
YMCA bike test protocol

1st stage	150 kgm/min (0.5 kg)			
	HR: <80	**HR: 80–89**	**HR: 90–100**	**HR: >100**
2nd stage	750 kgm/min (2.5 kg)	600 kgm/min (2.0 kg)	450 kgm/min (1.5 kg)	300 kgm/min (1.0 kg)
3rd stage	900 kgm/min (3.0 kg)	750 kgm/min (2.5 kg)	600 kgm/min (2.0 kg)	450 kgm/min (1.5 kg)
4th stage	1050 kgm/min (3.5 kg)	900 kgm/min (3.0 kg)	750 kgm/min (2.5 kg)	600 kgm/min (2.0 kg)

Directions:

1. Set the 1st work rate at 150 kgm/min (0.5 kg at 50 rpm)
2. If the HR in the third minute of the stage is: <80, set the 2nd stage at 750 kgm/min (2.5 kg at 50 rpm)
   80–89, set the 2nd stage at 600 kgm/min (2.0 kg at 50 rpm)
   90–100, set the 2nd stage at 450 kgm/min (1.5 kg at 50 rpm)
   >100, set the 2nd stage at 300 kgm/min (1.0 kg at 50 rpm)
3. Set the 3rd and 4th stages (if required) according to the work rates in the columns below the 2nd loads.

Note: HR = Heart rate

Note: Resistance settings shown here are appropriate for an ergometer with a flywheel of 6 m/revolution.

Note: Work rate is often expressed in watts; 1 watt = 6 kgm/min

American College of Sports Medicine (2010a). *ACSM's Guidelines for Exercise Testing and Prescription* (8th ed.). Philadelphia: Wolters Kluwer/Lippincott Williams & Wilkins.

with each specific column (e.g., if stage 2 is performed at 600 kgm/min, then follow that same column to 750 kgm/min and 900 kgm/min for the next two stages).

- Continue to record HR, RPE, and BP for each stage.
- The tension settings may loosen during the test. It is important for the tester to pay attention to both the settings and the cadence throughout the test to ensure consistent workloads. Additionally, discourage the client from talking during the test, as the effort to talk raises the heart rate, elevating the true HR response to the workload performed. The use and practice of signals should be encouraged.
- To ensure an accurate test, at least two stages must be completed to plot the appropriate HR response. These HR measurements must be between 110 and 155 bpm (and 85% of the age-predicted heart rate). Also, the exercise HR in the second and third minutes of stage 2 must be within 5 bpm of each other. This means that an HRss has been achieved for the particular stage/workload. If the HRs are >6 bpm apart between the second and third minutes, the client will continue for one more minute at the same workload in an effort to achieve HRss. *Note:* Approximately 10% of subjects will *not* achieve the HRss, so the test should be discontinued, as it will not be valid (ACSM, 2008).

Post-test procedure:

- The client should cool down at a work rate equivalent to, or lower than, the first stage.
- As the client cools down on the cycle, continue to observe him or her, as negative symptoms can arise immediately post-exercise.
- Plot HR against workload to estimate $\dot{V}O_2$max (Figure 8-12):
  - ✓ Determine the subject's MHR and draw a line across the graph at this value.
  - ✓ Plot two steady-state heart rates between 110 and 155 bpm against the respective workload performed.
  - ✓ Draw a line through the HR coordinates and extend the line to MHR. If more than two points are used, draw a line of best fit between the coordinates if necessary.
  - ✓ Drop a line perpendicular from this point to the baseline to determine the estimated $\dot{V}O_2$max indicated along the x axis.

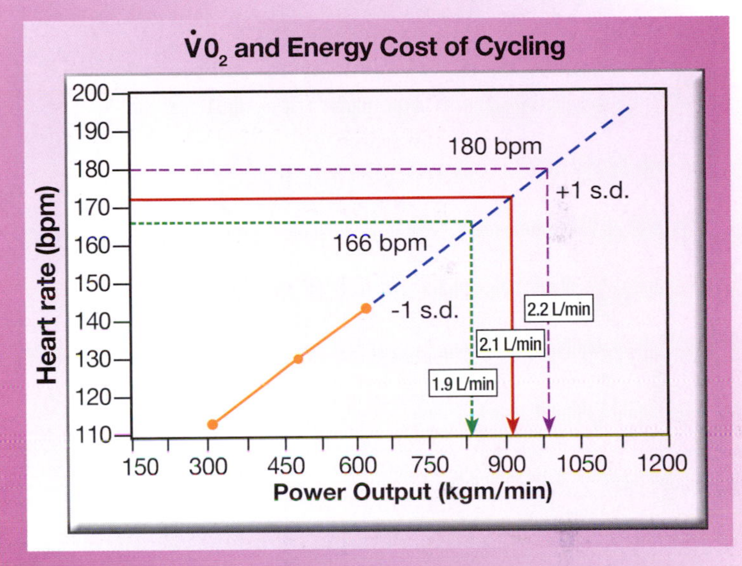

Figure 8-12
Heart-rate responses to three submaximal work rates for a 50-year-old, sedentary male weighing 79 kg (174 lb). $\dot{V}O_2$max was estimated by extrapolating the heart rate (HR) response to the age-predicted maximum HR of 173 beats per minute [based on 208 – (0.7 x Age)]. The work rate that would have been achieved at that HR was determined by dropping a line from that HR value to the x axis. $\dot{V}O_2$max is estimated to be 2.1 L/min. The other two lines estimate what the $\dot{V}O_2$max would have been if the subjects true maximum HR was ±1 standard deviation (s.d.) from the 173 beats/minute value.

$\dot{V}O_2$max Conversion

Oxygen uptake is dependent on the size of the individual being tested. To compare $\dot{V}O_2$max among individuals of different weights, oxygen uptake (in milliliters) must be divided by body weight (in kilograms). To calculate this conversion, perform the following steps:

- Convert L/minute to mL/minute by multiplying by 1,000
- Convert body weight in pounds to kg by dividing by 2.2
- Divide mL/kg

Oxygen uptake is always measured per minute, so the units become mL/kg/min.

Astrand-Ryhming (A-R) Cycle Ergometer Test

This test estimates $\dot{V}O_2max$ using a single-stage, six-minute submaximal cycling protocol. It is a single-stage test and relatively simple to perform. Because it is easier to administer than the YMCA bike test, this test may be a more appropriate choice for trainers who are new to cycle-ergometer testing. Consider, however, that inexperienced riders might find riding at a moderate-to-hard intensity for six minutes fatiguing.

Equipment:

- Cycle ergometer
- HR monitor with chest strap
- Metronome (optional)
- Stopwatch
- Sphygmomanometer
- RPE chart

Pre-test procedure:

- Estimate 85% of MHR [based on 208 – (0.7 x Age)] and record the value on the testing form. If an HR strap and monitor are unavailable, calculate a 10-second count for this value. For safety reasons, it is up to the tester to ensure that the client does not exceed this HR limit.
- Measure and record the client's weight and convert that value to kg by dividing the weight by 2.2.
- Measure and record a seated, resting BP.
- Discuss RPE and remind the client that he or she will be asked for perceived exertion levels throughout the test.
- Adjust the seat height and record the seat position for future tests to ensure consistency between tests:
  - ✓ Position the pedal at the bottom of a revolution so that the crank arm is orientated vertically. Have the client place the heel of the foot on the pedal. The knee should be almost straight (5 to 10 degrees of flexion) in this position, with the ankle held in neutral (i.e., the toes should not be pointed in either direction). Test results may be inaccurately low if the seat is set too low.
  - ✓ The seat and pedal position should be comfortable for the client.
- If a cadence meter is available on the bike, instruct the client to ride at 50 rpm. If it is unavailable, use a metronome set to 100 bpm to coincide with each pedal stroke.
- Allow for a two- to three-minute warm-up period at a low intensity (2- or 3-out-of-10 effort) to allow the client to practice and familiarize him- or herself with the cadence. There should be no tension on the cycle during the warm-up.
- Inform the client that the test will be six minutes in length, during which time he or she will attempt to maintain an HRss between 120 and 170 bpm to ensure test validity (ACSM, 2010a). The test can be stopped if the client exceeds 85% of age-predicted MHR or cannot maintain the cadence. The client can stop the test at any time and for any reason, but especially if he or she experiences chest pain, shortness of breath, dizziness, or nausea.

Test protocol and administration:

- Recommend a two- to three-minute warm-up to achieve an HRss slightly above 120 bpm to determine an appropriate test intensity.
- The workload should be determined by the client's gender and physical condition. The following workloads are used throughout the entire six minutes.
  - ✓ Male, unconditioned: 300 to 600 kilogram-meters per minute (kgm/min) (50 to 100 watts)
  - ✓ Male, conditioned: 600 to 900 kgm/min (100 to 150 watts)
  - ✓ Female, unconditioned: 300 to 450 kgm/min (50 to 75 watts)
  - ✓ Female, conditioned: 450 to 600 kgm/min (75 to 100 watts)
- After the first and second minutes, measure HR and adjust intensity accordingly:
  - ✓ Increase the exercise intensity/cycle resistance if the HR is below 120 bpm.
  - ✓ Decrease exercise intensity/cycle resistance if the HR is near 170 bpm.
- Instruct the client to maintain a steady pace throughout the test. Record RPE and HR at each minute to ensure the

client is staying within the recommended **target heart-rate range (THRR).** Blood pressure should be assessed and recorded at the four-minute mark. Record the client's HR at minute 5 and minute 6. These values will be averaged and used for determining $\dot{V}O_2$max.

- Once the test is completed, the client should cool down at a reduced workload for three to five minutes, until HR and breathing rate return to normal. The trainer should continue to observe the client, as negative symptoms can arise immediately post-exercise.
- Using the Astrand-Ryhming nomogram (Figure 8-13), draw a line from the averaged pulse rate through the $\dot{V}O_2$max and to the workload used for the test, either male or female. The place where the line intersects the $\dot{V}O_2$max is used to determine the client's maximum oxygen uptake.
- $\dot{V}O_2$max value must then be age-adjusted using the correction factors listed in Table 8-17. To calculate the estimated $\dot{V}O_2$max, the age correction factor is multiplied by the $\dot{V}O_2$max value from the nomogram.
- Record the value on the testing form.
- Convert to mL/kg/min and use Table 8-13 to rank the client's maximum oxygen uptake.

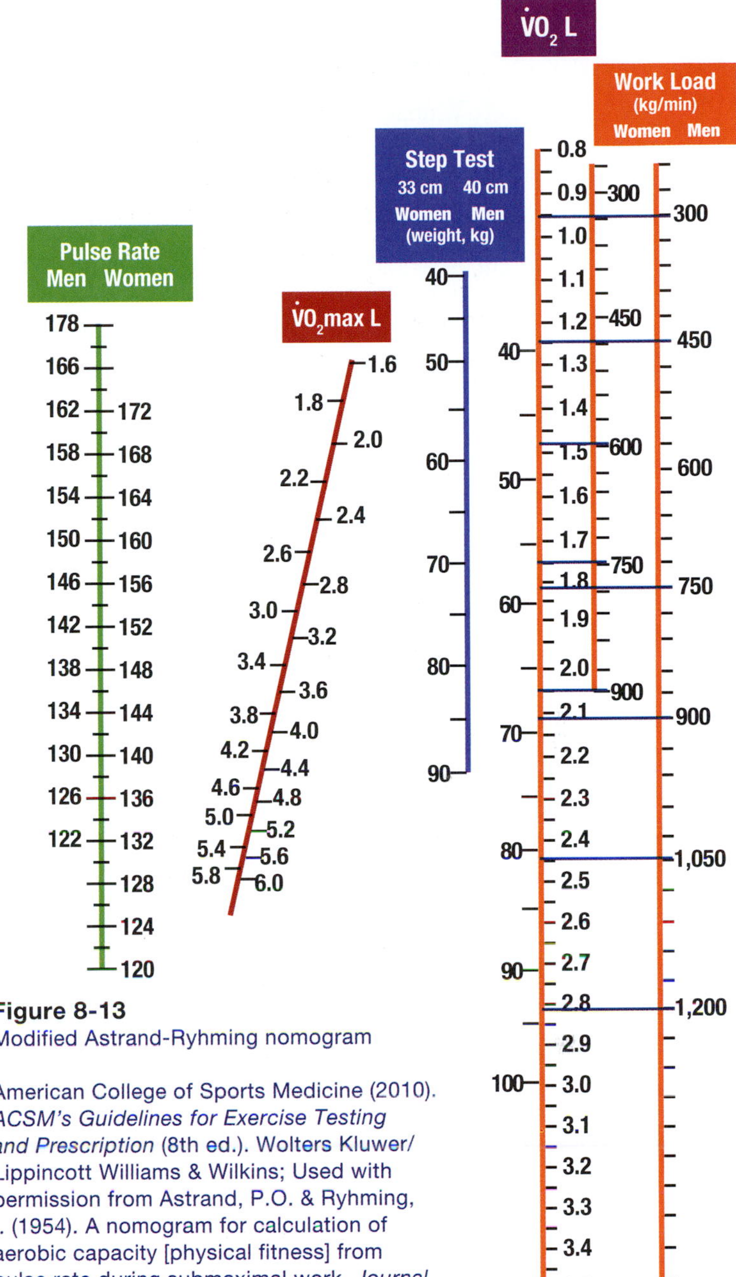

Figure 8-13
Modified Astrand-Ryhming nomogram

American College of Sports Medicine (2010). *ACSM's Guidelines for Exercise Testing and Prescription* (8th ed.). Wolters Kluwer/ Lippincott Williams & Wilkins; Used with permission from Astrand, P.O. & Ryhming, I. (1954). A nomogram for calculation of aerobic capacity [physical fitness] from pulse rate during submaximal work. *Journal of Applied Physiology*, 7, 218–221.

Table 8-17

$\dot{V}O_2$max Correction Factors

Age	Correction Factor
15	1.10
25	1.00
35	0.87
40	0.83
45	0.78
50	0.75
55	0.71
60	0.68
65	0.65

Sample $\dot{V}O_2$max Calculation

Determine $\dot{V}O_2$max for a 45-year-old female, weighing 115 pounds (52.3 kg), who completed the Astrand-Ryhming cycle ergometer test at 450 kgm/min (75 watts). Her exercise HR was 128 bpm at the fifth minute and 132 bpm at the sixth minute. The average HR is 130 bpm.

According the nomogram (use Figure 8-13), her $\dot{V}O_2$max is 3.4.

After multiplying by the age-correction factor (see Table 8-17), her adjusted $\dot{V}O_2$max is 2.028 L/min (2.6 x 0.78 = 2.028). To classify her effort, convert L/min to mL/min: 2.028 L/min x 1000 = 2,028 mL/min. Now divide 2,028 mL/min by her bodyweight of 52.3 kg to yield her $\dot{V}O_2$max in mL/kg/min:

2.028 L/min / 52.3 kg = 38.8 mL/kg/min, which ranks her in the 80th percentile for women of her age (see Table 8-13).

Ventilatory Threshold Testing

Ventilatory threshold testing is based on the physiological principle of ventilation. As exercise intensity increases, ventilation increases in a somewhat linear manner, demonstrating deflection points at certain intensities associated with metabolic changes within the body. One point, called the "crossover" point, or the **first ventilatory threshold (VT1),** represents a level of intensity where **lactic acid** begins to accumulate within the blood. Prior to this intensity, fats are a major fuel and only small amounts of lactic acid are being produced. The cardiorespiratory challenge to the body lies with **inspiration** and not with the **expiration** of additional amounts of carbon dioxide (associated with buffering lactic acid in the blood). The need for oxygen is met primarily through an increase in **tidal volume** and not respiratory rate. Hence, the ability to talk should not be compromised and should not appear challenging or uncomfortable to the individual. Past the crossover point, however, ventilation rates begin to increase exponentially as oxygen demands outpace the oxygen-delivery system and lactic acid begins to accumulate in the blood. Consequently, respiratory rates increase and talking becomes difficult.

Some trainers may have access to metabolic analyzers that will allow them to identify VT1 and the **second ventilatory threshold (VT2)** using the **respiratory exchange ratio (RER)** scores (approximately 0.85 to 0.87 for VT1 and approximately 1.00 for VT2). However, the majority of trainers will not have access to metabolic analyzers and will need valid field tests to identify these markers. This section reviews field tests for measuring HR at VT1 and VT2. This type of testing is also useful for athletes interested in estimating their **lactate threshold (LT)** (see page 204).

Contraindications

This type of testing is not recommended for:

- Individuals with certain breathing problems [**asthma** or other **chronic obstructive pulmonary disease (COPD)**]
- Individuals prone to panic/anxiety attacks, as the labored breathing may create discomfort or precipitate an attack
- Those recovering from a recent respiratory infection

> **Individualized Metabolic Markers**
>
> Ventilatory threshold tests for VT1 and VT2 provide heart-rate data based on a client's unique metabolic response to exercise, allowing for very individualized program design. The submaximal tests for VT1 and VT2 are part of cardiorespiratory training phases 2 through 4 of the ACE IFT Model.

Submaximal Talk Test for VT1

This test is best performed using HR **telemetry** (HR strap and watch) for continuous monitoring. To avoid missing VT1, the exercise increments need to be small, increasing steady-state HR by approximately 5 bpm per stage. Consequently, this test will require some preparation to determine the appropriate increments that elicit a 5 bpm increase (0.5 mph, 1% incline, or one to two levels on a bike/elliptical trainer are typical). Once the increments are determined, the time needed to reach steady-state HR during a stage must also be determined (60 to 120 seconds per stage is usually adequate).

The end-point of the test is not a predetermined heart rate, but is based on monitoring changes in breathing rate (technically metabolic changes) that are determined by the client's ability to recite the Pledge of Allegiance or a similar combination of phrases. *Note:* Reading as opposed to reciting from memory may not be advised if it compromises balance on a treadmill.

The objectives of the test are to measure the HR response at VT1 by progressively increasing exercise intensity and achieving steady-state at each stage, as well as to identify the HR where the ability to talk continuously becomes compromised. This point represents the intensity where the individual can continue to talk while breathing with minimal discomfort and reflects an associated increase in tidal volume that should not compromise breathing rate or the ability to talk. Progressing beyond this point where breathing rate increases significantly, making continuous talking difficult, is not necessary and will render the test inaccurate.

Equipment:

- Treadmill, cycle ergometer, elliptical trainer, or arm ergometer
- Stopwatch
- HR monitor with chest strap (optional)
- Cue cards, if needed; any 30- to 50-word paragraph will do

Pre-test procedure:

- As this test involves small, incremental increases in intensity specific to each individual, the testing stages need to be predetermined. The goal is to incrementally increase workload in small quantities to determine VT1. Large incremental increases may result in the individual passing through VT1, thereby invalidating the test:
    - ✓ Recommended workload increases are approximately 0.5 mph, 1% grade, or 15 to 20 watts.
    - ✓ The objective is to increase HRss at each stage by approximately 5 bpm.
    - ✓ Plan to complete this test within eight to 16 minutes to ensure HRss is achieved at each stage. The trainer should progress the client so that localized muscle fatigue from longer durations of exercise is not an influencing factor.
- Measure pre-exercise HR and BP (if necessary), both sitting and standing, and then record the values on the testing form.
- Describe the purpose of this graded exercise test, review the predetermined protocol, and allow the client the opportunity to address any questions or concerns. Each stage of the test lasts one to two minutes to achieve HRss at each workload.
- Toward the latter part of each stage (i.e., last 20 to 30 seconds), measure the HR and then ask the client to recite the Pledge of Allegiance or another predetermined passage or combination of phrases. The client's ability to talk without difficulty will be evaluated.
    - ✓ When fats are the primary fuel (below VT1), the demand for O_2 is met by increasing tidal volume. Therefore, the ability to talk continuously during expiration should not be compromised. This implies taking a noticeably deeper breath every five to 10 words, but not gasping due to the increased breathing rate.
    - ✓ However, when carbohydrates become the primary fuel (above VT1) the demand for CO_2 removal is met by increasing breathing rate. Therefore, the ability to talk continuously during expiration becomes compromised. This implies a noticeable increase in breathing rate where the ability to string five to 10 words together becomes challenging or difficult.
- Conversations with questions and answers are not suggested, as the test needs to evaluate the challenge of talking continuously, not in brief bursts as in conversation.
- Allow the client to walk on the treadmill or use the ergometer to warm up and get used to the apparatus. If using a treadmill, he or she should avoid holding the handrails. If the client is too unstable without holding onto the rails, consider using another testing modality, as this will invalidate the test.
- Take the client through a light warm-up (2- to 3-out-of-10 effort) for three to five minutes, maintaining a heart rate below 120 bpm.

Test protocol and administration:

- Once the client has warmed up, adjust the workload intensity so the client's HR is approximately 120 bpm, or an intensity level of 3 to 4 on a 10-point scale.
- Begin the test, maintaining the intensity until HRss is achieved. Record this value.
- Ask the client to recite something from memory or read out-loud continuously for 20 to 30 seconds.

- ✓Trainers should exercise caution if deciding to ask a client to read something while using a treadmill, given the potential risk of falling.
- Upon completion of the recital or reading, ask the client to identify whether he or she felt this task was easy, uncomfortable-to-challenging, or difficult.
- If VT1 is not achieved, progress through the successive stages, repeating the protocol at each stage until VT1 is reached.
- Once the HR at VT1 is identified, progress to the cool-down phase (matching the warm-up intensity) for three to five minutes.
- This test should ideally be conducted on two separate occasions with the same exercise modality to determine an average VT1 HR.
  - ✓HR varies between treadmills, bikes, etc., so it is important to conduct the tests with the exercise modality that the client uses most frequently.
  - ✓The VT1 HR will also be noticeably higher if the test is conducted after weight training due to fatigue and increased metabolism. Therefore, clients should be tested before performing resistance-training exercises.

Application

The HR at VT1 can now be used as a target HR when determining exercise intensity. Those interested in sports conditioning and/or competition would benefit from training at higher intensities, but those interested in health and general fitness are well-served to stay at or slightly below this exercise intensity.

VT2 Threshold Test

Another important metabolic marker is the determination of a client's **onset of blood lactate accumulation (OBLA),** the point at which lactic acid accumulates at rates faster than the body can buffer and remove it (blood lactate >4 mmol/L). This marker represents an exponential increase in the concentration of blood lactate, indicating an exercise intensity that can no longer be sustained. This point has historically been referred to as the lactate or **anaerobic threshold,** and corresponds with VT2. This is an important marker, as it represents the highest sustainable level of exercise intensity, a strong marker of exercise performance. Continually measuring blood lactate is an accurate method to determine OBLA and the corresponding VT2. However, the cost of lactate analyzers and handling of biohazardous materials make it impractical for most fitness professionals. Consequently, field tests have been created to challenge an individual's ability to sustain high intensities of exercise for a predetermined duration to *estimate* VT2. This method of testing requires an individual to sustain the highest intensity possible during a single bout of steady-state exercise. This obviously mandates high levels of conditioning and experience in pacing. Consequently, VT2 testing is *only* recommended for well-conditioned individuals with performance goals.

While laboratory testing (collecting blood samples) represents the most accurate method to assess OBLA (i.e., LT or VT2), limitations related to accessibility, equipment, technical expertise, cost, and functional application render this unfeasible in most cases. Consequently, field tests are commonly used to identify the HR response associated with VT2. The major disadvantages associated with field tests are that they do not assess any direct metabolic responses beyond heart rate and that they can be influenced by environmental variables (e.g., temperature, humidity, wind) that may potentially impact the actual numbers obtained. While several laboratory protocols have been validated through research over the past 30 years, relatively little research has evaluated or validated field-testing protocols.

Well-trained individuals can probably estimate their own HR response at VT2 during their training by identifying the highest sustainable intensity they can maintain for an extended duration. In cycling, coaches often select a 10-mile time trial or 60 minutes of sustained intensity, whereas in running, a 30-minute run is often used. Given that testing for 30 to 60 minutes is impractical in most fitness facilities, trainers can opt to use shorter single-stage tests of highest sustainable intensity to estimate the HR response at VT2.

In general, the intensity that can be sustained for 15 to 20 minutes is higher than what could be sustained for 30 to 60 minutes in conditioned individuals. To predict the HR response at VT2 using a 15- to 20-minute test, trainers can estimate that the corrected HR response would be equivalent to approximately 95% of the 15- to 20-minute HR average. For example, if an individual's average sustainable HR for a 20-minute bike test is 168 bpm, his or her HR at VT2 would be 160 bpm (168 bpm x 0.95).

This test is best performed using HR telemetry (HR strap and watch) for continuous monitoring. Individuals participating in this test need experience with the selected modality to effectively pace themselves at their maximal sustainable intensity for the duration of the bout. In addition, this test should only be performed by clients who are deemed low- to moderate-risk and who are successfully training in phase 3 of the ACE IFT Model.

Objective: To measure HR response at VT2 using a single-stage, sustainable, high-intensity 15- to 20-minute bout of exercise

Pre-test procedure:

- Briefly explain the purpose of the test, review the predetermined protocol, and allow the client the opportunity to address any questions or concerns.
- Take the client through a light warm-up (2- to 3-out-of-10 effort) for three to five minutes, maintaining a heart rate below 120 bpm.

Test protocol and administration:

- Begin the test by increasing the intensity to the predetermined level.
  ✓ Allow the individual to make changes to the exercise intensity as needed during the first few minutes of the bout. Remember, he or she needs to be able to maintain the selected intensity for 20 minutes.
- Record the HR response at the end of each of the last five minutes of the bout.
- Use the average HR collected over the last five minutes to account for any **cardiovascular drift** associated with fatigue, **thermoregulation,** and changing blood volume.
- Multiply the average HR attained during the 15- to 20-minute high-intensity exercise bout by 0.95 to determine the VT2 estimate.

Application

The lactate threshold and corresponding VT2 are commonly related to performance. For example, if two athletes with the same $\dot{V}O_2max$ are competing, the athlete with the higher lactate threshold will likely outperform the other athlete. Lactate threshold is improved by endurance training and high-intensity training (up to 105% of $\dot{V}O_2max$). At these intense training levels, the body can respond and adapt to the increased workloads, thereby "clearing" the blood lactate at a more efficient rate. In essence, lactate-threshold training shifts the lactate curve to the right (Figure 8-14).

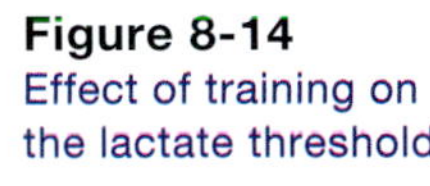

Figure 8-14
Effect of training on the lactate threshold

Note: LT = Lactate threshold

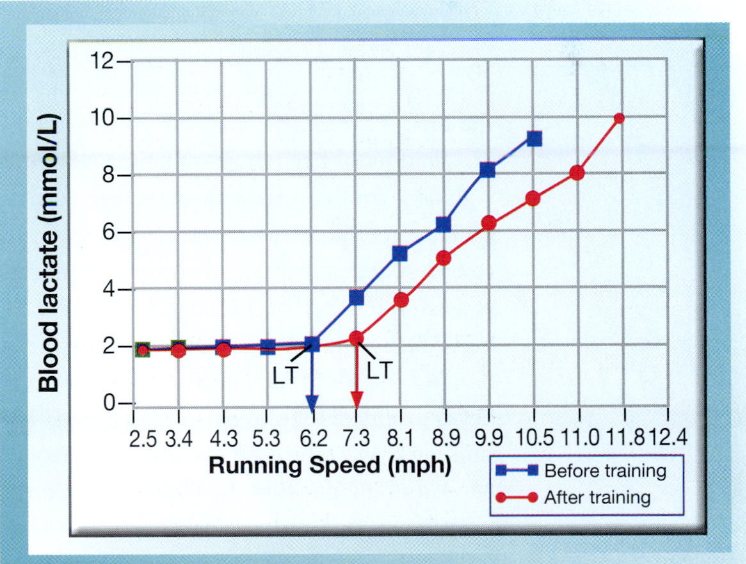

Field Testing

Most field tests are simple to administer, involve very little expense, and can be used for testing multiple clients. Many of the field tests described in this section can also be self-administered, allowing clients to periodically reassess their own progress. These assessments offer reliable testing methods for a personal trainer who does not have access to many of the traditional testing equipment found in a fitness center or health club.

Since many of the field tests can be performed outside, it is important to be mindful of extreme weather conditions and avoid exercise testing during extreme heat and humidity or when the weather turns cold.

Contraindications

Outdoor walk/run testing is not appropriate:

- In extreme weather conditions
- For individuals with health challenges that would preclude continuous walking (e.g., intermittent leg claudication, osteoarthritis of the knee or hip)
- For individuals with breathing difficulties exacerbated by pollution or outdoor allergens

Running tests are not recommended for those who are deconditioned.

Rockport Fitness Walking Test (1 Mile)

The purpose of the Rockport fitness walking test is to estimate $\dot{V}O_2$max from a client's HRss response. This test involves the completion of a 1-mile (1.6 km) walking course as fast as possible. The $\dot{V}O_2$max is calculated using the client's HRss, or immediate post-exercise HR, and his or her 1-mile walk time. This test is suitable for many individuals, easy to administer, and inexpensive to conduct. However, considering that walking may not elicit much of a cardiorespiratory challenge to conditioned individuals, this test will generally under-predict $\dot{V}O_2$max in fit individuals and is therefore not appropriate for that population group. A running track is the preferred testing surface. Most running tracks in the United States are a quarter-mile in distance, which means that walking four times around on the innermost lane will equal 1 mile. This test is also suitable for testing large groups of people, and clients can periodically reassess their own fitness levels by self-administering this test. This method of testing would also be preferred for a client who intends to walk/run outdoors as his or her mode of fitness training.

Research has shown that clients using a treadmill and walking on a track achieved similar $\dot{V}O_2$max results. When the weather is inclement and/or a track is not available, a treadmill test can be administered (Nieman, 2003).

Equipment:

- Quarter-mile track or suitable alternative (e.g., treadmill)
- Stopwatch
- RPE chart
- HR monitor with chest strap (optional)

Pre-test procedure:

- After explaining the purpose of the 1-mile Rockport fitness walking test, define the 1-mile course.
- The goal of the test is to walk as fast as possible for 1 mile. Running is not permitted for this test. Pacing is strongly recommended throughout the test.
- Discuss RPE and remind the client that he or she will be asked for perceived exertion levels throughout the test.

Test protocol and administration:

- Record the client's weight (in kg) and age.
- On the trainer's "go", the stopwatch is started and the client begins.
- The client's 1-mile (1.6-km) time, RPE, and immediate post-exercise heart rate (HRss), are recorded on the testing form. If an HR monitor is not used, a manual pulse count should be done for 15 seconds and then multiplied by four to determine an accurate HR immediately post-exercise.
- Encourage a three- to five-minute cool-down, followed by stretching of the lower extremities.

Evaluation of performance:

- The client's information is plugged into one of the following formulas (ACSM, 2008):
  - ✓ *Females:* $\dot{V}O_2$ (mL/kg/min) = 132.853 – (0.1692 x weight in kg) – (0.3877 x age) – (3.265 x walk time expressed in minutes to the nearest 100th) – (0.1565 x HR)
  - ✓ *Males:* $\dot{V}O_2$ (mL/kg/min) = 139.168 – (0.1692 x weight in kg) – (0.3877 x Age) – (3.265 x walk time expressed in minutes to the nearest 100th) – (0.1565 x HR)

- Record the values on the testing form. It is also important to include weather, surface conditions, or any other variables that may have an impact on overall time.
- Continue to observe the client, as negative symptoms can arise immediately post-exercise.
- Evaluate the client's score using Table 8-13 or use Table 8-18 to classify performance using normative data.
- *Example:* Jessica, a 26-year-old client weighing 125 lb (56.8 kg), completes the 1-mile walk in 16:40 with an HRss of 132 bpm.

  ✓ $\dot{V}O_2max$ = 132.853 – (0.1692 x body weight) – (0.388 x age) – (3.265 x time) – (0.1565 x HR)

  = 132.853 – (0.1692 x 56.8) – (0.388 x 26) – (3.265 x 16.67) – (0.1565 x 132)

  = 132.853 – 9.61 – 10.09 – 54.43 – 20.66

  = 38.06 mL/kg/min

Table 8-18
Normative Values for the Rockport Walking Test

Rating	Males (Age 30–69)	Females (Age 30–69)
	Time (minutes : seconds)	Time (minutes : seconds)
Excellent	<10:12	<11:40
Good	10:13–11:42	11:41–13:08
High average	11:43–13:13	13:09–14:36
Low average	13:14–14:44	14:37–16:04
Fair	14:45–16:23	16:05–17:31
Poor	>16:24	>17:32
Percentile	**Males (Age 18–30)**	**Females (Age 18–30)**
90%	11:08	11:45
75%	11:42	12:49
50%	12:38	13:15
25%	13:38	14:12
10%	14:37	15:03

Adapted with permission from Morrow, J.R. et al. (2005). *Measurement and Evaluation in Human Performance* (3rd ed.). Champaign, Ill.: Human Kinetics.

1.5-mile Run Test

The 1.5-mile (2.4-km) run test is used by the U.S. Navy to evaluate cardiovascular fitness levels of its personnel. The purpose of this test is to measure cardiovascular endurance and muscular endurance of the legs. Like the Rockport 1-mile (1.6-km) fitness walking test, the goal of this test is to cover the required distance in the least amount of time. A running track is the preferred setting. Due to the intense nature of running, this test is not suitable for less-conditioned individuals. Effective pacing is important for a successful outcome.

Equipment:

- Quarter-mile track or suitable alternative (e.g., treadmill)
- Stopwatch
- HR monitor with chest strap (optional)

Pre-test procedure:

- After explaining the purpose of the 1.5-mile (2.4-km) run test, define the course.
- The goal of the test is to run as fast as possible for 1.5-miles (2.4-km). Walking is permitted if necessary, though it will create an underestimation of the $\dot{V}O_2max$ score.

Test protocol and administration:

- Record the client's weight (in kg).
- On the trainer's "go", the stopwatch is started and the client begins.
- Record the client's time and immediate post-exercise HR (HRss) on the testing form.
- Encourage a three- to five-minute cool-down followed by stretching of the lower extremities.
- The client information is plugged into the following formula (ACSM, 2008):

  ✓ $\dot{V}O_2max$ (mL/kg/min) = 88.02 – (0.1656 x weight in kg) – (2.76 x time, expressed in minutes to the nearest 100th) + (3.716 x sex*)

  *1 for males, 0 for females
- Classify the client's score using Table 8-13 or the normative data presented in Table 8-19 and record the values on the testing form.
- Continue to observe the client, as negative symptoms can arise immediately post-exercise.

Table 8-19
Normative Values for the 1.5-mile (2.4-km) Run

Men	Age				
Percentile	20–29 (n = 1,675)	30–39 (n = 7,095)	40–49 (n = 6,837)	50–59 (n = 3,808)	60+ (n = 1,005)
90	9:09	9:30	10:16	11:18	12:20
80	10:16	10:47	11:44	12:51	13:53
70	10:47	11:34	12:34	13:45	14:53
60	11:41	12:20	13:14	14:24	15:29
50	12:18	12:51	13:53	14:55	16:07
40	12:51	13:36	14:29	15:26	16:43
30	13:22	14:08	14:56	15:57	17:14
20	14:13	14:52	15:41	16:43	18:00
10	15:10	15:52	16:28	17:29	19:15
Women	**Age**				
Percentile	**20–29 (n = 764)**	**30–39 (n = 2,049)**	**40–49 (n = 1,630)**	**50–59 (n = 878)**	**60+ (n = 202)**
90	11:43	12:51	13:22	14:55	14:55
80	12:51	13:43	14:31	15:57	16:20
70	13:53	14:24	15:16	16:27	16:58
60	14:24	15:08	15:57	16:58	17:46
50	14:55	15:26	16:27	17:24	18:16
40	15:26	15:57	16:58	17:55	18:44
30	15:57	16:35	17:24	18:23	18:59
20	16:33	17:14	18:00	18:49	19:21
10	17:21	18:00	18:31	19:30	20:04

Hoffman, J. (2006). *Norms for Fitness, Performance, and Health.* Champaign, Ill.: Human Kinetics.; Adapted from American College of Sports Medicine (1995). *ACSM's Guidelines for Exercise Testing and Prescription* (5th ed.). Philadelphia: Williams & Wilkins.

- *Example:* Todd, a 34-year-old client weighing 175 lb, completes the 1.5-mile (2.4-km) run in 11:20 with an HRss of 155 bpm.
  ✓ 175 lb/2.2 lb/kg = 79.54 kg
  ✓ $\dot{V}O_2max$ = 88.02 – (0.1656 x body weight) – (2.76 x time) + (3.716 x sex)
  = 88.02 – (0.1656 x 79.54) – (2.76 x 11.33) – (3.716 x 1)
  = 88.02 – 13.17 – 31.27 – 3.716
  = 39.86 mL/kg/min

Step Tests

Step tests are another tool used to assess cardiorespiratory fitness. In general, step tests require the subject to step continuously at a specific cadence or pace for a predetermined timeframe (usually three minutes). Fitness level is determined by the immediate post-exercise recovery heart rate. More fit individuals will (1) not work as hard during exercise and require less effort from their heart and (2) recover from exercise faster than those who are less fit. In essence, the *lower* the exercising or recovery HR, the *higher* the level of fitness. Given the relatively low cardio-respiratory challenge of these tests, they are not appropriate for fit individuals, as they do not differentiate fitness levels between fit and very fit individuals.

Step tests are very simple to administer, require very little investment in supplies, and take very little time. Another advantage of step tests is that they can be administered to large groups and even be self-administered.

Contraindications

Due to the nature of step testing, this assessment may not be appropriate for:

- Individuals who are extremely overweight
- Individuals with balance concerns
- Individuals with orthopedic problems (e.g., knee, low-back)
- Individuals who are extremely deconditioned, as the intensity of the test may require near-maximal effort
- Individuals who are short in stature, as they may have trouble with the step height, especially during the McArdle step test

YMCA Submaximal Step Test

The YMCA submaximal step test is one of the most popular step tests used to measure cardiorespiratory endurance and is considered suitable for low-risk, apparently healthy, non-athletic individuals between the ages of 20 and 59. This particular test uses any 12-inch (30.5 cm) step, with the Reebok® step being utilized most frequently in fitness settings (four risers plus the platform).

Equipment:

- 12-inch (30.5 cm) step
- Stopwatch
- Metronome
- Stethoscope (optional)

Pre-test procedure:

- After explaining the purpose of the YMCA submaximal step test, set the metronome to a cadence of 96 "clicks" per minute, which represents 24 steps/minute (or 96 foot placements).

- ✓ Describe and demonstrate the four-part stepping motion ("up," "up," "down," "down").
- ✓ Either foot can lead the step sequence.
- ✓ Permit a short practice to allow clients to familiarize themselves with the cadence.

- The goal of the test is to step up and down on a 12-inch riser for three minutes (Figure 8-15).
- Explain to the client that heart rate will be measured through **palpation** (or **auscultation**) for one full minute upon completion of the test, counting the number of beats during that first minute of recovery. It is important for the client to sit down immediately following the test and remain quiet to allow the trainer to accurately assess heart rate.

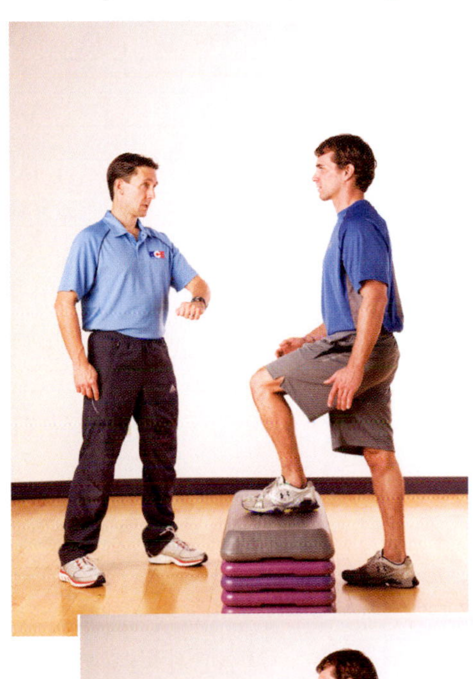
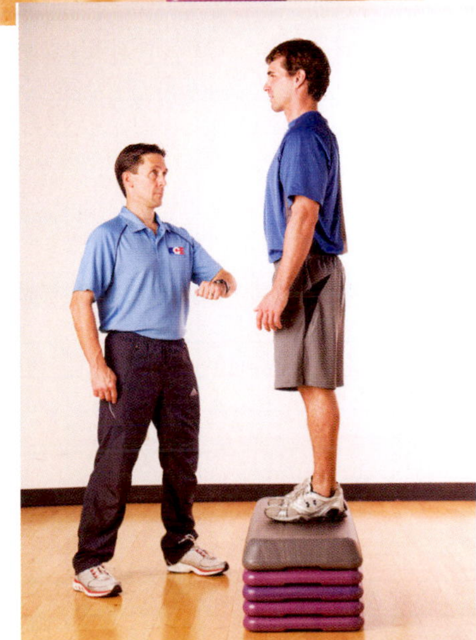

Figure 8-15
Three-minute step test—stepping cycle

Test protocol and administration:

- On the trainer's cue, the client begins stepping and the stopwatch is started.
- The trainer can coach the initial steps to make sure the client is keeping pace with the metronome. Cue the time remaining to allow the client to stay on task.
- At the three-minute mark, the test is stopped and the client immediately sits down. Count the client's HR for one entire minute, starting the count at "zero."
  - ✓ The test score is based on the fact that the immediate post-exercise HR will decrease throughout the minute cycle.
  - ✓ It is important that the HR check begin within five seconds of test completion. (Placing a stethoscope to the client's chest enhances the tester's ability to count the actual heartbeats. In some cases, the client may be uncomfortable with this procedure, in which case a radial pulse check will also suffice.)
- The client's one-minute post-exercise HR is recorded on the testing form.
- Encourage a three- to five-minute cool-down followed by stretching of the lower extremities. The client may experience post-exercise dizziness or other signs of distress if no cool-down is performed (i.e., blood pooling in the extremities and accelerated HR).
- Classify the client's score using Table 8-20 or 8-21 and record the values on the testing form.
- Continue to observe the client, as negative symptoms can arise post-exercise.

For those who score "below average" to "very poor," it will be necessary to be conservative in the initial exercise program. Keeping exercise duration and intensity to a minimum will be important. For those who score "above average" to "excellent," it would be appropriate to focus on exercise duration as well as intensity.

Table 8-20

Post-exercise Heart Rate Norms for YMCA Submaximal Step Test (Men)

		Age					
Rating	**% Rating**	**18–25**	**26–35**	**36–45**	**46–55**	**56–65**	**66+**
Excellent	100	50	51	49	56	60	59
	95	71	70	70	77	71	74
	90	76	76	76	82	77	81
Good	85	79	79	80	87	86	87
	80	82	83	84	89	91	91
	75	84	85	88	93	94	92
Above average	70	88	88	92	95	97	94
	65	90	91	95	99	99	97
	60	93	94	98	101	100	102
Average	55	95	96	100	103	103	104
	50	97	100	101	107	105	106
	45	100	102	105	111	109	110
Below average	40	102	104	108	113	111	114
	35	105	108	111	117	115	116
	30	107	110	113	119	117	118
Poor	25	111	114	116	121	119	121
	20	114	118	119	124	123	123
	15	119	121	124	126	128	126
Very poor	10	124	126	130	131	131	130
	5	132	134	138	139	136	136
	0	157	161	163	159	154	151

Reprinted with permission from *YMCA Fitness Testing and Assessment Manual*, 4th ed. © 2000 by YMCA of the USA. All rights reserved

Table 8-21

Post-exercise Heart Rate Norms for YMCA Submaximal Step Test (Women)

		Age (years)					
Rating	**% Rating**	**18–25**	**26–35**	**36–45**	**46–55**	**56–65**	**66+**
Excellent	100	52	58	51	63	60	70
	95	75	74	77	85	83	85
	90	81	80	84	91	92	92
Good	85	85	85	89	95	97	96
	80	89	89	92	98	100	98
	75	93	92	96	101	103	101
Above average	70	96	95	100	104	106	104
	65	98	98	102	107	109	108
	60	102	101	104	110	111	111
Average	55	104	104	107	113	113	116
	50	108	107	109	115	116	120
	45	110	110	112	118	118	121
Below average	40	113	113	115	120	119	123
	35	116	116	118	121	123	125
	30	120	119	120	124	127	126
Poor	25	122	122	124	126	129	128
	20	126	126	128	128	131	129
	15	131	129	132	132	135	133
Very poor	10	135	134	137	137	141	135
	5	143	141	142	143	147	145
	0	169	171	169	171	174	155

Reprinted with permission from *YMCA Fitness Testing and Assessment Manual*, 4th ed. © 2000 by YMCA of the USA. All rights reserved

McArdle Step Test

The McArdle step test is another field test used to measure cardiorespiratory endurance. Unlike the YMCA submaximal step test that evaluates recovery HR, this test measures exercising HR from which $\dot{V}O_2$max can be estimated. This is a useful test for clients with higher levels of aerobic fitness, but individuals who are short in stature may struggle with this test given that the step height is 16.25 inches (41.3 cm).

Equipment:

- 16.25-inch (41.3 cm) step (This is the common height of a bleacher; no configuration of the Reebok step will achieve this height.)
- Stopwatch
- Metronome
- Stethoscope (optional)

Pre-test procedure, test protocol, and administration:

- The pre-test procedures, test protocol, and administration are very similar to the YMCA submaximal step test, with the following changes:
  - ✓Women step at a cadence of 88 steps per minute (22 step cycles), while men will step at the same 96 steps-per-minute cadence used in the YMCA test ("up," "up," "down," "down").
  - ✓The post-exercise HR is counted for 15 seconds while the client remains standing (instead of the one-minute sitting count used in the YMCA test). Multiply the 15-second count by four to use in the appropriate formula.
- The client's 15-second post-exercise HR is recorded on the testing form.
- Encourage a three- to five-minute cool-down followed by stretching of the lower extremities. If there are concerns with post-exercise dizziness or other signs of distress from an abrupt cessation of exercise, allow the client to march in place during the HR measurement to prevent pooling of blood in the lower extremity.
- Use the following formulas to determine $\dot{V}O_2$max:
  - ✓Women: $\dot{V}O_2$max = 65.81 – (0.1847 x HR)
  - ✓Men: $\dot{V}O_2$max = 111.33 – (0.42 x HR)
- *Example:* Pete completes this three-minute step with a 15-second HR count of 35 beats.
  - ✓15-second count at 35 beats = 140 bpm
  - ✓$\dot{V}O_2$max (mL/kg/min)
    = 111.33 – (0.42 x HR)
    = 111.33 – (0.42 x 140)
    = 111.33 – 58.8
    = 52.53 mL/kg/min
- Have the client cool down for three to five minutes and continue to observe the client, as negative ymptoms can arise post-exercise.
- Classify the client's score using Table 8-13 and record the values on the testing form.

Application of Information from Cardiorespiratory Fitness Testing

If any negative signs or symptoms arise during exercise testing, the client's personal physician should be notified immediately. Emergency medical services (EMS) should be called when severe signs or symptoms arise, including the following:

- Unconsciousness
- Chest pain or other signs or symptoms of heart attack or cardiac distress
- Extreme difficulty in breathing that cannot be controlled with rest

If the cardiorespiratory testing was unremarkable, an appropriate fitness program can be initiated. For novice exercisers and those who score in the lowest percentiles, improving on cardiorespiratory fitness should be addressed in a twofold manner. The first goal is to gradually increase exercise duration. This allows the body to adapt to the new demands of exercise and respond accordingly (e.g., increase in capillary density, increase in mitochondrial size/number, enhanced ability to remove lactic acid). Initially, training volume can be increased by 10 to 20% per week, until the desired training volume is achieved.

For those who already have a solid cardiorespiratory fitness base, training should focus on increasing exercise intensity. As long as there are no **contraindications** to higher-intensity training, it is appropriate to incorporate higher-intensity steady-state training as well as interval training.

Cardiorespiratory fitness is a strong predictor of morbidity and mortality. Low levels of cardiorespiratory fitness have been linked to increased risk of premature death from all causes, especially from cardiovascular disease. High levels of cardiorespiratory fitness are associated with increased levels of regular physical activity, which translates to numerous health benefits.

Once the client's cardiorespiratory fitness level has been established, and any cardiovascular health risks have been ruled out, it is important to understand how to safely and efficiently improve upon his or her results. Trainers should keep in mind that physical fitness exists in a continuum, ranging from health to peak sports performance. The time and energy commitment required to improve sports performance is obviously much more involved than the requirements for improving overall health.

To achieve health-related benefits, physical activity recommendations from the Surgeon General, CDC, and ACSM suggest 30 minutes of moderate activity, most days of the week. The U.S. Department of Health & Human Services (2008) states that 150 minutes of weekly moderate-intensity activity is important for health, but these guidelines also add another dimension to the recommendations: 75 minutes of vigorous activity provides suitable health benefits. For clients who are not capable of achieving these recommendations at the outset, reaching this level of activity should be the primary goal during the initial conditioning stage. It is prudent for the personal trainer to encourage regular participation in cardiorespiratory activities. Chapter 11 provides details for developing safe and effective cardiorespiratory exercise plans.

Muscular-fitness Testing

Muscular fitness encompasses both muscular endurance and **muscular strength.** Muscular endurance represents a muscle's ability to resist fatigue and perform work for successive repetitions, while muscular strength defines a muscle's ability to overcome external resistance. Both are essential health-related fitness components. The following list describes the many health-related benefits of muscular fitness:

- Enhances the ability to carry out ADL, which translates to an increase in self-esteem and fosters a sense of independence
- Provides for musculoskeletal integrity, which translates to a reduction in common musculoskeletal injuries
- Enhances or maintains fat-free mass and ultimately positively impacts RMR, which is an important aspect of weight management
- Guards against osteoporosis by protecting or enhancing bone density
- Enhances **glucose** tolerance, which can protect against type 2 diabetes

Muscular-endurance Testing

Muscular-endurance testing assesses the ability of a specific muscle group, or groups, to perform repeated or sustained contractions to sufficiently invoke muscular fatigue. Assessment criteria are based on either the actual number of successful repetitions that can be performed (e.g., the push-up test) or the sustained holding of a particular position (e.g., McGill's trunk flexor endurance test). Simple field tests can measure muscular endurance without much equipment or advanced training. When considering assessments for muscular endurance, trainers should always determine the relevancy and appropriateness of the assessments for their clients. Given the function of the various muscle groups within the body, muscular endurance of the trunk and lower extremity is most relevant to optimal function. Lack of endurance of the trunk musculature also correlates well with low-back pain

(McGill, 2007). While the push-up and curl-up tests are included in this section, many experts favor assessments of trunk and lower-extremity endurance. Stuart McGill's battery of trunk-endurance tests evaluates balance between the trunk flexors, extensors, and lateral muscles and their relationships to each other. The following are some important things to consider prior to any muscle-endurance testing:

- Remember to *always* screen for low-back pain before performing any of these assessments.
- As with any test, any indication of pain during a test merits immediate termination of the test and referral to a more qualified professional.
- If a client has a history of diagnosed low-back pain or is currently experiencing pain and/or discomfort, these tests should not be performed until he or she has consulted with a doctor.

One of the most important things to observe during testing is that the client is maintaining the integrity of the repetition and/or the recommended posture for the specific exercise movement.

The following tests are described in this section:

- Push-up test
- Curl-up test
- McGill's torso muscular endurance test battery
- Bodyweight squat test

Push-up Test

The push-up test measures upper-body endurance, specifically of the pectoralis muscles, triceps, and anterior deltoids. Due to common variations in upper-body strength between men and women, women should be assessed while performing a modified push-up. The push-up is not only useful as an evaluation tool for measuring upper-body strength and endurance, but is also a prime activity for developing and maintaining upper-body muscular fitness.

Contraindications/Considerations

This test may not be appropriate for clients with shoulder or wrist problems. Alternate muscular-endurance tests or the Cooper 90-degree push-up test (where the elbows do not exceed a 90-degree angle) may be more appropriate. A major problem associated with tests that require performance to fatigue is that the point of "exhaustion" or fatigue is a motivational factor. Novice exercisers may not push themselves to the maximal point of exertion.

Equipment:

- Mat (optional)
- Towel or foam block

Pre-test procedure:

- After explaining the purpose of the push-up test, explain and demonstrate the correct push-up version (standard or modified) (Figure 8-16).

Figure 8-16
Push-up test

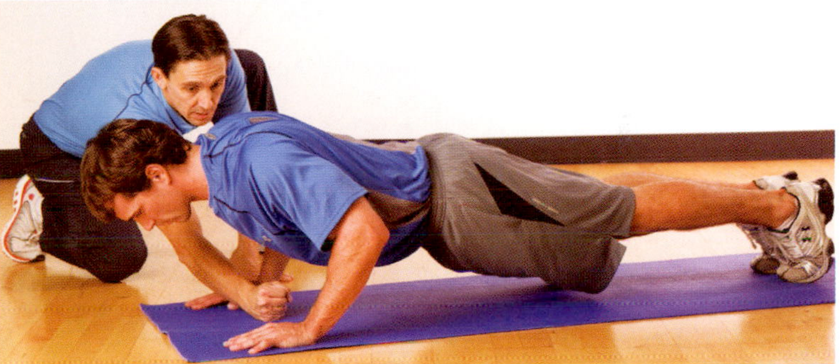

Standard push-up position

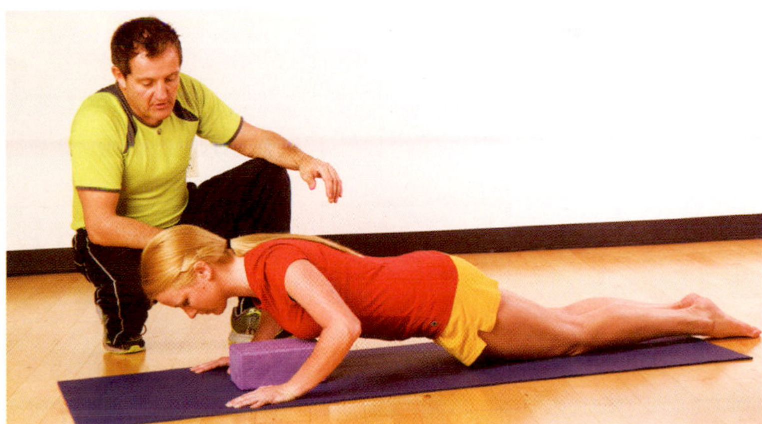

Modified bent-knee position

- The hands should point forward and be positioned shoulder-width apart, directly under the shoulders. The hips and shoulders should be aligned (i.e., rigid trunk) and the head should remain in a neutral to slightly extended position.
- The goal of the test is to perform as many consecutive and complete push-ups as possible before reaching a point of fatigue.

The push-ups must be steady, without any rest in between the repetitions. Explain that only correctly performed push-ups are counted.

- Encourage the client to perform a few practice trials before the test begins.

Test protocol and administration:

- The test starts in the "down" position and the client can begin the test whenever he or she is ready.
- Count each *complete* push-up until the client reaches fatigue. A complete push-up requires:
  - ✓Full elbow extension with a straight back and rigid torso in the "up" position
  - ✓The chest touching the trainer's fist, a rolled towel, or a foam block, without resting the stomach or body on the mat in the "down" position
- The test is terminated when the client is unable to complete a repetition or fails to maintain proper technique for two consecutive repetitions.
- Record the score on the testing form.
- Classify the client's score using Table 8-22. For example, if a 46-year-old female client completed a total of 23 modified push-ups, she would be classified as "good," which signifies that her upper-body muscular endurance scored very well.

Clients who are **sedentary** or unaccustomed to working the upper body are likely lacking in upper-body strength and endurance. If the muscles of the upper body are weak, this can lead to poor posture and problems ranging from low-back pain to poor digestion.

In the fitness setting, there are a variety of strength-training activities that can be incorporated into a client's training program that would help increase muscular fitness in the pectoralis, triceps, and deltoid muscle groups, individually or collectively. The push-up itself is a great exercise for developing muscular strength, endurance, and overall tone in the upper body. Push-ups do not require any equipment and can be performed virtually anywhere. For this reason, it is a beneficial exercise to add to any client's home exercise program.

Table 8-22

Push–up Fitness Test Norms

	Age				
Men	**20–29**	**30–39**	**40–49**	**50–59**	**60+**
Excellent	>54	>44	>39	>34	>29
Good	45–54	35–44	30–39	25–34	20–29
Average	35–44	24–34	20–29	15–24	10–19
Poor	20–34	15–24	12–19	8–14	5–9
Very Poor	<20	<15	<12	<8	<5
Women	**20–29**	**30–39**	**40–49**	**50–59**	**60+**
Excellent	>48	>39	>34	>29	>19
Good	34–48	25–39	20–34	15–29	5–19
Average	17–33	12–24	8–19	6–14	3–4
Poor	6–16	4–11	3–7	2–5	1–2
Very Poor	<6	<4	<3	<2	<1

Pollock, M.L. et al. (1984). *Health and Fitness Through Physical Activity.* New York: John Wiley & Sons.

Curl-up Test

The curl-up test is used to measure abdominal strength and endurance. Like the push-up test, this test requires the client to perform to fatigue. The curl-up is preferred over the full sit-up because it is a more reliable indicator of abdominal strength and endurance and is much safer for the exerciser. The full sit-up requires additional recruitment of the hip flexors, which places increased loads across the lumbar spine. Many clients are also inclined to pull on the neck in an effort to generate momentum during a full sit-up, potentially increasing the risk for injury in the cervical region. Most clients will be able to perform the curl-up test unless they suffer from low-back problems. The curl-up test is an easy and inexpensive method of evaluating abdominal strength and endurance.

Contraindications

The following issues should be considered prior to the performance of abdominal strength assessments:

- Clients with low-back concerns should check with their physicians prior to attempting this test.
- Clients with cervical neck issues may find that this exercise exacerbates their pain. All clients should be encouraged to relax the neck and rely on their abdominal muscles to do the work.

Equipment:

- Mat

Pre-test procedure:

- After explaining the purpose of the curl-up test, explain and demonstrate proper body position and movement technique. The starting position requires the client to be **supine,** with feet flat on the floor, both knees bent to a 90-degree angle, and arms crossed at the chest (Figure 8-17).
- Cue the client to perform a controlled curl-up to lift the shoulder blades off the mat (approximately 30 degrees of trunk flexion), and then to lower the torso back down to rest the shoulders completely on the mat (the head does not need to touch the mat).

Figure 8-17
Curl-up test

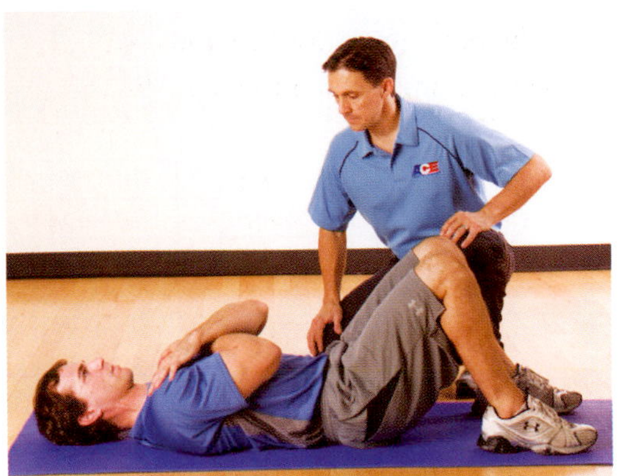

Curl-up test: Down position. Head support is optional.

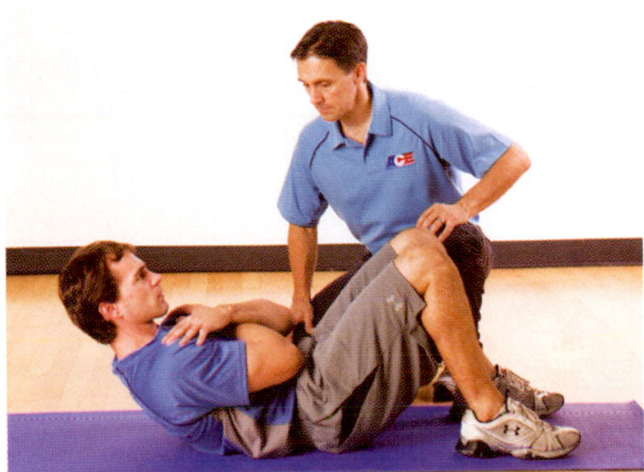

Curl-up test: Up position

- Instruct the client to exhale on the way up and inhale on the way down.
- Encourage the client to perform a few practice or warm-up repetitions prior to the test.

Test protocol and administration:

- The client starts in the "down" position and begins on the trainer's instruction.
- Count each *complete* curl-up until the client reaches fatigue.
- Make sure the client is not holding his or her breath during the test.
- The client must not flex the cervical spine by curling the neck.
- Record the client's score on the testing form as the maximum number of curl-ups completed.
- Classify the client's score using Table 8-23 or 8-24. For example, if a 27-year-old male client completes a total of 36 curl-ups, he would be classified in the upper range of "below average," signifying that his abdominal endurance needs improvement.

Table 8-23

Norms for Curl-up Test (Men)

		Age (years)					
Rating	**% Rating**	**18–25**	**26–35**	**36–45**	**46–55**	**56–65**	**66+**
Excellent	100	99	80	79	78	77	66
	95	83	68	65	68	63	55
	90	77	62	60	61	56	50
Good	85	72	58	57	57	53	44
	80	66	56	52	53	49	40
	75	61	53	48	52	48	38
Above average	70	57	52	45	51	46	35
	65	54	46	44	47	43	32
	60	52	44	43	44	41	31
Average	55	49	41	39	41	39	30
	50	46	38	36	39	36	27
	45	43	37	33	36	33	26
Below average	40	41	36	32	33	32	24
	35	40	34	31	32	31	23
	30	37	33	29	29	28	22
Poor	25	35	32	28	25	25	21
	20	33	30	25	24	24	19
	15	29	26	24	21	21	15
Very poor	10	27	21	21	16	20	12
	5	23	17	13	11	17	10
	0	14	7	6	6	5	5

Reprinted with permission from *YMCA Fitness Testing and Assessment Manual*, 4th ed. © 2000 by YMCA of the USA. All rights reserved

Table 8-24

Norms for Curl-up Test (Women)

		Age (years)					
Rating	**% Rating**	**18–25**	**26–35**	**36–45**	**46–55**	**56–65**	**66+**
Excellent	100	91	70	74	73	63	54
	95	76	60	60	57	55	41
	90	68	54	54	48	44	34
Good	85	64	50	48	44	42	33
	80	61	46	44	40	38	32
	75	58	44	42	37	35	31
Above average	70	57	41	38	36	32	29
	65	54	40	36	35	30	28
	60	51	37	35	33	27	26
Average	55	48	36	32	32	25	25
	50	44	34	31	31	24	22
	45	41	33	30	30	23	21
Below average	40	38	32	28	28	22	20
	35	37	30	24	27	20	18
	30	34	28	23	25	18	16
Poor	25	33	26	22	23	15	13
	20	32	24	20	21	12	11
	15	28	22	19	19	11	10
Very poor	10	25	20	16	13	8	9
	5	24	17	14	9	7	8
	0	11	7	4	2	1	0

Reprinted with permission from *YMCA Fitness Testing and Assessment Manual*, 4th ed. © 2000 by YMCA of the USA. All rights reserved

McGill's Torso Muscular Endurance Test Battery: Trunk Flexor Endurance, Trunk Lateral Endurance, Trunk Extensor Endurance

There is more to abdominal tone and core stability than showing off a "six pack." Possessing a strong core is important when performing simple ADL like lifting a heavy laundry basket or recreational activities like swinging a golf club. Core stability involves complex movement patterns that continually change as a function of the three-dimensional torque needed to support the various positions of the body. Even back pain and dysfunction can be reversed by having a strong core. Dr. Stuart McGill (2007) states that back problems can often be alleviated by improving and then grooving the motor patterns of the abdominal musculature. To evaluate balanced core strength and stability, it is important to assess all sides of the torso. The true benefit of each one of the following tests is in the assessment of the interrelationships among the results of the three torso tests. In other words, the tests are performed individually, but then evaluated collectively. Poor endurance capacity of the torso muscles or an imbalance between these three muscle groups is believed to contribute to low-back dysfunction and core instability.

Trunk Flexor Endurance Test

The flexor endurance test is the first in the battery of three tests that assesses muscular endurance of the deep core muscles (i.e., transverse abdominis, quadratus lumborum, erector spinae). It is a timed test involving a static, isometric contraction of the anterior muscles, stabilizing the spine until the individual exhibits fatigue and can no longer hold the assumed position.

> **Contraindications**
>
> This test may not be suitable for individuals who suffer from low-back pain, have had recent back surgery, and/or are in the midst of an acute low-back flare-up.

Equipment:
- Stopwatch
- Board (or step)
- Strap (optional)

Pre-test procedure:
- After explaining the purpose of the flexor endurance test, describe the proper body position.
  - ✓ The starting position requires the client to be seated, with the hips and knees bent to 90 degrees, aligning the hips, knees, and second toe.
  - ✓ Instruct the client to fold his or her arms across the chest, touching each hand to the opposite shoulder, lean against a board positioned at a 60-degree incline, and keep the head in a neutral position (Figure 8-18).
  - ✓ It is important to ask the client to press the shoulders into the board and maintain this "open" position throughout the test after the board is removed.
  - ✓ Instruct the client to engage the abdominals to maintain a flat-to-neutral spine. The back should never be allowed to arch during the test.
  - ✓ The trainer can anchor the toes under a strap or manually stabilize the feet if necessary.

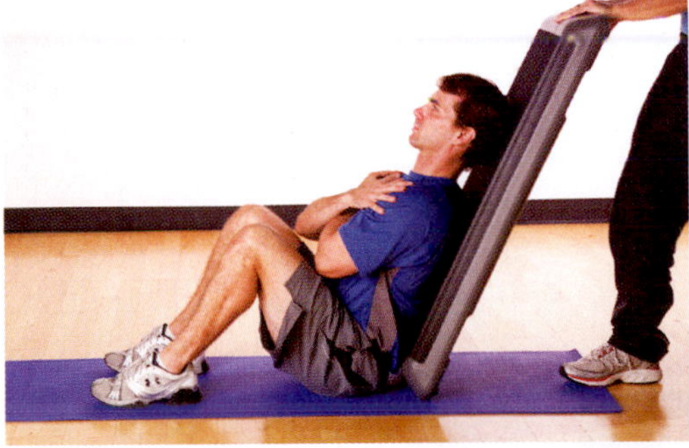

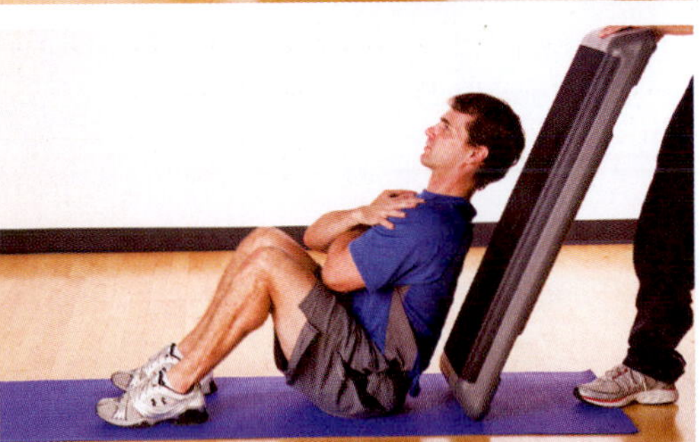

Figure 8-18
Trunk flexor endurance test

- The goal of the test is to hold this 60-degree position for as long as possible without the benefit of the back support.
- Encourage the client to practice this position prior to attempting the test.

Test protocol and administration:

- The trainer starts the stopwatch as he or she moves the board about 4 inches (10 cm) back, while the client maintains the 60-degree, suspended position.
- Terminate the test when there is a noticeable change in the trunk position:
  - ✓ Watch for a deviation from the neutral spine (i.e., the shoulders rounding forward) or an increase in the low-back arch.
  - ✓ No part of the back should touch the back rest.
- Record the client's time on the testing form.

Trunk Lateral Endurance Test

The trunk lateral endurance test, also called the side-bridge test, assesses muscular endurance of the lateral core muscles (i.e., transverse abdominis, obliques, quadratus lumborum, erector spinae). Similar to the trunk flexor endurance test, this timed test involves static, isometric contractions of the lateral muscles on each side of the trunk that stabilize the spine.

Contraindications

This test may not be suitable for individuals:

- With shoulder pain or weakness
- Who suffer from low-back pain, have had recent back surgery, and/or are in the midst of an acute low-back flare-up

Equipment:

- Stopwatch
- Mat (optional)

Pre-test procedure:

- After explaining the purpose of this test, describe the proper body position.
  - ✓ The starting position requires the client to be on his or her side with extended legs, aligning the feet on top of each other or in a tandem position (heel-to-toe).
  - ✓ Have the client place the lower arm under the body and the upper arm on the side of the body.
  - ✓ When the client is ready, instruct him or her to assume a full side-bridge position, keeping both legs extended and the sides of the feet on the floor. The elbow of the lower arm should be positioned directly under the shoulder with the forearm facing out (the forearm can be placed palm down for balance and support) and the upper arm should be resting along the side of the body or across the chest to the opposite shoulder.
  - ✓ The hips should be elevated off the mat and the body should be in straight alignment (i.e., head, neck, torso, hips, and legs). The torso should only be supported by the client's foot/feet and the elbow/forearm of the lower arm (Figure 8-19).
- The goal of the test is to hold this position for as long as possible. Once the client breaks the position, the test is terminated.
- Encourage the client to practice this position prior to attempting the test.

Test protocol and administration:

- The trainer starts the stopwatch as the client moves into the side-bridge position.
- Terminate the test when there is a noticeable change in the trunk position
  - ✓ A deviation from the neutral spine (i.e., the hips dropping downward)
  - ✓ The hips shifting forward or backward in an effort to maintain balance and stability
- Record the client's time on the testing form.
- Repeat the test on the opposite side and record this value on the testing form.

Trunk Extensor Endurance Test

The trunk extensor endurance test is generally used to assess muscular endurance of the torso extensor muscles (i.e., erector spinae, longissimus, ilicostalis, multifidi). This is a timed test involving a static, isometric contraction of the trunk extensor muscles that stabilize the spine.

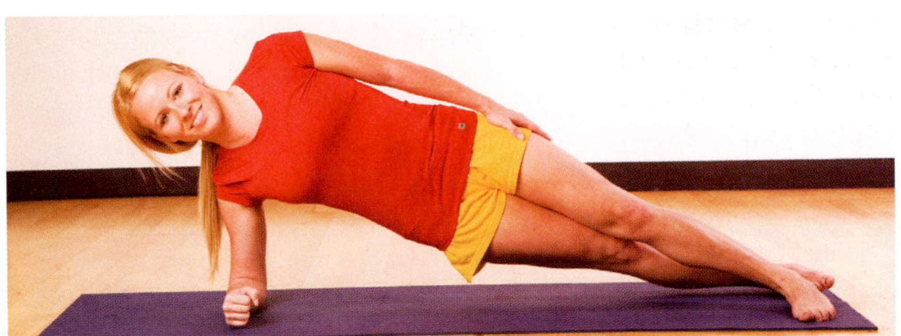

Figure 8-19
Trunk lateral endurance test

Contraindications

This test may not be suitable for:

- A client with major strength deficiencies, where the individual cannot even lift the torso from a forward flexed position to a neutral position
- A client with a high body mass, in which case it would be difficult for the trainer to support the client's suspended upper-body weight
- Individuals who suffer from low-back pain, have had recent back surgery, and/or are in the midst of an acute low-back flare-up

Equipment:

- Elevated, sturdy exam table
- Nylon strap
- Stopwatch

Pre-test procedure:

- After explaining the purpose of the test, explain the proper body position.
  - ✓ The starting position requires the client to be prone, positioning the iliac crests at the table edge while supporting the upper extremity on the arms, which are placed on the floor or on a riser.
  - ✓ While the client is supporting the weight of his or her upper body, anchor the client's lower legs to the table using a strap. If a strap is not used, the trainer will have to use his or her own body weight to stabilize the client's legs.
- The goal of the test is to hold a horizontal, prone position for as long as possible. Once the client falls below horizontal, the test is terminated.
- Encourage the client to practice this position prior to attempting the test.

Test protocol and administration:

- When ready, the client lifts/extends the torso until it is parallel to the floor with his or her arms crossed over the chest (Figure 8-20).
- Start the stopwatch as soon as the client assumes this position.
- Terminate the test when the client can no longer maintain the position.
- Record the client's time on the testing form.

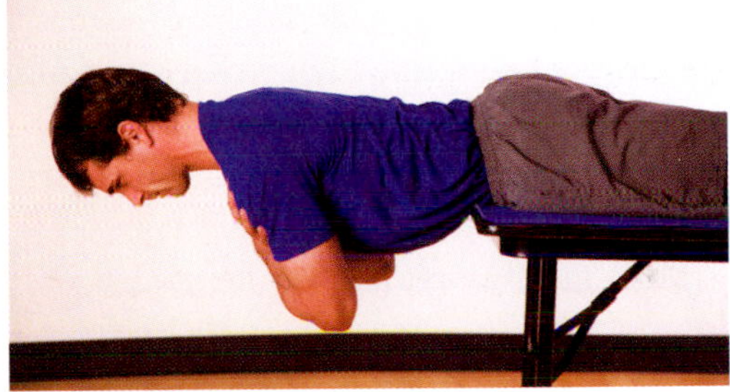

Figure 8-20
Trunk extensor endurance test

Evaluation and Application of Performance for McGill's Torso Muscular Endurance Test Battery

Each individual test in this testing battery is not a primary indicator of current or future back problems. McGill (2007) has proven that the *relationships* among the tests are more important indicators of muscle imbalances that can lead to back pain. In fact, even in a person with little or no back pain, the ratios can still be off, suggesting that low-back pain may eventually occur without diligent attention to a solid core-conditioning program. McGill (2007) suggests the following ratios indicate balanced endurance among the muscle groups:

- Flexion:extension ratio should be less than 1.0
  - ✓ For example, a flexion score of 120 seconds and extension score of 150 seconds generates a ratio score of 0.80

- Right-side bridge (RSB):left-side bridge (LSB) scores should be no greater than 0.05 from a balanced score of 1.0
  - ✓For example, a RSB score of 88 seconds and an LSB score of 92 seconds generates a ratio score of 0.96, which is within the 0.05 range from 1.0
- Side bridge (either side):extension ratio should be less than 0.75
  - ✓For example, a RSB score of 88 seconds and an extension score of 150 seconds generates a ratio score of 0.59

Demonstrated deficiencies in these core functional assessments should be addressed during exercise programming as part of the foundational exercises for a client. The goal is to create ratios consistent with McGill's recommendations. Muscular endurance, more so than muscular strength or even ROM, has been shown to be an accurate predictor of back health (McGill, 2007). Research shows that low-back stabilization exercises have the most benefit when performed daily. When working with clients with low-back dysfunction, it is prudent to include daily stabilization exercises in their home exercise plans.

Since most Americans will experience low-back pain at some point in their lives, a comprehensive fitness program should incorporate spinal stabilization exercises. Even when working with clients who have yet to develop an interest in the health of their back, core stability should still be a key element in any training program. For example, if the core is not strong, the back may be compromised during a dumbbell shoulder press, creating excessive lumbar **lordosis.** The same break in position can happen during a squat or a bench press, thus creating excess stress on the lumbar spine. Improper alignment can create a whole host of problems for the lower back, ranging from herniated discs to sciatic pain. Clients' training objectives can vary from rehabilitation or prevention of low-back pain to optimizing health and fitness or maximizing athletic performance. All clients will benefit from exercises targeting core stability. Refer to Chapter 9 for more information on training for core stability.

Bodyweight Squat Test

This test assesses muscular endurance of the lower extremity when performing repetitions of a squat and stand movement. This test is *only* suitable for individuals who demonstrate proper form when performing a squat movement. While this test lacks strong scientific validity, it can be used to effectively gauge relative improvements in a client's lower-extremity muscular endurance.

Contraindications

While this test mimics a primary movement that most individuals perform on a daily basis, it may not be suitable for:

- A deconditioned or frail client with lower-extremity weakness
- A client with balance concerns
- A client with orthopedic issues, especially in the knees
- A client who fails to demonstrate proper squatting technique

Equipment:

- None needed

Pre-test procedure:

- After explaining the purpose of the bodyweight squat test, explain and demonstrate the proper technique.
- Allow for adequate warm-up and stretching if needed.
- Evaluate the depth of the squat using either of the following criteria (Figure 8-21):
  - ✓The fingertips (held to the sides of the body) touch the floor
  - ✓The thighs reach parallel to the floor
- To enhance balance and stability, the client may extend his or her arms to the sides or front for balance.
- The goal of the test is to complete as many controlled and proper repetitions as possible. Once the client exhibits fatigue where he or she can no longer complete a full repetition, terminate the test. This includes an inability to fully lower into the down position, pausing to rest, or faltering as he or she stands.

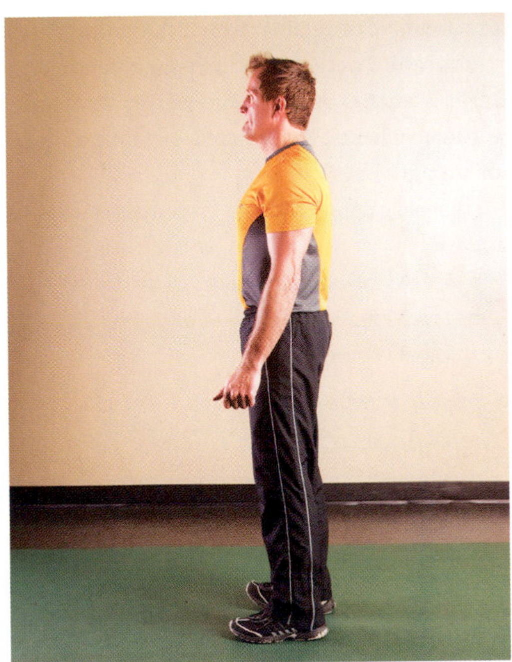

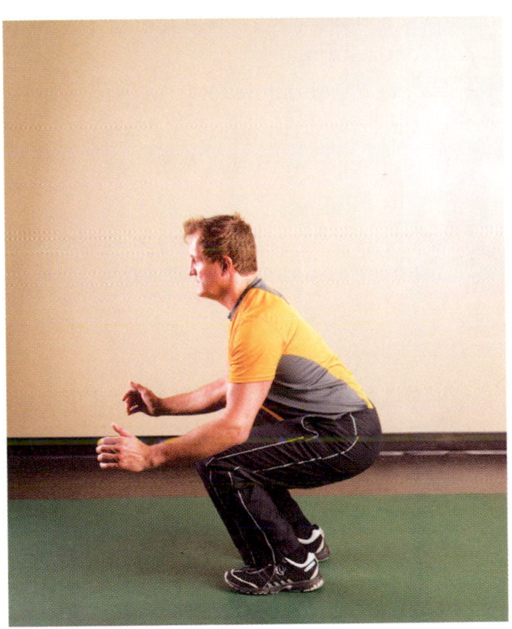

Figure 8-21
Bodyweight squat test

- Encourage the client to practice this movement prior to attempting the test.

Test protocol and administration:

- When ready, the client begins performing squat repetitions.
- Count only complete repetitions until any test-termination criteria is reached.
- Use the information presented in Table 8-25 to categorize the client's performance.

Table 8-25

Norms for Bodyweight Squats

Males	18–25	26–35	36–45	46–55	56–65	65+
Excellent	>49	>45	>41	>35	>31	>28
Good	44–49	40–45	35–41	29–35	25–31	22–28
Above average	39–43	35–39	30–34	25–38	21–24	19–21
Average	35–38	31–34	27–29	22–24	17–20	15–18
Below average	31–34	29–30	23–26	18–21	13–16	11–14
Poor	25–30	22–28	17–22	13–17	9–12	7–10
Very poor	<25	<22	<17	<9	<9	<7
Females	**18–25**	**26–35**	**36–45**	**46–55**	**56–65**	**65+**
Excellent	>43	>39	>33	>27	>24	>23
Good	37–43	33–39	27–33	22–27	18–24	17–23
Above average	33–36	29–32	23–26	18–21	13–17	14–16
Average	29–32	25–28	19–22	14–17	10–12	11–13
Below average	25–28	21–24	15–18	10–13	7–9	5–10
Poor	18–24	13–20	7–14	5–9	3–6	2–4
Very Poor	<18	<13	<7	<5	<3	<2

Mackenzie, B. (2005). *101 Performance Evaluation Tests.* London: Electric Word.

Muscular-strength Testing

Muscular strength is an important component of physical fitness. Strength is dependent on variables such as muscle size (diameter), limb length, and neurological adaptations. Maintaining muscular strength is important for everything from performance of ADL to sports performance. Strength can be expressed as either **absolute strength** or **relative strength.** Absolute strength is defined as the greatest amount of weight that can be lifted one time. In sports science, this is defined as a **one-repetition maximum (1 RM).** On the other hand, relative strength takes the person's body weight into consideration and is used primarily when comparing individuals.

> Relative strength is the maximum force a person is able to exert in relation to his or her body weight and is calculated using the formula:
>
> Relative strength = Absolute strength*/Body weight
>
> *Absolute strength equals the amount of weight lifted

Just as in previous assessments, it is important to understand the goals of the client being tested and then choose tests that are associated with those goals.

- Does the client want to improve overall function or is he or she interested in precise performance gains?
- Is the client interested in total-body fitness or is he or she interested in specific muscle fitness (e.g., to rehabilitate an injury)?
- Does the client need to enhance muscular power, strength, and/or endurance? For example, 1 RM is not well-correlated to muscular endurance.

When a personal trainer is deciding on an appropriate strength test, any 1-RM test should be chosen with thoughtful consideration. 1-RM tests should only be performed during phase 3 or 4 of the ACE IFT Model, as appropriate. A certain amount of risk is associated with maximal exertion, including musculoskeletal injury or worse. Submaximal strength testing can be used with a high amount of accuracy to determine a client's likely 1 RM.

There is no single assessment that evaluates total-body muscular strength. Therefore, a variety of tests would be appropriate to determine strength in different muscle groups. Strength testing is important to determine muscular fitness, identify areas of weakness or imbalances, monitor rehabilitation progress, and assess training effectiveness. The following strength tests are described in this section:

- Bench press
- Leg press
- Squat

Strength tests will likely be incorporated into a comprehensive assessment session. A client should warm up prior to strength testing to reduce the likelihood of injury and enhance overall strength. Prolonged static stretching prior to strength testing should be discouraged, as it may decrease performance.

Normative data are not available for all forms of 1-RM testing and, in most cases, this form of testing is most valuable as a source of baseline data against which the trainer can measure a client's future performance. Improvements in 1 RM can be very motivating for many clients, as they are a clear indication of strength development.

The following tests are presented in this section:

- 1-RM bench-press test
- 1-RM leg-press test
- 1-RM squat test

Considerations and Contraindications for 1-RM Testing

- Many strength tests are performed using free weights, so proper form and control are necessary elements. Novice exercisers may not have the familiarity or skill to handle the heavier free weights.
- Beginning exercisers are often unsure of their abilities and tend to quit before their true maximum.
- Proper breathing patterns are necessary. Clients should avoid the **Valsalva maneuver** or any other form of breath-holding.
- Individuals with hypertension and/or a history of **vascular disease** should avoid a 1-RM testing protocol.

1-RM Bench-press Test

This test assesses upper-extremity strength using a fundamental upper-extremity movement: the bench press. It is *only* suitable for individuals who demonstrate proper form in performing a bench press.

Equipment:

- Barbell and bench
- Weights, ranging from 2.5-lb plates to 45-lb plates
- Collars
- Spotter (in addition to the trainer is preferred)

Pre-test procedure:

- After explaining the purpose of the 1-RM bench-press test, explain and demonstrate the proper technique for the bench press (Figure 8-22).
  - ✓ The client is supine with both feet planted firmly on the floor or on a riser to accommodate a neutral or flat back.

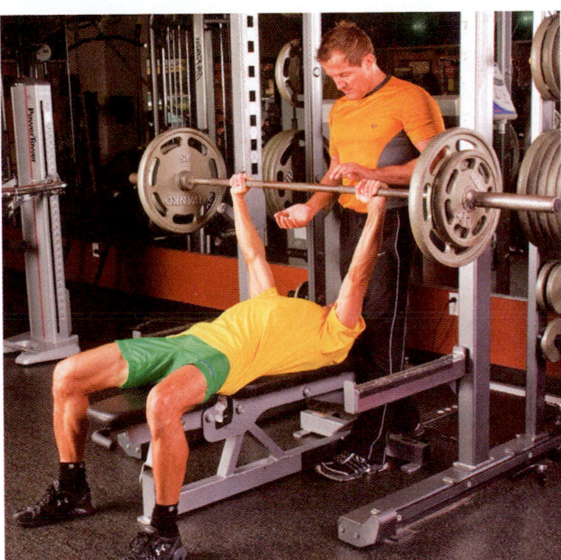

Starting and ending position

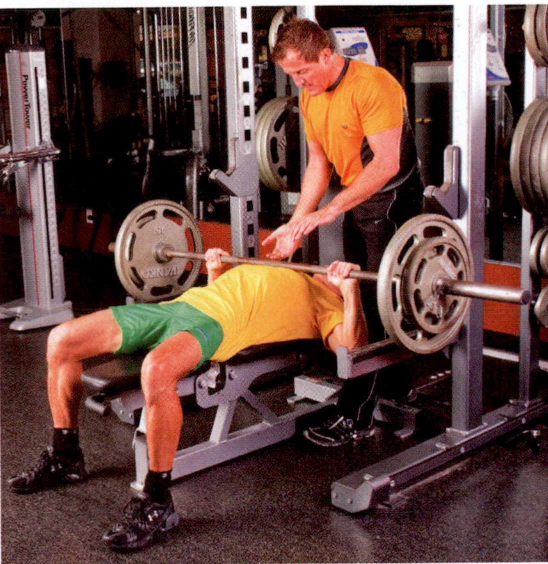

Mid-range position

Figure 8-22
Bench press test

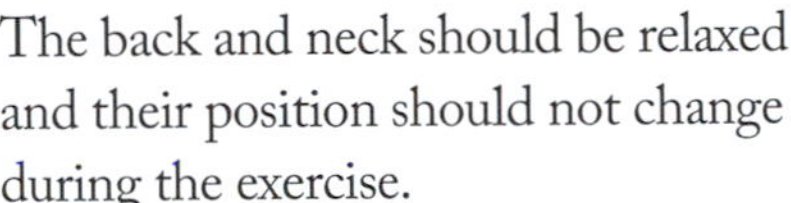

The back and neck should be relaxed and their position should not change during the exercise.

✓ The hands should be positioned slightly wider than shoulder-width apart, so that the elbows are at a 90-degree angle (or slightly less) at the bottom of the movement range.

✓ Proper ROM during the bench press is from arms fully extended (bar positioned above the chest) to the bar lightly touching the chest (bar located over the lower part of the sternum).

✓ The client should inhale while slowly lowering the bar and exhale while raising the bar. Breath-holding (or the Valsalva maneuver) should be avoided.

✓ It is important for the client to communicate with the spotter if he or she cannot complete the repetition.

✓ Instruct the client not to lock the elbows and not to bounce the bar off the chest. Poor technique can cause injuries, so the client should not contort his or her body in an effort to prove strength beyond his or her capabilities.

- Encourage the client to perform a few practice trials to ensure proper technique.
- The responsibilities of the spotter include providing assistance in racking and unracking the barbell, and raising the bar during an incomplete attempt.

✓ *Single spotting:* The spotter stands behind the client in a split-stance position with a dead-lift or alternate grip (i.e., a mix of an overhand grip and an underhand grip) on the bar with the hands placed in the area between the client's hands (see Figure 8-22).

✓ *Double spotting:* The two spotters grasp either end of the barbell.

- The goal of the test is to determine the maximum amount of weight that can be lifted one time (i.e., the 1 RM). It is important to avoid fatiguing the client by having him or her perform too many "unnecessary" repetitions. Finding a suitable starting weight is important.

Test protocol and administration:

- Administer the test protocol for a 1-RM bench press (Table 8-26).

Table 8-26

1-RM Bench Press Testing Protocol

Set	Repetitions	Intensity	Rest Interval
1	5–10	~50% of anticipated 1 RM	60 seconds
2	3–5	~70% of anticipated 1 RM	60 seconds
3	2–3	~85–90% of anticipated 1 RM	2 minutes
4+ (3–5 trials)	1	Attain actual 1-RM score	2–4 minutes between trials

Note: 1 RM = One-repetition maximum

✓ The client should warm up with one set of light resistance (~50% of anticipated 1-RM weight) that allows five to 10 repetitions, and then rest for one minute.

✓ Based on the client's warm-up effort, determine a suitable starting workload for the second set that allows for three to five repetitions (~70 to 75% of the anticipated 1-RM weight), and then allow the client to rest for one minute. Use the following guideline for determining workload increases throughout this test:

- In general, increase by approximately 5 to 10% or 5 to 20 pounds (1 to 9 kg).

✓ Next, have the client perform one heavy set of two to three repetitions at ~85 to 90% of the anticipated 1-RM weight and rest for two minutes.

- Based on the client's third set, determine the next workload to find the client's 1-RM effort. The 1-RM chart provided in Table 8-27 can be used to make these calculations.

Table 8-27

1 RM—Repetition Table

Repetitions	% 1 RM
1	100
2	95
3	93
4	90
5	87
6	85
7	83
8	80
9	77
10	75
11	70
12	67
15	65

Note: 1 RM = One-repetition maximum

Baechle, T.R. & Earle, R.W. (2008). *Essentials of Strength Training and Conditioning* (3rd ed.). Champaign, Ill.: Human Kinetics.

✓ For example, if Pete completes five repetitions at 185 pounds (84 kg), this represents 87% of his 1 RM. Therefore, the weight attempted for his first 1-RM trial could be set at 213 lb (97 kg) [(185 lb/0.87 = 213 lb (97 kg)].

- Allow the client to attempt this set. If the client is successful, he or she should rest for two to four minutes and repeat the 1-RM effort with a heavier load.
- If the attempt was unsuccessful, decrease the load accordingly [by 2.5 to 5% or 5 to 10 pounds (2 to 4 kg)] and have the client try again after resting for two to four minutes.
- Continue the up or down increments until a true 1 RM is achieved. *Ideally, the client should achieve his or her 1 RM in three to five testing sets.*
- Use the testing form to record the weight, progression, sets, repetitions, and any comments on the client's progress. The final weight/load is recorded as the absolute strength.
- Calculate relative strength and record that value as well.

  ✓ For example, if Pete's actual 1 RM was measured at 205 lb and he weighs 175 lb, then his strength-to-weight ratio, or relative strength, would be 1.17 (205/175).

- Use Table 8-28 or 8-29 to rank the client's ability, which should be recorded on the testing form as well.

While Table 8-27 provides useful information, keep in mind that its widespread application is limited for several reasons:

- Much of the research to establish the 1-RM repetition table was primarily based on research using trained male athletes.
- This table is based on single-set research and the values may need to be lowered with multiple-set training.
- This table is derived from bench press, squat, and power clean exercises and has not been effectively validated using other exercises.
- This table is based on free-weight exercises and the values may need to be adjusted for machine-based exercises.

Table 8-28
Upper-body Strength (Men)

One-repetition Maximum Bench Press (Bench Press Weight Ratio = Weight Pushed / Body Weight)							
		Age					
	%	< 20	20–29	30–39	40–49	50–59	60+
Superior	95	1.76	1.63	1.35	1.20	1.05	0.94
Excellent	80	1.34	1.32	1.12	1.00	0.90	0.82
Good	60	1.19	1.14	0.98	0.88	0.79	0.72
Fair	40	1.06	0.99	0.88	0.80	0.71	0.66
Poor	20	0.89	0.88	0.78	0.72	0.63	0.57
Very Poor	5	0.76	0.72	0.65	0.59	0.53	0.49

Reprinted with permission from The Cooper Institute, Dallas, Texas from *Physical Fitness Assessments And Norms For Adults And Law Enforcement*. Available online at www.cooperinstitute.org.

Table 8-29
Upper-body Strength (Women)

One-repetition Maximum Bench Press (Bench Press Weight Ratio = Weight Pushed / Body Weight)							
		Age					
	%	< 20	20–29	30–39	40–49	50–59	60+
Superior	95	0.88	1.01	0.82	0.77	0.68	0.72
Excellent	80	0.77	0.80	0.70	0.62	0.55	0.54
Good	60	0.65	0.70	0.60	0.54	0.48	0.47
Fair	40	0.58	0.59	0.53	0.50	0.44	0.43
Poor	20	0.53	0.51	0.47	0.43	0.39	0.38
Very Poor	5	0.41	0.44	0.39	0.35	0.31	0.26

Reprinted with permission from The Cooper Institute, Dallas, Texas from *Physical Fitness Assessments And Norms For Adults And Law Enforcement*. Available online at www.cooperinstitute.org.

- This table has demonstrated accuracy for loads greater than 75% 1 RM and is not as accurate for lower intensities.

1-RM Leg-press Test

This test assesses lower-extremity strength using a stable, supported movement: the leg press. It is *only* suitable for individuals who demonstrate proper form in performing a leg press and are free of low-back or knee pain.

Equipment:

- Leg-press machine

Pre-test procedure:

- After explaining the purpose of the 1-RM leg-press test, explain and demonstrate the proper technique for the leg press (Figure 8-23).
  - ✓ The client assumes a seated position with both feet planted firmly on the foot plate.

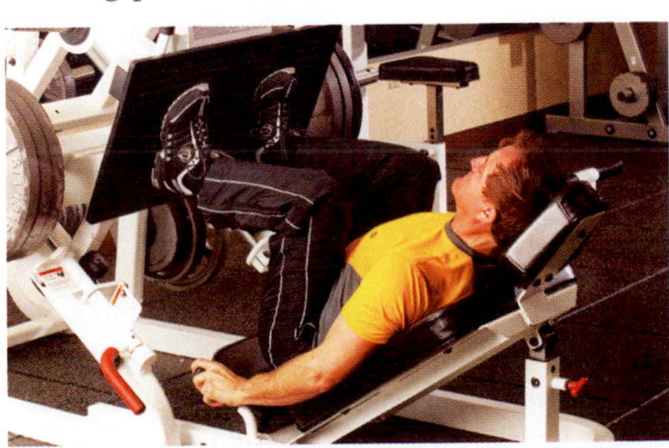

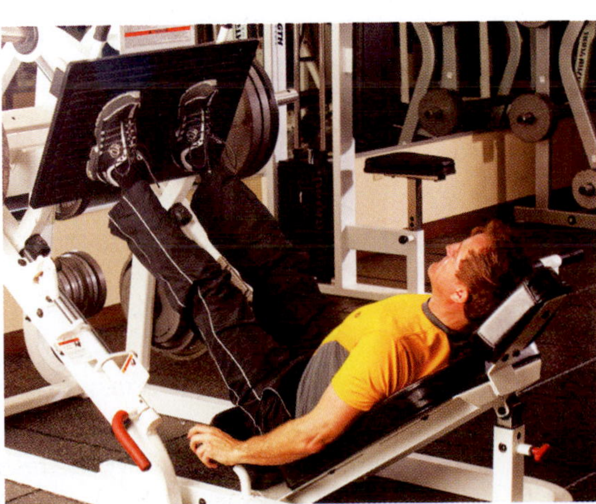

Figure 8-23
Leg press test

- ✓ The ROM during the leg press begins with the legs fully extended, but not hyperextended, with heels flat on the surface, and ends at a 90-degree bent-knee position with the knees aligned with or behind the toes.
- ✓ The client should inhale while slowly lowering the weight (to the bent-knee position) and exhale while extending the legs (pushing the weight). Breath-holding (or the Valsalva maneuver) should be avoided.
- ✓ Instruct the client to avoid locking the knees and not to exceed a bent-knee angle of 90 degrees. Ensure proper foot placement to avoid undue strain on the knees.

- Encourage the client to perform a few practice trials to ensure proper technique.
- The goal of the test is to determine the 1 RM. It is important not to fatigue the client by having him or her perform too many "unnecessary" repetitions. Finding a suitable starting weight is important.
- The responsibilities of the spotter include providing assistance with pushing the rack during an incomplete attempt.

Test protocol and administration:

- Explain the test protocol for a 1-RM leg press.
    - ✓ The client should warm up with one set of light resistance (~50% of anticipated 1-RM weight) that allows five to 10 repetitions, and then rest for one minute.
    - ✓ Based on the client's warm-up effort, determine a suitable workload for the second set that allows for three to five repetitions (~70 to 75% of anticipated 1-RM weight) and then allow the client to rest for one minute. Use the following guideline for determining workload increases throughout this test:
        - ◦ Increase the weight by 10 to 20% or 30 to 40 pounds (14 to 18 kg).
    - ✓ Next, have the client perform one heavy set of two to three repetitions at ~85 to 90% of the anticipated 1-RM weight and rest for two minutes.
- Based on the client's third set, determine the next workload to find the client's 1-RM effort. Table 8-27 can be used to make these calculations.
    - ✓ For example, if Pete completes three repetitions at 350 pounds (159 kg), this represents 93% of his 1 RM. Therefore, the weight attempted for his first 1-RM trial could be set at 376 pounds (171 kg) [350 lb/0.93 = 376 lb (171 kg)].
- Allow the client to attempt this set. If the client is successful, he or she should rest for two to four minutes and repeat the 1-RM effort with a heavier load.
- If the attempt was unsuccessful, decrease the load accordingly [by 2.5 to 5%] and have the client try again after resting for two to four minutes.
- Continue the up or down increments until a true 1 RM is achieved. *Ideally, the client should achieve his or her 1 RM in three to five testing sets.*
- The final successful load is recorded as the absolute strength.
- Record the weight, progressions, sets, repetitions, and any comments on the client's progress in the testing form.
- Calculate relative strength and record that value as well.
    - ✓ For example, if Pete's actual 1 RM was measured at 385 lb and he weighs 175 lb, then his strength-to-weight ratio, or relative strength, would be 2.20 (385/175).
- Use Table 8-30 or 8-31 to rank the client's ability, which should be recorded on the testing form as well.

The values in Tables 8-30 and 8-31 are valid for plate-loaded weight machines and do not provide comparable results for the variety of selectorized leg press machines available in the fitness market. The vast array of potential hip, knee, and ankle angles makes it difficult to standardize the 1 RM. If the test is being used to determine a baseline for future comparison, without the need to look at norms, any leg-press machine can be utilized, as long as the same machine is used for all assessments.

Table 8-30
Leg Strength (Men)

One-repetition Maximum Leg Press (Leg Press Weight Ratio = Weight Pushed / Body Weight)							
		Age					
	%	< 20	20–29	30–39	40–49	50–59	60+
Superior	95	2.82	2.40	2.20	2.02	1.90	1.80
Excellent	80	2.28	2.13	1.93	1.82	1.71	1.62
Good	60	2.04	1.97	1.77	1.68	1.58	1.49
Fair	40	1.90	1.83	1.65	1.57	1.46	1.38
Poor	20	1.70	1.63	1.52	1.44	1.32	1.25
Very Poor	5	1.46	1.42	1.34	1.27	1.15	1.08

Note: Values are most appropriate for tests using a plate-loaded leg-press machine.

Reprinted with permission from The Cooper Institute, Dallas, Texas from *Physical Fitness Assessments And Norms For Adults And Law Enforcement.* Available online at www.cooperinstitute.org.

Table 8-31
Leg Strength (Women)

One-repetition Maximum Leg Press (Leg Press Weight Ratio = Weight Pushed / Body Weight)							
		Age					
	%	< 20	20–29	30–39	40–49	50–59	60+
Superior	95	1.88	1.98	1.68	1.57	1.43	1.43
Excellent	80	1.71	1.68	1.47	1.37	1.25	1.18
Good	60	1.59	1.50	1.33	1.23	1.10	1.04
Fair	40	1.38	1.37	1.21	1.13	0.99	0.93
Poor	20	1.22	1.22	1.09	1.02	0.88	0.85
Very Poor	5	1.06	0.99	0.96	0.85	0.72	0.63

Note: Values are most appropriate for tests using a plate-loaded leg-press machine.

Reprinted with permission from The Cooper Institute, Dallas, Texas from *Physical Fitness Assessments And Norms For Adults And Law Enforcement.* Available online at www.cooperinstitute.org.

1-RM Squat Test

This test assesses lower-extremity strength using an unsupported, functional movement: the squat. It is *only* suitable for individuals who demonstrate proper form when performing a squat and are free of low-back or knee pain.

Equipment:

- Barbell and squat rack
- Weights, ranging from 2.5-pound plates to 45-pound plates
- Collars
- Spotter (in addition to the trainer is preferred)

Pre-test procedure:

- After explaining the purpose of the 1-RM squat test, explain and demonstrate the proper technique for the squat (Figure 8-24).

✓ The client should stand behind a racked bar that is positioned below the shoulders, but above the nipple line.

✓ He or she should grasp the bar with a closed, pronated grip, hands placed wider than shoulder-width apart, and step under the bar with the feet in a split-stance position (one foot on either side of the bar) to unrack the bar.

✓ Position the barbell in the high-bar position (i.e., the bar is placed above the posterior deltoids, resting on the upper trapezius at the base of the neck). *Note:* More experienced lifters may opt for the low-bar position, where the bar is placed across the posterior deltoids along the spine of the scapulae.

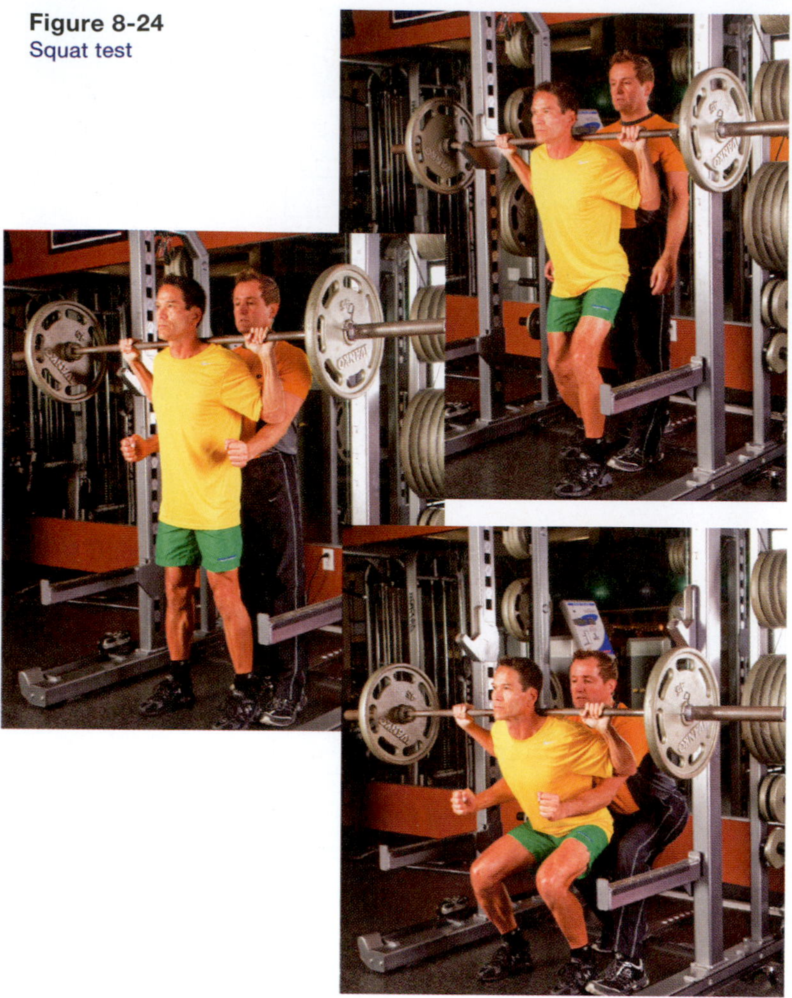

Figure 8-24
Squat test

✓ The client engages the core and abdominal muscles to brace the trunk, then uses the lower extremity to unrack the bar and move into the starting position.

✓ The client stands with the feet shoulder-width apart, back neutral, feet flat, chest up and out, and the head neutral or positioned facing slightly upward.

✓ The lowering phase is initiated with flexion at the hips first, pushing the buttocks backward prior to bending the knees. This ensures a more natural hinge motion at the knees, reducing the stresses across the joints.

✓ Range of motion during the squat is from standing with legs straight to a squatting position with the knees bent slightly more than 90 degrees, or until the thighs are parallel to the floor.

✓ The client inhales during the lowering phase and exhales during the lifting phase. Breath-holding (i.e., Valsalva maneuver) should be avoided.

✓ Throughout the movement, the heels must remain in contact with the floor, and the upward phase is performed pushing through the heels.

✓ It is important for the client to communicate with the spotter if he or she cannot complete the repetition.

✓ Instruct the client to avoid locking the knees and not to exceed a parallel-with-the-floor position with the thighs.

- Encourage the client to perform a few practice trials to ensure proper technique.
- The goal of this test is to determine the client's 1 RM. It is important not to fatigue the client by having him or her perform too many "unnecessary" repetitions. Finding a suitable starting weight is important.

Test protocol and administration:

- Explain the test protocol for a 1-RM squat.

✓ The client should warm up with one set of light resistance (~50% of the anticipated 1-RM weight) that allows five to 10 repetitions, and then rest for one minute.

✓ Based on the client's warm-up effort, determine a suitable workload for the second set that allows for three to five repetitions (~70 to 75% of the anticipated 1-RM weight), after which the client will rest for one minute. Use the following guidelines for determining workload increases throughout this test:

  ◦ Increase the weight by 10 to 20%, or 30 to 40 pounds (14 to 18 kg).

✓ Next, have the client perform one heavy set of two to three repetitions at ~85–90% of the anticipated 1-RM weight and rest for two minutes.

- Based on the client's third set, determine the next workload to find the client's

1-RM effort. Table 8-27 can be used to make these calculations.

✓ For example, if Pete completes two repetitions at 220 pounds (100 kg), this represents 95% of his 1 RM. Therefore, the weight attempted for his first 1-RM trial could be set at 232 pounds (105 kg) [220 lb/0.95 = 232 lb (105 kg)].

- Allow the client to attempt this set. If the client is successful, he or she should rest for two to four minutes and repeat the 1-RM effort with a heavier load.
- If the attempt was unsuccessful, decrease the load accordingly [by 2.5 to 5%] and have the client try again after resting for two to four minutes.
- Continue the up or down increments until a true 1 RM is achieved. *Ideally, the client should achieve his or her 1 RM in three to five testing sets.*
- The final successful load is recorded as the absolute strength.
- Record the weight, progression, sets, repetitions, and any comments on the client's progress in the testing form.
- Calculate relative strength and record that value as well.
  ✓ For example, if Pete's actual 1 RM was measured at 230 lb and he weighs 175 lb, then his strength-to-weight ratio, or relative strength, would be 1.31 (230/175).
- Record the client's performance and use the results as a baseline against which to measure future progress.

Special Considerations for 1-RM Testing

When working with inexperienced exercisers or individuals with health considerations that would preclude them from performing a 1-RM test, it is appropriate to assess strength using submaximal efforts. Table 8-32 provides prediction coefficients of 1 RM for a client completing anywhere between one and 10 repetitions at a maximal effort. Submaximal tests that exceed 10 repetitions assess muscular endurance and not muscular strength.

Table 8-32 offers personal trainers a way to estimate a client's 1 RM without requiring the client to perform an exercise with maximal effort. In fact, the client's 1 RM can be estimated by simply observing a workout and making the appropriate calculation. For example:

- A client is performing bench presses during his or her workout and the trainer observes that he or she consistently completes eight repetitions with 160 pounds (73 kg). Using the coefficient of 1.255, the client's 1 RM is calculated as follows:
  ✓ 1 RM = 160 pounds x 1.255 = 201 pounds (91 kg)

Table 8-32

One-repetition Maximum (1 RM) Prediction Coefficients

Number of repetitions completed	Squat or leg press coefficient	Bench or chest press coefficient
1	1.000	1.000
2	1.0475	1.035
3	1.13	1.08
4	1.1575	1.115
5	1.2	1.15
6	1.242	1.18
7	1.284	1.22
8	1.326	1.255
9	1.368	1.29
10	1.41	1.325

Brzycki, M. (1993). Strength testing: Predicting a one-rep max from reps-to-fatigue. *Journal of Physical Education, Recreation, and Dance,* 68, 88–90.

Submaximal Strength Testing

Testing protocol:

- Determine the number of repetitions that are appropriate for the client based upon his or her current training regimen or experience [e.g., Mary usually performs three sets of eight repetitions at 60 pounds (27 kg)].
- Sets:
  ✓ Have the client perform one or two warm-up sets at a lower intensity than the target weight and allow one to two minutes of recovery between the sets.
  ✓ Instruct the client to perform the first attempt at a personal best, completing the targeted number of repetitions

consistent with his or her current training [e.g., Mary completes one set of eight repetitions at 60 pounds (27 kg)].

✓ If the client is successful, he or she should rest for approximately two minutes and repeat the personal-best effort with a heavier load.

✓ If the client is unsuccessful at achieving the goal repetitions, simply use the actual number completed in the calculation [e.g., If Mary completes five squat repetitions with an increased load of 70 lb (32 kg), her predicted 1-RM would equal 84 lb (38 kg)].

Assessments can also be performed to determine left-to-right muscle balance or appropriate ratios of **agonist** to **antagonist** muscle strength. Muscle imbalances occur from improper training, overuse of one side of the body (e.g., tennis serves or golf swings), or from structural imbalances caused by injury or poor posture or body mechanics. Muscle balance is essential to prevent injury, enhance sports performance, and avoid chronic conditions later in life. Table 8-33 presents the recommended strength ratios between opposing muscle groups.

Sport-skill Assessments

Given the increased popularity of sports conditioning, some clients may desire or need assessments of the skill- or performance-related parameters of fitness, which include:

- Balance
- Power (anaerobic power and anaerobic capacity)
- Speed
- Agility
- Reactivity
- Coordination

Many of these assessments consist of dynamic, and perhaps ballistic, movements that involve rapid phases of acceleration and deceleration. This places significant stress across the joints and throughout the kinetic chain, which may be inappropriate for many individuals. Trainers should therefore determine whether these assessments are skill- and conditioning-level appropriate for clients beforehand.

Power Testing: Field Tests

Human power is defined as "the rate at which mechanical work is performed under a defined set of conditions" (ACSM, 2010b). Power correlates to the immediate energy available

Table 8-33

Appropriate Strength Ratios

Joint	Movements	Muscles	Ratio
Shoulder	Flexion:Extension	Anterior deltoids:Trapezius, posterior deltoids	2:3
Shoulder	Internal rotation: External rotation	Subscapularis:Supraspinatus, infraspinatus, teres minor	3:2
Elbow	Flexion:Extension	Biceps:Triceps	1:1
Lumbar spine	Flexion:Extension	Iliopsoas, abdominals:Erector spinae	1:1
Hip	Flexion:Extension	Iliopsoas, rectus abdominus, tensor fascia latae:Erector spinae, gluteus maximus, hamstrings	1:1
Knee	Flexion:Extension	Hamstrings:Quadriceps	2:3
Ankle	Plantarflexion:Dorsiflexion	Gastrocnemius:Tibialis anterior	3:1
Ankle	Inversion:Eversion	Tibialis anterior:Peroneals	1:1

Heyward, V.H. (2006). *Advanced Fitness Assessment and Exercise Prescription* (5th ed.). Champaign, Ill.: Human Kinetics.

through the anaerobic energy system, specifically the phosphagen energy system. Anaerobic power involves a single repetition or event and represents the maximal amount of power the body can generate, whereas anaerobic capacity represents the sustainability of power output for brief periods of time.

Strength and power are closely related, but for assessment purposes, they should be evaluated independently. Power is also sport- or activity-specific. Evaluation and subsequent correction of athletic performance is closely related to body mechanics and movement. Evaluation of fluid movements like a golf swing or a swimming stroke requires digital movement analysis or other technology. The power assessments covered in this section are also related to skills and performance in a variety of sports and are significant indicators of sports success.

Power Equations

Power = Force x Velocity

or

Power = Work/Time

Where:

Force = Mass x Acceleration

Velocity = Distance/Time

Work = Force x Distance

Field tests that assess power measure how fast the body can move in a short time period. The following tests are commonly used to assess power:

- Anaerobic power: Standing long jump test
- Anaerobic power: Vertical jump test
- Anaerobic power: Kneeling overhead toss
- Anaerobic capacity: Margaria-Kalamen test
- Anaerobic capacity: 300-yard shuttle run

Personal trainers must keep in mind that power tests are designed for clients interested in training at phase 4 of the ACE IFT Model, or for high-level athletic performance. Therefore, the majority of normative data presented with these test has been obtained from studies involving college and professional athletes. Little, if any, data exists for middle-aged or older adults. The results of these tests are perhaps best utilized as baseline data against which to measure a client's future performance.

Contraindications for Field Tests of Power, Speed, Agility, and Quickness

Because these tests are intended for athletes and those interested in advanced forms of training, individuals in "special populations" are not likely candidates. When working with a client who is still recovering from an injury, it is wise to omit these tests.

Anaerobic Power: Standing Long Jump Test

The standing long jump test is simple to administer and does not require much time or equipment. It is a valuable tool for assessing explosive leg power.

Equipment:

- A flat, stable jumping area at least 20 feet (6 meters) in length that provides good traction (e.g., gym floor)
- Tape measure
- Tape

Pre-test procedure:

- After explaining the purpose of the standing long jump test, describe and demonstrate the technique. Allow the client to perform a few practice trials before administering the test. Many clients may remember this test as part of the President's Council on Sports and Physical Fitness battery of tests performed during childhood.
- The goal of the test is to jump as far as possible from a standing/stationary position. The jumping distance is measured from the takeoff line to the back edge of the client's rearmost heel. If the person steps or stumbles backward, exclude this effort and repeat the test.
- A two-foot takeoff and landing are used. Since proper technique plays a role in achieving maximum distance, clients should be encouraged to use

their arms and legs for propulsion. Allow for some practice time before the test.

Test protocol and administration:

- Place a strip of tape across the floor and instruct the client to stand with his or her feet slightly apart, toes positioned just behind the takeoff line.
- Using the arms and legs for propulsion, the client attempts to jump as far as possible, landing on both feet.
- Measure the distance between the takeoff line and the rearmost point of contact. Allow three attempts and record the maximum distance achieved on the testing form.
- Use Table 8-34 to rank the client's performance.

Table 8-34
Standing Long Jump Test Norms

	Distance Jumped			
Ratings	**Males (in)**	**Males (cm)**	**Females (in)**	**Females (cm)**
Excellent	>97.5	>250	>78	>200
Very good	94–97.5	241–250	74.5–78	191–200
Above average	90–94	231–240	70.5–74.5	181–190
Average	86–90	221–230	66.5–70.5	170–180
Below average	82–86	211–220	63–66.5	161–170
Poor	74.5–82	191–210	55–63	141–160
Very poor	<74.5	<191	<55	<141

From www.topendsports.com.

Anaerobic Power: Vertical Jump Test

The vertical jump test is very simple and quick to administer. It is especially valuable when assessing the vertical jump height in athletes who participate in sports that require skill and power in jumping (e.g., basketball, volleyball, swimming).

Equipment:

- A smooth wall with a relatively high ceiling
- A flat, stable floor that provides good traction
- Chalk (different color than the wall)
- Measuring tape or stick
- Stepstool or small ladder
- Vertical jump tester (e.g., Vertec®) (optional)

Pre-test procedure:

- After explaining the purpose of the vertical jump test, describe and demonstrate the procedure. Allow the client to perform a few practice trials before administering the test.
- Instruct the client to stand adjacent to a wall, with the inside shoulder of the dominant arm approximately 6 inches (15 cm) from the wall. Measure the client's standing height by marking the fingers with chalk, extending the inside arm overhead, and marking the wall (Figure 8-25). This mark will then be compared to the maximum height achieved on a vertical jump.
- The goal of this test is to jump as high as possible from a standing position.
- Since proper technique plays a role in achieving maximum jump height, encourage the client to use the arms and legs for propulsion.

Test protocol and administration:

- The client stands adjacent to the wall, 6 inches (15 cm) away from the wall, with both arms extended overhead and feet flat on the floor.

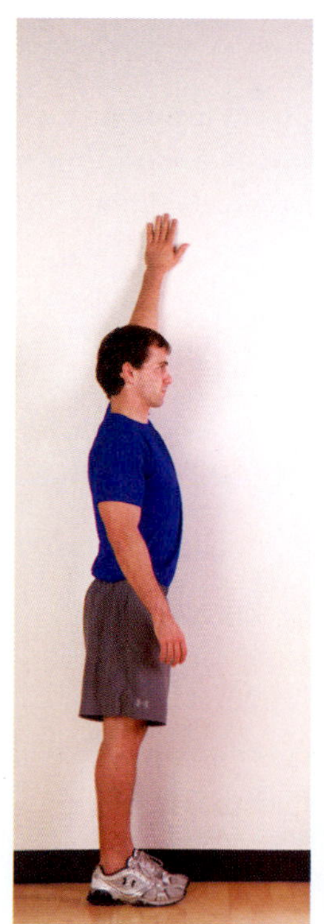
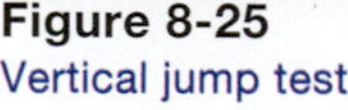
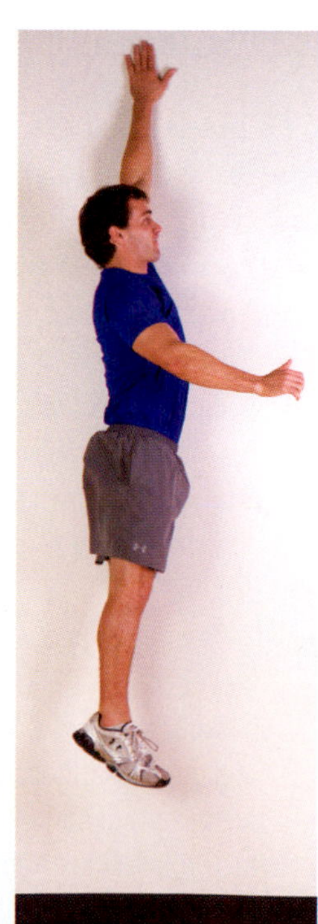

Figure 8-25
Vertical jump test

- The client then lowers the arms and, without any pause or step, drops into a squat movement before exploding upward into a vertical jump.
- At the highest point the athlete touches the wall, marking it with chalk.
- The vertical jump measurement is determined by the vertical distance between the new chalk mark and the starting height.
- Allow three repetitions and record the maximum height achieved on the testing form.
- Use Table 8-35 to rank the client's performance.

Table 8-35
Vertical Jump Test Norms

Rating	Males (in)	Males (cm)	Females (in)	Females (cm)
Excellent	>28 in	>70 cm	>24 in	>60 cm
Very good	24–28	61–70	20–24	51–61
Above average	20–24	51–60	16–20	41–50
Average	16–20	41–50	12–16	31–40
Below average	12–16	31–40	8–12	21–30
Poor	8–12	21–30	4–8	11–20
Very poor	<8	<21	<4	<11

From www.topendsports.com.

Anaerobic Power: Kneeling Overhead Toss

While previous tests assessed power of the lower extremities, this test measures power in the upper extremities. This test is especially appropriate for clients who take part in sports where upper-body power is important (e.g., volleyball, swimming, field events such as javelin and shot put). This is also an appropriate power test for wheelchair athletes, if modified.

The kneeling overhead toss test is simple to administer and does not require much time.

Supplies:
- 2-kg (4.4-lb) medicine ball for females
- 3-kg (6.6-lb) medicine ball for males
- Tape measure
- Foam pad
- Open area for throwing

Pre-test procedure:
- After explaining the purpose of the test, describe and demonstrate the procedure. Allow the client to perform a few practice trials before administering the test.
- The goal of the test is to throw the ball as far as possible using a two-handed overhead throw.
  - ✓The client must not rotate the spine or favor one arm over the other.
  - ✓The knees cannot leave the mat and the feet must stay in contact with the mat.
  - ✓The client thrusts the ball outward, allowing him- or herself to fall forward and land in a push-up position.
- Proper technique and trajectory both play important roles in achieving maximum distance. A 45-degree trajectory angle is optimal.

Test protocol and administration:
- The client kneels on the pad with the body upright. The upper legs are vertical and parallel to each other.
- Hand the client the medicine ball. The client grasps the ball from both sides, using wide, open hands for added control (Figure 8-26).
- The client holds the ball in front of the body with outstretched arms. He or she brings the ball back overhead, leaning backward from the knees and, without hesitation, launches the ball forward.

Figure 8-26
Kneeling overhead toss

- The spot where the ball initially lands is used for measurement. Measure from the outer edge of the launch line to the central point of the ball's landing point.
- Allow three trials and record the maximum distance achieved on the testing form. Measurements are recorded in feet and inches.
- Trainers should record the client's performance and use the results as a baseline against which to measure future progress.

Anaerobic Capacity: Margaria-Kalamen Stair Climb Test

The Margaria-Kalamen stair climb test is a classic test used to assess leg power and activation of the phosphagen energy system.

Equipment:

- Flight of stairs with the following:
  - ✓ A 20-foot (6-m) flat surface in front of the stairs.
  - ✓ Nine or more steps with the third, sixth, and ninth steps clearly marked with tape.
  - ✓ Measure the vertical height between the third and the ninth steps, as this value is used in the power calculation.
- Tape measure
- Stopwatch
- Marking tape
- Timing mats (optional). Timing mats allow for more accurate timing, as the clock starts and stops upon foot impact.

Figure 8-27 illustrates the setup for this test.

Pre-test procedure:

- After explaining the purpose of the stair-climb test, describe and demonstrate the procedure. Allow the client to warm up and perform a few practice trials before administering the test.
- The client will sprint toward the stairs from a standing start 20 feet (6 m) from the base of the stairs.
- He or she will run up the flight of stairs, taking three steps at a time. Measure the performance from the time it takes the client to get from the third step to the ninth step to the nearest 0.01 second. The goal of the test is to run up the stairs as quickly as possible.
- If timing mats are being used, one should be placed at the third step and the other on the ninth step.

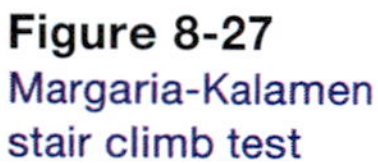

Figure 8-27
Margaria-Kalamen stair climb test

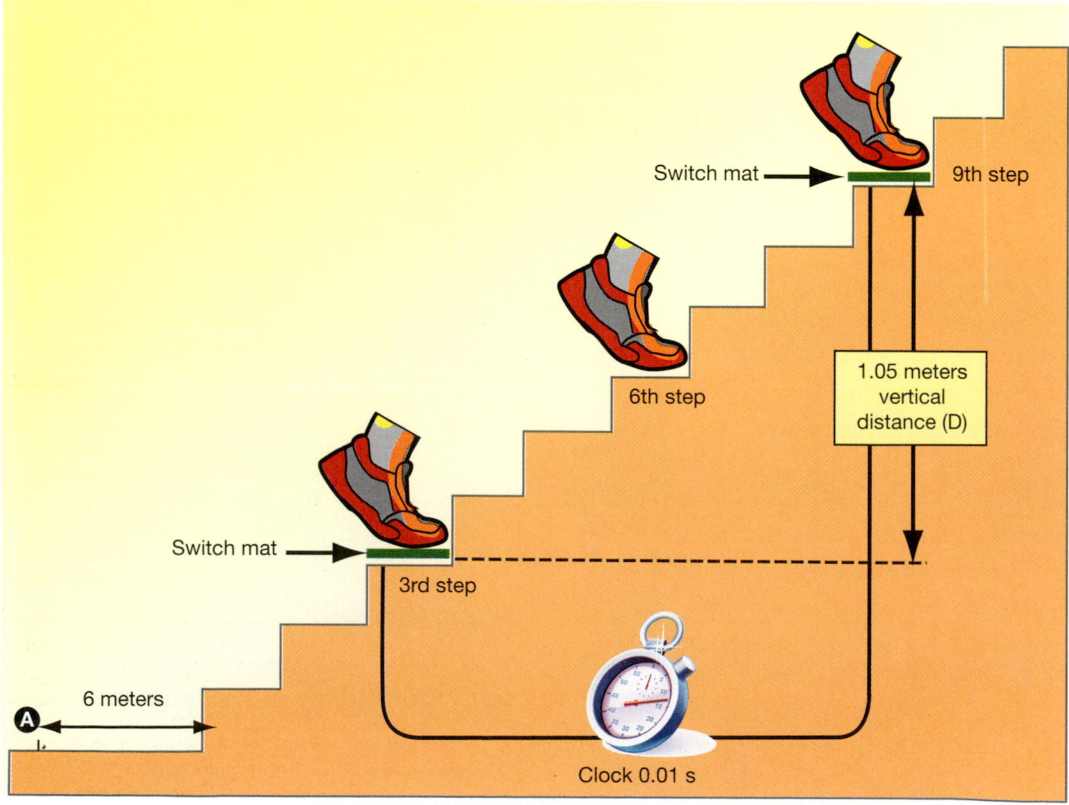

Calculating Power

Power = [(Body weight x 9.807) x Height]/Time

Weight in kg; Height = vertical distance between step 3 and step 9 in meters; Time = seconds

Example: John weighs 180 lb and scored a best attempt of 0.8 seconds when climbing six steps with a combined height of 49.5 inches.
180 lb = 81.8 kg; step height = 49.5 inches x 0.0254 = 1.26 m
Power = [(81.7 x 9.807) x 1.26]/0.8
Power = 1,262 watts

Test protocol and administration:

- Record the client's weight in kilograms.
- The client stands 20 feet (6 m) away from the base of the stairs and starts the test whenever he or she is ready.
- Start the stopwatch when the client's foot hits the third step and stop it when the client lands on the ninth step.
  ✓ To increase the accuracy of the test, it is recommended that a second person also time the client's performance. Use the average of the two times as the "actual" time for each attempt.
- Allow three trials, with two to three minutes recovery between attempts.
- The fastest time achieved is recorded on a testing form.
- The following formula is used to assess power.
- Use Table 8-36 to rank the client's performance.

Anaerobic Capacity: 300-yard Shuttle Run

This test assesses anaerobic capacity, or the highest rate of sustainable power over a predetermined distance.

Equipment:

- Cone or line markers
- 25 yards of flat surface (field or hardwood court)
- Stopwatch

Pre-test Procedure:

- After explaining the purpose of this test, describe the procedure. Allow the client to warm up and perform a practice trial (if necessary) before administering the test.
- Set two cones 25 yards (22.5 m) apart on a stable surface that provides good traction (e.g., gym floor, grass, or track).

Table 8-36
Margaria-Kalamen Stair Sprint Guidelines (watts)

	Age				
Men's Classification	**15–20**	**20–30**	**30–40**	**40–50**	**50+**
Excellent	>2,197	>2,059	>1,648	>1,226	>961
Good	1,844–2,197	1,726–2,059	1,383–1,648	1,040–1,226	814–961
Average	1,471–1,824	1,373–1,716	1,098–1,373	834–1,030	647–804
Fair	1,108–1,461	1,040–1.363	834–1,088	637–824	490–637
Poor	<1,108	<1,040	<834	<637	<490
Women's Classification	**15–20**	**20–30**	**30–40**	**40–50**	**50+**
Excellent	>1,785	>1,648	>1,226	>961	>736
Good	1,491–1,785	1,383–1,648	1,040–1,226	814–961	608–736
Average	1,187–1,481	1,098–1,373	834–1,030	647–804	481–598
Fair	902–1,177	834–1,089	637–824	490–637	373–471
Poor	<902	<834	<637	<490	<373

Adapted with permission from Hoffman, J. (2006). *Norms for Fitness, Performance, and Health.* Champaign, Ill.: Human Kinetics. Adapted from Fox, E., Bowers, R., & Foss, M. (1993). *The Physiological Basis for Exercise and Sport* (5th ed.). Dubuque, Iowa: Wm C. Brown, 676, with permission of The McGraw-Hill Companies; based on data from Kalamen, J. (1968). *Measurement of Maximum Muscular Power in Man,* Doctoral Dissertation, The Ohio State University, and Margaria, R., Aghemo, I., & Rovelli, E. (1966). Measurement of muscular power (anaerobic) in man. *Journal of Applied Physiology,* 21, 1662–1664.

- The client runs back and forth between the two cones, making foot contact with the line of the second cone, then turning and running as quickly as possible back toward the starting cone or line marker.
  - ✓ The goal of this test is to complete six continuous round trips without stopping in the quickest time possible.
  - ✓ After completing the test, the client should take a five-minute recovery interval.
  - ✓ After this rest interval, the client repeats the test a second time.
  - ✓ The average of the two times is noted as the final test score.

Test protocol and administration:

- Instruct the client to line up on one of the cone or line markers of the 25-yard (22.5-m) course.
- On the trainer's command, the client begins the test as the trainer starts the stopwatch.
- The client completes six consecutive round trips without stopping.
- It is helpful for the trainer to count each lap to help the client gauge his or her progress.
- Record the average of the two trials (to the nearest tenth of a second) on a testing form.
- Use Table 8-37 to rank the client's performance.

Table 8-37

Percentile Ranks for 300-yard Shuttle Run for NCAA Division I Athletes (time in seconds)

Percentile Rank	Baseball	Men's Basketball	Women's Basketball	Softball
90th	56.7	54.1	58.4	63.3
80th	58.9	55.1	61.8	65.1
70th	59.9	55.6	63.6	66.5
60th	61.3	56.3	64.7	67.9
50th	62.0	56.7	65.2	69.2
40th	63.2	57.2	65.9	71.3
30th	63.9	58.1	66.8	72.4
20th	65.3	58.9	68.1	74.6
10th	67.7	60.2	68.9	78.0

Hoffman, J. (2006). *Norms for Fitness, Performance, and Health.* Champaign, Ill.: Human Kinetics; Adapted from Gilliam, G.M. (1983). 300 yard shuttle run. *National Strength and Conditioning Journal,* 5, 46.

> As with power tests, tests of speed, agility, and quickness are designed for clients interested in training at phase 4 of the ACE IFT Model, or for high-level athletic performance. Therefore, the majority of normative data presented with these test has been obtained from studies involving college and professional athletes. Little, if any, data exists for middle-aged or older adults. The results of these tests are perhaps best utilized as baseline data against which to measure a client's future performance.

Speed, Agility, and Quickness Testing

Speed and agility tests are not only important for assessing speed and quickness, but are also useful in predicting athletic potential. In football, the 40-yard dash is often used as a measure of performance, while baseball coaches use a 60-yard sprint and volleyball coaches use a 20-yard test. Peak running speed is a strong predictor of running performance (regardless of distance), even more so than $\dot{V}O_2$max (Noakes, 1988). In events that require quick bursts of speed, quickness is obviously important, but technique is critical as well. For a trainer working with an individual interested in improving his or her performance in a timed sprint, it is important to not only focus on drills that will increase overall muscular speed, but to also work on sprinting techniques, including optimal start positioning, body position during acceleration and during the sprint itself, and breath control.

Speed and agility tests require maximal effort and swift limb movement. To perform well and avoid injury, it is imperative that the client warms up adequately. A sample warm-up includes a five- to 10-minute jog or light cardiovascular activity combined with some short sprints. Light, dynamic stretching should be included for the involved muscle groups (i.e., quadriceps, hamstrings, calves, hip flexors).

The following tests are described in this section:

- Pro agility test
- T-test
- 40-yard dash

Pro Agility Test

The pro agility test is sometimes called the 20-yard agility test or the 5-10-5 shuttle run. This test quickly and simply measures an individual's ability to accelerate, decelerate, change direction, and then accelerate again. The National Football League and USA Women's Soccer Team use this assessment as part of their battery of tests.

Equipment:

- A marked football field, but the test can be conducted on any hard, flat surface that offers good traction
- Measuring tape
- Cones or tape
- Stopwatch
- Timing gates (optional)

Pre-test procedure:

- Set up the cones as shown in Figure 8-28.
- After explaining the purpose of the test, describe and demonstrate the proper route and technique. Allow the client to warm up and perform a few practice trials before administering the test.
- The goal of the test is to complete the course as quickly as possible.
- The client does not need to touch the cone with his or her hand, but must touch the line with either foot. Proper technique must be followed or the test run will not count.

Test protocol and administration:

- The trainer is positioned as the timer/judge at the center cone or line marker.
- Ask the client to straddle the middle cone or line marker facing the trainer and assume a three-point stance (see Figure 8-30 on page 239).
- On the trainer's command, the client turns and sprints to the cone or line marker to the *left,* making foot contact with the marker before changing direction and sprinting 10 yards across the center marker to make foot contact with the cone or line marker on the right, then changes direction once again and sprints back through the center line.
- Record the time needed to complete the test to the nearest one-hundredth of a second.
  ✓ The pro agility test is then repeated two more times. The client can take a few minutes to recover between tests.
- The fastest of the three trials is noted as the final test score on the testing form.
- Use Table 8-38 to rank the client's performance. *Note:* The test can be run in either or both directions.

Table 8-38
Percentile Ranks for the Pro Agility Test for NCAA Division I Athletes (time in seconds)

Percentile Rank	Men's Basketball	Men's Baseball	Men's Football	Women's Volleyball	Women's Basketball	Women's Softball
90th	4.22	4.25	4.21	4.75	4.65	4.88
80th	4.29	4.36	4.31	4.84	4.82	4.96
70th	4.35	4.41	4.38	4.91	4.86	5.03
60th	4.39	4.46	4.44	4.98	4.94	5.10
50th	4.41	4.50	4.52	5.01	5.06	5.17
40th	4.44	4.55	4.59	5.08	5.10	5.24
30th	4.48	4.61	4.66	5.17	5.14	5.33
20th	4.51	4.69	4.76	5.23	5.23	5.40
10th	4.61	4.76	4.89	5.32	5.36	5.55

Adapted with permission from Hoffman, J. (2006). *Norms for Fitness, Performance, and Health.* Champaign, Ill.: Human Kinetics.

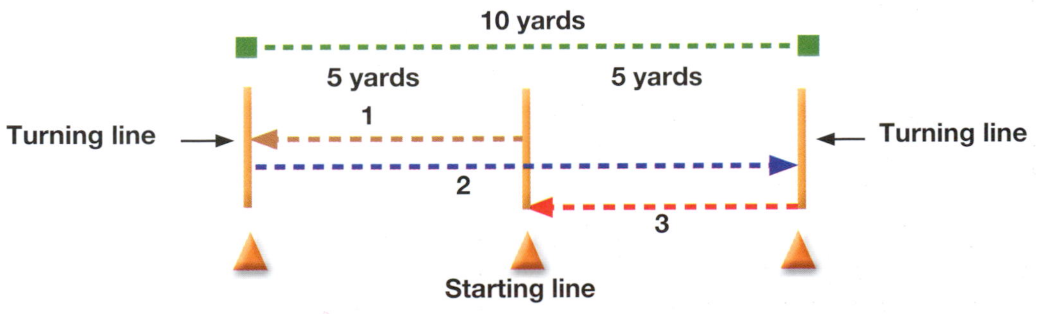

Figure 8-28
The layout for the pro agility test

T-Test

The T-test is a useful agility test for assessment of multidirectional movement (forward, lateral, and backward). It is a simple test to administer and does not require much time or investment in supplies.

Equipment:

- A marked football field, but the test can be conducted on any hard, flat surface that offers good traction
- Measuring tape
- Four cones
- Stopwatch
- Timing gates (optional)

Pre-test procedure:

Set up the cones as depicted in Figure 8-29.

- After explaining the purpose of the T-test, describe and demonstrate the proper route and technique. Allow the client to warm up and perform a few practice trials before administering the test.
- The goal of the test is to complete the course as quickly as possible.
- The client must keep his or her body facing forward at all times and must physically touch each cone with the correct hand.

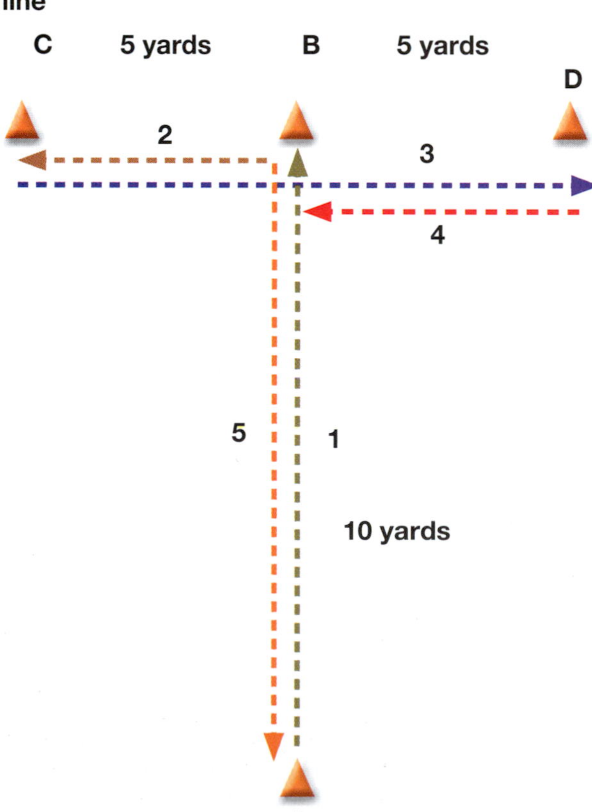

Figure 8-29
Layout for the T-test

The client shuffles through the course and cannot allow the feet to crossover at any time. Proper technique must be followed or the test run will not count.

Test protocol and administration:

- The client starts at cone A. On the trainer's command, the client sprints to cone B and touches the base of the cone with the right hand.
- He or she then shuffles left to cone C and touches the base of the cone with the left hand.
- He or she then shuffles right to cone D and touches the base of the cone with the right hand.
- He or she then shuffles back to cone B and touches the base with the right hand before running backward to the start (cone A).
- Stop the stopwatch as the client passes cone A.
- The T-test is performed three times with a few minutes of recovery between each test.
- Record the fastest time on a testing form.
- Use Table 8-39 to rank the client's performance. *Note:* The test can be run in either or both directions.

Table 8-39
T-test Performance Norms

Ranking	Males (seconds)	Females (seconds)
Excellent	<9.50	<10.50
Good	9.51–10.50	10.51–11.50
Average	10.51–11.50	11.51–12.50
Poor	>11.50	> 12.50

Adapted with permission from Hoffman, J. (2006). *Norms for Fitness, Performance, and Health.* Champaign, Ill.: Human Kinetics.

40-yard Dash

The purpose of the 40-yard dash is to determine acceleration and speed. This test is simple to administer and does not require much time or equipment. The 40-yard dash, or variations on the test that use other distances, are performed extensively in football and other sports that require quick bouts of speed.

Weather conditions and running surface can greatly affect the speed of the client. On follow-up assessments, it is important to test on the same running surface and in the same conditions as in the initial test.

Equipment:

- Running track, marked field, or measuring tape and unobstructed surface (of at least 60 yards)
- Stopwatch
- Cones
- Timing gates (optional)

Pre-test procedure:

- After explaining the purpose of the 40-yard dash, describe the test to the client. The client should warm up prior to the actual test and even perform some practice starts to work on acceleration techniques.
- The goal of the test is to run as quickly as possible. The client begins in a four-point (track start) or three-point stance if that is more comfortable, and runs past the 40-yard (37-m) mark (Figure 8-30).

Test protocol and administration:

- The client starts in a four-point (track start) or three-point stance with the front foot positioned on or behind the starting line. He or she should place the hands and feet on the line, but not beyond it. The client can lean across the line, but is not permitted to rock. This position must be held for at least three seconds prior to starting.
- Start the stopwatch at the first movement and stop it when the client's chest crosses the finish line.
- The time is measured to one-hundredth of a second.
- Have the client perform two trials with appropriate recovery (at least 2 minutes) between the trials and record the average of the two trials on the testing form.

Refer to Table 8-40 for descriptive data that can be used to show clients where their performance might rank among various groups of athletes.

Figure 8-30
Four-point stance (track start)

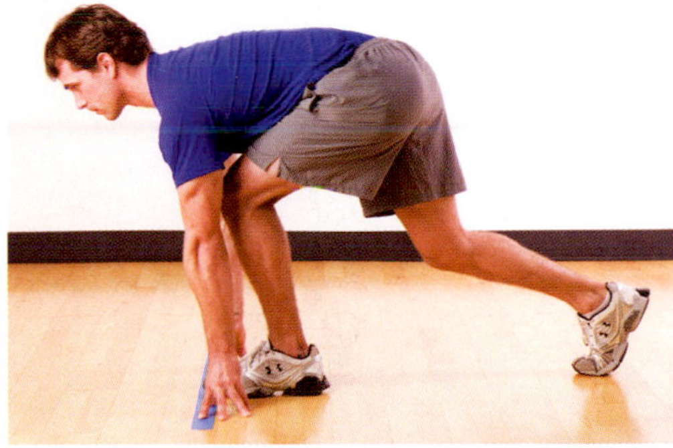

Three-point stance

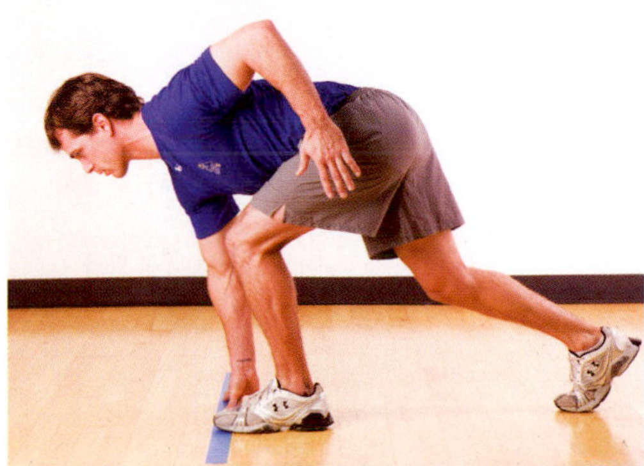

Table 8-40
40-yard Dash—Descriptive Data

Group, Sport, or Position	40-yard (37-m) sprint (seconds)
NCAA Division I college American football players:	
• Split ends, wide receivers, strong safeties, outside linebackers, and offensive and defensive backs	4.6–4.7
• Linebackers, tight ends, safeties, and quarterbacks	4.8–4.9
• Defensive tackles	4.9–5.1
• Defensive guards	5.1
• Offensive tackles	5.4
College American football players	5.35
Competitive college athletes:	
• Men	5.0
• Women	5.5–5.96
Recreational college athletes:	
• Men	5.0
• Women	5.8
Sedentary college students:	
• Men	5.0
• Women	6.4
High school American football players:	
• Backs and receivers	5.2
• Linebackers and tight ends	5.4
• Linemen	4.9–5.6

Note: The data listed are either means or 50th percentiles (medians). There was considerable variation in sample size among the groups tested. Thus, the data should be regarded as only descriptive, not normative.

Source: Baechle, T.R. & Earle, R.W. (2008). *Essentials of Strength Training and Conditioning* (3rd ed.). Champaign, Ill.: Human Kinetics.

Fitness Testing Accuracy

There are many causes of inaccuracy in fitness testing, ranging from equipment failure to human error (Table 8-41). Most personal-training clients are motivated by improvements in their fitness assessments. Clients like to see that the hard work and dedication to their health and fitness have paid off. There may be test inaccuracies, but repeating the same test, in the same environment, and at the same time of day, will ensure that test results can be compared to earlier test outcomes. For example, even if optimal results are not always attainable, a client who sees his or her performance assessment move from "below average" to "above average" will likely be thrilled with the results and motivated to maintain a regular exercise regimen.

Summary

Assessments are an integral part of any personal-training program. When conducted properly, a thorough assessment can provide valuable health, fitness, and performance information for the trainer to use in exercise program planning and implementation. Assessment information is important for goal setting, determining health risks, and even in helping to establish **rapport** with the client. Not all tests are suitable for all populations. It is up to the trainer to decide the timing and most appropriate battery of tests for each individual client. Periodic reassessments are also important to gauge progress and continue to foster the client–trainer relationship.

Table 8-41

Causes of Fitness Test Inaccuracy

Client Fatigue, lack of sleep Motivation, lack of conviction Excess activity prior to test Food intake prior to test Hydration level Chronic health condition(s) Medications or supplements	**Trainer or Test Technician** Inexperience with testing protocol Poor application of testing protocol Partiality; trying to affect results Level of encouragement
Equipment Improper calibration Mismatched to subject Failure, out of order	**Environment** Distractions Privacy Temperature Weather conditions

References

American College of Sports Medicine (2010a). *ACSM's Guidelines for Exercise Testing and Prescription* (8th ed.). Philadelphia: Wolters Kluwer/Lippincott Williams & Wilkins.

American College of Sports Medicine (2010b). *ACSM Resource Manual for Guidelines for Exercise Testing and Prescription* (6th ed.). Philadelphia: Lippincott Williams & Wilkins.

American College of Sports Medicine (2008). *ACSM's Health-Related Physical Fitness Assessment Manual* (3rd ed.). Philadelphia: Lippincott Williams & Wilkins.

American Council on Exercise (2007). *A pinch of fat: Practical tools for your trade: Body composition assessments.* San Diego, Calif.: American Council on Exercise.

Astrand, P.O. & Ryhming, I. (1954). A nomogram for calculation of aerobic capacity [physical fitness] from pulse rate during submaximal work. *Journal of Applied Physiology*, 7, 218–221.

Baechle, T.R. & Earle, R.W. (2008). *Essentials of Strength Training and Conditioning* (3rd ed.). Champaign, Ill.: Human Kinetics.

Blair, S.N. et al. (1995). Changes in physical fitness and all-cause mortality: A prospective study of healthy and unhealthy men. *Journal of the American Medical Association,* 273, 14, 1093–1098.

Bray, G.A. (2004). Don't throw the baby out with the bath water. *American Journal of Clinical Nutrition,* 70, 3, 347–349.

Bray, G.A. & Gray, D.S. (1988). Obesity: Part I: Pathogenesis. *Western Journal of Medicine,* 149, 429–441.

Brozek, J. et al. (1963). Densiometric analysis of body composition: Revisions of some quantitative assumptions. *Annals of the New York Academy of Sciences,* 110, 113–140.

Brzycki, M. (1993). Strength testing: Predicting a one-rep max from reps-to-fatigue. *Journal of Physical Education, Recreation, and Dance,* 68, 88–90

Centers for Disease Control and Prevention (2004). *National Health and Nutrition Examination Survey (NHANES), 2003–2004*. Hyattsville, Md.: U.S. Department of Health & Human Services, Centers for Disease Control and Prevention, National Center for Health Statistics.

Chobanian, A.V. et al. (2003). *JNC 7 Express: The Seventh Report of the Joint National Committee on Prevention, Detection, Evaluation, and Treatment of High Blood Pressure. NIH Publication No. 03-5233.* Washington D.C.: National Institutes of Health and National Heart, Lung, and Blood Institute.

Ebbeling, C.B. et al. (1991). Development of a single-stage sub-maximal treadmill walking test. *Medicine & Science in Sports & Exercise,* 23, 8, 966–973.

Fitness Canada (1986). *Canadian Standardized Test of Fitness (CSTF) Operations Manual* (3rd ed.). Ottawa: Fitness and Amateur Sport, Canada.

Foster, C. & Porcari, J.P. (2001). The risks of exercise training. *Journal of Cardiopulmonary Rehabilitation,* 21, 347–352.

Foster, C. et al. (1984). Generalized equations for predicting functional capacity from treadmill performance. *American Heart Journal,* 107, 1229–1234.

Fox, E., Bowers, R., & Foss, M. (1993). *The Physiological Basis for Exercise and Sport* (5th ed.). Dubuque, Iowa: Wm C. Brown.

Fox III, S.M., Naughton, J.P., & Haskell, W.L. (1971). Physical activity and the prevention of coronary heart disease. *Annuals of Clinical Research,* 3, 404–432.

Gallagher, D. et al. (2000). Healthy percentage body fat ranges: An approach for developing guidelines based on body mass index. *American Journal of Clinical Nutrition,* 72, 694–701.

Gilliam, G.M. (1983). 300 yard shuttle run. *National Strength and Conditioning Journal,* 5, 46.

Golding, L.A. (2000). *YMCA Fitness Testing and Assessment Manual* (4th ed.). Champaign, Ill.: Human Kinetics.

Heyward, V.H. (2006). *Advanced Fitness Assessment and Exercise Prescription* (5th ed.). Champaign, Ill.: Human Kinetics.

Hoffman, J. (2006). *Norms for Fitness, Performance, and Health*. Champaign, Ill.: Human Kinetics.

Jackson, A.S. & Pollock, M.L. (1985). Practical assessment of body composition. *Physician & Sports Medicine,* 13, 76–90.

Janssen, I. et al. (2004). Waist circumference and health risk. *American Journal of Clinical Nutrition,* 79, 379–384.

Kalamen, J. (1968). *Measurement of Maximum Muscular Power in Man,* Doctoral Dissertation, The Ohio State University.

Mackenzie, B. (2005). *101 Performance Evaluation Tests.* London: Electric Word.

Margaria, R., Aghemo, I., & Rovelli, E. (1966). Measurement of muscular power (anaerobic) in man. *Journal of Applied Physiology,* 21, 1662–1664.

McGill, S. (2007). *Low Back Disorders: Evidence Based Prevention and Rehabilitation* (2nd ed.). Champaign, Ill.: Human Kinetics.

Miller, T.D. (2008). The exercise treadmill test: Estimating cardiovascular prognosis. *Cleveland Clinic Journal of Medicine*, 75, 6.

Morrow, J.R. et al. (2005). *Measurement and Evaluation in Human Performance* (3rd ed.). Champaign, Ill.: Human Kinetics.

Nieman, D.C. (2003). *Exercise Testing and Prescription: A Health-Related Approach* (5th ed.). Mountain View,

Calif.: Mayfield Publishing Company.

Noakes, T.D. (1988). Implications of exercise testing for prediction of athletic performance: A contemporary perspective. *Medicine & Science in Sports & Exercise*, 20, 4, 319–330.

Olshansky, S.J. et al. (2005). A potential decline in life expectancy in the United States in the 21st century. *New England Journal of Medicine,* 352, 1103–1110.

Pollock, M.L. et al. (1982). Comparative analysis of physiologic responses to three different maximal graded exercise test protocols in healthy women. *American Heart Journal,* 103, 363–373.

Pollock, M.L. et al. (1976). A comparative analysis of four protocols for maximal treadmill stress testing. *American Heart Journal,* 92, 39–46.

Siri, W.E. (1961). Body composition from fluid space and density. In: J. Brozek & A. Henschel (Eds.). *Techniques for Measuring Body Composition* (pgs. 223–224. Washington, D.C.: National Academy of Sciences.

Tanaka, H., Monahan, K.D., & Seals, D.R. (2001). Age-predicted maximal heart revisited. *Journal of the American College of Cardiology,* 37, 153–156.

U.S. Department of Health & Human Services (2008). *2008 Physical Activity Guidelines for Americans: Be Active, Healthy and Happy.* www.health.gov/paguidelines/pdf/paguide.pdf

Wilmore, J.H., Costill, D., & Kenney, W.L. (2008). *Physiology of Sport and Exercise* (4th ed.). Champaign, Ill.: Human Kinetics.

Suggested Reading

American College of Sports Medicine (2007). *ACSM's Health/Fitness Facility Standards and Guidelines* (3rd ed.). Champaign, Ill.: Human Kinetics.

American College of Sports Medicine (2009). *ACSM's Exercise Management for Persons with Chronic Disease and Disabilities* (3rd ed.). Champaign, Ill.: Human Kinetics.

American Council on Exercise (2011). *ACE Lifestyle & Weight Management Coach Manual* (2nd ed.). San Diego, Calif.: American Council on Exercise.

Baechle, T.R. & Earle, R.W. (2008). *Essentials of Strength Training and Conditioning* (3rd ed.). Champaign, Ill.: Human Kinetics.

Bassett D.R. & Howley, E.T. (2000). Limiting factors for maximum oxygen uptake and determinants of endurance performance. *Medicine & Science in Sports & Exercise,* 32, 70–84.

Block, P. & Kravitz, L. (2005). The "talk test." *IDEA Fitness Journal*, 2, 2, 22–23.

Cooper Institute of Aerobic Research (2009). *Physical Fitness Assessments and Norms for Adults and Law Enforcement.* Dallas, Tex.: Cooper Institute.

Flávio, O. et al. (2008). Ventilation behavior in trained and untrained men during incremental test: Evidence of one metabolic transition point. *Journal of Sports Science and Medicine,* 7, 335–343.

Golding, L.A., Clayton, R.M., & Sinning, W.E. (1989). *Y's Way to Physical Fitness* (3rd ed.). Champaign, Ill.: Human Kinetics.

Heyward, V. (2006). *Advanced Fitness Assessments and Exercise Prescription* (5th ed.). Champaign, Ill.: Human Kinetics.

Londeree, B.R. (1997). Effect of training on lactate/ventilatory thresholds: A meta-analysis. *Medicine & Science in Sports & Exercise*, 29, 6, 837–843.

Maud, P.J. & Foster, C. (2006). *Physiological Assessment of Human Fitness*. Champaign, Ill.: Human Kinetics.

McArdle, W., Katch, F., & Katch, V. (2006). *Exercise Physiology: Energy, Nutrition, and Human Performance.* Philadelphia: Lippincott, Williams & Wilkins.

Neder, J.A. & Stein, R. (2006). A simplified strategy for the estimation of the exercise ventilatory thresholds. *Medicine & Science in Sports & Exercise,* 38, 5, 1007–1013.

Peirce, A. (1999). *The American Pharmaceutical Association Practical Guide to Natural Medicines.* New York: Stonesong Press.

Pressman, A. & Shelley, D. (2000). *Integrative Medicine.* New York: St. Martin's Press.

Riegelman, R.K. (2004). *Studying a Study and Testing a Test: How to Read the Medical Evidence*. Philadelphia: Lippincott, Williams & Wilkins.

U.S. Department of Health & Human Services (1996). *Physical Activity and Health: A Report of the Surgeon General.* Atlanta, Ga.: U.S. Department of Health & Human Services, Centers for Disease Control and Prevention, National Center for Chronic Disease Prevention and Health Promotion.

IN THIS CHAPTER:

Movement

- Length-tension Relationships
- Force-couple Relationships
- Neural Control

Phase 1: Stability and Mobility Training

- Proximal Stability: Activating the Core
- Proximal Stability: Core Function
- Proximal Mobility: Hips and Thoracic Spine
- Proximal Stability of the Scapulothoracic Region and Distal Mobility of the Glenohumeral Joint
- Distal Mobility
- Static Balance: Segmental
- Static Balance: Integrated (Standing)

Phase 2: Movement Training

- Bend-and-lift Patterns
- Single-leg Stand Patterns
- Pushing Movements
- Pulling Movements
- Rotational Movements

Summary

***FABIO COMANA, M.A., M.S.**, is an exercise physiologist and spokesperson for the American Council on Exercise and faculty at San Diego State University (SDSU) and the University of California San Diego (UCSD), teaching courses in exercise science and nutrition. He holds two master's degrees, one in exercise physiology and one in nutrition, as well as certifications through ACE, ACSM, NSCA, and ISSN. Prior to joining ACE, he was a college head coach and a strength and conditioning coach at SDSU. Comana also managed health clubs for Club One. He lectures, conducts workshops, and writes on many topics related to exercise, fitness, and nutrition both nationally and internationally. As an ACE spokesperson and presenter, he is frequently featured in numerous media outlets, including television, radio, Internet, and more than 100 nationwide newspaper and print publications. Comana has authored chapters in various textbooks.*

CHAPTER 9

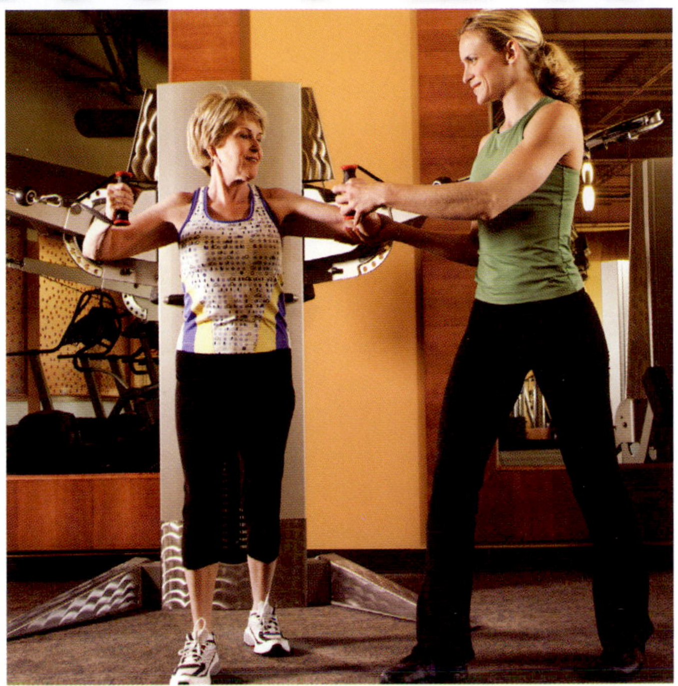

Functional Programming for Stability-Mobility and Movement

Fabio Comana

The human body is designed to move and develops in response to the loads placed on its individual systems. Decreasing levels of activity and a propensity toward poor posture and muscle imbalance alter normal physiological function within the neuromuscular systems. This changes joint loading and movement mechanics, triggering compensations in the way people exercise and perform their daily activities, which ultimately triggers breakdowns along the kinetic chain. These potential breakdowns raise concern regarding traditional programming models that largely ignore the need to re-establish appropriate levels of **stability** and **mobility** within the kinetic chain and train the body to move effectively. This chapter focuses on this need to reestablish stability and mobility across the joints, as well as how to train the five basic movement patterns—bend-and-lift movements (e.g., squatting), single-leg movements (e.g., single-leg stance and lunging), pushing movements (primarily in the vertical/horizontal planes), pulling movements (primarily in the vertical/horizontal planes), and rotational (spiral) movements.

Movement

One fundamental objective that trainers should all share is to improve clients' movement efficiency and ability to perform daily activities. This is one of many possible definitions of functional training. Movement is the result of muscle force, where actions at one body segment affect successive body segments along the kinetic chain. While an individual produces forces to move, the body must also tolerate the imposed forces of any external load, gravity, and **reactive forces** pushing upward through the body, if it is to remain stable. Consequently, the ability of an individual to move efficiently requires that his or her body possesses appropriate levels of both stability and mobility.

- Joint stability is defined as the ability to maintain or control joint movement or position. It is achieved by the synergistic actions of the components of the joint (e.g., muscles, **ligaments,** joint capsule) and the neuromuscular system, and must never compromise joint mobility (Houglum, 2005).
- Joint mobility is defined as the range of uninhibited movement around a joint or body segment. It is achieved by the synergistic actions of the components of the joint and the neuromuscular system, and must never compromise joint stability (Houglum, 2005).

Individuals who exhibit optimal levels of stability and mobility receive and interpret sensory information efficiently regarding movement (i.e., anticipate movement and stabilization needs), and then elicit the necessary motor responses (Sahrmann, 2002). Sensory input and motor output are contingent on collaborative contributions from the neurological and physiological systems, as well as proper joint mechanics (**arthrokinematics**) (Figure 9-1).

Movement efficiency involves a synergistic approach between stability and mobility where "**proximal** stability promotes **distal** mobility." For example, if the hips, trunk, and shoulder girdle are stable, it facilitates greater mobility of the legs and arms. While this is fundamentally true, the relationship between stability and mobility throughout the kinetic chain is slightly more complex. Trainers should understand this relationship, as it serves as the foundation from which all **flexibility** and resistance programming originate.

It is important to remember that while all joints demonstrate varying levels of stability and mobility, they tend to favor one over the other, depending on their function within the body (Figure 9-2) (Cook & Jones, 2007a; 2007b). For example, while the lumbar spine demonstrates some mobility (approximately 15 degrees of **rotation**), it is generally stable, protecting the low back from injury. On the other hand, the thoracic spine is designed to be more mobile to facilitate a variety of movements in the upper extremity. The scapulothoracic joint is a more stable joint formed by collective muscle action attaching the scapulae to the ribcage that provides a solid platform for pulling and pushing movements at the glenohumeral joint and must tolerate the reactive forces transferred into the body during these movements. The foot is unique, as its level of stability varies during the **gait** cycle. Given its need to provide a solid platform for force production against the ground during push-off (heel-off and toe-off **instants**), it is stable. However, as the foot transitions from the heel strike to accepting body weight on one leg (load-response instant), the ankle moves into **pronation** (with accompanying calcaneal **eversion** that increases the space between the tarsal and metatarsal bones), and the foot forfeits some stability in exchange for increased mobility to help absorb the impact forces. As the foot prepares to push off, the ankle moves back into **supination** (with accompanying calcaneal **inversion** that decreases the space between the tarsal and metatarsal bones), becoming more rigid and stable again to increase force transfer into motion.

Individuals who exhibit good posture generally demonstrate an improved relationship between stability and mobility throughout the kinetic chain, but concern arises when an individual exhibits bad posture. What happens

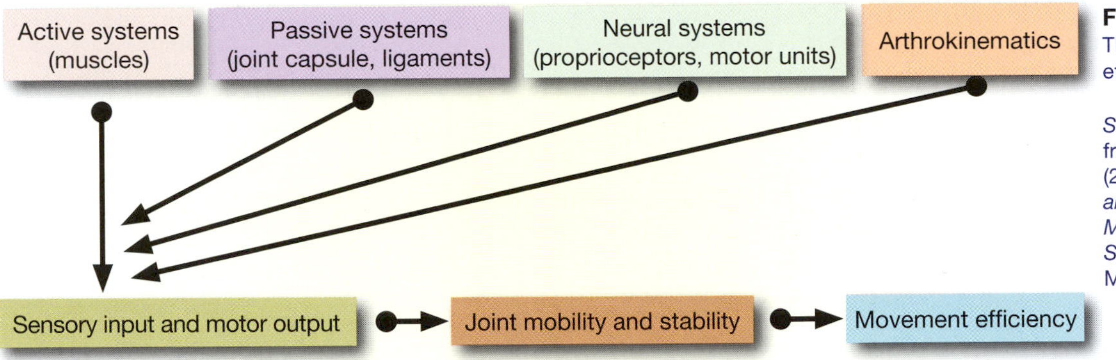

Figure 9-1
The movement efficiency model

Source: Adapted from Sahrmann, S.A. (2002). *Diagnosis and Treatment of Movement Impairment Syndromes.* St. Louis, Mo.: Mosby

when a joint lacks the appropriate level of mobility needed for movement? When mobility is compromised, the following movement compensations typically occur:

- The joint will seek to achieve the desired **range of motion (ROM)** by incorporating movement into another plane. For example, if a client performs a birddog exercise with hip extension (**sagittal plane** movement) (see page 512) and lacks flexibility in the hip flexors, it is common to see the extended leg and hips externally rotate into the **transverse plane,** thereby producing a compensated movement pattern.
- Adjacent, more stable joints may need to compromise some degree of stability to facilitate the level of mobility needed. For example, if a client exhibits **kyphosis** and attempts to extend the thoracic spine, an increase in lumbar **lordosis** often occurs as a compensation for the lack of thoracic mobility.

A lack of mobility can be attributed to numerous factors, including reduced levels of activity and actions and conditions that promote muscle imbalance (e.g., repetitive movements, habitually poor posture, side-dominance, poor exercise technique, imbalanced strength-training programs) (Kendall et al., 2005). This loss of mobility leads to compensations in movement and potential losses to stability at subsequent joints. Muscle imbalances alter the physiological and neurological properties of muscles in a way that ultimately contributes to dysfunctional movement (Figure 9-3). Technology is another contributing factor that promotes dysfunctional movement. As technology continues to advance the complexity of exercise equipment, many exercises and drills have become equally technical. For example, with the introduction of the free-standing, dual-stack, low-high pulley cable systems that move in multiple directions, advanced exercises like the wood chop (see page 305) are now common practice in most fitness settings. Individuals who exhibit limited mobility and stability will often resort to compensated movement when performing complex exercises or using advanced equipment. This raises the potential concern of whether exercise without regard for an individual's levels of stability and mobility throughout the kinetic chain is actually doing more harm than good, advancing the concept of "dysfunctional fitness."

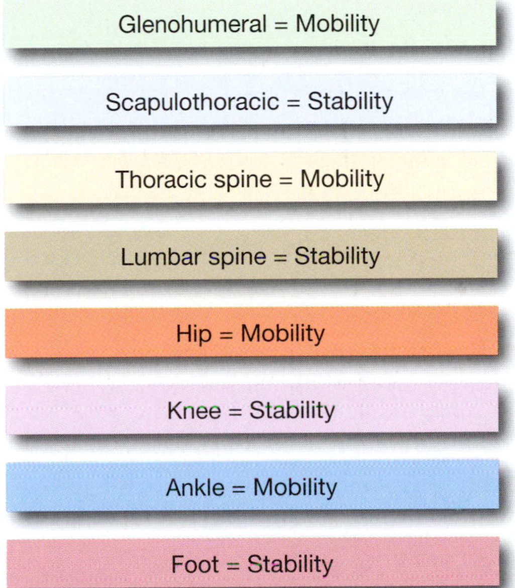

Figure 9-2
Mobility and stability of the kinetic chain

Movement compensations generally

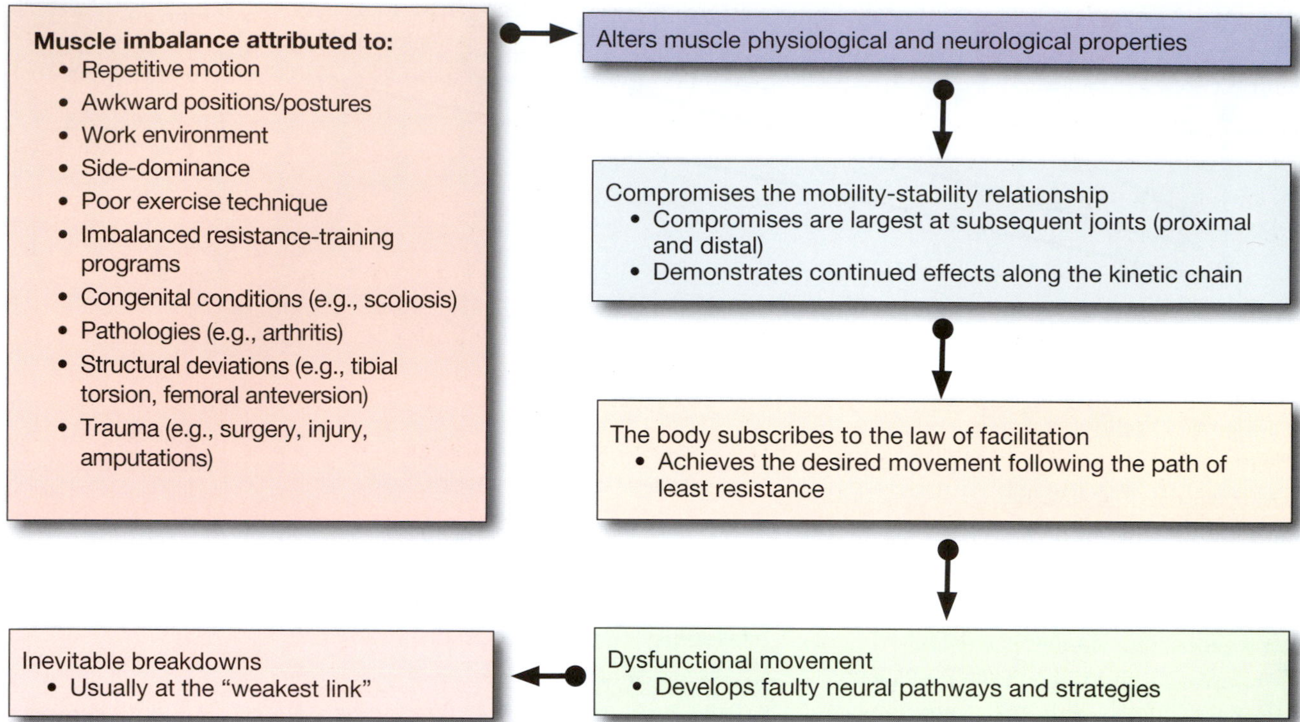

Figure 9-3
Dysfunctional movement

represent an inability to maintain muscle balance and neutrality at the joint (Kendall et al., 2005). Periods of inactivity when joints are held passively in shortened positions result in muscle shortening (e.g., prolonged periods of sitting without hip extension shortens the hip flexors). As one muscle (the **agonist**) shortens, the opposing muscle (the **antagonist**) at the joint tends to lengthen. Muscle shortening and lengthening alter both the physiological and neural properties within the muscle (i.e., length-tension and force-coupling relationships).

Length-tension Relationships

The length-tension relationship is the relationship between the **contractile proteins** (e.g., **actin** and **myosin**) of a **sarcomere** and their force-generating capacity. A slight stretching of the sarcomere beyond its normal resting length increases the spatial arrangement between the muscle's contractile proteins and increases its force-generating capacity (Figure 9-4). Further stretching of the sarcomere beyond optimal length, however, reduces the potential for

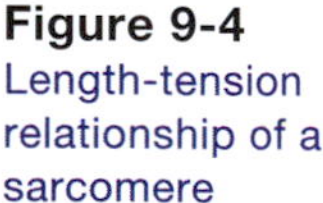

Figure 9-4
Length-tension relationship of a sarcomere

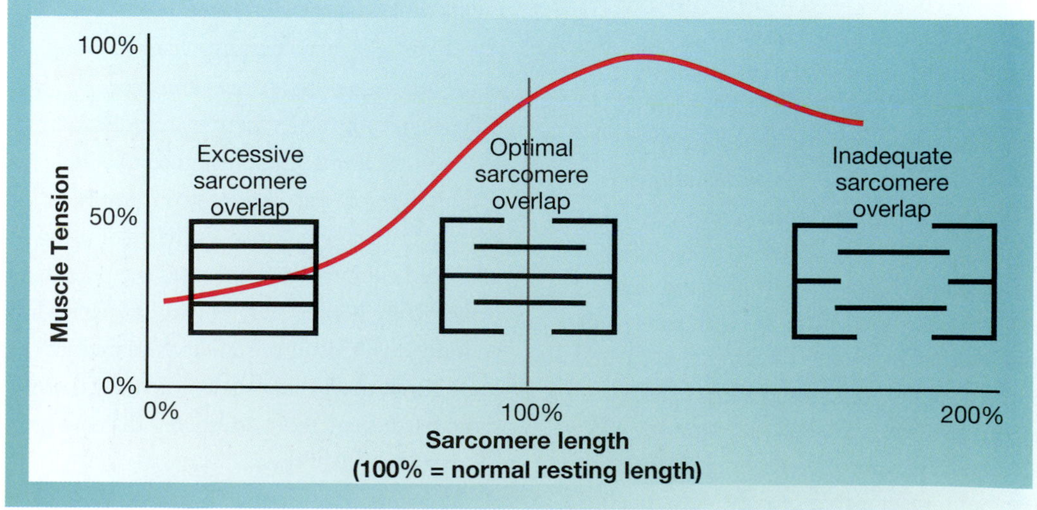

contractile protein binding and decreases the muscle's force-generating capacity (Wilmore, Costill, & Kenney, 2008). Similarly, shortening the sarcomere beyond resting length results in an overlap of contractile proteins, which also reduces the muscle's force-generating potential.

Muscle immobilization, passive shortening, trauma, and aging all shorten muscles, thereby shifting the length-tension curve to the left (Figure 9-5) (MacIntosh, Gardiner, & McComas, 2006; Lieber, 2002; Williams & Goldspink, 1978). This represents a loss in the number of sarcomeres within the **myofibril** of the muscle fiber (a typical muscle myofibril may have approximately 500,000 sacromeres arranged in series). While the muscle may demonstrate good force-generating capacity in the shortened position, it demonstrates reduced force-generating capacity in both the normal-resting-length (good posture) and lengthened positions. Muscles can shorten in as little as two to four weeks when held in passively shortened positions without being stretched or used through a full or functional ROM (e.g., continuous bouts of sitting hunched over a desk without extension activity within the upper thorax can shorten the pectoralis major). Simply stretching a tight muscle does not immediately restore its normal force-generating capacity due to the reduced number of sarcomeres present within the myofibril. Passive stretching or elongation of a tightened muscle will gradually add sarcomeres back in line and help restore the muscle's normal resting length and its length-tension relationship.

Also illustrated in Figure 9-5 is what happens to the lengthened muscles on the opposing side of the joint. These muscles undergo an adaptive change and add sarcomeres in series, shifting the length-tension curve to the right (MacIntosh, Gardiner, & McComas, 2006; Lieber, 2002; Williams & Goldspink, 1978). They demonstrate greater force-generating capacities in lengthened positions, but demonstrate reduced force-generating capacity in the normal-resting-length (good posture) or shortened positions. Restoring the normal resting length and the muscle's force-generating capacity requires a physiological adaptation best achieved by strengthening a muscle in normal-resting-length positions, but not in lengthened positions. For example, when a client exhibits protracted shoulders, performing high-back rows using a full ROM to strengthen the rhomboids and posterior deltoids is not recommended initially. As the rhomboids demonstrate good strength in the lengthened position, the momentum generated during a full-ROM row will carry the movement through the weaker region, essentially decreasing the ability to strengthen the muscle where it needs strengthening. A more appropriate approach is to perform this same exercise initially with either an **isometric** contraction in a good postural position or through a limited ROM.

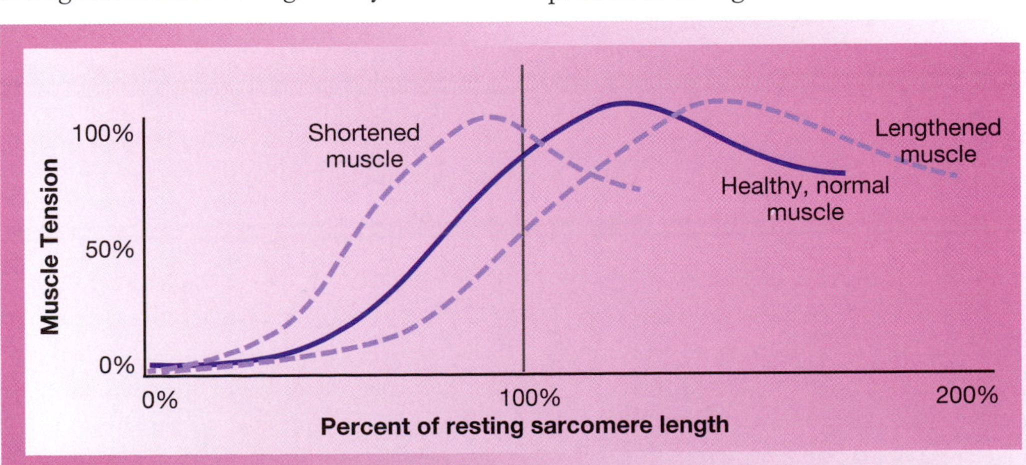

Figure 9-5 Alterations to the length-tension relationship of a sarcomere

Force-couple Relationships

Muscles rarely ever work in isolation, but instead function as integrated groups. Many function by providing opposing, directional, or contralateral pulls at joints (termed force-couples) to achieve efficient movement [American Council on Exercise (ACE), 2009; Houglum, 2005; Sahrmann, 2002]. For example, maintenance of a neutral pelvic position is achieved via opposing force-couples between four major muscle groups that all have attachments on the pelvis. The rectus abdominis pulls upward on the **anterior, inferior** pelvis, while the hip flexors pull downward on the anterior, **superior** pelvis (Figure 9-6). On the **posterior** surface, the hamstrings pull downward on the posterior, inferior pelvis, while the erector spinae pull upward on the posterior, superior pelvis. When these muscles demonstrate good balance, the pelvis holds an optimal position. However, when one muscle becomes tight, it alters this relationship and changes the pelvic position. Changes to pelvic position will affect the position of the spine above and the femur below, thereby altering posture and the loading on the joints along the kinetic chain (Panjabi, 1992).

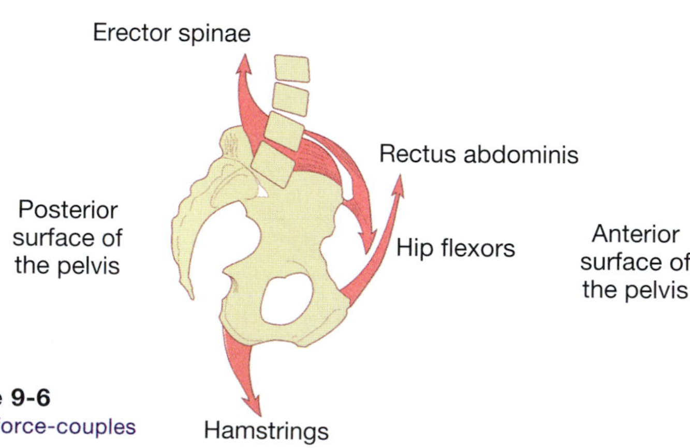

Figure 9-6
Pelvic force-couples

Another example of a force-couple occurs at the glenohumeral joint between the deltoids and rotator cuff muscles during arm **abduction.** While the deltoid acts as the **prime mover** in arm abduction, it is the collaborative action of the rotator cuff muscles, with respect to magnitude and timing of contraction, that counters the direct upward pull of the deltoid to produce rotation. Without the action of the rotator cuff muscles that allows the humeral head to glide inferiorly during rotation, the isolated, upward pull of the deltoid would impinge the humeral head upward against the coracoacromial arch (Cook & Jones, 2007a; Houglum, 2005).

Neural Control

Joint movement is dependent on nerve activity, in that impulses are transmitted to the intended muscles. To help stabilize and control movement within the joint, some degree of simultaneous **co-contraction** of the antagonist also occurs. However, when a muscle becomes shortened, this increases **tonicity** within that muscle (i.e., **hypertonicity**), implying that the muscle now only requires a smaller or weaker nerve impulse to activate a contraction (i.e., lowered irritability threshold) (Whittle, 2007). Thus, when an individual tries to activate the antagonist at a joint, the reduced irritability threshold of the agonist may prematurely activate the muscle and in turn inhibit the action of the antagonist (e.g., tight hip flexors will fire prematurely and may inhibit gluteus activation during hip extension). Consequently, hypertonic muscles decrease the neural drive to the opposing muscle via **reciprocal inhibition.** While both muscles on either side of the joint demonstrate weakness due to their altered length-tension relationship, the reciprocal inhibition of the opposing muscles contributes to further weakening of the antagonist, thereby reducing its ability to generate adequate levels of force to move the joint. When this occurs, the body has to call on other muscles at the joint (i.e., the synergists) that will assume the responsibility of becoming the prime mover, a process called **synergistic dominance** (Sahrmann, 2002). For example, a tight hip flexor may inhibit and weaken the gluteus maximus, forcing the hamstrings (a synergist) to assume a greater role in hip extension. Unfortunately, the hamstrings are not designed for this function and may suffer from overuse or overload, increasing the likelihood for tightness and injury. Additionally, as the hamstrings do not offer the same degree of movement control of the femoral head during hip extension as the gluteus maximus does, this also increases the likelihood for dysfunctional movement and injury to the hip over time. Compromised joint movement alters neuromuscular control and function, prompting additional postural misalignments and faulty loading at the joints that inevitably increases overload and the likelihood for further injury and pain (Figure 9-7). It is therefore imperative that trainers work to restore and maintain normal joint alignment, joint movement, muscle balance, and muscle function, all of which are critical for optimal health and longevity. Effective programming and attention to exercise technique will help the trainer achieve this goal.

Phase 1: Stability and Mobility Training

The objective of this first phase of functional movement and resistance training is to reestablish appropriate levels of stability and mobility within the body. This process begins by targeting an important proximal region of the body, the lumbar spine, which encompasses the body's **center of mass (COM)** and the core. As this region is primarily stable, programming should begin by first promoting stability of the lumbar region through the action and function of the core. Once an individual demonstrates the ability to stabilize this region, the program should then progress to the more distal segments. Adjacent to the lumbar spine are the hips and thoracic spine, both of which are primarily mobile. As thoracic spine mobility is restored, the program can target stability of the scapulothoracic region. Finally, once stability and mobility of the lumbo-pelvic, thoracic, and shoulder regions have been established, the program can then shift to enhancing mobility and stability of the distal extremities. Attempting to improve mobility within distal joints without developing more proximal stability only serves to compromise any existing stability within these segments. When a joint lacks stability, many of the muscles that normally mobilize that joint may need to alter their true functions to assist in providing stability. For example, if an individual lacks stability in the scapulothoracic joint, the deltoids, which are normally responsible for many glenohumeral movements, may need to compromise some of their force-generating capacity and assist in stabilizing glenohumeral movement (Cook & Jones, 2007a). This altered deltoid function decreases force output and may increase the potential for dysfunctional movement and injury.

It is also important to note that muscles that act primarily as stabilizers generally contain greater concentrations of **type I muscle fibers** (**slow-twitch muscle fibers**).

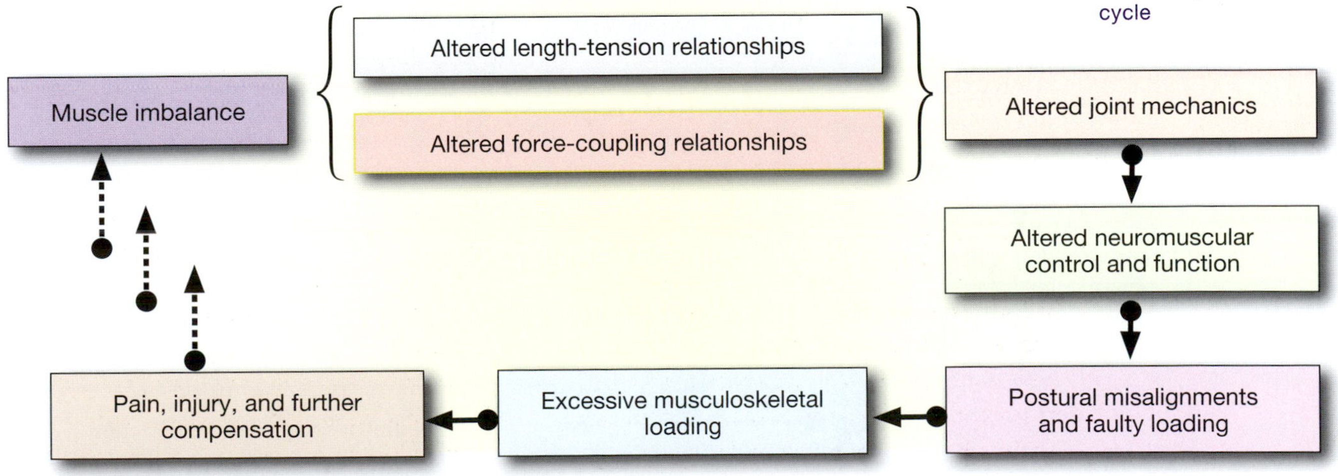

Figure 9-7
Pain-compensation cycle

Type I muscle fibers enhance a stabilizer muscle's capacity for endurance, which allows the muscle to efficiently stabilize the joint for prolonged periods without undue fatigue. For example, the core muscles that protect the spine during loading and movement throughout the day have higher concentrations of type I fibers (Arokoski et al., 2001). Consequently, these muscles are better suited for endurance-type training (higher-volume, lower-intensity). Muscles primarily responsible for joint movement and generating larger forces generally contain greater concentrations of **type II muscle fibers** (**fast-twitch muscle fibers**). These muscles are better suited for strength- and power-type training (higher-intensity, lower-volume).

Figure 9-8 illustrates a programming sequence to promote stability and mobility within the body. It adheres to the basic principle that proximal stability facilitates distal mobility. For each of the five sections of this figure, several exercise examples are provided later in this chapter to help trainers plan and implement programs. Trainers may opt to apply these same principles using different exercises and different programs individualized to a client's specific needs. Based on the postural and movement screen observations, trainers will identify potential problem areas of the body that need attention (i.e., improvements in stability or mobility). For example, if a client demonstrates a lack of trunk stability during the hurdle step test (see page 153), a lack of core function should be suspected. Likewise, if a client exhibits an anterior pelvic tilt during a static postural assessment due to tight hip flexors, the trainer will need to address a lack of hip flexor mobility.

Considering that much of this phase is devoted to improving muscle flexibility, the different stretching approaches need to be considered (e.g., **myofascial release, static stretching, proprioceptive neuromuscular facilitation, active isolated stretching,** and **dynamic** and **ballistic stretching**). Figure 9-9 provides a template, along with suggestions on which stretching technique is best to include before, during, and following exercise with individuals exhibiting poor or

Figure 9-8
Programming components of the stability and mobility training phase

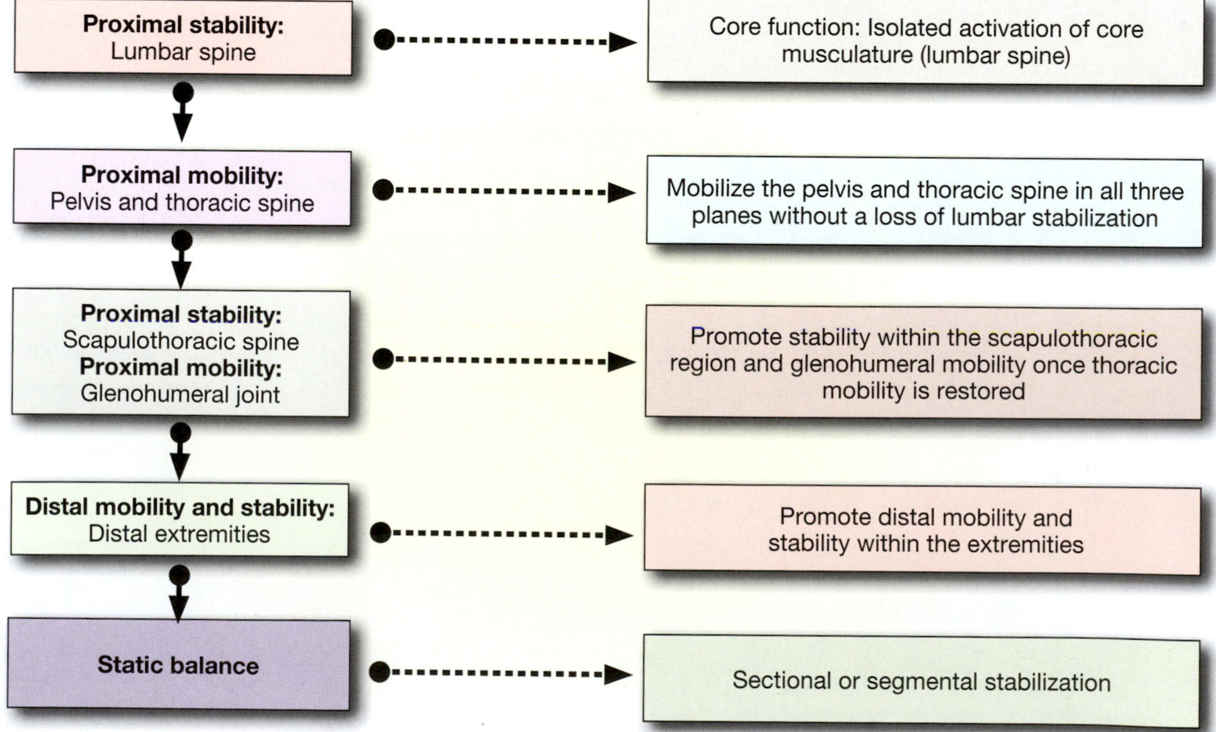

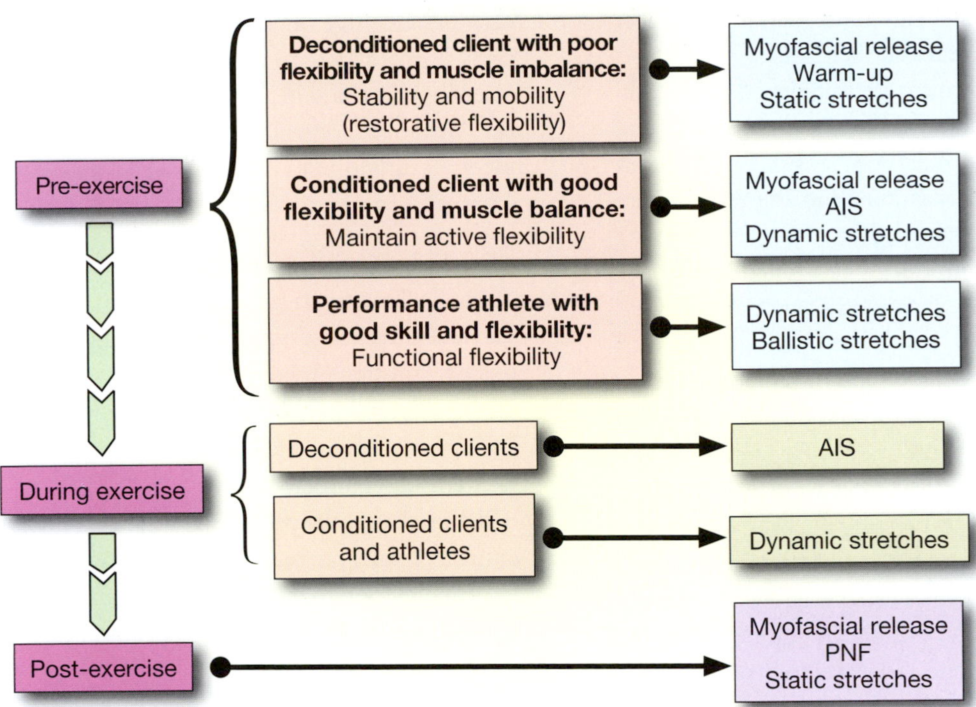

Note: AIS = Active isolated stretching; PNF = Proprioceptive neuromuscular facilitation

Figure 9-9
Stretching techniques during each phase of a workout session

good posture, as well as for well-conditioned athletes. The following are some general guidelines:

- *Myofascial release:* Clients perform small, continuous, back-and-forth movements (on a foam roller), covering an area of 2 to 6 inches (5 to 15 cm) over the tender region for 30 to 60 seconds (Cook & Jones, 2007b; Barnes, 1999).
  - ✓ As myofascial release realigns the elastic muscle fibers from a bundled position (called a knot or adhesion) into a straighter alignment with the muscle and fascia, and resets the proprioceptive mechanisms of the soft tissue, it should precede static stretching (Barnes, 1999). Myofascial release helps reduce hypertonicity within the underlying muscles.
- *Static stretches:* Static stretches should be taken to the point of tension, with clients performing a minimum of four repetitions and holding each repetition for 15 to 60 seconds [American College of Sports Medicine (ACSM), 2010].
- *Proprioceptive neuromuscular facilitation (PNF):* Clients can perform a hold-relax stretch, holding the isometric contraction of the agonist for a minimum of six seconds, followed by a 10- to 30-second assisted or passive static stretch (ACSM, 2010).
- *Active isolated stretches (AIS):* Clients can perform one or two sets of five to 10 repetitions at a controlled tempo, holding the end range of motion for one to two seconds (Alter, 2004).
- *Dynamic and ballistic stretches*: Perform one or two sets of 10 repetitions (Cook, 2003).

Strengthening muscles to improve posture should initially focus on placing the client in positions of good posture and begin with a series of low-grade isometric contractions [<50% of maximal effort or maximum voluntary contraction (MVC)], with the client completing two to four repetitions of five to 10 seconds each. The goal is to condition the postural (tonic) muscles that typically contain greater concentrations of type I fibers with volume as opposed to intensity (Kendall et al., 2005). Higher intensities that require greater amounts of force will generally evoke faulty recruitment patterns. The exercise volume can be gradually increased (overload) to improve strength and endurance, and to reestablish muscle balance at the joints.

Because many deconditioned individuals lack the ability to stabilize the entire kinetic chain, the initial emphasis should be placed on muscle isolation using supportive surfaces and devices (e.g., floor, wall, chair backrest) prior to introducing integrated (whole-body, unsupported) strengthening exercises. For example, to help a client strengthen the posterior deltoids and rhomboids, which are associated with forward-rounded shoulders, a trainer should start by having the client perform reverse flys in a supine position, isometrically pressing the backs of the arms into the floor, rather than sets of dynamic, high-back rows using external resistance. The use of support offers the additional benefit of kinesthetic and visual feedback, which is critical to helping clients understand the alignment of specific joints (e.g., when lying on the floor, the individual can feel and see the contact points with the floor when joints are placed in ideal postural positions). The strengthening exercises should ultimately progress to dynamic movement, initially controlling the ROM to avoid excessive muscle lengthening before introducing full-ROM movement patterns. Remember, while a muscle may be strong in a lengthened position, it needs strength at a normal and healthy resting length (MacIntosh, Gardiner, & McComas, 2006; Lieber, 2002; Williams & Goldspink, 1978). For example, to strengthen the rhomboids using more dynamic movements, the client should hold the scapulae in a good postural position and avoid scapular protraction and retraction during the movement. Again, remember that dynamic strengthening exercises for good posture do not involve heavy loads, but rather volume training to condition the type I fibers. Consequently, trainers should plan on one to three sets of 12 to 15 repetitions when introducing dynamic strengthening exercises. To summarize, the strengthening of weakened muscles follows a progression model beginning with two to four repetitions of isometric muscle contractions, each held for five to 10 seconds at less than 50% of MVC in a supported, more isolated environment. The next progression is to dynamic, controlled ROM exercises incorporating one to three sets of 12 to 15 repetitions.

Proximal Stability: Activating the Core

The goal of this stage is to promote stability of the lumbar spine by improving the reflexive function of the core musculature that essentially serves to stabilize this region during loading and movement. The core functions to effectively control the position and motion of the trunk over the pelvis, which allows optimal production, transfer, and control of force and motion to more distal segments during integrated movements (Willardson, 2007; Kibler, Press, & Sciascia, 2006). The term "core" generally refers to the muscles of the lumbo-pelvic region, hips, abdomen, and lower back. Rather than identify each muscle, it may be easier to categorize the muscles and structures by function and location (McGill, 2007; Golding & Golding, 2003; Sahrmann, 2002; Arokoski et al., 2001; Hodges & Richardson, 1996).

The **deep** or innermost layer of the core consists of vertebral bones and discs; spinal ligaments running along the front, sides, and back of the spinal column; and small muscles that span a single vertebra (e.g., rotatores, interspinali, intertransversarii) that are generally considered too small to offer significant stabilization of the spine (Figure 9-10). While they do offer some segmental stabilization of each individual vertebra, especially at end ranges of motion, these small muscles are rich in sensory nerve endings and provide continuous feedback to the brain regarding loading and position of the spine.

The middle layer consists of muscles and **fasciae** that encircle the lower regions of the spine. Envision a box spanning the vertebrae from the diaphragm to the sacroiliac joint and pelvic floor, with muscles enclosing the back, front, and sides. This box allows the spinal and sacroiliac joints to stiffen in anticipation of loading and movement, and provides a

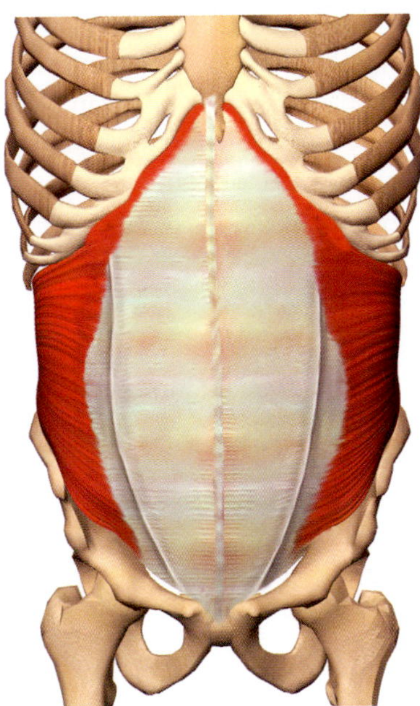

Figure 9-10
Muscles of the inner unit of the core

Source: LifeART image copyright 2008 Wolters Kluwer Health, Inc., Lippincott Williams & Wilkins. All rights reserved.

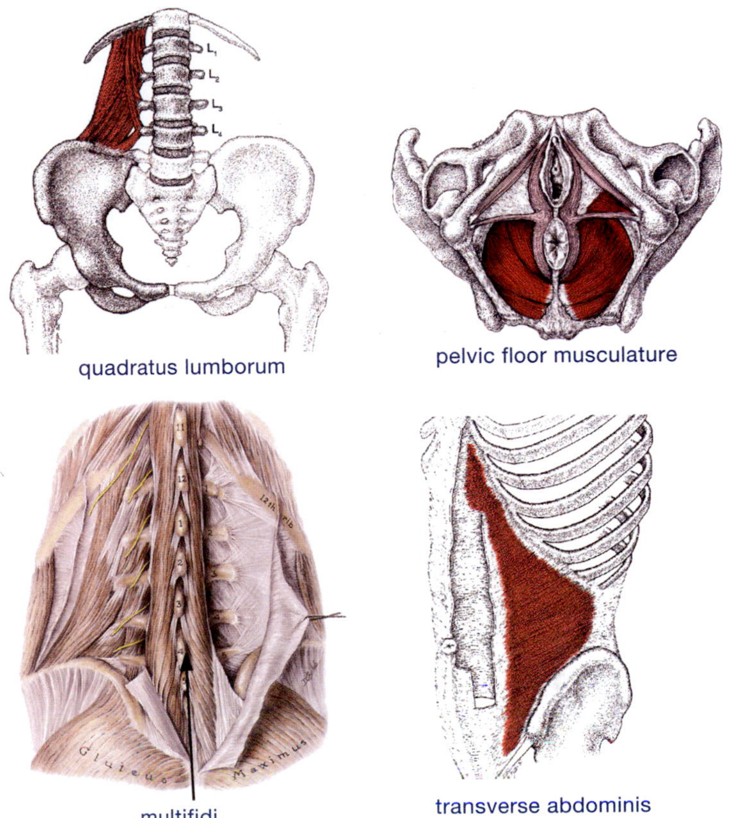

Figure 9-11
Middle layer of core muscles

Source: LifeART image copyright 2008 Wolters Kluwer Health, Inc., Lippincott Williams & Wilkins. All rights reserved.

solid, stable working foundation from which the body can operate. These muscles include the transverse abdominis (TVA), multifidi, quadratus lumborum, deep fibers of the internal oblique, diaphragm, pelvic floor musculature, and the adjoining fasciae (linea alba and thoracolumbar fascia). This is the muscular layer usually referred to as the core (Figure 9-11).

The outermost layer consists of larger, more powerful muscles that span many vertebrae and are primarily responsible for generating gross movement and forces within the trunk. Muscles in this region include the rectus abdominis, erector spinae, external and internal obliques, iliopsoas, and latissimus dorsi.

The relationship between the vertebrae and the core muscles can be likened to a segmented flagpole with guy wires controlled by the neural subsystem (Figure 9-12). The segmented pole represents the vertebrae, while the guy wires represent the core layer. Balanced tension within the guy wires increases tension to stiffen the flagpole and enhance spinal stability.

In healthy individuals free from low-back

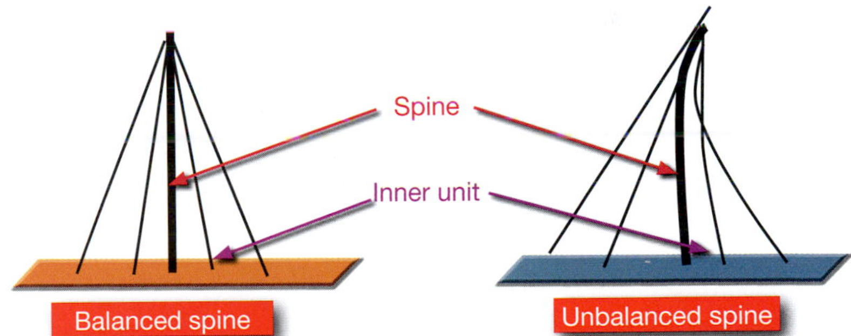

Figure 9-12
The relationship of the core layer and spine

pain, the core musculature functions reflexively to stabilize the spine in anticipation of, and during, voluntary or involuntary loading without any need for conscious muscle action (McGill, 2007; Cresswell & Thortensson, 1994). Creswell and Thortensson (1994) also discovered that the TVA is the key muscle that works reflexively with the neural system. Activation of the core muscles, primarily the TVA, produces a "hoop tension" effect similar to that of cinching a belt around the

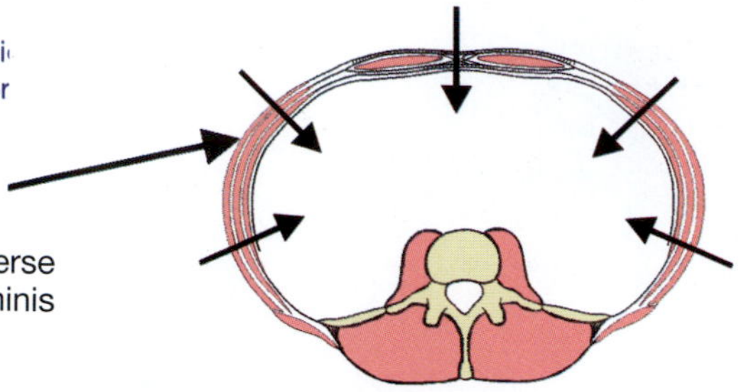

Figure 9-13
The hoop orientati
of the middle layer
of the core

Fibers of the transverse abdominis

waist (Figure 9-13). This contraction pulls on the linea alba, drawing the abdominal wall inward and upward, compressing the internal organs to push upward against the diaphragm and downward against the pelvic floor musculature (Cresswell & Thortensson, 1994). This increases intra-abdominal pressure, creating a lift pressure against the diaphragm that has attachments on the second and third lumbar vertebra, pulling them upward and increasing traction between the lumbar vertebrae (Cresswell & Thortensson, 1994). This reduces joint and disc compression in the lumbar discs by creating a rigid cylinder (spinal stiffening) to stabilize the spine against loading forces.

Hodges and Richardson (1996) found delayed or minimal activation of the TVA and limited co-contraction of core muscles in individuals suffering from low-back pain, indicating some form of neural control deficits. Delayed activation of the TVA may inadequately stabilize the lumbar spine during movements of the upper and lower extremities, increasing the potential for injury (Sahrmann, 2002). Individuals lacking appropriate TVA function may need to rely on synergistic muscles to assume the role of stabilizing the spine (e.g., rectus abdominis). Altering the roles of these muscles for purposes of stabilization increases the potential for compromised function. While low-back pain has been reported to affect 80% of the U.S. population, it is possible that a well conditioned core will reduce the incidence of low-back pain (McGill, 2007; Rasmussen-Barr, Nilsson-Wikmar, & Arvidsson, 2003). It is also speculated that deconditioned individuals who spend much of their time seated using supportive devices (e.g., backrests) may demonstrate similar neural-control deficits. Considering the prevalence of inactivity and **obesity** in adults, it is recommended that this training phase begin with the establishment of stability within the lumbar spine with exercises that emphasize TVA activation and the re-education of potentially faulty motor patterns.

Activation of the TVA draws the abdomen inward toward the spine, a movement termed "centering," "hollowing," or "drawing-in" in many training disciplines. Exercises performed during this stage are designed to achieve this isolated muscle action. McGill states, however, that while centering serves essential motor re-education purposes, it does not ensure the same degree of stability as an activation pattern he calls "bracing." Bracing is the co-contraction of the core and abdominal muscles to create a more rigid and wider **base of support (BOS)** for spinal stabilization (McGill, 2007). To better understand this point, clients can compare their BOS with the feet positioned close together to a stance with the feet wider apart, which provides greater stability. The co-contraction of the outer layer of trunk muscles during bracing movements widens the BOS. Ultimately, clients should implement bracing when loading the spine with external loads (e.g., lifting children or weights), as doing so provides greater stability to the spine. Analogous to learning how to walk before running, the concept of "centering" should be mastered first, reestablishing the core's reflexive function, before introducing the concept of "bracing."

As the body's COM is located within the region of the core, and controlling the COM within the BOS is critical to **balance** training, core conditioning and balance training are fundamentally the same thing. To effectively activate and condition the core—and train balance—trainers can utilize the progressive training program outlined in Figure 9-14. This program involves three stages, with stage 1 (core function) and the initial portions of stage 2 (**static balance**) encompassed within the first training phase (stability and mobility

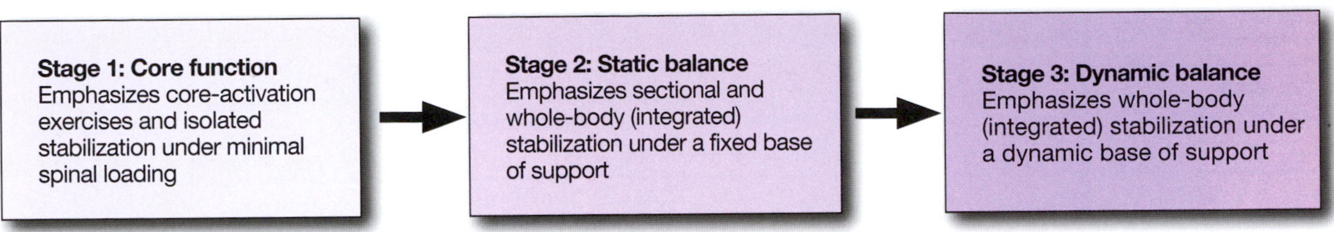

Figure 9-14
Three-stage model for core and balance training

training). The later portions of stage 2 (static balance) and all of stage 3 **(dynamic balance)** occur within the second training phase (movement training).

Proximal Stability: Core Function

Exercise 1: Supine Drawing-in (Centering)

- Ask the client to assume a supine, bent-knee position, align the knees and second toe with the anterior superior iliac spine (ASIS), and hold this position throughout the exercise (Figure 9-15).
  - ✓Instruct the client to place the hands immediately **medial** to the ASIS, in line with the umbilicus (belly button), and rest the fingers over the TVA.
- All muscle contractions should be of a moderate intensity (≤50% of maximal effort).
  - ✓Throughout these exercises, there should be no movement of the pelvis, low back, or ribcage.
  - ✓Movement of these joints indicates activation of the rectus abdominis and an inability to activate the TVA in an isolated manner.
- Have the client follow the exercise progression outlined in Table 9-1.
  - ✓During the TVA contractions, the client should feel some tension develop under the fingers. This may not be possible with heavier individuals.
  - ✓The purpose of these exercises is to re-educate faulty neural pathways. Thus, the appropriate exercise volume conducted via perfect exercise technique will help regain the reflexive function of the core musculature.
  - ✓Teach the client how to perform these exercises by providing a demonstration of the progressions and instructing him or her to perform them as frequently as possible for one to two weeks.

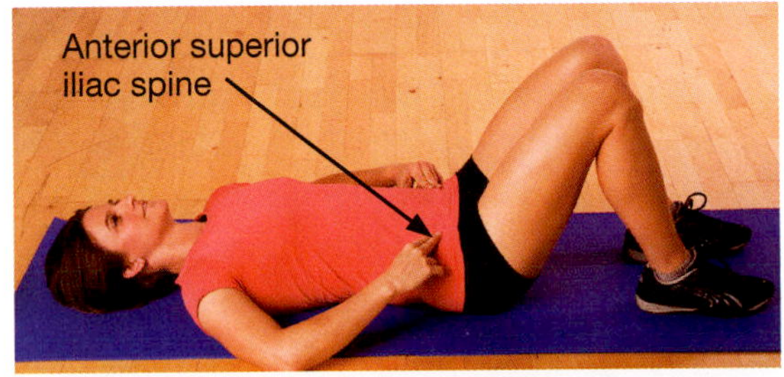

Figure 9-15
Supine drawing-in body position

Table 9-1
Exercise Progression for Core Activation

Pelvic floor contractions ("Kegels," or the contraction to interrupt the flow of urine)	Perform 1–2 sets x 10 repetitions with a 2-second tempo, 10–15 second rest intervals between sets
TVA contractions (drawing the belly button toward the spine)	Perform 1–2 sets x 10 repetitions with a 2-second tempo, 10–15 second rest intervals between sets
Combination of both contractions	Perform 1–2 sets x 10 repetitions with a 2-second tempo, 10–15 second rest intervals between sets
Contractions with normal breathing	Perform 1–2 sets x 5–6 repetitions with slow, 10-second counts while breathing independently, 10–15 second rest intervals between sets Progress to 3–4 sets x 10–12 repetitions, each with a 10-second count, 10–15 second rest intervals between sets

Note: TVA = Transverse abdominis

Exercise 2: Quadruped Drawing-in (Centering) With Extremity Movement

Once the client effectively demonstrates his or her ability to activate the core and pelvic floor muscles independent of the diaphragm (during breathing), the trainer can have him or her follow the exercise progression for core stabilization. These exercises train clients to stabilize the lumbar spine with minimal loading on the spine during movements of the hips and shoulders.

The purpose of this exercise sequence is to activate the core muscles by working against gravity while placing small loads on the spine by moving the hips and shoulders. Clients should activate the core muscles as demonstrated in the core-activation exercises (see Table 9-1) and continue to breathe independently.

- Have the client adopt the quadruped position with the knees under the hips and the hands under the shoulders. The client must maintain a neutral spine (Figure 9-16a).
  - ✓ Due to limb-length discrepancies between the arms and legs, the slope of the spine may range from parallel with the floor to a slight incline or decline.
  - ✓ The goal of this exercise is to elevate one arm and/or leg 0.5 to 1 inch (1.25 to 2.5 cm) off the floor and perform slow, controlled extremity movements using a short lever (i.e., with a bent knee and bent elbow) without losing control of the lumbar spine (Figure 9-16b). Extending the limbs too far may result in a loss of lumbar stability (increased lordosis) or force hip and shoulder rotation due to a lack of mobility within those joints, and therefore should be avoided.
  - ✓ Encourage clients to perform this exercise adjacent to a mirror and use visual feedback to monitor and control changes in spinal position (e.g., increased lordosis), which indicate a loss of core control.
- Have clients follow the exercise progression outlined in Table 9-2.
- The purpose of these exercises is to reestablish core control with minimal loading on the spine during hip and shoulder movements. Thus, appropriate exercise volume conducted via perfect exercise technique will help clients regain reflexive control of loading along the lumbar spine.
  - ✓ Teach the client how to perform these exercises by providing a demonstration of the progressions and instructing him or her to perform them as frequently as possible for one to two weeks.

Figure 9-16
Quadruped drawing-in with extremity movement

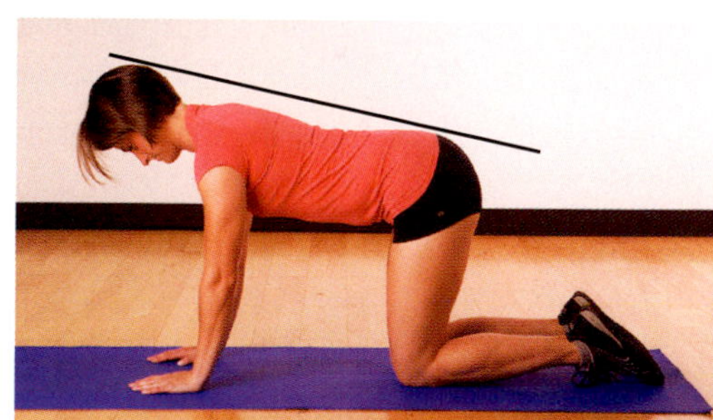
a.

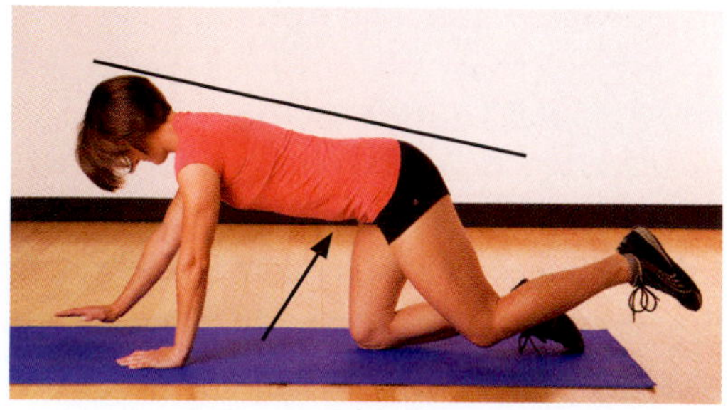
b.

Proximal Mobility: Hips and Thoracic Spine

The goal of this stage is to improve mobility of the two joints immediately adjacent to the lumbar spine. Based on observations made during the postural assessments and movement screens, limitations in mobility within these two areas in any of the three planes should become the focus. Trainers should follow some fundamental principles when programming to improve mobility in these body regions:

- Although these two regions should exhibit good mobility in all three planes, they are typically prone to poor mobility. Consequently, some static stretching to improve muscle flexibility (or extensibility) should precede dynamic mobilization exercises.
- When attempting to improve muscle flexibility or joint mobility, clients must avoid undesirable or compensated movements at successive joints (e.g., avoid

Table 9-2
Exercise Progression for Core Stabilization

1. Raise one arm 0.5 to 1 inch (1.25 to 2.5 cm) off the floor and perform the sequence of controlled shoulder movements: • 6–12 inch (15–30 cm) sagittal plane shoulder movements (flexion/extension) • 6–12 inch (15–30 cm) frontal plane shoulder movements (abduction/adduction) • 6–12 inch (15–30 cm) transverse plane shoulder movements (circles or circumduction)	Perform 1–2 sets x 10 repetitions with a 2-second tempo, use 10–15 second rest intervals between sets
2. Raise one knee 0.5 to 1 inch (1.25 to 2.5 cm) off the floor and perform the sequence of controlled hip movements: • 6–12 inch (15–30 cm) sagittal plane hip movements (flexion/extension) • 6–12 inch (15–30 cm) frontal plane hip movements (abduction/adduction) • 6–12 inch (15–30 cm) transverse plane hip movements (circles)	Perform 1–2 sets x 10 repetitions with a 2-second tempo, use 10–15 second rest intervals between sets
3. Raise contralateral limbs (i.e., one arm and the opposite knee) 0.5 to 1 inch (1.25 to 2.5 cm) off the floor and perform the sequence of movements: • Repeat the above movements in matching planes (i.e., simultaneous movement in the same plane with both limbs) or alternating planes (i.e., mixing the planes between the two limbs). • This contralateral movement pattern mimics the muscle-activation patterns used during the push-off phase portion of walking and is an effective exercise to train this pattern.	Perform 1–2 sets x 10 repetitions with a 2-second tempo, use 10–15 second rest intervals between sets

any increases in lumbar lordosis associated with a tight latissimus dorsi muscle during an overhead stretch).

- Trainers should familiarize themselves with muscle anatomy and differentiate between mono- or uniarticulate muscles and biarticulate muscles.
  - ✓A monoarticulate muscle crosses one joint (e.g., soleus muscle), whereas a biarticulate muscle crosses two joints (e.g., hamstrings).
  - ✓When stretching a biarticulate muscle, joint movement must be controlled at both ends of the muscle to avoid any compromise to stability at adjacent joints. For example, when performing a passive straight-leg raise to stretch the hamstrings, posterior tilting of the pelvis must be avoided when the hamstrings reach their limit of flexibility, because further stretching forces pelvic rotation and a flattening of the low back, which compromises the stability of the lumbar spine.
- Because the body still lacks the ability to effectively stabilize the entire kinetic chain, supportive surfaces should be utilized while promoting mobility (e.g., floor, benches, backrests).
  - ✓Once an individual effectively demonstrates the ability to stabilize the more proximal regions of the body (i.e., the lumbar spine and scapulothoracic region), exercises can become more unsupported in nature. This transition should coincide with a shift from more isolated exercises to more integrated multijoint and multiplanar movements.
- Because muscles contribute to movement in all three planes, trainers should incorporate flexibility exercises that lengthen the muscles in all three planes. It is important, however, to focus on the muscle's primary plane of movement before adding complexity by introducing movement in other planes. For example, when stretching the hip flexors using a half-kneeling lunge

stretch, the client should stretch the muscle in the sagittal plane before incorporating any frontal or transverse plane movements into the stretch (e.g., a lateral trunk lean or trunk rotation).

Exercises and Stretches

Because many individuals exhibit tightness in the low back, trainers should consider including the two exercises presented in Figures 9-17 and 9-18 during the core-activation phase. When working with individuals with a tight low back, but with no limitations or restrictions to exercise, trainers can begin with the supine 90-90 neutral back exercise. When the individual demonstrates a marked improvement in the low-back flexibility, he or she can progress to the cat-camel exercise, but continue to use the 90-90 neutral back exercise occasionally for maintenance. When performing each exercise, clients should follow the repetition and duration guidelines listed.

The exercises presented in Figures 9-19 through 9-30 promote mobility of the hips and thoracic spine.

Figure 9-17
Supine 90-90 neutral back

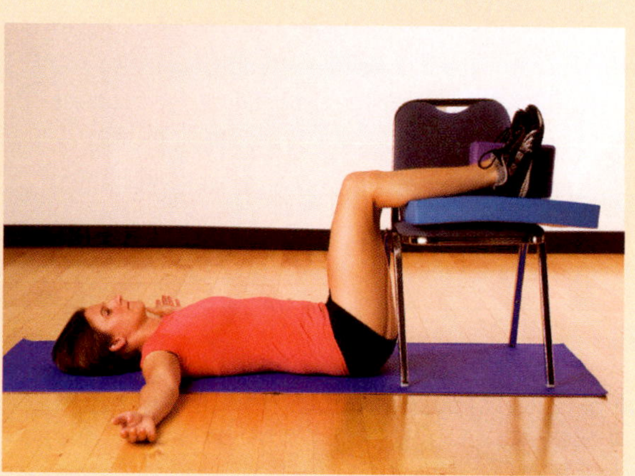

Objective: To unload the low-back extensor muscles and reduce muscle tension in the lumbar spine

Preparation and position:

- Lie supine on the floor with both legs draped over a chair or riser. The height of the chair or riser should allow the knees and hips to flex to 90 degrees without elevating the hips off the floor.
- Align the anterior superior iliac spine (ASIS) with the knee and second toe and use supports to hold the feet in this position (e.g., pillows), preventing any external or internal rotation of the feet and lower legs (this alters pelvic and low-back position).
- Externally rotate the arms (palms facing upward) and abduct to shoulder level, resting them on the floor.
- Attempt to relax the neck and rest the head on the floor (if necessary, place a small pillow under the head).

Exercise:

- Relax in this position for three to 10 minutes, or as needed to allow the head, body, and more specifically, the muscles of the low back, to relax.
- As the muscles around the hips and pelvis and along the spine relax, the body should return to a more neutral, symmetrical position.

Source: Carey, A. (2005). *The Pain Free Program.* Hoboken, N.J.: John Wiley & Sons.

Figure 9-18
Cat-camel

Objective: To improve extensibility within the lumbar extensor muscles

Preparation and position:

- Assume the quadruped position with the hands positioned directly under the shoulders (shoulder-width apart) and the knees positioned directly under the hips (shoulder-width apart).
- Engage the core muscles to create a neutral spine in this starting position.
- The elbows should remain extended throughout the exercise.

Exercise:

- From this starting position, exhale slowly while contracting the abdominals [draw the belly button toward the spine (i.e., "hollowing")], gently pushing and rounding the entire back upward. Drop the head, bringing the chin toward the chest (a).
- Hold this position for 15 seconds.
- Slowly inhale, relax, and return to the starting position, but allow the stomach and spine to sag toward the floor. Allow the shoulders to collapse (adduct) toward the spine, and tilt the head upward (b).
- Hold this position for 15 seconds.
- Perform two to four repetitions.

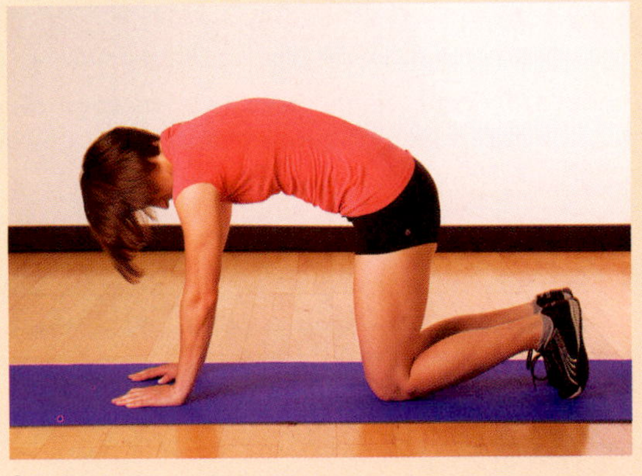
a.

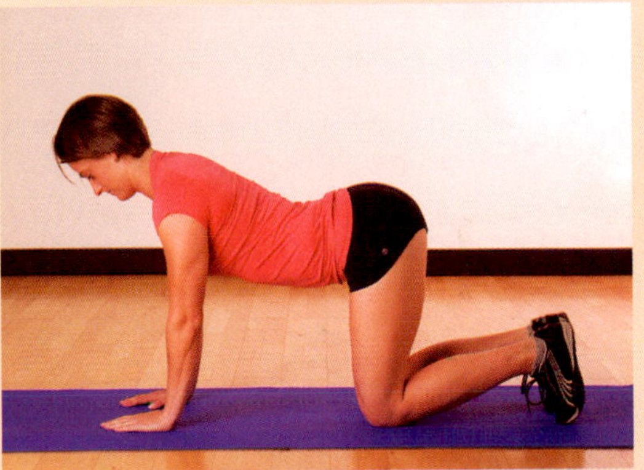
b.

Figure 9-19
Pelvic tilts

Objective: To improve hip mobility in the sagittal plane

Preparation and position:

- Lie supine with the knees bent and the feet placed flat on the floor, aligning the anterior superior iliac spine (ASIS) with the knee and second toe.
- Abduct the arms to shoulder height, resting them on the floor with the arms externally rotated (palms facing upward) (a).

Exercise:

- Slowly contract the abdominals to tilt the pelvis posteriorly, hold briefly, relax and then contract the erector spinae muscles and hip flexors to tilt the pelvis anteriorly (b).
- Perform one or two sets of five to 10 controlled repetitions, holding the end position for one or two seconds with 30-second rest intervals between sets.

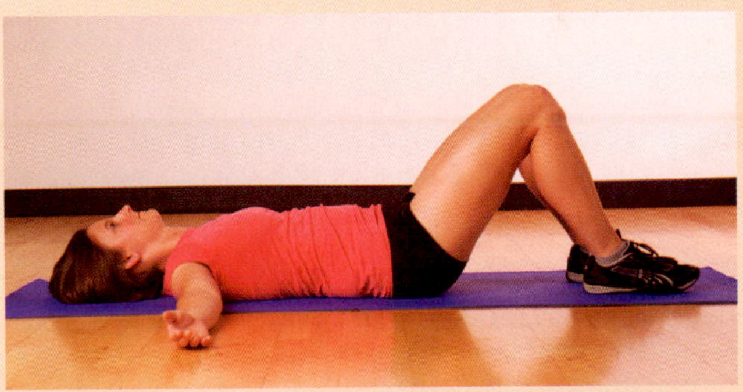
a.

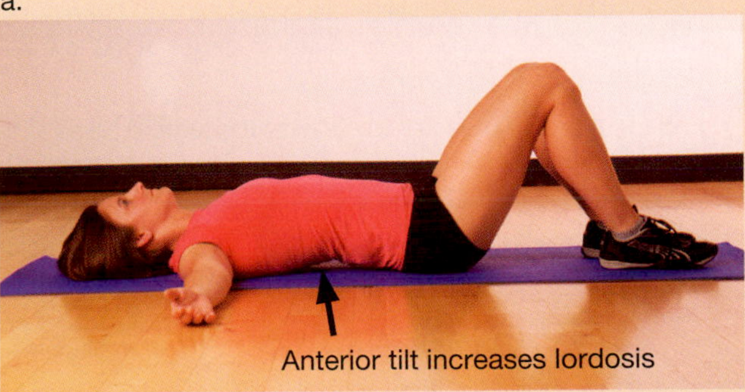

b.

Figure 9-20

Pelvic tilts progressions: Supine bent-knee marches

Objective: To improve hip mobility in the sagittal plane without compromising lumbar stability during lower-extremity movement

Preparation and position:

- Lie supine with the knees bent and the feet placed flat on the floor, aligning the anterior superior iliac spine (ASIS) with the knee and second toe.
- Abduct the arms to shoulder height, resting them on the floor with the arms externally rotated (palms facing upward).
- Engage the core muscles to stabilize the lumbar spine in the neutral position (a).

Exercise:

- Slowly raise one leg, maintaining a bent-knee position, and drive the knee toward the chest, stopping when the thigh is perpendicular to the ground (b).
- Hold this position briefly before returning to the starting position.
- Repeat this same movement with the opposite leg.
- Perform one or two sets of five to 10 controlled repetitions per leg, holding the end range of motion for one or two seconds, with 30-second rest intervals between sets.

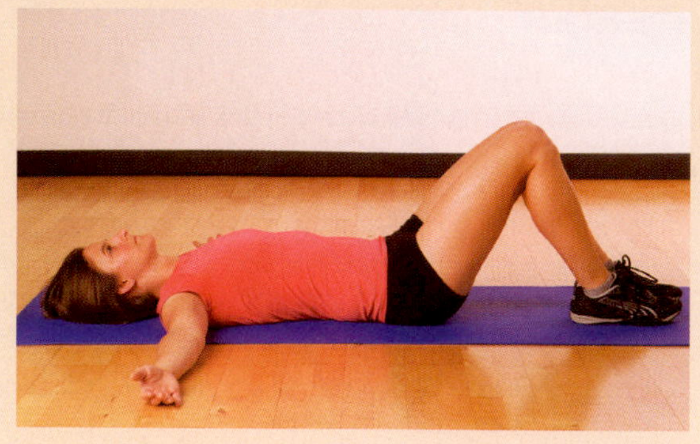

a.

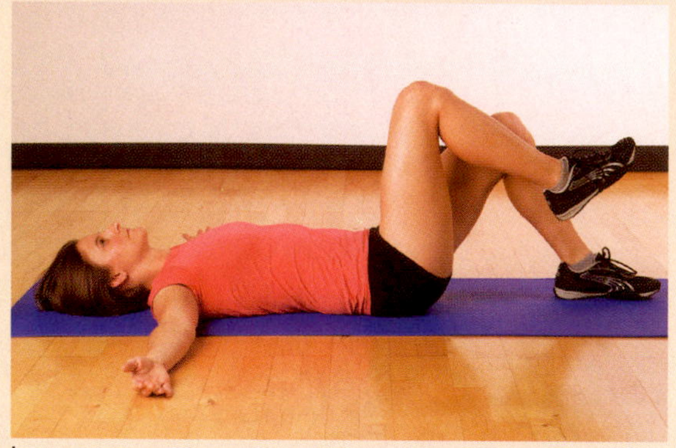

b.

Figure 9-21

Pelvic tilts progressions: Modified dead bug with reverse bent-knee marches

Note: Introduce this exercise as a progression to the exercise presented in Figure 9-20.

Objective: To improve hip mobility in the sagittal plane without compromising lumbar stability during lower-extremity movement

Preparation and position:

- Lie supine and place a rolled-up towel under the low back, which can be used by the client to monitor any changes in the low-back position kinesthetically during this exercise (a). An alternative option is to place one hand in the natural curve under the low back to control changes in the low-back position.
- Engage the core muscles to stabilize the lumbar spine in the neutral position.
- Raise both legs until the hips and knees are flexed to approximately 90 degrees (feet in the air), aligning the anterior superior iliac spine (ASIS) with the knee and second toe (b).

Continued on next page

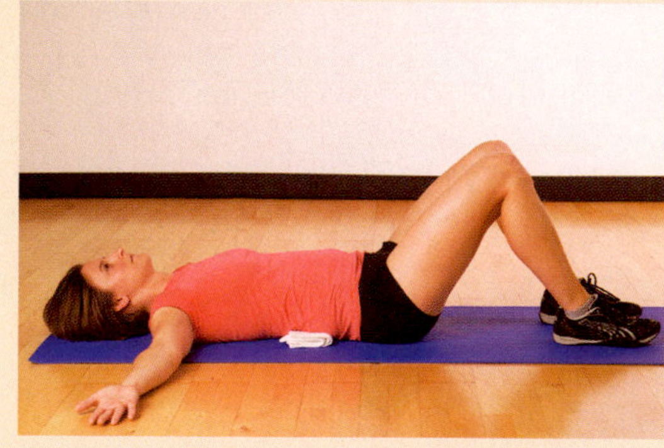

a.

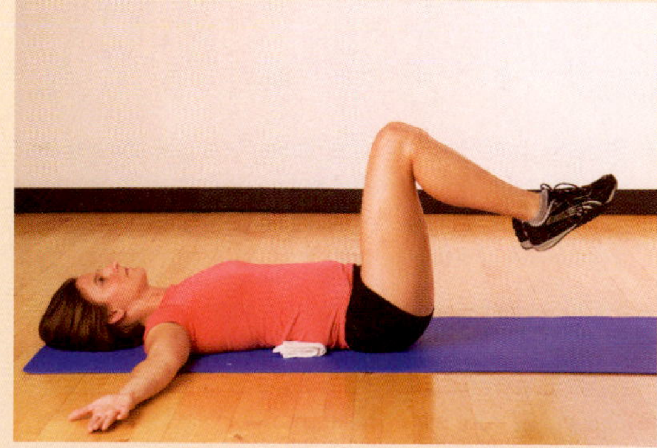

b.

Exercise:

- Exhale while slowly lowering one leg toward the floor and maintaining a bent-knee position. Avoid any loss of lumbar stability throughout the movement.
- Hold this position briefly before returning to the starting position.
- Repeat this same movement with the opposite leg.
- Perform one or two sets of five to 10 controlled repetitions per leg, holding the end range of motion for one or two seconds, with 30-second rest intervals between sets.

Progression—Dead bug with reverse bent-knee and arm movements: Assume the same starting position, but flex both shoulders to raise the arms perpendicular to the floor in line with the shoulders (c). Exhale while simultaneously lowering one leg and the same-side (ipsilateral) arm toward the floor and maintaining a bent-knee position (d). Avoid any loss of lumbar stability throughout the movement. Hold this position briefly before returning to the starting position. Additional progressions include moving contralaterally (opposite arm and leg) or bilaterally (both arms and legs simultaneously).

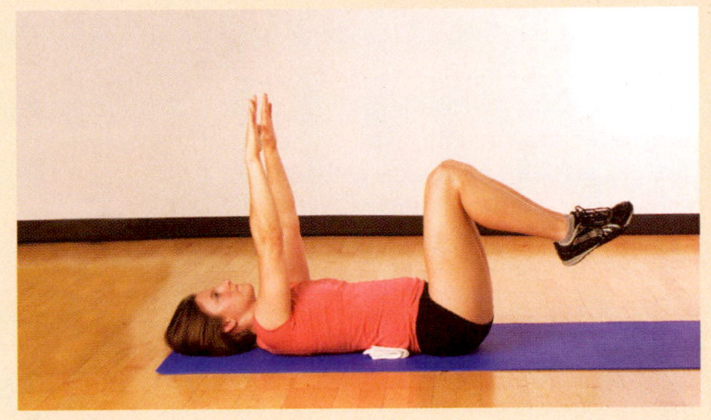

c.

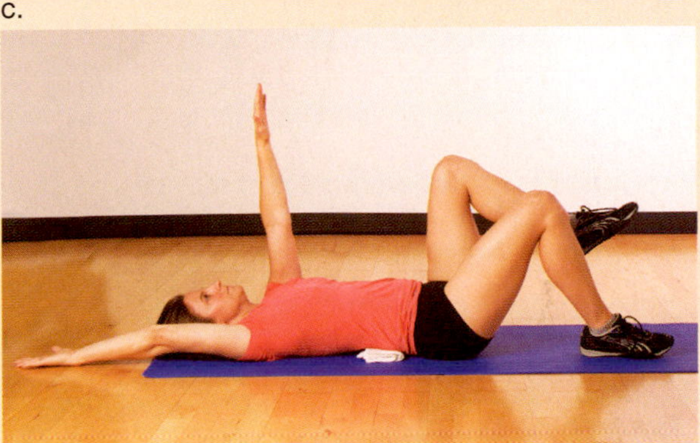

d.

Figure 9-22
Hip flexor mobility: Lying hip flexor stretch

Objective: To improve mobility of the hip flexors in the sagittal plane without compromising lumbar stability

Preparation and position:

- Lie supine with the knees bent and the feet placed flat on the floor, aligning the anterior superior iliac spine (ASIS) with the knee and second toe.
- Engage the core muscles to stabilize the lumbar spine in the neutral position and maintain this position throughout the exercise.

Exercise:

- Reach both hands behind one knee and gently pull the knee toward the chest (a).
- Slowly extend the opposite leg until it is either fully extended or lumbar stability is compromised (b).
- Perform two to four repetitions per side, each for a minimum of 15 seconds.

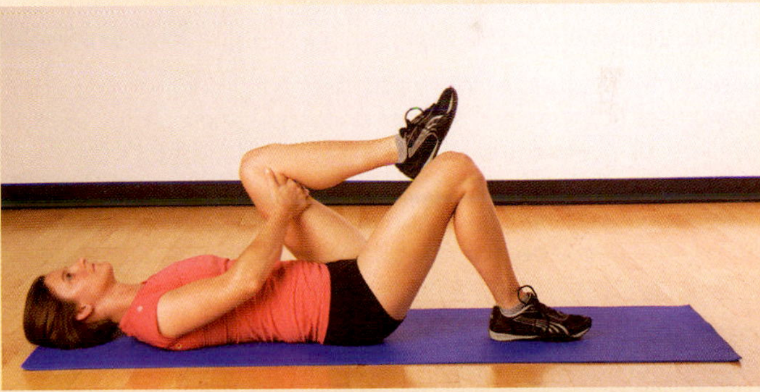

a.

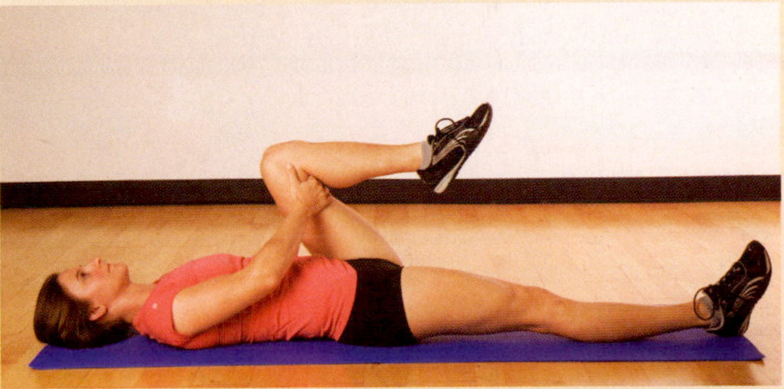

b.

Figure 9-23
Hip flexor mobility progression: Half-kneeling triplanar stretch

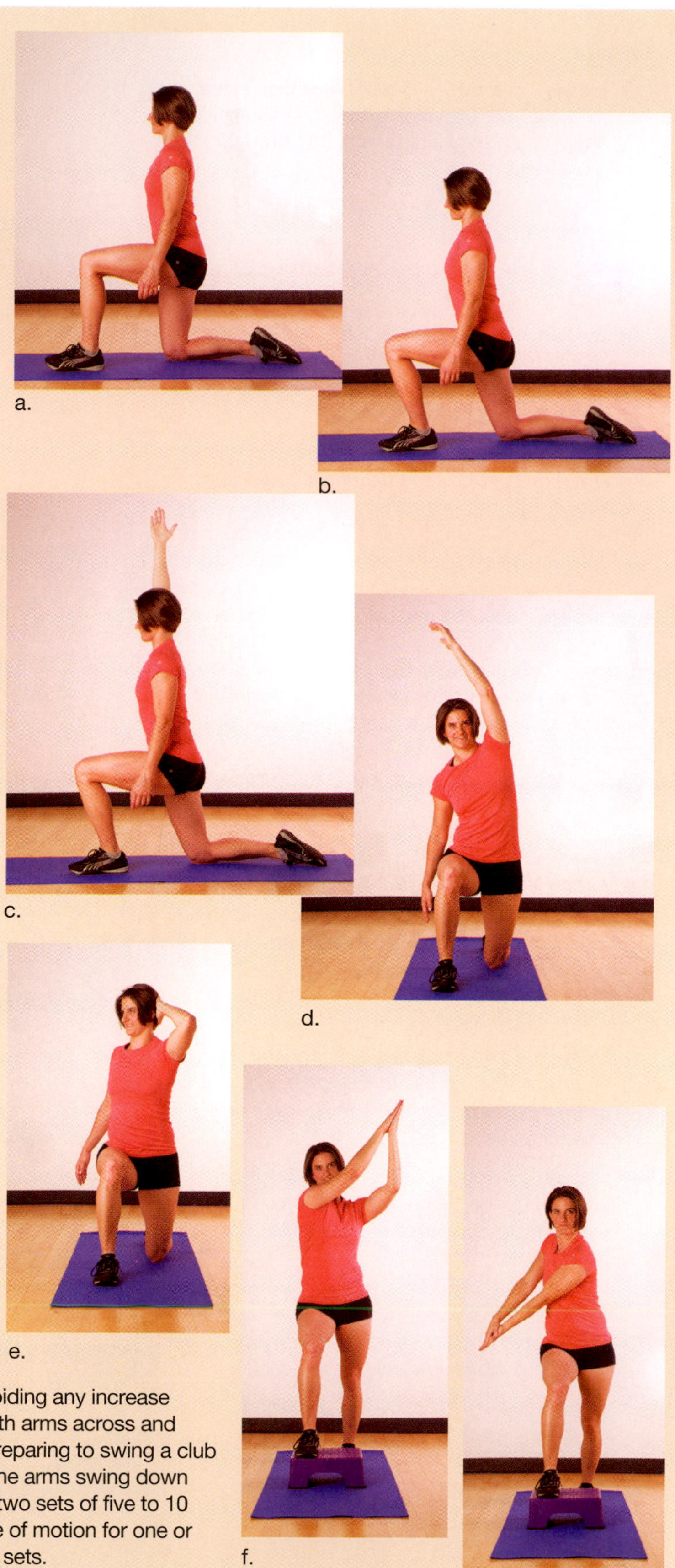

Objective: To improve mobility of the hip flexors in all three planes without compromising lumbar stability

Preparation and position:

- Assume a half-kneeling lunge position, placing the rear leg directly under the hips and torso (a).
- Engage the core muscles to stabilize the lumbar spine in the neutral position. Maintain this position throughout the exercise.

Exercise:

- Exhale and slowly lunge forward to stretch the hip flexors. Avoid any forward tilt of the pelvis that increases lordosis in the low back (b).
- Perform two to four repetitions per side.
- Hold each stretch for a minimum of 15 seconds.

Progression—sagittal plane: While maintaining a neutral lumbar spine, extend the arm opposite the forward leg overhead (c). Slowly reach the arm behind the head while slowly lunging forward, avoiding any increase in lumbar lordosis. Perform two to four repetitions per side and hold each stretch for a minimum of 15 seconds.

Progression—frontal plane: While maintaining a neutral lumbar spine, extend the arm opposite the forward leg overhead. Laterally flex the torso over the leading leg while slowly lunging forward, avoiding any increase in lumbar lordosis (d). Perform two to four repetitions per side and hold each stretch for a minimum of 15 seconds.

Progression—transverse plane: While maintaining a neutral lumbar spine, place the arm opposite the leading leg behind the head (prisoner position). Rotate the torso over the leading leg while slowly lunging forward, avoiding any increase in lumbar lordosis (e). Perform two to four repetitions per side and hold each stretch for a minimum of 15 seconds.

Progression—spiral pattern: Assume a staggered-stance position, elevating the front leg and placing the foot on a riser or chair. Slowly lunge forward, avoiding any increase in lumbar lordosis, while simultaneously reaching both arms across and behind the body to the side of the leading leg as if preparing to swing a club or axe (f). Return to the starting, upright position as the arms swing down and across the front of the body (g). Perform one or two sets of five to 10 controlled repetitions per side, holding the end range of motion for one or two seconds, with 30-second rest intervals between sets.

a. b. c. d. e. f. g.

Figure 9-24
Hamstrings mobility: Lying hamstrings stretch

Objective: To improve mobility of the hamstrings in the sagittal plane without compromising lumbar stability

Preparation and position:

- Lie supine inside a door jamb or beside a sturdy table with one knee bent and the foot placed flat on the floor, aligning the anterior superior iliac spine (ASIS) with the knee and second toe.
- Engage the core muscles to stabilize the lumbar spine in the neutral position, and maintain this position throughout the exercise.
- Raise the opposite leg to rest it on the table or door jamb with slight flexion in the knee and plantarflexion at the ankle (to remove any limitation from the gastrocnemius during the stretch) (a).

Exercise:

- Exhale and slowly extend the raised leg, stretching the hamstrings.
- The objective is to promote hamstrings flexibility with the extended leg positioned at an 80- to 90-degree angle with the floor.
- Perform two to four repetitions per side, each for a minimum of 15 seconds.

Progression: Perform a series of pelvic tilts, holding the anterior pelvic tilt to increase the magnitude of he stretch (b).

Progression: Extend the lower leg for the duration of the stretch without compromising lumbar stability (c).

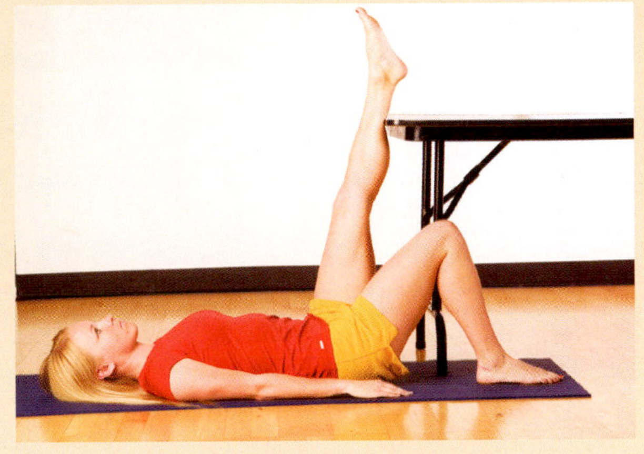
a.

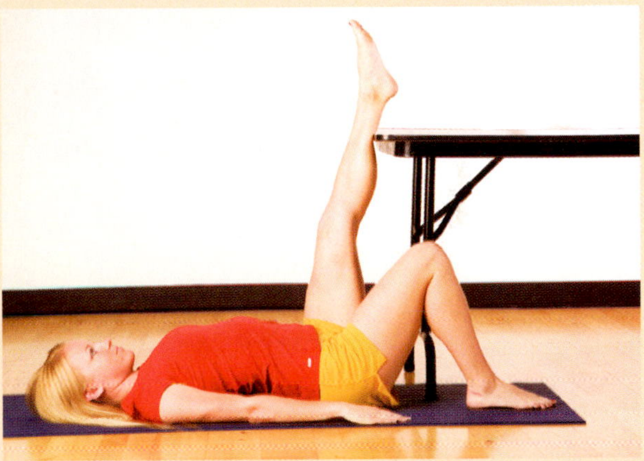
b.

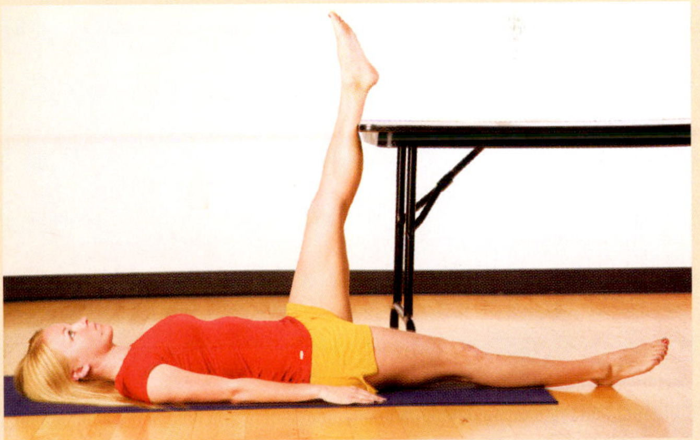
c.

Figure 9-25

Hip mobilization with glute activation: Shoulder bridge (glute bridge)

Objective: To improve hip mobility and stability and core stability by activating the gluteal muscle groups

Preparation and position:

- Lie supine with knees bent and the feet placed flat on the floor, aligning the anterior superior iliac spine (ASIS) with the knee and second toe (a).
- Engage the core muscles to stabilize the lumbar spine in the neutral position and maintain this position throughout the exercise. A common mistake made during this exercise is an increased lordosis in the up or "bridge" position due to a lack of lumbar stability. Recognizing the frequency of this compensation, full activation of the abdominals to tilt the pelvis posteriorly may be needed initially to prevent any increase in lordosis.

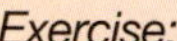

Exercise:

- Exhale and activate the gluteal muscles to elevate the hips off the floor into hip extension without increasing lordosis (b).
- Perform one or two sets of five to 10 controlled repetitions per side, holding the end range of motion for one or two seconds, with 30-second rest intervals between sets.

Progression: From the starting position, gently pull one knee toward the chest, tilting the pelvis posteriorly, and hold this knee to the chest while raising the body into the bridge position (c).

Progression: Place a riser or pad under the thoracic spine. This permits additional thoracic extension and increases the core challenge (d).

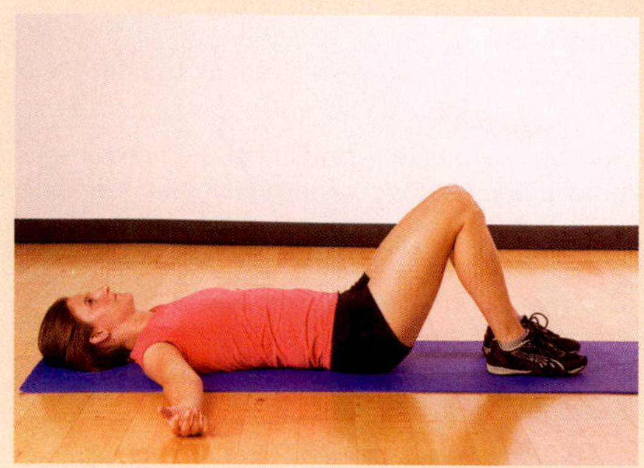

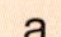

a.

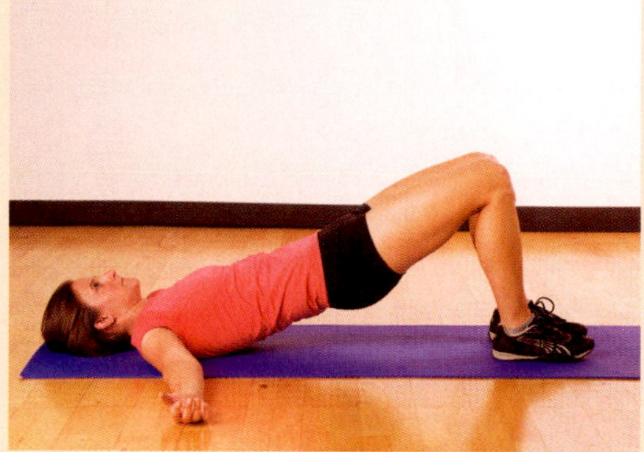

b.

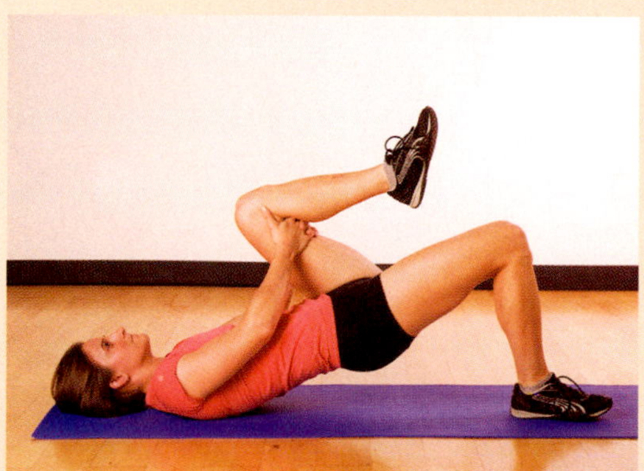

c.

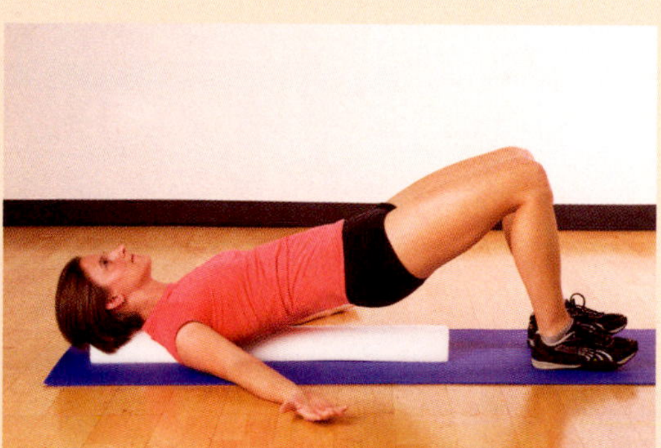

d.

Figure 9-26
Hip mobilization: Supine 90-90 hip rotator stretch

Objective: To improve hip mobility in the transverse plane

Preparation and position:

- Lie supine with both feet placed against a wall, with an approximately 90-degree bend at the knees and 60 to 80 degrees of flexion at the hips (a).
- Cross one leg over the opposite knee, resting that ankle on the knee.
- Engage the core muscles to stabilize the lumbar spine in the neutral position and maintain this position throughout the exercise.
- Place one hand on the crossed knee.

Exercise:

- Exhale and gently push the crossed knee away from the body while simultaneously lifting the opposite foot off the wall, increasing the degree of hip flexion (b).
- Perform two to four repetitions per side.
- Hold each stretch for a minimum of 15 seconds.

Progression: Assume the quadruped position, crossing the lower part of the left leg over the right leg (externally rotating the left leg). Position the right arm 1 to 2 feet (30 to 61 cm) out to the side of the body (c). Slowly lean the body out to that side, supporting the weight on the outspread hand (d). Perform two to four repetitions per side and hold each stretch for a minimum of 15 seconds (Tumminello, 2007).

Progression: Assume the quadruped position, engaging the core muscles to stabilize the lumbar spine. Lift the left leg slightly, extend it backward while sliding it across the left leg and behind the body, and drop the hips toward the floor during the movement while avoiding hip rotation (e) (Tumminello, 2007). Perform one or two sets of five to 10 controlled repetitions per side, holding the end range of motion for one or two seconds, with 30-second rest intervals between sets.

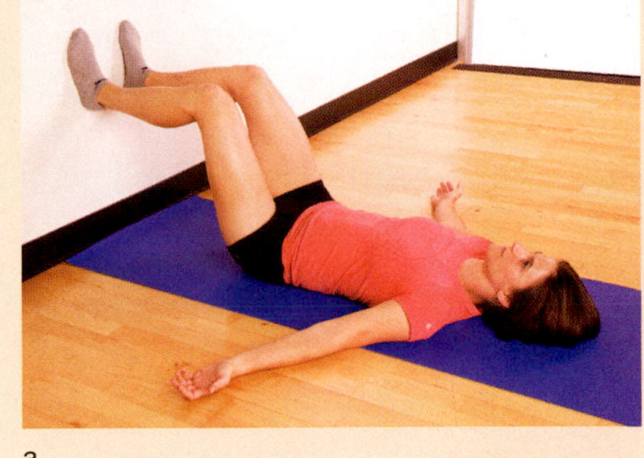
a.

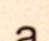

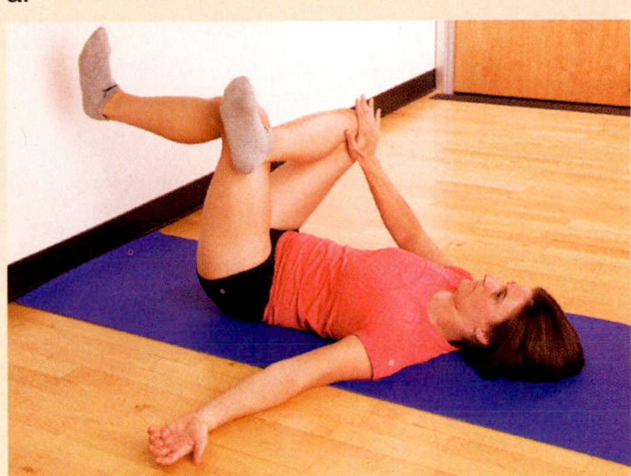
b.

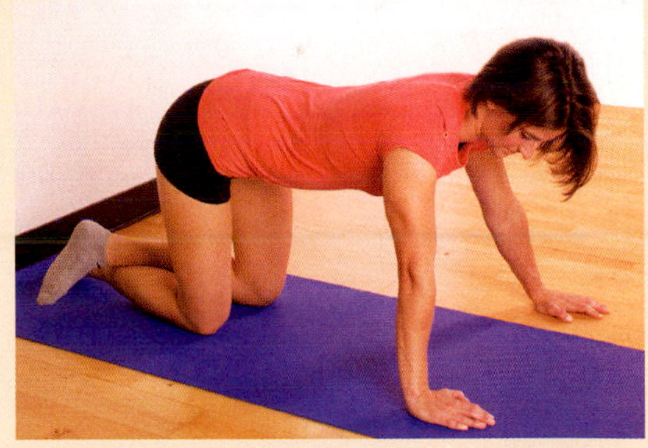
c.

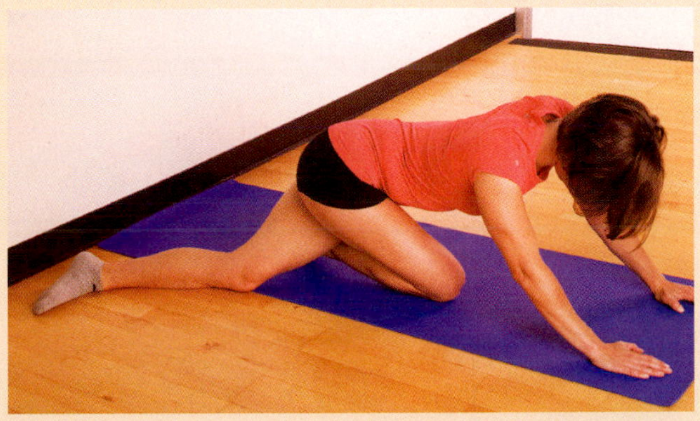
e.

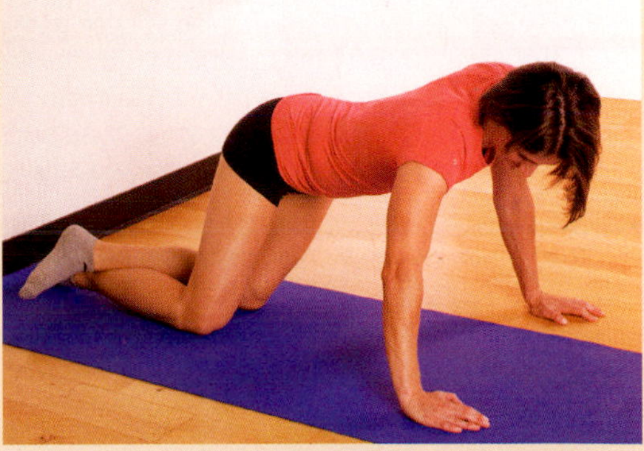
d.

Figure 9-27
Posterior compartment mobilization: Table-top kneeling lat stretch

Objective: To improve flexibility in the latissimus dorsi to facilitate mobility between the hips and shoulders

Preparation and position:

- Kneel facing a low table, couch, or chair, bending forward to place both extended arms on the object (resting the forearms) (a).
- Engage the core to stabilize the spine in neutral and prevent any lordosis.
- Start with arms internally rotated (thumbs pointing inward).

Exercise:

- Exhale and gently collapse the trunk and head toward the floor, maintaining a neutral spine while externally rotating the arms (thumbs point toward the ceiling) (b).
- Hold this position for a minimum of 15 seconds and then perform a series of slow anterior and posterior pelvic tilts.
- Relax and repeat two to four times.

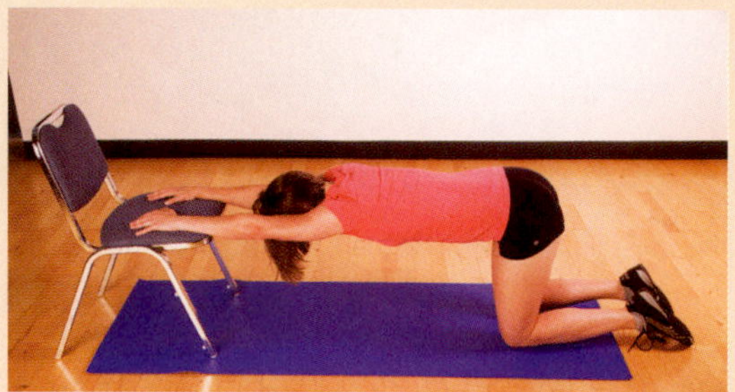
a.

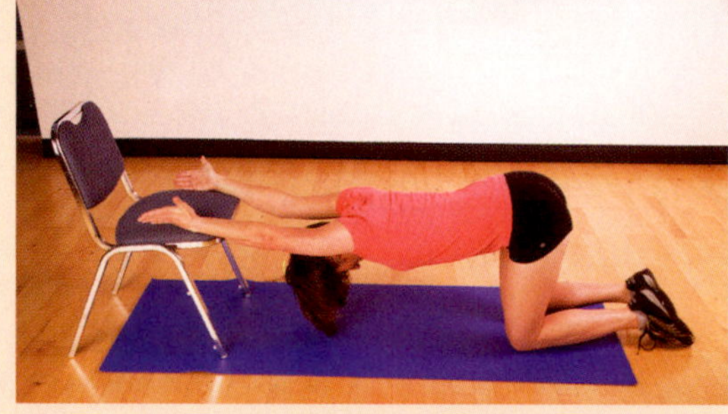
b.

Figure 9-28
Thoracic spine (T-spine) mobilization exercises: Spinal extensions and spinal twists

Spinal Extensions

Objective: To promote thoracic extension

Preparation and position:

- Lie supine with the knees bent and feet placed flat on the floor, aligning the anterior superior iliac spine (ASIS) with the knee and second toe.
- Position the arms at the sides with elbows extended.
- Engage the core muscles to stabilize the lumbar spine (avoiding increased lordosis during the exercise) and maintain this contraction throughout the exercise.
- Depress and retract the scapulae while stabilizing the low back (a).

Exercise:

- Exhale and slowly flex the shoulders, raise both arms overhead, and attempt to bring both hands to touch the floor overhead ("I" position) (b). Since the arms tend to internally rotate during shoulder flexion, and shrugging of the shoulders often occurs, attempt to depress the scapulae and keep the arms in a neutral or externally rotated position.
- Slowly return to the starting position.
- Perform one or two sets of five to 10 controlled repetitions, holding the end range of motion for one to two seconds, with 30-second rest intervals between sets.
- Repeat the entire movement from the starting position, but move into a "Y" formation, abducting the arms to 135 degrees (c).

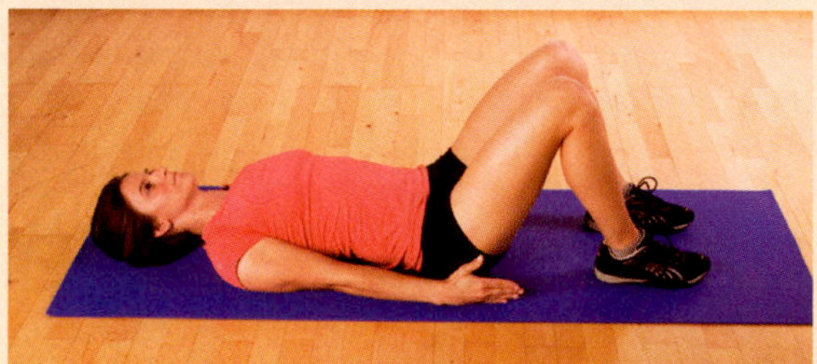
a.

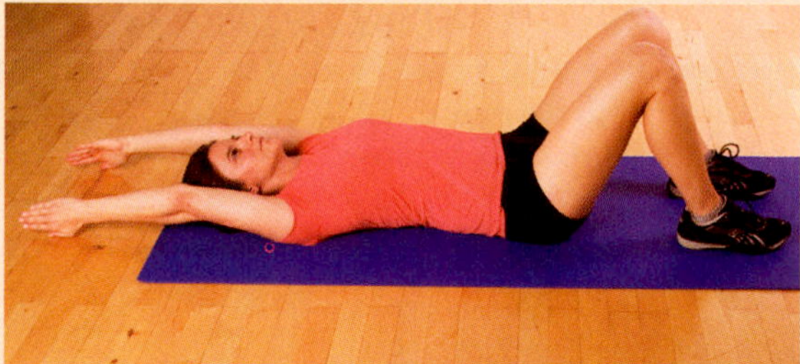
b.

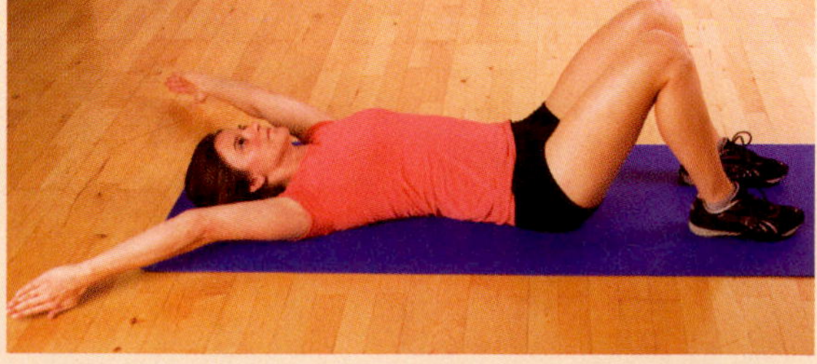
c.

Continued on next page

- Repeat the entire movement from the starting position, but move in a "T" formation, sliding the arms along the floor and abducting them to 90 degrees (d).
- Repeat the entire movement from the starting position, but, with the elbows bent, move in a "wiper formation," sliding the arms along the floor from the sides to an overhead position.

Spinal Twists

Objective: To promote trunk rotation, primarily through the thoracic spine with some lateral hip mobility

Preparation and position:

- Lie on one side, bending both knees to 90 degrees, flexing the hips to 90 to 100 degrees, and aligning both knees together, resting them on a ball or riser. Keep the lower knee on the ball or riser throughout this first exercise progression and keep both knees aligned. Engage the core muscles to stabilize the lumbar spine (avoiding increased lordosis) and maintain this contraction throughout the exercise.
- Reach the upper arm across and in front of the body, grasping the rib-cage on the opposite side of the trunk (e).

Exercise:

- Exhale and slowly rotate the torso by pulling on the ribcage. Attempt to avoid any rotational movement of the hips and knees.
- Perform two to four repetitions to each side.
- Hold each pull for 15 to 30 seconds.

Progression: Repeat the same stretch, but place a squeezable object (e.g., a soft ball or yoga block) between the knees, positioning the lower knee on the floor.

Progression: Repeat the same stretch, but extend the lower leg and rest the inside of the upper knee on a squeezable object.

Progression: Repeat the same stretch, but change the upper arm from the rib-grab position to abducting the arm to 90 degrees with an extended elbow, and attempt to bring the upper arm down to touch the floor (f).

Progression—push-pull: Assume any of the starting positions for the lower extremity on one side. Depress and retract both scapulae, then move the upper arm to the start position of a press movement (e.g., bench press), while the lower arm moves into the start position of a pull movement (without protracting the scapula) (g & h). Simultaneously perform an upward press with the upper arm and a high-back row with the lower arm. Perform one or two sets of five to 10 controlled repetitions per side, holding the end range of motion for one or two seconds, with 30-second rest intervals between sets.

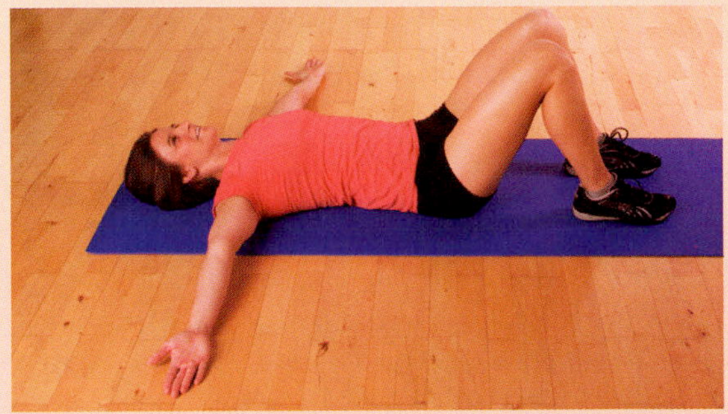

d.

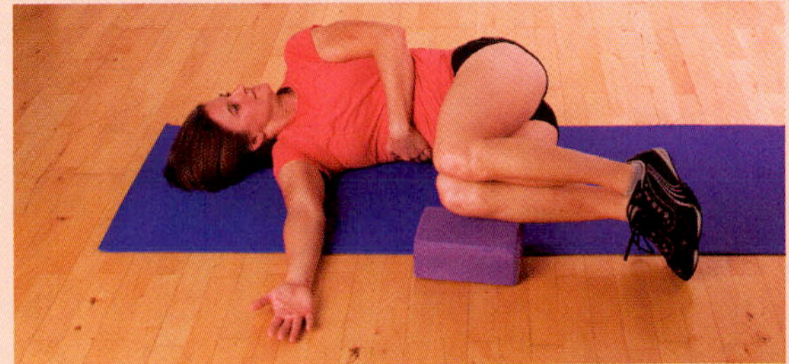

e.

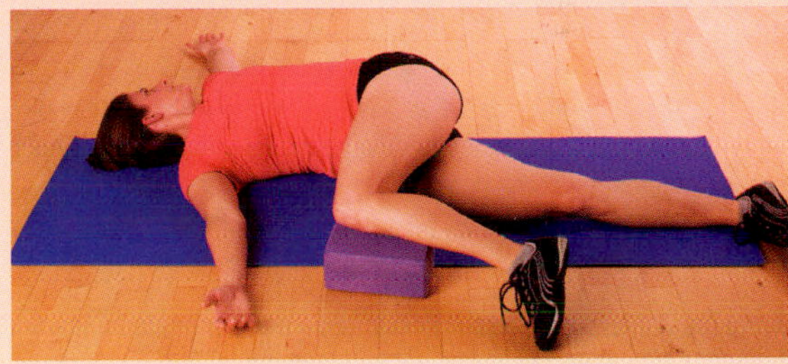

f.

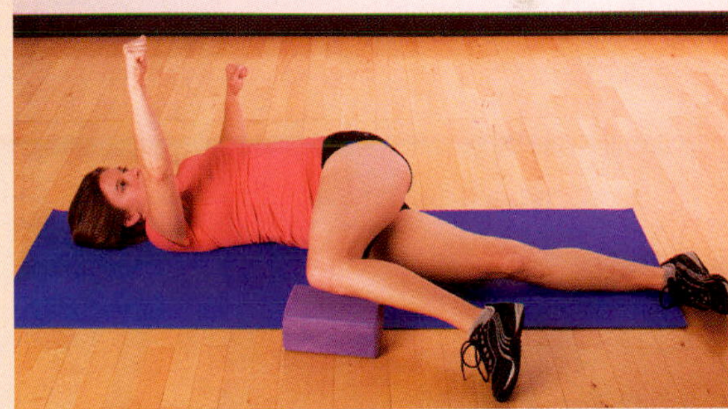

g.

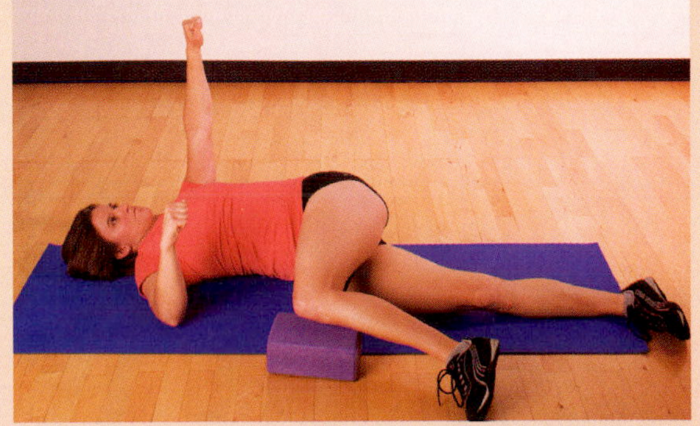

h.

Figure 9-29
Thoracic spine (T-spine) mobilization: Prisoner rotations

Objective: To promote thoracic spine mobility in the transverse plane

Preparation and position:

- Assume a kneeling position and interlock the hands lightly behind the head without pulling the head forward into neck flexion (a).
- Engage the core muscles to stabilize the lumbar spine, and maintain this contraction throughout the exercise.
- The exercise objective is to promote trunk rotation, primarily within the thoracic spine without rotating the hips.

Exercise:

- Exhale and slowly rotate the arms to the right until a point of resistance is reached (no bouncing movement) (b). Avoid rotating the hips.
- Hold this position for 15 seconds and then laterally flex the trunk, pointing the right elbow toward the floor (c). Hold this position for five seconds.
- Return to an upright position and then laterally flex in the opposite direction (d). Hold this position for five seconds.
- Return to the upright position and allow the trunk to rotate further into the movement.
- Perform two to four repetitions to each side.

Source: Tumminello, N. (2007). *Warm-up Progressions—Volumes 1 and 2*. Baltimore, Md.: Performance University.

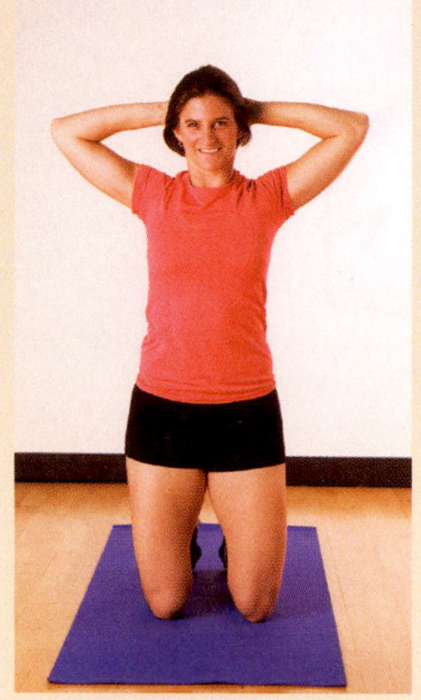
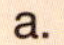
a.

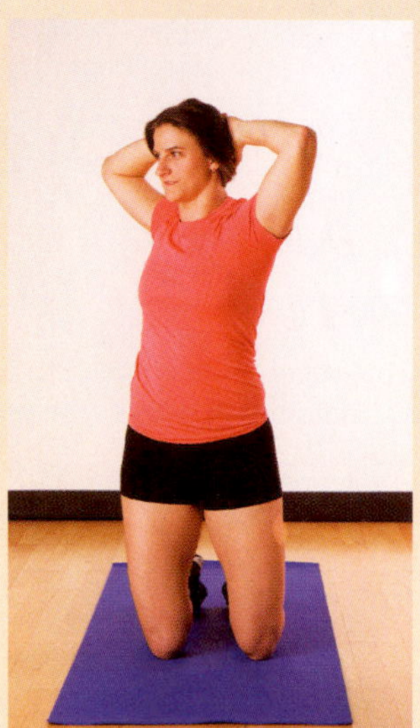
b.

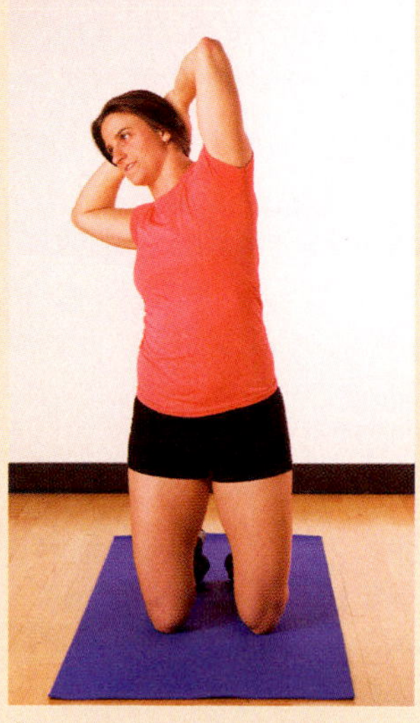
c.

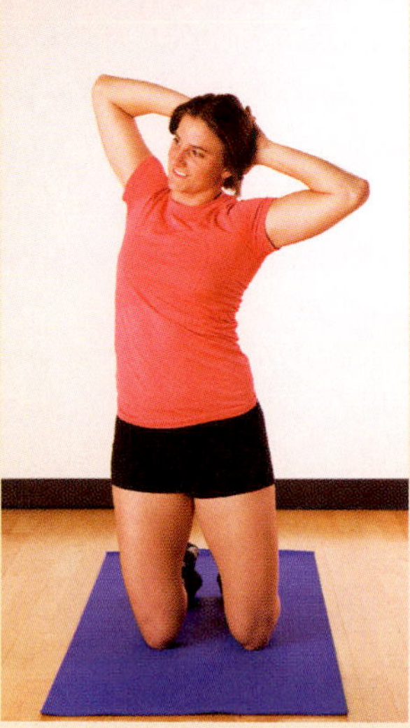
d.

Figure 9-30
Posterior mobilization: Rocking quadrupeds

Objective: To promote hip and thoracic mobility while simultaneously maintaining lumbar stability

Preparation and position:

- Assume the quadruped position adjacent to a mirror, placing both hands directly under the shoulders (shoulder-width apart) and knees directly under the hips (hip-width apart) (a).
- Engage the core muscles to create a neutral spine. Maintain this flat or neutral spine throughout the exercise.

Exercise:

- While focusing on the spine, slowly rock backward and forward using visual feedback to control the range of movement, as dictated by a changing position of the spine (rounding during the backward roll and arching into lordosis during the forward rock) (b & c).
- Perform one or two sets of five to 10 controlled repetitions, holding the end range of motion for one or two seconds, with 30-second rest intervals between sets.

Progression: While maintaining a bent-knee and bent-elbow position, slowly extend the contralateral limbs (hip extension and shoulder flexion) away from the trunk during the backward rock, bringing them toward each other under the body during the forward rock (d & e). Attempt to minimize the changes in the lumbar spine. Perform one or two sets of five to 10 controlled repetitions per side, holding the end range of motion for one or two seconds, with 30-second rest intervals between sets.

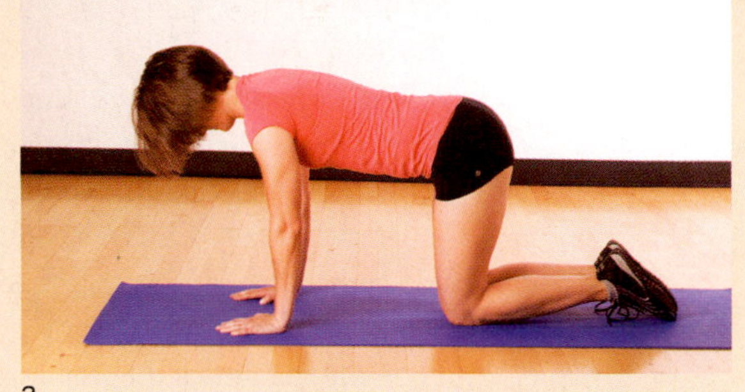

a.

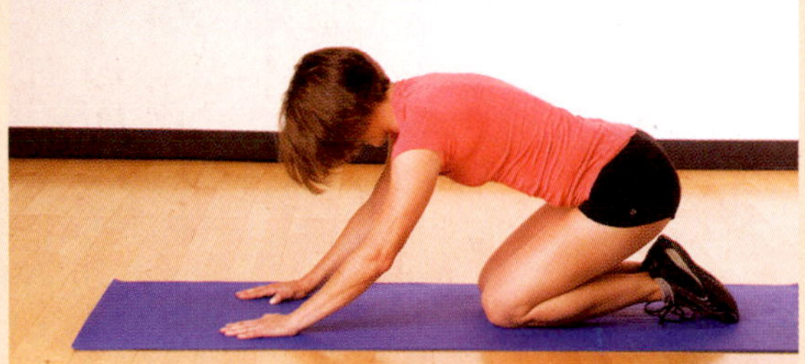

b.

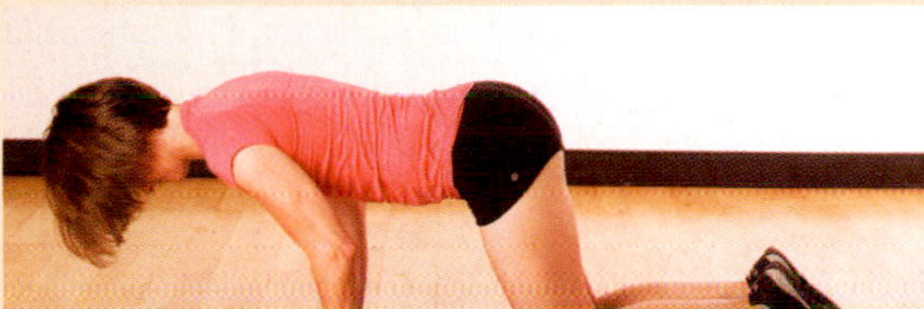

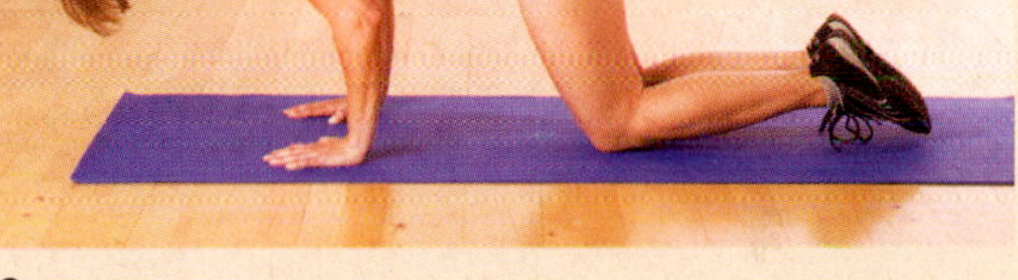

c.

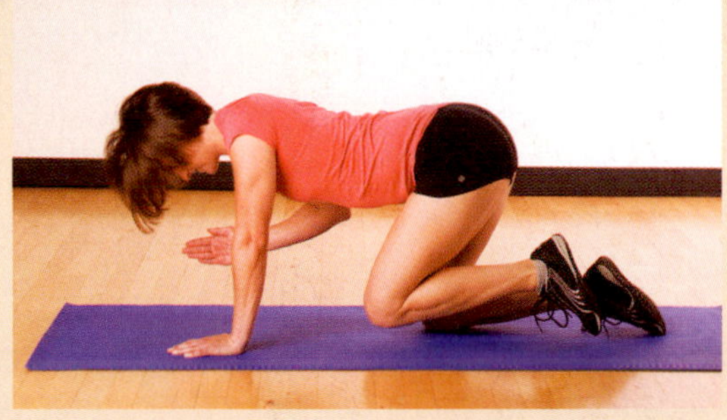

d.

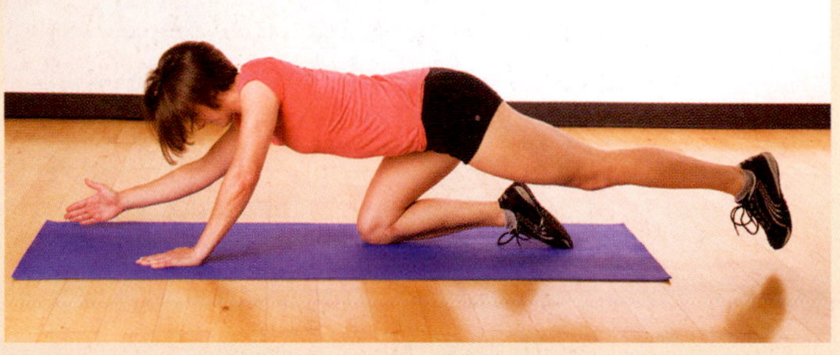

e.

Proximal Stability of the Scapulothoracic Region and Distal Mobility of the Glenohumeral Joint

This stage is designed to improve stability within the scapulothoracic region during upper-extremity movements (e.g., push- and pull-type motions). The glenohumeral joint is a highly mobile joint and its ability to achieve this degree of movement is contingent upon the stability of the scapulothoracic region (i.e., the ability of the scapulae to maintain appropriate proximity against the ribcage during movement) (Houglum, 2005; Sahrmann, 2002). It is the synergistic actions of muscle groups working through force-couples in this region that help achieve this stability, considering that the scapulae only attach to the axial skeleton via the clavicles. Promoting stability within this joint, therefore, requires muscle balance within the force-couples of the joint. Additionally, as many of these muscles also cross the glenohumeral joint, they require substantial levels of mobility. This implies that a program promoting scapulothoracic stability may need to include stretches to promote extensibility of both the muscle and joint structures. Therefore, static stretches to improve tissue extensibility should precede dynamic movement patterns and strengthening exercises.

A normally positioned scapula promotes muscle balance and effective force-coupling relationships. However, given the design of the shoulder girdle (favoring mobility at a cost of stability) and the propensity toward bad posture in the upper extremity due to a myriad of lifestyle-related positions and activities, compensated movement and shoulder injuries occur very frequently. Perhaps the most problematic movements are associated with arm abduction and a lack of scapular stability during horizontal push-and-pull movements.

During abduction, the rotator cuff muscles play an important role in initiating movement and facilitating an inferior glide of the humeral head (Houglum, 2005). This glide is critical, as the articular surface of the humeral head is almost twice the size of the glenoid fossa, and therefore cannot operate as a true ball-and-socket joint. The rotator cuff muscles contract in anticipation of deltoid action. It is the collaborative action of the supraspinatus acting as the primary abductor for the first 15 degrees of abduction and the infraspinatus, subscapularis, and teres minor depressing the head of the humerus inferiorly within the glenoid fossa that permit rotation to occur (in this case, abduction of the shoulder) (Figure 9-31) (Cook & Jones, 2007a; Kendall et al., 2005). After approximately 15 degrees of abduction, the deltoid takes over as the primary abductor, while the rotator cuff muscles continue to depress and stabilize the humeral head, along with the anterior and posterior deltoid. If the deltoid acted alone, pure superior glide would occur, which would impinge the humeral head against the coracoacromial arch at approximately 22 degrees of abduction.

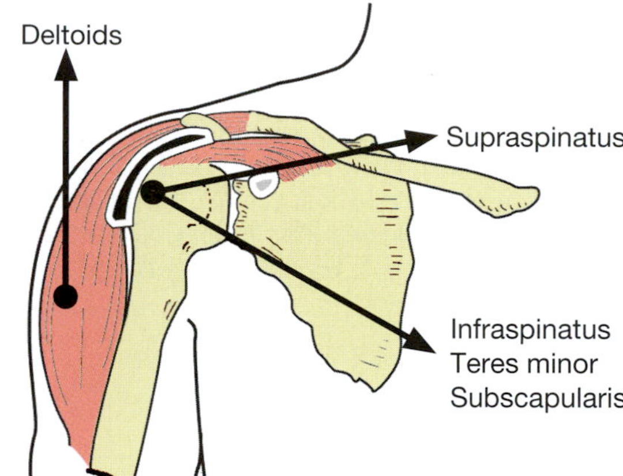

Figure 9-31
Muscle action involved in abducting (raising) the arm

During pushing and pulling movements, key parascapular muscles (i.e., serratus anterior, rhomboids, and lower trapezius) co-contract to permit movement of the scapulae, yet help it maintain proximity against the ribcage. When the thoracic spine lacks appropriate mobility, what often results is compensation to stability within the scapulothoracic region, which in turn affects mobility within the glenohumeral joint and muscle action within that joint. However, with good thoracic mobility and muscle balance in the scapulothoracic region to effectively stabilize the scapula and control its movement, the more distal mobilizers (e.g., deltoid) can generate larger amounts of force. It therefore appears that promoting stability within the scapulothoracic region requires thoracic mobility in addition to other key factors:

- Tissue extensibility (both active and passive structures)
- Healthy rotator cuff muscle function
- Muscle balance within the parascapular muscles
- The ability to resist upward glide and impingement against the coracoacromial arch during deltoid action

To enhance tissue extensibility, trainers can employ several different stretching modalities. Myofascial release using a stick or foam roller—moving across the tender spots—will help realign the elastic fibers and reduce hypertonicity (Barnes, 1999). This should precede static stretching of the shoulder capsule and of specific muscles of the scapulae. When stretching the shoulder capsule with a client, trainers must address the inferior, posterior, anterior, and superior components.

- Stretch the inferior capsule using an overhead triceps stretch (Figure 9-32).
- Stretch the posterior capsule by bringing the arm across and in front of the body (Figure 9-33a). An alternative position for this stretch is to stand adjacent to a wall, flexing the arm in front of the body to 90 degrees and resting the full length of the arm against the wall, then slowly rotate the trunk inward toward the wall (Figure 9-33b & c). Since this movement also produces scapular abduction, and since it is common for clients to have abducted scapulae as a postural deviation, it should be a minimal focus during shoulder stretching.
- Stretch the anterior capsule using a pectoralis stretch (Figure 9-34a & b).
- Stretch the superior capsule by placing a rolled-up towel 2 inches (5.1 cm) above the elbow against the trunk (bent-elbow position at the side of the body), grasping the base of the elbow and pulling it downward and inward (Figure 9-35).

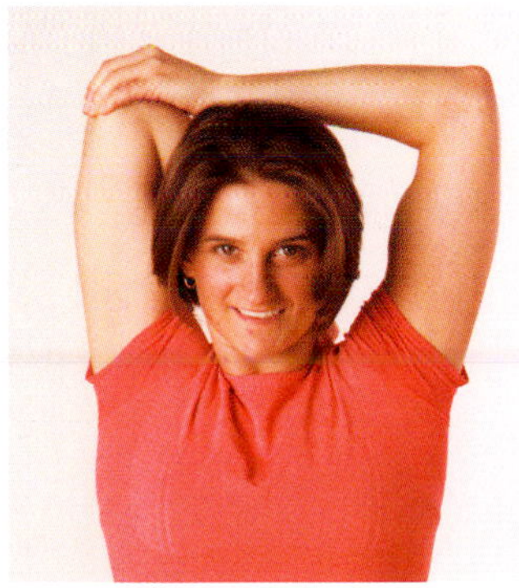

Figure 9-32
Inferior capsule stretch

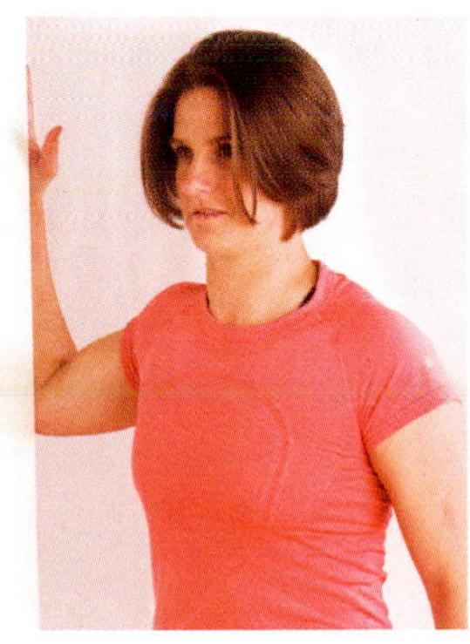

a.

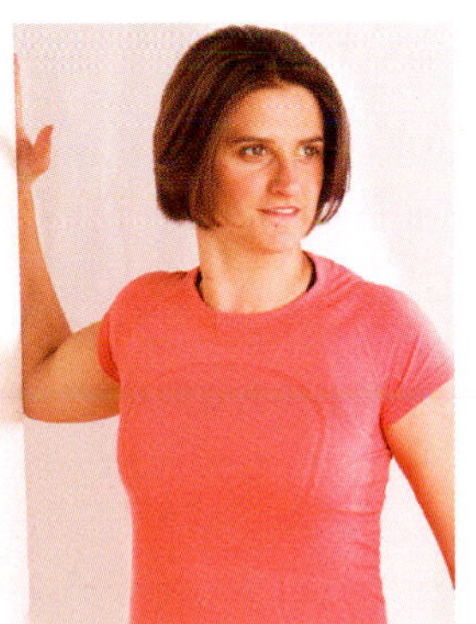

b.

Figure 9-34
Anterior capsule (pectoralis) stretch

Figure 9-35
Superior capsule stretch

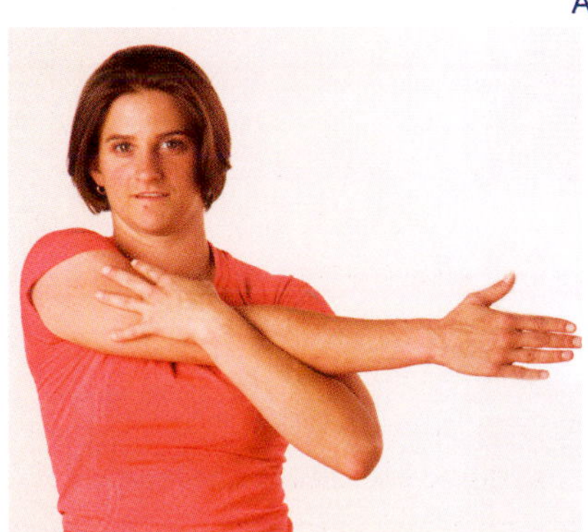

a.

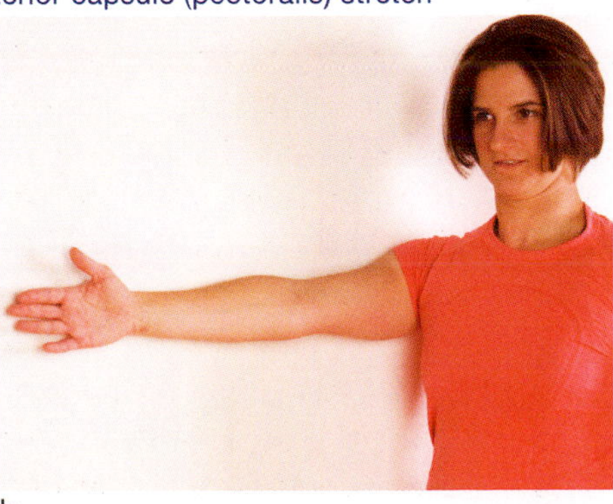

b.

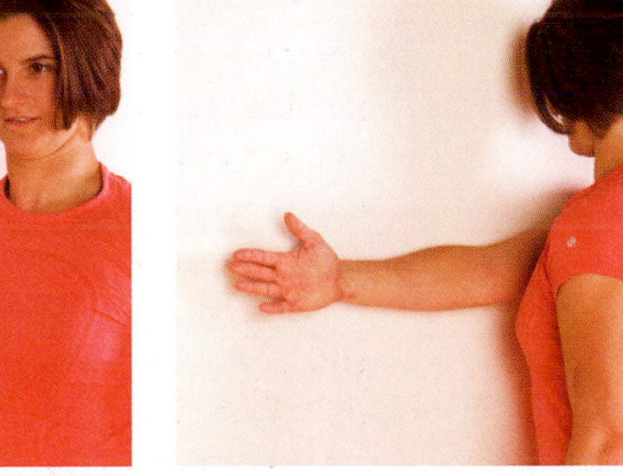

c.

Figure 9-33
Posterior capsule stretches

One important consideration for promoting scapulothoracic stability revolves around the type of exercises selected (i.e., closed-chain or open-chain exercises). During closed kinetic chain (CKC) movements where the distal segment is more fixed (e.g., pull-ups and push-ups), a key role of the serratus anterior is to move the thorax toward a more fixed, stable scapulae (Cook & Jones, 2007a; Houglum, 2005). During open kinetic chain (OKC) movements, however, a key role of the serratus anterior is to control movement of the scapulae against a more fixed ribcage (Cook & Jones, 2007a; Houglum, 2005). OKC movements are generally considered more functional, as they closely mimic daily activities. CKC exercises load and compress joints, increasing kinesthetic awareness and **proprioception,** which translates into improved parascapular and shoulder stability (Cook & Jones, 2007a). Isolated OKC exercises, on the other hand, are not as effective in restoring coordinated parascapular control. One challenge with CKC exercises is that many are too challenging for deconditioned individuals. Thus, it is important to initially use the floor to provide kinesthetic feedback and OKC movements to improve control and movement efficiency and increase kinesthetic awareness of shoulder position. Trainers can start by first helping the individual recognize the normal resting position of the scapulae kinesthetically (i.e., feel the correct scapulae position against the floor). The exercise presented in Figure 9-36 helps achieve this awareness by instructing the client on how to "pack" the scapulae.

A variety of exercises can be used to condition the rotator cuff muscles, but whichever exercises the trainer and client select, the client must perform them from the packed shoulder position. Figures 9-37 through 9-42 provide examples of OKC and CKC rotator cuff exercises that promote scapulothoracic stability.

Figure 9-36
Shoulder packing

Objective: To kinesthetically improve awareness of good scapular position, improving flexibility and strength of key parascapular muscles

Preparation and position:

- Lie supine on a mat with knees bent to 90 degrees and the feet placed flat on the floor, aligning the anterior superior iliac spine (ASIS) with the knee and second toe.
- Position the arms at the sides of the trunk with the palms facing upward.
- Engage the core muscles to stabilize the lumbar spine in the neutral position. Maintain this position throughout the exercise (a).

Exercise:

- Exhale and perform two to four repetitions of each of the following, holding each contraction for five to 10 seconds (b):
  - ✓ Scapular depression
  - ✓ Scapular retraction
- Using passive assistance from the opposite arm, gently push down on the shoulder (posterior tilt on scapula) without losing lumbar stability. Hold this position for 15 to 60 seconds.
- Relax and repeat two to four times on each shoulder.

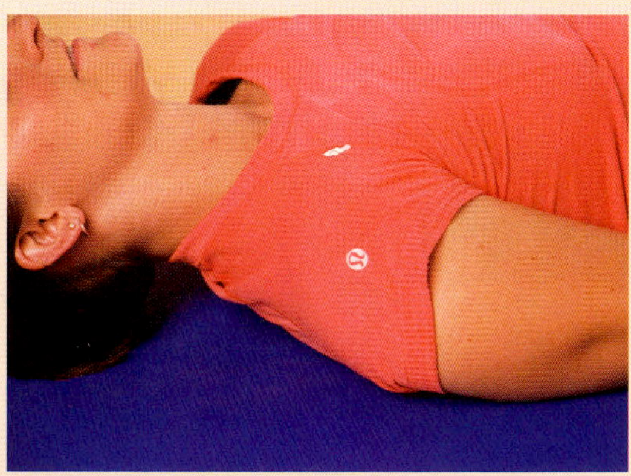

a.

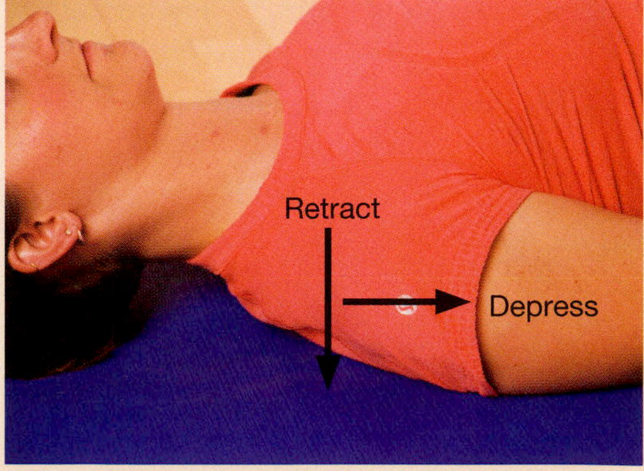

b.

Figure 9-37
Internal and external humeral rotation

Objective: To improve rotator cuff function while maintaining good scapular position

Preparation and position:

- Lie supine on a mat with knees bent and feet placed flat on the floor, aligning the anterior superior iliac spine (ASIS) with the knee and second toe.
- Engage the core muscles to stabilize the lumbar spine in the neutral position and maintain this position throughout the exercise.
- Pack both scapulae and maintain this position throughout the exercise.
- Abduct the arms to 90 degrees (shoulder height), resting the backs of the upper arms on the mat, and bend the elbows 90 degrees so that the forearms are perpendicular to the floor (a).

Exercise:

- *External rotation:* Slowly externally rotate the arms backward, bringing the forearms toward the floor. The ultimate goal is to achieve movement so that the back of the forearm rests on the floor (90 degrees of movement) (b).
- Hold this position for 15 to 60 seconds and repeat two to four times.
- *Internal rotation:* From the starting position, internally rotate the arms forward, bringing the forearms toward the floor. The ultimate goal is to achieve movement so that the forearms reach an angle of 20 to 30 degrees above the floor (60 to 70 degrees of movement) (c).
- Hold this position for 15 to 60 seconds, and repeat two to four times.

Progression: Once the end ranges can be reached, add resistance to condition these muscles (d & e). Remember, these are small muscles with higher concentrations of type 1 fibers, so they respond best to volume training. Add no more than 5 pounds (2.3 kg) of external resistance (cable or dumbbell) and build volume toward three sets of 12 to 15 repetitions with 30-second rest intervals between sets.

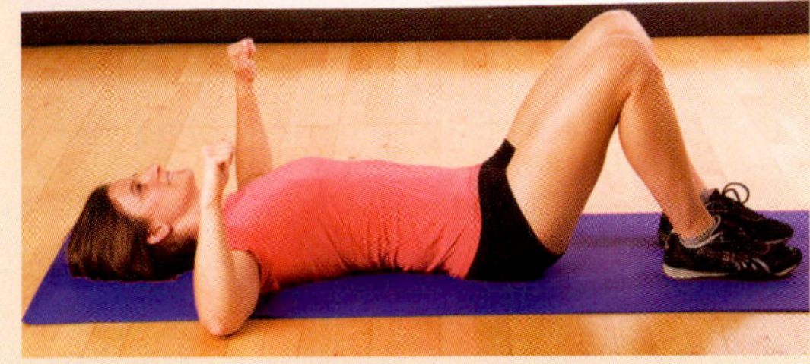
a.

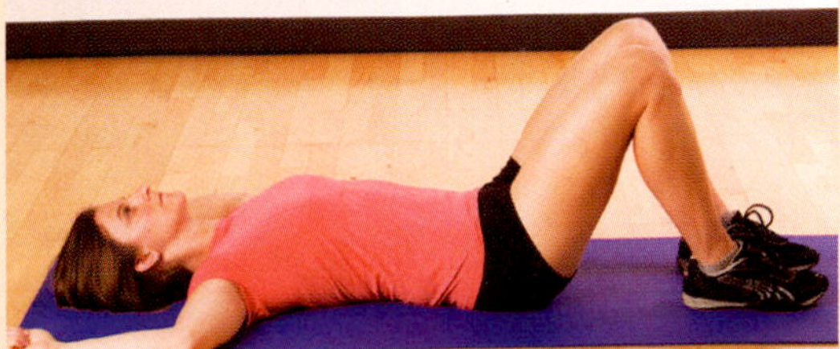
b.

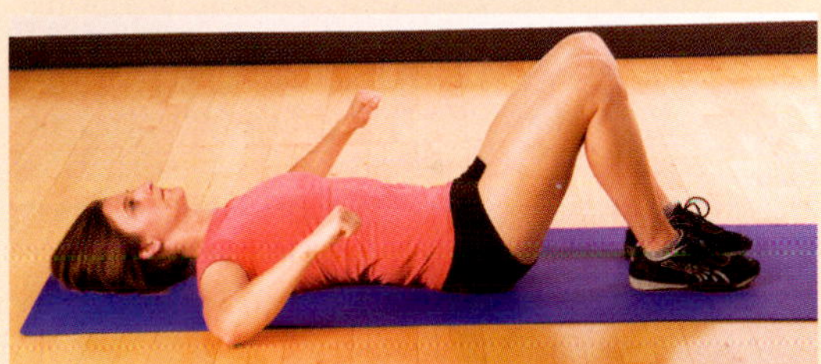
c.

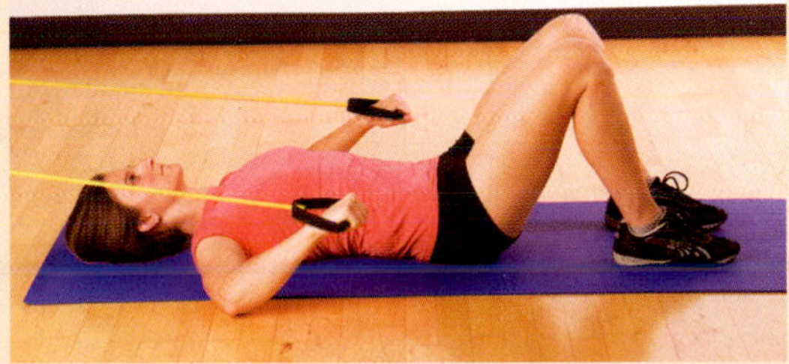
d.

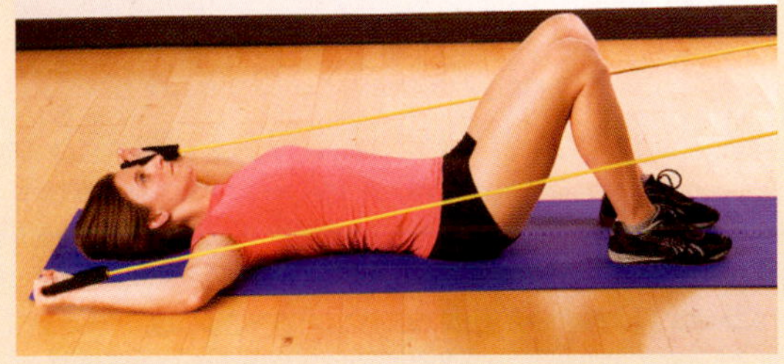
e.

Figure 9-38
Diagonals

Objective: To improve rotator cuff function with four integrated movements (in two diagonal patterns) at the glenohumeral and scapulothoracic joints

Preparation and position:

- Lie supine on a mat with knees bent and feet placed flat on the floor, aligning the anterior superior iliac spine (ASIS) with the knee and second toe.
- Engage the core muscles to stabilize the lumbar spine in the neutral position and maintain this position throughout the exercise.
- Pack both scapulae and maintain this position throughout the exercise.

Exercises:

- *Diagonal 1:* Start with one arm extended and placed across the body in an internally rotated position (as if reaching across to withdraw a sword from its sheath) (a). Pull the arm back across the body, externally rotating and abducting the arm to 90 degrees (b). This movement combines elevation, adduction, and upward rotation of the scapulae with extension, abduction, and external rotation of the glenohumeral joint. Perform the opposite movement to return to the starting position. Perform one or two sets of five to 10 controlled repetitions per arm, holding the end range of motion for one or two seconds, with 30-second rest intervals between sets.
- *Diagonal 2:* Start with one arm extended and placed at the side of the body in an internally rotated position (c). Pull the arm across the body, toward the opposite shoulder, externally rotating and adducting the arm as it moves toward that shoulder (with the palm toward the face) (d). This movement combines elevation, abduction, and upward rotation of the scapulae with flexion, adduction, and external rotation of the glenohumeral joint. Perform the opposite movement to return to the starting position. Perform one or two sets of five to 10 controlled repetitions per arm, holding the end range of motion for one or two seconds, with 30-second rest intervals between sets.

Progression: Repeat the four diagonal movements, but add light cable resistance. Remember, these are small muscles with higher concentrations of type I fibers, so they respond best to volume training. Add no more than 5 pounds (2.3 kg) of external resistance (cable or dumbbell) and build volume toward three sets of 12 to 15 repetitions, with 30-second rest intervals between sets.

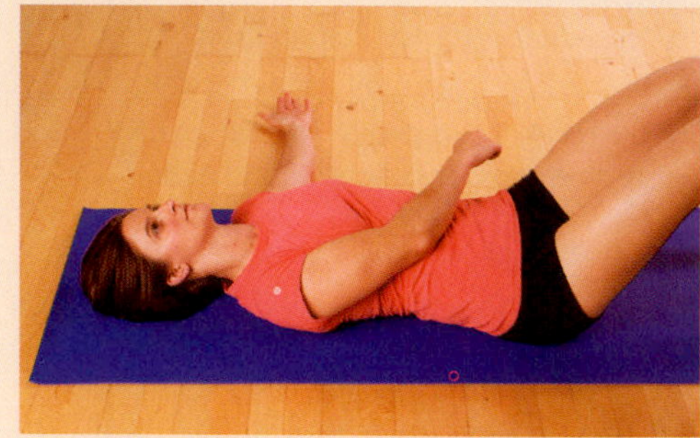
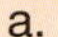
a.

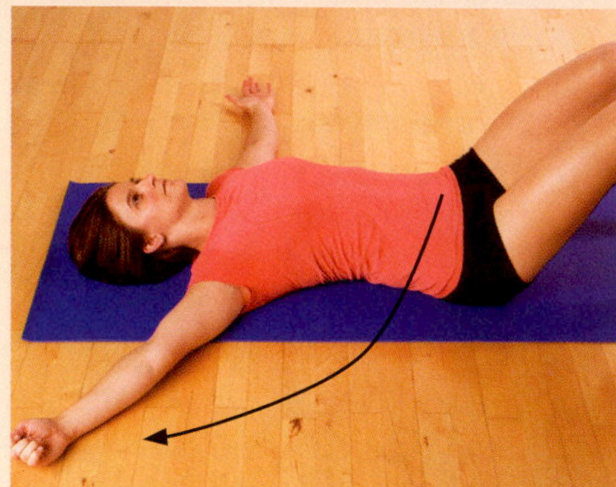
b.

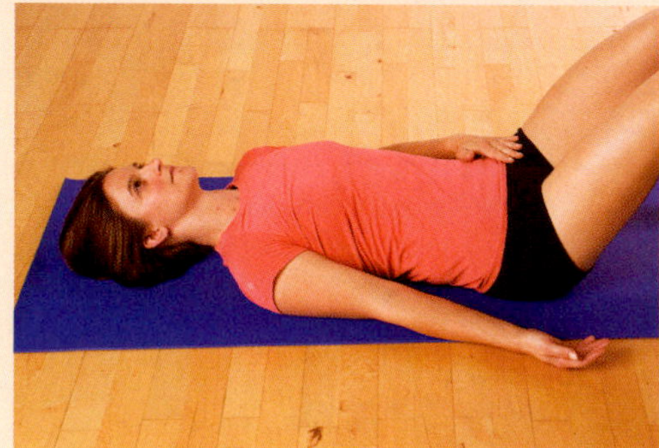
c.

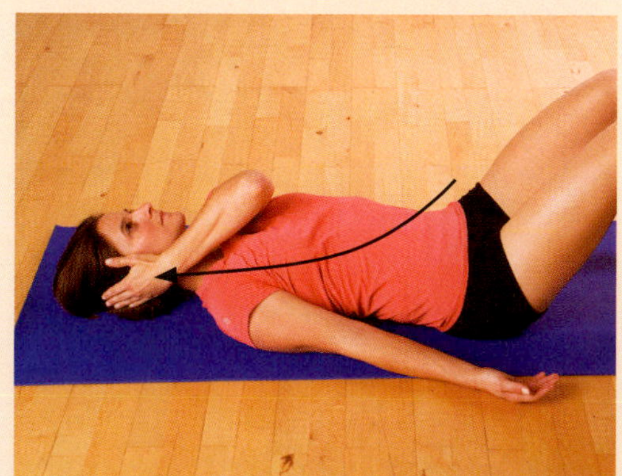
d.

Figure 9-39
Reverse flys with supine 90-90

Objective: To strengthen the posterior muscles of the shoulder complex

Preparation and position:

- Lie supine on the floor with both legs draped over a chair or riser. The height of the chair or riser should allow the knees and hips to flex to 90 degrees without elevating the hips off the floor.
- Align the anterior superior iliac spine (ASIS) with the knee and second toe and use supports to hold the feet in this position (e.g., pillows), preventing any external or internal rotation of the feet and lower legs, which would alter pelvic and low-back position.
- Abduct the arms to 90 degrees (shoulder height), resting the backs of the upper arms on the mat and bending the elbows 90 degrees so that the forearms are perpendicular to the floor.
- Engage the core muscles to stabilize the lumbar spine in the neutral position and maintain this position throughout the exercise (a).
- Pack both scapulae and maintain this position throughout the exercise.

Exercise:

- Exhale and press the back of the arms into the floor with less than 50% of maximum voluntary contraction, without altering the position of the lumbar spine.
- Perform two to four repetitions, holding each isometric contraction for five to 10 seconds.

Progression: Lying supine, build exercise volume toward three sets of 12 to 15 repetitions, with 30-second rest intervals between sets.

Progression: Seated with the back flat against a wall and knees bent, perform three sets of 12 to 15 repetitions, with 30-second rest intervals between sets. Maintain contact between the sacrum, low back, scapulae, and back of the head and the wall (b).

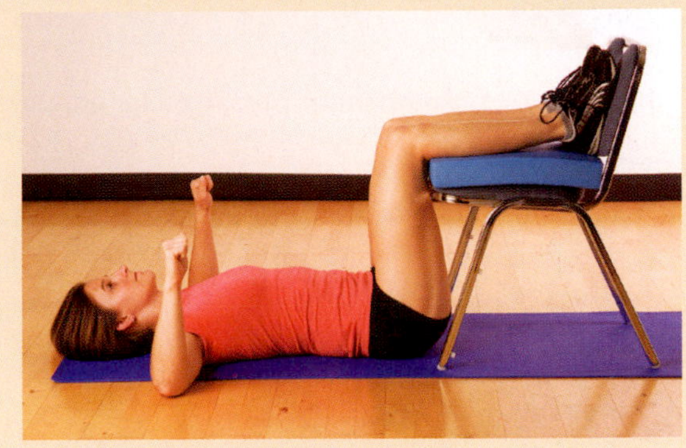

a.

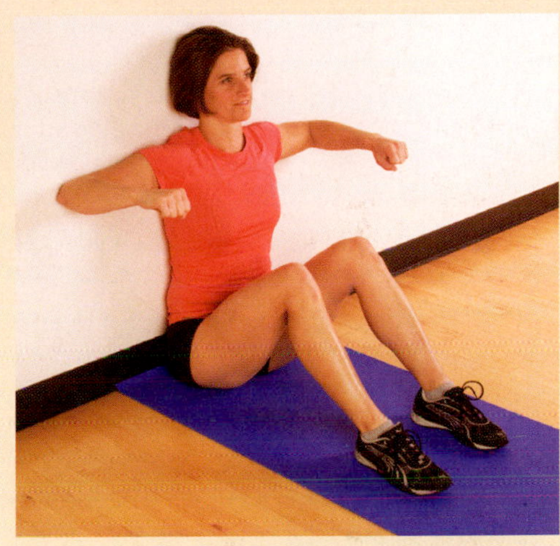

b.

Figure 9-40
Prone arm lifts

Objective: To strengthen the parascapular muscles

Preparation and position:

- Lie prone on a mat with both legs extended and arms positioned overhead with bent elbows, resting the back of the upper arms on a mat.
- Engage the core muscles to stabilize the lumbar spine in the neutral position and maintain this position throughout the exercise.
- Pack both scapulae and maintain this position throughout the exercise (a).

Exercise:

- *"I" formation:* Exhale and lift both arms 2 to 4 inches (5 to 10 cm) off the floor (keeping the elbows bent), while maintaining a depressed scapular position (avoiding scapular elevation) (b).
- Perform two to four repetitions, holding each repetition for five to 10 seconds.
- *"Y" formation:* Slide both arms out to a 135-degree position, keeping the elbows bent, but resting the arms on the mat (forming the letter "Y"). Exhale and lift both arms 2 to 4 inches (5 to 10 cm) off the floor while maintaining a depressed scapular position (avoiding scapular elevation) (c).
- Perform two to four repetitions, holding each repetition for five to 10 seconds.
- *"W" formation*: Slide both arms out to 90 degrees (shoulder height), resting the arms on the mat (forming the letter "W"). Exhale and lift both arms 2 to 4 inches (5 to 10 cm) off the floor while maintaining a depressed scapular position (avoiding scapular elevation) (d).
- Perform two to four repetitions, holding each repetition for five to 10 seconds.
- *"O" formation:* Reach behind the back and interlock the fingers, forming a giant letter "O" on the back, resting both forearms on the back. Exhale and lift both arms 2 to 4 inches (5 to 10 cm) off the back, while maintaining a depressed scapular position (avoiding scapular elevation) (e).
- Perform two to four repetitions, holding each repetition for five to 10 seconds.

Progression: Repeat the "I", "Y," and "W" formations with fully extended arms (note that the "W" formation becomes a "T" formation with the arms fully extended). Build the exercise volume toward three sets of 12 to 15 repetitions with 30-second rest intervals between sets. These exercises can ultimately be progressed to an incline position on a stability ball, standing, or in a hip-hinge or forward-bending position (hips flexed 90 degrees).

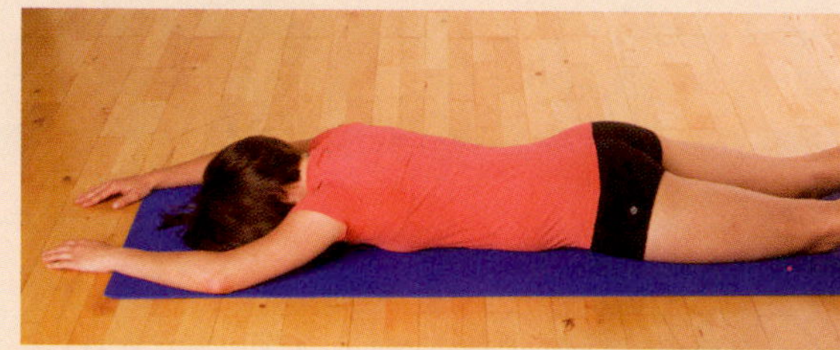
a.

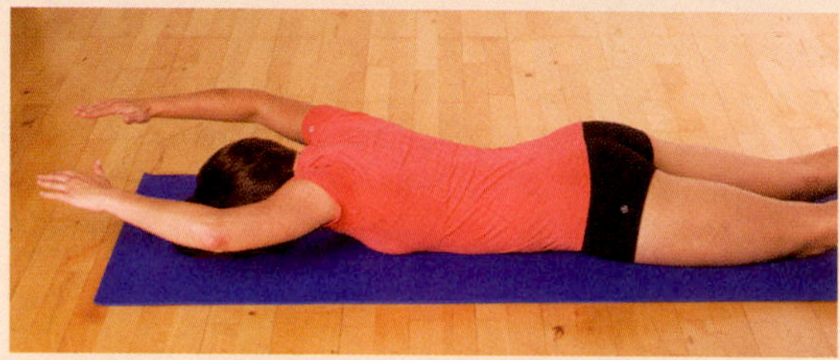
b.

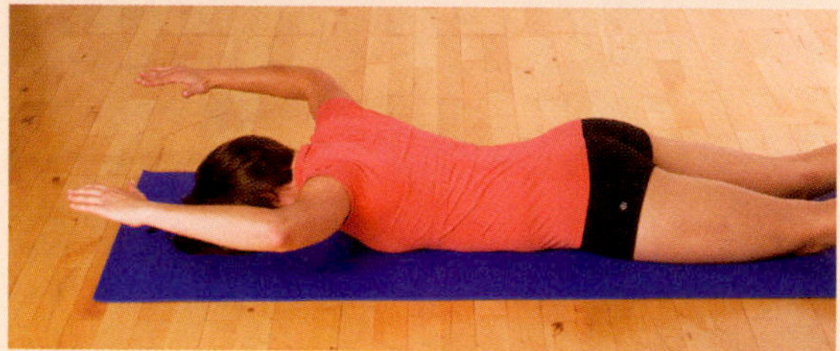
c.

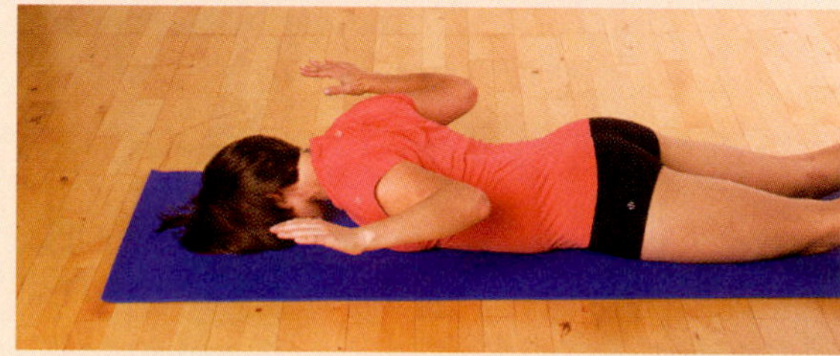
d.

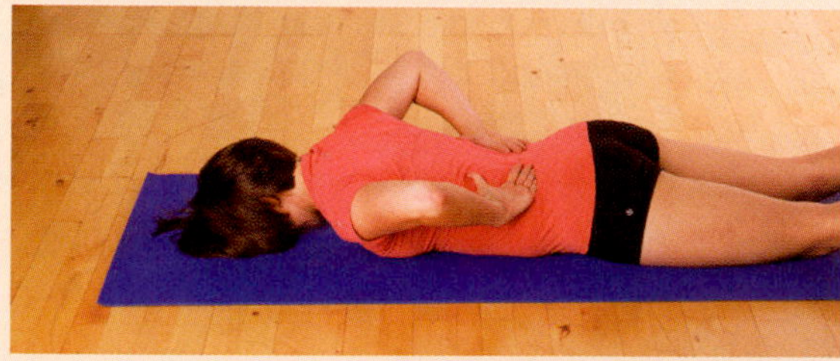
e.

Figure 9-41
Closed kinetic chain weight shifts

Objective: To stabilize the scapulothoracic joint and lumbar spine in a closed kinetic chain (CKC) position

Preparation and position:

- Lie prone on a mat, placing the hands directly under the shoulders and extending both legs.
- Engage the core muscles to stabilize the lumbar spine in the neutral position. Maintain this position throughout the exercise.
- Pack the shoulders (see Figure 9-36) and maintain this position throughout the exercise (a).
- Press the body upward to assume a full or bent-knee press-up position (b).

Exercise:

- Slowly shift the body weight 3 to 6 inches (8 to 15 cm) in all three directions without moving the hands (c).
- Perform two to four repetitions, holding each for five to 10 seconds.

Progression: Offset one hand into a staggered position by moving it 6 to 12 inches (15 to 30 cm) forward of the shoulder and repeat the movement (d). Perform two to four repetitions, holding each for five to 10 seconds. Repeat to the opposite side.

Progression: Drop the shoulder of the hand positioned under the shoulder toward the floor (e). Perform one or two sets of five to 10 repetitions to each side.

Progression: Perform side shuffles, moving the hands 6 to 12 inches (15 to 30 cm) side-to-side (f & g). Perform one or two sets of five to 10 repetitions to each side.

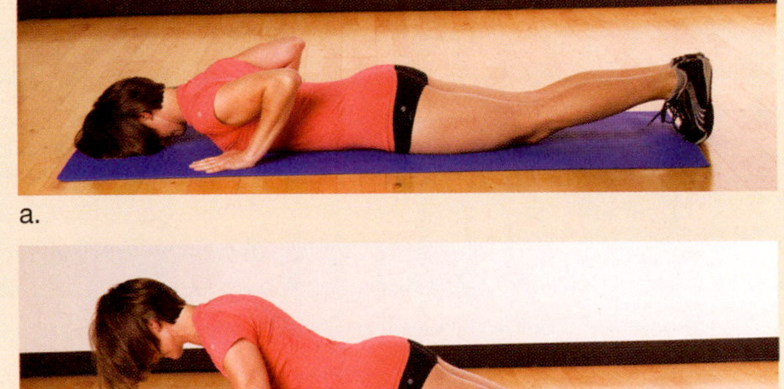
a.

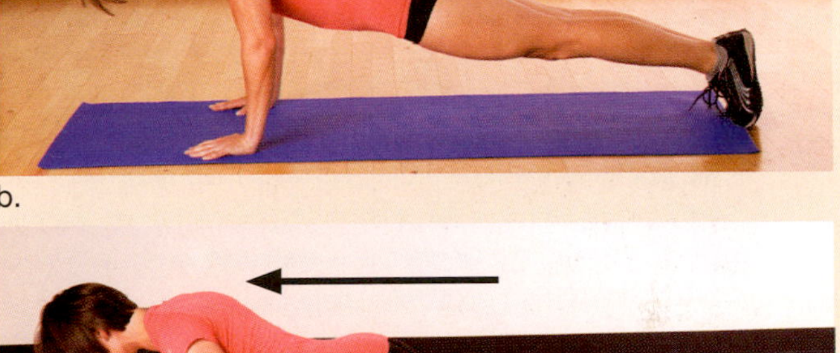
b.

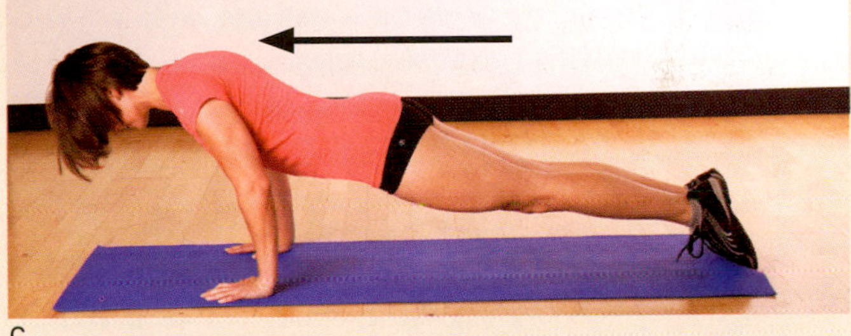
c.

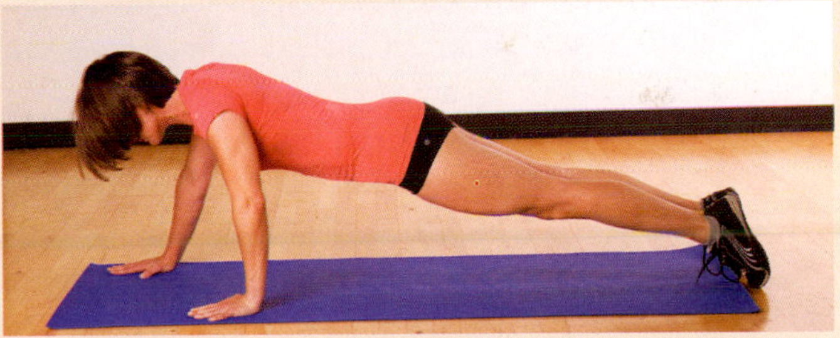
d.

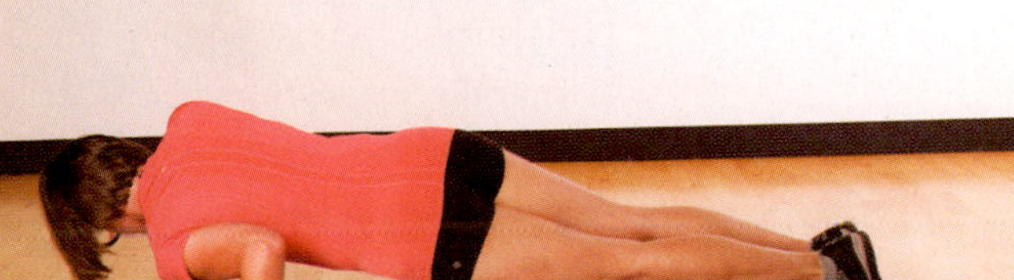
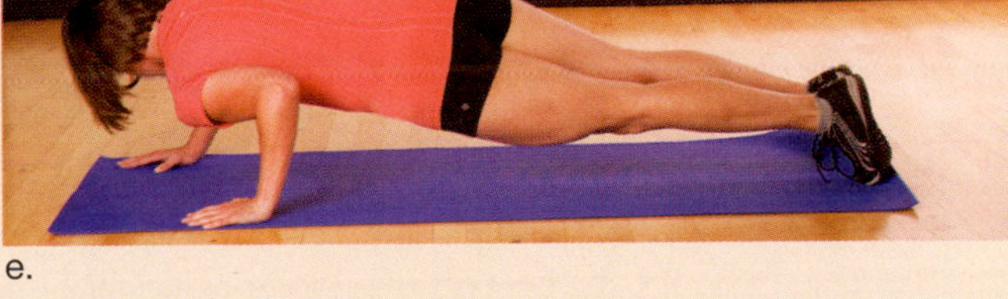
e.

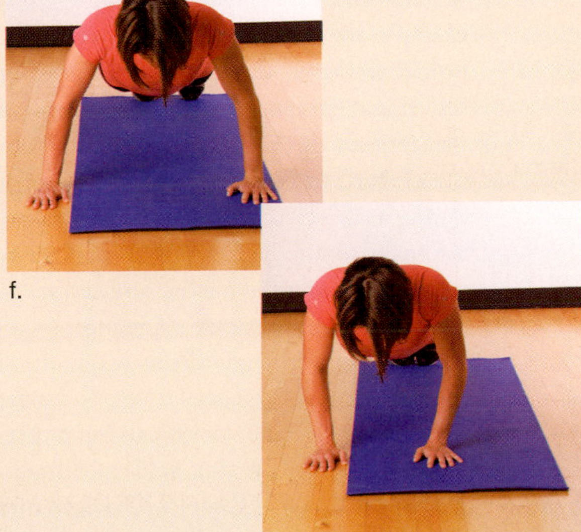
f.

g.

Figure 9-42
Arm roll

Objective: To promote scapular stabilization during dynamic movement

Preparation and position:

- Lie on one side, with the hips and knees in slight flexion. Hold a light dumbbell [5 to 10 lb (2.3 to 4.5 kg)] in the hand of the upper arm.
- Engage the core muscles to stabilize the lumbar spine in the neutral position. Maintain this position throughout the exercise (a).
- Pack the shoulders (see Figure 9-36) and maintain this position throughout the exercise.
- Abduct the arm, holding the dumbbell so that it is perpendicular to the ground.

Exercise:

- Slowly roll forward, bringing the front of the body toward the mat, but keep the arm in the vertical position (b).
- Perform one or two sets of five to 10 repetitions to each side, holding the end position for one or two seconds, allowing 30 seconds of recovery between sets.

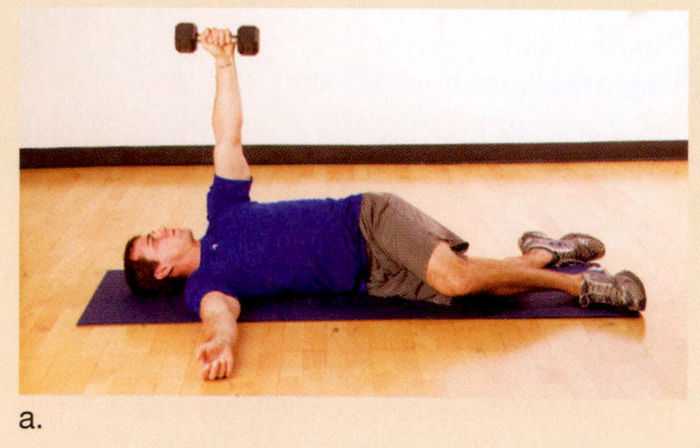
a.

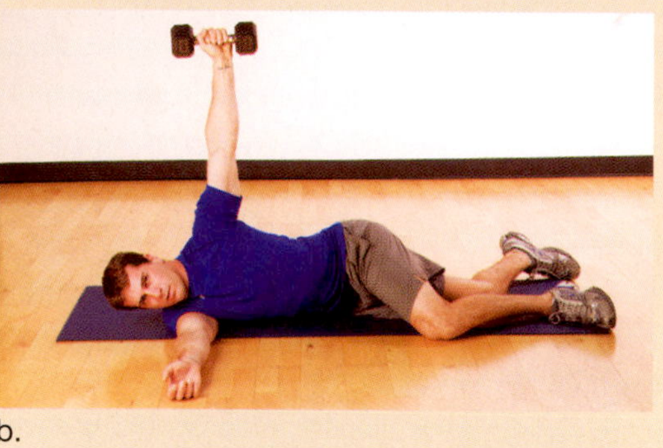
b.

Distal Mobility

Within the distal segments of the body, the gastrocnemius and soleus muscles (triceps surae) are often problematic, exhibiting tightness and limited mobility. During a squatting movement, many individuals demonstrate a lack of adequate ankle **dorsiflexion** and are unable to keep their heels down during the lowering phase. In terms of the structure of the ankle and the relationship of the talus bone to the calcaneus, tightness within the triceps surae or a foot positioned in pronation may often exhibit calcaneal eversion (Gray & Tiberio, 2007). To better understand this point, remove the shoes and stand with the feet shoulder-width apart. Next, force the foot into pronation (collapse the arch of the foot) while observing the outside heel. Notice the slight lifting of the heel off the floor, or calcaneal eversion, as the heel moves out and up. This lifting of the heel promotes shortening of the soleus and gastrocnemius muscles, which will pose problems during a bend-and-lift or squatting movement (Gray & Tiberio, 2007). As a significant number of individuals stand in pronation, the probability of tightness within these muscles is quite high. During the bend and lift movement screen (see page 151), an individual who is unable to keep the heels down will need to improve ankle mobility and calf flexibility, which will promote stability within the foot (if he or she stands in a pronated position).

When a stretch reaches the muscle's limit of flexibility, the likelihood of compensated movement with further stretching increases. When a client is stretching tight calf muscles with a forward lean against a wall, for example, the trainer should be aware of ankle pronation during the stretch. This represents movement compensation, yet may create the perception that the client is stretching the muscle further. To avoid ankle pronation during a calf stretch, the client can either internally rotate the feet slightly or place a small riser under the medial surfaces of each foot (both promote ankle supination).

After reestablishing flexibility within the calf muscles through myofascial release and static stretching techniques, individuals can progress to performing the dynamic ankle mobilization exercise presented in Figure 9-43, which mimics the ankle's role during walking and running activities (Gray & Tiberio, 2007).

Figure 9-43
Standing ankle mobilization

Objective: To promote ankle mobility during a dynamic movement pattern

Preparation and position:
- Remove shoes and stand in front of a wall with the feet placed a few inches apart. Lean forward and support the upper extremity with the arms by placing the hands on the wall while stretching the calf muscles.
- Engage the core muscles to stabilize the lumbar spine in the neutral position. Maintain this position throughout the exercise.

Exercise:
- Slowly lift one foot off the ground, flexing the hip and bending the knee close to 90 degrees.
- While stabilizing the body over the stance leg and continuing to lean forward, swing the raised leg across the front of the body in the transverse plane (a), and then swing that same leg back out in the opposite direction (b).
- Perform one or two sets of five to 10 repetitions with each leg, holding each end position for one or two seconds.

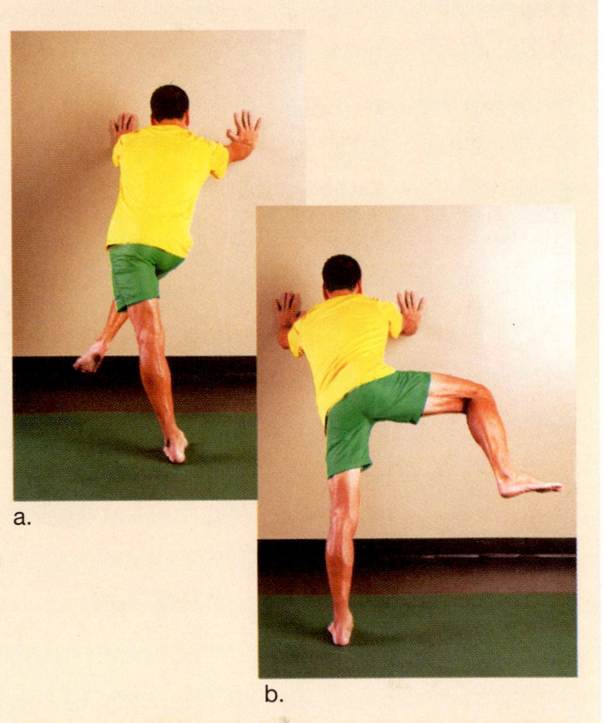
a. b.

Static Balance: Segmental

Movement is essential to complete all **activities of daily living (ADL),** and the ability to move efficiently requires control of the body's postural alignment or balance. Balance is the foundational element of all programming and should be emphasized early in the training program once core function is established and an individual shows improvements in mobility and stability throughout the kinetic chain. Balance not only enhances physical performance, but also contributes to improving the psychological and emotional states by building **self-efficacy** and confidence (Rose, 2003). Balance is subdivided into static balance, or the ability to maintain the body's COM within its BOS, and dynamic balance, or to the ability to move the body's COM outside of its BOS while maintaining postural control and establishing a new BOS (Whiting & Rugg, 2006; Shumway-Cook & Woollacott, 2001).

COM, or **center of gravity (COG),** represents that point around which all weight is evenly distributed (Kendall et al., 2005). It is generally located about 2 inches (5.1 cm) anterior to the spine in the location of the first and second sacral joints (S1 and S2), but varies in individuals by body shape, size, and gender, being slightly higher in males due to greater quantities of musculature in the upper body (Kendall et al., 2005; Rose, 2003). A person's COM constantly shifts as he or she changes position, moves, or adds external resistance (Figure 9-44). BOS is defined as the two-dimensional distance between and beneath the body's points of contact with a surface (Figure 9-45) (Houglum, 2005).

Moving the feet closer together reduces this area, and consequently the BOS, thereby reducing balance control. The body is considered stable when its **line of gravity (LOG)** falls within its BOS. As illustrated in Figure 9-44, the LOG is a theoretical vertical line passing through the COM, dissecting the body into two hemispheres (in the sagittal and **frontal planes**). When the LOG or the COM falls near, or outside of, the BOS, or when one challenges the body's **limits of stability (LOS),** maintaining balance becomes more challenging. LOS is the degree of allowable sway away from the

Figure 9-44
Center of gravity

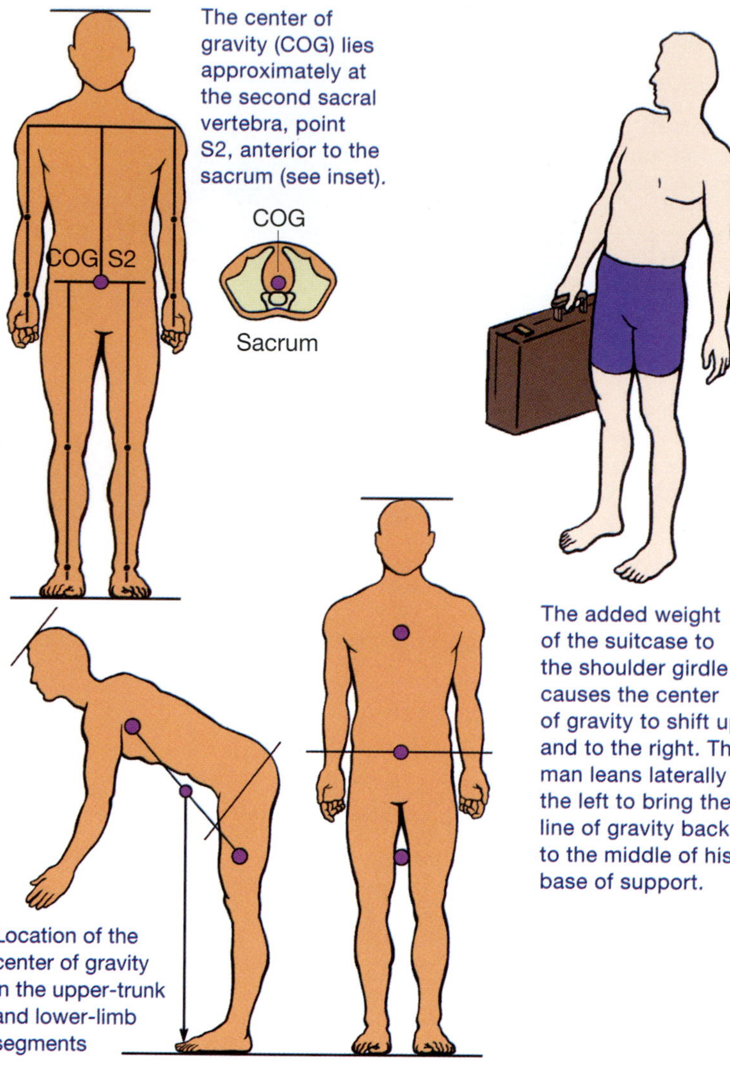

Figure 9-45
A wide base of support allows a wide excursion of the line of gravity (LOG) without permitting it to fall outside the base of support.

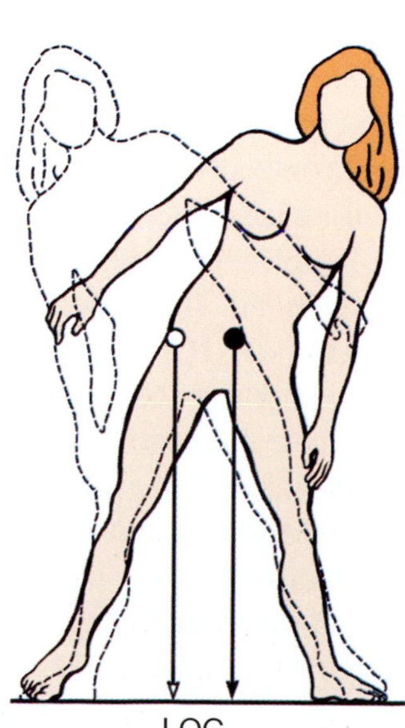

line of gravity that can be tolerated without a need to change the BOS.

After the client performs exercises to reestablish core function, the trainer can introduce static balance training, beginning with segmental or sectional stabilization training (see Figure 9-14). This entails the use of specific static-balance exercises performed over a fixed BOS that impose small balance challenges on the body's core.

- These exercises engage the core musculature (centering, hollowing, or drawing-in) when performing each exercise.
- The exercises are performed in seated positions using stable surfaces (e.g., chair) or unstable surfaces (e.g., Airex® pad or air disc on a chair or stability ball) to impose small challenges to the balance centers.
- The exercises progressively manipulate training variables to challenge the body's balance centers and LOS.
- The exercises are more static in nature, implying that once the balance challenge is imposed, postural control must be maintained for approximately five to 10 seconds.

The client adopts a seated position and engages the core musculature. By following the training guidelines and manipulating the variables and conditions listed in Table 9-3, trainers can gradually progress balance exercises by increasing the balance challenge until the client experiences difficulty in maintaining postural control without falling (Rose, 2003). As each variable or condition is introduced, the trainer may need to remove others temporarily until the client regains postural control (Rose, 2003). Remember, balance is a trainable skill and improvements are evident within a few weeks.

After incorporating the variables and conditions covered in Table 9-3, trainers can introduce two more challenging variables, but only if they are considered appropriate and consistent with the client's goals:

- Reduce the points of contact (e.g., move from balancing on two feet to one foot).

Table 9-3

Training Guidelines for Static Balance

Training Variables	Training Conditions
2–3 times per week Perform exercises toward the beginning of workouts before the onset of fatigue (which decreases concentration) Perform 1 set of 2–4 repetitions, each for 5–10 seconds	Narrow BOS (e.g., wide to narrow) Raise COM (e.g., raising arms overhead) Shift LOG (e.g., raising arms unilaterally, leaning or rotating trunk) Sensory alteration [e.g., shifting focal point to a finger 12 inches (30 cm) in front of one's face, performing slow hand-eye tracking, or performing slow head movements such as looking up and down] Sensory removal (e.g., closing eyes)

Note: BOS = Base of support; COM = Center of mass; LOG = Line of gravity

- Add additional unstable surfaces (e.g., foot placement on Airex pad, foam roller, air discs, or medicine ball).

Trainers should introduce each of these challenges separately, gradually increasing the exercise difficulty by manipulating the variables and conditions provided in Table 9-3 under this new challenge. Next, trainers can introduce the second challenge in a similar manner (e.g., move to one foot and reintroduce the variables listed in Table 9-3 before implementing additional unstable surfaces, which should be introduced with two feet).

Static Balance: Integrated (Standing)

The natural progression from seated exercises is to standing exercises, thereby integrating the entire kinetic chain, which represents more function and mimics many ADL. During integrated movements, the effects of external loads, gravity, and reactive forces all increase, thereby necessitating a greater need to stabilize the spine. McGill (2004) introduced the concept of bracing discussed previously, explaining how it improves spinal stability by providing a wider BOS.

To teach a client how to brace, a trainer can simply have the client stand in a relaxed position and engage the core muscles. The client can then imagine a person standing in front of him or her who is about to deliver a quick jab to the stomach. In anticipation of the jab, the individual should stiffen up the trunk region by co-contracting both layers of muscles. This represents bracing, which, unlike centering that acts reflexively, is a conscious contraction used for short time periods during external loading on the spine (e.g., when performing a weighted squat or picking up a box).

The trainer can introduce standing static-balance training on stable surfaces before progressing to static unstable (e.g., Airex pad, BOSU®, iStep®) or dynamic unstable surfaces (e.g., Coretex®), both of which gradually increase the balance challenge. While the ground and many unstable, static balance-training devices are considered proactive (i.e., where one can generally anticipate balance needs), there are also dynamic, unstable devices that are considered reactive and can be utilized to train balance (i.e., where the body has to react to the changing surface). These surfaces obviously offer a greater challenge to training balance. Both forms of training are important to developing efficiency within the proprioceptive (somatosensory), vestibular, and ocular (visual) systems, but the decision regarding which training surfaces to use depends primarily on the client's needs and goals. Regardless, all balance exercises should ultimately incorporate some form of dynamic balance training on stable surfaces (e.g., movement on the ground) to mimic ADL. When designing static balance-training programs, trainers should follow the stance-position progressions illustrated in Figure 9-46. The trainer should identify which stance position challenges the client's balance threshold and then repeat the exercises outlined in Table 9-3.

Although the single-leg stance represents the final stance position, trainers should delay introducing balance exercises in this position until the next training phase, after the client has learned how to correctly perform a single-leg stand. Failure to do so may only promote further dysfunctional or compensated movement.

While phase 1 (stability and mobility training) includes some static-balance training (segmental and static whole-body stabilization), it is during the next level of training (phase 2: movement training) that the entire kinetic chain is integrated into more dynamic movement. During this phase, the dynamic nature of the movement patterns, especially when adding external resistance, will demand a greater need for bracing.

Phase 2: Movement Training

As discussed previously, technology continues to advance the complexity of exercise equipment and many of the exercises people perform. This appears to be advancing the concept of "dysfunctional fitness," where individuals, many of whom are deconditioned and have poor posture, demonstrate compensated movement. This increases the likelihood for musculoskeletal overload and the potential for pain and injury (see Figure 9-7).

Human movement can essentially be broken down into five primary movements that encompass all ADL. Movements can be as simple as one primary movement or as complex as the integration of several of them into a single motion. The five primary movements are as follows:

- Bend-and-lift movements (e.g., squatting)
- Single-leg movements (e.g., single-leg stance and lunging)
- Pushing movements (primarily in the vertical/horizontal planes)
- Pulling movements (primarily in the vertical/horizontal planes)
- Rotational (spiral) movements

For example, a woman picking up her child, then turning to place the child in a highchair for dinner, performs the following: a bend-and-lift movement; a rotational movement; a single-leg movement to walk; a pushing movement while extending her arms to place her child in the highchair; and a pulling movement to resist gravity while lowering her child into the highchair. A track-and-field athlete executing a shot put performs the following: bend-and-lift and rotation movements coupled with a pushing movement while coming out of his or her explosive stance; and a single-leg movement to slow down after the release.

What is universal to all clients is the need to train these movement patterns as a prerequisite to all exercises. In essence, if a client can perform these five primary movements effectively and possesses the appropriate levels of stability and mobility throughout the kinetic chain, it improves his or her potential for efficient movement and decreases the likelihood for compensation, pain, or injury (Gray & Tiberio, 2007). This phase of training follows stability and mobility training and involves teaching patterns for these five movements, using body weight as resistance and the **levers** within the body (e.g., the arms) as drivers to increase exercise intensity (Gray & Tiberio, 2007).

The timeframe needed to successfully train these movements depends on individual differences, including current conditioning level, past experiences, body type, abilities, attitudes, motivational levels, emotional make-up, learning styles, and maturation levels (Schmidt & Wrisberg, 2007).

Figure 9-46
Stance-position progressions

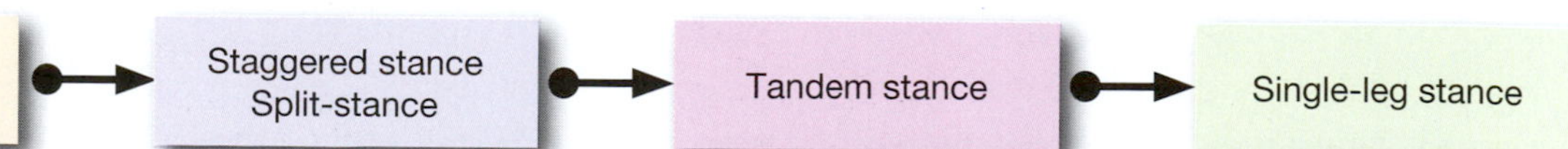

Although these movements are teachable, trainers should differentiate between abilities and skills when establishing the timeframes needed to teach movement patterns. Abilities are inherited traits that are stable and enduring, and underlie the performance of many skills, whereas skills are developed and modified with practice (Schmidt & Wrisberg, 2007). While two to four weeks is usually adequate, trainers might need to exercise patience and devote extra time when teaching these movement patterns.

Before teaching the movement patterns, it is also important to understand certain **kinematics** within the body, specifically within the lower extremity, to understand the logic behind some of the exercises presented here. An important relationship exists among the ankle, knee, and hip. During the heel-strike instant of gait, chain reactions originating from the ankle dissipate forces upward through the knee and beyond. To help tolerate these forces, the foot normally moves into pronation as a person bears weight onto that foot. Pronation forces internal rotation of the tibia, which in turn drives the femur into a greater and faster internal rotation (Figure 9-47) (Gray & Tiberio, 2007). To better understand this point, perform a basic movement pattern with shoes off. Stand comfortably with the feet hip-width apart and place the palms of the hands on the fronts of the upper thighs, and then slowly pronate (collapse inward) and supinate (roll outward) the ankles. Observe how both the tibia and femur rotate during the ankle movements by watching the directional movements of the hands.

The different rate and degree of internal rotation between the femur and tibia places stresses on the medial surface of the knee and forces the knee into abduction, also known as **valgus** stress. To demonstrate this point, walk a few steps slowly, observing how the knee collapses slightly inward as weight is loaded onto a particular leg. This increases the strain placed on the **anterior cruciate ligament (ACL),** given its orientation. The ACL connects from a posterior-lateral part of the femur to an anterior-medial part of the tibia within the knee joint, is a very important stabilizer of the femur on the tibia during knee extension, and prevents the tibia from sliding forward (anterior translation) and rotating excessively inward during walking (Kendall et al., 2005). While the body is designed to resist this stress by having a large **medial collateral ligament (MCL)** on the medial surface of the knee, a key mechanism to protect the knee is directly related to a group of powerful and large

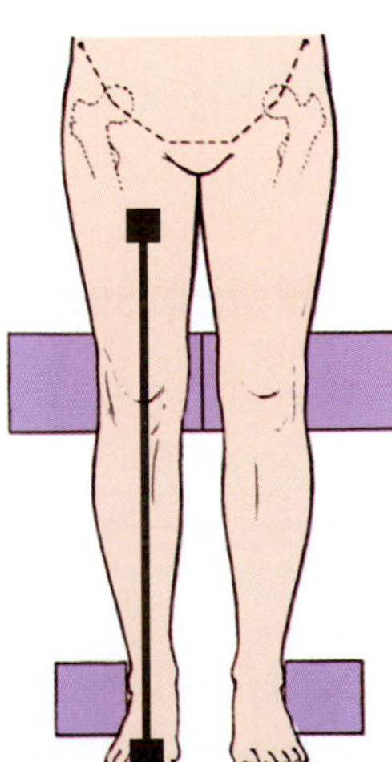
Neutral subtalar position with neutral knee alignment

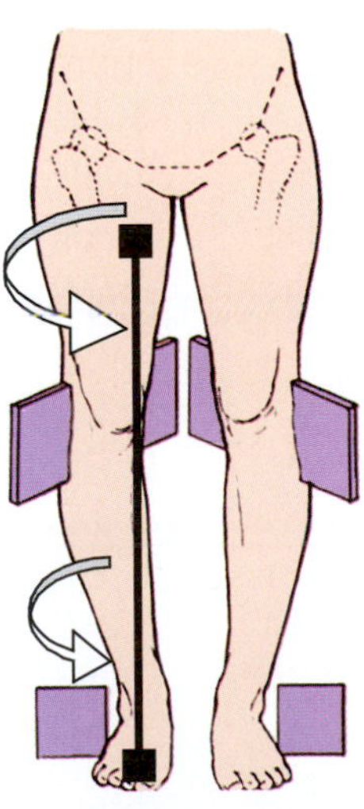
Pronation with internal rotation of the knee

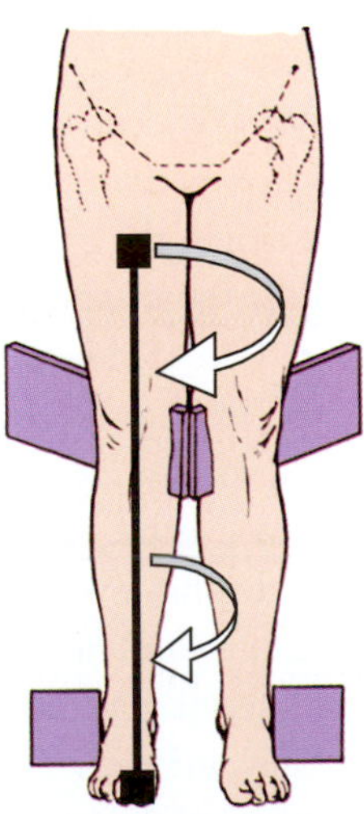
Supination with external rotation of the knee

Figure 9-47
Ankle pronation and supination and the effects up the kinetic chain

Source: LifeART image copyright 2008 Wolters Kluwer Health, Inc., Lippincott Williams & Wilkins. All rights reserved.

posterior-lateral muscles at the hips, the gluteal group, that functions to decelerate internal hip rotation. When walking, gluteal activity is critical to decelerate the internal rotation associated with each step. Since a common postural deviation is to stand in pronation, there is concern that a lack of adequate gluteal activity may fail to protect the integrity of the knee as this muscle becomes lengthened and weakened. To illustrate this point, repeat the previous exercise, but place the hands over the gluteus maximus, and notice how the gluteus maximus alternates between being active and relaxed during the rotation (contracting concentrically during supination and relaxing during pronation). An individual demonstrating excessive foot pronation during standing may lengthen this muscle and weaken it.

The gluteals also play an important role in the bend-and-lift movement, during which individuals exhibit either "glute dominance" or "quad dominance."

- *Glute dominance:* This implies reliance on eccentrically loading the gluteus maximus during a squat (bend-and-lift) movement. The first 10 to 15 degrees of the downward phase are initiated by pushing the hips backward, creating a hip-hinge movement. In the lowered position, this maximizes the eccentric loading on the gluteus maximus to generate significant force during the upward, concentric phase.
- *Quad dominance:* This implies reliance on loading the quadriceps group during a squat (bend-and-lift) movement. The first 10 to 15 degrees of the downward phase are initiated by driving the tibia forward, creating shearing forces across the knee as the femur slides over the tibia. In this lowered position, the gluteus maximus does not eccentrically load and cannot generate much force during the upward phase. Quad-dominant individuals transfer more pressure into the knees, placing greater loads on the ACL (Wilthrow et al., 2005).

Glute dominance also helps activate the hamstrings, which pull on the posterior surface of the tibia and help unload the ACL to protect it from potential injury (Hauschildt, 2008). To better understand this point, a trainer can place his or her hands on the hamstrings and perform the following two movements:

- Perform a quad-dominant squat and feel for any tension development in the hamstrings.
- Perform a glute-dominant squat and feel for any tension development in the hamstrings. The trainer should feel increased tension during this squat, indicating an eccentric load placed on the hamstrings that helps stabilize the knee.

While these mechanics are important to preserving the integrity of the knee, they are even more critical to women given their larger **Q-angle** (the angle formed by the longitudinal axis of the femur and the line of pull of the patellar ligament), increased joint **laxity** associated with **hormones** (e.g., **estrogen**), smaller ligaments and surface area for attachment, and weaker muscles (Gary & Tiberio, 2007; Houglum, 2005; Kendall et al., 2005).

Trainers should also consider the issue of weight transference onto the stance-leg during gait. As the body moves to accept weight onto one leg, this requires a weight shift over the stance-leg while preserving optimal alignment among the hip, knee, and foot. This weight transference normally involves a 1- to 2-inch (2.5- to 5.1-cm) lateral shift of the hips over the stance-leg, coupled with a small change in hip angle, tilting that hip upward by approximately 4 to 5 degrees (i.e., hip adduction) (Whiting & Rugg, 2006). In Figure 9-48a, the line of gravity passes vertically through the vertebrae and sacrum, whereas in Figure 9-48b, the right hip is elevated (as it would be during gait when one accepts weight onto the right leg). The line of gravity now passes through the midline at an angle following the angle of the vertebrae and sacrum, shifting the LOG toward the right femur.

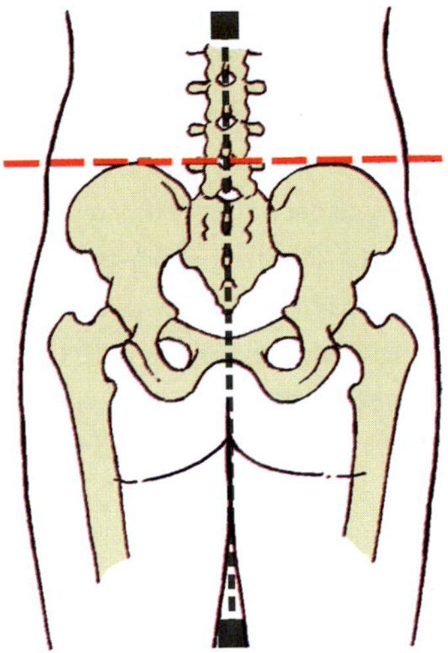
a. Normal hip position

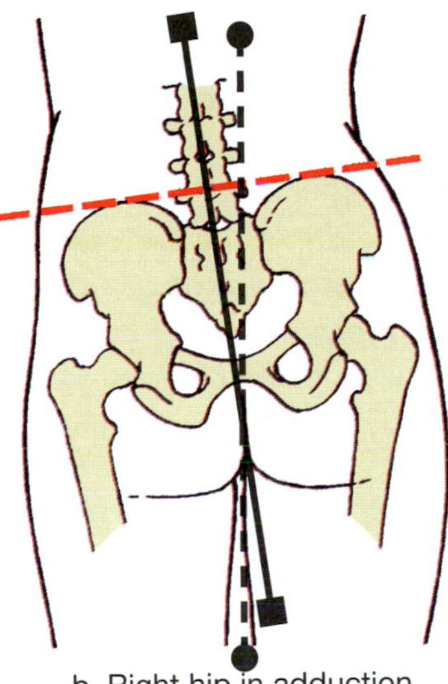
b. Right hip in adduction

Figure 9-48
Normal hip position versus right hip adduction (posterior view)

Source: LifeART image copyright 2008 Wolters Kluwer Health, Inc., Lippincott Williams & Wilkins. All rights reserved.

As the right hip and femur are positioned closer to the midline, they are classified as moving into adduction. This movement involves the collaborative actions of the right gluteal group to control excessive hip adduction (the lateral shift) and the left quadratus lumborum to prevent excessive hip tilting (by holding the left hip up). Weakness in any of these muscle groups can create potential knee issues by allowing excessive hip adduction that increases the Q-angle and places stress on the ACL and medial knee structures.

Bend-and-lift Patterns

The bend-and-lift movement associated with the squat is perhaps one of the most prevalent activities used in strength training and throughout most individuals' ADL, yet this movement is subject to much controversy given its potential for harm to the knees and low back. Faulty movement patterns associated with poor technique will disrupt muscle function and joint loading, compromising performance and ultimately leading to overload and potential injury (Kendall et al., 2005, Sahrmann, 2002). Proper technique is therefore the key differentiator. One limiting factor to good technique is a lack of ankle mobility, which, according to Kendall et al. (2005), is normally between 15 and 20 degrees of ankle dorsiflexion. To evaluate this limitation, the trainer can have the client place one foot on a low riser [<12 inches (30 cm)], positioning the tibia perpendicular to the floor. The client leans slowly forward, dorsiflexing the ankle until the heel lifts off the floor or the ankle falls into pronation. The trainer can then determine the degree of motion achieved. Mobility of less than 15 degrees merits a need to improve ankle flexibility prior to teaching the full bend-and-lift movement.

While the hips typically exhibit between 100 and 135 degrees of flexion, the amount of hip flexion required during a squat averages approximately 95 degrees (Hemmerich et al., 2006; Kendall et al., 2005). Hence, it is important to shift the pelvis posteriorly during the downward phase to facilitate adequate hip flexion. The hip-hinge exercise discussed later in this section teaches clients how to shift their hips backward, not only to promote additional hip flexion, but more importantly to reduce the shearing forces across the knee joint.

During a squat movement, the inability to stabilize the lumbar spine or maintain a straight or slightly extended thoracic spine increases compressive and shear forces on the lumbar vertebrae (McGill, 2004; Broomfield, 1998). When a client lacks adequate mobility in the thoracic spine, what frequently occurs is a movement compensation that involves increased lumbar extension (increased lordosis).

Squatting (with external loads) with excessive lumbar extension dramatically increases the compressive forces on the lumbar spine (Walsh et al., 2007). A 2-degree increase in lumbar extension from neutral can increase compressive forces on the vertebral discs by 16% over a neutral spine (Walsh et al., 2007). The pelvic tilts and back alignment and figure-4 exercises discussed later in this section promote optimal spinal alignment.

The bend-and-lift maneuver begins with a solid platform of good posture and bracing of the abdominal region (when using external loads). As the exercises in this training phase (phase 2, movement training) utilize body weight as the only form of resistance, bracing may not be necessary, but trainers should remind clients to brace the core when lifting external loads. The movement-training sequence presented in Figures 9-49 through 9-52 follows the **part-to-whole teaching strategy.**

Throughout their daily activities, people often find themselves bending down to lift objects off the floor, and rarely do they use proper dead-lift technique. Split- or staggered-stance positions, internal or external foot rotation, and even variations in arm position are common. Considering that these variations represent most individuals' daily movements, clients should be trained functionally to mimic these patterns. Therefore, once a client demonstrates proficiency with the bend-and-lift movement, progress the movement patterns to incorporating variations in foot position coupled with various arm movements (Figure 9-53). From a standpoint of functionality, people normally bend down to lift objects with their hands by their sides, so trainers should teach these variations beginning with the most simplistic position (i.e., arms at the sides) prior to moving into high-arm positions (e.g., front squat, back squat, or overhead positions). Keep in mind that these high-arm positions require a greater degree of thoracic mobility, which many clients may lack. Trainers should teach the bend and lift in the dead-lift position first (i.e., arms at sides), before introducing the front-squat position and then the back and overhead positions.

Figure 9-49
Hip-hinge

Objective: To emphasize "glute dominance" over "quad dominance" during the initial 10 to 15 degrees of movement

Preparation and position:

- Stand in a neutral stance position with the feet hip-width apart and place a light bar or dowel along the back that makes contact with the head, thoracic spine, and sacrum (three-point contact).
- Hold the bar above the head in one hand and around the low-back region with the other hand.
- Engage the core muscles to stabilize the lumbar spine in the neutral position and maintain this position throughout the exercise (a).

Exercise:

- While pressing the dowel into the three points, slowly perform a forward bend, pushing the hips backward with slight knee flexion, while maintaining contact with the dowel on all three points at all times (b).
- The goal is to emphasize moving backward while minimizing the downward movement of the hips toward the floor.
- Perform one to three sets of 15 repetitions.

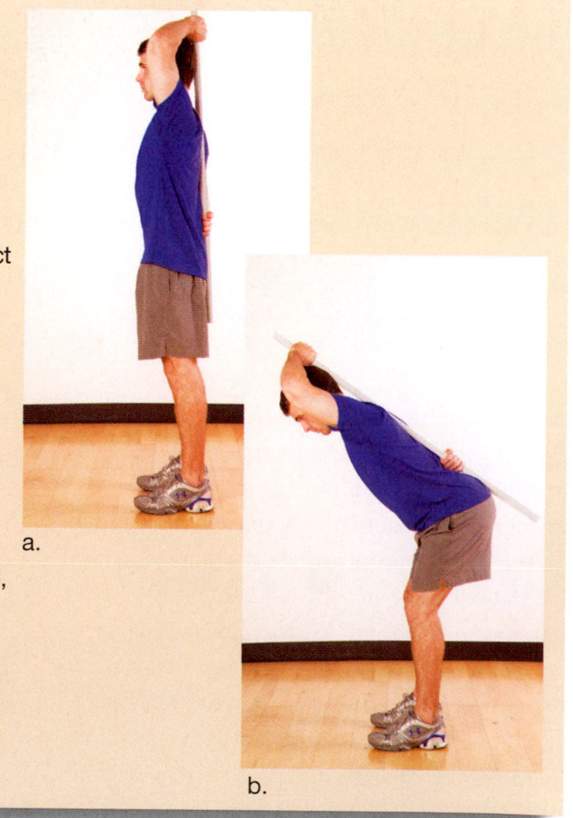
a.
b.

Figure 9-50
Pelvic tilts and back alignment

Objective: To promote pelvic control and lumbar stability throughout the lowering phase

Preparation and position:

- Stand in a neutral position with the feet hip-width apart, and, with the hands on the upper thighs, hip-hinge 10 to 15 degrees (not shown).
- Engage the core muscles to stabilize the lumbar spine in the neutral position.

Exercise:

- While holding this position, perform a series of pelvic tilts, changing the low-back position between flexion (rounding) and extension (arching).
- Perform one or two sets of five to 10 repetitions, holding each end position for one to two seconds.
- Move the hands down to rest on the knees, dropping deeper into the bend, and perform the same number of repetitions (a & b).
- Lower the body further, resting the elbows on the lower thighs and perform the same number of repetitions.
- Lower the hands toward the floor or to a low riser [<12 inches (30 cm)] and perform the same number of repetitions.
- Lower the hands to the floor to touch the underside of the front of the feet or shoes. (*Note:* Some heavier clients may not be physically able to achieve this position.) Once this position is achieved, perform full repetitions pushing through the heels to a full standing position, then return to this lowered position. Perform the same number of repetitions.

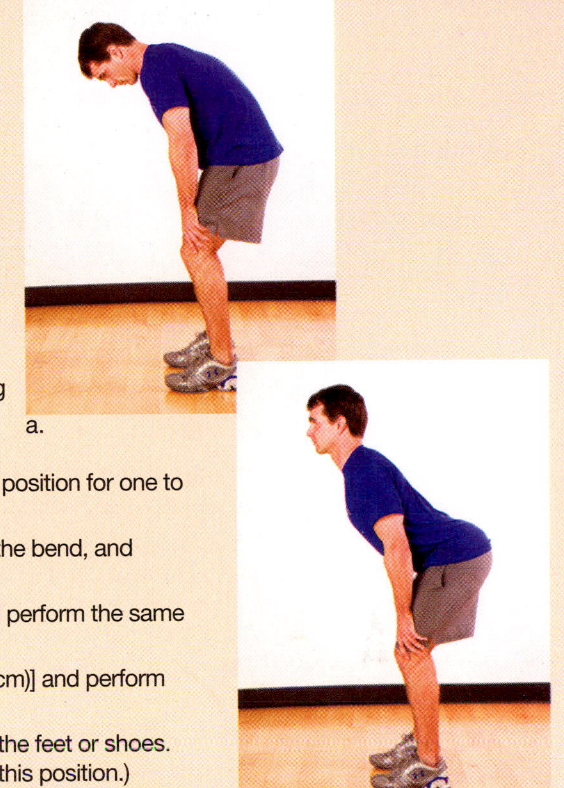
a.
b.

Figure 9-51
Lower-extremity alignment

Note: Based on the bend and lift screen (see page 151), trainers can determine the need to strengthen the hip abductors or adductors.

Objective: To promote alignment among the hips, knees, and feet during a bend-and-lift movement

Preparation and position:

- Start seated in a chair, aligning the anterior superior iliac spine (ASIS) with the knee and second toe.
- Clients who need to strengthen the hip adductors can place a soft squeezable ball between the knees (a).
- Clients who need to strengthen the hip abductors can wrap an elastic band around the knees (b).
- Engage the core muscles to stabilize the lumbar spine in the neutral position and maintain this position throughout the exercise.

Exercise:

- Perform one or two sets of five to 10 contractions, holding each contraction in the specific direction for one or two seconds.

Progression: Hold the isometric contraction while standing up out of the chair to full-standing position and returning into the chair. Perform one or two sets of 10 repetitions, holding the contraction in the specific direction throughout the movement.

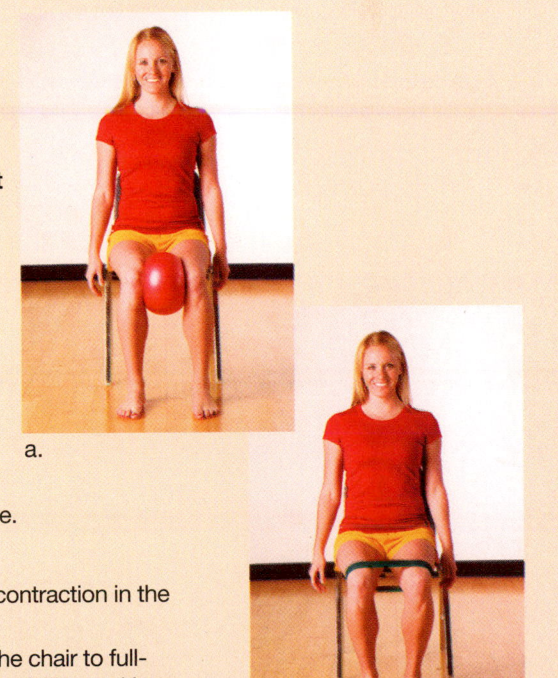
a.
b.

Figure 9-52
Figure-4 position

Objective: To promote optimal alignment between the trunk and tibia, as well as optimal position of the spine

Preparation and position:

- Start in the standing position adjacent to a mirror, with a low bench or chair behind if needed. Keep the feet hip-width apart, shoulders packed (see Figure 9-36), head neutral, and weight distributed toward the heels.
- Engage the core muscles to stabilize the lumbar spine in the neutral position and maintain this position throughout the exercise.

Exercise:

- Hip-hinge and drop into a squat, ideally lowering the body to an end-range where the thighs are parallel to the floor or the fingertips touch the floor. Use a higher position if experiencing difficulty in squatting to this depth.
- Using a pair of plastic or wooden dowels, the trainer can evaluate the alignment of the tibia against the torso. The goal is to achieve parallel between the two body segments while achieving the desired squat depth (figure-4 position) (a & b).
- With consent from the client and using both visual (mirror) and kinesthetic feedback (touch), the trainer can coach the client to parallel.
- If the tibia is too vertical, the trainer can slowly cue the client to shift forward by raising the heels.
- If the torso is too flat, the trainer can cue the client to raise the entire torso toward vertical from the hips by first stabilizing the lumbar and thoracic spine, then extending the entire torso as a unit. Clients must avoid only extending the thoracic spine, which hyperextends the low back.
- Trainers can continue coaching the client with tibia and torso adjustments until the desired parallel position is achieved.

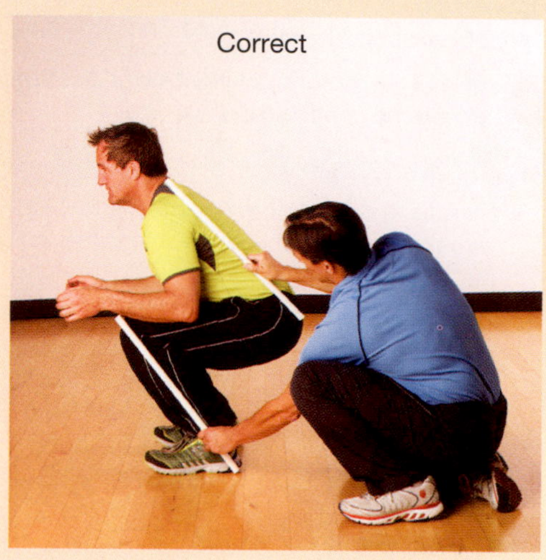
Correct

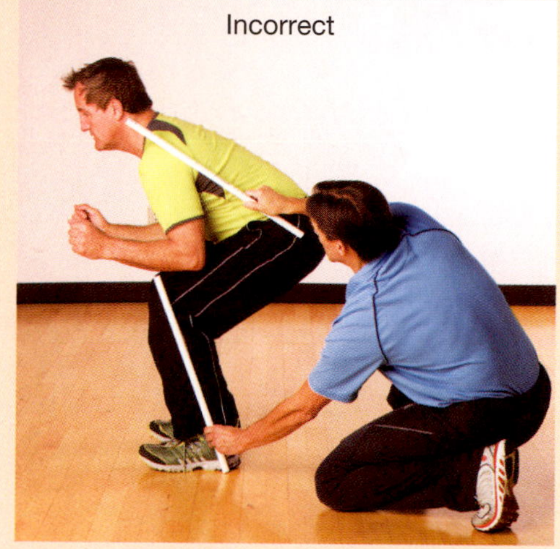
Incorrect

Figure 9-53
Squat variations

Note: Trainers should progress to these exercises only when a client demonstrates good technique with a standard squat.

Objective: To promote stability and mobility throughout the kinetic chain with variations of the standard squat movement

Preparation and position:

- Start in the standing (neutral) position with the feet hip-width apart, but vary the position of the feet as follows:
  - ✓ *Staggered stance:* Right or left foot forward (a)
  - ✓ *Internal rotation:* Right or left foot rotated inward from neutral (always maintain knee alignment over the second toe) (b)
  - ✓ *External rotation:* Right or left foot rotated outward from neutral (always maintain knee alignment over the second toe) (c)
- Engage the core muscles to stabilize the lumbar spine in the neutral position. Maintain this position throughout the exercise.

Exercise:

- Hip-hinge and drop into a squat, ideally lowering the body to an end-range where the thighs are parallel with the floor or where the fingertips touch the floor.
- Perform one to three sets of 10 to 15 repetitions at a controlled tempo, varying foot positions.

Progressions: Adding the arms as drivers (bilaterally or unilaterally) increases the exercise intensity and the need for additional stability and mobility along the kinetic chain. For example, begin by driving the arms toward the floor during the lowering phase prior to driving the arms in all three planes with a high-arm position.

- Add the following drivers:
  - ✓ *Sagittal plane:* Drive both arms toward the floor or toward the ceiling during the lowering phase (d).
  - ✓ *Frontal plane:* Drive both arms to either side (lateral lean) during the lowering phase (e).
  - ✓ *Transverse plane:* Drive both arms in rotation to either side during the lowering phase (f).

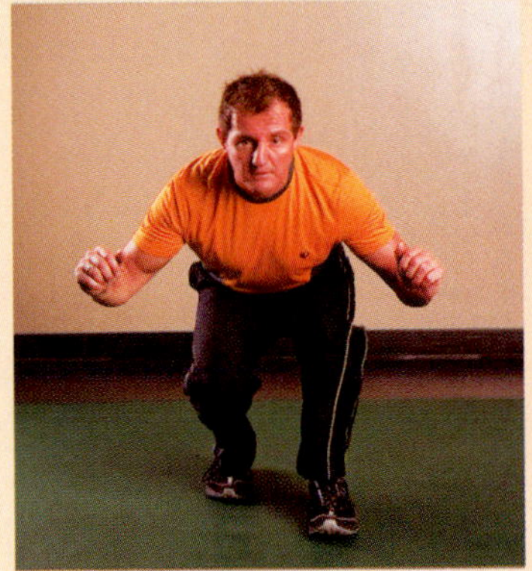

a.

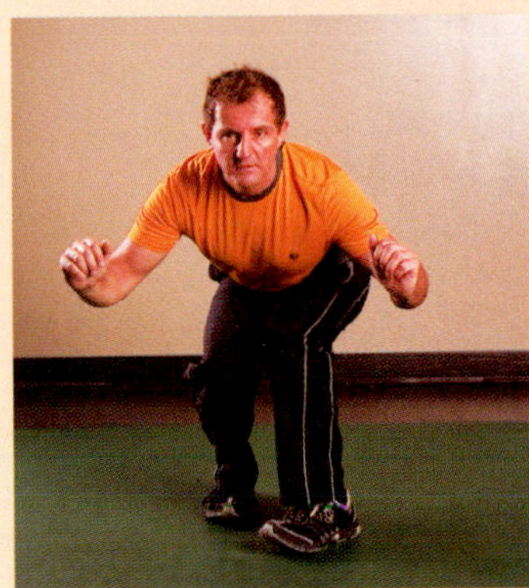

b.

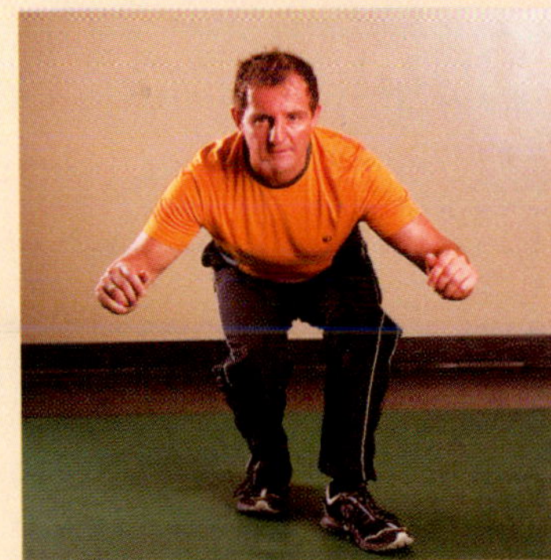

c.

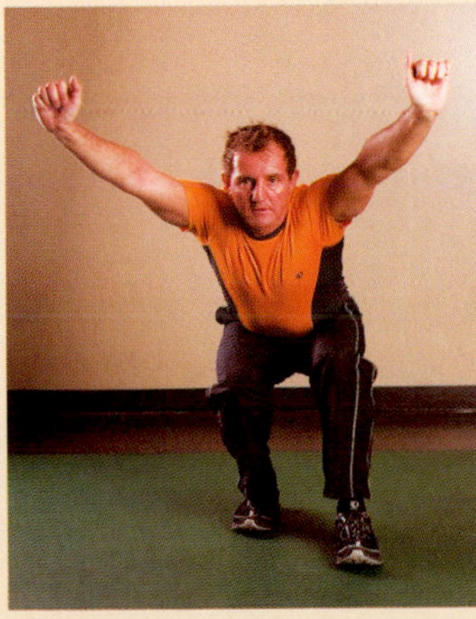

d.

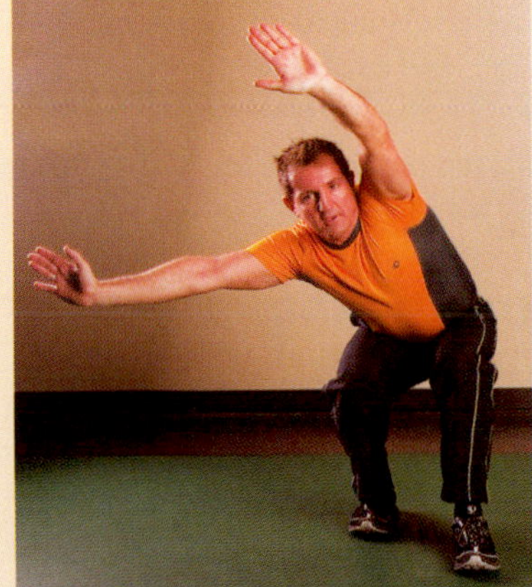

e.

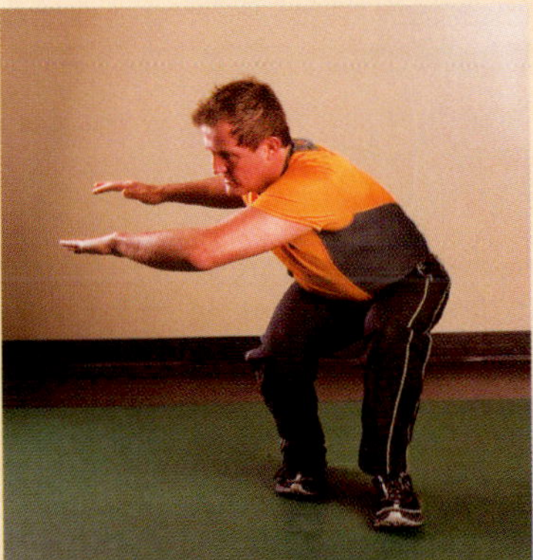

f.

Single-leg Stand Patterns

While most individuals can stand on a single leg, there is the possibility that they achieve this position with some form of compensation. As identified with the hurdle step screen (see page 153), standing efficiently on a single leg mandates stability in the stance-leg, hip, and torso, while simultaneously exhibiting mobility in the raised leg if stepping is involved. Weakness in the hip abductors reflects an inability to control lateral hip shift, placing additional stress on the knee. Clients should first strengthen these muscles in isolation (e.g., side-lying leg raise) before integrating full-body, weightbearing movements. Before learning any single-leg movements (e.g., lunges), clients should learn how to effectively control hip adduction. Ultimately, individuals should demonstrate control of this lateral shift during gait, where the feet are positioned approximately 3.0 to 3.5 inches (7.6 to 8.9 cm) apart. However, trainers should teach this exercise from a feet-together position before progressing to the normal gait-width distance (Figure 9-54).

Figure 9-54

Single-leg stands

Objective: To promote stability within the stance-leg and hip during a single-leg stand

Preparation and position:

- The trainer hangs a plumb line from the ceiling or high fixed point, attaching a small weighted object (e.g., washer, nut) to the other end and suspending it 1 to 2 inches (2.5 to 5.1 cm) from the floor.
- Stand facing a mirror with feet together, positioning the right hip immediately adjacent to the plumb line (the plumb line should lightly touch the right hip).
- Engage the core muscles to stabilize the lumbar spine in the neutral position and maintain this position throughout the exercise (a).

Exercise:

- Hip-hinge 10 to 15 degrees, transferring the body weight into the heels.
- Contract the adductor and abductor muscle groups in the left thigh, then slowly raise the right heel 1 inch (2.5 cm) off the floor (do not raise the entire foot yet) (b).
- Briefly hold this position, then slowly unload the entire foot, lifting it 1 to 3 inches (2.5 to 7.6 cm) off the floor while watching the hip position in the mirror. Attempt to control the lateral hip shift away from the plumb line (to the right). The goal is to prevent the space that appears between the line and hips from exceeding 2 inches (5.1 cm) [smaller individuals should aim for approximately 1 inch (2.5 cm) of space, while taller individuals should aim for 2 inches (5.1 cm)].
- Briefly hold this position, then slowly extend the hips and stand vertically, again controlling the spacing. The torso should not move and the stance-leg should remain stable.
- Perform one or two sets of five to 10 repetitions per leg, resting for 30 seconds between sets. Repeat with the opposite leg.

Progression: Perform a leg swing to mimic gait (i.e., from the hip-hinge position, swing the leg with each standing vertical stand) (c & d).

Progression: Repeat the same exercise with the feet positioned at the normal gait-width distance.

Note: This exercise can be performed without a plumb line if one is not available.

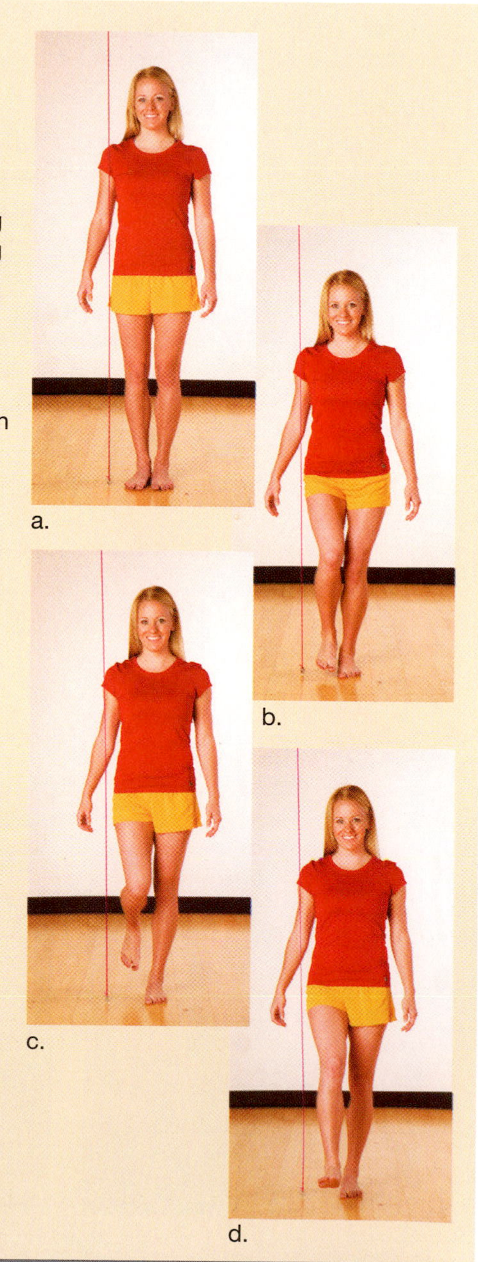

a. b. c. d.

Static Balance on a Single Leg

Once an individual demonstrates the ability to effectively stand on one leg, the trainer can introduce dynamic movements of the upper and lower extremity over a static base of support. Next, the trainer can introduce various forms of resistance (e.g., medicine balls, cables, or bands) that increase the stabilization demands and the potential need for bracing during movement. This is where the trainer's creativity in programming becomes important—to heighten the fun factor. Trainers can be creative, but should always exercise common sense and keep the drills and exercises skill- and conditioning-level appropriate, and purposeful. The basic, but very functional, series of movement patterns presented in Table 9-4 and Figure 9-55 is based off the Balance Matrix created by Gary Gray, and

Table 9-4

Dynamic Movement Patterns Over a Static Base of Support

Introduce upper-extremity movements • Movements: ✓ Arms can move unilaterally (one arm at a time) ✓ Arms can move bilaterally (both arms move together) ✓ Arms can move reciprocally (alternating arm directions) ✓ Position the feet in any stance indicated in Figure 9-46 (except single-leg stance) • Directions: ✓ Move arm(s) in the sagittal plane (flexion/extension) ✓ Move arm(s) in the frontal plane (lateral flexion from an overhead position) ✓ Move arm(s) in the transverse plane (rotation from the shoulder-height position with a bent elbow)	**Perform the following:** • 1–2 sets of 10–20 repetitions per side • Slow, controlled tempos [avoid bouncing at the end-ROM—the transition zone between movement in one direction and movement in another direction (also known as the transformational zone)] • <30-second rest intervals between sets
Introduce lower-extremity movements • Movements: ✓ Assume a single-leg stand ✓ Start by swinging the leg forward and backward, touching the toes to the floor at each end-ROM (transformational zone), then progress to unsupported leg swings. • Directions: ✓ Move the leg in the sagittal plane (flexion/extension) ✓ Move the leg in the frontal plane (abduction/adduction) ✓ Move the leg in the transverse plane (rotation in front or behind the stance leg)	**Perform the following:** • 1–2 sets of 10–20 repetitions per side • Slow, controlled tempos (avoid bouncing at the end-ROM—the transformational zone) • <30-second rest intervals between sets
Integrate upper- and lower-extremity movements: • Move limbs ipsilaterally (same side) or contralaterally (opposite side) • Move limbs "in synch"—moving in the same direction (e.g., the leg and arm move forward together) • Move limbs "out of synch"—moving in opposite directions	**Perform the following:** • 1–2 sets of 10–20 repetitions per side • Slow, controlled tempos (avoid bouncing at the end-ROM—the transformational zone) • <30-second rest intervals between sets

Note: ROM = Range of motion

Figure 9-55
Dynamic movement patterns

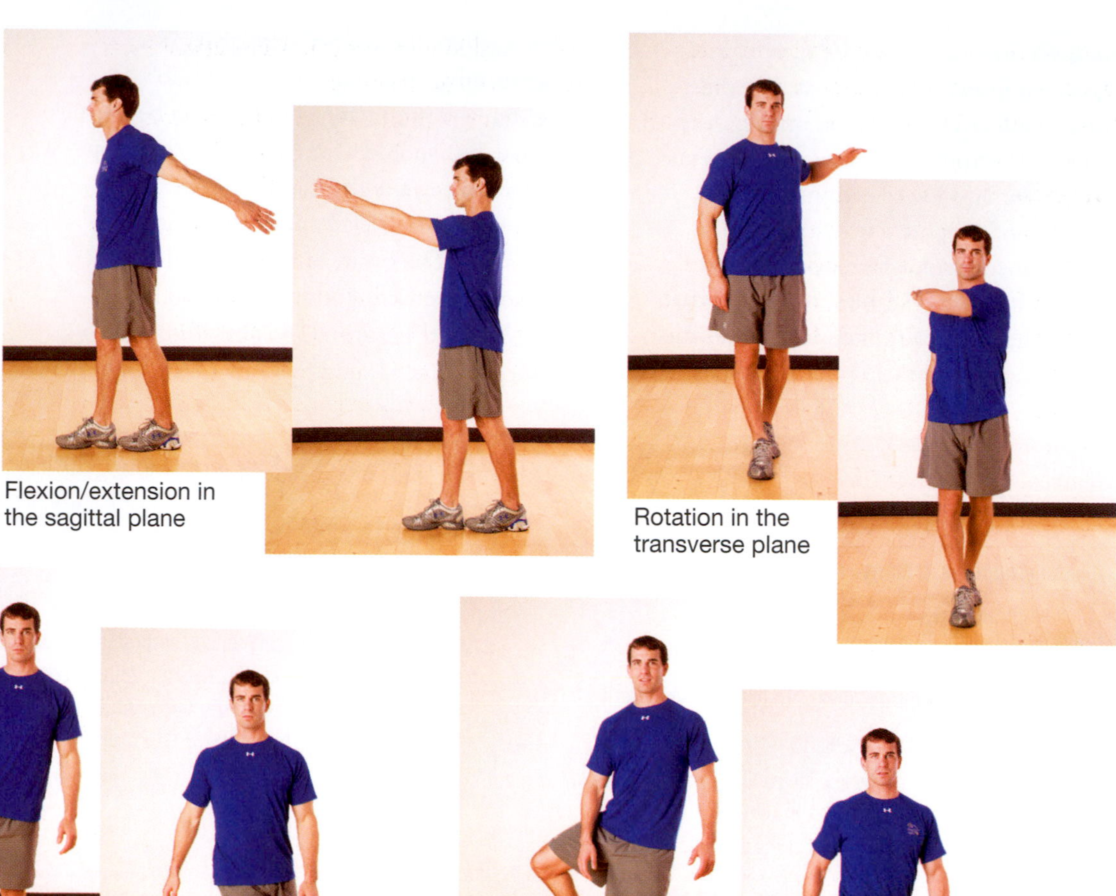
Flexion/extension in the sagittal plane

Rotation in the transverse plane

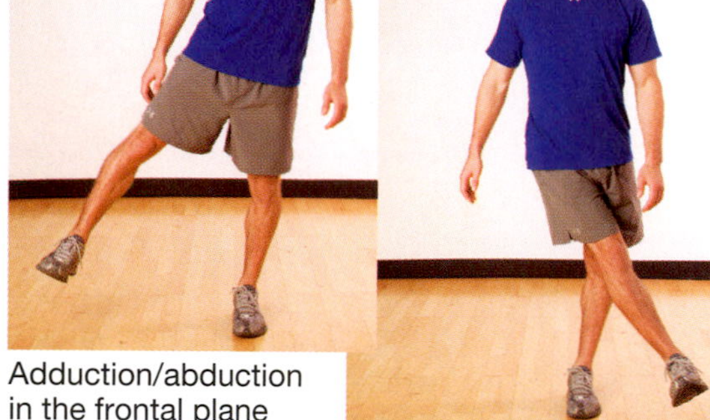
Adduction/abduction in the frontal plane

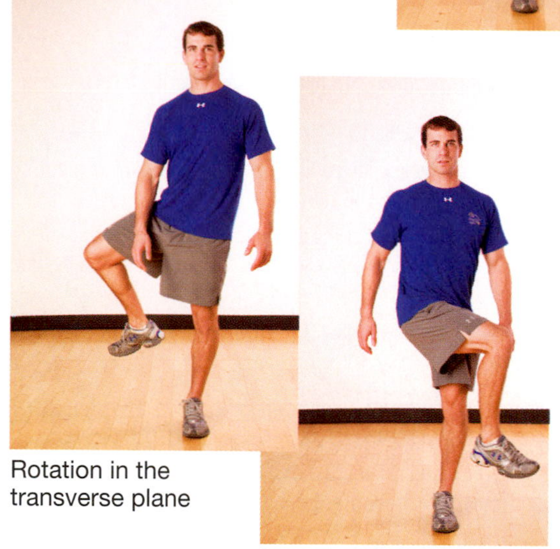
Rotation in the transverse plane

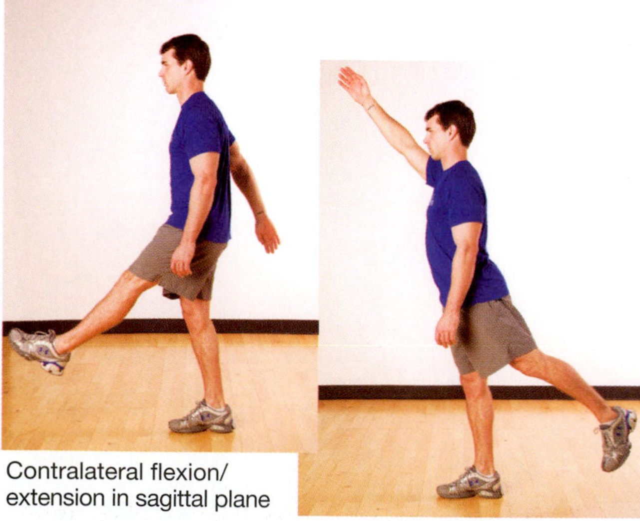
Contralateral flexion/extension in sagittal plane

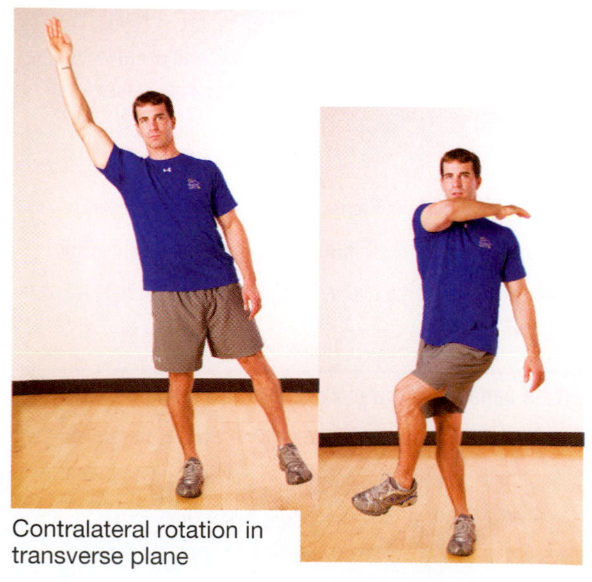
Contralateral rotation in transverse plane

incorporates both isolated and integrated upper- and lower-extremity movement in all three planes, all over a static base of support (Gray, 2008).

Progression for the single-leg stance involves adding external resistance and increasing the balance challenge. Holding a medicine ball or dumbbell, or introducing partial single-leg squats, adds resistance to the kinetic chain and increases the balance challenge. If adding resistance, the increased load merits a reduction in volume (e.g., one or two sets of eight to 12 repetitions per side), and longer rest intervals between sets (e.g., 30 to 60 seconds).

A primary single-leg pattern involves teaching clients how to lunge effectively, a movement pattern that is often performed poorly in any plane. While lunge mechanics are very similar to the squat or bend-and-lift mechanics, many individuals deviate from basic movement principles (Cook & Jones, 2007b). The exercises presented in Figure 9-56 and 9-57 teach the mechanics of the lunge and variations to the basic lunge.

As with squats, people often find

Figure 9-56
Half-kneeling lunge rise

Objective: To teach the proper mechanics of the rising portion of the lunge

Preparation and position:

- Assume a half-kneeling position, placing the back knee directly under the hips (held in a neutral position).
- Position the tibia of the leading leg in a slight forward-leaning position (anterior translation over the foot), aligning the anterior superior iliac spine (ASIS) and knee over the second toe.
- Assume a stable, but slightly forward, lean of the torso to parallel the angle of the tibia (this is the same torso lean used when climbing stairs). Avoid a vertical torso, as this position forces increased lumbar lordosis with tight hip flexors.
- Engage the core muscles to stabilize the lumbar spine in the neutral position and maintain this position throughout the exercise (a).

Exercise:

- *Upward movement:* While the adductor and gluteus medius/minimus group generally stabilize the hips, the gluteus maximus, hamstrings, and leading-leg adductor group function to propel the body upward (b).
- Emphasize both the glute "push" and hamstrings/leading-leg adductor "pull," with the forward leg rising from the lunge position.
- Use any necessary balance supports.
- Perform one to three sets of 12 to 15 repetitions with a controlled tempo, allowing 30-second rest intervals between sets. Repeat with the opposite leg.

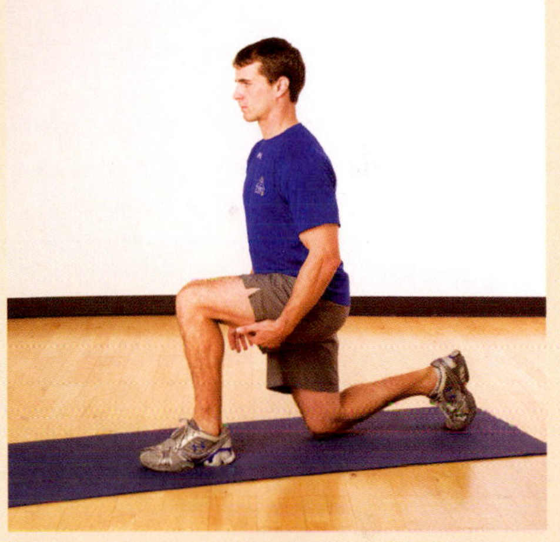
a.

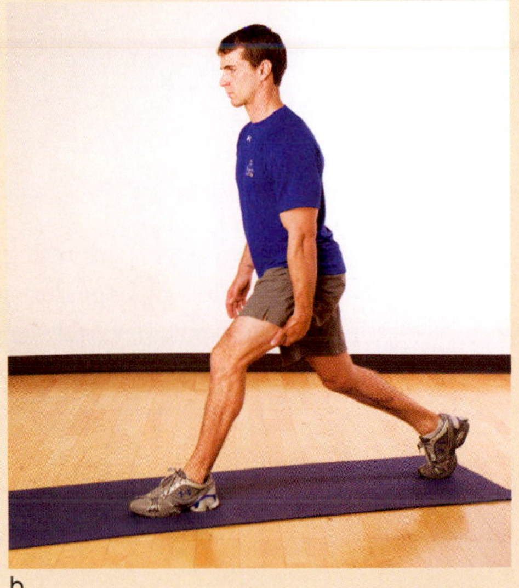
b.

Figure 9-57

Lunges

Objective: To teach the proper mechanics of the full lunge

Preparation and position:

- Start in the standing position, with the feet hip-width apart, shoulders packed (see Figure 9-36), head neutral, and weight distributed toward the heels.
- Engage the core muscles to stabilize the lumbar spine in the neutral position and maintain this position throughout the exercise.

Exercise:

- Slowly lift one leg, controlling the lateral hip shift and reaching forward to take a small step [<24 inches (61 cm)], lightly touching the heel on the floor. Briefly hold this position (a).
- Allow the entire foot to make contact. Once it is firmly positioned on the ground, initiate a hip-hinge movement to begin the downward phase of the lunge (b). This allows for a more natural hinge motion at the knee and reduces the shearing forces.
- Lower the hips and shoulder together, allowing a slight forward torso lean, but maintain strong core engagement to avoid lumbar lordosis (c).
- Avoid any misalignment of the knee over the foot, as well as hip adduction and torso rotation.
- In the lowered position, the trainer can check for the following:
  - ✓ Alignment in the frontal plane of the anterior superior iliac spine (ASIS), knee, and second toe
  - ✓ The figure-4 position with the leading leg and torso in parallel, with the leading leg near perpendicular to the floor (exhibiting a slight forward lean—tibial translation)
  - ✓ No lateral weight shifting or torso rotation
- Perform one to three sets of 12 to 15 repetitions with a controlled tempo, allowing 30-second rest intervals between sets.
- Use the glute "push" and hamstrings "pull" to rise out of the lunge.

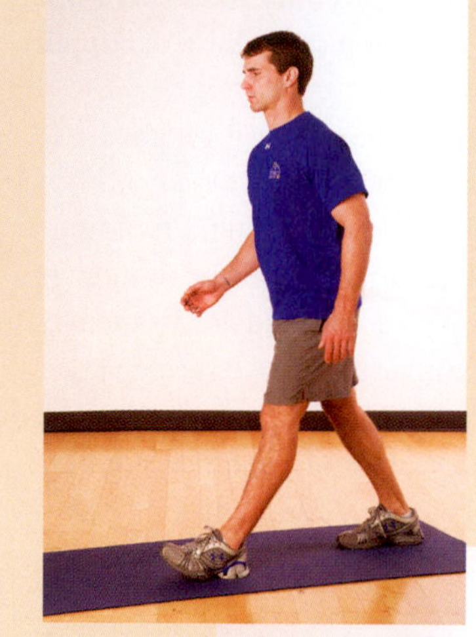

a.

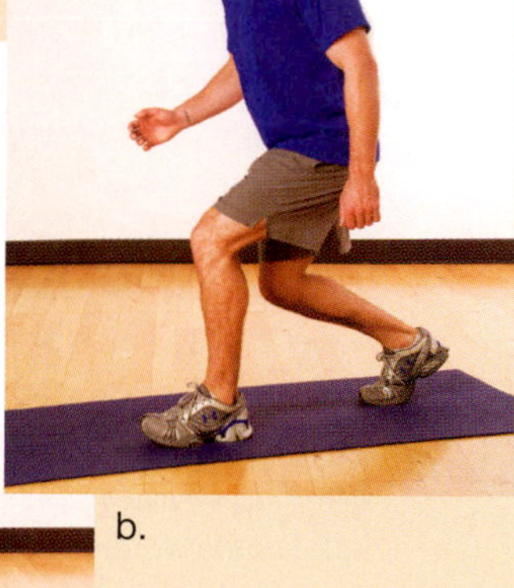

b.

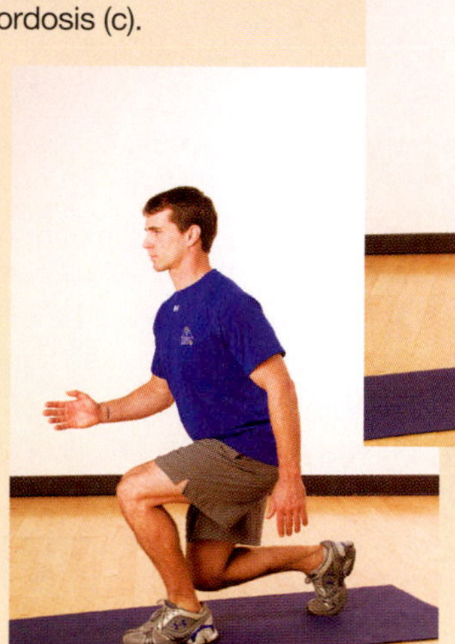

c.

themselves performing variations to the traditional lunge during their daily activities, workouts (e.g., side lunges), or even during sports (e.g., cutting and sidestepping). These variations involve directional lunges, foot-position variations, and movements with the upper extremities in all three planes of movement. Considering these variations represent daily movements, clients should be trained functionally to mimic these patterns. Once a client demonstrates proficiency with the standard lunge pattern, progress the exercise to include directional changes, different foot positions, and upper-extremity movement (Figure 9-58). Bear in mind that high-arm positions require a greater degree of thoracic and hip mobility, which a client may lack. Therefore, clients should begin by driving the arms in the low position prior to incorporating the high-arm-position movements.

When working with more athletic individuals, these same movement patterns can progress to jumps, hops, or bounds. However, individuals should never begin jumping, bounding, or hopping activities until they can effectively demonstrate correct landing technique and the ability to decelerate the impact forces of landing.

Figure 9-58
Lunge matrix

Note: Trainers should progress to this exercise only after a client demonstrates good technique with a standard forward lunge.

Objective: To promote stability and mobility throughout the kinetic chain using variations of the standard lunge movement

Preparation and position:

- Using the grid presented in Figure 9-59, the trainer can teach the client to move in all eight directions, starting and ending each repetition from the center position.
- Engage the core muscles to stabilize the lumbar spine in the neutral position and maintain this position throughout the exercise.

Exercise:

- The trainer teaches the directional movements with stepping prior to introducing lunges.
- When lunging forward, backward, and sideways, align the feet and hips forward (a, c, e, & g).
- When lunging to the oblique angles, align the feet and hips in that direction (b, d, f, & h).
- Follow the same technique instructions outlined in Figure 9-57.
- Perform one to three sets to each direction with each leg.

Source: Gray, G. & Tiberio, D. (2007). *Chain Reaction Function.* Adrian, Mich.: Gray Institute.

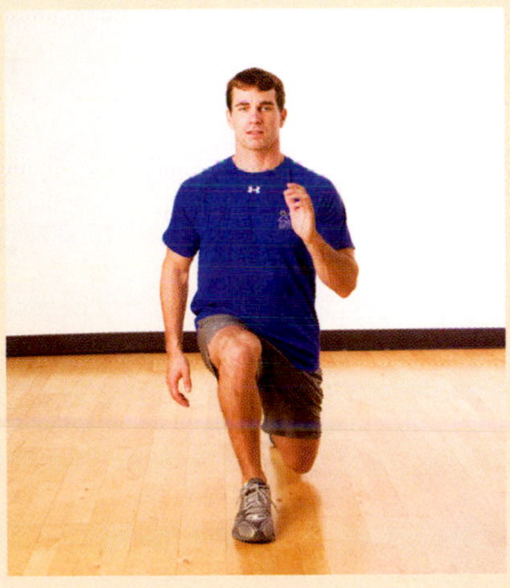
a.

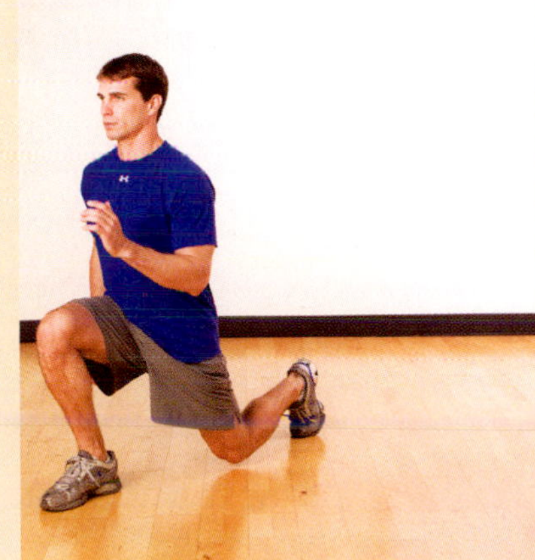
b.

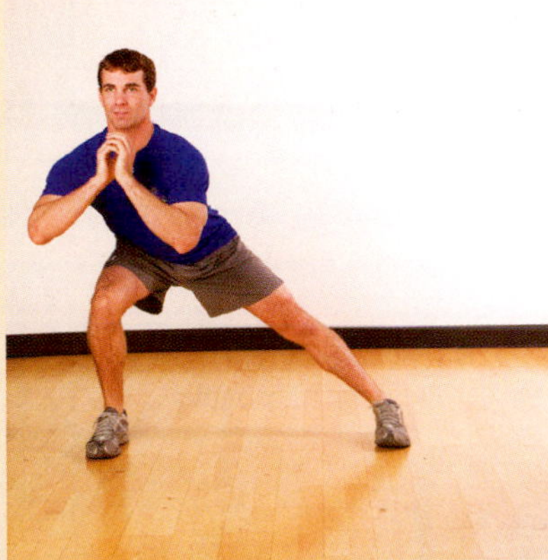
c.

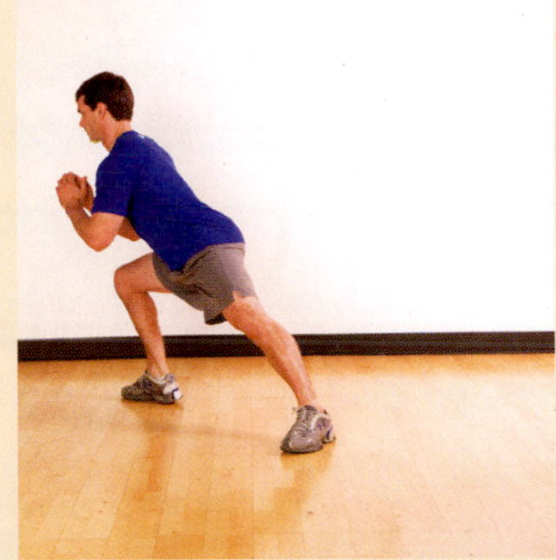
d.

Continued on next page

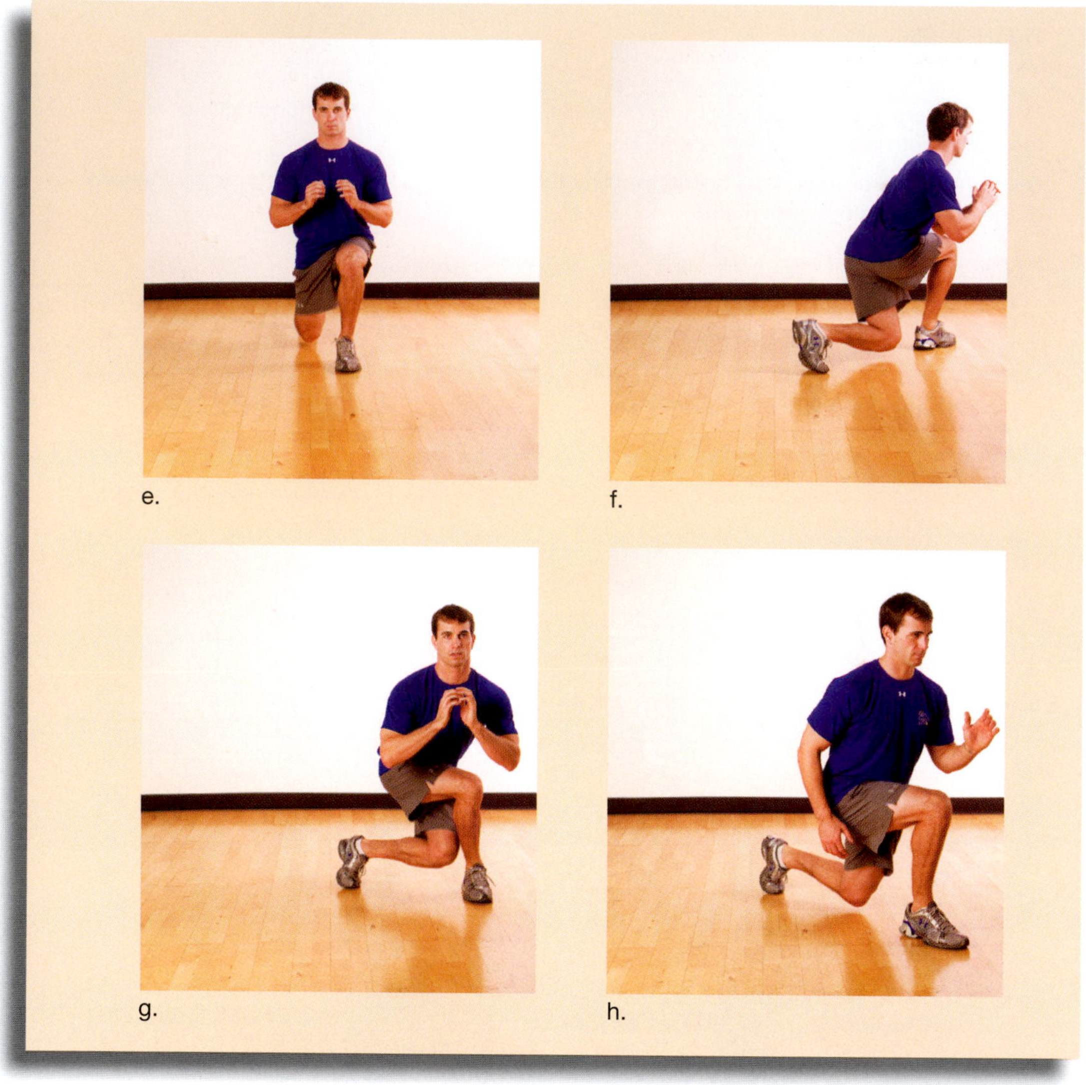

e.

f.

g.

h.

Figure 9-59
Directional movements for the lunge

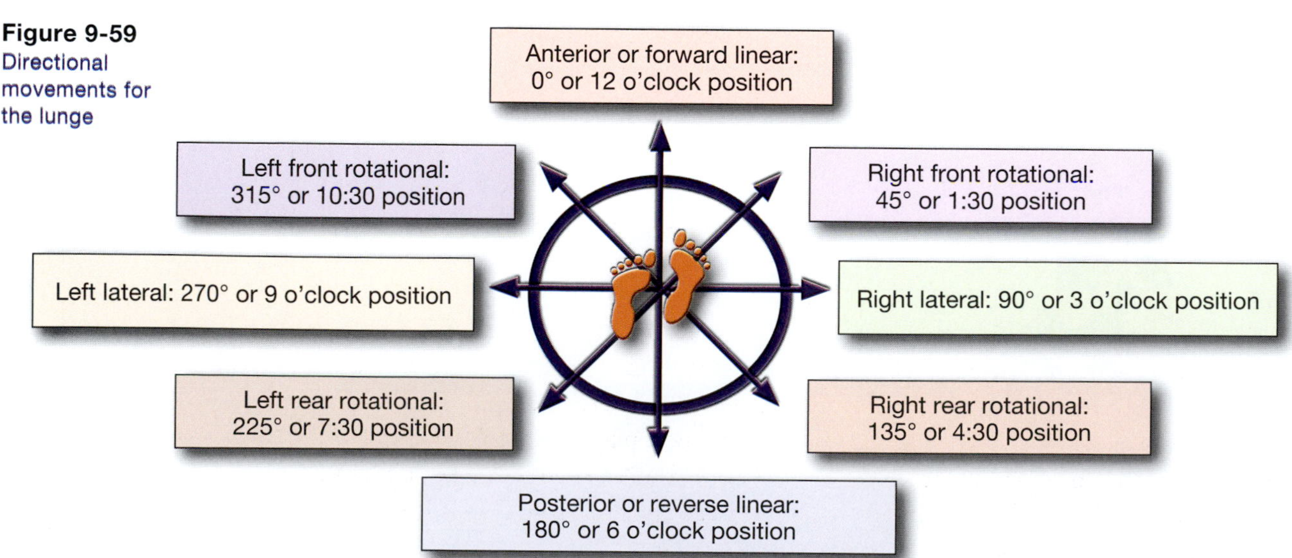

Pushing Movements

During shoulder flexion (e.g., front raise) and overhead presses (e.g., dumbbell press), movement to 180 degrees is achieved by the collaborative effort of the scapulae rotating against the ribcage and the humerus rotating within the glenoid fossa. The movement generally requires approximately 60 degrees of scapular rotation and 120 degrees of glenohumeral rotation (Figure 9-60) (Sahrmann, 2002). While the scapulae require some degree of mobility to perform the various movements of the arm, they fundamentally need to remain stable to promote normal mobility within the glenohumeral joint. During these movements, insufficient, premature, or excessive activation of specific scapular muscles (e.g., dominant rhomboids resisting upward scapular rotation, overactive upper trapezius forcing excessive scapular elevation) will compromise scapular stability, which in turn affects the ability of the muscles around the glenohumeral joint to execute their function effectively. For example, if the scapulae cannot sink slightly while the arms extend overhead, this may interfere with scapular rotation and scapular stability. This forces the glenohumeral joint to assume greater loads, reducing its force-generating capacity and increasing the potential for injury (Cook & Jones, 2007a). This illustrates the importance of setting or packing the scapulae prior to shoulder flexion or abduction movements.

The need for thoracic mobility, scapulothoracic stability, and glenohumeral mobility during pushing and pulling movements is presented in "Proximal Stability of the Scapulothoracic Region and Distal Mobility of the Glenohumeral Joint" (page 272), along with a menu of exercises to promote the appropriate levels of stability and mobility at those respective joints. While many of those exercises focused on isolated action at and around those joints, the emphasis during this phase of training must shift toward integrating whole-body movement patterns. Exercises can begin

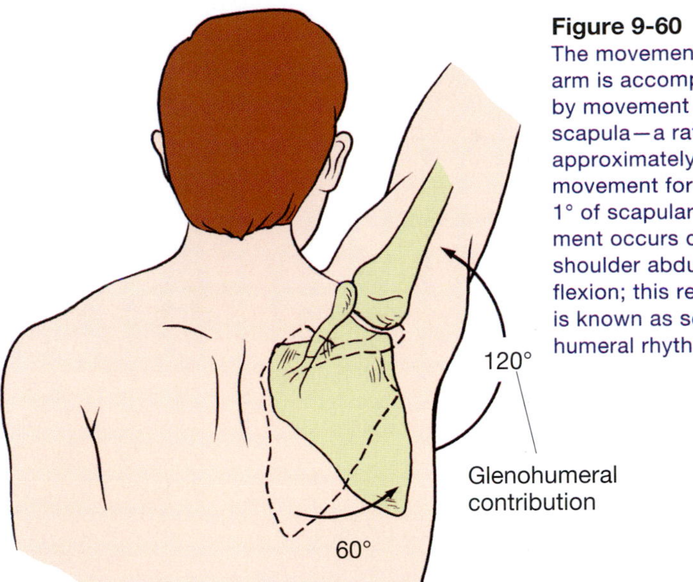

Figure 9-60
The movement of the arm is accompanied by movement of the scapula—a ratio of approximately 2° of arm movement for every 1° of scapular movement occurs during shoulder abduction and flexion; this relationship is known as scapulohumeral rhythm.

with more traditional pushing and pulling movements that primarily target the shoulder girdle in a bilateral or unilateral fashion, using supported backrests, then progress to becoming unsupported (e.g., standing in a normal or split-stance position), which better mimics most ADL (Figure 9-61).

To facilitate scapular stability during pushing and pulling movements, mobility within the thoracic spine must first be established. Gary Gray uses his Thoracic Matrix exercise, moving the thoracic spine three-dimensionally and driving the movement through each plane with the arms or by using a dowel or light bar in various standing or lunging positions to integrate the entire kinetic chain (Figure 9-62) (Gray, 2008). Gray utilizes individual and simultaneous movement between planes—moving the body in multiple planes in the same direction (e.g., rotating to the right while simultaneously flexing laterally to the right) or moving the body in multiple planes in opposite directions (e.g., rotating to the right while simultaneously flexing laterally to the left). To simplify terminology for instructional purposes, trainers can use the term "undifferentiated" for same-side movements and "differentiated" for opposite-side movements.

Another common mistake made when performing overhead presses is the tendency

Figure 9-61
Bilateral and unilateral presses

Objective: To execute open-chain pushing movements in unsupported environments without compromising stability in the scapulothoracic joint and lumbar spine

Preparation and position:

- Assume a seated position on a seat or bench of any weightstack or cable-press machine, making contact with the backrest. Progress by repeating the movement without any contact against the backrest.
- Grasp the machine or cable handles firmly in both hands, positioning the hands close to the chest in a starting press position.
- Pack both shoulders (see Figure 9-36) and brace the core, holding these positions throughout the exercise.

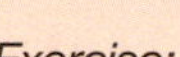

Exercise:

- Exhale and gently press the load away bilaterally from the chest, preventing any change to the position of the lumbar spine or scapulae (do not perform a push-plus by protracting the scapulae when the elbows fully extend or elevate the scapulae). The goal is to reach full elbow extension, yet maintain a stable trunk and shoulder girdle (a).
- Slowly return to the starting position by adducting the scapulae (maintain the same starting position).
- Perform one or two sets of 12 to 15 repetitions with a controlled tempo, allowing 30-second rest intervals between sets.

Progression—Standing press: Repeat the same bilateral movement, but from a standing, split-stance position, alternating the forward leg with each set (b). A cable press or TRX® are suitable pieces of equipment to introduce for these progressions.

Progression—Single-arm press with a contralateral stance: Repeat the same movement, but pushing unilaterally with one arm, while the opposite leg is positioned forward in the split-stance position (c).

Progression—Single-arm press with an ipsilateral stance: Repeat the same movement, but pushing unilaterally with one arm, while the same-side leg is positioned forward in the split-stance position (d). The challenge is to resist the body's tendency to rotate during the push movement.

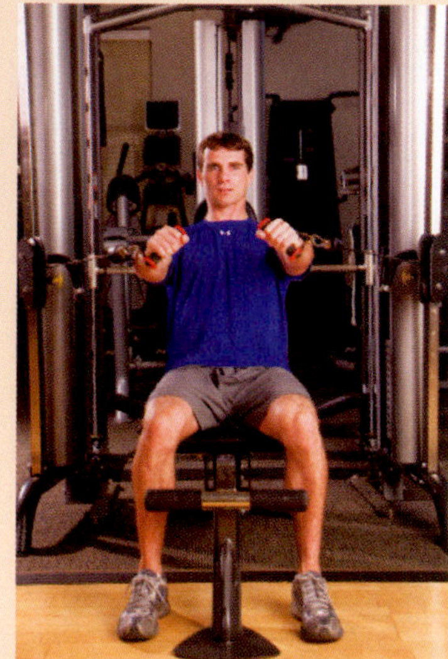

a.

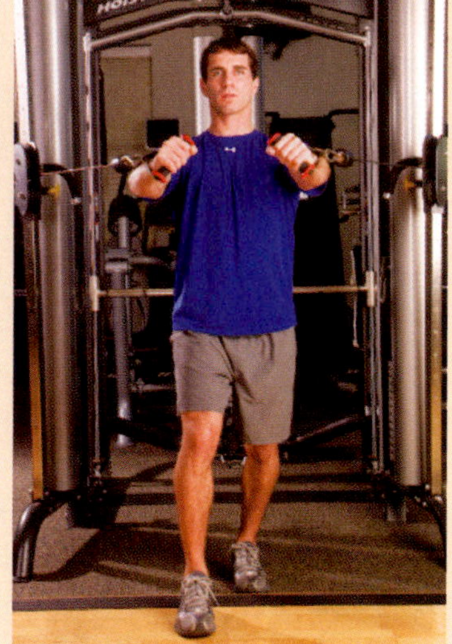

b.

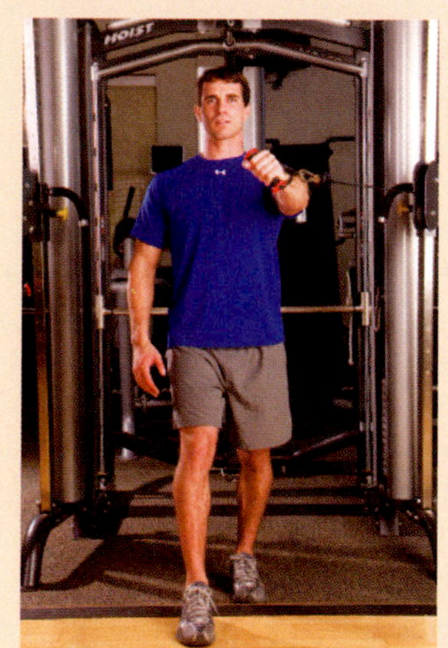

c.

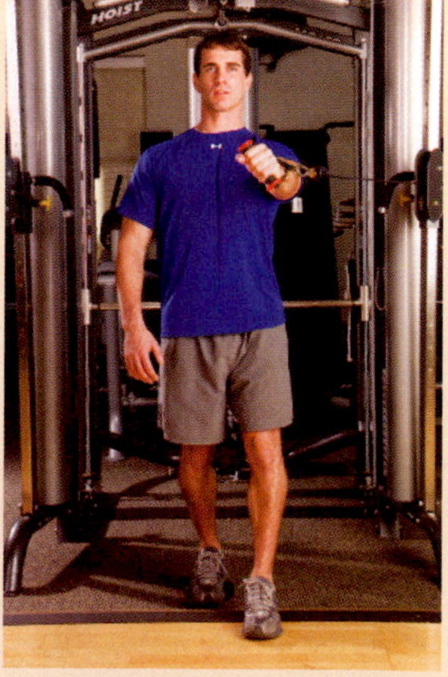

d.

Figure 9-62
Thoracic matrix

Objective: To promote multiplanar thoracic mobility with drivers (e.g., arms or a dowel or lightly weighted bar) while stabilizing the kinetic chain

Preparation and position:

- Stand in a neutral stance position with the feet hip-width apart.
- Pack both shoulders (see Figure 9-36) and brace the core, and hold these positions throughout the exercise.

Exercise:

- Move the arms in all three planes as follows (a & b):
  - ✓ Unilaterally in all three planes, promoting thoracic and hip mobility while avoiding any loss of lumbar stability
  - ✓ Bilaterally in all three planes, promoting thoracic and hip mobility while avoiding any loss of lumbar stability
  - ✓ Multiple planes, mixing movement in differentiated or undifferentiated patterns promoting thoracic and hip mobility while avoiding any loss of lumbar stability

Stance progression:

- Progress from neutral-stance to staggered-stance, and then perform the movements in various lunge and squat positions (c, d, & e).
- Perform one or two sets of 12 to 15 repetitions with each arm with a controlled tempo, allowing 10- to 15-second rest intervals between sets.

Source: Gray, G. (2008). *The Thoracic Spine*. Adrian, Mich.: Gray Institute.

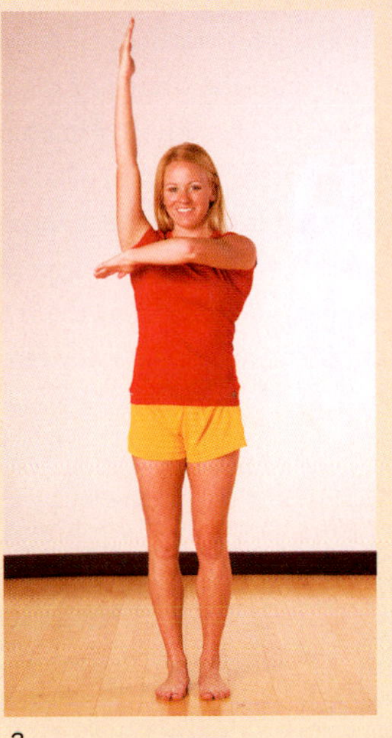
a.

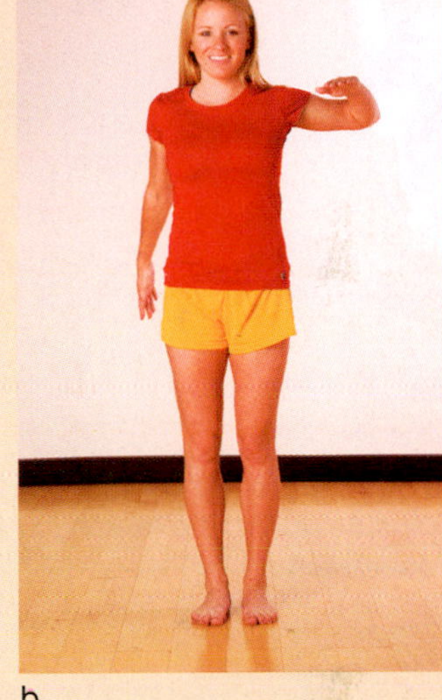
b.

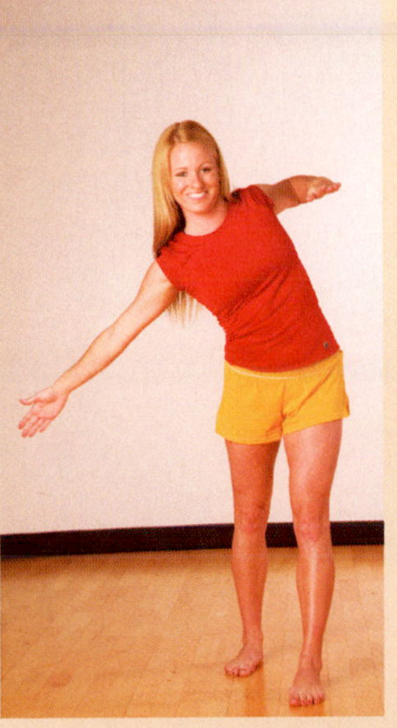
c.

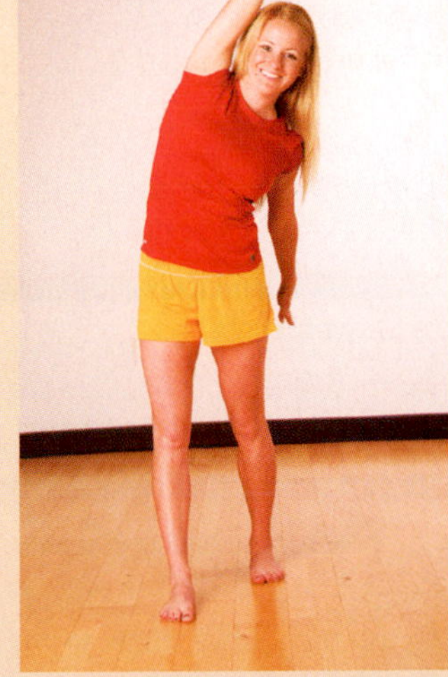
d.

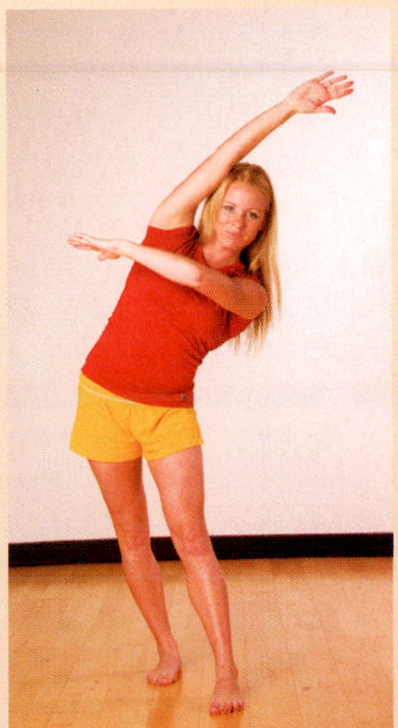
e.

to simply yield to gravity during the eccentric or downward phase of a shoulder press. This creates instability within the shoulder joint, given the changing roles of the deltoids between the starting and overhead position (Cook & Jones, 2007a). To better illustrate this point to a client, a trainer can place the index finger of one hand on the deltoid tuberosity (the insertion point of the deltoids muscle, which is located approximately midway or slightly behind the midline of the humerus and a few inches below the shoulder), and place the thumb of the same hand along the clavicle. This represents the position of the anterior deltoid, which acts to stabilize the anterior shoulder capsule during overhead lifting. The client performs an overhead press, noticing how the trainer's fingers will roll backward and away from the anterior portion of the shoulder as the arm moves overhead, abducting and externally rotating the humerus.

This overhead shoulder press position may increase the potential for anterior displacement of the humerus, given the lack of support from the anterior deltoid in the overhead position. However, the latissimus dorsi wraps around the anterior capsule from behind and, when elongated or loaded, can offer stability to the anterior shoulder (Cook & Jones, 2007a). Therefore, if the latissimus dorsi is engaged to begin the lowering phase, anterior containment is provided to help stabilize the shoulder and precipitate greater force production during the lifting phase. Trainers should therefore coach clients to engage the latissimus dorsi during the lowering phase and not simply yield to gravity (Figure 9-63).

Figure 9-63
Overhead press

Objective: To provide additional stability to the shoulder capsule during the lowering phase of overhead pressing movements

Preparation and position:

- Using a dowel or lightly weighted bar, assume a seated position to perform a seated overhead press.
- Pack both shoulders (see Figure 9-36) and brace the core, holding these positions throughout the exercise.
- Press the bar overhead to the fully extended arm position, ensuring that the scapulae are not elevated (a).

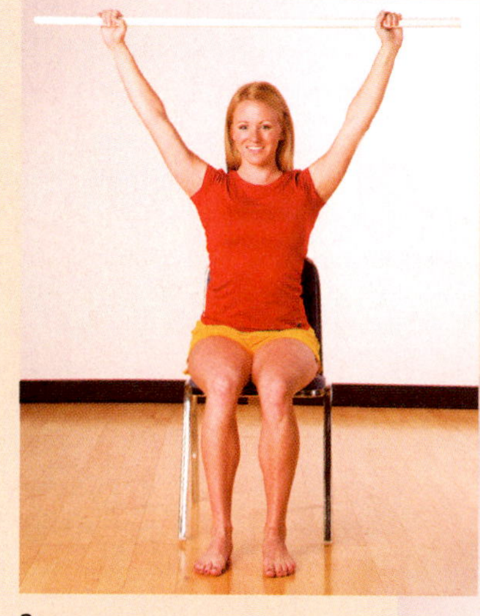

a.

Exercise:

- Actively engage the latissimus dorsi to initiate the pull-down sequence, lowering the bar to the starting position.
- Perform one or two sets of 12 to 15 repetitions with a controlled tempo, allowing 30-second rest intervals between sets.

Progression: Holding dumbbells, perform a variety of shoulder-press movements while introducing changes in the plane of movement:

- Add a trunk rotation, pressing upward across and even behind the body (b).
- Add lateral trunk movements (e.g., side lunge) and press overhead or across the front of the body.
- Assume a squat position, holding the dumbbells closer to waist level, and perform a series of uppercuts, driving the dumbbells across and behind the body to an end-point just above shoulder level.

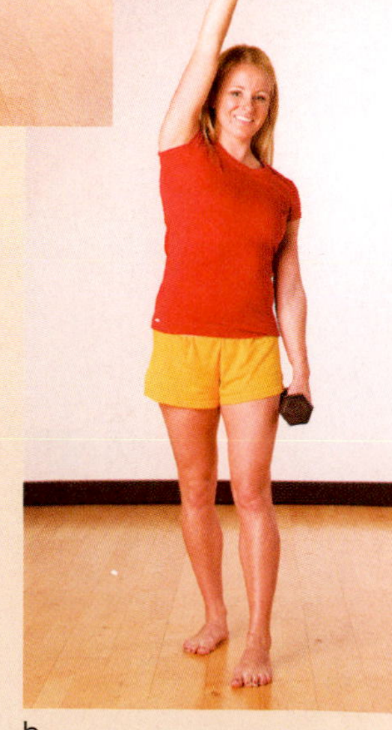

b.

Pulling Movements

Pulling movements follow many of the same principles as pressing movements with regard to stabilizing the scapulothoracic region, which helps promote effective glenohumeral function (Figure 9-64). Trainers need to identify whether they want to train a client to pull from a position of scapular stability, implying that the movement is purely from the shoulder (i.e., glenohumeral or shoulder extension/ horizontal extension), or whether they are intentionally incorporating scapular retraction into the pulling motion.

Figure 9-64
Bilateral and unilateral rows

Objective: To execute open-kinetic-chain pulling movements in unsupported environments without compromising stability of the scapulothoracic joint and lumbar spine

Preparation and position:

- Assume a seated position on a seat or bench of any weightstack or cable machine, making contact with a chest plate or rest. Progress by repeating the movement without any contact against a rest.
- Pack both shoulders (see Figure 9-36) and brace the core, holding these positions throughout the exercise.
- Grasp the machine or cable handles firmly in both hands, in a shoulder-flexed, elbow-extended position without protracting the scapulae.

Exercise:

- Exhale and gently pull the load bilaterally toward the body, preventing any change to the position of the lumbar spine or scapulae (avoid retracting or squeezing the shoulder blades together). The goal is to continue pulling until the elbows are bent 90 degrees, yet maintain a stable trunk and shoulder girdle.
- Slowly return to the starting position by extending the arms.
- Perform one or two sets of 12 to 15 repetitions with a controlled tempo, allowing 30-second rest intervals between sets.

Progression—Standing pull: Repeat the same bilateral movement, but from a standing, split-stance position, alternating the forward leg with each set (a). A cable pull or TRX are suitable pieces of equipment to introduce for these progressions.

Progression—Single-arm pull with a contralateral stand: Repeat the same movement, but pulling unilaterally with one arm while the opposite leg is positioned forward in the split-stance position (b).

Progression—Single-arm pull with an ipsilateral stand: Repeat the same movement, but pulling unilaterally with one arm, while the same-side leg is positioned forward in the split-stance position (c). The challenge is to resist the body's temptation to rotate during the pulling movement.

a.

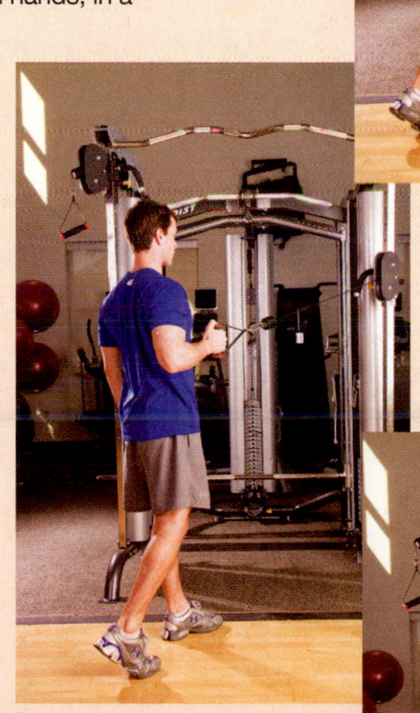

b.

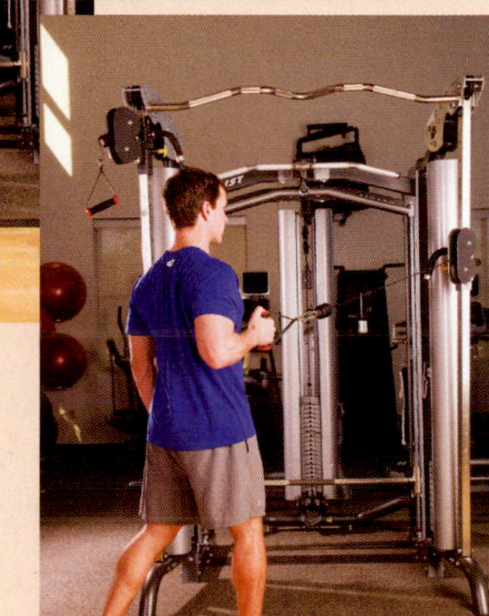

c.

Exercises to promote effective pulling can begin with more traditional movements that primarily target the shoulder girdle in a bilateral or unilateral fashion, using supported backrests, then progress to becoming unsupported (e.g., standing in a normal, split-stance or lunge position), which better mimics most ADL.

Rotational Movements

Rotational movements represent the last of the primary movements and are perhaps some of the most complex movements, given how many follow spiral or diagonal patterns throughout the body. These patterns involve a series of muscle and tissue arrangements called anatomy trains or **myofascial slings.** Given the complexity of knowledge required to fully understand myofascial slings, they are not discussed in this manual. However, four key slings pertaining to gait are discussed in greater detail in the *ACE Advanced Health & Fitness Specialist Manual,* or more detail can be found in *Anatomy Trains* by Thomas Myers (ACE, 2009; Myers, 2001).

These movements generally incorporate movement into multiple planes simultaneously (e.g., a golf backswing requires transverse plane rotation, thoracic and lumbar extension, and some lateral flexion). Many of these movements increase the forces placed along the vertebrae, so trainers must exercise care when teaching these movements and only do so after the client has conditioned the core effectively. Consideration of good technique and appropriate levels of mobility and stability in the thoracic and lumbar spine is critical in facilitating synchronous movement and dissipating the generated ground and reactive forces over larger surface areas (e.g., upward toward the cervical vertebra and downward toward the hips, knees, and ankles) (Gray & Tiberio, 2007). The ability to dissipate ground and reactive forces reduces the impact on local areas and decreases the potential for injury.

Two key movements involving diagonal or spiral patterns of movement within the arms, shoulders, trunks, hips, and legs are the wood chop and the hay bailer:

- *Wood chops:* This exercise involves a pulling action to initiate the movement down across the front of the body, followed by a pushing action in the upper extremity as the arms move away from the body (Figure 9-65). In addition, it requires stabilization of the trunk in all three planes (i.e., during flexion, rotation, and side-bending), and weight transference through the hips and between the legs to gain leverage and maintain balance (Cook & Jones, 2007b). Concentric action during the downward chop is achieved by using a high anchor point (e.g., high cable pulley or band).
- *Hay bailers:* This exercise involves a pulling action to initiate the movement up across the front of the body, followed by a pushing action in the upper extremity as the arms move away from the body (Figure 9-66). In addition, it requires stabilization of the trunk in all three planes (extension, rotation, and side-bending), and weight transference through the hips and between the legs to gain leverage and maintain balance (Cook & Jones, 2007b).

The need for thoracic mobility is greater during these movements than with pushing and pulling movements, given the three-dimensional nature of the movement patterns. Performing these exercises without thoracic mobility or lumbar stability may compromise the shoulders and hips, and increase the likelihood for injury.

The instructions provided for the wood chop are similar to those for performing the hay bailer. Although the mechanics are similar, the differences involve moving from a low starting position to a high ending position, and assuming a staggered stance with the opposite leg forward.

Given the directional pull of gravity, the intensity of the hay bailer is perhaps greater due to the need to lift against the force of gravity (concentric) versus resisting or slowing the effects of gravity (eccentric),

Figure 9-65

Wood-chop spiral patterns

Note: Given the complexity of the wood-chop movement, the individual should first learn basic spiral patterns without placing excessive loads upon the spine.

Objective: To introduce basic spiral patterns with small, controlled forces placed along the spine

Preparation and position:

- Assume a half-kneeling position, placing the rear knee directly under the hips. This position engages both the hip flexors and extensors to help stabilize the spine.
- An unstable surface may be placed under the rear knee to increase the stability demands on the core.
- Pack both shoulders (see Figure 9-36) and brace the core, holding these positions throughout the exercise.
- Imagine holding a short handle that positions the hands 6 to 12 inches (15 to 30 cm) apart and raise the handle toward the shoulder on the same side as the leading leg, keeping both hands close to the body (a).
- The hips and torso (chest) should remain aligned forward.

Exercise:

- Exhale and slowly perform a downward movement across the front of the body, moving the handle toward the opposite hip and keeping both arms close to the body to shorten the length of the lever (called the moment arm) (b).
- The hips and torso (chest) should remain aligned forward.
- Return to the starting position and repeat.
- Perform one or two sets of 12 to 15 repetitions in each direction, alternating the knee position with each directional change.

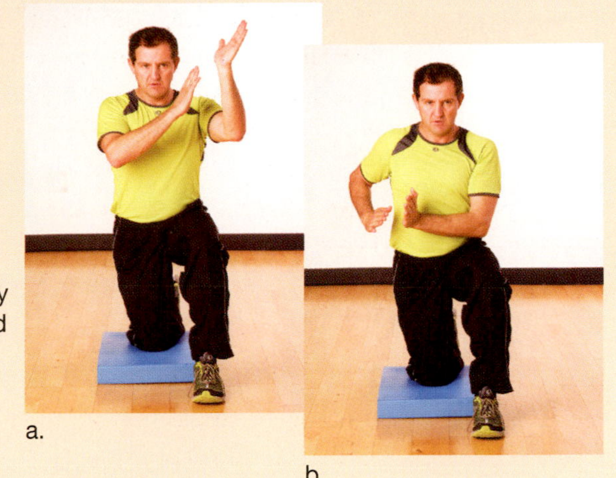

a. b.

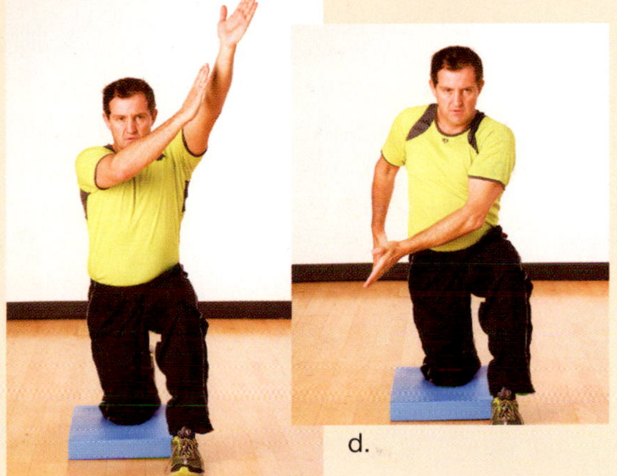

c. d.

Progression—Long moment arm: Repeat the same movement, but extend the arms (acting as a driver) to increase the range of motion and leverage, but keep both arms close the body during the movement (c & d). The hips and torso (chest) should remain aligned forward.

Progression—Standing short moment arm: Assume a split-stance position, placing the leg on the same side as the chop start position forward. Bend both elbows, placing the hands 6 to 12 inches (15 to 30 cm) apart and raise the handle toward the shoulder on the same side as the leading leg, keeping both hands close to the body (e & f). Repeat the same chopping movement with bent elbows. The hips and torso (chest) should remain aligned forward.

Progression—Standing long moment arm: Assume the same split-stance position and repeat the same chopping movement, but extend the arms (g & h). The hips and torso (chest) should remain aligned forward.

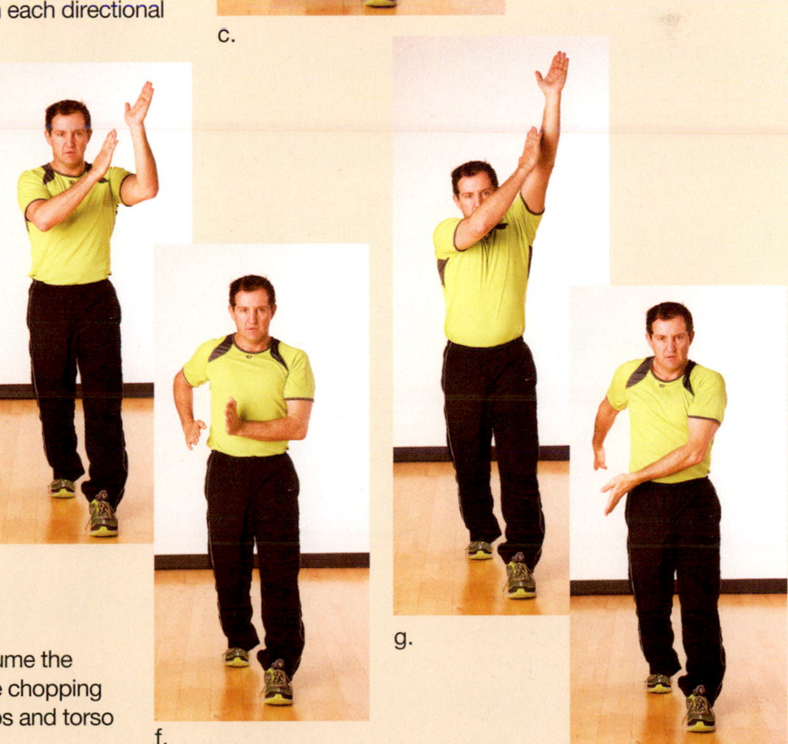

e. f. g. h.

Figure 9-66

Full wood-chop and hay-bailer patterns

Objective: To introduce the full multiplanar wood-chop and hay-bailer movement patterns while controlling forces placed along the spine

Preparation and position (a & b):

- Assume a staggered position, placing the inside leg 6 to 12 inches (15 to 30 cm) forward.
- Pack both shoulders (see Figure 9-36) and brace the core, holding these positions throughout the exercise.
- Imagine holding a short handle that positions the hands 6 to 12 inches (15 to 30 cm) apart and raise the handle toward the inside shoulder on the same side as the leading leg, keeping both hands close to the body.
- Load 60 to 70% of the body weight onto the inside leg.

Exercise:

- Exhale, hip-hinge (hip flex), and squat while rotating the hips outward, transferring 60 to 70% of the body weight onto the outside leg.
- While the hips rotate, the chest and shoulders should remain aligned over the pubis (center of the pelvis).
- Return to the starting position and repeat.
- Perform one or two sets of 12 to 15 repetitions in each direction, alternating the stance position with each directional change.

Progression—Long moment arm: Repeat the same movement, but extend the elbows and move the hands 2 to 3 feet (0.6 to 0.9 m) apart (the use of a dowel might prove useful). A wide, extended grip concentrates force-generation from the hips and not from the shoulder or arms. Repeat the movement and, while the hips rotate, the chest and shoulders should remain aligned over the pubis (center of the pelvis).

Progression—Full chop (c & d): Repeat the same movement, but allow the torso to rotate further into the start position and rotate past the hips at the end position. Allow the unloaded leg to pivot during the movement to help transfer and dissipate forces.

Progression: Add external resistance in the form of a medicine ball, kettle bell, cable, or elastic tubing (e & f).

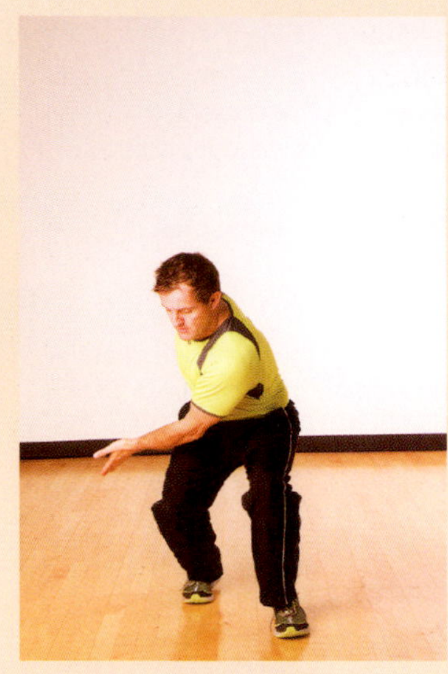

a.

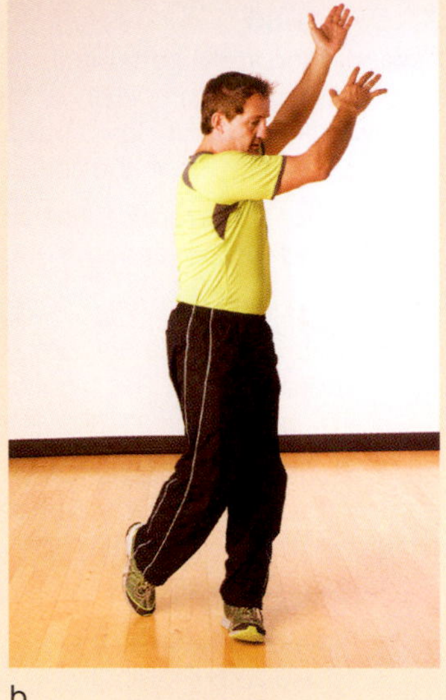

b.

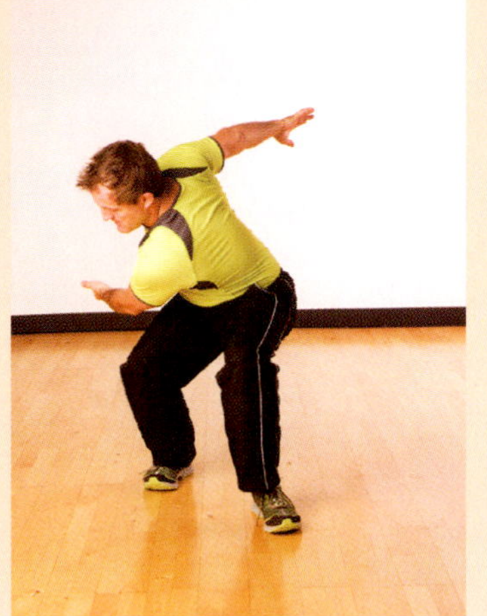

c.

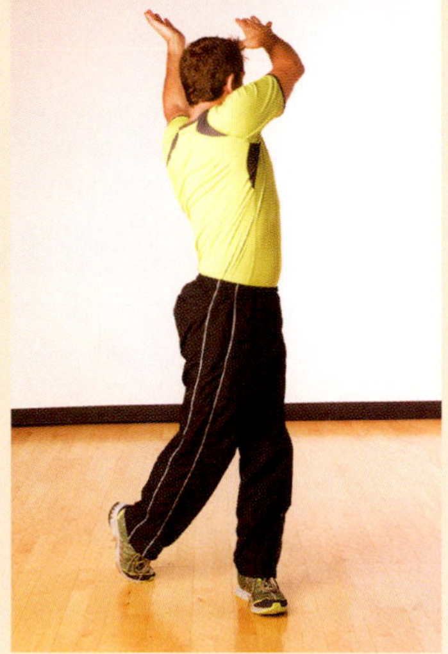

d.

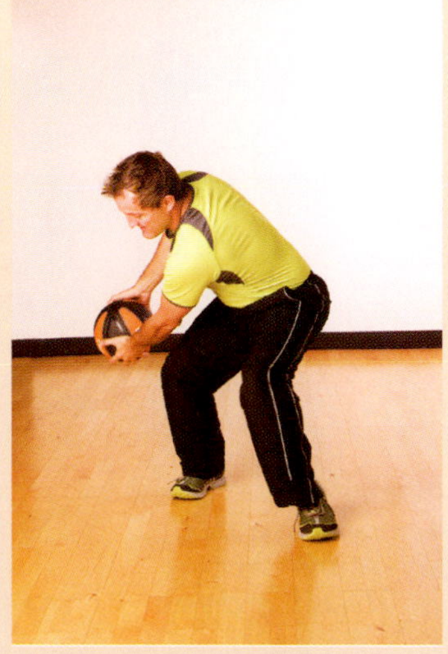

e.

f.

as is done during the wood chop. Trainers need to remember that the thoracic spine offers greater mobility than the lumbar spine. Therefore, they need to emphasize lumbar stability and control of lumbar rotation while promoting movement within the thoracic spine.

Summary

This chapter introduces two essential prerequisite stages to training clients that are frequently overlooked. Traditional training focuses on strengthening muscles or improving their endurance capacity in isolation and generally disregards the relationship of the entire kinetic chain (stability-mobility relationship) with reference to postural alignment of the joints. Trainers should always emphasize these two stages during the initial phase of a client's training program to "straighten the body before strengthening it," and restore good joint alignment and muscle balance across joints. Good joint alignment facilitates effective muscle action and joint movement, serving as the platform from which good exercise technique is built. Given the complexity of current exercise equipment and the advanced nature of many exercises, trainers must stress the importance of learning how to perform the five primary movement patterns correctly, as they represent the foundation to all movement. Proper execution of these movements enhances the potential to promote movement efficiency, as well as long-term maintenance and integrity of the joint structures, muscles, connective tissues, and nerves of the musculoskeletal system.

References

Alter, M.J. (2004). *Science of Flexibility* (3rd ed.). Champaign, Ill.: Human Kinetics.

American College of Sports Medicine (2010). *ACSM's Guidelines for Exercise Testing and Prescription* (8th ed.). Philadelphia, Pa.: Wolters Kluwer/Lippincott Williams and Wilkins.

American Council on Exercise (2009). *ACE Advanced Health & Fitness Specialist Manual.* San Diego, Calif.: American Council on Exercise.

Arokoski, J.P. et al. (2001). Back and abdominal muscle function during stabilization exercises. *Archives Physical Medicine and Rehabilitation,* 82, 1089–1098.

Barnes, J.F. (1999). Myofascial release. In: Hammer, W.I. (Ed.) *Functional Soft Tissue Examination and Treatment by Manual Methods* (2nd ed). Gaithersburg, Md.: Aspen Publishers.

Broomfield, J. (1998). Posture and proportionality in sport. In: Ellito, B. (Ed.) *Training in Sport: Applying Sport Science*. Hoboken, N.J.: John Wiley & Sons.

Carey, A. (2005). *The Pain Free Program*. Hoboken, N.J.: John Wiley & Sons.

Cook, G. (2003). *Athletic Body in Balance*. Champaign, Ill.: Human Kinetics.

Cook, G. & Jones, B. (2007a). *Secrets of the Shoulder.* www.functionalmovement.com

Cook, G. & Jones, B. (2007b). *Secrets of the Hip and Knee*. www.functionalmovement.com

Cresswell, A.G. & Thorstensson, A. (1994). Changes in intra-abdominal pressure, trunk muscle activation and force during isokinetic lifting and lowering. *European Journal of Applied Physiology,* 68, 315–321.

Golding, L.A. & Golding, S.M. (2003). *Fitness Professional's Guide to Musculoskeletal Anatomy and Human Movement*. Monterey, Calif.: Healthy Learning.

Gray, G. (2008). *The Thoracic Spine.* Adrian, Mich.: Gray Institute.

Gray, G. & Tiberio, D. (2007). *Chain Reaction Function*. Adrian, Mich.: Gray Institute.

Hauschildt, M. (2008). Landing mechanics: What, why and when? *NSCA's Performance Training Journal,* 7, 1, 13–16.

Hemmerich, A. et al. (2006). Hip, knee and ankle kinematics of high range of motion activities of daily living. *Journal of Orthopedic Research,* 24, 770–781.

Hodges, P.W. & Richardson, C.A. (1996). Inefficient muscular stabilization of the lumbar spine associated with LBP: A motor control evaluation of the TVA. *Spine,* 21, 2640–2650.

Houglum, P.A. (2005) *Therapeutic Exercise for Musculoskeletal Injuries* (2nd ed.). Champaign, Ill.: Human Kinetics.

Kendall, F.P. et al. (2005). *Muscles Testing and Function with Posture and Pain* (5th ed.). Baltimore, Md.: Lippincott Williams & Wilkins.

Kibler, W.B., Press, J., & Sciascia, A. (2006). The role of core stability in athletic function. *Sports Medicine,* 36, 3, 189–198.

Lieber, R.L. (2002). *Skeletal Muscle Structure, Function, and Plasticity: The Physiological Basis of Rehabilitation*. Baltimore, Md.: Lippincott Williams & Wilkins.

MacIntosh, B.R., Gardiner, P.F., & McComas, A.J. (2006). *Skeletal Muscle Form and Function* (2nd ed.). Champaign, Ill.: Human Kinetics.

McGill, S.M. (2007). *Low Back Disorders: Evidence-based Prevention and Rehabilitation* (2nd ed.). Champaign, Ill.: Human Kinetics.

McGill, S.M. (2004). *Ultimate Back Fitness and Performance* (3rd ed.). Waterloo, Canada: Backfitpro.com

Myers, T. (2001). *Anatomy Trains: Myofascial Meridians for Manual and Movement Therapists.* Edinburgh: Churchill Livingstone.

Panjabi, M.M. (1992). The stabilizing system of the spine. Part I: Function, dysfunction, adaptation and enhancement. *Journal of Spinal Disorders,* 5, 380–389.

Rasmussen-Barr, E., Nilsson-Wikmar, L., & Arvidsson, I. (2003) Stabilizing training compared with manual treatment in sub-acute and chronic low back pain. *Manual Therapy,* 8, 4, 233–241.

Rose, D.J. (2003). *Fall Proof.* Champaign, Ill.: Human Kinetics.

Sahrmann, S.A. (2002). *Diagnosis and Treatment of Movement Impairment Syndromes*. St. Louis, Mo.: Mosby.

Schmidt, R.A. & Wrisberg, C.A. (2007). *Motor Learning and Performance* (4th ed.). Champaign, Ill.: Human Kinetics.

Shumway-Cook, A. & Woollacott, M.H. (2001). *Motor Control: Theory and Practical Applications* (2nd ed.). Philadelphia: Lippincott Williams & Wilkins.

Tumminello, N. (2007). *Warm-up Progressions—Volumes 1 and 2.* Baltimore, Md.: Performance University.

Walsh, J.C. et al. (2007). Three-dimensional motion analysis of the lumbar spine during "free squat" weight lift training. *American Journal of Sports Medicine*, 35, 6, 927–932.

Whiting, W.C. & Rugg, S. (2006). *Dynatomy: Dynamic Human Anatomy*. Champaign, Ill.: Human Kinetics.

Whittle, M.W. (2007). *Gait Analysis: An Introduction* (4th ed.). Edinburgh: Heineman Elsevier.

Willardson, J.M. (2007). Core stability training: Applications to sports conditioning programs. *Journal of Strength and Conditioning Research,* 21, 3, 979–985.

Williams, P. & Goldspink, G. (1978). Changes in sarcomere length and physiologic properties in immobilized muscle. *Journal of Anatomy,* 127, 459.

Wilmore, J.H., Costill, D.L., & Kenney, W.L. (2008). *Physiology of Sport and Exercise* (4th ed.). Champaign, Ill.: Human Kinetics.

Wilthrow, T.J. et al. (2005). The relationship between quadriceps muscle force, knee flexion and anterior cruciate ligament strain in an *in vitro* simulated jump landing. *American Journal of Sports Medicine*, 34, 2, 269–274.

Suggested Reading

American Council on Exercise (2009). *ACE Advanced Health & Fitness Specialist Manual.* San Diego, Calif.: American Council on Exercise.

Carey, A. (2005). *The Pain Free Program*. Hoboken, N.J.: John Wiley & Sons.

Kreighbaum, E. & Barthels, K.M. (1996). *Biomechanics: A Qualitative Approach for Studying Human Movement* (4th ed.). Needham, Mass.: Pearson Education.

Myers, T. (2001). *Anatomy Trains: Myofascial Meridians for Manual and Movement Therapists*. Edinburgh: Churchill Livingstone.

Sahrmann, S.A. (2002). *Diagnosis and Treatment of Movement Impairment Syndromes*. St. Louis, Mo.: Mosby.

IN THIS CHAPTER:

Benefits of Resistance Training

- Physical Capacity
- Physical Appearance and Body Composition
- Metabolic Function
- Injury Risk and Disease Prevention

Physiological Adaptations to Resistance Training: Acute and Long-term

- Factors That Influence Muscular Strength and Hypertrophy

Muscular Strength/Power/Endurance Relationships

Training Variables: Factors Affecting Strength Development and Program Design

- Needs Assessment
- Training Frequency
- Exercise Selection and Order
- Training Volume
- Training Intensity
- Training Tempo
- Rest Intervals

Training Principles

- Progression
- Specificity
- Overload
- Reversibility
- Diminishing Returns

Resistance-training Periodization Models

- Periodization Program—Sample Protocols

Program Design Using the ACE Integrated Fitness Training™ Model

- Phase 1: Stability and Mobility Training
- Phase 2: Movement Training
- Phase 3: Load Training
- Phase 4: Performance Training

Special Considerations for Youth and Older Adults

- Youth Strength Training
- Older Adult Strength Training

Strength-training Equipment Options

- Selectorized Equipment
- Cables
- Free Weights
- Tubing
- Medicine Balls
- Bodyweight Training

Ergogenic Aids and Supplements

- Protein and Amino-acid Supplements
- β-Alanine (Carnosine) and Sodium Bicarbonate
- Caffeine
- Creatine
- Vitamins and Minerals
- Anabolic-androgenic Steroids and Related Compounds

Common Resistance-training Myths and Mistakes

Summary

***WAYNE WESTCOTT, Ph.D.**, teaches exercise science and directs fitness research at Quincy College in Quincy, Mass. Dr. Westcott was a member of the original ACE Personal Trainer Certification Exam Committee. He has authored or co-authored 24 books on physical fitness, including the* ACE Youth Fitness *and* ACE Youth Strength Training *books.*

ACE would like to acknowledge the contributions to this chapter made by Sabrena Merrill, M.S., fitness-industry consultant, author, and educator, and Natalie Digate Muth, M.D., MPH, R.D., a freelance nutrition author who is currently completing her pediatrics residency at UCLA Mattel Children's Hospital.

CHAPTER 10

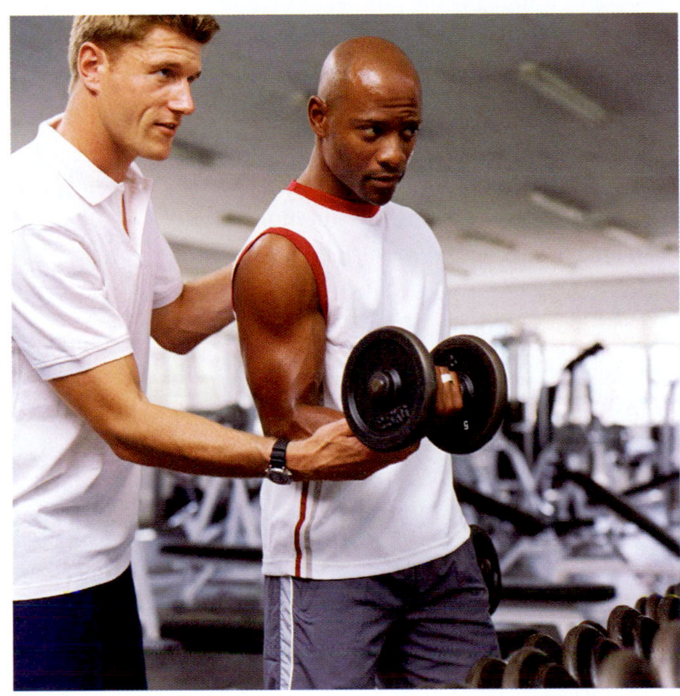

Resistance Training: Programming and Progressions

Wayne Westcott

Every bodily movement is a result of the muscular system acting on the skeletal system. Muscles are unique in their ability to produce force, which they can do through **concentric** actions as they shorten, **eccentric** actions as they lengthen, and **isometric** actions without changing their length. Muscle is metabolically active tissue that is highly responsive to the stimuli of progressive resistance exercise. With appropriate training, muscles grow and become stronger; without appropriate training, muscles diminish and become weaker. This chapter presents information about the benefits of sensible strength training, as well as research-based recommendations for safe and effective muscle development.

Benefits of Resistance Training

Strength training is the process of exercising with progressively heavier resistance to stimulate muscle development. The primary outcome of regular resistance exercise is an increase in muscle fiber size and contractile strength. Secondary outcomes include increased tensile strength in **tendons** (which attach muscles to bones) and **ligaments** (which attach bones to bones), as well as increased **bone mineral density (BMD).** Properly performed resistance training has a positive impact on the entire musculoskeletal system. While strength training has obvious implications for improving power production and sports performance, it is equally important from a health and fitness perspective.

Physical Capacity

Physical capacity is the ability to perform work or exercise. Muscles utilize energy to produce the forces that enable people to move their body parts and any external resistance, thereby functioning as the engines of the body. Resistance training results in stronger muscles that increase the physical capacity for force production. For example, progressive resistance exercise enables an individual to perform a single lift with a heavier weightload (**muscular strength**), and to perform more repetitions with a submaximum weightload (**muscular endurance**). On average, previously untrained youth, adults, and older adults increase their muscle mass by 2 to 4 pounds (0.9 to 1.8 kg) and their muscular strength by 40 to 60% after eight to 12 weeks of standard strength training (Westcott et al., 2009; Westcott, Tolken, & Wessner, 1995; Campbell et al., 1994; Fiatarone et al., 1994).

Physical capacity decreases dramatically with age in non–strength training adults due to an average 5-pound (2.3-kg) per decade loss of muscle tissue (disuse **atrophy**). Consequently, men and women who want to maintain their physical capacity and performance abilities must make resistance exercise a regular component of an active lifestyle.

Physical Appearance and Body Composition

The human body is composed of two primary components—fat weight and fat-free weight, or lean weight. Lean weight consists of muscle, bone, blood, skin, organs, and **connective tissue,** with muscle contributing about half of the lean weight (a little more than half in men and a little less than half in women). Lean mass is subject to progressive decreases associated with aging and with a lack of training. A woman who does not strength train loses about 0.5 pounds (0.23 kg) of muscle each year. For example, if Susan is 30 years old, weighs 120 pounds (54 kg), and has 20% **body fat,** she has 24 pounds (11 kg) of fat weight and 96 pounds (44 kg) of lean weight [about 45 lb (20 kg) of muscle).

- Susan's weight: 120 lb (54 kg), with 20% body fat
- Fat mass: 120 lb x 0.2 = 24 lbs (11 kg)
- Lean mass: 120 lb x 0.8 = 96 lbs (44 kg) [and approximately 45 lb (20 kg) of muscle]

At age 50, if Susan weighs the same [120 lb (54 kg)], her **body composition** would change by 20 pounds (9 kg):

- Loss of 0.5 lb muscle/year = 10 lb (4.5 kg) less muscle in 20 years
- Gain of 10 lb (4.5 kg) of fat in 20 years

Her new body composition is as follows:

- Fat mass: 34 lb (15.5 kg)
- Lean mass: 86 lb (39.1 kg)
- Percent body fat: (34 lb/120 lb) x 100 = 28.3%

Of course, this increase in percent body fat has a negative impact on her appearance, fitness, and health.

Fortunately, a basic program of resistance exercise can reverse this situation. Numerous strength-training studies have shown that several weeks of traditional strength training result in about 3 pounds (1.4 kg) more muscle and 4 pounds (1.8 kg) less fat in adults and older adults (Westcott et al., 2009; Campbell et al., 1994; Pratley et al., 1994), and this rate of body-composition improvement appears to continue for several months (Westcott et al., 2008).

Metabolic Function

Muscle tissue is constantly active for purposes of maintenance and remodeling of muscle **proteins.** Even during sleep, resting skeletal muscles are responsible for more than 25% of the body's calorie use. Logically, the decrease in muscle tissue that results from disuse atrophy is accompanied by a decrease in **resting metabolic rate (RMR),** and the increase in muscle tissue that results from resistance exercise is accompanied by an increase in RMR. More specifically, the 5-pound (2.3-kg) per decade muscle loss experienced by non–strength training adults leads to a 3% per decade reduction in RMR. This gradual decrease in metabolism is associated with the gradual increase in body fat that typically accompanies the aging process. When less energy is required for daily metabolic function, calories that were previously used by muscle tissue (that has since atrophied) are stored as fat.

In contrast, strength training raises RMR and results in more calories burned on a daily basis. Several studies have demonstrated a 7 to 8% increase in resting metabolism following several weeks of regular resistance exercise (Hunter et al., 2000; Van Etten et al., 1997; Campbell et al., 1994; Pratley et al., 1994). More recently, Hackney, Engels, and Gretebeck (2008) reported an average 9% increase in resting metabolism for three days after an intense resistance workout in untrained individuals, and an average 8% increase in resting metabolism for three days after an intense resistance workout in trained individuals. Apparently, the micro-trauma-repair and muscle-remodeling processes require increased energy for at least 72 hours following a challenging strength-training session. As most trainees perform resistance exercise at least every third day, the elevated metabolism would seem to be a continuous physiological response to regular strength training.

Given a typical RMR of about 1,500 calories per day, an 8% elevation represents 120 additional calories burned at rest on a daily basis. Other things being equal, this would total 3,600 more calories used every 30 days, for a 1-pound (0.5-kg) fat loss per month and a 12-pound (5.4-kg) fat loss per year. While other factors seldom remain the same, it is clear that resistance exercise can increase muscle mass, decrease fat mass, and raise RMR, effectively countering primary degenerative processes of **sedentary** aging. Additionally, the calories used during the strength-training session and in the post-exercise muscle-remodeling period contribute to fat loss and provide associated health benefits.

Injury Risk and Disease Prevention

Muscles serve as shock absorbers and balancing agents. Strong muscles help dissipate the repetitive landing forces experienced in weightbearing activities such as running and step exercise. Balanced muscle development reduces the risk of overuse injuries that result when one muscle group is relatively strong and the opposing muscle group is relatively weak. For example, jogging places greater stress on the posterior leg muscles than the anterior leg muscles, leading to a muscle imbalance that may cause knee injuries.

To reduce the risk of unbalanced muscle development, personal trainers should include resistance exercises for all of the major muscle groups, paying special attention to opposing muscles at the joints (e.g., gastrocnemius and anterior tibialis, quadriceps and hamstrings, erector spinae and rectus abdominis). A comprehensive program of resistance exercise that addresses all of the major muscle groups may be the most effective means of preventing various musculoskeletal injuries and reducing the risk of many degenerative diseases.

One of the most direct benefits of regular strength training is increased BMD (Menkes et al., 1993), which may reduce the risk of **osteoporosis** (Nelson et al., 1994). Other benefits of resistance training include:

- Improved body composition (more muscle, less fat), which reduces the risk of **type 2 diabetes** (Gordon et al., 2009) and **cardiovascular disease** (Braith & Stewart, 2006). With respect to diabetes, resistance exercise has been shown to improve **insulin** response (Ryan et al., 2001) and **glucose** utilization (Holten et al., 2004). With respect to cardiovascular disease, strength training has been demonstrated to lower resting **blood pressure** (Cornelissen & Fagard, 2005), improve blood **lipid** profiles (Kelley & Kelley, 2009), enhance vascular condition (Olson et al., 2006), and decrease the risk of developing the **metabolic syndrome** (Wijndaele et al., 2007).

- Facilitation of the movement of food and waste through the gastrointestinal system. Four months of basic resistance exercise increases gastrointestinal transit speed by 56% in older men (Koffler et al., 1992), which may reduce the risk of colon cancer (Hurley, 1994).
- Stronger muscles, which appears to be particularly important for low-back health. Strong erector spinae muscles enhance low-back support, control, function, and shock absorption. After 10 weeks of performing full-range resistance exercise for the lumbar spine muscles, many individuals with low-back pain reported significantly less discomfort and some were pain-free (Risch et al., 1993).
- Reduced pain of **osteoarthritis** and **rheumatoid arthritis** (Jan et al., 2008; Lange, Vanwanseele, & Fiatarone-Singh, 2008)
- A decrease in **depression** in older men and women (Annesi & Westcott, 2007; Singh, Clements, & Fiatarone, 1997)
- Improved functional ability in older adults (Kalapotharakos et al., 2005)
- Increased mitochondrial content and oxidative capacity of muscle tissue (Phillips, 2007; Parise, Brose, & Tarnopolsky, 2005). In one study, older subjects who performed six months of circuit strength training experienced positive adaptations in 179 genes associated with age and exercise, giving their muscles mitochondrial characteristics similar to those of young adults (Melov et al., 2007).

Research has demonstrated numerous health and fitness benefits resulting from regular resistance exercise. Taken together, these benefits enhance the quality of life and lower the risk of premature all-cause **mortality** (Ruiz et al., 2008; Hurley & Roth, 2000).

Physiological Adaptations to Resistance Training: Acute and Long-term

To perform resistance exercise, a number of acute physiological responses must take place. First, nerve impulses must be transmitted from the **central nervous system** to activate the appropriate **motor units** and muscle fibers in the **prime mover** muscles. As the muscle fibers contract to provide the necessary movement force, they use fuel sources such as **creatine phosphate** and **glycogen** for **anaerobic** energy production. These cellular combustion processes result in metabolic by-products such as hydrogen ions and **lactic acid.** Acute adaptations to resistance exercise also occur within the endocrine system. Concentrations of **catabolic** hormones (**cortisol** and **epinephrine**) and **anabolic** hormones (**growth hormone** and **testosterone**) increase during a resistance-training session.

There are two principal long-term physiological adaptations to progressive resistance exercise: increased muscular strength and increased muscle size (**hypertrophy**). During the first several weeks of training, strength gains are largely the result of neurological factors, which is known as **motor learning.** Repeat performances of a resistance exercise result in more efficient activation of the motor units involved in the exercise movement. Motor units that produce the desired movement are facilitated, and motor units that produce the opposing movement are inhibited, thereby resulting in stronger contractions of the prime mover muscles.

Some of the strength gains are the result of muscle hypertrophy. Resistance exercise causes varying degrees of muscle tissue microtrauma, depending on the intensity and volume of the training session. During the days following a challenging resistance-training session, muscle tissue remodeling results in growth of muscle fibers coupled with small increases in muscular strength. Satellite cells within the muscle are largely responsible for building larger and stronger muscle fibers.

Strength trained muscle fibers increase in cross-sectional area as a result of two tissue adaptations. One response to progressive resistance exercise is an increase in the number of **myofibrils** (**contractile proteins**) within the muscle fiber. This is referred to as **myofibrillar hypertrophy** and results in greater muscle contraction force.

Another response to progressive resistance exercise is an increase in the muscle cell **sarcoplasm** that surrounds the myofibrils, but is not directly involved in contractile processes. This is known as **sarcoplasmic hypertrophy** and does not result in greater muscle contraction force, but does increase the cross-sectional area, or size, of the muscle. This form of hypertrophy should not be confused with **transient hypertrophy,** a term denoting the "muscle pump" experienced by many people immediately following resistance training. It is caused by fluid accumulation in the spaces between cells (due to muscle contraction) and it quickly diminishes soon after exercise as the fluid balance between the various tissues and compartments returns to normal.

For most people and for most practical purposes, standard resistance exercise produces both myofibrillar and sarcoplasmic hypertrophy in the trained muscle fibers (Zatsiorsky & Kraemer, 2006). Some experts believe that resistance-training protocols that feature heavy weightloads, low repetitions, and long rests between sets favor myofibrillar hypertrophy, whereas resistance-training protocols that emphasize moderate weightloads, moderate repetitions, and short rests between sets favor sarcoplasmic hypertrophy (Zatsiorsky & Kraemer, 2006).

Research indicates that the muscle-remodeling processes following a challenging session of resistance exercise may continue for 72 hours (Hackney, Engels, & Gretebeck, 2008). In a well-designed study of training frequency, muscular strength did not reach or exceed baseline levels until 72 hours after a standard workout (eight exercises, three sets, 10 repetitions per set) (McLester et al., 2003).

Factors That Influence Muscular Strength and Hypertrophy

There are several factors that influence the development of muscular strength and size, most of which are genetically determined. These include **hormone** levels, gender, age, muscle fiber type, muscle length, limb length, and tendon **insertion** point.

Hormone Levels

Hormones are produced in the endocrine glands and transported throughout the body by blood circulation. Two hormones associated with tissue growth and development (anabolic processes) are growth hormone and testosterone. Higher levels of these anabolic hormones are advantageous for increasing muscular strength and size. Growth hormone levels are highest during youth and decrease with advancing age. Testosterone is the principal male sex hormone and is largely responsible for the greater size and strength of male muscles compared to female muscles. Testosterone concentrations also decrease with age, which, together with lower growth hormone levels, lead to reduced muscle mass and strength in older adults. Individuals who have higher levels of growth hormone and testosterone typically have enhanced potential for muscle development.

Sex

Male and female muscle tissue is essentially the same with respect to strength production, as each square centimeter of cross-sectional area is capable of developing 1 to 2 kilograms of contractile force. However, while an individual's sex does not affect muscle quality, it does influence muscle quantity. Due to larger body size, higher lean weight percentage, and more anabolic hormones (testosterone), men typically have greater muscle mass and overall muscular strength than women. For example, in a study of more than 900 men and women, the men were 50% stronger than the women on a standard assessment of quadriceps muscle strength (Westcott, 2003). However, when compared on a pound-for-pound basis of lean (muscle) weight, the average quadriceps muscle force production was almost identical for the male and female subjects.

Age

Advancing age is associated with less muscle mass and lower strength levels, at least partly due to lower levels of anabolic hormones. Cross-sectional assessments of strength performance on standard weightstack machine exercises show an average strength loss of 10% per decade in adults between 20 and 80 years of age (Westcott, 2003). Nonetheless, in a study of more than 1,700 men and women, the younger adults (20 to 44 years old), middle-aged adults (45 to 64 years old), and older adults (65 to 80 years old) all added statistically similar amounts of lean (muscle) weight after 10 weeks of strength training (Westcott et al., 2009). It would therefore appear that people of all ages respond favorably to progressive resistance exercise and gain muscle at approximately the same rate during the initial training period. However, the potential for total-body muscle mass diminishes during the older-adult years.

Muscle Fiber Type

Muscles are composed of two categories of contractile proteins, known as **type I muscle fibers** (**slow-twitch muscle fibers**) and **type II muscle fibers** (**fast-twitch muscle fibers**), which are further broken down into type IIa and type IIx fibers. Type I fibers are typically smaller with more aerobic capacity (lower levels of force production for larger periods of time), whereas type II fibers are typically larger with more **anaerobic capacity** (higher levels of force production for shorter periods of time). Both type I and type II fibers are involved in resistance exercise, with the slow-twitch fibers activated at lower force levels and the fast-twitch fibers activated at higher force levels. Likewise, both type I and type II muscle fibers increase in cross-sectional area as a result of strength training. Because type II muscle fibers experience greater size increases than type I muscle fibers, it would appear that fast-twitch fibers play a larger role than slow-twitch fibers in muscle hypertrophy. This being the case, individuals who are born with higher percentages of type II muscle fibers (e.g., sprinters) may have more potential for muscle hypertrophy than individuals who are born with higher percentages of type I muscle fibers (e.g., marathoners). Adaptations to endurance and resistance training can create small shifts (<10%) in fiber composition, shifting the number of type IIx fibers to type IIa fibers, while more explosive anaerobic training causes an adaptation where type IIa fibers change to function more like type IIx fibers. Trainers should be aware that type I fibers also have the potential for modest hypertrophy. As a result, they should target all muscle fiber types when designing resistance-training programs (Wilmore, Costill, & Kenney, 2008; Shoepe, 2003; Pette, 2001).

Muscle Length

Perhaps the most important factor for attaining large muscle size is muscle length relative to bone length. Muscles typically attach to bones by connective tissues called tendons. Some people have relatively short muscles with long tendon attachments, whereas other people have relatively long muscles with short tendon attachments. Those with relatively long muscles possess greater potential for muscle development than those with relatively short muscles. For example, an individual who has relatively long gastrocnemius muscles with short Achilles tendons possesses more potential to develop large calf muscles than an individual who has relatively short gastrocnemius muscles with long Achilles tendons.

Limb Length

Although limb length does not influence muscle hypertrophy, it definitely affects strength performance. Other things being equal, shorter limbs provide leverage advantages over longer limbs. The relationship between muscle force and resistance force is mediated by leverage factors, as expressed in the following formula:

Muscle force x Muscle force arm =
Resistance force x Resistance force arm

The muscle force arm is the distance from the joint **axis of rotation** to the muscle–tendon insertion point, and the resistance force arm is the distance from the joint axis of rotation to the resistance application point. Longer limbs provide longer resistance force arms and require more muscle force to move a given resistance. Conversely, shorter limbs provide shorter resistance force arms and require less muscle force to move a given resistance. Assuming equal biceps muscle strength and tendon insertion points, a person with a shorter forearm can curl a heavier dumbbell than a person with a longer forearm.

Tendon Insertion Point

Like limb length, the point where the tendon inserts on the bone does not influence muscle hypertrophy, but definitely affects strength performance. Based on the formula presented in the previous section, a longer muscle force arm provides a leverage advantage for moving a heavier resistance. Assuming equal biceps muscle strength and forearm lengths, an individual with a tendon insertion point farther from the elbow joint axis can curl a heavier dumbbell than an individual with a tendon insertion point closer to the elbow joint.

Muscular Strength/Power/ Endurance Relationships

Muscular strength is the foundation of all physical activities. Every movement humans make requires a certain percentage of maximum muscular strength. The standard measure of muscular strength is the highest resistance that can be moved through the full movement range at a controlled movement speed, which is referred to as the **one-repetition maximum (1 RM). Muscular endurance** is closely related to muscular strength, and is typically assessed by the number of repetitions that can be performed with a given submaximal resistance. Most people can complete approximately 10 repetitions with 75% of their 1-RM weightload. For example, if a client's maximum bench press is 100 pounds (45 kg), he or she can probably perform 10 repetitions with 75 pounds (34 kg) (75% of the 1 RM). If training increases this client's 1-RM bench press to 120 pounds (54 kg), he or she can most likely complete 10 repetitions with 90 pounds (41 kg) (75% of his new 1 RM). That is, this client's "relative muscular endurance" maintains the same ratio to his or her maximum strength. However, when the client's 1-RM bench press increases to 120 pounds (54 kg), he or she can perform approximately 15 repetitions with 75 pounds (34 kg), because this weightload is now only 62.5% of his or her maximum strength. Therefore, this client's "absolute muscular endurance" increases as muscular strength increases.

Muscular power is the product of muscular strength and movement speed. Assuming that an individual's movement speed remains the same, an increase in muscular strength is accompanied by a proportional increase in muscular power. However, the relationship between the exercise weightload and muscular power is somewhat complex, and is best represented by an inverted U curve (Figure 10-1). Training with light resistance enables fast movement speed, but results in a relatively low power output due to the low strength component. Training with heavy resistance enables a high strength component, but requires slow movement speed, and therefore results in a relatively low power output. Training with medium resistance and moderate-to-fast movement speeds produces the highest power output and is the most effective means for increasing muscular power.

Figure 10-1
The relationship between the exercise weightload and muscular power

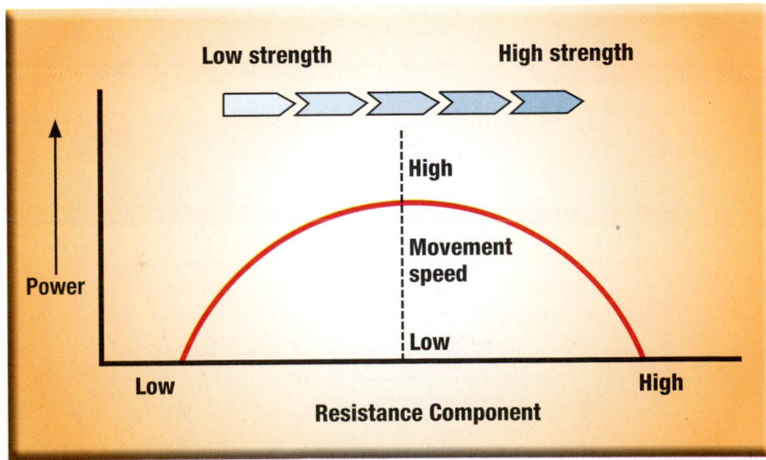

Training Variables: Factors Affecting Strength Development and Program Design

There are several exercise performance factors that affect the rate and degree of strength development. These training variables include volume, intensity, tempo, rest intervals, and frequency. The design of effective programs requires consideration of several factors and programming variables, including the following:

- A thorough needs assessment on the client
- Appropriate exercise frequency consistent with the client's goals, training experience, current conditioning level, and necessary recovery periods between sessions
- Appropriate exercises and exercise order consistent with program needs and goals, equipment availability, client experience, technique, and conditioning level
- The exercise volume and load—sets, repetitions, and intensity
- The appropriate rest intervals between sets selected according to the client's needs and goals

Needs Assessment

One of the trainer's initial responsibilities during the planning stage of program design is to complete a detailed needs assessment on each client to determine what the appropriate program will entail. The trainer must identify what physiological parameters need to be included in the program to achieve success with respect to the client's goals (Table 10-1).

Table 10-1
Health- and Skill-related Parameters

Health-related Parameters	Skill-related Parameters
Aerobic capacity	Power
Muscular endurance	Speed
Muscular strength	Balance
Flexibility	Agility
Body composition	Coordination
	Reactivity

To complete the needs assessment, the trainer should consider the following:

- Evaluation of the activity or sport
  - ✓ Movement analysis (What movement patterns, speeds, and muscle involvements are needed?)
  - ✓ Physiological analysis (Which energy systems are utilized? Does the activity require muscular endurance, hypertrophy, strength, or power?)
  - ✓ Injury analysis (What are prevalent injuries associated with participation in this activity or sport?)
- Individual assessment
  - ✓ Current conditioning level
  - ✓ Training history and technique
  - ✓ History of injury or fear of injury
  - ✓ Tolerance for discomfort

Trainers unfamiliar with a particular activity or sport would be best served establishing communication with some higher-level coaches and athletes, as well as a medical support staff that can provide valuable insight and information into completing the needs assessment.

Training Frequency

Training frequency is inversely related to both training volume and training intensity. Less vigorous exercise sessions produce less muscle microtrauma, require less time for tissue remodeling, and can be performed more frequently. More vigorous exercise sessions produce more muscle microtrauma, require more time for tissue remodeling, and must be performed less frequently for optimum results. Research has revealed that a challenging resistance workout elevates RMR by 8 to 9% for three days following the exercise session, presumably due to muscle-building processes (Hackney, Engels, & Gretebeck, 2008). Other studies have shown that standard strength-training sessions (eight exercises, three sets of 10 repetitions) require at least 72 hours for muscular strength to attain or exceed baseline levels (McLester et al., 2003).

It would therefore appear that advanced exercisers who perform high-volume/

high-intensity strength workouts should not train the same muscle groups more frequently than every third day. For example, they could perform workouts that emphasize pushing movements with the chest, shoulders, and triceps on Mondays and Thursdays, workouts that focus on pulling movements with the back, biceps, and trunk on Tuesdays and Fridays, and squatting and lunging movements with the legs on Wednesdays and Saturdays.

On the other hand, a large-scale study on exercise frequency demonstrated similar muscular development for beginning participants who trained two or three days per week. After 10 weeks of basic resistance exercise, both training frequencies increased the subjects' lean (muscle) weight by 3.1 pounds (1.4 kg) (Westcott et al., 2009). Based on these results, two or three weekly strength-training sessions work equally well for new exercisers, and the choice should be a matter of personal preference. The same study examined the effects of one weekly resistance workout on muscle development. Although marginally productive, the one-day-per-week training frequency resulted in significantly less lean (muscle) weight gain than the two-days-per-week and three-days-per-week training frequencies. It is therefore recommended that new exercisers perform resistance training two or three days a week for best results. Table 10-2 provides general guidelines that a trainer can follow to determine appropriate training frequencies for beginner, intermediate, and advanced exercisers.

Table 10-2

General Training Frequency Guidelines

Training Status	Frequency Guidelines (sessions per week)
Beginner—not currently training or just beginning with minimal skill	2–3
Intermediate—basic skill	3–4
Advanced—advanced skill	4–7

Baechle, T.R. & Earle, R.W. (2008). *Essentials of Strength Training and Conditioning* (3rd ed.). Champaign, Ill.: Human Kinetics.

Exercise Selection and Order

Exercise selection and order is a complex process that requires consideration of the individual's experience and exercise technique, movement and physiological demands of the activity or sport, equipment availability, and time availability. While hundreds of resistance exercises exist, one effective method of exercise selection is to group exercises based on body area (e.g., legs or shoulders) or function (e.g., push versus pull), or by relevance to the activity or sport.

- Primary exercises involve multiple muscles from one or more of the larger muscle areas (e.g., chest, thigh) that span two or more joints (i.e., multijoint exercises) and are generally performed in a linear fashion (i.e., integrated muscle action and joint movements working in the same direction—squat, shoulder press, etc.).
- Assisted exercises involve smaller muscle groups from more isolated areas that span one joint (i.e., single-joint).

Trainers often design programs by grouping specific muscles into a session. While various strategies exist, the muscle grouping should ultimately reflect the specific needs of the client and his or her availability for training. Guidelines from the American College of Sports Medicine (ACSM) recommend targeting each major muscle group two to three days a week, allowing a minimum of 48 hours of recovery between sessions (ACSM, 2010). Therefore, training twice per week may require the use of circuits that target all the major muscle groups within a session, whereas training with greater frequency allows the trainer flexibility to divide sessions into body parts.

Trainers can select from a variety of methods to enhance muscle hypertrophy or improve muscular endurance, strength, and power. Some of these options include:

- Performing primary exercises followed by assisted exercises within a targeted area

- ✓ May entail performing multijoint linear exercises (e.g., movement collaboration of several joints moving resistance in one direction—squats, chest press, shoulder press), followed by single-joint rotary exercises (e.g., movements around one joint—leg extensions, flys, lateral raises).
- Alternating upper- and lower-extremity exercises within or between training sessions
- Grouping pushing and pulling muscles within a session (e.g., chest, shoulders, and triceps in a session)
- Alternating pushing and pulling movements or targeting joint **agonists** and **antagonists** within a session (e.g., chest muscles and back muscles or biceps and triceps)
- Performing supersets or compound sets where exercises are done in sequence with little or no rest between them, before an appropriate rest interval is taken. Two common methods include:
  - ✓ Supersets where two or more sequentially performed exercises that target opposing muscles are completed (e.g., agonist–antagonist)
  - ✓ Compound sets where two or more sequentially performed exercises that target the same muscle group are completed (e.g., dumbbell flys followed by chest presses).

Trainers should also consider exercise progression relative to the client's conditioning status and ability to stabilize the entire kinetic chain. Given the advancements made in technology and equipment design, trainers should avoid making the mistake of prematurely progressing clients to equipment that is too challenging for their current abilities. Figure 10-2 provides an example of an appropriate exercise progression for trainers to follow.

Training Volume

During each resistance-training session, a certain amount of work is performed. The cumulative work completed is referred to as the training volume. Training volume is calculated in several ways:

- *Repetition-volume calculation:* Volume = Sets x Repetitions (for either the muscle group or the session)
- *Load-volume calculation:* Volume = Exercise weightload x Repetitions x Sets (and then summing the total for each muscle group or the entire session)

Although training volume is an excellent measure of how much work was performed, it may not be an accurate assessment of how hard a person truly worked. For example, Mary can complete four leg presses with 90 pounds, eight leg presses with 80 pounds, and 12 leg presses with 70 pounds. Although each set requires a high effort and produces similar levels of muscle fatigue (e.g., no additional repetitions can be performed), the training volume varies considerably.

- 1 set x 4 repetitions with 90 pounds = 360 pounds
- 1 set x 8 repetitions with 80 pounds = 640 pounds
- 1 set x 12 repetitions with 70 pounds = 840 pounds

Training volume provides a reasonably good indication of the energy used in a workout, as there is a correlation between the total amount of weight lifted and the total number of calories burned. It is recommended that training volume be changed periodically for physiological and psychological purposes. Training volume is typically lower for competitive powerlifters who perform fewer exercises, repetitions, and sets with heavier weightloads as they focus on improving the muscle's ability to maximally recruit fibers to generate higher amounts of force. Competitive bodybuilders, on the other hand, perform higher-volume workouts with more exercises, repetitions, and sets with moderate weightloads as they focus on increasing the amount of time the muscle spends under tension performing work to stimulate hypertrophy.

While each individual's training goals dictate the training volume needed, his or her fitness status provides a good indicator of the appropriate volume. Therefore, trainers

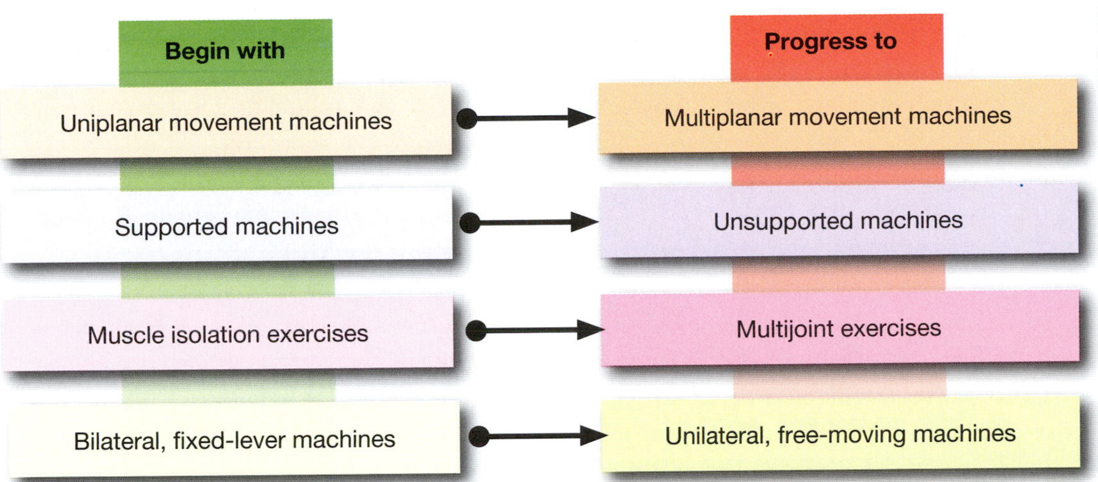

Figure 10-2
Appropriate program progressions

should consider starting deconditioned or novice clients with manageable volumes prior to progressing their volume to the ranges outlined in Table 10-3 (Baechle & Earle, 2008; Westcott, 2003).

As a client begins a resistance-training program and is in the transition from the **preparation** to the **action** stages of behavior change, the total training volume should be kept relatively low to allow for adaptation and accommodation to the training stress. Another benefit of keeping the training volume low during the initial stages of an exercise program is to allow the client to feel successful after accomplishing the goal of performing a specific volume of training. Training volume can be gradually increased as the client develops **adherence** to the program, becoming stronger as a result.

Training Intensity

Training intensity has two different applications in the area of resistance exercise. Some strength experts define training intensity as the percentage of maximum resistance used in an exercise. They would consider four repetitions with 90 pounds to be a higher-intensity training bout than eight repetitions with 80 pounds, even if each exercise set produced similar levels of muscle fatigue (no additional repetitions could be performed), based purely on the amount of weight lifted. Other strength experts define training intensity as the effort level achieved during an exercise set. They would consider four repetitions with 90 pounds and eight repetitions with 80 pounds to be equal in training intensity, as long as each exercise bout produced similar levels of muscle fatigue (no additional repetitions could be performed).

Table 10-3
Recommended Training Volumes Based on Training Goals

Training Goal	Sets	Repetitions
General muscle fitness	1–2	8–15
Muscular endurance	2–3	≥12
Muscular hypertrophy	3–6	6–12
Muscular strength	2–6	≤6
Power:		
Single-effort events	3–5	1–2
Multiple-effort events	3–5	3–5

Sources: Baechle, T.R. & Earle, R.W. (2008). *Essentials of Strength Training and Conditioning* (3rd ed.). Champaign, Ill.: Human Kinetics; Westcott, W.L. (2003). *Building Strength & Stamina* (2nd ed.). Champaign, Ill.: Human Kinetics.

Using either definition, training intensity varies inversely with training volume. For most individuals, higher-intensity training sessions require lower exercise volumes, and higher-volume exercise sessions require lower training intensities. Most **periodization** models for strength-training programs begin with higher-volume/lower-intensity workouts, progress to moderate-volume/moderate-intensity workouts, and conclude with lower-volume/higher-intensity workouts. Although both volume and intensity are key components of progressive resistance exercise, the more important factor for strength development appears to be the training effort.

When developing an exercise program for a client who is new to resistance training, the initial stage should feature exercises with a low level of intensity. A client who is new to resistance training may perceive exercise as painful and uncomfortable. An exercise program with a high level of intensity relative to the client's experience could create **delayed onset muscle soreness (DOMS)** and impede the client's adherence to regular exercise. Intensity can be used to help foster adherence to an exercise program for a client with limited or no resistance-training experience. Designing an exercise program to begin with a low level of intensity in the initial phase, allowing the client to physically and psychologically adapt to the training stress, and gradually progressing the intensity will help the client experience results while developing long-term adherence to exercise. Progressing intensity too quickly could lead to muscle soreness or injury, providing reasons for a client to quit the exercise program.

Training Tempo

Research has not identified a particular training tempo that is most effective for increasing muscular strength and size. For example, Olympic lifters perform their competitive exercises at fast movement speeds, bodybuilders generally train at moderate movement speeds, and powerlifters do their competitive exercises at slow movement speeds. Controlled movement speeds require a relatively even application of muscle force throughout the entire movement range. Conversely, fast movement speeds require a high level of muscle force to initiate the lift, with momentum mostly responsible for the remainder of the movement.

When momentum is minimized, as is the case with **isokinetic** resistance equipment, muscle force decreases as movement speed increases. The same effect may be seen with **isotonic** training, such as free weights and weightstack machines. The heavier the weightload, the longer the time required to complete 10 repetitions of an exercise (Westcott, 1991).

The commonly recommended movement speed of six seconds per repetition is consistent with the repetition speed long recommended for weightstack (or selectorized) machine training (Brzycki, 1995; Westcott, 1991; Darden, 1988). The concentric muscle action should be performed in two to three seconds and the eccentric muscle action should be performed in three to four seconds. Although other controlled movement speeds may be equally effective for strength development, six-second repetitions represent an excellent introductory training speed for new exercisers. The trainer should emphasize the performance of all exercises through a full **range of motion (ROM).** However, as previously discussed, trainers may need to consider muscle soreness when planning the duration of the eccentric phase of contraction with new exercisers, as it is this phase that triggers DOMS, which may create a negative experience.

Rest Intervals

Rest intervals refer to the recovery periods between successive exercises or between successive sets of the same exercise. The length of the rest interval is dependent on the training goal, the client's conditioning status, and the load and amount of work performed. The heavier the load, the longer the rest interval needed for recovery to replenish the muscle's energy pathways. The recommended rest intervals for endurance, hypertrophy, strength, and power are outlined in Table 10-4. A high-effort set of resistance exercise reduces the muscle's internal energy stores of creatine phosphate. Replenishment of these local energy substrates is relatively rapid, with 50% renewal within the first 30 seconds, 75% renewal

Table 10-4

Rest Intervals Based on Training Goals

Training Goal	Rest Interval
General fitness	30–90 seconds
Muscular endurance	≤30 seconds
Muscle hypertrophy	30–90 seconds
Muscular strength	2–5 minutes
Power: Single-effort events Multiple-effort events	 2–5 minutes 2–5 minutes

Sources: Baechle, T.R. & Earle, R.W. (2008). Essentials of Strength Training and Conditioning (3rd ed.). Champaign, Ill.: Human Kinetics; Westcott, W.L. (2003). *Building Strength & Stamina* (2nd ed.). Champaign, Ill.: Human Kinetics.

within the first minute, and 95% renewal within the first two minutes. For most practical purposes and general muscular conditioning, one-minute rest intervals between successive exercise sets are sufficient.

Competitive Olympic lifters and powerlifters typically take longer rest intervals between sets to ensure complete muscle recovery and energy replenishment. The longer recovery periods permit the use of relatively heavy weightloads throughout the training session. Exercisers interested in maximizing muscular strength typically take several minutes of rest between sets of the same exercise.

Competitive bodybuilders are less concerned about the exercise resistance and more concerned about "pumping up" their muscles. Therefore, they take relatively short rests between sets to keep the blood congested in the prime mover muscles. Individuals interested in maximizing muscle size typically take 30 to 90 seconds between successive exercise sets.

Rest intervals are an important component of an exercise program because they allow a client to recover after each particular exercise and maintain a consistent level of energy throughout the workout. Clients new to resistance training should have rest intervals long enough to allow them to maintain their comfort levels, but not so long that their **heart rate** and body temperature return to normal resting levels.

When performing a strength-training circuit in which each exercise addresses a different muscle group, the recovery interval has more impact on the cardiovascular system than on the exercise performance. Shorter rest intervals increase cardiovascular and metabolic responses both during and after the exercise session (Haltom et al., 1999; Westcott, 1991). This format of resistance training, coupled with higher volumes of resistance work that increase metabolism, is becoming more popular with individuals seeking to lose or manage their weight.

Training Principles

When muscles are stressed beyond their normal demands, they respond in some way to the imposed stress. If the training stress is much greater than normal, the muscles react negatively to high levels of tissue microtrauma. The resulting (large-scale) cell damage requires several days of muscle repair and rebuilding to regain pre-training strength and functional abilities. Although exceptionally challenging training sessions are typically associated with several days of muscle weakness, fatigue, and discomfort, known as DOMS, they may not lead to larger and stronger muscles. On the other hand, when muscles are systematically stressed in a progressive manner, they gradually increase in size and strength. That is, if the training stress is slightly greater than normal, the muscles respond positively to low levels of tissue microtrauma. The resulting (small-scale) cell damage elicits muscle-remodeling processes that lead to larger and stronger muscles. Research indicates that muscular strength increases significantly above baseline levels 72 to 96 hours after an appropriately stressful session of resistance exercise (McLester et al., 2003). However, when the training program no longer produces gains in muscular strength or size, the exercise protocol should be changed in some way to again elicit the desired neuromuscular adaptations.

As mentioned previously, when people with limited resistance-training experience first encounter DOMS, it can create the negative perception that exercise is uncomfortable or painful. It is important to remember to gradually progress exercise intensity and training volume and to not push a new client past his or her current fitness and comfort limits until an ability to adhere to the exercise program has been demonstrated.

Progression

There are two principal approaches to strength-training progression. The first and simplest method is to increase the number of repetitions performed with a given resistance (progressive repetitions). This is the standard means for improvement with bodyweight exercises, such as push-ups, chin-ups, and bar dips. This method works well when a client is working within the repetition ranges specified for each training goal in Table 10-3, as well as for exercise sets that can be completed using the anaerobic energy system (less than 90 seconds). However, if a client is capable of performing 40 trunk curls in two minutes, increasing the repetitions to 60 in three minutes will have a relatively small effect on abdominal muscle strength.

To maximize strength development, the resistance should be heavy enough to fatigue the target muscles within the limits of the anaerobic energy system. This is best achieved by the second method of training progression, which gradually increases the exercise workload (progressive resistance). By systematically increasing the training resistance, the trainer ensures that the exercise set is always completed within the limits of the anaerobic energy system. For example, whenever John can perform incline presses for 90 seconds, his weightload is increased by 5%, which reduces his time to muscle fatigue.

Because it is cumbersome to time each exercise set, repetition ranges provide a more practical means for progressive resistance training. For example, at a movement speed of six seconds per repetition, 10 repetitions would be completed in 60 seconds and 15 repetitions would be completed in 90 seconds. Recommended repetition ranges enable clients to use a double-progressive training protocol that is effective for strength development and reduces the risk of doing too much too soon.

Assuming a repetition range of 10 to 15 repetitions per set, a double-progressive training protocol would be applied in the following manner. Joan can presently perform 10 leg presses with 100 pounds (45 kg). She continues to train with this weightload until she can complete 15 repetitions with the same weightload. At that point, her exercise resistance is increased by 5% to 105 pounds (48 kg). The heavier weightload reduces the number of leg presses that she can perform to 12 repetitions. She continues to train with 105 pounds (48 kg) until she can again complete 15 repetitions, at which point she increases the weightload another 5% to 110 pounds (50 kg).

The double-progressive strength-training protocol may be used with any repetition range. The first progression is adding repetitions, and the second progression is adding resistance in 5% increments. There is no time limit on double-progressive protocol training. Whether it takes one week or one month, the resistance is increased only when the end-range number of repetition can be completed with proper form.

As a general guideline, many strength authorities recommend a training range of eight to 12 repetitions (ACSM, 2010). Most people can complete eight repetitions with approximately 80% of maximum resistance and 12 repetitions with about 70% of maximum resistance. Progressively training to muscle fatigue with 70 to 80% of maximum resistance represents an anaerobic exercise bout that provides an effective strength-building stimulus. Another benefit of progression is that a properly organized program allows a client to experience strength gains, which is critical for developing **self-efficacy** and long-term adherence.

Specificity

The principle of training **specificity** has many applications for achieving desired strength-training objectives. The most obvious aspect of training specificity is to exercise the appropriate muscles. For example, if a client wants to improve his or her rope climbing ability, the prime mover muscles for this activity based on the pulling movement are the latissimus dorsi, teres major, biceps, and forearm flexors. Specific resistance exercises for strengthening these muscles include lat pull-downs, chin-ups, dumbbell bent-over rows, and seated rows. Of course, to maintain balanced muscle development, these muscles should not be trained to the exclusion of exercises for the opposing muscle groups responsible for pushing movements (e.g., pectoralis major, deltoids, triceps, forearm extensors). While it is essential to emphasize the specific movements and muscles used in a particular activity, it is equally important to train all of the major muscle groups to reduce the risk of muscle imbalance and overuse injuries.

Another aspect of training specificity is to use appropriate resistance-repetition protocols. For example, a shot putter, whose event requires a one-time maximum effort, should typically train with heavier weightloads and fewer repetitions to emphasize muscular strength development. On the other hand, a rower whose event requires several minutes of strenuous muscular activity should typically train with moderate weightloads and more repetitions to emphasize the development of muscular endurance. Although there is a strong, positive relationship between muscular strength and endurance, specifically designed training protocols are advisable for athletes whose events require greater emphasis on either end of the strength–endurance continuum. The resistance-repetition protocol also affects the energy system that is most prominent during the exercise set. For example, a set of two repetitions performed in 10 seconds primarily uses creatine phosphate for energy, whereas a set of 15 repetitions performed in 75 seconds attains most of the energy from **anaerobic glycolysis.**

Overload

Muscular endurance can be increased by performing more repetitions with a given resistance, such as by doing more push-ups with bodyweight. However, to maximize strength development, muscles must be subjected to progressively heavier training loads. The process of gradually adding more exercise resistance than the muscles have previously encountered is referred to as **overload.** While the degree of overload should be individually determined, a general guideline is to increase the resistance in gradations of about 5%. As presented earlier, a range of eight to 12 repetitions represents approximately 70 to 80% of maximum resistance, which provides an effective training overload, assuming the exercise is continued to the point of muscle fatigue. Once 12 repetitions can be completed, it is advisable to add about 5% more resistance to provide progressive overload and facilitate further strength development. Of course, the overload principle may be applied to other resistance–repetition protocols. Clients training with four to eight repetitions per set should add about 5% more resistance after completing eight repetitions, and those training with 12 to 16 repetitions per set should increase the weightload by 5% after completing 16 repetitions.

Reversibility

Muscle tissue has an amazing ability to make relatively rapid changes in size and strength. Due primarily to a lack of resistance exercise, adults lose about 3 pounds (1.4 kg) of muscle every six years. However, a basic strength-training program can add 3 pounds (1.4 kg) of muscle tissue in three months (Westcott et al., 2009; Campbell et al., 1994; Pratley et al., 1994).

On the other hand, a client who stops performing resistance exercise will lose strength at about one-half the rate that it was gained (Faigenbaum et al., 1996). That is, if an individual increased his or her leg press strength by 50% over a 10-week training period, he or she would lose half of that strength gain after 10 weeks of no resistance exercise, and all of his strength gain after 20 weeks without training.

The principle of muscle **reversibility** reinforces the importance of resistance training as a lifestyle component, rather than as a short-term process for attaining a temporary objective. Without strength training, muscles gradually become smaller and weaker. With progressive resistance exercise, regardless of age, muscles increase in size and strength at relatively rapid rates (Westcott et al., 2009; Westcott, Tolken, & Wessner, 1995; Fiatarone et al., 1994).

Diminishing Returns

As clients approach their genetic potential for muscle size and strength, the rate of development decreases accordingly. Regardless of the quality and quantity of training, genetic limitations leave little room for further improvement. The phenomenon of **diminishing returns** can be discouraging to clients who want to attain additional strength gains. One means for addressing this situation, sometimes referred to as a strength plateau, is to change the training exercise. The introduction of a new exercise involves a new neuromuscular response and motor-unit activation pattern that facilitates a period of progressive strength gains. For example, if a client encounters a strength plateau in the bench press exercise, it may be helpful to switch to the incline press exercise. Although both exercises target the pectoralis major, anterior deltoid, and triceps muscles, the motor learning factor should enable the client to use progressively heavier weightloads during the first few weeks of training with the new exercise.

Resistance-training Periodization Models

Periodization refers to a planned progression of resistance exercise that intentionally varies the training stimuli, especially with respect to intensity and volume. Systematically changing the exercise variables (e.g., resistance, repetition, sets) appears to be more effective for attaining both strength development and peak performance than standardized resistance-training protocols (Kraemer et al., 2000; Fleck, 1999). According to Brooks (2003), the advantage of periodization over non-periodized exercise programs is the frequently changing demands on the neuromuscular system that require progressively higher levels of stress adaptation.

Periodized training is divided into time segments referred to as **macrocycles, mesocycles,** and **microcycles** (Figure 10-3). The overall time frame for a specific periodization program is called the macrocycle, which may cover a training period of six to 12 months. The long-range goal to be attained by the end of the macrocycle is divided into shorter-term goals that are addressed in time segments of less duration. For example, a six-month macrocycle may consist of two three-month mesocycles. Each mesocycle would provide sequential goals leading to the ultimate goal of the six-month macrocycle.

Because even three-month mesocycles represent a relatively long period for goal attainment, these are divided into more manageable microcycles. Microcycles are typically two to four weeks in length and provide regular reinforcement for making small steps toward the larger goals.

Periodized programs may be performed in either a linear manner or an undulating approach (Figure 10-4). Basically, **linear periodization** provides a consistent training protocol *within* each microcycle and changes the training variables *after* each microcycle. On the other hand, **undulating periodization** provides different training

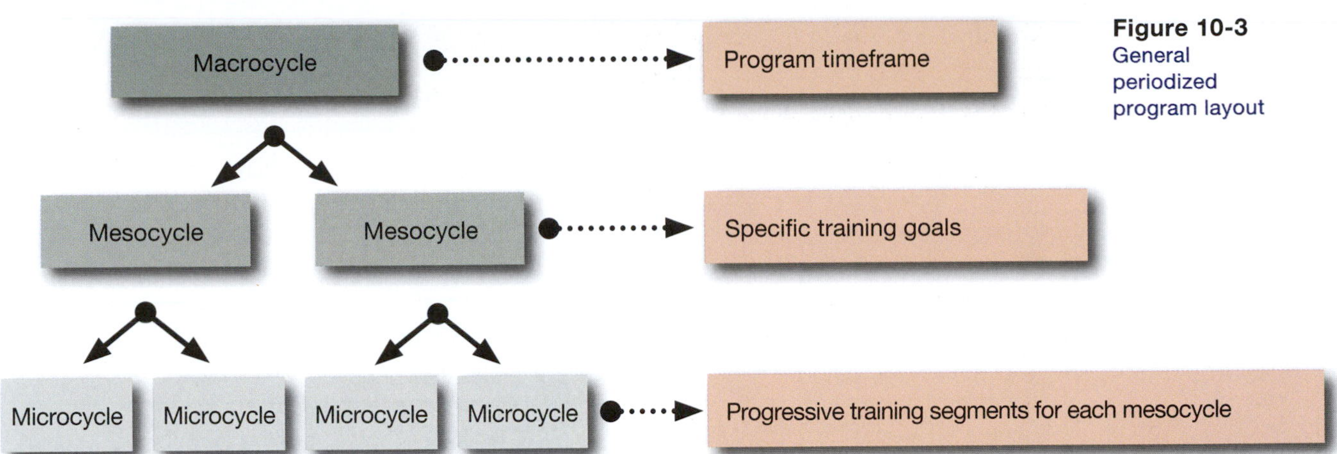

Figure 10-3 General periodized program layout

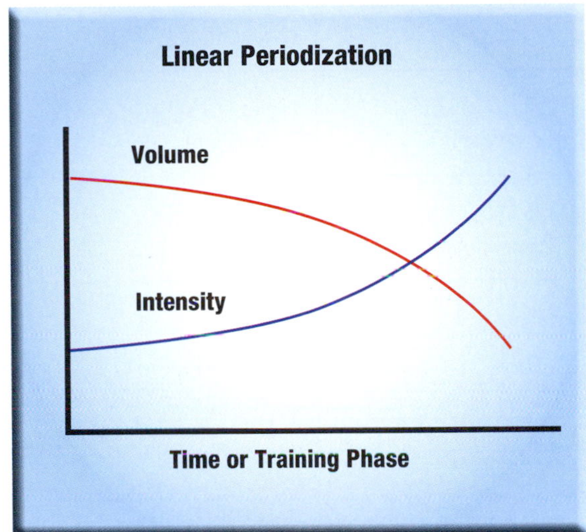

Figure 10-4 Linear vs. undulating periodization

protocols *during* the microcycles in addition to changing the training variables *after* each microcycle.

Periodization Program—Sample Protocols

John has a goal of bench pressing 250 pounds (114 kg). He can presently perform a maximum bench press of 200 pounds (91 kg). The following is a sample bench press training program using a linear periodization model.

- One macrocycle with a six-month goal of bench pressing 250 pounds (114 kg)
- Two mesocycles of three months each. The goal of the first mesocycle is to bench press 230 pounds (104 kg). The goal of the second mesocycle is to bench press 250 pounds (114 kg).
- Twelve microcycles of two weeks each. A linear periodization model is presented in Table 10-5, while an undulating periodization model is presented in Table 10-6. Although the strength-training program includes exercises for all of the major muscle groups, only the bench press protocols are presented here. The training weightload progressions are consistent with research data, but the recommended number of repetitions may not apply to all individuals. John should perform as many repetitions as possible with each exercise set, even if this is slightly lower or higher than the target number. John is advised to perform two progressive bench press warm-up sets, followed by two sets with the training weightload.

Table 10-5

Linear Periodization Model—Six-month Macrocycle

Mesocycle 1 (3 months)	Monday	Wednesday	Friday
Microcycle 1 (2 weeks)	140 lb (64 kg) x 12 repetitions	140 lb (64 kg) x 12 repetitions	140 lb (64 kg) x 12 repetitions
Microcycle 2 (2 weeks)	160 lb (73 kg) x 8 repetitions	160 lb (73 kg) x 8 repetitions	160 lb (73 kg) x 8 repetitions
Microcycle 3 (2 weeks)	180 lb (82 kg) x 4 repetitions	180 lb (82 kg) x 4 repetitions	180 lb (82 kg) x 4 repetitions
Microcycle 4 (2 weeks)	155 lb (70 kg) x 12 repetitions	155 lb (70 kg) x 12 repetitions	155 lb (70 kg) x 12 repetitions
Microcycle 5 (2 weeks)	175 lb (79 kg) x 8 repetitions	175 lb (79 kg) x 8 repetitions	175 lb (79 kg) x 8 repetitions
Microcycle 6 (2 weeks)	195 lb (89 kg) x 4 repetitions	195 lb (89 kg) x 4 repetitions	195 lb (89 kg) x 4 repetitions
Interim Week	230 lb (104 kg) x 1 repetition (goal assessment)	Rest	Rest
Mesocycle 2 (3 months)	**Monday**	**Wednesday**	**Friday**
Microcycle 1 (2 weeks)	170 lb (77 kg) x 12 repetitions	170 lb (77 kg) x 12 repetitions	170 lb (77 kg) x 12 repetitions
Microcycle 2 (2 weeks)	190 lb (86 kg) x 8 repetitions	190 lb (86 kg) x 8 repetitions	190 lb (86 kg) x 8 repetitions
Microcycle 3 (2 weeks)	210 lb (95 kg) x 4 repetitions	210 lb (95 kg) x 4 repetitions	210 lb (95 kg) x 4 repetitions
Microcycle 4 (2 weeks)	180 lb (82 kg) x 12 repetitions	180 lb (82 kg) x 12 repetitions	180 lb (82 kg) x 12 repetitions
Microcycle 5 (2 weeks)	200 lb (91 kg) x 8 repetitions	200 lb (91 kg) x 8 repetitions	200 lb (91 kg) x 8 repetitions
Microcycle 6 (2 weeks)	220 lb (100 kg) x 4 repetitions	220 lb (100 kg) x 4 repetitions	220 lb (100 kg) x 4 repetitions
Interim Week	250 lb (114 kg) x 1 repetition (goal assessment)	Rest	Rest

Table 10-6

Undulating Periodization Model—Six-month Macrocycle

Mesocycle 1 (3 months)	Monday	Wednesday	Friday
Microcycle 1 (2 weeks)	140 lb (64 kg) x 12 repetitions	160 lb (73 kg) x 8 repetitions	180 lb (82 kg) x 4 repetitions
Microcycle 2 (2 weeks)	140 lb (64 kg) x 12 repetitions	160 lb (73 kg) x 8 repetitions	180 lb (82 kg) x 4 repetitions
Microcycle 3 (2 weeks)	140 lb (64 kg) x 12 repetitions	160 lb (73 kg) x 8 repetitions	180 lb (82 kg) x 4 repetitions
Microcycle 4 (2 weeks)	155 lb (70 kg) x 12 repetitions	175 lb (79 kg) x 8 repetitions	195 lb (89 kg) x 4 repetitions
Microcycle 5 (2 weeks)	155 lb (70 kg) x 12 repetitions	175 lb (79 kg) x 8 repetitions	195 lb (89 kg) x 4 repetitions
Microcycle 6 (2 weeks)	155 lb (70 kg) x 12 repetitions	175 lb (79 kg) x 8 repetitions	195 lb (89 kg) x 4 repetitions
Interim Week	230 lb (104 kg) x 1 repetition (goal assessment)	Rest	Rest
Mesocycle 2 (3 months)	**Monday**	**Wednesday**	**Friday**
Microcycle 1 (2 weeks)	170 lb (77 kg) x 12 repetitions	190 lb (86 kg) x 8 repetitions	210 lb (95 kg) x 4 repetitions
Microcycle 2 (2 weeks)	170 lb (77 kg) x 12 repetitions	190 lb (86 kg) x 8 repetitions	210 lb (95 kg) x 4 repetitions
Microcycle 3 (2 weeks)	170 lb (77 kg) x 12 repetitions	190 lb (86 kg) x 8 repetitions	210 lb (95 kg) x 4 repetitions
Microcycle 4 (2 weeks)	180 lb (82 kg) x 12 repetitions	200 lb (91 kg) x 8 repetitions	220 lb (100 kg) x 4 repetitions
Microcycle 5 (2 weeks)	180 lb (82 kg) x 12 repetitions	200 lb (91 kg) x 8 repetitions	220 lb (100 kg) x 4 repetitions
Microcycle 6 (2 weeks)	180 lb (82 kg) x 12 repetitions	200 lb (91 kg) x 8 repetitions	220 lb (100 kg) x 4 repetitions
Interim Week	250 lb (114 kg) x 1 repetition (goal assessment)	Rest	Rest

Program Design Using the ACE Integrated Fitness Training Model

Phase 1: Stability and Mobility Training

The primary goal during this phase of functional movement and resistance training is to facilitate the development of the stability–mobility relationship within the kinetic chain. As discussed in Chapter 9, trainers may need to promote appropriate levels of stability or mobility at the joints without compromise (i.e., promote stability without compromising mobility and vice versa).

The programming model presented for this phase illustrates a progression model that begins by promoting **proximal** stability within the lumbar spine, then moves through the **axial skeleton** toward proximal mobility of the more **distal** segments. The strategies aim to reestablish proper neuromuscular function and balance within the muscles acting at and across the joints.

- To promote tissue extensibility and mobility at the joint, trainers should utilize a variety of flexibility methods that include **static stretching, proprioceptive neuromuscular facilitation (PNF),** and **myofascial release.**
- To improve a muscle's ability to maintain good joint position and function (endurance and strength), trainers should follow the ACE-recommended general progression sequence. This sequence begins with the implementation of low-grade isometric contractions of the targeted muscle (with the joint positioned in good posture), followed by controlled dynamic movements that increase the muscular volume and load.

Phase 2: Movement Training

Once a client demonstrates improvements to the stability-mobility relationship, illustrated by improved posture and awareness, enhanced core function, and a general improvement in his or her overall physical, emotional, and psychological status, trainers should progress to phase 2 of the ACE Integrated Fitness Training™ (ACE IFT™) Model. Movement training focuses on developing movement efficiency, essentially teaching clients to perform the five primary movements effectively in all three planes. Training these movements three-dimensionally will improve the client's ability to perform his or her daily activities.

- *Bend-and-lift movements:* Bend-and-lift, or squatting, movements are performed many times throughout the day as a person sits or stands from a chair or squats down to lift an object off of the floor.
- *Single-leg movements:* Single-leg movements, including lunging, are performed during the alternating leg action of the **gait** cycle as well as when a person steps forward to reach down with one hand to pick something small up off the floor or walks down or up a flight of stairs.
- *Pushing movements:* Pushing movements occur either in a forward direction (e.g., during a push-up exercise or when pushing open a door), in an overhead direction (e.g., during a shoulder press or when putting an item on a high shelf), or in a lateral direction (e.g., pushing open double sliding doors or lifting one's torso when getting up from a side-lying position).
- *Pulling movements:* Pulling movements occur during an exercise such as a bent-over row or pull-up or during a movement like pulling open a car door.
- *Rotational (spiral) movements:* **Rotation** occurs during many common movements, such as the rotation of the thoracic spine during gait or reaching across the body to pick up an object on the left side and placing it on the right side.

Most pushing, pulling, and squatting motions can be performed either unilaterally or bilaterally, while lunges require combined acyclical unilateral movements of the legs. Most everyday pushing, pulling, and squatting movements also have a rotational component that requires either motion or stabilization to prevent motion in the

transverse plane, yet traditional exercise selection emphasizes linear movements that do not require individuals to produce or control torque (i.e., rotational force). A client who learns how to perform the basic movement patterns with control and without compensation will address asymmetries of limb strength and muscle imbalance, reducing the risk of injury as the intensity of the exercise program is progressed through repetition and the addition of external loads.

Resistance-training Focus

When the five primary movements can be performed with proper form, external resistance may be applied for progressive strength development. It is essential that the external loads are increased gradually so that correct movement patterns are not altered during the exercise performance.

- *Squat:* External loading may be applied with various types of resistance equipment. A client may begin by holding a medicine ball while doing squats. Another resistance option is placing an elastic band under the feet and holding each end of the band while performing squats. A third resistance tool is free weights, beginning with dumbbells and progressing to barbell squats when the legs can handle more resistance than the hands can hold. An alternative exercise to the barbell squat is the leg press, which trains the same pattern of movement without the influence of gravity, while strengthening the quadriceps, hamstrings, and gluteus maximus muscles.
- *Lunge:* Lunge movements (in any direction) may be performed with external loads by holding a medicine ball or dumbbells. Resistance bands and barbells are not recommended tools for lunge movements.
- *Pushing movements:* Pushing movements may be performed with added resistance by using resistance bands or cables in a standing position, by performing machine chest presses from a seated position, or by lifting free weights (dumbbells or barbells) from a lying (**supine**) position. Medicine balls may also be used for pushing movements from a supine position, and from a standing position by performing a chest pass (releasing the medicine ball).
- *Pulling movements:* Pulling movements may be performed with external loads by using resistance bands or cables in a standing position, by performing machine rows and pull-downs from a seated position, and by lifting dumbbells from a bent-over standing position with the torso parallel to the floor and supported by one arm (bent-over row exercise). Medicine balls and barbells are not recommended for beginners for rowing exercises, because one arm is not free for torso support.
- *Rotational movements:* External resistance may be applied to rotational movements by using resistance bands or cables in a standing position, by using machines from a seated position, or by lifting medicine balls from a variety of positions (standing, seated, lying). It can be difficult to use barbells in rotational movements, but dumbbells can be used in movements that directly oppose gravity's line of pull.

Assessments

Assessments performed during this phase should include protocols such as movement screens to identify a client's ability to control mobility through specific ranges of motion. As previously sedentary clients enter this phase of training, personal trainers should do a comparison of baseline data from a battery of movement screens to data collected during the stability and mobility training phase (phase 1). At this point, core muscular-endurance assessments should be implemented if they were not conducted during the prior phase. Movement-training phase assessments should be conducted on a monthly basis until the client has mastered the squat, lunge, push, pull, and rotation movements.

Program Design

The acronym FIRST may be used to designate the five key components of resistance-training program design: frequency, intensity, repetitions, sets, and type of exercise. During the movement-training phase of training, motor learning plays a major role in the desired physical development and movement patterns. Consequently, during this training period, exercise repetition should be emphasized over exercise intensity.

Frequency: Beginning exercisers experience excellent results by strength training two to three days a week, and this is the recommended training frequency during the movement-training phase.

Intensity: Due to the emphasis on proper movement patterns, the training intensity is lower during this phase. Progress intensity for movement-training exercises as described in Chapter 9.

Repetitions: The number of repetitions performed varies inversely with the intensity of the exercise set. That is, fewer repetitions can be performed with a higher resistance and more repetitions can be completed with a lower resistance. During the movement-training phase, the lower training intensity permits more repetitions in each exercise set. Repetition recommendations for exercises in phase 2 can be found in Chapter 9.

Sets: Studies have demonstrated that one set of resistance exercise is as effective as multiple training sets (Carpinelli & Otto, 1998; Starkey et al., 1996), especially for beginning exercisers. For movement-training phase workouts, one set of each exercise is certainly a good starting point. As training progresses, more sets of each exercise may be performed as determined by the client's desire to do so. During the first 10 to 12 weeks of resistance exercise, both single- and multiple-set training have been shown to increase lean (muscle) weight by approximately 3 pounds (1.4 kg) (Westcott et al., 2009; Campbell et al., 1994). Single-set programs are an effective way to help previously sedentary clients become comfortable with the challenges of resistance training. When the client demonstrates consistent adherence and initial adaptations to a single-set program, the volume of sets can increase.

Type: The type of exercise should be selected with respect to the client's movement efficiency as described in Chapter 9. Clients with less muscular strength and training experience should begin with basic exercises performed without external resistance and in relatively stable conditions, and progress as recommended in Chapter 9. Once a client demonstrates progress with motor control and muscular strength, he or she can begin performing ground-based standing exercises that emphasize muscle integration. As strength increases, emphasis may be placed on multiplanar movements that require higher levels of muscle integration. Movements may be performed from unsupported postures, with closed-kinetic-chain exercises for the lower-body muscles and open-kinetic-chain exercises for the upper-body muscles. Free-moving lever-action exercises are appropriate during movement training.

Appropriate Rates of Progression

The standard recommendation for progression is a 5% resistance increase whenever the end range number of repetitions can be completed. However, during the early stages of resistance training, the motor-learning effect enhances strength gains by facilitating muscle-fiber recruitment and contraction efficiency. Therefore, during the movement-training phase, resistance increases may be more than 5% if the exerciser experiences a relatively fast rate of progression. Movement training is progressed through increased repetitions and sets, then adding more advanced movement-training exercise and some initial external loads such as tubing, medicine balls, or cables (see Chapter 9 for detailed exercise progressions).

Once the exercises can be executed with correct movement patterns while maintaining a neutral posture, a stable **center of gravity,** and controlled movement speed, clients may progress to the loading phase (phase 3). The timeframe for movement training is two weeks to two months, depending on each client's initial level of movement ability and his or her rate of progression.

Phase 3: Load Training

In the load-training phase, the training emphasis progresses from stability and mobility and movement training to muscle force production, which can be addressed in different ways to attain specific developmental objectives. The training objectives may include increased muscular endurance, increased muscular strength, increased muscle hypertrophy, as well as improved body composition, movement, function, and health. Regardless of the specific objective of the load-training program, it is recommended that stability and mobility exercises be included in the warm-up and cool-down activities.

During the load-training phase, muscular strength and endurance should be periodically assessed to facilitate program design and to quantify training effectiveness. If, for some reason, the client has a significant period without exercise, it may be prudent to conduct postural and movement assessments to determine if any postural deviations, muscle imbalances, or movement errors have reappeared due to lack of training. If so, these should be addressed and corrected before reintroducing load training.

Program Design for Improving Muscular Endurance, Fitness, and Health

Muscular endurance is typically assessed by an increased number of repetitions performed with a submaximal resistance. For example, if a client increases his or her leg press performance with 200 pounds (91 kg) from 10 repetitions to 15 repetitions, that client's muscular endurance has improved by 50%. While an increase in muscular endurance is positively related to an increase in muscular strength (1-RM weightload), the percentage improvement in muscular strength is typically less than the percentage improvement in muscular endurance.

The recommended frequency, intensity, repetitions, sets, and type of exercise for improving muscular endurance with external loading are as follows:

- *Frequency:* At this point, the variables of program design can be adjusted to provide varying levels of training stimulus. During the initial months of a standard strength-training program, two or three weekly workouts appear to be equally effective for improving muscular fitness (Westcott et al., 2009). However, as clients become more advanced and train at higher effort levels, more recovery time is needed between successive exercise sessions (McLester et al., 2003). While appropriate recovery time is essential for both muscular-strength and muscular-endurance training, the use of lighter weightloads and more repetitions with endurance exercise emphasizes the type I (slow-twitch) muscle fibers. Type I fibers fatigue more slowly and recover more quickly than type II (fast-twitch) muscle fibers. Consequently, three weekly exercise sessions may be effective for muscle-endurance training in advanced clients. If an equal or greater number of repetitions cannot be completed in subsequent workouts, the training frequency should be reduced to two weekly exercise sessions.
- *Intensity:* There is an inverse relationship between the amount of resistance used and the number of repetitions completed. One objective of muscular-endurance training is to work the targeted muscles to fatigue in the end range of the anaerobic energy system. For most individuals, this requires an exercise set that continues for about 75 to 100 seconds. Given a training speed of six seconds per repetition, this is a range of 12 to 16 controlled repetitions. Generally, 12 repetitions can be completed with about 70% of maximum resistance and 16 repetitions can be completed with about 60% of maximum resistance. It is therefore recommended that the training intensity for muscular endurance development be between 60 and 70% of maximum resistance.
- *Repetitions:* The recommended repetition range for enhancing muscular endurance is between 12 and 16 controlled repetitions that fatigue the targeted muscles within 75 to 100 seconds. Rather than train outside

the normal anaerobic energy system, the resistance should be increased by approximately 5% when 16 controlled repetitions can be completed. This weightload increase typically shortens the set by two to four repetitions, and permits application of the double-progressive training protocol (see "Progression" on page 324).

- *Sets:* Inherent in the development of muscular endurance is repeated performance of the training bouts. Therefore, most programs designed for increasing muscular endurance incorporate multiple sets of each training exercise. Another application of muscular-endurance training is to take relatively brief rest periods between successive exercise sets. Unlike muscular-strength training, which emphasizes full recovery between exercise sets, muscular-endurance training is typically characterized by one- to two-minute rest periods between exercise sets, or 30–60 seconds or less in higher-intensity circuits. It is therefore recommended that clients training for muscular endurance perform two to four sets of each exercise with one to two minutes of rest between successive sets.
- *Type:* There are many types of resistance that are effective for improving muscular endurance. While these include bands, medicine balls, and other forms of resistance, standard free-weight and machine exercises are well-suited for muscular-endurance training because the weightloads can be progressed with consistency and in small increments. Although all of the major muscles groups should be included, it is not necessary to train each muscle group independently. For example, a workout that includes bench presses, shoulder presses, and bar dips may not require a specific triceps exercise, as the triceps are targeted in all of these multimuscle exercises. In fact, exercise selection during the initial phase of load training can develop integrated strength-endurance by continuing to emphasize the five basic movement patterns.

Traditional training for muscular endurance features a total-body workout beginning with exercises for the larger muscle groups of the legs, followed by exercises for the trunk, then exercises for the upper body and arms. Generally, three sets of 12 to 16 repetitions are performed for each exercise, with a one- to two-minute rest between successive sets. Assuming a total of 10 exercises, this workout would require about 90 minutes for completion (3 sets x 10 exercises x 90 seconds performance plus 30 x 90 seconds recovery time). While traditional training is highly effective for increasing muscular endurance, it requires a relatively large time commitment. A more time-efficient means for improving muscular endurance, as well as cardiovascular endurance, is known as circuit strength training (Westcott, 1998; Messier & Dill, 1985; Gettman, Ward, & Hagan, 1982).

Circuit strength training involves a series of resistance exercises that are arranged to work different muscle groups, thereby eliminating the need to rest between exercises. For example, a 10-station strength-training circuit could consist of the following machine exercises: (1) leg **extension,** (2) abdominal **flexion,** (3) chest press, (4) leg curl, (5) low-back extension, (6) seated row, (7) leg press, (8) trunk rotation, (9) shoulder press, and (10) lat pull-down. With a 10-second transition between successive exercises and 90 seconds to perform each exercise, one circuit of 10 machines would take less than 17 minutes, two circuits would require about 33 minutes, and three circuits would be completed in less than 50 minutes. The performance of three circuits provides three sets of each exercise, but in about half the time required for traditional training.

The major disadvantage of circuit strength training is the use of lower weightloads (typically 40 to 60% of maximum) due to the cumulative effects of fatigue from nearly continuous resistance exercise. The advantages of circuit strength training are shorter training sessions and moderate aerobic conditioning from sustaining relatively high heart rates throughout the exercise session (Messier & Dill, 1985; Gettman, Ward, & Hagan, 1982). To further emphasize cardiovascular conditioning, some research programs have alternated strength training with aerobic activity, such as doing a resistance exercise for 60 seconds, followed by stationary cycling for 60 seconds, followed by a different resistance exercise for 60 seconds, and so on throughout the combined strength-endurance training circuit (Westcott et al., 2007).

Appropriate Rates of Progression

With traditional training methods for muscular endurance, progression to heavier weightloads should be done in 5% increments whenever the end-range repetitions (e.g., 16 repetitions) can be completed in all of the sets (e.g., three sets) for a given exercise. This is simply a higher-repetition-range application of the double-progressive training protocol. With circuit strength training, the first progression is to increase the number of circuits (e.g., from two to three circuits). When the desired number of circuits can be completed (e.g., three circuits), the weightloads may be increased by approximately 5%.

Program Design for Improving Muscular Strength

Muscular strength is a measure of the maximum force that can be produced by one or more muscle groups, and is typically assessed by the 1-RM weightload in an exercise (e.g., leg press, bench press). If a client increases his or her 1-RM bench press from 200 pounds (91 kg) to 250 pounds (114 kg), he or she has experienced a 25% improvement in bench press strength. Although some of the weightload increase may be attributed to motor learning, much of the improvement is due to strength development in the pushing muscles—pectoralis major, anterior deltoids, and triceps—as a result of a progressively challenging training program. Although increases in muscular strength are accompanied by increases in muscular endurance, preferred protocols for strength development place more emphasis on training intensity.

The FIRST recommendations for improving muscular strength are as follows:

- *Frequency:* High-intensity resistance training causes significant tissue microtrauma that typically requires 72 hours for muscle remodeling to higher strength levels (McLester et al., 2003). Consequently, clients who complete total-body workouts should schedule two training sessions per week. Clients who prefer to perform split routines (working different muscle groups or movement patterns on different days) should take at least 72 hours between workouts for the same muscles. For example, clients who do pushing movements for the chest, shoulders, and triceps on Mondays and Thursdays, pulling movements for the upper back and biceps on Tuesdays and Fridays, and squat, lunge, and rotational movements for the legs and trunk on Wednesdays and Saturdays have six weekly workouts, but provide at least 72 hours recovery time between exercises for the same muscle groups.
- *Intensity:* The initial stages of muscular-strength training may be successfully conducted with a range of weightloads (e.g., 70 to 90% of maximum resistance). However, for optimal strength development, most authorities recommend weightloads between 80 and 90% of the 1 RM. Exercises with near-maximum weightloads that allow one to three repetitions with more than 90% of maximum resistance are highly effective for developing muscular strength. However, these exercises are not appropriate for the average client unless he or she has a training goal directly related to increased strength. Because these are relatively heavy weightloads, a periodized approach that progressively increases the training intensity over several weeks is recommended.
- *Repetitions:* Repetition ranges are essentially determined by the exercise resistance. Because exercises with relatively high exercise weightloads

cannot be performed for many repetitions, training for muscular strength involves fewer repetitions than training for muscular endurance. Most individuals can complete about four repetitions with 90% of maximum resistance and about eight repetitions with 80% of maximum resistance. Therefore, the general recommendation for muscular strength development is four to eight repetitions. When nine repetitions can be completed with correct training technique, the weightload should be increased by approximately 5%.

- *Sets:* Muscular strength can be significantly increased through either single-set or multiple-set training (Carpinelli & Otto, 1998; Starkey et al., 1996). It may be prudent to start clients with one hard set of each exercise (after performing progressively challenging warm-up sets), and increase the number of stimulus sets in accordance with clients' interest and ability to perform additional sets. Generally, muscular-strength programs do not exceed three to four stimulus sets of each training exercise. To perform repeated exercise sets with relatively heavy weightloads, clients must take longer recovery periods between successive sets. Unlike muscular-endurance training, which features one- to two-minute rests between sets, muscular-strength training generally features three- to four-minute recovery periods between sets of the same exercise. The longer rests lead to longer workouts for muscular-strength training programs. For example, a standard 10-exercise workout could require about two hours (125 minutes) for completion (3 sets x 10 exercises x 40-second performance plus 30 x 210 seconds recovery time).
Fortunately, single-set training programs can effectively increase muscular strength in much shorter exercise sessions. For example, a single set of 10 exercises would require about 20 to 25 minutes for completion, and the inclusion of a warm-up set for each exercise would make the workout about 45 to 50 minutes in duration. Single-set programs using an appropriate warm-up and a challenging training intensity are effective means of helping clients maintain adherence to their programs when they have other demands for their time, such as a hectic schedule at work or managing the needs of a busy household.
- *Type:* Muscular-strength training may be performed with many types of resistance equipment. However, like muscular-endurance training, the consistency and incremental weightloads provided by standard machine and free-weight exercises make these the preferred training modes for developing higher strength levels. Generally, linear exercises that involve multiple muscle groups utilized in the basic movements are the preferred method for increasing total-body strength. These exercises include squats, deadlifts, or leg presses for the squat pattern, step-ups and lunges for the lunge pattern, bench presses, incline presses, shoulder presses, and bar dips for the push pattern, and seated rows, lat pull-downs, and pull-ups for the pulling pattern. Rotary exercises that isolate specific muscle groups (e.g., leg extensions, leg curls, hip adductions, hip abductions, lateral raises, chest crosses, pull-overs, arm extensions, arm curls, trunk extensions, and trunk curls) should not be excluded from muscular-strength workouts, but these typically play a lesser role than the movement-based exercises that challenge multiple muscles at the same time.

Due to the relatively lengthy time requirements of multiple-set training, it may be advisable for clients to consider split-routine exercise programs for muscular strength development. Although some strength enthusiasts work only one major muscle group during each training session (e.g., Monday—legs; Tuesday—chest; Wednesday—upper back; Thursday—shoulders; Friday—arms; Saturday—trunk), most split routines are characterized by two weekly workouts for the major muscle groups responsible for producing the basic movement patterns. As presented earlier, a standard split routine targets the chest, shoulders, and triceps (pushing muscles) on Mondays and Thursdays, the upper back and biceps (pulling muscles) on Tuesdays and Fridays, and the leg muscles responsible for squats and lunges and the trunk muscles that control rotation on Wednesdays and Saturdays.

Basically, total-body strength training involves fewer weekly exercise sessions with longer workout durations, whereas split-routine strength training involves more weekly exercise sessions with shorter workout durations. Both methods of resistance training are effective for muscle development, so the choice is largely a matter of lifestyle, logistics, and personal preference when developing an exercise program to help a client achieve his or her goals. When a client is first being progressed into load-based strength training, total-body workouts are an effective means of producing a desired overload. However, as the client demonstrates adherence and adaptation to the program, split routines are the best way to increase the total training volume.

A time-saving training method is referred to as supersets. Instead of simply resting between successive sets of the same exercise, it is possible to train a different muscle group while the first muscle group is recovering. Using this method, the exercise session duration can be reduced by almost 50%. For example, immediately after a set of a push exercise like bench presses (chest, shoulders, and triceps) the client can perform a set of pull exercises like seated rows (upper back and biceps). In addition to saving time, superset training maintains a higher metabolic response because muscular activity is occurring throughout the entire workout. Supersets typically pair opposing movement patterns and muscle groups (e.g., pectoralis major responsible for pushes and latissimus dorsi for pulls), but may involve different areas of the body as well (e.g., shoulders and abdominals).

Appropriate Rates of Progression

The recommended procedure for improving muscular strength is the double-progressive training protocol. There are numerous factors that affect the rate of strength development, and progress varies considerably among individuals. Consequently, it is not practical to suggest weekly weightload increases, as some clients will progress more quickly and others will progress more slowly than the recommended resistance increments. To facilitate individual stimulus–response relationships and to reduce the risk of doing too much too soon, trainers should factor both repetitions and resistance into the training progression. First, the trainer must establish the client's repetition range, such as four to eight repetitions per set. Second, the client can continue training with the same exercise resistance until the terminal number of repetitions (eight repetitions) can be completed with proper technique. When this is accomplished, the trainer should raise the resistance by approximately 5%, which will reduce the number of repetitions the client can perform. The trainer can continue to train the client with this resistance until eight repetitions can again be completed, then increase the weightload by another 5%. Although a relatively conservative approach to resistance exercise, the double-progressive training protocol is a highly effective means for developing muscular strength.

Program Design for Muscle Hypertrophy (Bodybuilding)

Muscle hypertrophy is the physiological process of muscle-fiber enlargement (increased contractile proteins and cell sarcoplasm) that results from progressive resistance exercise. While standard strength training produces some degree of muscle enlargement, greater hypertrophy may be experienced with more specialized exercise protocols. Generally, muscle hypertrophy is facilitated by exercise sessions that favor relatively high training volumes and relatively brief rests between sets.

Consequently, muscle hypertrophy training typically involves lower weightloads and higher repetitions than muscular-strength training, but higher weightloads and lower repetitions than muscular-endurance training. Consider the following FIRST recommendations for developing muscle hypertrophy.

- *Frequency:* Bodybuilders generally perform high-volume workouts that include several sets of many exercises for each major muscle group. Therefore, split routines are typically employed for hypertrophy training. Most bodybuilding routines feature a six-day split, working one or two major muscle groups during each session. It is essential to give each muscle group 72 hours of recovery and remodeling time between successive training sessions. Clients who perform pushing exercises for their chest, shoulders, and triceps on Mondays and Thursdays, pulling exercises for their upper back and biceps on Tuesdays and Fridays, and squats or lunges for their legs and rotational movements for the trunk on Wednesdays and Saturdays should have sufficient rest and remodeling time for each muscle group with a six-day-per-week training frequency.
- *Intensity:* The recommended training intensity for muscle hypertrophy is about 70 to 80% of maximum resistance. This is a higher intensity than that recommended for muscular-endurance training (60 to 70% of 1 RM), and a lower intensity than that recommended for muscular-strength training (80 to 90% of 1 RM). Due to the overlapping intensities, it should not be surprising that muscle hypertrophy training is associated with both increased muscular strength and increased muscular endurance. Essentially, bodybuilding workouts use moderate training weightloads that can be performed for a moderate number of repetitions with little rest between successive exercise sets. Training with approximately three-quarters of maximum resistance is highly effective for enhancing muscle hypertrophy.
- *Repetitions:* Most people can perform about eight repetitions with 80% of maximum resistance and about 12 repetitions with 70% of maximum resistance. Therefore, the eight to 12 repetition range is generally recommended for muscle hypertrophy training, which is standard practice among bodybuilders. Assuming an exercise speed of about six seconds per repetition, each set of eight to 12 repetitions would be completed within the anaerobic energy system range of 50 to 70 seconds.

  In addition to the muscle-building stimulus provided by this productive training protocol, eight to 12 repetitions to fatigue with moderately heavy resistance causes blood congestion in the prime mover muscles, resulting in their temporary enlargement (i.e., transient hypertrophy). Successive sets with short rests further enhance the "pumped-up" effect, which appears to facilitate muscle hypertrophy, although the precise physiological process is not fully understood.
- *Sets:* Bodybuilders typically complete more exercise sets for each muscle group than people who perform resistance exercise for other purposes. This is due to two training factors. First, bodybuilders may perform four (or more) different exercises for each major muscle group (e.g., bench presses, incline presses, chest flys, and bar dips for the pectoralis major muscles). Second, bodybuilders may perform three to four sets of each exercise. Consequently, each muscle group may be trained for 12 to 16 sets of eight to 12 repetitions with approximately 75% of maximum resistance. This constitutes a relatively high-volume training protocol that seems to be especially effective for increasing muscle size (hypertrophy). Given the large number of exercises performed for each body part, three to

four sets of each exercise is a reasonable training recommendation for muscle hypertrophy workouts. As mentioned earlier, bodybuilders attempt to attain and maintain a muscle pump (blood congestion within the muscle tissue) by taking relatively brief recovery breaks between exercise sets. For most exercises, bodybuilders rest only 30 to 60 seconds between successive training sets. Many personal-training clients express an interest in improving their muscular definition, so it is tempting to design exercise programs that will help them achieve this goal. However, trainers must keep in mind that these clients might not have the time to commit to the high training volumes required for muscle hypertrophy. If a training program takes too long to complete (e.g., over an hour), then it might impact the client's ability to adhere to the program. Trainers must help each client set realistic goals based on his or her time availability (both in terms of the number of sessions per week and the duration of each session), and then use those goals to develop a total-body training program that will help the client achieve meaningful results within those time constraints.

- *Type:* Most bodybuilders use a combination of free weights and machines to target all of their muscle groups with an emphasis on isolation exercises. Although bodybuilders perform many multimuscle exercises, they also attempt to isolate each muscle to intensify the training stimulus and enhance the hypertrophy response. For example, bodybuilders generally perform barbell squats and leg presses to concurrently work the quadriceps, hamstrings, and gluteus maximus muscles against heavy weightloads. However, to train these muscles individually, they typically perform leg extensions (quadriceps), leg curls (hamstrings), hip extensions (gluteus maximus), and hip adductions for the hip adductor muscles and hip abductions for the hip abductor muscles. For the upper body, they may perform several free-weight pulling exercises that concurrently work the upper back and biceps muscles (e.g., bent-over rows, pull-downs, weighted pull-ups), followed by machine pull-overs that better isolate the latissimus dorsi muscles and machine back crosses that facilitate more complete contraction of the rhomboid muscles.

In addition to free weights and machines, bodybuilders frequently perform a variety of cable exercises for purposes of muscle isolation and intensification. It is not uncommon for bodybuilders to finish a training routine with bodyweight exercises such as pull-ups, bar dips, push-ups, and bench dips to fully fatigue the targeted muscles.

In years past, most bodybuilders completed a full-body exercise program three days per week and rested as much as possible on their non-training days. Total-body training was soon replaced by an every-other-day split routine that featured all pushing and pulling exercises (using the chest, upper back, shoulder, arm, and forearm muscles) on Mondays, Wednesdays, and Fridays, and all lower-body/trunk exercises such as squats, lunges, and rotational movements (targeting the hips, thighs, calves, lower back, and abdominals) on Tuesdays, Thursdays, and Saturdays. The cumulative effects of fatigue from everyday training made it very difficult to achieve full muscle recovery in 48 hours. Consequently, most bodybuilders work each major muscle group twice a week (e.g., pushing movements for the chest, shoulders, and triceps on Mondays and Thursdays, pulling exercises for the upper back and biceps on Tuesdays and Fridays, and squats and lunges for the legs and rotational movements for the trunk on Wednesdays and Saturdays). This is an excellent training protocol for enhancing muscle hypertrophy, as it provides two weekly workouts for each muscle group and provides at least 72 hours of recovery/remodeling time between similar training sessions.

At higher levels of competitive bodybuilding, each body part is trained with very high-volume workouts just one day a week. For example, these athletes may work legs on Mondays, chest on Tuesdays, upper back on Wednesdays, shoulders on Thursdays, arms on Fridays, and trunk on Saturdays.

Bodybuilders typically train with two types of supersets. In one approach, they alternate exercises for opposing muscle groups with little rest between sets. For example, they may alternate four sets of leg extensions with four sets of leg curls, moving quickly between the leg extension machine and leg curl machine. In the other approach, they may perform two or more exercises for the same muscles in rapid succession. For example, they may alternate three sets of triceps press-downs and three sets of bench dips to push the triceps to a high level of fatigue and muscle pump.

Another advanced training approach used to enhance muscle hypertrophy is extending each exercise set with a few post-fatigue repetitions. One method, known as **breakdown training,** requires the exerciser to train to muscle fatigue, then immediately reduce the resistance by 10 to 20% and perform as many additional repetitions as possible (typically three to five repetitions) to attain a deeper level of muscle fatigue. Another method, called **assisted training,** requires the exerciser to train to muscle fatigue, then receive manual assistance from a trainer on the lifting phase (concentric muscle action) for three to five post-fatigue repetitions. Because people are about 40% stronger on eccentric muscle actions than on concentric muscle actions, the exerciser does not receive assistance on the lowering phase. When the exerciser has difficulty controlling the lowering action, the post-fatigue repetitions are terminated. It is important to remember that these are advanced program-design techniques that might be appropriate for clients in the maintenance stage of behavior change, but are not recommended for new clients learning to exercise in the action stage.

Appropriate Rates of Progression

While it is tempting to recommend progressing by a 5% weightload increase whenever 12 repetitions can be completed, this approach is not as effective with bodybuilding routines. There are many reasons for this, such as the large number of exercises, short recovery periods, and modified training methods used by most bodybuilders. It is recommended that muscle-hypertrophy training be assessed in accordance with the exercise volume performed by the targeted muscle group. While bodybuilding is as much art as science, a good indication for increasing the training resistance is an average of 10 to 12 repetitions for all of the exercises completed in the body-part workout. Of course, fewer repetitions will be completed in the latter exercises, especially when advanced methods for fatiguing the targeted muscle are incorporated.

Because bodybuilding is essentially about attaining larger muscles, periodic measurements of body composition and body-part circumferences also provide practical assessment information. Increases in muscle mass and circumference measurements (e.g., upper arms, thighs) indicate that the exercise progression is effective, whereas lack of improvement indicates that a change in the training program is necessary. Most often, a progress plateau (or regression) is the result of overtraining rather than undertraining. If this occurs, the client should reduce the training volume and take more recovery/remodeling time between exercise sessions for the same muscle groups.

Prerequisite Muscular Strength Prior to Performance Training

Some athletically oriented clients will want to progress to performance-enhancement training to prepare for a specific athletic event or competition. The performance phase (phase 4) of training focuses specifically on enhancing athletic skills for sports through the application of power exercises that emphasize the speed of force production. Clients who progress to performance training should have successfully completed both the movement- and load-training phases (phases 2 and 3). They should demonstrate good postural stability, proper movement patterns, and relatively high levels of muscular strength before initiating the performance-training phase. To facilitate maintenance and progress of posture techniques and movement training, these exercises can be incorporated in dynamic warm-up activities prior to performing performance-training workouts.

> It is important that personal trainers understand that power training for performance involves advanced exercise techniques that can place greater stress on the musculoskeletal system than standard strength training. Consequently, trainers should be certain that their clients have both the movement abilities and muscular strength to properly and safely perform the performance-training progressions.

Phase 4: Performance Training

This phase of training emphasizes specific training related to performance enhancement. Power training during the performance phase is an important component of sports-conditioning programs that prepares athletes for the rigors of their specific sport. Typically, this type of program is not appropriate for the average personal-training client who is interested in improving general health and fitness. However, there are individuals who could benefit from adding power training to their fitness programs, such as middle-aged clients who have been exercising for months and are looking to improve their performance in competitive or recreational sport activities. Older-adult clients can also benefit from certain forms of power training that emphasize power and quickness to help avoid falls. Furthermore, if designed and progressed appropriately, power training can add interest and fun to an existing exercise program.

If a client has progressed through the other stages of training to improve his or her posture, movement technique, and strength, this final stage of training can provide the appropriate overload to create adaptations from training stimuli. An effective strategy to help clients advance their weight loss is to progress them to an advanced level of training where they can safely perform power-based movements, since this can be one of the most efficient methods of expending energy during a training session. When they are ready to progress, power training can be implemented, for those who are ready, as an effective way to enhance weight loss by maximizing energy expenditure per unit of training time. An additional benefit of training for performance is the development of lean muscle, since type II muscle fibers are responsible for high-force, short-duration contractions and for enhancing muscle size and definition.

While there is a lack of evidence for the safety and effectiveness of performance training in mid-life adults, personal trainers can program this form of conditioning for their clients, as long as the clients have demonstrated appropriate postural stability and movement abilities (see Chapters 7 and 9), as well as muscular strength. Of course, all clients who progress to the performance phase of training should continue to maintain good postural stability and proper movement patterns. Personal trainers can facilitate this progress by incorporating the techniques of stability and mobility training along with movement training (phases 1 and 2) as dynamic warm-ups.

Strength training performed during the load-training phase (phase 3) increases muscular force production, but does not specifically address the period of time during which the force is produced. Power training enhances the velocity of force production by improving the ability of muscles to generate a large amount of force in a short period of time. Power is needed in all sports and activities that require repeated acceleration and deceleration. Power can be defined as both the velocity of force production and the rate of performing work:

Power Equations

Power = Force x Velocity

Power = Work/Time

Where:

- Force = Mass x Acceleration
- Velocity = Distance/Time
- Work = Force x Distance

Client Prerequisites for Performance Training

Effective sports conditioning, or performance training, requires that clients demonstrate movement proficiency and control during loading and against reactive forces. Specifically, clients must be proficient at acceleration, deceleration, and stabilization during the powerful movements required for performance training. To ensure program safety and success, clients should have the following prerequisites:

- A foundation of strength and joint integrity (joint mobility and stability)
- Adequate static and dynamic balance
- Effective core function
- Anaerobic efficiency (training of the anaerobic pathways)
- Athleticism (sufficient skills to perform advanced movements)
- No **contraindications** to load-bearing, dynamic movements
- No medical concerns that affect balance and motor skills

Resistance-training Focus

As explained earlier in the chapter, muscular power is the product of muscular strength and movement speed and is best represented by an inverted U curve (see Figure 10-1). That is, training with light resistance enables explosive movement speed, but results in a relatively low power output due to the low strength component. Training with heavy resistance enables a high strength component but requires slow movement speed, and therefore results in a relatively low power output. Training with medium resistance and fast movement speeds produces the highest power output and is the most effective means for increasing muscular power.

Speed is the ability to achieve high velocity and incorporates reaction time and speed of travel over a given distance. Agility is the ability to decelerate an explosive movement and reactively couple it with acceleration. For example, a basketball player who sprints down the court at a high velocity (speed), quickly brakes (decelerates), and cuts to the left and jumps (accelerates) to make the shot is a perfect example of an athlete using speed and agility to his or her advantage.

Fast movement speeds require a high level of muscle force to initiate the movement, with momentum mostly responsible for the remainder of the movement. Given the element of momentum in high-velocity movements, a personal trainer must be certain that his or her clients have the postural stability and muscular strength to effectively execute these types of sports-conditioning activities. Once a client achieves an appropriate level of conditioning and expresses a desire to improve athletic skills, techniques to improve power, speed, agility, and reactivity can help the client reach his or her performance goals.

Prior to starting each performance-training session, a personal trainer should plan on having the client perform a specific low-intensity warm-up that incorporates movements that are similar to the high-intensity exercises that are planned during the training session. For example, exaggerated marching (with high knees and pumping arms) mimics running and emphasizes the posture and movement techniques involved in running. This type of pattern-specific warm-up readies the client's neuromuscular system for a more intense version of the movement, while simultaneously preparing the client mentally for the challenge ahead. Similarly, adding low-intensity activity-specific movements to a client's cool-down is a good practice because it can contribute to the recovery and relaxation process at the end of a performance-training session. The more power necessary for a given sport or activity, the more important the warm-up and cool-down.

Powerlifting versus Olympic Lifting

To prevent confusion, it is worth noting that a misnomer exists in weight-lifting sports. High muscular force combined with relatively slow movement speed characterizes the sport of powerlifting, in which participants attempt to test the limits of their strength. Powerlifting focuses on three lifts—the bench press, squat, and dead lift—to see who can lift the most weight both in each individual lift and as a combination of all three lifts. While relatively large amounts of load are lifted, the movements are relatively slow. Thus, the amount of mechanical power produced in power lifting is less than in other sports, such as Olympic lifting. In Olympic lifting, the participants attempt to quickly lift as much weight as possible using movements that test their speed-strength, such as the clean and jerk and the snatch. Clearly, more power production is produced in Olympic lifting than in power lifting. While most personal-training clients will not be interested in these activities, it is important to understand the fundamental concepts of these two sports.

Assessments of Power, Speed, Agility, and Reactivity

Information gleaned from a client's functional assessments should be used to determine the appropriate course of programming for performance training. Clients who exhibit problems with postural stability and movement mechanics are not appropriate candidates for power training. Furthermore, clients who are deconditioned in terms of muscular strength and endurance should not incorporate performance-training techniques into their programs until they have completed several months of muscular conditioning in the form of resistance training. Please refer to Chapter 8 for detailed explanations of assessments for power, speed, agility, and reactivity.

If a client meets all of the prerequisites for performance training and expresses an interest in amplifying his or her training regimen through high-intensity sports conditioning, the next step is to determine the purpose of the program. That is, the trainer must learn which fitness parameters or sports skills the client hopes to improve and then set out to design a safe and effective program to meet the client's goals. Answering the following questions may be helpful in determining an appropriate power-based performance-training program for a client:

- Which movement patterns and activities (aerobic vs. anaerobic) are required for the client to be successful in reaching his or her performance goals?
- What are the athletic skills and abilities the client currently lacks?
- What are the common injuries associated with the activity? For example, lateral ankle sprains are common in soccer, especially if the athlete has high arches, so incorporating drills designed to enhance a client's ankle reactivity, and thus stability, would be appropriate.

Program Design for Improving Power

To improve the production of muscular force and power, a conditioning format called **plyometric** exercise can be implemented. Plyometric exercise incorporates quick, powerful movements and involves the **stretch-shortening cycle** [an active stretch (eccentric contraction) of a muscle followed by an immediate shortening (concentric contraction) of that same muscle].

Muscles and tendons experience an increase in their elastic energy when they are rapidly stretched (eccentric action). When immediately followed by a concentric muscle action, this stored energy is released, resulting in an increased total force production. The period of time between the eccentric and concentric actions is called the **amortization phase** and should be kept to a minimum to produce the greatest amount of muscular force. The production of muscular power can also be explained in terms of the stretch reflex (the body's reflexive response to concentrically contract a muscle after it has been rapidly stretched). **Muscle spindles** sense differences in the rate and magnitude of stretching imposed on a muscle. When a quick stretch is detected (such as the pre-stretch performed in plyometric exercise), the muscle spindles respond by invoking an involuntary concentric contraction (stretch reflex), thus increasing the activity in the agonist muscle and increasing muscular force production.

Timing is another important factor in the stretch-shortening cycle, such that if the concentric muscle action does not occur immediately following the pre-stretch (a prolonged amortization phase), or if the eccentric phase is too long, the stored musculotendinous energy dissipates and is lost as heat, and the reflexive potential is negated. Thus, an individual's ability to quickly perform dynamic activity is a strong determinant of his or her potential for power output. This phenomenon explains the increase in vertical jump height experienced by an athlete who squats down (incorporating a pre-stretch) immediately prior to jumping, versus an athlete who jumps up after holding a static squat position for several seconds.

Plyometrics for the Lower and Upper Body

Plyometric training can be programmed specifically for either the lower body or upper body. Lower-body plyometrics are appropriate for clients who play virtually any sport, as well as for those who want to enhance their reaction and balance abilities. Lower-body plyometric exercises include jumps and bounds (involving one leg or both legs) (Table 10-7). Upper-body plyometrics are appropriate for individuals interested in improving upper-body power for sports such as softball, tennis, or golf that require rapid force production with an implement like a bat, racquet, or club. Other sports requiring upper-body power include crew, volleyball, American football, lacrosse, and rugby. Upper-body plyometric exercises include medicine-ball throws and catches and various types of push-ups.

Movement-pattern progression is another consideration for programming plyometric exercise. Patterns should begin with forward movements and then progress to lateral, then backward, then rotational, and then crossover, cutting, or curving movements (Figure 10-5).

Precautionary Guidelines

Given the ballistic nature of plyometric-training drills, appropriate strength, flexibility, and postural mechanics are required to avoid injury. The following recommendations are provided to reduce the potential for injury and increase the likelihood of performance-related goal achievement for clients.

Personal trainers should introduce clients to high-intensity, lower-body plyometric drills only after the clients have demonstrated their ability to successfully squat 1.5 times their body weight

Table 10-7
Lower-body Plyometric Exercises

Type of Jump	Description
Jumps in place	Jumps require taking off and landing with both feet simultaneously. Jumps in place emphasize the vertical component of jumping and are performed repeatedly with no rest between jumps.
Single linear jumps or hops	These exercises emphasize the vertical and horizontal components of jumping and are performed at maximal effort with no rest between actions.
Multiple linear jumps or hops	These exercises move the client in a single linear direction, emphasize the vertical and horizontal components of jumping or hopping, and are performed repeatedly with no rest between actions.
Multidirectional jumps or hops	These exercises move the client in a variety of directions, emphasize the vertical and horizontal components of jumping, and are performed repeatedly with no rest between actions.
Hops and bounds	Hops involve taking off and landing with the same foot, while bounds involve the process of alternating feet during the take-off and landing (e.g., taking off with the right foot and landing with the left foot). Hops and bounds emphasize horizontal speed and are performed repeatedly with no rest between actions.
Depth jumps or hops	These exercises involve jumping or hopping off of a box, landing on the floor, and immediately jumping or hopping vertically, horizontally, or onto another box.

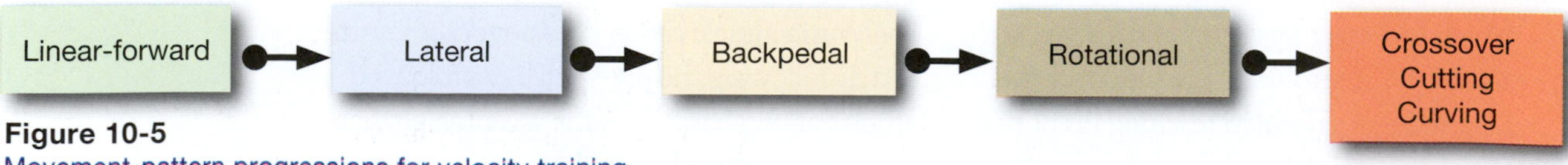

Figure 10-5
Movement-pattern progressions for velocity training

or complete five squat repetitions with 60% of their own body weight in five seconds (Baechle & Earle, 2008).

Plyometric drills should be performed at the beginning of a training session after the completion of a dynamic warm-up (while clients are not fatigued) to reduce the risk of injury.

Clients should not jump unless they know how to land. Ensure that clients are capable of landing correctly by initially teaching small, low-intensity jumps and using appropriate landing techniques.

Jumping and Hopping Tips

- Clients should land softly on the midfoot, and then roll forward to push off the ball of the foot. Landing on the heel or ball of the foot must be avoided, as these errors increase impacting forces. Landing on the midfoot also shortens the time between the eccentric and concentric actions (i.e., the amortization phase), thus increasing the potential for power development if another jump follows.
- Ensure alignment of the hip, knees, and toes due to the potential for injury, especially in women.
- Encourage clients to drop the hips to absorb the impact forces and develop gluteal dominance. Clients must avoid locking out the knees upon landing, which leads to the development of quadriceps dominance. Poor landing technique may lead to knee injuries. Proper hip mechanics during flexion and extension, along with the requisite muscular strength, is extremely important for developing lower-body power, which is why it is recommended that a client go through both the movement- and load-training phases (phases 2 and 3) before progressing to power-based exercises in the performance phase.
- Instruct clients to engage the core musculature, which stiffens the torso, protects the spine during landing, and allows for increased force transfer during the subsequent concentric contraction (or jump).
- Clients should land with the trunk inclined slightly forward, the head up, and the torso rigid. Trainers can cue clients to keep their "chests over their knees" and their "nose over their toes" during the landing phase of jumps.

Frequency

The number of plyometric-training workouts per week should range between one and three. The relatively low frequency underscores the importance of recovery time between plyometric exercise sessions. The recommended recovery period between high-intensity plyometric workout sessions is 48 to 72 hours.

Intensity

The most important aspect of determining plyometric exercise intensity is to understand the amount of stress placed on the muscles, connective tissues, and joints. Factors such as points of contact (e.g., one foot or both feet), speed, vertical height of the movement, the participant's body weight, and the complexity of the movement all contribute to the forces experienced by the body, thus affecting intensity (Table 10-8). Intensity of plyometric drills should be progressed from light, to moderate, to high intensity as indicated in Figure 10-6.

Table 10-8
Intensity Factors Related to Lower-body Plyometric Drills

Points of contact	The feet are the points of contact for lower-body drills. Single-leg drills impart more stress on the body than double-leg drills.
Speed	Faster movements increase intensity more than slower movements.
Vertical height	The higher the body's center of gravity, the greater the forces of impact upon landing.
Body weight	The greater the client's weight, the more intense the drill. Additional external weight (e.g., medicine ball, weighted vest) can be added to increase the drill's intensity.
Complexity of the exercise	Increasing the complexity, such as adding more body segments or increasing the balance challenge, increases the intensity of the drill.

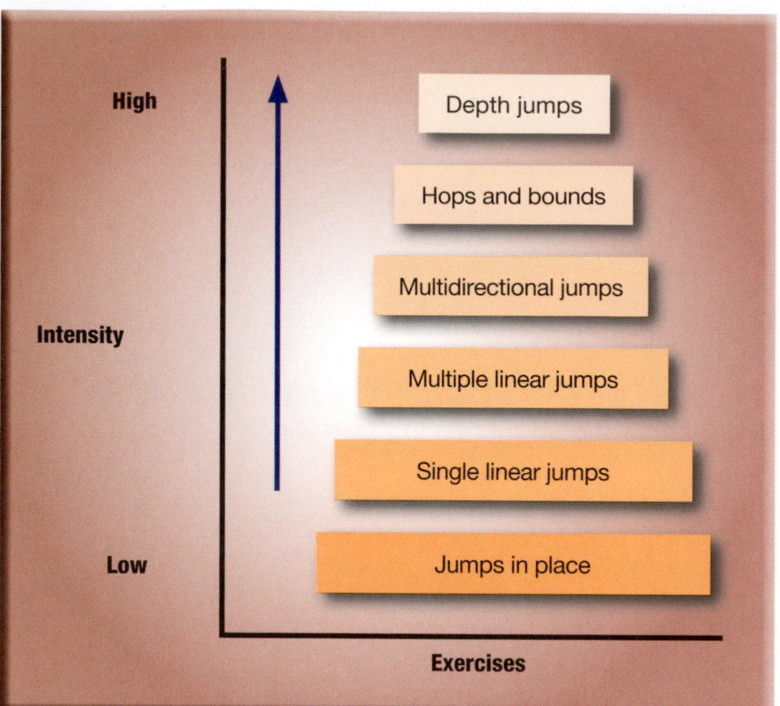

Figure 10-6
Plyometric drill classification model

Repetitions and Sets

Volume in plyometric training is expressed as the number of repetitions and sets performed in a given workout. Repetitions for lower-body plyometric training are normally counted as the number of foot contacts (i.e., each time one foot or both feet together make contact with the training surface) per session. For example, four sets of 10 repetitions of knee-tuck jumps equal 40 foot contacts. Upper-body plyometric-training repetitions are counted as the number of hand contacts (push-up exercises), as well as the number of throws or catches per workout. A progressive-volume format should be followed when programming plyometric workouts for clients (Table 10-9). Generally, as intensity increases, volume should decrease.

Table 10-9
Plyometric Volume Guidelines (Given in Contacts per Session)

Athletic Level	Low-intensity Drills	Moderate-intensity Drills	High-intensity Drills
Beginner (no experience)	80–100	60 (100–120 total*)	40 (100–120 total*)
Intermediate (some experience)	100–150	80–100 (150–200 total*)	60–80 (150–200 total*)
Advanced (vast experience)	140–200	100–120 (180–220 total*)	80–100 (180–220 total*)

*Includes some low-intensity drills as movement preparation for the more advanced drills

Type

Plyometric exercises consist of quick, powerful movements for the lower and upper body. Tables 10-10 and 10-11 list common plyometric drills.

Program Design for Improving Speed, Agility, and Reactivity

Terms used to describe functional-movement speed include quickness, reactivity, and explosive strength. An individual's ability to move quickly while simultaneously overcoming the forces imposed by his or her own body weight or an external load is determined by the rate of muscle shortening (or concentric action). Speed-strength is the ability to develop force at high velocities and relies on a person's **reactive ability.** Speed-endurance refers to the ability of an individual to maintain maximal velocity over an extended time period, such as a sprinter running at all-out velocity for 20 seconds. Both speed-strength and speed-endurance are important components of agility training. A client's reactive ability can be improved through training that applies explosive force to specific movements, such as the movements performed in speed and agility drills.

Agility training involves the components of acceleration, deceleration, and balance, and requires the client to control the **center of mass (COM)** over the **base of support (BOS)** while rapidly changing body position. Speed training incorporates moving rapidly

Table 10-10
Lower-body Plyometric Drills

Drill	Description
Jumps in place	Jumps require taking off and landing on both feet simultaneously. Jumps in place require multiple explosive jumps with no rest between repetitions.
Jumping jacks	Jumping jacks involve simultaneous lower- and upper-body movements. The traditional jumping jack involves both the arms and legs moving in the frontal plane. However, arm and leg actions can take place in all three planes and could occur either in-synch (where the arms and legs move the same direction at the same time), or out-of-synch (where the arm and leg actions occur during opposing movements).
Alternating push-off [<12-inch (30-cm) box]	Clients begin with the right foot on the top of a step or small box and the left foot placed behind on the floor. The client explosively pushes off with the right leg and switches feet in the air to land with the left foot on the box and the right foot on the floor.
Single linear jumps	These exercises emphasize the vertical and horizontal components of jumping and are performed at maximal effort with rest between jumps.
Standing long/vertical jumps	These exercises emphasize an explosive action in either the horizontal (long jumps) or vertical direction and are performed with little to no rest between repetitions.
Single front/lateral box jumps	These exercises require an explosive action to move either forward or laterally to land on top of a stable box or platform. The client should explosively jump to the top of the box, and then step back down to perform the next repetition.
Multiple jumps	These exercises move the client in a single linear direction, emphasize the vertical and horizontal components of jumping, and are performed repeatedly with no rest between jumps.
Knee tucks	These exercises challenge the client to pull the knees up to the chest during the flight time in the air. They can be performed one at a time, or repeatedly with no rest between jumps.
Front/lateral cone jumps	These exercises require jumping over cones in either a forward or lateral direction. The height of the cones can vary to change the intensity of the jumps.
Multidirectional jumps	These exercises move in a variety of directions, emphasize the vertical and horizontal components of jumping, and are performed repeatedly with no rest between jumps.
Hexagon drill	The trainer marks off a hexagon on the ground using 18-inch (46-cm) lines. The drill involves jumping in and out of the hexagon and moving from one line to the next to complete two full revolutions around the hexagon.
Diagonal cone jumps	These exercises require jumping over cones in a diagonal direction. The height of the cones can vary to change the intensity of the jumps.

Table 10-11

Upper-body Plyometric Drills

Drill	Description
Push-ups	
Power push-up (Figure 10-7)	• Adopt a push-up position with the hands slightly wider than shoulder-width apart. • Flex the elbows to approximately 90 degrees and then explosively extend the elbows so that the hands lift off the floor slightly. • Land with the elbows slightly flexed.
Medicine ball power push-up (Figure 10-8)	• Adopt a push-up position with both hands on top of a 5- to 8-lb (~2- to 3.5-kg) medicine ball. • Quickly remove the hands and drop them to the floor slightly wider than shoulder-width apart. • Make sure to land with the elbows slightly flexed. • Continue to flex the elbows and drop the chest to almost touch the medicine ball. • Explosively extend the elbows and push up so that the hands return to the top of the ball. *Note:* This exercise is appropriate for elite-level clients only.
Throws and catches	
Horizontal chest pass* (Figure 10-9)	• Hold a 2- to 8-lb (~1- to 3.5-kg) medicine ball with both hands directly in front of the chest with the elbows flexed. • Throw the ball to a partner or a rebounder by extending the elbows and releasing the ball through the fingertips. • Upon return, catch the ball at chest level and immediately repeat the pass.
Supine vertical chest toss (Figure 10-10)	• Lie supine on a mat with the arms extended upward (shoulders at approximately 90 degrees of flexion). • A partner stands on top of a box and holds a 2- to 8-lb (~1- to 3.5-kg) medicine ball above the exerciser's arms. • When the partner drops the ball, catch the ball using both arms and immediately toss the ball back up to the partner.

*Can be performed sitting, kneeling, or standing

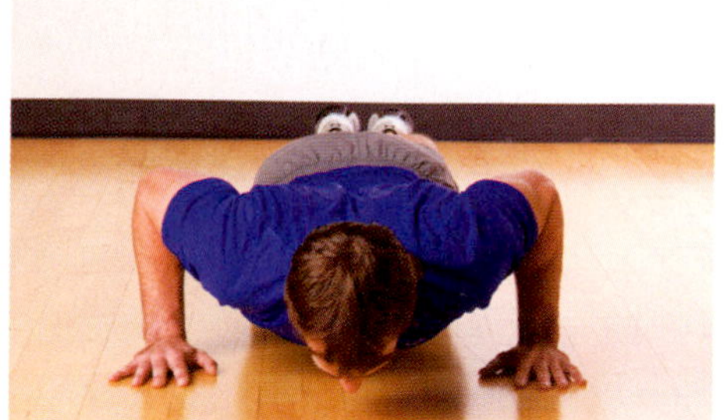

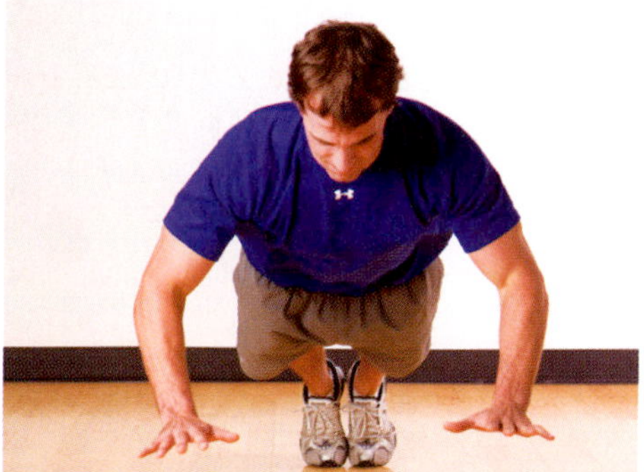

Figure 10-7
Power push-up

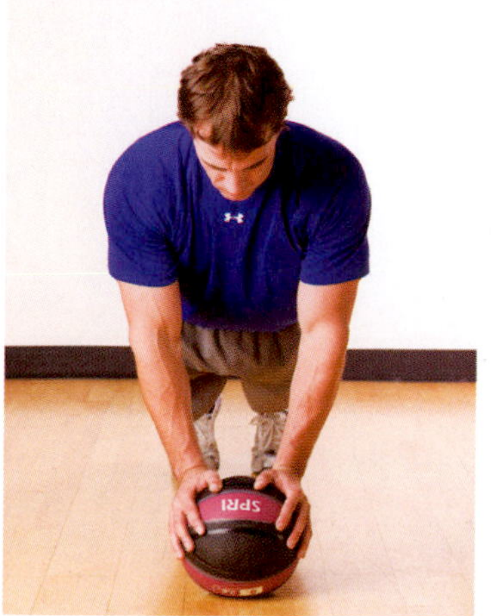

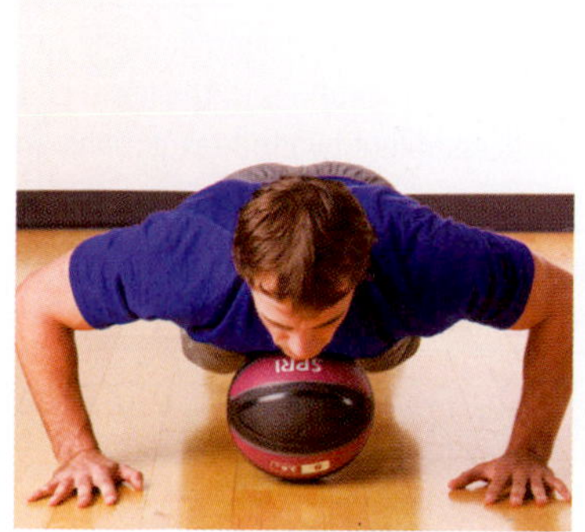

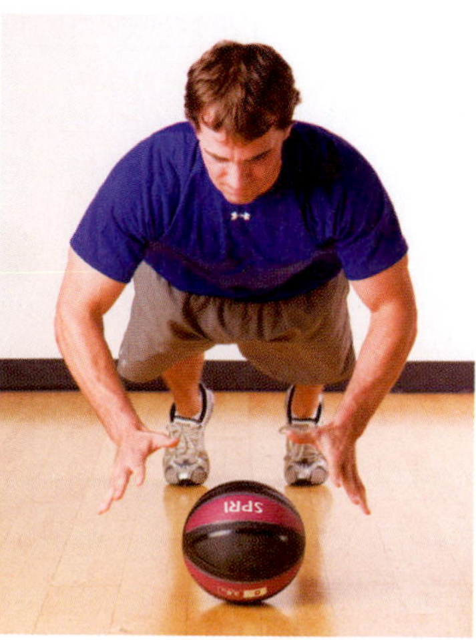

Figure 10-8
Medicine ball power push-up

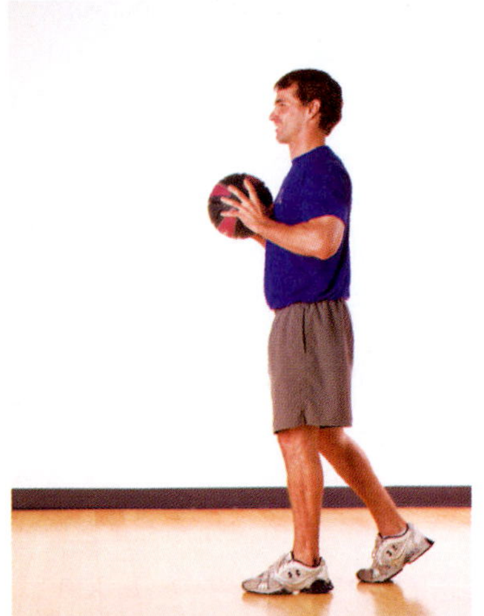
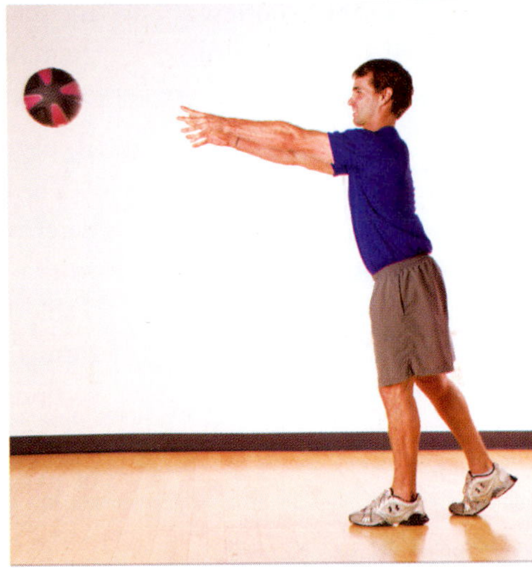

Figure 10-9
Horizontal chest pass

Figure 10-10
Supine vertical chest toss

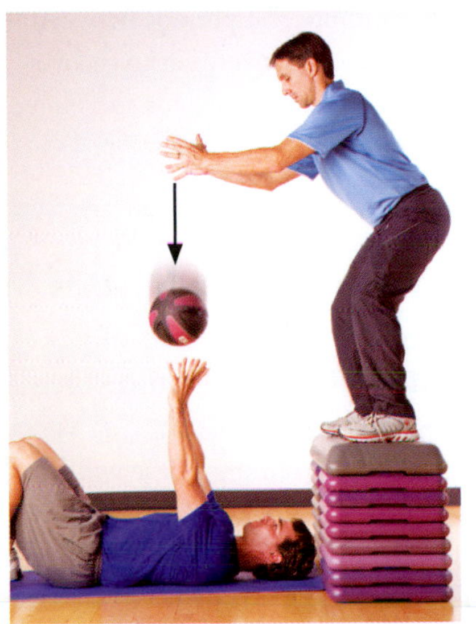
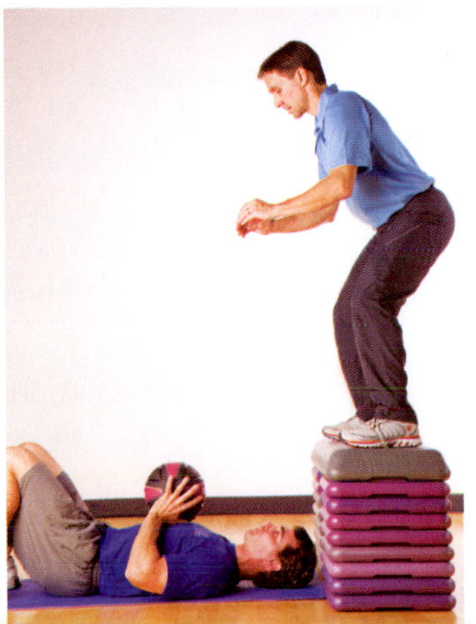
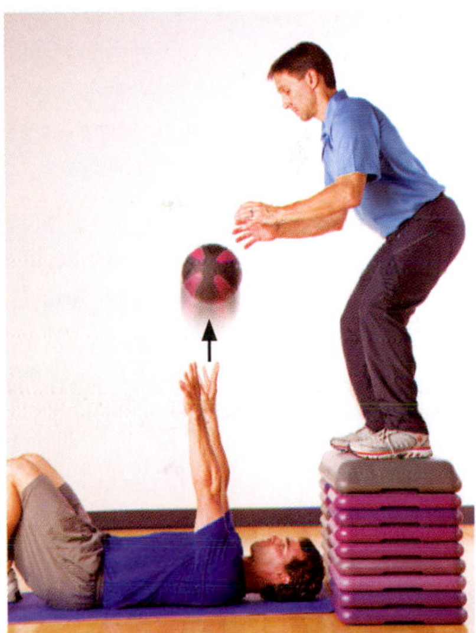

Training Tips for Speed Drills

- Body position or lean
  - ✓ Maintain a slight forward lean during the acceleration phase.
  - ✓ Transition to a more vertical position with top speed to facilitate hip and knee extension for stride length.
- Head position
  - ✓ Assume a relaxed, neutral position.
- Arm action
  - ✓ Drive from the shoulders, not the elbows.
  - ✓ Short strokes (or pumping actions) are utilized during the acceleration and deceleration phases.
  - ✓ Long strokes are utilized during top speed and sustained speed phases.
  - ✓ Relax the hands and maintain an open hand position.
- Leg action
  - ✓ At toe-off, kick upward explosively and directly under the buttocks while simultaneously driving the knee forward and upward until the thigh is parallel to the ground.
  - ✓ The foot then swings below the knee, moving to a fully extended knee position while maintaining a dorsiflexed ankle position.

from one point to another in the shortest timeframe possible. Speed and agility drills should be preceded by practice drills that are initially performed at submaximal speed to ensure proper technique.

Training Tips for Agility Drills

- Progress drills by increasing the speed of movement, complexity of tasks, and direction of movement, and by introducing resistance (e.g., bands and ankle weights).
- Drills can be predetermined (i.e., the client is informed of the expected task) or reactive (i.e., the client reacts to unexpected verbal or visual cues).
- Aim to progressively narrow the BOS to improve agility.

Frequency

The same guidelines for safe and effective plyometric training can be used for programming speed and agility training (see page 345). The number of speed and agility training workouts should range between one and three non-consecutive days per week.

Intensity

The high-intensity, explosive nature of speed and agility drills requires that these activities be performed early in a training session, after an appropriate warm-up but before other fatiguing exercises. Intensity is determined by the energy system that predominates during a drill, which is influenced by the duration of a drill. Table 10-12 lists the training variables to consider when programming speed and agility drills for clients of different fitness levels.

Table 10-12

Training Variables for Speed and Agility Drills

	Duration	Intensity
Beginner	15–30 seconds	<70% maximal intensity or effort (glycolytic system)
Intermediate	<10 seconds	>90% of maximal intensity or effort (phosphagen system)
Advanced	10–60 seconds	>75–90% of maximal intensity or effort (glycolytic and phosphagen systems)

Repetitions and Sets

Volume for speed and agility training is determined by the duration of time spent working in each of the energy systems (see Table 10-12). Stationary drills can be performed for one to three sets for 10 to 15 seconds per repetition, eventually progressing to 20 to 30 seconds. Dynamic drills can be performed for one to three sets for 20 to 30 yards per repetition, eventually progressing to 100 yards. Training sessions should be planned to include a minimum duration of two- to three-minute rest periods between repetitions to allow the exerciser to recover and produce maximum power for successive repetitions.

Type

Various speed and agility drills are presented in Tables 10-13 through 10-15.

Periodization of Power, Speed, and Agility Training for Peak Performance in Key Competitions

The performance-training phase will last at least four weeks, with the total duration often determined by the segment of a client's annual training plan that is dedicated to the production of power. During performance training, the focus should be on rate of force production with a taper in the volume and intensity of exercises in exchange for this velocity of movement.

For example, a client preparing for a recreational tennis tournament would benefit from a progression of both lower- and upper-body power-training exercises. If the tournament is three months away, then that provides a macrocycle of approximately 12 weeks. The 12-week macrocycle can be organized into three mesocycles of four weeks each. Each of the four week mesocycles can be further divided into two two-week microcycles (Table 10-16). Refer to Chapter 12 for additional examples of long-term training programs.

Table 10-13	
Speed Drills	
Basic Arm Drills*	**Description**
Arm squeeze and rear drive (Figure 10-11)	• Position one arm in rear-cocked position, forming a triangle with 90 degrees of elbow flexion (place the hand "in a side pocket"). • Squeeze the arm to side of the body moving only in the sagittal plane. • Allow the upper arm to move slowly forward to align with the torso, then pop back explosively. • Minimal torso rotation is allowable. • Perform 1–2 sets x 10–15 repetitions per arm.
Arm squeeze and forward drive (Figure 10-12)	• Position one arm at the side of the body, forming 90 degrees of elbow flexion. • Squeeze the arm to side of the body moving only in the sagittal plane. • Short strokes drive the arm to align the fingertips with the clavicle/chin level. • Long strokes drive the arm to align the fingertips with the nose level. • Minimal torso rotation is allowable. • Perform 1–2 sets x 10–15 repetitions per arm.
Arm squeeze and full cycles	• Integrate the previous two drills into full cycles. • Minimal torso rotation is allowable.
Basic Leg Drills	**Description**
ABC drills	• These drills improve leg mechanics for stride length and leg turnover. Perform 1–2 sets x 20–30 yards of each drill. • During each of these drills, assume a slight forward lean (5°), maintaining a rigid torso, but a relaxed head position.
A: High knees (Figure 10-13)	• While incorporating arm cycles, march in place, driving each knee high while maintaining dorsiflexed ankles. • Progress to walking, skipping, and then slow running, attempting to explode off the stance leg (extension of the ankle, knees, and hips) with each step.
B: High marches (Figure 10-14)	• While incorporating arm cycles, march in place, driving each knee high while maintaining dorsiflexed ankles. • Once the knee reaches peak height, quickly kick the knee out (knee extension) before returning to the ground. Hip flexion must precede knee extension. Avoid the "soccer kick" movement (i.e., swinging the entire leg forward from the ground). • Progress to walking, skipping, and then slow running, attempting to explode off the stance leg (extension of the ankle, knees, and hips) with each step.
C: Butt kicks (Figure 10-15)	• Drive the stance leg positioned under the hips directly upward to strike the heel of the foot under the butt. • Return the leg to the ground slightly in front of the body, attempting to "paw" the ground with the mid-foot, cycling the leg backward under the hip, before driving the knee upward again. Avoid the "mule kick" movement (i.e., swinging the leg behind the body); performing this exercise while standing against a wall will help clients avoid this movement. • Start with single leg cycles before progressing to walking, slow running, and then incorporating the arm cycles.

*Can be performed sitting, kneeling, or standing

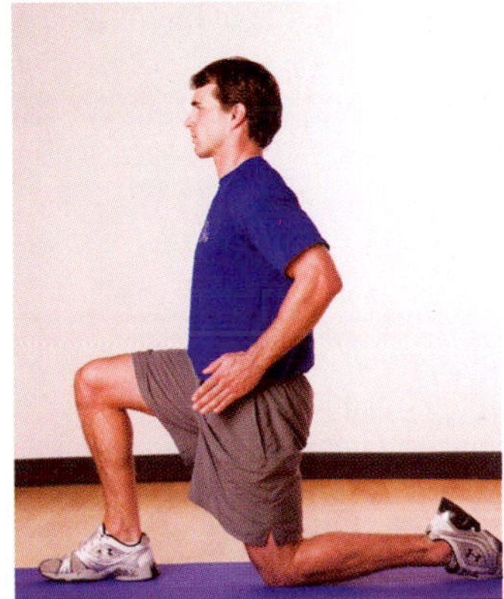

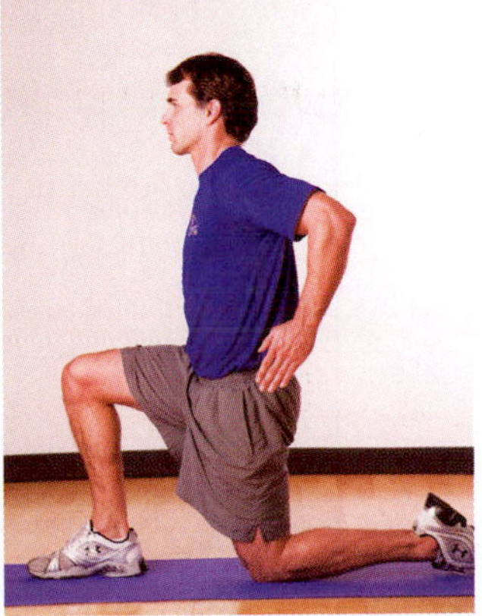

Figure 10-11
Arm squeeze and rear drive

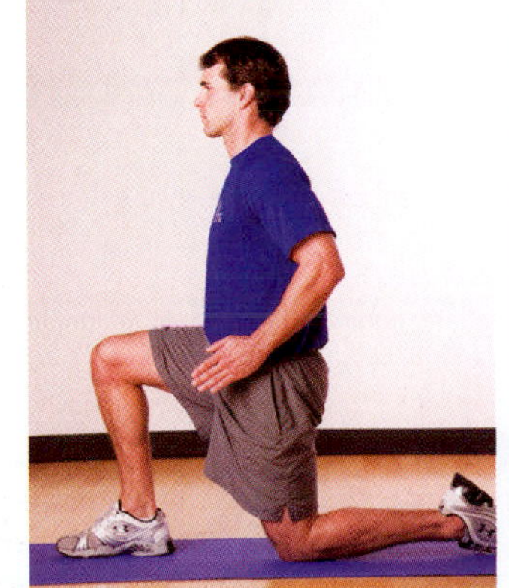

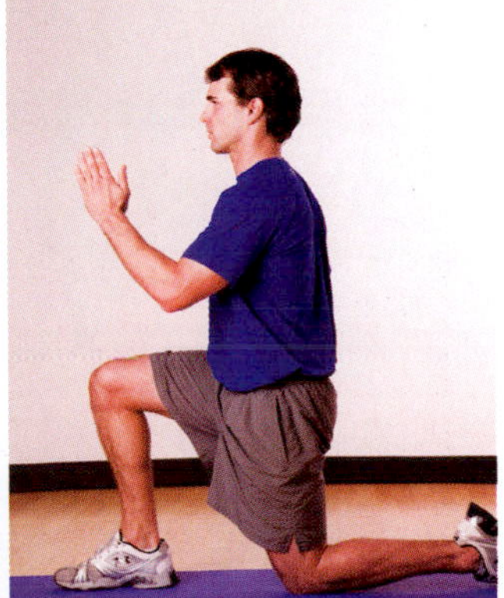

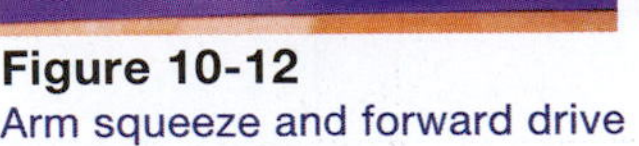

Figure 10-12
Arm squeeze and forward drive

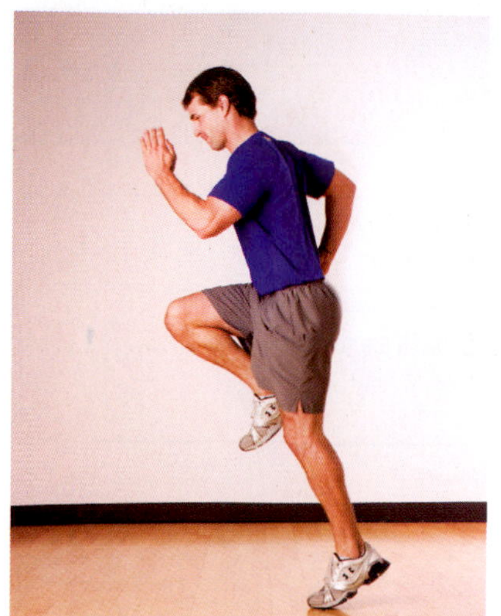
Figure 10-13
High knees

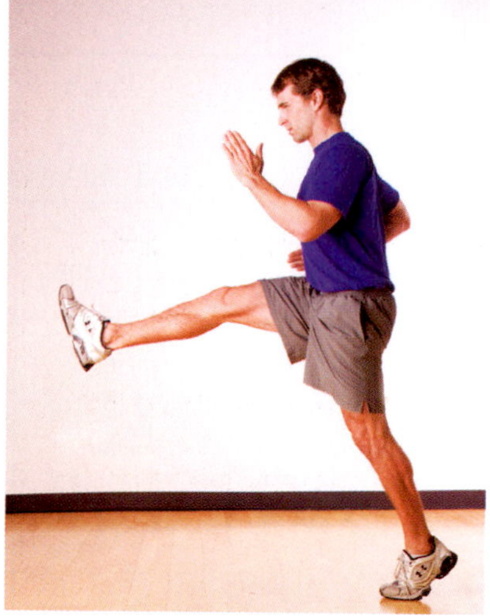
Figure 10-14
High marches

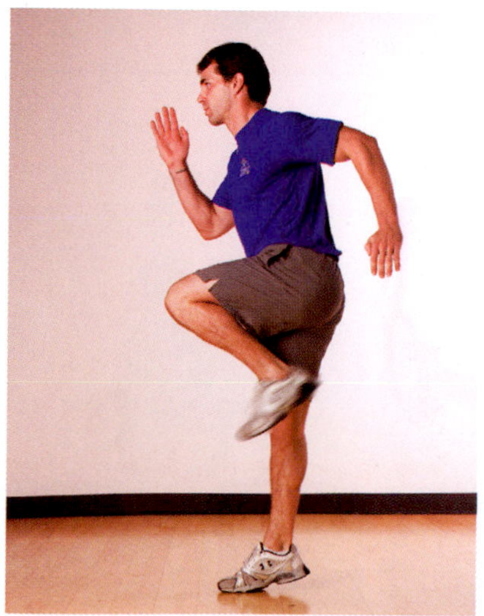
Figure 10-15
Butt kicks

Table 10-14
Agility—Ladder/Hurdle Drills

Agility Ladder/Hurdle Drills	Examples (Complete 30 feet per drill/leg)
Forward (Figure 10-16a)	• Single step-in ✓One foot in each rung • Double step-in ✓Two feet in each rung
Forward jumps/hops	• Double foot (jumps) • Jumping jacks (side-straddle jumps) ✓Both feet inside one rung, then on either side of the following rung • Hopscotch • Single foot (hops)
Lateral (Figure 10-16b)	• Basic shuffle ✓Both feet in each rung • Carioca (grapevines)
Lateral jumps/hops	• Double foot (jumps) • Single foot (hops) • Crossovers ✓Moving left-to-right, start with one foot in each rung (left in 1st rung, right in 2nd rung) ✓Jump laterally, moving the left foot into the 3rd rung, keeping the right foot in the 2nd rung ✓Jump, moving the right foot into the 4th rung, while the left foot remains in the 3rd rung ✓Repeat the sequence
Backpedal	• Steps • Jumps and hops
Multidirectional (Figure 10-16c)	• Single side-ins (zigzags or slalom) ✓One foot contacts outside the rung on each side • Double slalom ✓Two-feet contact outside the rung on each side • W's ✓Lateral-diagonal movements forming the letter "W" ✓Moving left-to-right, step back into the rung with the right, follow with the left ✓Step forward out of the rung with the right, follow with the left ✓Repeat • M's ✓Opposite movement to form the letter "M" (i.e., start moving forward) • James Bonds ✓Alternating push-jumps—moving left-to-right, start with the right foot in the rung and the left foot out ✓Perform alternating push-jumps, switching foot positions, moving down the ladder • Machine gunners ✓Rapid fire, forward-backward stepping (>2x/foot) in each rung, moving down the ladder

Figure 10-16
Agility ladder/hurdle drills

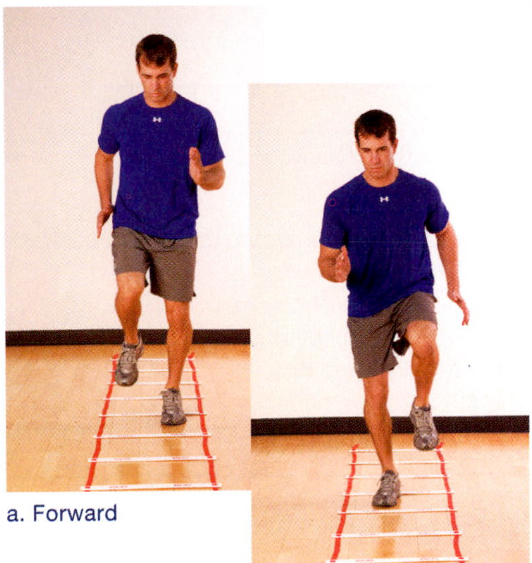

a. Forward

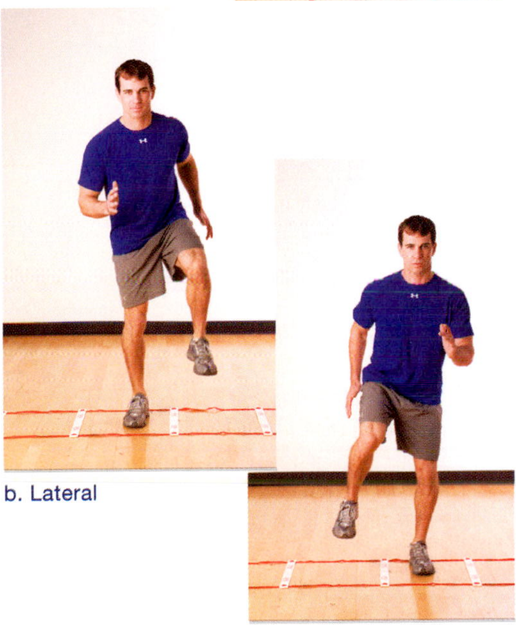

b. Lateral

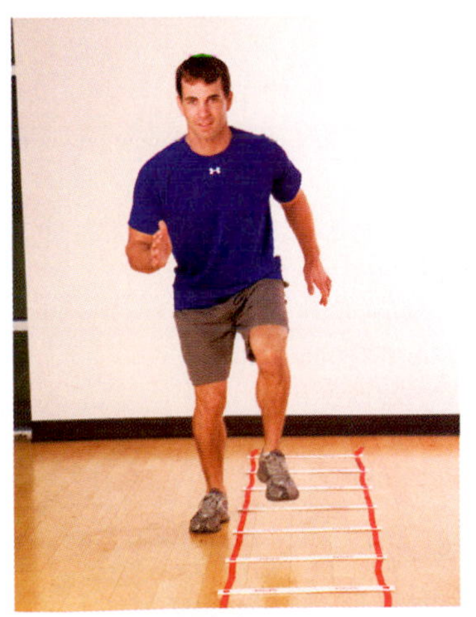
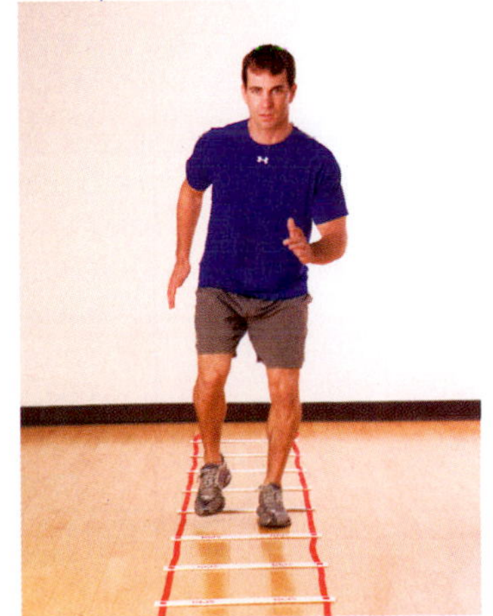
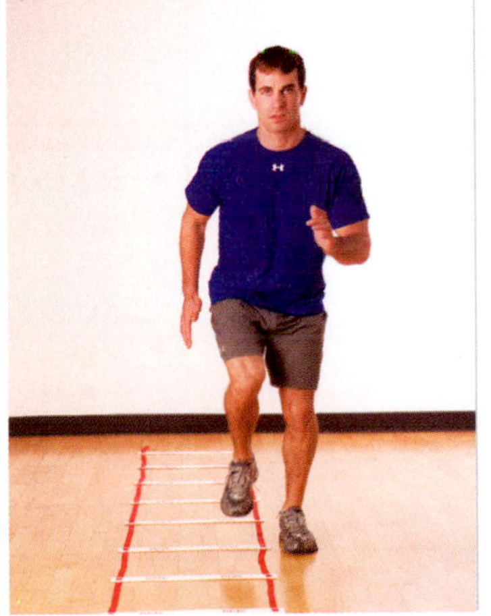

c. Multidirectional

Table 10-15
Agility—Cone/Marker Drills

Cone/Marker Drills	Description (1–2 sets x 5–15 seconds)
Lateral shuffles	• Set two cones 5–10 yards apart ✓Shuffle back and forth, touching each cone with the outside hand ✓Do not cross feet over
Pro agility drill	• Set three cones in a line, 5 yards apart ✓Start by straddling the center cone ✓On a cue, turn and run right (5 yards) to touch the right cone with the outside hand ✓Turn and run left to the far left cone (10 yards), touching it with the outside hand ✓Turn again and run through the middle cone (5 yards)
Multidirectional drill	• Hexagon drill ✓Predetermined—where directions are structured in advance ✓Reactive—the individual moves to the cone markers identified by the trainer • T-drill ✓Set three cones in a line, 5 yards apart, and one cone 10 yards from the middle cone to form the letter "T" ✓Start on the baseline, run to the middle cone, touch it with the left hand, then shuffle right to the right cone, touching it with the outside hand ✓Proceed to shuffle to the left cone, touching it with the outside hand ✓Shuffle back to the middle cone, touching it with the outside hand, then run backward through the line ✓Run the course in both directions
Curved or cutting drills	• Figure 8s ✓Use the same cone configuration as the T-drill ✓Individual starts on the baseline and completes the course outline ✓Run the course in both directions

Table 10-16

Sample 12-week Program for a Tennis Player

Macrocycle (12 weeks)	Lower-body Exercises	Upper-body Exercises
Mesocycle 1 (4 weeks)		
Microcycle 1 (2 weeks)	• Jumps in place: 3 sets x 6 repetitions • Jumps to 12-inch (30-cm) box: 3 sets x 6 repetitions	• Explosive modified push-ups: 3 sets x 6 repetitions
Microcycle 2 (2 weeks)	• Long jumps: 3 sets x 6 repetitions • Jumps to 18-inch (46-cm) box: 2 sets x 6 repetitions • Lateral jumps to 12-inch (30-cm) box: 2 sets x 6 repetitions	• Explosive push-ups: 3 sets x 6 repetitions • Medicine ball chest passes: 3 sets x 6 repetitions
Mesocycle 2 (4 weeks)		
Microcycle 3 (2 weeks)	• Long jump to knee-tuck jumps: 2 sets x 6 repetitions • Jumps to 18-inch (46-cm) box: 3 sets x 6 repetitions • Lateral jumps to 12-inch (30-cm) box: 2 sets x 6 repetitions • Lateral hops to 12-inch (30-cm) box: 3 sets x 4 repetitions	• Explosive push-ups: 3 sets x 6 repetitions • Medicine ball throw-downs: 3 sets x 6 repetitions
Microcycle 4 (2 weeks)	• Long jumps to knee-tuck jumps: 3 sets x 8 repetitions • Long jump to lateral jump: 3 sets x 4 repetitions • Lateral hops to 12-inch (30-cm) box: 3 sets x 6 repetitions	• Explosive push-ups: 3 sets x 8 repetitions • Medicine ball chest passes: 3 sets x 8 repetitions • Medicine ball rotational throws: 3 sets x 8 repetitions • Medicine ball overhead throws: 2 sets x 6 repetitions
Mesocycle 3 (4 weeks)		
Microcycle 5 (2 weeks)	• Long jumps to lateral jumps: 3 sets x 6 repetitions • Lateral hops to 18-inch (46-cm) box: 3 sets x 4 repetitions • Depth jumps off 12-inch (30-cm) box: 3 sets x 6 repetitions	• Explosive push-ups: 3 sets x 8 repetitions • Medicine ball chest passes: 3 sets x 8 repetitions • Medicine ball rotational throws: 3 sets x 8 repetitions • Medicine ball overhead throws: 3 sets x 8 repetitions
Microcycle 6 (2 weeks)	• Long jumps to lateral jumps: 3 sets x 8 repetitions • Lateral hops to 18-inch (46-cm) box: 3 sets x 6 repetitions • Depth jumps off 18-inch (46-cm) box: 3 sets x 4 repetitions	• Explosive push-ups: 3 sets x 8 repetitions • Medicine ball chest passes: 3 sets x 8 repetitions • Medicine ball rotational throws: 3 sets x 8 repetitions • Medicine ball overhead throws: 2 sets x 6 repetitions

Special Considerations for Youth and Older Adults

Youth Strength Training

Youth increase their muscular strength and size through normal growth and maturation processes. However, preadolescents who perform regular resistance exercise make significantly greater strength gains than their non-training peers. In the classic study by Faigenbaum and associates (1993), boys and girls who performed five basic resistance exercises twice a week for eight weeks experienced five times as much strength development as matched control students (65% vs. 13% strength gains). A follow-up study demonstrated that resistance-trained youth were still significantly stronger than their untrained counterparts after eight weeks of detraining (no resistance exercise) (Faigenbaum et al., 1996).

In addition to stronger muscles, strength training has been shown to enhance skeletal development in children. Research has revealed up to four times as much increase in BMD among preadolescent girls who did 10 months of resistance training and aerobic exercise compared to a matched control group (Morris et al., 1997). Strength training has also been shown to enhance psychosocial health, motor skills, and sports performance in preadolescent participants (Faigenbaum et al., 2009).

The NSCA guidelines for youth resistance training include the following exercise-program recommendations (Faigenbaum et al., 2009):

- Qualified instruction and supervision
- Safe exercise environment
- Pre-training warm-up period of dynamic exercise
- One to three sets of each resistance exercise
- Resistance that permits six to 15 repetitions per set
- Variety of upper- and lower-body strength exercises
- Resistance increases by 5 to 10% increments
- Two or three non-consecutive training days per week
- Post-training cool-down with less intense calisthenics and static stretching
- Individual training logs to monitor progress

Because no serious injuries have been reported in supervised studies of preadolescent strength training, resistance exercise should be a key component of youth fitness programs. When performed properly, progressive resistance training provides many health, fitness, and performance benefits for children, including enhanced musculoskeletal development, improved body composition, reduced injury risk, and increased physical self-concept (Faigenbaum & Westcott, 2009; Annesi et al., 2005).

Older Adult Strength Training

Older adults respond in the same manner as young and middle-aged adults to standard strength-training programs. In a study of more than 1,700 men and women between 21 and 80 years old, all of the age groups added approximately 3 pounds (1.4 kg) of lean (muscle) weight after 10 weeks of regular resistance exercise (Westcott et al., 2009). Although the physiological effects are similar, the exercise protocols for older adults should be modified during the initial training period. Most fitness authorities agree that older adults should begin strength training with more repetitions, and therefore less resistance, than their younger counterparts. ACSM (2010) recommends that older adults use a resistance that can be performed for between 10 and 15 repetitions. This corresponds to about 60 to 75% of maximum resistance, which provides a productive training range without putting excessive stress on joint structures.

To prevent unnecessary increases in blood pressure, older adults should avoid holding their breath and holding the resistance in a static position (isometric contraction). The proper breathing pattern is to exhale during concentric muscle actions (lifting movements) and to inhale during eccentric muscle actions (lowering movements).

Research indicates that older adults recover more slowly from their strength-training workouts than younger adults (McLester et al., 2003). Consequently, two resistance-exercise sessions per week may be advisable for older trainees to attain ample muscle-remodeling time between training days.

It is advisable for previously inactive older adults to begin training with a few basic resistance exercises, and progress to about a dozen exercises that cumulatively address all of the major muscle groups. Older clients should start with a single set of each exercise, performed through full movement ranges with controlled movement speed. A warm-up set of each exercise with 50 to 60% of the training weightload is recommended. Clients who desire higher training volumes may progress to two or three sets of each exercise as they become capable of doing so.

Older adults who have general **frailty,** weak muscles, or balance issues should begin with stable/supported resistance exercises before gradually progressing to less stable/unsupported resistance exercises. As their strength increases, their ability to perform more challenging training exercises should improve accordingly.

Because older adults may have a more extensive medical history than younger adults, they should complete a health questionnaire that reveals any exercise cautions or contraindications. It is also recommended that older adults have their **resting heart rate** and blood pressure monitored periodically. During exercise, older adults should be monitored using heart rate and **ratings of perceived exertion (RPE).** They should also be asked to give feedback on how they are feeling, especially if they are experiencing any aches, pains, or physical problems.

Finally, it is advisable to provide plenty of positive reinforcement to older exercisers, particularly during the initial training period. Once they develop competence and confidence in their exercise performance, they are likely to make a lifetime commitment to physical fitness.

Strength-training Equipment Options

There are many types of strength-training equipment that may be used to stimulate muscle development. The most important factor for increasing muscular strength is progressive resistance that is systematically applied through appropriate training equipment. Incremental increases in resistance elicit gradual improvements in contraction force. The key is for clients to use proper exercise technique and be patient in terms of progression to avoid doing too much too soon.

Selectorized Equipment

Selectorized machines are particularly well-suited for beginning exercisers, because they provide body support and predetermined movement patterns. The weightstacks always move vertically to provide a consistent resistance force throughout the lifting and lowering actions. Some selectorized machines provide 1-pound weightstack increments for gradual resistance progression, as well as cam devices to automatically vary the resistance forces in accordance with the biomechanical factors inherent in the joint actions. Well-designed and properly engineered selectorized machines provide safe, time-efficient, and highly effective resistance exercise that facilitates strength development in the prime mover muscles.

Exercises particularly well-suited to selectorized resistance machines include trunk flexion, trunk extension, trunk rotation, knee flexion, knee extension, hip adduction, and hip abduction, as it is difficult to isolate these joint actions with free weights.

Cables

Like selectorized equipment, cables are attached to weightstacks that move vertically against the force of gravity. Therefore, the resistance force remains constant during all of the exercise actions. Unlike selectorized equipment, cables permit considerable freedom of movement and typically require contraction of many stabilizer muscles to maintain proper posture and positioning during the exercise performance. Some of the more popular cable exercises include triceps press-downs, lat pull-downs, chest crossovers, and overhead chops.

Free Weights

Free-weight exercises include both barbell and dumbbell exercises, and the name reflects the freedom of movement that characterizes free-weight movements. Barbell exercises typically permit heavier weightloads that can be supported by racks such as barbell squats, bench presses, and incline presses. Due to the possibility of being trapped under a heavy weight, all of these barbell exercises should be performed with a spotter. Dumbbell exercises require equal force application from both arms and permit various wrist positions. Conversely, barbells can be leveraged to favor one side and require either a fully pronated or fully supinated wrist position. In some cases, such as the bent-over row, performing a dumbbell exercise with one arm while supporting the body with the other arm provides important back support and reduces the risk of injury compared to the barbell alternative. In other cases, such as the overhead press, performing alternating dumbbell presses provides excellent resistance exercise for the deltoid muscles with less potential for shoulder impingement than barbell presses. The numerous combinations of barbell and dumbbell exercise make free-weight training a relatively comprehensive and highly versatile means of developing muscular strength and size.

Tubing

Unlike selectorized equipment, cables, and free weights, elastic bands and rubberized tubing provide a softer form of resistance that can be easily adapted to almost any exercise. Tubing is inexpensive and requires little space for exercise performance, making it particularly accommodating for resistance training in a hotel room or at the office. Elastic bands work especially well for pushing exercises such as chest presses, shoulder presses, and squats. This is because the bands provide greater resistance force as they are stretched and the muscles (working together) produce greater force as the pressing movement nears completion.

Medicine Balls

Medicine balls are available in 1-pound increments and can be used for a variety of seated, standing, and moving exercises. If dropped, they are not as damaging to the feet or floors as other types of free-weight equipment, and they may be passed safely from person to person. Perhaps the most important feature of medicine balls is that they may be moved very fast and be released (e.g., tossed or thrown). That is, they permit a powerful exercise action that does not stress joint structures at the end of the movement because the resistance is released. Medicine balls are therefore ideal for performing fast movements against resistance to enhance muscle power, with a relatively low risk of injury.

Bodyweight Training

The most practical resistance to use is bodyweight. Some bodyweight exercises can be performed without equipment (squats, planks, push-ups), and others require only a chair (chair dips), parallel bars (bar dips), or an overhead bar (chin-ups). With these bodyweight exercises, progression is accomplished by performing more repetitions rather than by adding resistance. The progressive-repetition approach works well until the exercise set exceeds 100 seconds, after which the strength-building stimulus diminishes.

One way to enhance bodyweight exercise is to wear a weighted vest or strap on one or more weight plates by a means of a rope over the hips. This works particularly well for bar dips and chin-ups. Other ways to vary the amount of bodyweight resistance used in an exercise involve pushing and pulling the body at different angles (more horizontal to more vertical). This may be done with stable equipment such as Total Gym® or Gravity Power Tower®, or through suspension training, such as with TRX® cords. Bodyweight resistance is also used in **Pilates** exercise with relatively simple to more complex equipment options.

Ergogenic Aids and Supplements

The information that follows is meant to provide education about research on some of the more popular ergogenic aids and supplements and is not intended to serve as an endorsement of these substances by the American Council on Exercise. Refer to Appendix C for ACE's Position Statement on Nutritional Supplements.

Protein and Amino-acid Supplements

Many people use protein supplements to boost protein intake and ensure consumption of a particular protein type or amino acid. To aid in efficient **digestion** and **absorption,** most protein supplements are sold as **hydrolysates,** which are short amino-acid chains of partially digested protein. **Whey** and **casein** tend to be the most popular.

Whey, the liquid remaining after milk has been curdled and strained, is a high-quality protein that contains all of the **essential amino acids.** There are three varieties of whey—whey protein powder, whey protein concentrate, and whey protein isolate—all of which provide high levels of the essential and **branched-chain amino acids (BCAAs), vitamins,** and **minerals.** Whey powder is 11 to 15% protein and is used as an additive in many food products. Whey concentrate is 25 to 89% protein, while whey isolate is 90+% protein; both forms are commonly used in supplements. Notably, while the isolate is nearly pure whey, the proteins can become denatured during the manufacturing process, decreasing the supplements' usefulness. Unlike the other whey forms, the isolate is lactose-free (Hoffman & Falvo, 2004). Studies of whey protein have found that whey offers numerous health benefits, including increased muscular strength (when combined with resistance training) and bone growth (Hayes & Cribb, 2008).

Casein, the source of the white color of milk, accounts for 70 to 80% of milk protein. Casein exists in what is known as a **micelle,** a compound similar to a soap sud that has a water-averse inside and water-loving outside. This property allows the protein to provide a sustained slow release of amino acids into the bloodstream, sometimes lasting for hours. Some studies suggest that combined supplementation with casein and whey offers the greatest muscular strength improvements following a 10-week intensive resistance-training program (Kerksick et al., 2006).

Some research supports that BCAAs (leucine, isoleucine, and valine) may enhance endurance by delaying the onset of central nervous system fatigue and contributing to increased energy availability (American Dietetic Association, Dietitians of Canada, & American College of Sports Medicine, 2000). Others have found that following exercise, the BCAAs, especially leucine, increase the rate of protein synthesis and decrease the rate of protein catabolism (Blomstrand et al., 2006).

Glutamine, a popular nonessential amino-acid supplement, is marketed for its potential to increase strength, speed recovery, decrease frequency of respiratory infections, and prevent overtraining. While glutamine does play a role in each of these functions, research has failed to find a performance-enhancing benefit to glutamine supplementation (Phillips, 2006).

β-Alanine (Carnosine) and Sodium Bicarbonate

β-alanine, a nonessential amino-acid precursor of the dipeptide **carnosine,** and **sodium bicarbonate** both act as pH buffers in muscle tissue. It is widely believed that acid accumulation in muscle cells during a strenuous exercise bout is responsible for the development of muscle fatigue; thus, compounds such as β-alanine and sodium bicarbonate that contribute to a less acidic environment may delay fatigue and enhance muscle force and power output. Several studies have shown performance-enhancing benefits of β-alanine and sodium bicarbonate, especially during high-intensity activities. However, other studies have found little benefit. It appears that the supplements have few harmful side effects, though much more research is needed to better understand their risks and benefits (Van Thienen et al., 2009; Jenkinson & Harbert, 2008).

Caffeine

Research findings are clear: Caffeine enhances athletic performance. Caffeine sustains duration, maximizes effort at 85% **$\dot{V}O_2$max** in cyclists, and quickens speed in an endurance event (Keisler & Armsey, 2006). Perceived exertion decreases and high-intensity efforts seem less taxing (Armstrong et al., 2007). Personal trainers should be aware that there is a catch: Performance-enhancing benefits of caffeine are stronger in non-users (<50 mg/day) than regular users (>300 mg/day) (Bell, McLellan, & Sabiston, 2002). This is because the brain adapts to chronic caffeine use by producing more adenosine receptors for adenosine binding. Caffeine's effects are lessened and the same dose produces fewer desirable physiological changes. Chronic caffeine use contributes to high blood pressure, high blood sugar, decreased bone density in women, jittery nerves, and sleeplessness (Doheny, 2006), and for many users, there are withdrawal symptoms after a brief respite from the stimulant, including headache, irritability, increased fatigue, drowsiness, decreased alertness, difficulty concentrating, and decreased energy and activity levels (Keisler & Armsey, 2006).

Creatine

Creatine is naturally stored in the muscle tissue in small amounts. It supplies a rapid burst of energy for an all-out athletic endeavor lasting about five to 10 seconds. A meta-analysis of 100 studies found increased performance following creatine supplementation in the context of repetitive bursts of exercise lasting less than 30 seconds each, but no improvement in running or swimming ability. Few adverse effects of creatine supplementation have been reported (Jenkinson & Harbert, 2008).

Vitamins and Minerals

The best sources of vitamins and minerals are whole food products. The following vitamins and minerals are particularly important for optimal athletic performance:

- Iron is necessary for the synthesis of **hemoglobin** and **myoglobin,** iron–protein complexes that deliver oxygen from the lungs to the working muscles. Athletic training combined with low dietary intake can lead to a depletion of iron stores and subsequently hampered athletic performance, though iron-deficiency **anemia** is rare among athletes (Venderley & Campbell, 2006).
- Zinc is important for immune function, protein synthesis, and blood formation. It is readily lost from the body following strenuous exercise, especially in hot, humid environments.
- Vitamin B12 is important for the normal metabolism of nerve tissue, protein, fat, and carbohydrate.
- Riboflavin is an essential nutrient for energy production. The nutrient is stored in muscles and used most in times of muscular fatigue.
- Vitamin D is necessary for calcium absorption, bone growth, and mineralization.
- While necessary for maintaining bone structure and vitamin D metabolism, calcium is also important for blood clotting, nerve transmission, and muscle stimulation (Venderley & Campbell, 2006).

Anabolic-androgenic Steroids and Related Compounds

Anabolic-androgenic steroids (AAS) include all synthetic derivatives of testosterone. AAS improve performance by increasing muscle protein synthesis, which leads to increased strength and body weight from increased lean mass. Harmful consequences of AAS use include aggression, acne, testicular atrophy, hair loss, decreased libido, menstrual irregularities in women, elevated blood pressure, and increased premature death, mostly from suicide and **myocardial infarction** (Graham et al., 2008; Jenkinson & Harbert, 2008). AAS use is prohibited by the International Olympic

Committee (IOC) and the National Collegiate Athletic Association (NCAA).

Androstenedione and **dehydroepiandrosterone (DHEA)** are intermediary compounds in the conversion of cholesterol to testosterone. Both are marketed as being able to increase muscle mass and increase strength by increasing blood testosterone levels. However, they cause such a minimal increase in testosterone that supplementation fails to markedly increase testosterone levels, overall strength, or performance in men. Supplementation may lead to a small increase in performance in females. Harmful effects include hormonal changes of unknown significance; decreased **high-density lipoprotein (HDL)** cholesterol; and, in one reported case, priapism, a prolonged and painful erection (Jenksinson & Harbert, 2008). Both supplements are prohibited by the IOC and NCAA. Androstenedione is illegal under the Anabolic Steroid Control act of 2004.

Common Resistance-training Myths and Mistakes

There are a number of misconceptions and myths regarding resistance exercise. This section addresses some of the most common misconceptions and training mistakes.

Fat deposits in certain areas (e.g., the abdomen or thighs) can be targeted with strength training via spot reduction.

Building muscle is extremely exercise-specific. Only the muscles that are exercised against progressive resistance experience the training effects of increased size and strength. For example, biceps curls impact the biceps muscles, but have essentially no training effect on the triceps muscles. However, reducing fat is not necessarily exercise-specific. That is because people lose fat from **adipose** deposit areas in the reverse order that they accumulated that fat. Adipose deposit areas are genetically determined, as evidenced by the fact that men preferentially store fat in their abdominal region, whereas women preferentially store fat in their hips and thighs. Thus, the body loses fat in specific areas due to overall genetic factors, *not* specific spot-reduction exercises.

For example, John first adds fat to his midsection area, then to his hip area. He decides to do abdominal exercise to reduce the fat that is stored there. However, assuming John burns enough calories through his abdominal workouts to decrease his adipose deposits, he will lose fat first in his hip area, as this was the last place it was stored. He will lose fat last in his midsection area, regardless of the exercises performed, as this was the first place it accumulated. Although people can spot train muscles, they cannot necessarily spot reduce fat.

Women will build bulky muscles through weight training.

A very small percentage of women possess the genetic potential to experience significant muscle hypertrophy, or bulk-up. This is because women are typically smaller in size, have less muscle tissue, and have lower levels of anabolic hormones (e.g., testosterone) than their male counterparts. Even with these physiological advantages, most men are unable to add large amounts of muscle mass. Consequently, women should not be fearful of "bulking up" as a result of regular resistance exercise. Under natural training conditions, women can enhance their muscular strength and size within genetic limitations but, with rare exceptions, they will not develop unusually large, muscular physiques. For example, a training program that includes three days a week of a total-body strength-training circuit with loads of 70% 1RM for three sets of each exercise for the squat, lunge, push, pull, and rotation movements is not enough volume to develop excessive muscular hypertrophy in most women.

Individuals should use light weights and high repetitions to improve muscle tone, and heavy weights and low repetitions to increase muscle mass.

Due to the unfounded fear of bulking up, many women restrict their strength training to light weights and high repetitions to emphasize muscle toning over muscle building. On the other hand, many men who want to add muscle mass train exclusively with heavy weights and low repetitions to facilitate muscle development.

First, it should be restated that genetic factors are largely responsible for individual muscular responses to resistance exercise.

Second, several studies have demonstrated similar improvements in muscular endurance, strength, and size from high-repetition and low-repetition training (Behm et al., 2002; Bemben et al., 2000; Chestnut & Docherty, 1999; Taaffe et al., 1996).

Based on these research results, it would appear that resistance training with lighter weights and higher repetitions or heavier weights and lower repetitions produces similar muscular responses, as long as the exercise set fatigues the targeted muscles within the limits of the anaerobic energy system (less than 90 seconds). The effects on muscular endurance, strength, and size are approximately the same whether the individual performs five repetitions to fatigue in 30 seconds, 10 repetitions to fatigue in 60 seconds, or 15 repetitions to fatigue in 90 seconds.

That said, it is essential to use enough resistance to produce a reasonable degree of muscle fatigue within the limits of the anaerobic energy system. Training with very light weights that can be performed for two minutes or more is an inefficient exercise technique that has limited benefit for muscle development.

At some point, people get too old to lift weights.

One of the most amazing aspects of resistance exercise is that it works about equally well for people of all ages. In a 10-week strength-training study with more than 1,700 men and women between 21 and 80 years old, the muscle gains were statistically similar for those between ages 21 and 44 [2.5 lb (1.1 kg)], those between ages 45 and 54 [3.1 lb (1.4 kg)], those between ages 55 and 64 [2.9 lb (1.3 kg)], and those between 65 and 80 [3.2 lb (1.5 kg)] (Westcott et al., 2009). Fortunately, older muscles are very responsive to progressive resistance exercise, as evidenced by the nearly 90-year-old nursing home residents who added 4 pounds (1.8 kg) of muscle in just 14 weeks of basic and brief strength training (Westcott, 2009a).

Children are too young to lift weights.

On the other end of the age continuum, some people believe that preadolescents are too young to strength train and that doing so will damage their bones. Nothing could be further from the truth. Numerous studies have shown that children can significantly increase their muscular strength and physical abilities through properly designed programs of progressive resistance exercise (Faigenbaum et al., 2009).

In fact, strength training is the most effective means for young people to build bone density. In one study, nine-year old girls who performed 10 months of simple resistance exercise increased their BMD four times as much as nine-year old girls who did not strength train (6.2% increase vs. 1.4% increase) (Morris et al., 1997).

With respect to safety, there has never been a report of growth retardation, skeletal damage, or even substantial injury in any published research on youth strength training. In a study of sports-related injuries, strength training had a much better safety record than other athletic activities (Hamill, 1994). Youth who perform regular strength exercise may experience numerous health and fitness benefits, including improved cardiovascular risk profile, better body composition and weight control, stronger bones, more proficient motor-skill performance, reduced injury risk, and positive psychosocial outcomes (Faigenbaum et al., 2009).

Free weights are always better than machines.

Both free weights and weightstack machines provide isotonic exercise that involves dynamic concentric and eccentric muscle actions. Both free weights and weight-stack machines provide progressive resistance training that fatigues the prime mover muscle groups using the anaerobic energy system, and thereby stimulate strength development.

One difference between these training modes is that machines have fixed movement patterns, whereas free weights may be moved without restraint. For example, on a machine bench press, the handles automatically move vertically above the chest in a predetermined path. With free weights, the vertical movement of the barbell or dumbbells must be controlled by the exerciser. While this has little bearing on the prime mover muscles, it does require greater activation of the joint-stabilization muscles.

Another difference between machines and free weights can be seen in the supportive structures. Whereas both free-weight and machine bench presses offer similar body support, free-weight standing exercises (e.g., dumbbell squats) require more body balance and stabilization than their machine counterparts (e.g., leg presses).

Unlike free weights, most machines provide automatically variable resistance by means of a cam device or linkage mechanism, thereby varying the resistance in accordance with the normal strength curve for that joint action. That is, the machine provides proportionately more resistance in positions of higher muscle force production and proportionately less resistance in positions of lower muscle force production. Providing better matching of resistance forces to muscular forces throughout the movement range may be an advantage for machine training.

Another possible advantage of machine training may be the ability to isolate specific muscle groups. For example, it is difficult to isolate the quadriceps, hamstrings, hip adductors, hip abductors, and erector spinae muscles with free weights. However, all of these muscle groups can be worked independently with specific rotary-movement resistance machines.

Machine training typically reduces workout duration and injury risk by means of a shielded weightstack or other type of resistance that can be quickly changed by inserting a pin or turning a dial. There is no possibility of being trapped under a barbell or being injured by a dropped barbell plate.

On the other hand, free-weight training is more cost-efficient than machine training. Free-weight training is also more space-efficient than machine training, with the possible exception of multistation and cable-type machines that permit a variety of exercises on a single apparatus.

While there are definite differences between free-weights and machines, both training modes are highly effective for increasing muscular strength in the prime mover muscle groups. The choice of exercise equipment is primarily a matter of personal preference based on a variety of training factors and considerations.

After a person stops resistance training, the muscle turns to fat.

This statement is not only untrue, but impossible. Muscle and fat are separate and unique tissues and one cannot transform into the other. What often occurs is a gain in muscle (hypertrophy) and a reduction in fat during the training period. Then, if the exercise program is discontinued for a significant period of time, muscle mass decreases (atrophy) and fat stores increase as a result of the lower (non-training) energy expenditure. It therefore appears as though the muscle turned to fat, but in reality there is simply less muscle and more fat rather than a conversion of tissues.

One way to avoid this problem is to make strength training a lifestyle commitment, periodically varying the exercise program but not quitting. If injury, illness, or unforeseen circumstances require a lengthy period of program discontinuation, calorie intake should be reduced accordingly. While this will not prevent muscle loss, it will reduce the likelihood of adding unwanted adipose tissue.

Strength training is bad for the exerciser's blood pressure.

Straining against an immovable object can elevate blood pressure to excessive levels. Therefore, long bouts of isometric exercise are not recommended for older adults or hypertensive individuals. Holding one's breath can also raise blood pressure to undesirable levels, which is why trainees are always advised to breathe continuously when performing resistance exercise (preferably exhaling during concentric muscle actions and inhaling during eccentric muscle actions).

However, resistance training that involves continuous movement and continuous breathing does not cause large increases in blood pressure. Depending on the exercise, a set of 10 repetitions to muscle fatigue will raise **systolic blood pressure (SBP)** about 35 to 50% above the resting level (Westcott & Howes,

1983). For example, if a client's resting SBP is 120 mmHg, it may reach 180 mmHg on the last repetition of leg presses during a 10-repetition set to muscle fatigue. This is well below the 250 mmHg caution level for exercise SBP advised by ACSM (2010).

More importantly, the long-term effects of circuit strength training on resting blood pressure are profoundly positive (Cornelissen & Fagard, 2005; Kelley & Kelley, 2000). Research has demonstrated that several weeks of circuit resistance exercise leads to approximately 4% reduction in resting **diastolic blood pressure (DBP)** and 3% reduction in resting SBP (Westcott, 2009b; Kelley, 1997).

Consequently, properly performed resistance exercise does not adversely affect blood pressure, and circuit strength training has been shown to significantly reduce resting SBP and DBP in as little as 10 weeks.

Summary

Traditional strength-training program designs for muscle hypertrophy, strength, or endurance all require external loads to enhance muscular force production. The progressive loading of external resistance will improve motor-unit recruitment and increase the potential of a muscle to generate a maximal force, while the progressive accumulation of repetitions will train a muscle to generate a lower level of force over an extended period of time. Therefore, during load training, program-design variables are applied in a manner consistent with the standard application of training for increasing muscular hypertrophy, enhancing muscular endurance, or improving muscular strength. Exercise selection is consistent with traditional strength-training exercises and is dictated by the client's specific goals and needs. Resistance, or loading, can be applied through a number of different options, including selectorized equipment, plate-loaded machines, barbells, dumbbells, kettlebells, medicine balls, elastic tubing, chains, or other non-traditional strength-training equipment such as tires or water-filled containers. Regardless of the exercise selected or the type of load used, the focus during load training is increasing the ability of a muscle to generate force against an external resistance.

Functional movement and resistance training are often treated as two separate training methodologies. Yet, resistance training is defined as the application of an external load to linear, isolated, total-body, and functional movements. The ACE IFT Model provides a comprehensive and integrated training approach that spans from initial programming for a long-time sedentary client who has to build a foundation of health before moving on to working on fitness, all the way to a highly skilled client striving to enhance athletic performance.

Load training is the third phase of progression in the ACE IFT Model, because in order for a client to receive the greatest benefit from strength training, he or she should first address muscle imbalances and improve movement skill and coordination. If a client begins an exercise program with the application of external loading before addressing postural or movement issues, the client will be at an increased risk of injury from the application of too much training stress before his or her body is conditioned to accommodate it. This is especially important for new clients inexperienced with resistance training, because if a client develops an injury related to a muscular imbalance or poor movement technique, he or she has a much higher chance of quitting the exercise program before it can yield the desired results.

The initial program-design phases of stability and mobility training and movement training focus on addressing postural imbalances and muscle motor control to help clients develop the prerequisite postural stability and proper movement sequences to allow for external loading during full-body movements. However, some clients will already have good coordination and muscular strength and will not need to spend much, if any, time in the initial phases. Clients who have experience with strength training, demonstrate good movement skills, maintain good posture, and have no adverse health risks can begin in the load-training phase (phase 3) if it is consistent with their stated goals. Strength training during the load-training phase of program design improves the client's fitness level by placing emphasis on muscle force production and manipulating the variables of training to address a variety of specific exercise goals.

Clients' specific goals may include changes in body composition to increase lean muscle; improve muscular strength, muscle hypertrophy, or muscular endurance; or simply develop a more "toned" look. It is during the load-training phase that personal trainers will apply the current understanding of exercise science related to strength training to create and progress exercise programs to meet the many different needs of their clients.

The client's specific training goals will dictate the exact application of the variables and the length of time of training during the loading phase, with programs lasting a minimum of four weeks, and well into the maintenance stage of change for clients who are not interested in progressing on to power-based performance training (phase 4). If the client has a significant lapse during this phase of training, the personal trainer should conduct postural and movement assessments to ensure that the client has not developed new, or reestablished previous, postural deviations, muscle imbalances, or movement errors before reintroducing external loads to the exercise program. Before progressing to performance training, clients should develop the prerequisite strength necessary to move into training for power, speed, agility, and quickness. If the client moves on to power-based performance training before this base is developed, he or she will be at a high risk for injuries.

While strength training has obvious implications for improving muscle force production and sports performance, it is equally important from a health and fitness perspective. For the apparently healthy adult, the benefits of strength training far outweigh the risks, especially if he or she is following a resistance-training program designed for his or her specific needs. This chapter covers the science and principles of resistance training and their application to building muscular endurance, muscular strength, hypertrophy, power, speed, agility, quickness, and functional strength for everything from **activities of daily living (ADL)** to athletic performance. During the load-training phase of the ACE IFT Model, the behavioral strategies should build on those implemented during the previous stages, with a specific focus on enhancing the intrinsic motivational strategies that were implemented during the previous phase. **Intrinsic motivation** and good self-efficacy are necessary for individuals to move into the **maintenance** stage of behavior change. Effective strategies for preventing and coping with **lapses** are also necessary for an individual to make it to the maintenance stage. For many clients, the load-training phase will be the final phase they will reach in their exercise programming, as the performance-training phase of the ACE IFT Model involves training techniques and methods designed to enhance athletic performance. While a number of clients will welcome the challenge of incorporating athletic-training techniques into their programs for variety and possibly improved performance in team or individual competitions, many clients will not want to take this extra step.

To help facilitate client progress during the load-training phase, the personal trainer should reassess fitness, goals, and training systems on a regular basis and make appropriate adjustments to the exercise program. This is important to facilitate continued goal achievement and new goal setting, thereby avoiding burnout and keeping a good mix of challenge and fun to keep motivation high. Finally, as clients improve their strength, movement skill, and aerobic fitness levels, they could incorporate group exercise as additional workouts and be encouraged to try strength training, boot camp, or sports-conditioning classes to add variety to their routines.

References

American College of Sports Medicine (2010). *ACSM's Guidelines for Exercise Testing and Prescription* (8th ed.). Philadelphia: Wolters Kluwer/Lippincott William & Wilkins.

American Dietetic Association, Dietitians of Canada, & American College of Sports Medicine (2000). Position of the American Dietetic Association, Dietitians of Canada, and the American College of Sports Medicine: Nutrition and athletic performance. *Journal of the American Dietetic Association*, 100, 12, 1543–1556.

Annesi, J.J. & Westcott, W.L. (2007). Relations of physical self-concept and muscular strength with resistance exercise-induced feeling state scores in older women. *Perceptual and Motor Skill,* 104, 183–190.

Annesi, J.J. et al. (2005). Effects of a physical activity protocol delivered by YMCA after-school counselors (Youth Fit for Life) on fitness and self-efficacy changes in 5- to 12-year-old boys and girls. *Research Quarterly for Exercise and Sports,* 76, 468–476.

Armstrong, L.E. et al. (2007). Caffeine, fluid-electrolyte balance, temperature regulation, and exercise-heat tolerance. *Exercise and Sports Science Reviews*, 35, 3, 135–140.

Baechle, T.R. & Earle, R.W. (2008). *Essentials of Strength Training and Conditioning* (3rd ed.). Champaign, Ill.: Human Kinetics.

Behm, D. et al. (2002). The effect of 5, 10, and 20 repetition maximums on the recovery of voluntary and evoked contractile properties. *Journal of Strength and Conditioning Research,* 16, 2, 209–218.

Bell, D.G., McLellan, T.M., & Sabiston, C.M. (2002). Effect of ingesting caffeine and ephedrine on 10-km run performance. *Journal of Applied Physiology*, 93, 1227–1234.

Bemben, D. et al. (2000). Musculoskeletal response to high and low intensity resistance training in early postmenopausal women. *Medicine & Science in Sports & Exercise,* 32, 11, 1949–1957.

Blomstrand, E. et al. (2006). Branched-chain amino acids activate key enzymes in protein synthesis after physical exercise. *Journal of Nutrition*, 136, 1 Suppl., 269S–273S.

Braith, R. & Stewart, K. (2006). Resistance exercise training: Its role in the prevention of cardiovascular disease. *Circulation,* 113, 2642–2650.

Brooks, D.S. (2003). Strength training program design. In: American Council on Exercise. *ACE Personal Trainer Manual* (3rd ed.). San Diego, Calif.: American Council on Exercise.

Brzycki, M. (1995). *A Practical Approach to Strength Training* (3rd ed.). Indianapolis, Ind.: Masters Press.

Campbell, W. et al. (1994). Increased energy requirements and changes in body composition with resistance training in older adults. *American Journal of Clinical Nutrition,* 60, 167–175.

Carpinelli, R.N. & Otto, R.M. (1998). Strength training: Single versus multiple sets. *Sports Medicine*, 26, 2, 73–84.

Chestnut, I. & Docherty, D. (1999). The effects of 4 and 10 repetition maximum weight training protocols on neuromuscular adaptations in untrained men. *Journal of Strength and Conditioning Research,* 13, 353–359.

Cornelissen, V. & Fagard, R. (2005). Effect of resistance training on resting blood pressure: A meta-analysis of randomized controlled trials. *Journal of Hypertension,* 23, 251–259.

Darden, E. (1988). *The Nautilus Book.* Chicago: Contemporary Books.

Doheny, K. (2006). Pros and cons of the caffeine craze. *WebMD.* www.webmd.com/diet/features/pros-and-cons-caffeine-craze?page=4. Retrieved March 23, 2009.

Faigenbaum, A.D. & Westcott, W.L. (2009). *Youth Strength Training.* Champaign, Ill: Human Kinetics.

Faigenbaum, A.D. et al. (2009). Youth resistance training: Updated position paper from the National Strength and Conditioning Association. *Journal of Strength and Conditioning Research,* 23, 4, 1–20.

Faigenbaum, A.D. et al. (1996). The effects of strength training and detraining on children. *Journal of Strength and Conditioning Research,* 10, 2, 109–114.

Faigenbaum, A.D. et al. (1993). The effects of a twice-per-week strength training program on children. *Pediatric Exercise Science,* 5, 339–346.

Fiatarone, M.A. et al. (1994). Exercise training and nutritional supplementation for physical frailty in very elderly people. *New England Journal of Medicine,* 330, 25, 1769–1775.

Fleck, S.J. (1999). Periodized strength training: A critical review. *Journal of Strength and Conditioning Research,* 13, 1, 82–89.

Gettman, L., Ward, P., & Hagan, R. (1982). A comparison of combined running and weight training with circuit weight training. *Medicine & Science in Sports & Exercise,* 14, 229–234.

Gordon, B. et al. (2009). Resistance training improves metabolic health in type 2 diabetes: A systematic review. *Diabetes Research and Clinical Practice,* 83, 157–175.

Graham, M.R. et al. (2008). Anabolic steroid use: Patterns of use and detection of doping. *Sports Medicine*, 38, 6, 505–525.

Hackney, K., Engels, H., & Gretebeck, R. (2008). Resting energy expenditure and delayed-onset muscle soreness after full-body resistance training with an eccentric concentration. *Journal of Strength and Conditioning Research,* 22, 5, 1602–1609.

Haltom, R. W. et al. (1999). Circuit weight training and its effects on excess postexercise oxygen consumption.

Medicine & Science in Sports & Exercise, 31, 11, 1613–1618.

Hamill, B. (1994). Relative safety of weight lifting and weight training. *Journal of Strength and Conditioning Research,* 8, 53–57.

Hayes, A. & Cribb, P.J. (2008). Effect of whey protein isolate on strength, body composition, and muscle hypertrophy during resistance training. *Current Opinions in Clinical Nutrition and Metabolic Care*, 11, 40–44.

Hoffman, J.R. & Falvo, M.J (2004). Protein: Which is best? *Journal of Sports Science and Medicine*, 3, 118–130.

Holten, M. et al. (2004). Strength training increases insulin-mediated glucose uptake, GLUT4 content, and insulin signaling in skeletal muscle in patients with type 2 diabetes. *Diabetes,* 53, 294–305.

Hunter, G. et al. (2000). Resistance training increases total energy expenditure and free-living physical activity in older adults. *Journal of Applied Physiology*, 89, 977–984.

Hurley, B. (1994). Does strength training improve health status? *Strength and Conditioning,* 16, 7–13.

Hurley, B. & Roth, S. (2000). Strength training in the elderly: Effects on risk factors for age-related diseases, *Sports Medicine,* 30, 249–268.

Jan, M. et al. (2008). Investigation of clinical effects of high- and low-resistance training for patients with knee osteoarthritis: A randomized controlled trial. *Physical Therapy,* 88, 427–436.

Jenkinson, D.M. & Harbert, A.J. (2008). Supplements and sports. *American Family Physician*, 78, 9, 1039–1046.

Kalapotharakos, V. et al. (2005). Effects of heavy and moderate resistance training on functional performance in older adults. *Journal of Strength and Conditioning Research,* 19, 652–657.

Keisler, B.D. & Armsey, T.D. (2006). Caffeine as ergogenic acid. *Current Sports Medicine Reports*, 5, 215–219.

Kelley, G. (1997). Dynamic resistance exercise and resting blood pressure in healthy adults: A meta-analysis. *Journal of Applied Physiology,* 82, 1559–1565.

Kelley, G. & Kelley, K. (2009). Impact of progressive resistance training on lipids and lipoproteins in adults: A meta-analysis of randomized controlled trials. *Preventive Medicine,* 48, 9–19.

Kelley, G. & Kelley, K. (2000). Progressive resistance exercise and resting blood pressure: A meta-analysis of randomized controlled trials. *Hypertension,* 35, 838–843.

Kerksick, C.M. et al. (2006). The effects of protein and amino acid supplementation on performance and training adaptations during ten weeks of resistance training. *Journal of Strength and Conditioning Research*, 20, 3, 643–653.

Koffler, K.H. et al. (1992). Strength training accelerates gastrointestinal transit in middle-aged and older men. *Medicine & Science in Sports & Exercise,* 24, 415–419.

Kraemer, W.J. et al. (2000). Influence of resistance training volume and periodization on physiological and performance adaptations in collegiate women tennis players. *The American Journal of Sports Medicine,* 28, 5, 626–633.

Lange, A., Vanwanseele, B., & Fiatarone-Singh, M. (2008). Strength training for treatment of osteoarthritis of the knee: A systematic review. *Arthritis and Rheumatism*, 59, 1488–1494.

McLester, J. et al. (2003). A series of studies: A practical protocol for testing muscle endurance recovery. *Journal of Strength and Conditioning Research,* 17, 2, 259–273.

Melov, S. et al. (2007). Resistance exercise reverses aging in human skeletal muscle. *PLoS ONE,* 2, e465.

Menkes, A. et al. (1993). Strength training increases regional bone mineral density and bone remodeling in middle-aged and older men. *Journal of Applied Physiology,* 74, 2478–2484.

Messier, S. & Dill, M. (1985). Alterations in strength and maximal oxygen uptake consequent to Nautilus circuit weight training. *Research Quarterly for Exercise and Sport,* 56, 345–351.

Morris, F. et al. (1997). Prospective ten-month exercise intervention in premenarcheal girls: Positive effects on bone and lean mass. *Journal of Bone and Mineral Research,* 12, 9, 1453–1462.

Nelson, M.E. et al. (1994). Effects of high-intensity strength training on multiple risk factors for osteoporotic fractures. *Journal of the American Medical Association,* 272, 24, 1909–1914.

Olson, T.P. et al. (2006). Moderate resistance training and vascular health in overweight women. *Medicine & Science in Sports & Exercise,* 38, 9, 1558–1564.

Parise, G., Brose, A., & Tarnopolsky, M. (2005). Resistance exercise training decreases oxidative damage to DNA and increases cytochrome oxidase activity in older adults. *Experimental Gerontology,* 40, 173–180.

Pette, D. (2001). Historical perspectives: Plasticit yof mammalian skeletal muscle. *Journal of Applied Physiology,* 90, 3, 1119–1124.

Phillips, S. (2007). Resistance exercise: Good for more than just Grandma and Grandpa's muscles. *Applied Physiology, Nutrition and Metabolism,* 32, 1198–1205.

Phillips, S.M (2006). Dietary protein for athletes: From requirements to metabolic advantage. *Applied Physiology, Nutrition, & Metabolism*, 31, 647–654.

Pratley, R.B. et al. (1994). Strength training increases resting metabolic rate and norepinephrine levels in healthy 50–65 year-old men. *Journal of Applied Physiology,* 76, 1, 133–137.

Risch, S. et al. (1993). Lumbar strengthening in chronic low-back pain patients. *Spine,* 18, 232–238.

Ruiz, J. et al. (2008). Association between muscular strength and mortality in men: Prospective cohort study. *British Medical Journal,* 337, a439.

Ryan, A. et al. (2001). Insulin action after resistance training in insulin resistant older men and women. *Journal of the American Geriatric Society,* 49, 247–253.

Shoepe, T. et al. (2003). Functional adaptability of muscle fibers to long-term resistance exercise. *Medicine & Science in Sports & Exercise,* 35, 6, 944–951.

Singh, N., Clements, K., & Fiatarone, M. (1997). A randomized controlled trial of progressive resistance training in depressed elders. *Journal of Gerontology,* 52A, M27–M35.

Starkey, D. et al. (1996). Effect of resistance training volume on strength and muscle thickness. *Medicine & Science in Sports & Exercise,* 28, 10, 1311–1320.

Taaffe, D. et al. (1996). Comparative effects of high and low intensity resistance training on thigh muscle strength, fiber area, and tissue composition in elderly women. *Clinical Physiology,* 16, 4, 381–392.

Van Etten, L. et al. (1997). Effect of an 18-week weight-training program on energy expenditure and physical activity. *Journal of Applied Physiology,* 82, 1, 298–304.

Van Thienen, R. et al. (2009). ß-alanine improves sprint performance in endurance cycling. *Medicine & Science in Sports & Exercise*, 41, 4, 898–903.

Venderley, A.M. & Campbell, W.W. (2006). Vegetarian diets: Nutritional considerations for athletes. *Sports Medicine*, 36, 4, 293–305.

Westcott, W.L. (2009a). ACSM strength training guidelines: Role in body composition and health enhancement. *ACSM's Health & Fitness Journal,* 13, 4, 14–22.

Westcott, W. (2009b). Strength training for frail older adults. *Journal on Active Aging,* 8, 4, 52–59.

Westcott, W.L. (2003). *Building Strength & Stamina* (2nd ed.). Champaign, Ill.: Human Kinetics.

Westcott, W.L. (1998). Circuit training. In: Burke, E. (Ed.). *Precision Heart Rate Training.* Champaign, Ill.: Human Kinetics.

Westcott, W.L. (1991). *Strength Fitness* (3rd ed.). Dubuque, Iowa: Wm. C. Brown Publishers.

Westcott, W.L. & Howes, B. (1983). Blood pressure response during weight training exercise. *National Strength and Conditioning Association Journal,* 5, 67–71.

Westcott, W.L., Tolken, J., & Wessner, B. (1995). School-based conditioning programs for physically unfit children. *Strength and Conditioning,* 17, 5–9.

Westcott, W. et al. (2009). Prescribing physical activity: Applying the ACSM protocols for exercise type, intensity, and duration across 3 training frequencies. *Physician and Sportsmedicine,* 37, 2, 51–58.

Westcott, W.L. et al. (2008). Protein and body composition. *Fitness Management,* 24, 5, 50–53.

Westcott, W.L. et al. (2007). Comparison of two exercise protocols on fitness score improvement in poorly conditioned Air Force personnel. *Perceptual Motor Skills,* 104, 629–636.

Wijndaele, K. et al. (2007). Muscular strength, aerobic fitness, and metabolic syndrome risk in Flemish adults. *Medicine & Science and Sports & Exercise,* 39, 2, 233–240.

Wilmore, J.H., Costill, D.L., & Kenney, W.L. (2008). *Physiology of Sport and Exercise* (4th ed.). Champaign, Ill.: Human Kinetics.

Zatsiorsky, V. & Kraemer, W. (2006). *Science and Practice of Strength Training* (2nd ed.) Champaign, Ill.: Human Kinetics.

Suggested Reading

Aaberg, E. (2006). *Resistance Training Instruction* (2nd ed.). Champaign, Ill.: Human Kinetics.

Baechle, T. & Earle, R. (Eds.) (2008). *Essentials of Strength Training and Conditioning* (3rd ed.). Champaign, Ill.: Human Kinetics.

Baechle, T. & Earle, R. (2005). *Fitness Weight Training* (2nd ed.). Champaign, Ill.: Human Kinetics.

Brooks, D. (2001). *Effective Strength Training.* Champaign, Ill.: Human Kinetics.

Brown, L.E. (Ed.) (2007). *Strength Training*. Champaign, Ill.: Human Kinetics.

Chu, D. (1996). *Explosive Power and Strength.* Champaign, Ill.: Human Kinetics.

DeLavier, F. (2006). *Strength Training Anatomy* (2nd ed.). Champaign, Ill.: Human Kinetics.

Earle, R. & Baechle, T. (Eds.). (2004). *NSCA's Essentials of Personal Training.* Champaign, Ill.: Human Kinetics.

Faigenbaum, A. & Westcott, W. (2009). *Youth Strength Training* (2nd ed.). Champaign, Ill.: Human Kinetics.

Fleck, S. & Kraemer, W. (2004). *Designing Resistance Training Programs* (3rd ed.). Champaign, Ill.: Human Kinetics.

Kraemer, W. & Fleck, S. (2007). *Optimizing Strength Training*. Champaign, Ill.: Human Kinetics.

National Strength and Conditioning Association (2008). *Exercise Techniques Manual for Resistance Training* (2nd ed.). Champaign, Ill.: Human Kinetics.

Philbin, J. (2004). *High-Intensity Training.* Champaign, Ill.: Human Kinetics.

Sandler, D. (2003). *Weight Training Fundamentals.* Champaign, Ill.: Human Kinetics.

Stoppani, J. (2006). *Encyclopedia of Muscle and Strength*. Champaign, Ill.: Human Kinetics.

Westcott, W. (2003). *Building Strength and Stamina* (2nd ed.). Champaign, Ill.: Human Kinetics.

Westcott, W. & Baechle, T. (2007). *Strength Training Past 50* (2nd ed.). Champaign, Ill.: Human Kinetics.

IN THIS CHAPTER:

Physiological Adaptations to Acute and Chronic Cardiorespiratory Exercise
- Muscular System
- Cardiovascular System
- Respiratory System
- Time Required for Increases in Aerobic Capacity
- Physiological Adaptations to Steady-state and Interval-based Exercise

Components of a Cardiorespiratory Workout Session
- Warm-up
- Conditioning Phase
- Cool-down

General Guidelines for Cardiorespiratory Exercise for Health, Fitness, and Weight Loss
- Frequency
- Intensity
- Duration
- Exercise Progression

Modes or Types of Cardiorespiratory Exercise
- Equipment-based Cardiovascular Exercise
- Group Exercise
- Circuit Training
- Outdoor Exercise
- Seasonal Exercise
- Water-based Exercise
- Mind-body Exercise
- Lifestyle Exercise

ACE Integrated Fitness Training™ Model—Cardiorespiratory Training Phases
- Phase 1: Aerobic-base Training
- Phase 2: Aerobic-efficiency Training
- Phase 3: Anaerobic-endurance training
- Phase 4: Anaerobic-power Training

Recovery and Regeneration

Special Considerations for Youth and Older Adults
- Youth
- Older Adults

Summary

CARL FOSTER, Ph.D., *is a professor in the Department of Exercise and Sports Science and director of the Human Performance Laboratory at the University of Wisconsin–La Crosse (UWL). He is a fellow of the American College of Sports Medicine (ACSM) and of the American Association of Cardiovascular and Pulmonary Rehabilitation. He was the 2005–2006 President of ACSM. Dr. Foster's research interests range from high-performance physiology (he is the head of sports science for U.S. Speedskating) to clinical exercise physiology (he is the research director for the Clinical Exercise Physiology graduate program at UWL). He has published more than 250 scientific papers and book chapters and 22 longer works (e.g., books, monographs, position stands, videos).*

JOHN P. PORCARI, Ph.D., *is a professor in the Department of Exercise and Sports Science and executive director of the La Crosse Exercise and Health Program at the University of Wisconsin–La Crosse. He is a fellow of the American College of Sports Medicine and of the American Association of Cardiovascular and Pulmonary Rehabilitation (AACVPR) and was the President of AACVPR in 2002–2003. Dr. Porcari's research interests have focused on the acute and training responses to exercising on a variety of exercise modalities, particularly new fitness products. He has authored more than 75 peer-reviewed publications and made more than 150 national presentations dealing with health and fitness.*

CHAPTER 11

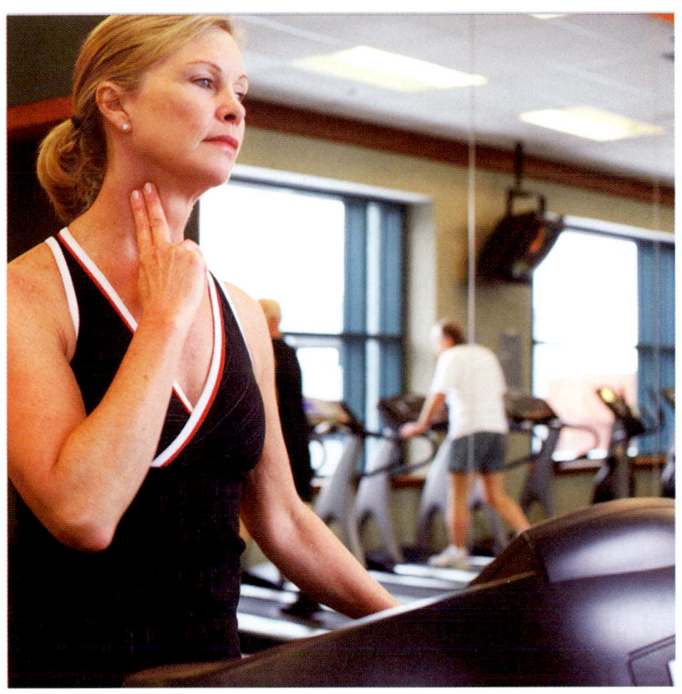

Cardiorespiratory Training: Programming and Progressions

Carl Foster & John P. Porcari

Humans are designed to move. Since emerging as a distinct species, humans moved (exercised) to secure food, escape from dangerous situations, attract mates, and do a variety of other activities that have allowed the species to thrive. In the small groups of hunter-gatherers that still exist, everyday levels of physical activity are extraordinarily high, essentially equivalent to walking/running 10 to 12 miles per day (Booth & Roberts, 2008; Cordain, Gotshall, & Eaton, 1998). The so-called "diseases of civilization" (e.g., heart disease, **diabetes,** many cancers) are very uncommon in these groups (Booth et al., 2002). Since physical movement is essential for human survival, the organ systems involved in energy metabolism (muscular, cardiorespiratory) function best when subjected to regular physical challenges.

Physical activity leads to improvements in work capacity (e.g., **cardiorespiratory fitness**), the sense of well-being, and overall health, as well as to fewer diseases. However, the obligatory need for physical activity is very low in modern society. Most people can do their jobs and feed themselves with a minimum of exertion. Accordingly, the need for people to structure their lives in a way that intentionally includes either higher levels of physical activity or even any exercise at all has risen dramatically.

Physiological Adaptations to Acute and Chronic Cardiorespiratory Exercise

Muscular System

The organ systems stressed during physical activity and exercise adapt in a way that is very specific to the type of exercise performed. In other words, the muscle fibers that are recruited to perform exercise are the only ones stimulated to adapt. During low-intensity endurance exercise, this usually means adaptations in the **type I muscle fibers** (i.e., the **slow-twitch muscle fibers**). These adaptations involve increasing the size and number of **mitochondria** within the cell to augment aerobic **adenosine triphosphate (ATP)** generation. There is also a growth of more **capillaries** around the recruited muscle fibers, which enhances the delivery of oxygenated blood to the muscle fibers. If the recruitment is near the upper limit of a given muscle fiber's capacity to generate force, there may also be adaptations in the contractile mechanism (i.e., the **actin** and **myosin** filaments), leading to **hypertrophy** of those muscle fibers. During higher-intensity exercise, the **type II muscle fibers** (i.e., the **fast-twitch muscle fibers**) may also be recruited. They adapt primarily by increasing the number of anaerobic **enzymes** so that **anaerobic** energy production will be enhanced. With increased training intensity, there may also be hypertrophy of the contractile proteins within the muscle fiber.

Cardiovascular System

Due to the expansion of blood volume that occurs with endurance training, the heart muscle will hypertrophy, enlarging its chambers and becoming a bigger and stronger muscle that is able to deliver a higher **cardiac output** to the muscles. These adaptations are primarily in the form of a larger **stroke volume** (i.e., the amount of blood pumped per beat), as a number of studies suggest that the **maximum heart rate (MHR)** does not increase with training. This increase in stroke volume is due to chamber enlargement, greater amounts of chamber filling (**end-diastolic volume**) and greater chamber emptying (**ejection fraction**) of the heart with each beat. There is also some evidence that the redistribution of the cardiac output to the active muscles (via **vasodilation**) may improve after training, thus making the increase in cardiac output more effective in terms of delivering oxygen where it is needed.

Respiratory System

Although somewhat less adaptable than the heart and circulatory system, the muscles of the respiratory system will adapt as exercise is performed regularly to allow for increased ventilation of the **alveoli,** which is where the cardiovascular system interfaces with the respiratory system. The muscles involved in respiration span the thorax and abdomen and include the following:

- The diaphragm, which is the body's key breathing muscle, and the external intercostals used during passive (resting) **inspiration**
- The group of muscles that pull the ribcage upward (i.e., sternocleidomastoid, scalene, portions of the serratus anterior) during active (exercise) inspiration
- The group of muscles that pull the ribcage downward (i.e., rectus abdominis, quadratus lumborum) during active **expiration**

There is little evidence that the structures of the pulmonary system actually increase in size. However, both the strength and fatigue resistance of the respiratory muscles improve with training, allowing greater ventilation for longer periods than existed before training. This stronger musculature may allow the ventilation to increase by leading to an increase in **tidal volume,** which delivers more oxygen to the alveoli and reduces the relative amount of respiratory dead space (i.e., air trapped in the bronchial tubes that never reaches the alveoli) at high breathing frequencies, thus making ventilation more efficient.

Time Required for Increases in Aerobic Capacity

Cardiovascular adaptations to exercise begin with the first exercise bout, but are usually not readily measureable for a couple of weeks. $\dot{V}O_2$**max,** which is the traditional standard marker of the aerobic-training effect, increases with training, but reaches a peak and plateaus within about six months (Foster, Porcari, & Lucia, 2008). However, changes in **ventilatory threshold (VT),** a significant marker of metabolism that permits prediction of **lactate threshold (LT)** from the **minute ventilation** ($\dot{V}_E$) response during progressive exercise, may continue for years. This change is attributed primarily to capillary growth and increased mitochondrial density (size and number) in the active muscles (Figure 11-1). To support these cardiorespiratory adaptations, the capacity of the muscle to store additional **glycogen** increases and the ability to mobilize and use **fatty acids**

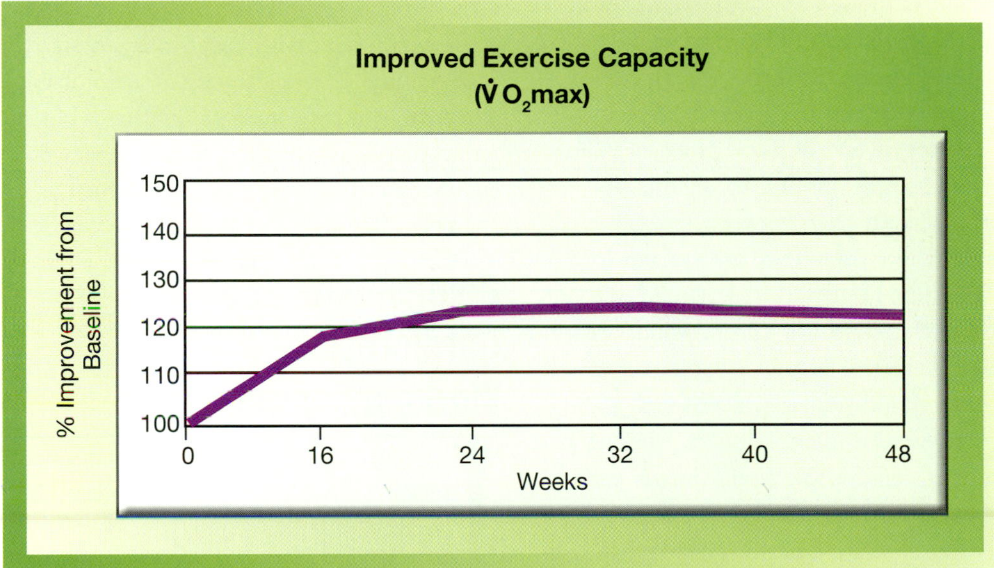

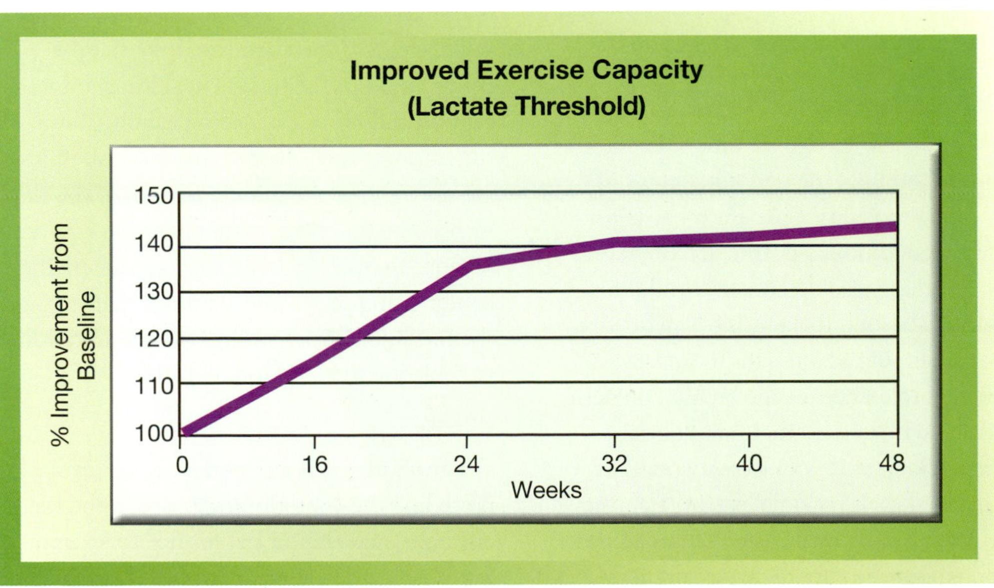

Figure 11-1
Schematic pattern of changes in $\dot{V}O_2$max and metabolic markers (e.g., lactate threshold) with a progressive training program in a formerly sedentary individual. Note that the improvement in $\dot{V}O_2$max is essentially complete after four to six months of training, but that the more sustainable exercise capacity represented by lactate threshold continues to improve for a much longer period of time.

as a fuel source is also enhanced. This ability increases for some time beyond the primary increase in $\dot{V}O_2$max.

Physiological Adaptations to Steady-state and Interval-based Exercise

The primary adaptations to exercise training typically occur during steady-state exercise at moderate intensity. The term **steady state** refers to that intensity of exercise where the energy and physiological demands of the exercise bout are met by the delivery of the physiological systems in the body. At steady state, the rate of **oxygen uptake ($\dot{V}O_2$), heart rate (HR),** cardiac output, ventilation, blood **lactate** concentration, and body temperature reach stable (although elevated) levels after a short period of exercise. That exercise duration is primarily limited by the willingness to continue or by the availability of oxygen, muscle glycogen, and/or blood **glucose.** When an exercise bout begins or exercise intensity changes, the body takes between 45 seconds and three to four minutes to achieve steady state. The time needed to achieve this level, sometime referred to as a "second wind," varies according to several factors, including fitness level (more fit individuals achieve steady state faster) and exercise intensity (when working at higher intensities, people require longer periods to achieve steady state).

There are several studies suggesting that **interval training** (a few repetitions of higher-intensity exercise followed by recovery periods) promotes similar improvements in $\dot{V}O_2$max and fitness as steady-state exercise. While this may prove to be a more time-efficient method of training, the appropriateness of this training modality must always be considered for deconditioned clients. Research on interval training also demonstrates additional adaptations beyond the **aerobic** benefits that include anaerobic adaptations to improve an individual's tolerance for the buildup of **lactic acid** (lactate threshold) that may continue to increase long after $\dot{V}O_2$max adaptations have reached their maximal extent (Laursen et al., 2002; Stepto et al., 1998). This adaptation enhances one's ability to sustain higher intensities of exercise for longer periods (Foster, Porcari, & Lucia, 2008).

A universal principle to training is that it is necessary to progressively perform higher intensities of exercise to effectively challenge or overload the cardiorespiratory system. Since muscle fibers that are not recruited are not likely to adapt, it is probable that there is little or no adaptation of type II muscle fibers during moderate-intensity aerobic training, whereas there would be with higher-intensity training. Generally, these intensities are not sustained through steady-state exercise. The overload on the heart to deliver blood to the exercising muscles during higher-intensity or non-steady-state exercise likely provokes adaptations that allow stroke volume to increase to levels that are not achievable with lower-intensity steady-state training. These adaptations are probably attributable to large increases in venous blood return that occur with very high-intensity exercise that increases end-diastolic volume (i.e., chamber filling).

Components of a Cardiorespiratory Workout Session

There are basically three components of any training session: the warm-up phase, the conditioning phase, and the cool-down phase. In some exercise bouts, the intensity of exercise may be very gradually increased, stabilized, and then decreased, so that the components of the session are almost imperceptibly different. For example, going for a run during which the first and last half miles are slower than the middle portion of the run incorporates all three components of a workout session. In other training sessions, where the conditioning phase may be more challenging, the transitions from warm-up to conditioning to cool-down may be quite distinct.

Warm-up

The warm-up is a period of lighter exercise preceding the conditioning phase of the exercise bout, and should last for five to 10 minutes for most healthy adults. It should begin with low- to moderate-intensity exercise or activity that gradually increases in intensity.

If higher-intensity intervals are planned during the conditioning phase, the latter portion of the warm-up could include some brief higher-intensity exercise to prepare the exerciser for the more intense elements of the stimulus phase. As a general principle, the harder the conditioning phase and/or the older the exerciser, the more extensive the warm-up should be (see Chapter 14 for specific recommendations for various populations). However, the warm-up should not be so demanding that it creates fatigue that would reduce performance, especially when working with competitive athletes.

There is some controversy regarding stretching as part of the warm-up. It probably does no harm to do some brief stretching at the end of the warm-up, although if very high-intensity elements are to be included in the workout, stretching may actually inhibit the ability to achieve full intensity. This is attributed to the fact that stretching improves muscle **elasticity** (decreasing tissue viscosity), which lowers the force-generating capacity of the contractile proteins of the muscle. Moreover, the practice of stretching *before* performing any warm-up is not justified and may potentially be harmful. The warm-up may be subdivided into a more general cardiovascular warm-up followed by a more exercise- or event-specific dynamic warm-up (if unique muscular elements are to be performed during the training session).

Conditioning Phase

The conditioning phase, which must be appropriate for the client's current fitness level and consistent with his or her training goals, should be planned in terms of frequency, duration, intensity (utilizing steady-state or interval-training formats), and modality. Although definitive evidence is lacking, empirical evidence suggests that the higher-intensity elements of a session should take place fairly early in the conditioning phase, and that the conditioning phase should conclude with more steady-state exercise, even if the intensity is still in the range likely to serve as a stimulus.

When utilizing steady-state bouts of exercise, trainers should be conscious of **cardiovascular drift,** a cardiovascular phenomenon that represents a gradual increase in heart-rate response during a steady-state bout of exercise (Wilmore, Costill, & Kenney, 2008). Causes for this drift include the following:

- Small reductions in blood volume that occur during exercise due to fluid lost to sweat and fluid moving into the spaces between cells, which results in a compensatory increase in heart rate to maintain cardiac output, offsetting the small decrease in stroke volume (Cardiac output = Heart rate x Stroke volume)
- Increasing core temperature that directs greater quantities of blood to the skin to facilitate heat loss, consequently decreasing blood return to the heart and blood available for the exercising muscles

Aerobic-interval training generally involves bouts of steady-state exercise performed at higher intensities for sustained periods (typically a minimum of three minutes), followed by a return to lower aerobic intensities for the recovery interval. These intervals often utilize exercise-to-recovery ratios between 1:2 and 1:1 (e.g., a four-minute steady-state bout is followed by an eight-minute recovery period at a lower intensity when following a 1:2 exercise-to-recovery ratio).

It should also be noted that higher-intensity intervals of 15 to 30 seconds may effectively recruit (and thus stimulate) type II muscle fibers, and are essentially aerobic from the standpoint of the overall metabolic response to training (Gorostiaga et al., 1991). Assuming that aerobically trained type II muscle fibers may serve as "lactate sinks" (structures that are proficient at using lactate for energy) during hard steady-state exercise, the aerobic-training stimulus should include at least some higher-intensity segments in programs for clients with goals that go beyond basic cardiorespiratory conditioning.

Cool-down

The cool-down should be of approximately the same duration and intensity as the warm-up (i.e., five to 10 minutes of low- to moderate-intensity activity). This phase is directed primarily toward preventing the tendency for blood to pool in the extremities, which may occur when exercise ends. The cessation of significant venous return from the "muscle pump" experienced during exercise can cause blood to accumulate in the lower extremity, reducing blood flow back to the heart and out to vital organs (e.g., the brain, potentially causing symptoms of light-headedness). An active cool-down also helps remove metabolic waste from the muscles so that it can be metabolized by other tissues. A stretching routine following the cool-down period can improve flexibility and reduce the potential for muscles soreness.

General Guidelines for Cardiorespiratory Exercise for Health, Fitness, and Weight Loss

The *2008 Physical Activity Guidelines for Americans* released by the U.S. Department of Health & Human Services provide comprehensive science-based recommendations to reduce the risk of many adverse health outcomes. Many of the recommendations are derived from the knowledge that most health benefits occur with at least 150 minutes a week of moderate-intensity physical activity and that the benefits of physical activity far outweigh the possibility of adverse outcomes. Specific guidelines for adults aged 18 to 64 include the following:

- Perform 150 minutes per week of moderate-intensity aerobic physical activity, or 75 minutes per week of vigorous-intensity aerobic physical activity, or a combination of both.
- Additional health benefits are obtained from performing greater amounts of activity than those quantities.
- Perform aerobic bouts that last at least 10 minutes, preferably spread throughout the week.
- Participate in muscle-strengthening activities involving all major muscle groups at least two days per week.

Specific guidelines for children and adolescents aged 6 to 17 include the following:

- Perform at least 60 minutes of moderate-to-vigorous physical activity every day.
- Include vigorous-intensity activity a minimum of three days per week.
- Participate in muscle-strengthening and bone-strengthening activity a minimum of three days per week.

With regard to cardiovascular programming, however, the most widely accepted guidelines for physical activity and basic fitness training are those presented by the American College of Sports Medicine (ACSM) and the American Heart Association (AHA). These guidelines frequently use the F.I.T.T. acronym to discuss cardiovascular programming guidelines (ACSM, 2010; Haskell et al., 2007). This acronym represents frequency, intensity, time (duration), and type (modality), but trainers should also consider including an "E" (i.e., F.I.T.T.E.) to represents "enjoyable" or "experience." Clients should always enjoy the exercise experience, as this influences the thoughts and emotions that can ultimately dictate participation and **adherence** rates. Frequency, intensity, and duration collectively represent the exercise volume, load, or magnitude of training that is likely to provoke the physiological adaptations to the training response. A dose-response relationship exists between volume and the health/fitness benefits achieved, implying that greater benefits are achieved with increased volumes.

Trainers generally progress their clients' programs by manipulating these variables. The rate of program progression depends on each client's individual health status, exercise tolerance, available time, and program goals. Improvement in cardiorespiratory fitness occurs most quickly from progressive increases in exercise intensity, and fades when training intensity is reduced. Changes in fitness are more sensitive to changes in intensity than to changes in the frequency or duration of training.

Frequency

While minimal health benefits can be attained in as little as one to two sessions per week, current guidelines recommend physical activity on most days of the week (U.S. Department of Health & Human Services, 2008). ACSM recommendations are presented in Table 11-1. For the beginning adult exerciser, the balance should be in the direction of more moderate-intensity exercise, since higher-intensity exercise has been associated with a risk of exercise-related complications, injury, and a poor experience in beginning exercisers (Foster et al., 2008).

Intensity

Exercise intensity is arguably the most important element of the exercise program to monitor. At the same time, it is the most difficult element to present quantitatively.

Table 11-1
Cardiorespiratory Recommendations for Healthy Adults

Exercise Type	Weekly Frequency
Moderate-intensity aerobic exercise • 40% to <60% $\dot{V}O_2R$ or HRR	Minimum of 5 days per week
Vigorous-intensity aerobic exercise • ≥60% $\dot{V}O_2R$ or HRR	Minimum of 3 days per week
Combination of moderate- and vigorous-intensity aerobic exercise	3–5 days per week

Note: $\dot{V}O_2R$ = $\dot{V}O_2$ reserve; HRR = Heart-rate reserve

Source: American College of Sports Medicine (2010). *ACSM's Guidelines for Exercise Testing and Prescription* (8th ed.). Wolters Kluwer/Lippincott Williams & Wilkins.

There are numerous methods by which the trainer can program and monitor exercise intensity:

- Heart rate [% MHR; % **heart-rate reserve (HRR)**]
- RPE
- $\dot{V}O_2$ or **metabolic equivalents (METs)**
- Caloric expenditure
- Talk test
- Blood lactate and VT2

Heart Rate

Using percentage of MHR or HRR is probably the most widely used approach for programming and monitoring exercise intensity. While there is a very large body of evidence supporting this approach, accuracy in using these methods requires knowledge of the individual's MHR. Without a maximal-effort exercise test, which is generally not considered appropriate for most individuals, this marker is not definable. Given the risk associated with conducting a maximal-effort test, MHR is normally determined via mathematical formulas (e.g., 220 – age). While these calculations are usually easy to compute and provide an easy marker from which trainers can anchor exercise intensity (e.g., %MHR), estimated MHR is less than useful as an exercise anchor for individual exercise programming and should be questioned due to its inherent error (see page 190). Numerous variables impact MHR, including the following:

- Genetics
- Exercise modality (e.g., MHR varies between running and cycling due to the involvement of upper-body musculature)
- Medications
- Body size. MHR is generally higher in smaller individuals who have smaller hearts, and hence lower stroke volumes, which explains why females often have higher **resting heart rates (RHR)** than males.
- Altitude. Altitude can lower the MHR reached due to most individual's inability to train at higher intensities.
- Age. MHR does not show a consistent 1-bpm drop with each year in all individuals.

MHR does not correlate strongly with performance and is generally not influenced by training. In fact, it may even become lowered with training given the training adaptation of expanded blood and stroke volume. Most importantly, MHR varies significantly among people of the same age. For example, the popular formula devised by Fox, Naughton, and Haskell (220 – age), which was never intended for use with the general population, demonstrates a standard deviation (s.d.) of approximately 12 beats per minute (Fox, Naughton, & Haskell, 1971). This implies that for 68% of a population (or one standard deviation assuming a normal distribution of data), the true MHR would differ from the estimated mathematical calculation by 12 beats on either side of that value (Figure 11-2). The remaining 32% would fall even further outside of this range (e.g., for 95%, or two standard deviations of the population, the true MHR would fall within 24 beats on either side of the calculated value).

Another concern with the 220 – age formula is the fact that it also tends to overestimate MHR in younger adults and underestimate MHR in older adults [e.g., a 25 year old may never reach 195 bpm (i.e., 220 – 25), while a 60 year old may exceed 160 bpm (i.e., 220 – 60) quite comfortably].

Figure 11-2
The standard deviation (i.e., 12 beats per minute) for the 220 – age maximum heart rate prediction equation for 20 year olds

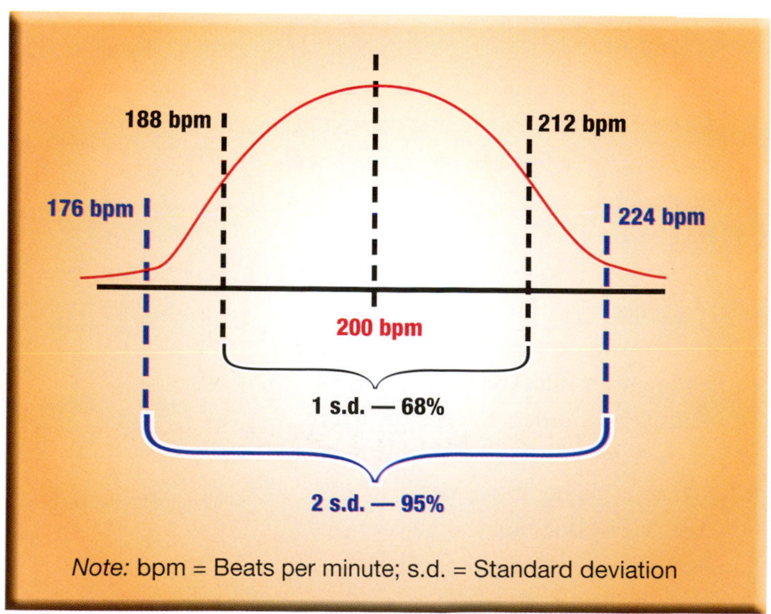

Beyond the invalidity of MHR, a significant concern with using a straight percentage of MHR to design and monitor training intensities stems from the fact that discrepancies in individual RHRs are not taken into consideration and may therefore lead the trainer to over- or underestimate appropriate exercise intensities.

Overtraining a client increases the risk of injury and creates a potentially negative experience, whereas undertraining can quickly disengage the individual from the exercise experience due to boredom and perhaps insufficient challenge. Given that the risk of serious cardiovascular complications during exercise in **sedentary** individuals is strongly related to inappropriately high exercise intensities (Foster et al., 2008), guiding exercise on the basis of a percentage of estimated age-based MHR is discouraged very strongly.

Regardless, ACSM provides guidelines for using %MHR (Table 11-2), but does make a strong recommendation against using the standardized 220 – age formula (ACSM, 2010). ACSM suggests formulas with standard deviations closer to 7 bpm (Gellish et al., 2007; Tanaka, Monahan, & Seals, 2001):

- Tanaka, Monahan, and Seals formula: 208 – (0.7 x Age)
- Gellish et al. formula: 206.9 – (0.67 x Age)

Another popular method for monitoring training intensity follows the Karvonen, or heart-rate reserve, formula. Given the concern with RHR discrepancy, the HRR method is more appropriate, as it does consider potential RHR differences by determining an HRR from which training intensities are calculated. This method reduces discrepancies in training intensities between individuals with different RHR and accommodates the training adaptation that lowers RHR, therefore expanding HRR (Table 11-3 and Figure 11-3).

While the HRR model does reduce the error in estimation, it still has limitations regarding its accuracy and appropriateness:

Table 11-2
Recommended Framework for Exercise Intensity for Apparently Healthy Adults

Activity/Exercise Level	Fitness Classification	%MHR	%HRR/$\dot{V}O_2$max or $\dot{V}O_2$R
Sedentary: No habitual activity or exercise, extremely deconditioned	Poor	57–67%	30–45%
Minimal activity: No exercise, moderately to highly deconditioned	Poor/fair	64–74%	40–55%
Sporadic physical activity: No or suboptimal exercise, moderately to mildly deconditioned	Fair/average	74–84%	55–70%
Habitual physical activity: Regular moderate-to-vigorous intensity	Average/good	80–91%	65–80%
High amounts of habitual activity: Regular vigorous-intensity exercise	Good/excellent	84–94%	70–85%

Note: MHR = Maximum heart rate; HRR = Heart-rate reserve; $\dot{V}O_2$max = $\dot{V}O_2$ maximum; $\dot{V}O_2$R = $\dot{V}O_2$ reserve

Adapted, with permission, from American College of Sports Medicine (2010). *ACSM's Guidelines for Exercise Testing and Prescription* (8th ed.). Philadelphia: Wolters Kluwer/Lippincott Williams & Wilkins.

Table 11-3
Comparing %HRR Estimations in Two 30 Year Olds With Different Resting Heart Rates

	Person A (bpm)	Person B (bpm)
MHR (220 – 30)	190	190
RHR	50	80
HRR (MHR – RHR)	140	110
60% HRR	84	66
Adding RHR	84 + 50	66 + 80
Training HR	134 (12 beat difference)	146

Note: HRR = Heart-rate reserve; MHR = Maximum heart rate; RHR = Resting heart rate; HR = Heart rate; bpm = Beats per minute

Karvonen Method

Target HR (THR) = (HRR x % Intensity) + RHR
HRR = MHR – RHR

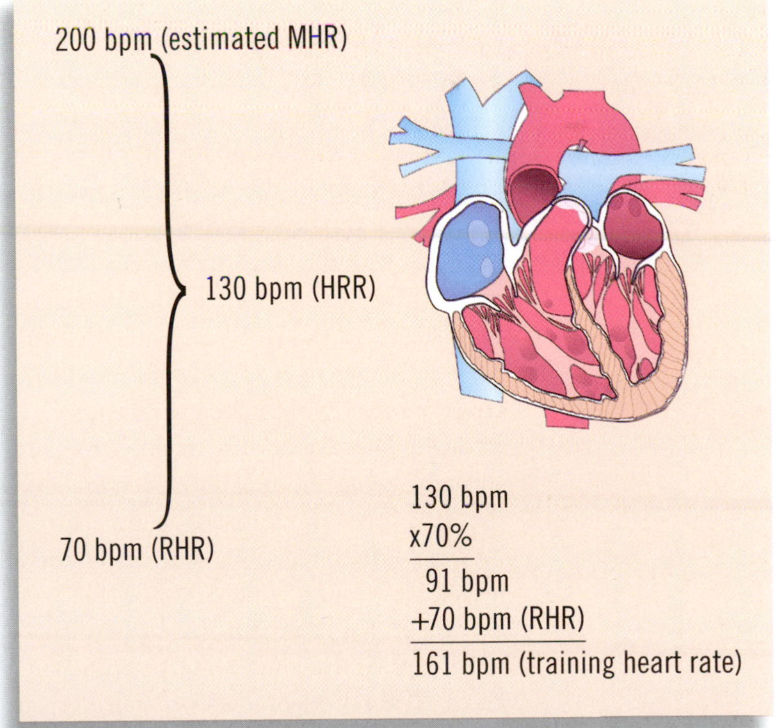

Figure 11-3
Use of the Karvonen formula for a 20-year-old man (average shape; resting heart rate = 70 bpm)

Note: bpm = Beats per minute; MHR = Maximum heart rate; HRR = Heart-rate reserve; RHR = Resting heart rate

- It utilizes a mathematical estimation for MHR. *Note:* Ideally, the Karvonen technique should be based on measured maximum heart rate to yield the most accurate results.
- There is some debate over the body position in which RHR is measured. This formula was created measuring true RHR, taken in the morning in a reclining position. RHR varies by approximately five to 10 beats when a person transitions from lying to standing, thereby altering the size of the HRR. Given the concern with some inconsistencies with clients measuring their own HR, ACE recommends measuring RHR in the body position in which the client will exercise. This may necessitate the need for two sets of training zones; one for seated/recumbent positions and another for standing activities.

Table 11-4

Ratings of Perceived Exertion (RPE)

RPE	Category Ratio Scale
6	0 Nothing at all
7 Very, very light	0.5 Very, very weak
8	1 Very weak
9 Very light	2 Weak
10	3 Moderate
11 Fairly light	4 Somewhat strong
12	5 Strong
13 Somewhat hard	6
14	7 Very strong
15 Hard	8
16	9
17 Very hard	10 Very, very strong
18	* Maximal
19 Very, very hard	
20	

Adapted, with permission, from American College of Sports Medicine (2010). *ACSM's Guidelines for Exercise Testing and Prescription* (8th ed.). Philadelphia: Wolters Kluwer/Lippincott Williams & Wilkins.

Ratings of Perceived Exertion

RPE emerged in the late 1970s and early 1980s as a subjective method of gauging exercise intensity. It has since gained wide acceptance as a method of monitoring exercise intensity. There are two versions of the RPE scale: the classical (6 to 20) scale and the more contemporary category ratio (0 to 10) scale, which was developed to remedy inconsistencies with the use of the classical RPE scale (Table 11-4) (Borg, 1998). Although fully subjective, the RPE scale (in both forms) has been shown to be capable of defining the ranges of objective exercise intensity associated with effective exercise training programs. In simple terms, a rating of "moderate" on the RPE scale is more or less equivalent to 70% of MHR, a rating of "somewhat hard" is more or less equivalent to 80% of MHR, and a rating of "hard" is more or less equivalent to 85% of MHR. Thus, for all practical purposes, RPE ratings of moderate to hard span the range of recommended exercise training intensities. The RPE system works well for about 90% of people. Very sedentary individuals often find it difficult to use, as they find any level of exercise fairly hard. However, in the very sedentary, even a small amount of low-intensity exercise is effective in terms of producing some exercise training benefits and improved health outcomes. At the other end of the continuum, individuals who have high muscular strength may under-rate the intensity of exercise if they focus on the muscular tension requirement of exercise rather than on the breathing elements. With practice during cardiorespiratory exercise, these individuals can usually learn to use the scale fairly effectively.

$\dot{V}O_2$ or Metabolic Equivalents

The traditional reference standard for exercise intensity is expressed in terms of percentages of $\dot{V}O_2$max or **$\dot{V}O_2$reserve ($\dot{V}O_2$R).** The great volume of experimental studies conducted in the 1960s and 1970s suggested that there are minimal improvements in VO_2max if the intensity of training is below a threshold of 40/50% of $\dot{V}O_2$max or $\dot{V}O_2$R (Foster, Porcari, & Lucia, 2008). While acknowledging that lower-intensity exercise can result in improvements in aerobic capacity in very sedentary or unfit individuals, there does seem to be a lower-limit intensity below which exercise is of minimal benefit.

Session RPE

Selecting an appropriate intensity is always a major challenge for trainers who seek proper levels of overload, yet want to create an optimal experience, especially when working with newer, deconditioned clients, clients who are apprehensive about undergoing cardiorespiratory fitness testing, and individuals for whom heart-rate measures are invalid (e.g., those taking beta blockers).

The "session RPE" was developed as a method of monitoring the combined intensity and duration of an exercise session (Herman et al., 2006; Foster et al., 1995). If an individual is asked to rate the overall intensity of an exercise bout about 30 minutes after the conclusion of that bout using the category ratio (0 to 10) scale, and then multiplies this rating by the duration of the bout, a score representing the combined intensity and duration of the bout is generated (i.e., the training load) (Foster et al., 2001a; Foster, Daniels, & Seiler, 1999; Foster et al., 1996). In practice, this daily score can be summated on a weekly basis, generating a weekly training load for self-monitoring purposes. This is an effective programming and monitoring tool that promotes appropriate initial exercise intensities, creates some ownership of programming on the part of the client, and allows a limited degree of training flexibility to facilitate adherence.

This model can be used exclusively and indefinitely to monitor exercise intensity, or trainers may opt to use it during only the initial stage of a clients' program, perhaps before conducting any cardiorespiratory tests for aerobic fitness.

Trainers should adhere to the following guidelines when using the session RPE model:

- Spend time helping the client becoming familiar with the 0 to 10 RPE scale.
- Determine appropriate RPE intensities for each exercise session based on the client's current activity levels, while providing a small overload challenge (e.g., a 5-out-of-10 effort for someone who has been exercising at a 4-to-4½ effort).
- Identify the frequency and duration that is appropriate for the client's current conditioning level and feasible within his or her schedule (e.g., three times a week for 15 minutes).
- Implement a RPE-training volume model (i.e., RPE x frequency x duration).
  - ✓For example, Joe's key goal is to improve his cardiorespiratory fitness, and he and his trainer mutually decide that a feasible start is for him to participate in cardiovascular training sessions three times each week for approximately 20 minutes each, at a 5-out-of-10 effort.
  - ✓His total weekly training volume is 3 x 20 minutes = 60 minutes, and his target goal for week one = 60 minutes x RPE of 5 = 300 points.
  - ✓Joe's progression over three weeks at a 10% progression rate per week:
    - Week 1 = 300 points
    - Week 2 = 330 points
    - Week 3 = 365 points
  - ✓ The trainer can provide Joe options on how he can achieve his target number by manipulating any of the three variables (i.e., intensity, frequency, and duration) (Table 11-5). While allowing Joe some flexibility and ownership of his program, the trainer should subscribe to the K.I.S.S. principle (keep it simple and short) to avoid confusion and potential drop-out.

Table 11-5

Training Progression and Options Using Frequency x Duration x Intensity (RPE)

	Frequency	Duration	Intensity (RPE)	Total Points
Week 1 goal				300
Options	3 sessions	x 20	x 5	**= 300**
	2 sessions 1 session	x 20 x 18	x 5 x 5.5	= 200 = 99 **299**
	2 sessions 2 sessions	x 16 x 13	x 5 x 5.5	= 160 = 143 **303**
Week 2 goal				330
Options	3 sessions	x 22	x 5	**= 330**
	2 sessions 1 session	x 22 x 18	x 5 x 6	= 220 = 108 **328**
	2 sessions 2 sessions	x 19 x 16.5	x 4 x 5.5	= 152 = 181 **333**

Note: RPE = Ratings of perceived exertion

Although the evidence base for percentage of $\dot{V}O_2max$ or $\dot{V}O_2R$ is very deep, the very large range of acceptable percentages creates the concern that a given percentage is not very specific in terms of recommending exercise. Katch and colleagues (1978) suggested that the "relative percent concept" was essentially flawed, and did not take into account the individual metabolic responses to exercise that might more properly represent the lowest effective training stimulus. Although contemporary guidelines for exercise training are still presented in terms of the relative percent concept, the two-decades-old comments of Professor Katch are still remarkably convincing. Although experimental evidence is lacking, this lowest effective training intensity at which adaptations might be provoked is probably better defined in terms of a metabolic marker called the **first ventilatory threshold (VT1)**, which is discussed in great detail later in this chapter. Although training below this threshold may have some benefit, it is highly probable that training very much below this threshold will yield minimal cardiorespiratory fitness benefits (Meyer et al., 2005). It is arguable that very extensive low-intensity training is important in terms of expending energy in programs designed for weight loss, although there does appear to be a lower limit of exercise intensity that is critical when training for cardiorespiratory fitness. Thus, basing the training program on metabolic or ventilatory responses is much more meaningful than using arbitrary ranges of $\%\dot{V}O_2max$ or $\%\dot{V}O_2R$.

Training programs based on $\%\dot{V}O_2max$ or $\%\dot{V}O_2R$ depend on a maximal exercise test to be accurate, or on some estimate of $\dot{V}O_2max$ derived from a submaximal test. Given that maximal tests are rarely available, and that equations for estimating $\dot{V}O_2max$ are not exceedingly accurate, particularly if any handrail support is allowed during treadmill testing or training (Berling et al., 2006; McConnell et al., 1991), recommending exercise on the basis of this "gold standard" technique probably is much less useful than is widely assumed.

In cases where $\dot{V}O_2$ is not directly measured during either testing or training, an alternative method for expressing exercise intensity is in terms of METs, which are multiples of an assumed average metabolic rate at rest of 3.5 mL/kg/min. This is very easy and intuitive for many people to understand (e.g., at 5.0 METs, they are working five times harder than resting). It is important to recognize, however, that the resting metabolic rate is not exactly 3.5 mL/kg/min in every individual, or even in the same person at all times. Nevertheless, the utility of using METs rather than directly measured $\dot{V}O_2$ is so substantial that it more than makes up for any imprecision (Table 11-6).

Caloric Expenditure

When the human body burns fuel (e.g., **fats, carbohydrates**), oxygen (O_2) is consumed, which yields calories to perform work. While the number of calories produced per liter of O_2 consumed varies according to the fuel utilized (i.e., 4.69 kcal per liter of O_2 for fats; 5.05 kcal per liter of O_2 for glucose), a value of 5 kcal per liter of O_2 is sufficiently accurate considering the fact that people burn a combination of fuels throughout their daily activities.

Caloric expenditure is usually calculated in terms of the gross or absolute $\dot{V}O_2$ during an activity by measuring or estimating the total quantity of O_2 consumed per minute and multiplying it by 5 kcal/liter O_2. If the quantity of O_2 consumed is provided or measured in relative terms (i.e., mL/kg/min), this value must first be converted to gross or absolute terms to determine the total amount of O_2 consumed before the caloric value can be calculated. For example, a relative $\dot{V}O_2$ of 40 mL/kg/min for a 220-lb (100-kg) individual is converted to gross or absolute terms as follows:

- If this individual consumes 40 mL/kg/min, then his or her entire body consumes 40 mL x 100 kg = 4,000 mL/min, or 4.0 L/min (1,000 mL = 1 L)

Table 11-6

MET Values of Common Physical Activities Classified as Light, Moderate, or Vigorous Intensity

LIGHT (<3 METs)	MODERATE (3–6 METs)	VIGOROUS (>6 METs)
Walking	**Walking**	**Walking, jogging, and running**
Walking slowly around home, store, or office = 2.0*	Walking 3.0 mph = 3.0*	Walking at very, very brisk pace (4.5 mph) = 6.3*
	Walking at a very brisk pace (4 mph) = 5.0*	Walking/hiking at moderate pace and grade with no or light pack (<10 pounds; 4.5 kg) = 7.0
		Hiking at steep grades and pack 10–42 pounds (4.5–19 kg) = 7.5–9.0
		Jogging at 5 mph = 8.0*
		Jogging at 6 mph = 10.0*
		Running at 7 mph = 11.5*
Household and occupation	**Household and occupation**	**Household and occupation**
Sitting—using computer, work at desk, using light hand tools = 1.5	Cleaning, heavy—washing windows, washing car, cleaning garage = 3.0	Shoveling sand, coal, etc. = 7.0
Standing performing light work, such as making bed, washing dishes, ironing, preparing food, or working as store clerk = 2.0–2.5	Sweeping floors or carpet, vacuuming, mopping = 3.0–3.5	Carrying heavy loads, such as bricks = 7.5
	Carpentry—general = 3.6	Heavy farming, such as bailing hay = 8.0
	Carrying and stacking wood = 5.5	Shoveling, digging ditches = 8.5
	Mowing lawn—walk power mower = 5.5	
Leisure time and sports	**Leisure time and sports**	**Leisure time and sports**
Arts and crafts, playing cards = 1.5	Badminton—recreational = 4.5	Basketball game = 8.0
Billiards = 2.5	Basketball—shooting around = 4.5	Bicycling on flat—moderate effort (12–14 mph) = 8; fast (14–16 mph) = 10
Boating—power = 2.5	Bicycling on flat—light effort (10–12 mph) = 6.0	Cross-country skiing–slow (2.5 mph) = 7.0; fast (5.0–7.9 mph) = 9.0
Croquet = 2.5	Dancing—ballroom slow = 3.0; ballroom fast = 4.5	Soccer—casual = 7.0; competitive = 10.0
Darts = 2.5	Fishing from riverbank and walking = 4.0	Swimming—moderate/hard = 8–11†
Fishing—sitting = 2.5	Golf—walking pulling clubs = 4.3	Tennis singles = 8.0
Playing most musical instruments = 2.0–2.5	Sailing boat, wind surfing = 3.0	Volleyball—competitive at gym or beach = 8.0
	Swimming leisurely = 6.0†	
	Table tennis = 4.0	
	Tennis doubles = 5.0	
	Volleyball—noncompetitive = 3.0–4.0	

Note: MET = Metabolic equivalent; mph = Miles per hour

*On flat, hard surface

†MET values can vary substantially from person to person during swimming as a result of different strokes and skill levels.

American College of Sports Medicine (2010). *ACSM's Guidelines for Exercise Testing and Prescription* (8th ed.). Philadelphia: Wolters Kluwer/Lippincott Williams & Wilkins; Adapted and modified from Ainsworth, B. et al. (2000). Compendium of physical activities: An update of activity codes and MET intensities. *Medicine & Science in Sports & Exercise,* 32 (suppl), S498–S504.

Example: Caloric Expenditure During Exercise

Caloric expenditure = [$\dot{V}O_2$ (mL/kg/min) x body weight (kg) / 1000] x 5 kcal/L/min

For example, if Mary weighs 154 lb and exercises for 25 minutes and maintains an average $\dot{V}O_2$ of 35 mL/kg/min, what would be her total caloric expenditure for the entire exercise bout?

- Convert 154 lb to kg by dividing by the conversion factor of 2.2 (1 kg = 2.2 lb):
  ✓154 lb/2.2 = 70 kg
- Mary's relative $\dot{V}O_2$ = 35 mL/kg/min. To calculate her gross or absolute $\dot{V}O_2$, multiply her $\dot{V}O_2$ by her body weight:
  ✓35 mL/kg/min x 70 kg = 2,450 mL/min or 2.45 L/min
- If Mary consumes 5 kcal/liter O_2, her caloric expenditure each minute is calculated as follows:
  ✓2.45 L/min x 5 kcal/L = 12.25 kcal/min
- If Mary exercised for 25 minutes, her total caloric expenditure during the entire exercise bout is calculated as follows:
  ✓12.25 kcal/min x 25 minutes = 306 kcal

Most pieces of commercial cardiovascular exercise equipment provide estimates of caloric expenditure in this same manner. While they may not always be 100% accurate, they calculate caloric expenditure by estimating gross or absolute $\dot{V}O_2$ based on the amount of work being performed (i.e., speed, grade, watts).

If direct measurement of $\dot{V}O_2$ during activity is not available, the trainer can use published MET estimates for a variety of activities (see Table 11-6). Online caloric-expenditure calculators are available for a variety of physical activities on the ACE website (www.acefitness.org/calculators).

Talk Test

Following up on suggestions from a generation ago, several groups have explored the value of the talk test as a method of monitoring (and controlling) exercise training intensity (Cannon et al., 2004; Persinger et al., 2004; Voelker et al., 2002; Recalde et al., 2002; Porcari et al., 2001; Dehart et al., 2000). The usual experience with the talk test is that if two people are exercising and having a conversation, one of them will eventually turn to the other and say something like, "If we are going to keep talking, you are going to have to slow down." The talk test works on the premise that at about the intensity of VT1, the increase in ventilation is accomplished by an increase in breathing frequency. One of the requirements of comfortable speech is to be able to control breathing frequency. Thus, at the intensity of VT1, it is no longer possible to speak comfortably.

Studies in a variety of populations (e.g., healthy individuals, cardiac patients, athletes) have demonstrated that the talk test is a very good marker of VT1. Typically, below the VT1, people will respond to any of a number of speech-provoking stimuli (normal conversation, a structured interview, reciting a standard paragraph) by stating that they can speak comfortably.

Above VT1, but below a second metabolic marker called the **second ventilatory threshold (VT2),** they will be able to speak, but not comfortably. VT2 represents the point at which high-intensity exercise can no longer be sustained given the accumulation of lactic acid that begins to overwhelm the blood's buffering system. While researchers define this point as the **onset of blood lactate accumulation (OBLA),** it is commonly referred to as the anaerobic or lactate threshold by athletes and fitness professionals. Exercise immediately below this marker represents the highest sustainable intensity for an individual and is considered an excellent marker of performance. Above the intensity of the VT2, speech is not possible, other than single words.

A variety of speech-producing strategies—collectively called the talk test—have been shown to work fairly well as an index of the exercise intensity at VT1 (see Chapter 8 for more information on the submaximal talk test for VT1). Options include asking clients to recite something familiar, such as the Pledge of Allegiance, the Lord's Prayer, or "A is for apple, B is for boy, etc.," or having them read from text, then answer the question, "Can you speak comfortably?" If the answer is yes, the intensity is below the VT1. At the first response that is less than an unequivocal "yes," the intensity is probably right at that of the VT1, and if the answer is "no," the intensity is probably above or nearer to VT2. Trainers should exercise caution if asking a client to read from text while using a treadmill, given the potential risk of falling.

Another option is to compare the number that an individual can count to during the expiration phase of one breath during exercise against the number that can be counted to during the expiration phase at rest. Normally, when the number that can be counted to during exercise drops to about 70% of the number that is possible at rest, the intensity is approximately equal to the VT1. For example, if an individual can count to 14 during the expiration phase at rest, 70%—the indicator of VT1—represents the exercise intensity at which he or she can no longer count past 10.

The talk test has several advantages as a method of programming and monitoring exercise compared to a given %$\dot{V}O_2$max or %MHR, since it is based off an individual's unique metabolic or ventilatory responses.

Thus, for most people, training at intensities at which the answer to the question, "Can you speak comfortably?" becomes less than an unequivocal "yes" may represent the ideal training intensity marker. Therefore, the talk test is an appropriate marker to use for many individuals, especially for those seeking to lose weight or develop their aerobic efficiency. At VT1, fats continue to contribute significantly to the number of calories burned (caloric quality). Additionally, training at or near this intensity (unique to the individual's own metabolism) increases the likelihood of a better exercise experience. Higher-intensity training for those individuals with performance goals can be regulated in terms of the VT2.

Blood Lactate and VT2

Although the increase in HR during exercise is somewhat linear, at least up to fairly high intensities, and although exercise is classically programmed in terms of %MHR, the metabolic response to exercise is generally nonlinear (Foster & Cotter, 2006). Accordingly, it is more reasonable to program exercise in terms of the metabolic response to exercise, which is easily marked by either blood lactate or the ventilatory responses of VT1 and VT2.

Lactate is produced at a higher rate as exercise intensity increases. At approximately 50% of an individual's power output during incremental exercise, the ability to remove lactate from the circulation starts to become limited, and a net accumulation of lactate in the blood begins. With the use of relatively simple and inexpensive portable lactate analyzers and small capillary blood samples (similar to a person with diabetes monitoring blood sugar), it is possible to evaluate the break in the pattern of blood lactate accumulation with increasing exercise intensity. From a scientific standpoint, this can be thought of as the first threshold, correctly defined as the blood lactate threshold. As discussed previously, this point is referred to here as VT1 to avoid confusion. Because of the need to prevent the accumulation of lactate from causing disturbances in the blood pH (i.e., acid–base) balance of the body, the acid associated with lactate is buffered by the bicarbonate buffering system in the blood. This produces extra carbon dioxide (CO_2), which causes a subsequent increase in the amount of breathing (VT1) and the subsequent challenge to talking continuously. Thus, this increase in blood lactate and VT1 occur at about the same exercise intensity.

Understanding the Ventilatory Response to Exercise

During exercise, higher intensities increase respiratory rates, moving larger volumes of air into and out of the lungs. This volume of air, called minute ventilation ($\dot{V}_E$), reflects the body's metabolism and defines the volume of air moved through the lungs on a minute-by-minute basis. As exercise intensity progressively increases, the air moving into and out of the respiratory tract increases linearly, or similarly. As the intensity of exercise continues to increase, there is a point at which ventilation starts to increase in a non-linear fashion (i.e., VT1). This point where ventilation deviates from the progressive linear increase corresponds (but is not identical) with the development of muscle and blood acidosis. Blood buffers, which are compounds that help to neutralize acidosis, work to reduce the muscle fiber acidosis. This leads to an increase in carbon dioxide [due to the added CO_2 to $\dot{V}_E$ that originates from a change in the predominant fuel being utilized (fats to carbohydrates)], which the body attempts to eliminate with the increase in ventilation (Figure 11-4).

- Lactic acid manufactured within muscle cells dissociates into lactate$^-$ + hydrogen (H^+).
- The blood's bicarbonate buffer (predominantly $NaHCO_3$) dissociates into $Na^+ + HCO_3^-$.
- H^+ and HCO_3^- combine to form H_2CO_3 (carbonic acid), which is transported to the lungs and dissociated into H_2O and CO_2, both of which be removed from the body during expiration, increasing $\dot{V}_E$.
- Na^+ and lactate combine to form Na-lactate, some of which enters the mitochondria within the muscle cell for energy use, some of which is shuttled to the heart tissue for energy use, and some of which is shuttled to the liver for reconversion back to usable forms of energy.

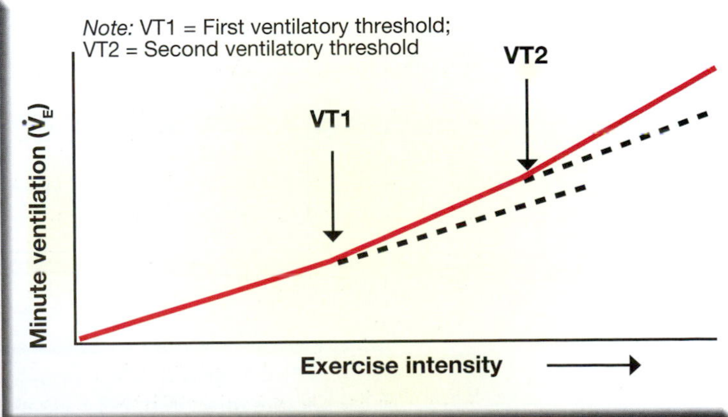

Figure 11-4
Ventilatory response to increasing exercise intensity

At higher intensities, when the buffering mechanism cannot keep up with the extra acid production, and the pH of the blood begins to fall (due to accumulating lactic acid), the respiratory center is strongly stimulated, and there is yet another increase in breathing (VT2) (see Figure 11-4). This is usually associated with a blood lactate concentration of about 4 mmol/L (this blood lactate concentration is equivalent to the OBLA) (Sjodin et al., 1982; Sjodin & Jacobs, 1981). This is the point that most fitness professionals identify as the anaerobic or lactate threshold, although scientifically speaking, it is correctly termed the OBLA. This point represents the intensity at which the body can no longer sustain an activity, given the accumulation of lactate, and begins to shut down. In most healthy people, this marker is associated with a flattening of the HR response to increasing intensity, referred to as the **HR turnpoint (HRTP)** (Figure 11-5).

Key Definitions

Lactate threshold (LT) technically refers to the point at which lactate production becomes greater than lactate removal, resulting in an initial rise in blood lactate values.

Onset of blood lactate accumulation (OBLA) technically refers to the point at which lactate levels begin to rise exponentially due to an accumulation within the blood and an inability to buffer the influx of acid. Blood lactate levels at this point rise above 4.0 mmol/L—a standard value to designate OBLA adopted by researchers. This intensity represents the "shutdown" point—what many fitness professionals call the LT. Intensities immediately below this marker represent the highest sustainable intensities of exercise, usually lasting 20 to 30 minutes in duration.

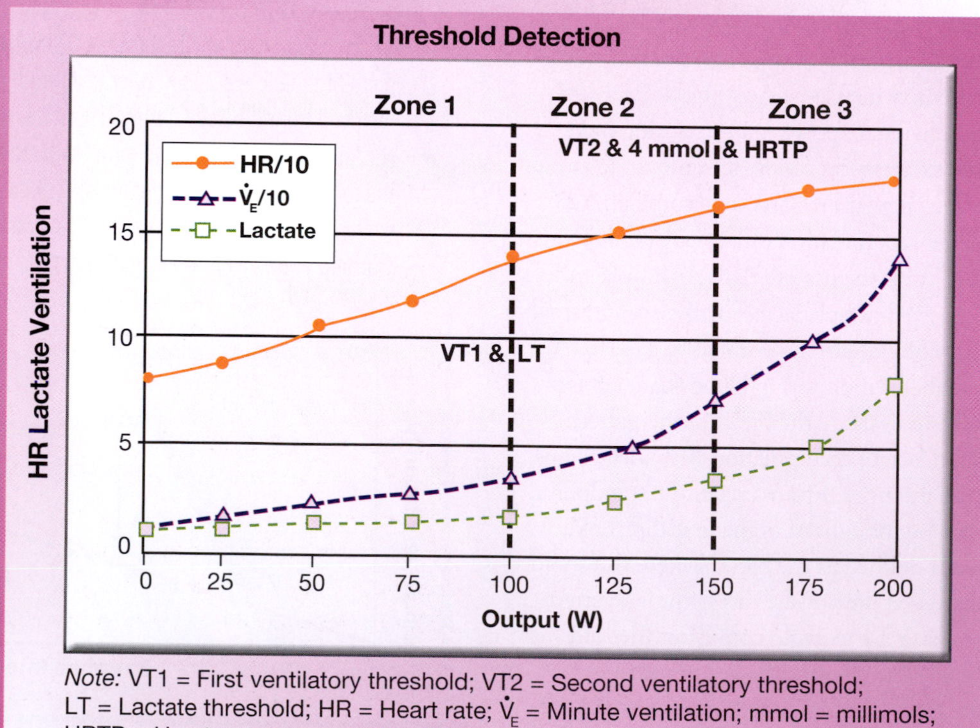

Note: VT1 = First ventilatory threshold; VT2 = Second ventilatory threshold; LT = Lactate threshold; HR = Heart rate; $\dot{V}_E$ = Minute ventilation; mmol = millimols; HRTP = Heart rate turnpoint; W = Watts

Figure 11-5
Schematic of the detection of the first and second thresholds based on increases in ventilation (VT1 and VT2), on lactate (LT and 4 mmol/L), and on the non-linearity of the HR increase. This provides for the possibility of three effective training zones based on two thresholds.

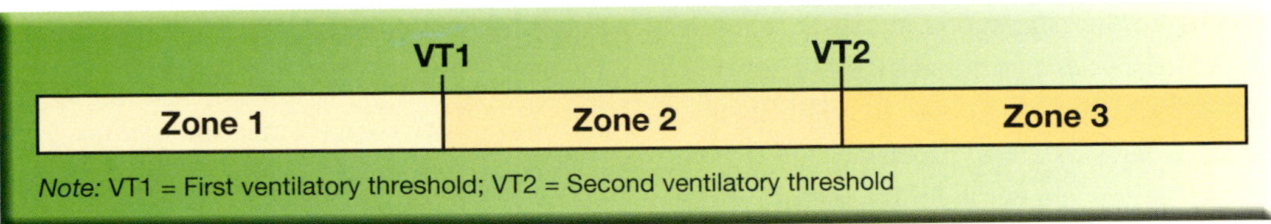

Figure 11-6
Three-zone training model

These two metabolic markers—VT1 and VT2—whether based on respiratory responses or blood lactate responses, provide a convenient way to divide intensity into training zones that are determined without any use of, or reference to, MHR (Figure 11-6):

- Zone 1 (relatively easy exercise) reflects heart rates below VT1.
- Zone 2 reflects heart rates from VT1 to just below VT2.
- Zone 3 reflects heart rates at or above VT2.

> Stated simply, if a client can talk comfortably, he or she is training in zone 1. If the client is not sure if he or she can talk comfortably, he or she is working in zone 2. If the client definitely cannot talk comfortably while training, he or she is working in zone 3.

Subsequent sections of this chapter introduce the four training phases of the ACE Integrated Fitness Training™ (ACE IFT™) Model, which follows this three-zone system. While this model presents a chronological progression beginning with aerobic-base training, moving through aerobic-efficiency training and anaerobic-endurance training, and culminating with anaerobic-power training (for those with goals that demand this phase), trainers should understand that each client will have a unique point of entry into this model based on his or her individual needs, goals, and current conditioning level. Deconditioned individuals and those seeking to lose weight by building their aerobic base and ability to efficiently burn more fats (caloric quality) will spend much of their initial training in zone 1, before being introduced to aerobic intervals that progress from the higher end of zone 1 to the lower end of zone 2. Although most data are observational, there is an appreciable body of literature suggesting that even among athletes, 70 to 80% of training occurs in zone 1, and about 10 to 20% of training is in zone 3 (Seiler & Kjerland, 2006; Esteve-Lanao et al., 2005). Many serious athletes seem to spend minimal time (less than 10%) training in zone 2 because of a belief that it is not hard enough to provoke significant anaerobic adaptations to training, but is hard enough to be particularly fatiguing.

Duration

Exercise duration generally defines the amount of time spent performing the physical activity, or it can be expressed in terms of exercise quantity (e.g., run two miles, take 5,000 steps, or burn 250 kcal). ACSM (2010) presents guidelines on recommended intensities that reduce the risks for **mortality** and **morbidity,** and improve overall fitness, but trainers should consider the following points:

- The quantity of exercise or physical activity may be performed in one continuous bout, or be performed intermittently and accumulated throughout the day in bouts lasting a minimum of 10 minutes each.
- While the guidelines provide recommended quantities to improve overall health and fitness, trainers should always place the needs and abilities of their clients first. Trainers should select suitable durations and progressions that fit each client's current conditioning level, tolerance, and availability, and aspire only to attain the recommendations when appropriate.

Benefits gained from exercise and physical activity are dose-related (i.e., greater benefits are derived from greater quantities of activity). For example, physical activity expending ≤1,000 kcal/week generally only produces improvements to health (e.g., lower **blood pressure** and **cholesterol**). This is considered a minimal recommendation for activity, whereas greater quantities expending ≥2,000 kcal/week promote effective weight loss and significant improvements to overall fitness.

Exercise guidelines call for the following (U.S. Department of Health & Human Services, 2008):

- Moderate-intensity exercise or activity performed for at least 30 minutes a session, a minimum of five days per week for a total of 150 minutes per week, *or*
- Vigorous-intensity exercise or activity performed for at least 20 to 25 minutes a session, a minimum of three days per week for a total of 75 minutes per week, *or*
- A combination of both (e.g., 20 to 30 minutes of moderate-to-vigorous exercise or activity performed three-to-five days per week).
- Overweight and obese individuals, or those seeking to manage their weight, should perform 50 to 60 minutes of moderate-intensity exercise or activity each day, five to seven days a week, for a total of 300 minutes, *or*
- A total of 150 minutes of vigorous exercise or activity per week, performed a minimum of three days a week, *or*
- A combination of both.

Trainers must bear in mind that beginner exercisers will generally not be able to complete 30 minutes of moderate-intensity cardiorespiratory exercise, nor will they be capable of achieving the recommended frequency (Table 11-7).

Exercise Progression

While exercise needs to create an enjoyable and positive experience for clients, the trainer will need to determine how to progress each client's program. Progression follows some basic training principles, including the following:

- The principle of **overload** states that when additional stresses are placed on the organs or systems (e.g., cardiorespiratory, muscular) in a timely and appropriate manner, physiological adaptations and improvement will occur. The rate of progression in a program depends on the individual's current conditioning level, program goals, and tolerance for the slight discomfort associated with raising training load or volume.
- The principle of **specificity** states that the physiological adaptations made within the body are specific to demands placed upon that body—sometimes referred to as the SAID principle: specific adaptations to the imposed demands. This implies that if a client's goals are consistent with running a half-marathon, the training program should progress to mimic the demands of that activity, to provide the specific stimuli that elicit appropriate adaptations within the body. The decision to progress to event- or sports-specific modalities should be made with

Table 11-7

Recommendations for Exercise Duration and Quantity

Physical Fitness Classification	Weekly Expenditure (kcal)	Duration/Day (minutes)	Weekly Duration (minutes)
Poor	500–1,000	20–30	60–150
Poor-fair	1,000–1,500	30–60	150–200
Fair-average	1,500–2,000	30–90	200–300
Average-good	>2,000	30–90	200–300
>Good-excellent	>2,000	30–90	200–300

Source: Adapted from American College of Sports Medicine (2010). *ACSM's Guidelines for Exercise Testing and Prescription* (8th ed.). Wolters Kluwer/Lippincott Williams & Wilkins.

consideration for the individual's skills and abilities, as well as his or her current conditioning level.

✓ Even among aerobic exercises, the transfer of benefits from one type of exercise to another is far from 100%. Research demonstrates that activities that use similar muscles (e.g., cycling performed by runners) have about 50% of the value of performing specific training (e.g., running) on a minute-by-minute basis. Muscularly non-similar training (e.g., swimming performed by runners) has about 25% of the value of performing specific training on a minute-by-minute basis (Foster et al., 1995; Loy, Holland, & Mutton, 1993).

Exercise duration is probably the most appropriate variable to manipulate initially, building the exercise session by 10%, or five to 10 minutes every week or two over the first four to six weeks. Thereafter, and once adherence is developed, trainers can implement progressions by increasing exercise frequency and then exercise intensity, but the progressions should always remain consistent with the client's goals (ACSM, 2010). It may be particularly important to include multiple modalities of exercise (e.g., **cross-training,** walking, cycling, elliptical training) and even variations within a modality (e.g., steady-state exercise, interval training, **Fartlek training**) to limit the risk of burnout or orthopedic injury from overuse as the volume of exercise builds.

Fartlek Training

Fartlek training was developed in Sweden in the 1930s and its name is derived from a Swedish term that means "speed play." This training format provides a sequence of different intensities that stress both the aerobic and anaerobic systems, something rarely achieved with exclusive steady-state training (aerobic), and different from traditional interval training (anaerobic with specific work-to-rest ratios). Consequently, this training format can be adapted to meet the needs of intermittent-sport athletes by essentially mimicking the changes of pace that occur during these events (e.g., rugby, soccer, football, hockey, lacrosse).

For example, Fartlek running involves varying the pace throughout the run, alternating between fast segments and slow jogs. Unlike traditional interval training that involves specific timed or measured segments, Fartleks are more unstructured. Work-rest intervals can be based on how the body feels. With Fartlek training, the exerciser can experiment with pace and endurance. Many runners, especially beginners, enjoy Fartlek training because it involves speed work, but is more flexible and not as demanding as traditional interval training.

Modes or Types of Cardiorespiratory Exercise

Virtually any type of activity that involves a large amount of muscle and can be performed in a rhythmic fashion and sustained for more than a few minutes can be classified as cardiorespiratory exercise. If this type of exercise is performed regularly, there are adaptations in the various organ systems (heart, lungs, blood, muscles) that improve the ability of the person to move around or otherwise perform sustained exercise (i.e., the cardiorespiratory training effect). Because of the unique muscular requirements of ambulatory exercises (e.g., walking, running, cycling, rowing, skating), these exercises are usually considered to be the primary cardiorespiratory exercises. Other related exercises (e.g., stair climbing, elliptical exercise, arm cranking) can also be classified as aerobic, or cardiorespiratory, exercise. Even game-type activities, assuming that they require sustained bodily movement, can be considered cardiorespiratory exercise. In this regard, the cardiorespiratory benefit of game-type exercise is proportional to the amount and intensity of ambulatory activity involved. Thus, golf can be beneficial if it involves walking for approximately 3 miles (4.8 km) (the average length of a standard 18-hole course), but is less beneficial than a steady walk of the same duration (because of the lower intensity of the intermittent walking during golf). Similarly, singles tennis is probably more valuable from the standpoint of cardiorespiratory exercise than doubles, because of the more extensive running required to cover the entire court. Table 11-8 provides a list of physical activities that promote improvement or maintenance of cardiorespiratory fitness.

Equipment-based Cardiovascular Exercise

Exercise equipment designed for cardiorespiratory training is a prominent feature in most fitness facilities, as well as in the home exercise market. This can include treadmills, cycle ergometers, elliptical machines, rowing machines, arm ergometers, and a variety of other devices. The aerobic value of any of these equipment-based approaches is largely based on how the machine is used. Sustained moderate-intensity exercise (i.e., more than 10 or 15 minutes in duration) is the key to cardiorespiratory exercise training. Many pieces of higher-end exercise equipment have programs designed to estimate the MET or caloric cost of exercise. If they also have an input feature that allows the exerciser to enter body weight, the caloric cost of exercise may be estimated. However, the accuracy of estimates for the MET cost of exercising on a particular device is only as good as the research supporting the equation. In many cases, these data are quite good. In other cases, the numbers are much less reliable. Common sense is required when using the MET or caloric values generated by exercise equipment. In many cases, the data are based on university students who are already fairly fit and are exercising without the benefit of handrail support. Thus, in less-fit individuals, and particularly if handrail support is required, the values suggested by the exercise device may overestimate the actual value attained. It is important to understand that the calorie counts on exercise machines (or those obtained from formulas) are simply estimates and will never be 100% accurate. Therefore, it is best to use them as rough benchmarks from workout to workout.

Group Exercise

Group exercise classes have been one of the hallmarks of the exercise industry since the beginning of organized gymnastics programs in Europe a century and a half ago. Group gymnastic routines and calisthenics were once the dominant modes of group exercise. The latter represented a significant portion of the physical fitness exercises of the military in the time period beginning before World War I, and its use

Table 11-8

Physical Activities That Promote Improvement or Maintenance of Cardiorespiratory Fitness

Exercise Description	Recommended Group	Activity Examples
Endurance activities requiring minimal skill or fitness	All adults	Walking, slow-dancing, recreational cycling or swimming
Vigorous-intensity endurance activities requiring minimal skill	Adults participating in regular exercise or having better than average fitness	Jogging, rowing, elliptical training, stepping, indoor cycling, fast-dancing
Endurance activities requiring higher skill levels	Adults with acquired skill and higher fitness levels	Swimming, cross-country skiing
Recreational sports	Adults participating in regular training with acquired fitness and skill levels	Soccer, basketball, racquet sports

continues even now. In the early 1970s, with the emergence of choreographed "aerobic dance" programs, the group exercise focus shifted significantly toward using dance-type movements, very often with music, as the dominant mode of group exercise. During the past few decades, an enormous variety of exercise types, with almost every focus imaginable, has emerged. Common to all these activities is the use of music to drive the tempo of exercise and to make the exercise more enjoyable. The choreography of group exercise can vary enormously, as can the exercise intensity. Studies have shown that some group exercise programs (e.g., group indoor cycling) can be very strenuous, often requiring workloads that elicit $\dot{V}O_2$ or HR values greater than those achieved during exercise tests. At the other end of the continuum, group exercise designed for older individuals or individuals with heart disease can be very low intensity (e.g., chair aerobics). When working with small groups, the personal trainer should always keep in mind the effect of music on the exercise intensity. A variety of studies have shown that exercisers will tend to follow the tempo or percussive beat of music. If fast-tempo music is used, the exercise intensity may be higher than intended.

Circuit Training

Because of the specificity principle of exercise, resistance-training programs designed to improve muscular strength and endurance are not intrinsically suited to producing cardiorespiratory training effects. As an adaptation of military training exercises, the concept of circuit weight training emerged in the 1950s and 1960s, based on the premise that sequential exercises using different muscle groups might allow the exerciser to focus on one muscle group while a previously used group is recovering (e.g., squats followed by chest presses, leg extensions, shoulder presses, leg curls, and arm curls). The logic behind this practice was that the overall metabolic rate might remain high enough to allow cardiorespiratory training effects, while still focusing the exercises on muscular components. Early controlled studies of this concept produced disappointing results, with improvements in aerobic capacity averaging only 5 to 7%. In attempts to find a way to improve circuit training, there were a variety of industry-sponsored research studies in the early- and mid-1970s. These studies demonstrated that alternating muscular strength and endurance activities with classical aerobic training (e.g., running, cycling, stepping, rowing) in rapid sequence allowed for significant cardiorespiratory training effects to be observed (i.e., super circuits). Depending on equipment availability, circuit training can be performed either by a single individual or by groups of people rotating in an organized manner through several exercise stations.

Outdoor Exercise

Over the past few decades, a wide variety of outdoor exercises have emerged out of recreational activities, many with the promise of providing cardiorespiratory fitness. Activities that require a lot of walking or running are, of course, very likely to provide cardiorespiratory training. Other outdoor activities (e.g., climbing, canoeing) are much more variable in their cardiorespiratory training effects and depend almost entirely on how they are conducted.

Seasonal Exercise

Many activities, particularly outdoor activities, are very seasonal in their application. To the degree that they require the exerciser to perform physical activity, they are likely to have a large cardiorespiratory training effect. Thus, cross-country skiing and snowshoeing in the winter months are similar to walking and running in the warmer months. Although there are clearly highly specific benefits of each type of exercise, the enjoyment and enthusiasm related to performing different types of activities during different seasons, and the underlying commonality of cardiorespiratory fitness, suggests the value of seasonal variation.

Water-based Exercise

Aquatic exercise can provide a convenient alternative form of exercise that is pleasant, reduces orthopedic loading, and is capable of training different muscle groups than those used during ambulatory activities. While the classical water-based exercise is swimming, group classes (e.g., water aerobics) and games (e.g., water polo, water volleyball) can be effective methods of exercise as well. Water-based exercise is particularly valuable for older or obese individuals or those who may have orthopedic issues, as the buoyancy provided by the water unloads the traditional targets of ambulatory exercise. It is important to remember that the energy cost of ambulatory activity in the water (e.g., walking in thigh-deep or chest-deep water) is very strongly related to the depth of the water and can increase markedly with only very slight increases in the speed of ambulating in the water. Secondly, immersion in water causes the blood to be redistributed to the central circulation, away from the limbs. In people with compromised circulatory function, this can lead to complications (e.g., breathlessness, heart failure). The energy cost of swimming is highly variable and depends not only on swimming velocity, but on the stroke, technique, and skill of the swimmer.

Mind-body Exercise

Mind-body exercises are often performed for reasons other than cardiorespiratory training, but cardiorespiratory training effects may still be achieved. The main concepts behind mind-body exercise is that it is performed with focus, with attempts to control and regulate the breathing, with a conscious intent to follow a specific form, and as a means of linking the physical and emotional aspects of the person (see Chapter 13). As such, mind-body exercise is generally not associated with high-intensity aerobic activity. Nevertheless, as a regular feature of an exercise program, it may provide an intensity comparable to that of walking. **Pilates, hatha yoga, Nia,** and **tai chi** are representative types of mind-body exercise.

Lifestyle Exercise

Normally, when people think of exercise, they think of an activity that is a "time out" from real life, something that they specifically have to plan to do, which their hunter-gatherer ancestors, or even their grandparents who were farmers, did not have to worry about doing. However, it is important to remember that humans once got ample amounts of exercise by simply performing daily chores around the house. The best examples of this are the reports of health variables among the Amish who, because of their religious beliefs, live a life that is much like that of a 19th-century farmer in the U.S. These reports suggest that domestic activities can be more than enough to make people quite fit and contribute to excellent health (Bassett, Schneider, & Huntington, 2004). Accordingly, activities like working in the yard should be viewed in the context of the total exercise load, and be considered comparable to walking for exercise.

ACE Integrated Fitness Training Model—Cardiorespiratory Training Phases

The basic concept of program design is to create an exercise program with appropriate frequency, intensity, and duration to fit the client's current health and fitness, with adequate progressions to help the client safely achieve his or her goals. Exercise intensity can be monitored using a variety of methods that have generally been developed through university-based research that included actual measurement of MHR, $\dot{V}O_2$max, blood lactate concentrations and HR at VT1 and VT2, power output (wattage), and other variables. These assessments provide accurate individualized data for use in exercise programming, but they are often not practical or available to most fitness professionals or consumers. As such, personal trainers generally have to rely on submaximal fitness assessments and prediction equations derived from these studies to predict variables such as MHR and $\dot{V}O_2$max, and then use these predicted values to set appropriate training intensities. Exercise guidelines based upon predictions of MHR or $\dot{V}O_2$max can help clients reach their goals (see Table 11-2), but they have a lot of room for error that must be accounted for when setting and modifying exercise intensities.

The submaximal talk test for VT1 and the VT2 threshold test provide personal trainers with submaximal cardiorespiratory fitness tests that give fairly precise HR data that relates directly to the metabolic markers of the first and second ventilatory thresholds. The submaximal talk test for VT1 can provide the personal trainer with the client's HR at VT1 to use when designing programs for weight loss and improving general fitness. The higher-intensity VT2 threshold test allows the personal trainer to establish the client's HR at VT2 for use in more advanced programming with clients who have advanced-fitness and endurance sports–performance goals.

The ACE IFT Model has four cardiorespiratory training phases:

- Phase 1: Aerobic-base training
- Phase 2: Aerobic-efficiency training
- Phase 3: Anaerobic-endurance training
- Phase 4: Anaerobic-power training

Clients are categorized into a given phase based on their current health, fitness levels, and goals. By utilizing the assessment and programming tools in each phase, personal trainers can develop individualized cardiorespiratory programs for clients ranging from sedentary to endurance athletes. Programming in each phase will be based on the three-zone training model shown in Figure 11-6, using HR at VT1 and VT2 to develop individualized programs based on each client's metabolic responses to exercise. It is important to note that training principles in the ACE IFT Model's cardiorespiratory training phases can be implemented by trainers using various exercise intensity markers, including ones based on predicted values such as %HRR or %MHR, but the exercise intensities will not be as accurate for individual clients as when they utilize measured HR at VT1 and VT2 (Table 11-9).

Table 11-10 provides an overview of the cardiorespiratory training phases of the ACE IFT Model. Detailed descriptions are provided that explain the training focus of each stage and strategies for implementing and progressing exercise programs to help clients reach their goals within the phase, and advance to the next phase if desired. It is important to note that not every client will start in phase 1, as many clients will already be regularly participating in cardiorespiratory exercise, and only clients with very specific performance or speed goals will reach phase 4. In addition, the submaximal talk test for VT1 is recommended for introduction in phase 2, while the VT2 threshold test should ideally be introduced during phase 3. Also, clients may be in different phases for cardiorespiratory training and functional movement and resistance training based on their current health, fitness, exercise-participation levels, and goals.

Phase 1: Aerobic-base training

Training Focus

Phase 1 has a principal focus of getting clients who are either sedentary or have little cardiorespiratory fitness to begin engaging in regular cardiorespiratory exercise of low- to moderate-intensity with a primary goal of improving health and a secondary goal of building fitness. These clients may have long-term goals for fitness and possibly even sports performance, but they need to progress through phase 1 first. The primary goal for the trainer during this phase should be to help the client have positive experiences with cardiorespiratory exercise and to help him or her adopt exercise as a regular habit. The intent of this phase is to develop a stable aerobic base upon which the client can build improvements in health, endurance, energy, mood, and caloric expenditure.

Table 11-9
Three-zone Training Model Using Various Intensity Markers

Intensity Markers	Zone 1	Zone 2	Zone 3	Advantages/Limitations
Metabolic markers: VT1 and VT2* (HR relative to VT1 and VT2)*	Below VT1 (HR <VT1)	VT1 to just below VT2 (HR ≥VT1 to <VT2)	VT2 and above (HR ≥VT2)	• Based on measured VT1 and VT2 • Ideally, VT1 and VT2 are measured in a lab with a metabolic cart and blood lactate • Field tests are relatively easy to administer, require minimal equipment, and provide accurate corresponding HRs at VT1 and VT2 • Programming with metabolic markers allows for individualized programming
Talk test*	Can talk comfortably	Not sure if talking is comfortable	Definitely cannot talk comfortably	• Based on actual changes in ventilation due to physiological adaptations to increasing exercise intensities • Very easy for practical measurement • No equipment required • Can easily be taught to clients • Allows for individualized programming
RPE (terminology)*	"Moderate" to "somewhat hard"	"Hard"	"Very hard" to "extremely hard"	• Good subjective intensity marker • Correlates well with talk test, metabolic markers, and measured $\%\dot{V}O_2max$ • Easy to teach to clients
RPE (0 to 10 scale)*	3 to 4	5 to 6	7 to 10	• Good subjective intensity marker • Correlates well with talk test, metabolic markers, and measured $\%VO_2max$ • 0 to 10 scale is easy to teach to clients
RPE (6 to 20 scale)	12 to 13	14 to 16	17 to 20	• Good subjective intensity marker • Correlates well with talk test, metabolic markers, and measured $\%\dot{V}O_2max$ • 6 to 20 scale is not as easy to teach to clients as the 0 to 10 scale • *Note:* An RPE of 20 represents maximal effort and cannot be sustained as a training intensity.
$\%\dot{V}O_2R$	40 to 59%	60 to 84%	≥85%	• Requires *measured* $\dot{V}O_2max$ for most accurate programming • Impractical due to expensive equipment and testing • Increased error with use of *predicted* $\dot{V}O_2max$ or *predicted* MHR • Relative percentages for programming are population-based and not individually specific
%HRR	40 to 59%	60 to 84%	≥85%	• Requires *measured* MHR and RHR for most accurate programming • Measured MHR is impractical for the vast majority of trainers and clients • Use of RHR increases individuality of programming vs. strict %MHR • Use of *predicted* MHR introduces potentially large error; the magnitude of the error is dependent on the specific equation used (see page 376) • Relative percentages for programming are population-based and not individually specific

Continued on next page

Table 11-9 *continued*

Three-zone Training Model Using Various Intensity Markers

Intensity Markers	Zone 1	Zone 2	Zone 3	Advantages/Limitations
%MHR	64 to 76%	77 to 93%	≥94%	• Requires *measured* MHR for accuracy in programming • Measured MHR is impractical for the vast majority of trainers and clients • Use of *predicted* MHR introduces potentially large error; the magnitude of the error is dependent on the specific equation used (see page 376) • Does not include RHR, as is used in %HRR • Relative percentages for programming are population-based and not individually specific
METs	3 to 6	6 to 9	>9	• Requires *measured* $\dot{V}O_2$max for most accurate programming • Can use in programming more easily than other intensity markers based off $\dot{V}O_2$max • Limited in programming by knowledge of METs for given activities and/or equipment that gives MET estimates • Relative MET ranges for programming are population-based and not individually specific (e.g., a 5-MET activity might initially be perceived as vigorous by a previously sedentary client)
Category terminology for exercise programming	Low to moderate	Moderate to vigorous	Vigorous to very vigorous	

Note: VT1 = First ventilatory threshold; VT2 = Second ventilatory threshold; HR = Heart rate; RPE = Ratings of perceived exertion; $\dot{V}O_2R$ = VO_2 reserve; HRR = Heart-rate reserve; MHR = Maximum heart rate; RHR = Resting heart rate; METs = Metabolic equivalents

*These are the preferred intensity markers to use with the three-zone model when designing, implementing, and progressing cardiorespiratory training programs using the ACE Integrated Fitness Training Model.

The training focus of phase 1 is establishing a regular exercise pattern, with relatively low- to moderate-intensity exercise of only moderate duration, in order to establish an aerobic base. Zone 1 training, where the training HR is below the VT1 level, may not be strenuous enough to provoke significant changes in $\dot{V}O_2$max (the classical definition of the cardiorespiratory training effect), but will contribute in a general way to improved health. Once regularity of exercise habits is established, the duration of exercise is extended until the exerciser progresses to phase 2 and is able to exercise for 30 to 60 minutes on most days with little residual fatigue. This approach to training ensures the safety of exercise, while at the same time allowing some of the potential physiologic adaptations and most of the health benefits to occur. In individuals desiring or requiring higher levels of fitness, higher-intensity training may then be incorporated as they progress to phase 2. Within this general design is recognition that the benefit-to-risk ratio of low-intensity zone 1 training is very high for the beginning exerciser, with the possibility for very large gains in health and basic fitness and almost no risk of either cardiovascular or musculoskeletal injury. As the exerciser develops more ambitious goals, more demanding training (either longer or more intense) can be performed.

The underlying base of most training programs is the development of aerobic power. Indeed, a consensus statement from the World Health Organization in 1968 defined endurance as equivalent to $\dot{V}O_2$max. Based on the large body of controlled training studies performed in the 1970s, the term "training effect" can be thought of as equivalent to the increase in $\dot{V}O_2$max that occurs during the first three to six months of an aerobic-endurance exercise program.

Table 11-10

Cardiorespiratory Training Phase Overview

Phase 1—Aerobic-base Training

- The focus is on creating positive exercise experiences that help sedentary clients become regular exercisers.
- No fitness assessments are required prior to exercise in this phase.
- Focus on steady-state exercise in zone 1 (below HR at VT1).
- Gauge by the client's ability to talk (below talk test threshold) and/or RPE of 3 to 4 (moderate to somewhat hard).
- Progress to phase 2 once the client can sustain steady-state cardiorespiratory exercise for 20 to 30 minutes in zone 1 (RPE of 3 to 4) and is comfortable with assessments.

Phase 2—Aerobic-efficiency Training

- The focus is on increasing the duration of exercise and introducing intervals to improve aerobic efficiency, fitness, and health.
- Administer the submaximal talk test to determine HR at VT1. There is no need to measure VT2 in phase 2.
- Increase workload at VT1 (increase HR at VT1), then introduce low zone 2 intervals just above VT1 (RPE of 5) to improve aerobic efficiency and add variety in programming.
- Progress low zone 2 intervals by increasing the time of the work interval and later decreasing the recovery interval time.
- As client progresses, introduce intervals in the upper end of zone 2 (RPE of 6).
- Many clients will stay in this phase for many years.
- If a client has event-specific goals or is a fitness enthusiast looking for increased challenges and fitness gains, progress to phase 3.

Phase 3—Anaerobic-endurance Training

- The focus is on designing programs to help clients who have endurance performance goals and/or are performing seven or more hours of cardiorespiratory exercise per week.
- Administer the VT2 threshold test to determine HR at VT2.
- Programs will have the majority of cardiorespiratory training time in zone 1.
- Interval and higher-intensity sessions will be very focused in zones 2 and 3, but will make up only a small amount of the total training time to allow for adaptation to the total training load.
- Many clients will never train in phase 3, as all of their non-competitive fitness goals can be achieved through phase 2 training.
- Only clients who have very specific goals for increasing speed for short bursts at near-maximal efforts during endurance or athletic competitions will move on to phase 4.

Phase 4—Anaerobic-power Training

- The focus is on improving anaerobic power to improve phosphagen energy pathways and buffer large accumulations of blood lactate in order to improve speed for short bursts at near-maximal efforts during endurance or athletic competitions.
- Programs will have a similar distribution to phase 3 training times in zones 1, 2, and 3.
- Zone 3 training will include very intense anaerobic-power intervals.
- Clients will generally only work in phase 4 during specific training cycles prior to competition.

Note: HR = Heart rate; VT1 = First ventilatory threshold; RPE = Ratings of perceived exertion; VT2 = Second ventilatory threshold

As long ago as the 1950s, the concept of a minimal-intensity threshold for provoking the training effect was articulated by Karvonen, who made the observation that training at intensities of less than 50% of HRR (approximately 60% of MHR) failed to cause reductions in RHR (Karvonen, 1957). This concept was confirmed in randomized training studies during the 1970s with $\dot{V}O_2$max as the outcome measure. A variety of studies have shown that there is a larger increase in $\dot{V}O_2$max with more intense training. Thus, the aerobic benefits of training increase markedly with training intensity. However, training is much less comfortable as intensity increases, which means there is an increased risk of clients dropping out during the first few weeks of training. Furthermore, in previously sedentary adults who might have an underlying risk of cardiovascular disease, more high-intensity exercise is associated with a greater risk of cardiovascular complications. Thus, an important rule of exercise training for sedentary adults is to start slowly during the beginning weeks of an exercise program. This guideline is sometimes frustrating, as many clients are enthusiastic at the beginning of a program and want rapid gains, and the personal trainer may want to impress clients with challenging, creative workouts. Clearly, restraint, proper education, and careful planning are essential during the early stages of any training program.

Improvements in $\dot{V}O_2$max may continue for six to 12 months after the beginning of a regular exercise program. This increase may be accentuated if there is significant weight loss, since the most appropriate expression of $\dot{V}O_2$max is when it is normalized for body weight (e.g., mL/kg/min). Lower-intensity exercise programs have been shown to be associated with a variety of beneficial health outcomes, although there may be smaller increases in $\dot{V}O_2$max at low exercise intensities than can be achieved with higher-intensity training. Nevertheless, outcomes related to longevity and a reduced incidence of many of the "diseases of civilization" have been well documented with exercise that is not sufficient to cause large increases in $\dot{V}O_2$max (Booth et al., 2002). In any case, with any beginning exerciser, this approach will ensure that not only are there significant gains in health and functional status, but there will be a minimum of injuries (i.e., a very high benefit/risk ratio).

Program Design for Phase 1: Aerobic-base Training

The primary goal of this phase is to help clients have positive experiences with exercise to facilitate program adherence and success. Cardiorespiratory fitness assessments are not necessary at the beginning of this phase, as they will only confirm low levels of fitness and potentially serve as negative reminders about why the sedentary client with low levels of fitness may not have good **self-efficacy** regarding exercise. All cardiorespiratory exercise during this phase falls within zone 1 (sub-VT1), so the trainer can use the client's ability to talk comfortably as the upper exercise-intensity limit. The trainer can also teach the client to use the 0 to 10 category ratio scale, with the client exercising at an RPE of 3 to 4 (moderate to somewhat hard). It is not necessary to conduct the submaximal talk test assessment to determine HR at VT1 until phase 2.

As a general principle, exercise programs designed to improve the aerobic base begin with zone 1–intensity exercise with HR below VT1 performed for as little as 10 to 15 minutes two to three times each week. However, this should be progressed as rapidly as tolerated to 30 minutes at moderate intensity (zone 1; below "talk test" with HR below VT1), performed at least five times each week. Changes in duration from one week to the next should not exceed a 10% increase versus the week prior. Once this level of exercise can be sustained on a regular basis, the primary adaptation of the aerobic base will be complete.

For the most part, early training efforts should feature continuous exercise at zone 1 intensity. Depending on how sedentary a person was prior to beginning the program, this level of easy exercise may be continued for as little as two weeks or for more than six weeks. The beginning duration of exercise should match what the client is able to perform. For some, this might be 15 continuous minutes, while for others it might be only 5 to 10 continuous minutes. From that point, duration should be increased at a rate of no more than 10% from one week to the next until the client can perform 30 minutes of continuous exercise. Once the client is comfortable with assessments and can sustain steady-state cardiorespiratory exercise for 20 minutes in zone 1 (RPE of 3 to 4), he or she can move on to phase 2.

A sample cardiorespiratory-training progression for a client exercising four days per week in zone 1 is illustrated in Table 11-11. This sample shows appropriate progressions for weekly duration with different options for session duration during most weeks to add variety and accommodate other program goals.

Phase 2: Aerobic-efficiency Training

Training Focus

Phase 2 has a principal training focus of increasing the time of cardiorespiratory exercise while introducing intervals to improve aerobic efficiency, fitness, and health. Clients who exercise sporadically will progress to this phase only after they have become consistent with their cardiorespiratory exercise and can comfortably perform a minimum of 20 to 30 minutes of steady-state cardiorespiratory exercise in zone 1 (RPE of 3 to 4). During phase 2, the trainer will be able to program more variety in terms of exercise frequency and duration. The trainer will also be able to challenge the client through the introduction of intervals, first in the lower end of zone 2 and eventually in the upper end of zone 2. For the highly motivated client who is interested in progressing toward performance goals, intervals that reach just above VT2 (into zone 3) can be introduced as an advanced challenge, often just before the client moves into phase 3 of cardiorespiratory training.

Once the aerobic base is developed, the exerciser may want to consider the value of additional gains in fitness that will result from increases in exercise intensity, frequency, or duration. However, it is important to understand that after an aerobic base has been achieved, additional gains in fitness

Table 11-11

Sample Phase 1 Cardiorespiratory-training Progression

Training Parameter	Week 1	Week 2	Week 3	Week 4	Week 5
Frequency	4 times/week	4 times/week	4 times/week	4 times/week	4 times/week
Duration— Total for Week: (10% weekly increase)	60 min/week	66 min/week	72 min/week	80 min/week	88 min/week
Duration of Sessions (continuous)	4 x 15 min	4 x 16.5 min or 2 x 15 min 2 x 18.5 min	4 x 18 min or 2 x 17 min 2 x 19 min	4 x 20 min or 2 x 18 min 2 x 22 min	4 x 22 min or 2 x 20 min 2 x 24 min
Intensity	<VT1 HR RPE = 3	<VT1 HR RPE = 3	<VT1 HR RPE = 3	<VT1 HR RPE = 3 to 4	<VT1 HR RPE = 3 to 4
Zone	1	1	1	1	1
Training Format	Steady state	Steady state	Steady state	Steady state	Steady state
Work-to-Recovery Intervals (active recovery)	None	None	None	None	None

Note: VT1 = First ventilatory threshold; RPE = Ratings of perceived exertion

will become progressively smaller, or require disproportionately large increases in training intensity, frequency, or duration. This is the time when the personal trainer needs to carefully evaluate the goals of each client. What are the client's exercise goals—health and basic fitness benefits, improved appearance, and/or weight-loss benefits? Or does he or she want to complete competitive challenges? Competitive competence at the biological limit of the exerciser requires significantly higher training loads, which are addressed in phases 3 and 4. Athletes may have to train at very high loads for only a 1 to 2% increase in performance, with matching increases in the time requirement of training and the risk of injury (Foster et al., 1996).

Within the context of aerobic training, the trainer must consider the relative proportion of different intensities of exercise. Early studies suggested that training at about the intensity of the "threshold" (i.e., zone 2) was the most effective intensity. Subsequent studies have suggested that very well-trained non-athletes tend to perform a high proportion of their training (approximately 50%) at this intensity (Seiler & Kjerland, 2006; Esteve-Lanao et al., 2005). Interestingly, much of this training can be categorized by the verbal anchor "hard," or an RPE of 6 on the 0 to 10 scale. Extensive training at this level requires a motivated exerciser, so this phase of training is reserved for the already motivated and committed client. However, once the volume of cardiorespiratory training goes over approximately seven hours per week, a different pattern of training distribution seems to appear. This training distribution for clients and athletes training seven or more hours per week is discussed in phase 3.

Phase 2 is the primary cardiorespiratory training phase for regular exercisers in a fitness facility who have goals for improving or maintaining fitness and/or weight loss. Cardiorespiratory training in this phase includes increasing the workload by modifying frequency, duration, and intensity, with intervals introduced that go into zone 2 and eventually approach HR at VT2. The zone 2 intervals in this phase provide a stimulus that will eventually increase the HR at VT1, resulting in the client being able to exercise at a lower HR when at the same level of intensity, and also allowing the client to exercise at higher intensities while at the VT1 HR.

Clients training in phase 2 who have a one-time goal to complete an event, such as a 10K run, can reach their goal of completing the event within the training guidelines of this phase. Once a client begins working toward multiple endurance goals, trains to improve his or her competitive speed, begins training seven or more hours per week, or simply wants to take on the challenge of training like an athlete, the client should move on to phase 3 of cardiorespiratory training.

For the many clients who never develop competitive goals or the desire to train like an endurance athlete, training in phase 2 will provide very adequate challenges to help them improve and maintain cardiorespiratory fitness for many years. The workouts in most non-athletically focused group exercise classes fall into this phase. Phase 2 covers the principles for building aerobic efficiency that are implemented with most personal-training clients and fitness enthusiasts.

Program Design for Phase 2: Aerobic-efficiency Training

At the beginning of phase 2, the trainer should have the client perform the submaximal talk test to determine HR at VT1. This HR will be utilized for programming throughout the phase, and will need to be reassessed periodically as fitness improves to see if the HR at VT1 has increased and training intensities need to be adjusted.

This phase of cardiorespiratory training is dedicated to enhancing the client's aerobic efficiency by progressing the program through increased duration of sessions, increased frequency of sessions when possible, and the introduction of zone 2 intervals. In phase 2, the warm-up, cool-down, recovery intervals, and steady-state cardiorespiratory exercise segments are performed at or just below VT1 HR (RPE of 3 to 4 on the 0 to 10 scale) to continue advancing the client's aerobic base. Aerobic intervals are introduced at a level that is just above VT1 HR, or an RPE of 5 (0 to 10 scale). The goal of these intervals is to improve aerobic efficiency by raising the intensity of exercise performed at VT1, improve the client's ability to utilize fat as a fuel source at intensities just below VT1, improve exercise efficiency at VT1, and add variety to the exercise program.

As a general principle, intervals should start out relatively brief (initially about 60 seconds), with an approximate hard-to-easy ratio of 1:3 (e.g., a 60-second work interval followed by a 180-second recovery interval), eventually progressing to a ratio of 1:2 and then 1:1. The duration of these intervals can be increased in regular increments, depending on the goals of the exerciser, but should be increased cautiously over several weeks depending on the client's fitness level. As a general principle, the exercise load (calculated from the session RPE or the integrated time in the zone) should be increased by no more than 10% per week. Early in phase 2, exercise bouts with a session RPE greater than 5 (e.g., hard exercise) should be performed infrequently. As the client's fitness increases, steady-state exercise bouts with efforts just above VT1 (RPE of 5) can be introduced.

Low zone 2 intervals should first be progressed by increasing the time of each interval and then moving to a 1:1 work-to-recovery (hard-to-easy) interval ratio. As the client progresses, intervals can progress into the upper end of zone 2 (RPE of 6) at a 1:3 work-to-recovery ratio, progressing first to longer intervals and then eventually moving to intervals with a 1:1 work-to-recovery ratio. Well-trained and motivated non-athletes can progress to where they are performing as much as 50% of their cardiorespiratory training in zone 2. Once the well-trained non-athlete reaches seven or more hours of training per week or develops performance goals, he or she should progress to phase 3. Clients with advanced fitness who are training for a one-time event or are preparing to advance to phase 3, can perform brief intervals (30 seconds) that go just above VT2 (RPE of 7) to further develop aerobic capacity and provide additional variety.

It is not necessary to measure VT2 during this phase, as an RPE of 5 to 6 (0 to 10 scale) can be used to represent intensities in zone 2, and an RPE of 7 (very hard) can be used to identify efforts just above VT2. Programming variables and variety during phase 2 are diverse enough for clients who do not have competitive goals to train in this phase for many years. A sample cardiorespiratory-training progression for a client in phase 2 is presented in Table 11-12. This sample shows appropriate progressions during a five-week microcycle during phase 2.

Phase 3: Anaerobic-endurance Training

Training Focus

Phase 3 is designed for clients who have endurance-performance goals and/or are performing seven or more hours of cardiorespiratory training per week. The training principles in phase 3 are for clients who have one or more endurance-performance goals that require specialized training to ensure that adequate training volume and appropriate training intensity and recovery are included to create performance changes that help the client reach his or her goals. Clients do not need to be highly competitive athletes to train in zone 3. They need only to be motivated clients with endurance-performance goals and the requisite fitness from phase 2 to build upon.

A variety of studies with different types of athletes, including Nordic skiers, cyclists, and runners, have suggested that 70 to 80% of training is performed at intensities lower than the VT1 (zone 1) (Seiler & Kjerland, 2006; Esteve-Lanao et al., 2005). These same studies suggest that athletes typically perform 5 to 10% of their training above the VT2 (zone 3). Thus, even though zone 3 training can be very effective in terms of provoking improvements, only a small amount is tolerable, even in competitive athletes. Surprisingly, very little training is actually performed in the intensity zone between the two thresholds (zone 2). This intensity has been called "the black hole"

Table 11-12

Sample Phase 2 Cardiorespiratory-training Progression

Training Parameter	Week 1	Week 2	Week 3	Week 4	Week 5
Frequency	3 times/week	3–4 times/week	3–4 times/week	4 times/week	4–5 times/week
Duration (10% weekly increase)	"X" minutes	10% increase	10% increase	10% increase	10% increase
Intensity	<VT1 HR	Below and above VT1 HR	Below and above VT1 HR	Below and above VT1 HR	Above VT1 HR
Zone	1	1 and 2	1 and 2	1 and 2	1 and 2
Training Format	Steady state	Aerobic intervals	Aerobic intervals	Aerobic intervals	Aerobic intervals
Work-to-Recovery Intervals (active recovery)	None	1:2 2–3 minute intervals	1:2 3–4 minute intervals	1:1½ 3–4 minute intervals	1:1 4–5 minute intervals

Note: VT1 = First ventilatory threshold; HR = Heart rate

(where there is a psychological push to do more, but a physiologic pull to do less), since it is the zone where exercise is hard enough to make a person fatigued, but not hard enough to really provoke optimal adaptations (Seiler & Kjerland, 2006).

Most of the studies with training loads have simply observed what athletes spontaneously do during training. In a very well-controlled study of training distribution, researchers randomized cross-country runners into groups, where the total training load was controlled and equalized (Esteve-Lanao et al., 2007). High-intensity (zone 3) training was limited to approximately 10% of total training time in both groups. One group increased the amount of easy (zone 1) training from the spontaneous 70% to about 85%, and decreased the amount of moderately hard (zone 2) training from the spontaneous 20% to about 5%. The other group, conversely, decreased zone 1 training to from the spontaneous 70% to about 60% and increased zone 2 training to from 20% to about 30%. After five months, the improvement in performance favored those who had performed more zone 1 training. Despite zone 1 being relatively easier training, the results supported the contention that zone 2 training is essentially a "black hole" (Seiler & Kjerland, 2006). It may be that there is an important interaction of the distribution of training with the total volume of training, but the best evidence is that in individuals who are already routinely exercising and who desire to move toward their optimal biological potential, most training (approximately 80%) should be performed at intensities where speech is comfortable (zone 1), and about 10% of training should be performed at intensities above VT2 (zone 3), where the physiological provocation to make large gains is present.

It is unclear at this time whether the dominant training intensity within a zone matters. It is easy to speculate that zone 1 training should, for the most part, be performed relatively high in zone 1. Similarly, it would seem to make sense that, except for training designed to augment anaerobic pathways, most zone 3 training should be performed relatively low in zone 3, with progression by duration rather than by intensity. This remains an area in need of controlled studies.

With the increase in training load during phase 3, consideration must also be given to the amount of recovery training. It can be taken as axiomatic that training hard enough to provoke adaptations requires recovery before subsequent training can be performed. Thus, where the regular recreational exerciser in the aerobic-base phase of training (phase1) can safely and comfortably perform essentially the same training bout every day, the competitive-level exerciser will need to use a decidedly hard/easy approach to training, or he or she will be at risk for problems from accumulating fatigue and loss of training benefit from the inability to repeatedly do really hard training sessions. Studies have indicated that maladaptations to training (e.g., **overtraining syndrome**) are almost exclusively attributable to a failure to incorporate appropriate recovery days, particularly if they are coupled with extensive travel or other occupational or social stressors (Meeusen et al. 2006). The concept of training monotony is important (not the degree to which training is boring, but the degree to which it does not change on a day-to-day basis). Many illnesses, as well as stagnation of training performances, can be attributed to high training monotony (Foster, 1998). This is probably only an issue when the training load is fairly high relative to the capacity of the person (30 minutes at moderate intensity performed daily does not create a risk of overtraining for most exercisers). An example of equivalent training loads performed in a high-monotony manner versus a low-monotony manner is presented in Figure 11-7. Extensive experience relative to preventing illnesses and other subtle markers of overtraining, as well as the results of experimental studies, suggest that alternating "hard" and "easy" training days is more effective than training that is more or less the same every day (Hansen et al., 2005). In any case, even in the most seriously trained athlete, it is probably not productive to perform more than three or four high-intensity or very long training sessions per week. Interestingly, studies performed with athletes working under the direction of a coach have indicated that athletes almost always work harder and longer than the coach intended for them to on designated recovery days. And, because they were not adequately recovered, they almost always trained less hard and for less time than the coach intended on training days (Foster et al., 2001b). This finding has helped greatly in the understanding of why overtraining syndrome occurs so frequently in athletes (who have the best inherent physical talent) while working under coaches (who are usually very well educated and motivated to enhance the success of their athletes).

Program Design for Phase 3: Anaerobic-endurance Training

Program design during this phase should be focused on helping the client enhance his or her aerobic efficiency to ensure completion of goal events, while building anaerobic endurance to achieve endurance-performance goals. Improved anaerobic endurance will help the client perform physical work at or near VT2 for an extended period, which will result in improved endurance, speed, and power to meet primary performance goals.

To program effective intervals for improving anaerobic endurance, the personal trainer should have the client perform the VT2 threshold test to determine the client's HR at VT2. Once the personal trainer has current values for the client's HR at VT1 and VT2, the trainer can establish a three-zone model that is specific to the client. For example, if a client's HR at VT1 is 143 bpm and HR at VT2 is 162 bpm, the client's HR zones would be as follows:

- Zone 1 = less than 143 bpm
- Zone 2 = 143 to 161 bpm
- Zone 3 = 162 bpm and above

These HR zones can then be used as intensity markers to help the client stay within the correct zone for the desired training outcome of a given workout.

Training intensity should be varied, with 70 to 80% of training in zone 1, approximately 10% to 20% of training in zone 3, and only brief periods (less that 10%) in zone 2. This large volume of zone 1 training time is critical to program success for clients with endurance-performance goals, as exercise frequency, intensity, and time all add to the total load. Individuals who increase each of these variables too quickly are at risk for

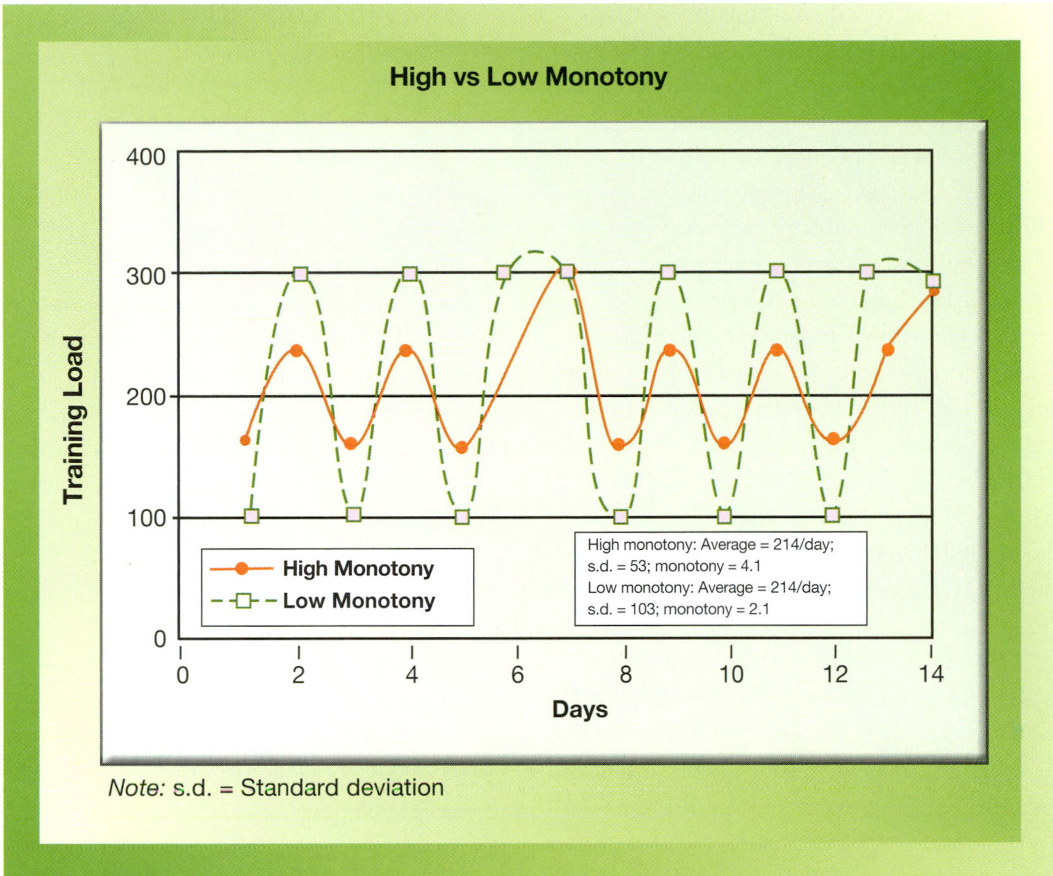

Figure 11-7
Schematic of low- and high-monotony training programs with the same average loading per day. In the low-monotony program, the higher standard deviation of training loads leads to a lower calculated training monotony, which is defined by the average divided by the standard deviation during each week. At a given level of training load, programs with lower monotony (e.g. more day-to-day variability in loading) are usually more effective at producing training results and less provocative of maladaptations to training.

burnout and overuse injuries. The trainer can help clients avoid overtraining by distributing zone 1 training time across warm-ups, cool-downs, moderate-intensity workouts focused on increasing distance and/or exercise time, recovery intervals following zone 2 and 3 work intervals, and recovery workouts on days following higher-intensity workouts. By completing adequate zone 1 training time, clients will have the mental and physical energy required to perform their zone 2 and 3 intervals as planned. The frequency of zone 2 and 3 interval workouts will be client-specific, based on the client's goals, available training time, available recovery time, and outside stressors. Highly fit competitive clients with adequate recovery time may be able to successfully complete and recover from three to four workouts with zone 2 or 3 intervals during weeks where the goal is to increase the load. If the client is not highly fit, has minimal recovery time, or is lacking in total training time, the trainer should design a program that has only one or two total zone 2 or 3 interval days. In recreation-level competitors, almost all of this training is performed in zone 1, with the exception of perhaps a single zone 3 training session per week.

The volume of training should be progressively increased (<10% per week) until the total weekly volume reaches a maximum of three times the anticipated duration of the target event for which the exerciser is training. This "rule of threes" is a classic concept from marathon running. Although there is a lack of direct experimental evidence, the concept is generally well-supported. Using running events as a model, the volume of high-intensity interval training performed on hard days will vary with the duration of the event. Thus, a person preparing for a 1-mile race might do about 2.5 times the racing distance (e.g., performing 10 x 400 m intervals is a very reasonable training load), whereas someone preparing for a 10K might do approximately equal to the race distance in his or her higher-intensity intervals (6 x 1 mile intervals might be appropriate). Someone preparing for a marathon might have a multiplier of approximately 0.25 (6 x 1 mile intervals might be appropriate) (Figure 11-8). Obviously, these kinds of volume multipliers are highly empirical, and probably best fit serious competitive athletes. Scaled-down versions, based more on common sense and time available rather than on experimentally derived data, are appropriate for more recreational competitors.

Intervals performed in zone 2 will generally be of longer duration than intervals performed in zone 3. This is due to the inability to sustain long intervals at zone 3 intensities where HR equals or exceeds HR at VT2 (RPE ≥7 on the 0 to 10 scale), as compared to zone 2 intervals where HR will be between HR at VT1 and VT2 (RPE of 5 or 6). Higher-intensity zone 3 work will also require greater recovery intervals relative to work intervals when compared to those used in zone 2. Table 11-13 illustrates the work in zones 1, 2, and 3 that might be performed by a client training for a marathon during a four-week training **mesocycle** (see "Recovery and Regeneration" on page 404, as well as Chapter 10 for more information on **periodization**).

If the client begins showing signs of overtraining (e.g., increased RHR, disturbed sleep, or decreased hunger on multiple days), the personal trainer should decrease the frequency and/or intensity of the client's intervals and provide more time for recovery. Also, if the client cannot reach the desired intensity during an interval, or is unable to reach the desired recovery intensity or heart rate during the recovery interval, the interval session should be stopped and the client should recover with cardiorespiratory exercise at an RPE of 3, and no more than 4, to prevent overtraining.

Phase 4: Anaerobic-power Training

Training Focus

The fourth phase of the ACE IFT Model for cardiorespiratory training focuses on anaerobic power. Only highly fit and competitive clients with very specific goals related to high-speed performance during endurance events will require exercise programming in phase 4. Some examples of athletes who might perform phase 4 training include runners and cyclists who compete in events that require repeated sprinting and recovery throughout the race and during the final sprint finish, competitive

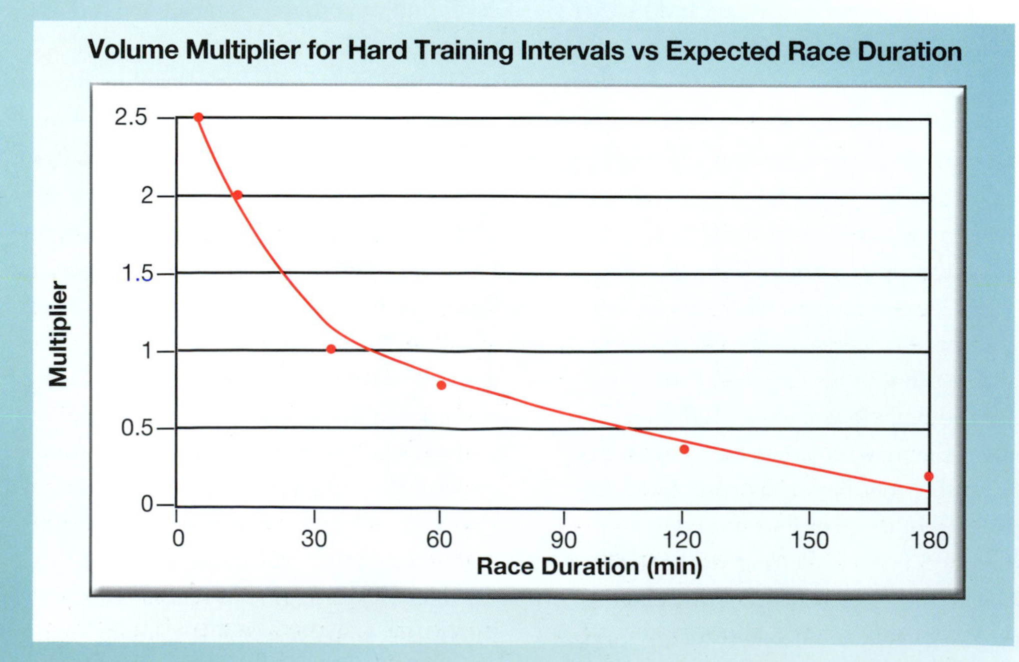

Figure 11-8
Schematic volume multiplier for the amount of high-intensity training within a "hard day" in relation to the expected duration of a competitive event. When preparing for a short event (e.g., running 1 mile), it might be appropriate to perform 2.5 times the race distance or duration (with appropriate recovery interval) (e.g., 10 x 400 m/400 m jog). For a longer event, such as a marathon (for a three-hour competitor), the multiplier might be quite low (0.25) (e.g., 6 x 1 mile). Although experimental evidence for such a multiplier is absent, it does represent a consensus of opinion.

Table 11-13

Sample Phase 3 Cardiorespiratory-training Program: Four-week Mesocycle for Marathon Training

Training Parameter	Week 1—Increase Intensity	Week 2—Increase Intensity	Week 3—Increase Intensity	Week 4—Recovery Week
Training Volume	Total training time = 9 hours	Total training time = 9.5 hours	Total training time = 10 hours	Total training time = 6.5 to 7.5 hours
Zone 1 (~80% of volume) 3 workouts per week plus warm-up, cool-down, and rest intervals during zone 2 and 3 workouts	1 time/week Long run = 2 hours 30 min 1 time/week 90-min run (RPE = 4) 1 time/week 60-min run (RPE = 3–4)	1 time/week Long run = 2 hours 45 min 1 time/week 90-min run (RPE = 4) 1 time/week 60-min run (RPE = 3–4)	1 time/week Long run = 3 hours 1 time/week 90-min run (RPE = 4) 1 time/week 60-min run (RPE = 3–4)	1 time/week Long run = 2 hours 1 time/week 60-min run (RPE = 4) 1 time/week 45-min run (RPE = 3)
Zone 2 (~10% of volume) 1 workout per week	3 x 5-min intervals 1:1½ work:rest ratio 60-min workout with long warm-up and cool-down	4 x 5-min intervals 1:1½ work:rest ratio 70-min workout with long warm-up and cool-down	5 x 5-min intervals 1:1½ work:rest ratio 75-min workout with long warm-up and cool-down	2 x 8-min intervals 1:2 work:rest ratio 60-min workout with long warm-up and cool-down
Zone 3 (~10% of volume) 1 workout per week	2 sets: 3 x 60-second intervals 1:3 work:rest ratio 10 min between sets 60-min workout with long warm-up and cool-down	3 sets: 3 x 45-second intervals 1:3 work:rest ratio 10 min between sets 70-min workout with long warm-up and cool-down	3 sets: 3 x 60-second intervals 1:3 work:rest ratio 10 min between sets 75-min workout with long warm-up and cool-down	2 sets: 3 x 30-second intervals 1:3 work:rest ratio 10 min between sets 45-min workout with long warm-up and cool-down
Strength Training	Circuit training 2 days/week 1 hour/session	Circuit training 2 days/week 1 hour/session	Circuit training 2 days/week 1 hour/session	Circuit training 1–2 days/week 1 hour/session

kayakers who need to paddle vigorously for short periods to navigate through difficult sections of rapids, and athletes in sports such as basketball and soccer where success requires both cardiorespiratory endurance and the ability to sprint repeatedly.

This anaerobic-power training phase can essentially be thought of as strength training, although it is specific to the mode of activity (e.g., running, cycling). The intent is to perform very high-intensity training of nearly maximal muscular capacity, but with enough recovery to prevent the rapid accumulation of fatigue, so that the muscular system can be taxed maximally.

This is very specialized training intended to be performed by individuals preparing for competition. It is intended to increase the tolerance for the metabolic by-products of high-intensity exercise, including exercise performed at intensities greater than $\dot{V}O_2max$. Since this kind of training is very uncomfortable and, in older individuals, potentially dangerous, it should be performed only after a long period of training accommodation.

The underlying physiologic principle of this type of training is that if there is substantial and sustained depletion of the **phosphagen** stores and accumulation of lactate (and other acid metabolites), the body will adapt with a larger phosphagen pool and potentially larger buffer reserves. Studies have suggested that adaptations of this sort can take place, but are relatively modest in magnitude (10%) (Tabata et al., 1996). For reasons that are not well understood, men seem to improve their anaerobic capacity more than women. Although there are not a lot of well-controlled studies, it appears that interval training with relatively brief (30-second) high-intensity elements is just as effective in terms of producing gains in anaerobic capacity as longer high-intensity bursts (where phosphagen depletion and lactate accumulation might be larger, and thus be expected to be more provocative of change). Although controlled studies demonstrating the best way to improve anaerobic capacity are not available, it is generally assumed that high-intensity bouts with relatively short recovery periods, that provoke larger disturbances in **homeostasis** are preferred. Thus, a training session of 10 x 70 seconds at 115% of $\dot{V}O_2max$, with a new repetition beginning every two minutes, might be typical. This kind of training session requires an extended warm-up and cool-down, and is tolerable only once or twice weekly.

Program Design for Phase 4: Anaerobic-power Training

Most clients will never reach phase 4 training, as only clients with very specific goals for achieving high sprinting speed and/or short bursts of very high levels of power for challenges such as short hills, will require anaerobic-power training. Some trainers who work with more highly competitive clients may work with several clients per year who train in phase 4, while other trainers may not work with anyone in phase 4 for several years. Even elite athletes will only spend part of a given year performing phase 4 training cycles to prepare for specific competitions.

Obviously, this kind of training is only designed for individuals interested in competition, and can be tolerated only on a limited basis. Examples might include 6 x 100-meter acceleration runs, where the middle 40 meters are performed at absolute maximal intensity. There might be five minutes of recovery between runs, allowing for full recovery. This type of training should not generally be viewed as cardiorespiratory training. It is entirely supplemental and designed for muscular accommodation.

The total weekly exercise program for a client training in phase 4 will look similar to a client training in phase 3, with 70 to 80% of the training time in zone 1, approximately 10% to 20% of training in zone 3, and only brief periods (less that 10%) in zone 2. The difference will be in the types of intervals performed during some of the zone 3 workout time. Intervals for the phase 4 client will be very short sprints or hill sprints designed to tax the phosphagen stores in the muscles and create a rapid rise in blood lactate levels. These short, highly intense intervals (RPE of 9 to 10) will be followed by long recovery intervals that may be 10 to 20 times longer than the work intervals. For example, a trainer may have a client perform 5 x 10-second accelerations while cycling on a relatively flat road with little traffic, with each acceleration followed by a 2- to 3-minute recovery interval. These anaerobic-power intervals are supplementary to the full training program performed by a client who has endurance-performance goals. As such, these intervals should be performed only once per week as a complement to the full endurance-training program. This type of anaerobic-power training is different than the speed, agility, and quickness training for power athletes that is discussed in Chapter 10.

Recovery and Regeneration

As a general principle, training should be periodized. This means that there should be a regular cycle of hard and easy days, hard and easy weeks, and hard and easy months. The point of training is to gradually progress the overload, but then to allow the body to recover and adapt to the changes provoked by hard training sessions. The more challenging the training program, the more that recovery and regeneration become important. A person interested only in basic fitness, who is performing 30 minutes of moderate-intensity training daily, hardly needs to worry about periodization. However, even in these individuals, there is an advantage to periodically adding a hard day, taking a day completely off, or changing the mode of exercise. The biggest mistakes made, once the training load starts to go up to accomplish more ambitious goals, are to take too few recovery days, to try to do something other than recover on recovery days, and to try to progress the training load on recovery days (when it should only be progressed on hard days). The bottom line is that recovery days are for recovery. If a client does not recover fully and properly, he or she will not be able to work hard enough on the hard training days to provoke further adaptations. Although there is a lack of well-controlled data about exactly how to periodize training plans, it is fair to say that even in the most serious athletes, there should be no more than four hard-training days per week. Even in this group, there is good data to suggest that it is much better to perform three really intense workouts per week rather than to do the same workload over seven days. In less serious competitors, two or three hard days per week are probably adequate to allow progress toward most goals. However, as mentioned earlier, it is common for athletes to train too hard on days the coach thinks are devoted to recovery. If there is a secret to athletic success, it is in the creative use of rest—really recovering on recovery days.

Special Considerations for Youth and Older Adults

Youth

In youth, there are two primary considerations: to prevent early overspecialization and to protect against orthopedic trauma from training too much. Prior to the age of puberty, children should engage in as much lightly structured activity as possible, preferably more than an hour per day. There should be very little focus on exercise per se, but instead on performing a variety of activities to allow for the development of motor skills and fitness in the most general sense. Observation of the play of children suggests that they typically perform intermittent activity rather than the more sustained activity that is typical of fitness exercise. For social-demographic reasons, the amount of exercise performed by children beginning at about the time of puberty and continuing into young adulthood diverges significantly, and either increases (athletes) or decreases (non-athletes) markedly. It is probably fair to say that the training of young athletes should be as general and diverse as possible for as long as possible. Although many young athletes have the time and motivation to perform serious training, there is broad agreement that even in youth who are destined to become good athletes, the longer more diverse training can be performed, the better the eventual level of performance is likely to be. Thus, a youth soccer player who is doing nothing but playing soccer 12 months a year is probably sacrificing his or her long-term best level of play for improvement in the early teen years. About the age at which high school is completed is likely the best time to truly specialize in one activity.

Youth are still growing, and their skeletons are maturing, so very heavy training loads may provide challenges to energy balance and bone and joint integrity. Accordingly, it makes little sense for youth to perform very heavy training too early in life. On the other hand, the development of a high incidence of **obesity** among non-athletic youth is of sufficient threat that all possible efforts should be made to increase activity in this group. While under ordinary circumstances performing systematic fitness exercise might not be the best policy in youth and adolescents, the benefit-to-risk ratio is strongly in the favor of more activity. At the same time, it is important to remember that short-term fitness gains should be sacrificed if the prospect of exercising is not attractive enough to help establish a long-term enjoyment of exercise. This suggests that the intensity of structured fitness training should be low enough that exercise is fairly comfortable (zone 1). Since energy expenditure is of primary importance, the goal duration of exercise should probably be an hour or more. Refer to Chapter 14 for more information on exercise and youth.

Older Adults

In older individuals, there are four overriding considerations that dictate modification of the exercise program (Foster et al., 2007):

- Avoiding cardiovascular risk
- Avoiding orthopedic risk
- The need to preserve muscle tissue
- The rate at which older individuals adapt to training

Even in apparently healthy older individuals, there is always a concern regarding the presence of subclinical cardiovascular disease. Data from the renowned Framingham Heart Study have shown that the first presentation of heart disease is fatal in approximately 35% of men and 17% of women. Together with the data demonstrating that the triggering event for **myocardial infarction** is often unaccustomed heavy exercise in sedentary individuals, the Framingham data suggest that those leading exercise sessions for older adults (over 45 for men and 55 for women) should behave as if there is underlying heart disease and restrict the exerciser to relatively low-intensity (zone 1) exercise for the first several weeks of an exercise program. The same data that suggest that unaccustomed heavy exercise can trigger a heart attack in sedentary individuals also convincingly demonstrate that individuals who routinely exercise will very rarely trigger a heart attack via exercise. Prior to beginning an exercise program, the personal trainer should take a careful health history and keep this document in each client's file. Individuals with answers indicating the presence of multiple risk factors or symptoms suggesting an inappropriate response to exercise should be referred back to their primary physicians prior to beginning an exercise program (Balady et al., 1998).

Although less likely to present traumatically, as with a heart attack, older individuals often have more pre-existing orthopedic problems, may have lost much of the elasticity from their musculotendinous system, or may even have reduced **bone mineral density** (particularly women). As such, this group is less tolerant of heavy training loads, rapid increases in training load, single-mode exercise, and stop-and-go game-type activities. Fortunately, the preliminary period of slowly progressed training that is performed to reduce the risk of cardiovascular catastrophes will also, to some degree, protect against musculoskeletal injuries.

Beyond about the age of 50, there is a tendency for older individuals to lose muscle mass (**sarcopenia**). This is especially pronounced in women, who do not have enough **testosterone** to support the muscle mass, but becomes a problem in men as well, since testosterone concentrations decrease progressively with age. For this reason, the overriding need for cardiorespiratory training that is present in younger individuals needs to be balanced by exercise designed to support muscle mass, muscular strength, and balance. For the most part, such musculoskeletal training can be performed as a brief addition after the main body of the cardiorespiratory training bout. At the simplest level, half a dozen exercises performed either against bodyweight or with light dumbbells or resistance tubing or bands can form the basis for this type of training. More advanced training models are also available. While there are no universally recognized guidelines, if 10 minutes were "stolen" from a 40-minute cardiorespiratory training bout to allow for 10 minutes of resistance exercise, the trade-off might be very favorable.

Lastly, both in the beginning and more serious exerciser, the response to training is probably slower in older individuals, and they can probably better tolerate and respond to fewer hard training days per week. To some degree, this is a function of the presence of prior musculoskeletal injuries and the generally increased fragility of older individuals. At another level, at least in men, it may be attributable to lower testosterone concentrations, which are involved in the rapidity with which new **protein** is synthesized after an exercise bout. Simply put, intense training causes microdamage to the body. The process of repairing this damage causes the adaptations that are generally considered the training response. Given that older people are generally more fragile and heal more slowly than younger people, the frequency of hard training must be reduced. Thus, even in very athletic older individuals, it is probably unwise to do more than two hard or long training sessions per week. Refer to Chapter 14 for more information on exercise and older adults.

Summary

Cardiorespiratory training can be thought of as being simultaneously simple and complex. At the simplest level, the saying "walk daily, walk far" is remarkably good advice and actually incorporates most of the accepted training principles. On a more complex level, training can be reduced to the saying "train really hard every two or three days, doing what it is you want to get better at, and spend the other days recovering." While these comments are overly simplistic, they demonstrate that there is an amazing generality to cardiorespiratory training, grounded as it is in the ambulatory activities that humans' distant hunter-gatherer ancestors had to perform just to survive. Physical activity or structured exercise, which can be thought of in terms of the FITT acronym, performed with regularity causes adaptation in the heart, lungs, blood, and muscle tissue and promotes the ability to perform even more exercise. This is the classical cardiorespiratory training effect. This training effect displays a pattern of diminishing returns, in that there are initially large gains in both health and fitness for even modest amounts of exercise training (30 minutes a day, at moderate intensity, on most days of the week), but progressively smaller gains as the individual's biological potential for exercise is approached. In athletic individuals, very hard individual training sessions may be necessary to promote gains in performance, but these need to be balanced by appropriate recovery efforts for the gains to be safely and fully realized.

References

American College of Sports Medicine (2010). *ACSM's Guidelines for Exercise Testing and Prescription* (8th ed.). Philadelphia: Wolters Kluwer/Lippincott Williams & Wilkins.

Balady, G.J. et al. (1998). Recommendations for cardiovascular screening, staffing and emergency policies at health/fitness facilities: A Joint Position Statement by the American College of Sports Medicine and the American Heart Association. *Medicine & Science in Sports & Exercise,* 30, 1009–1018.

Bassett, D.R., Schneider, P.L., & Huntington, G.E. (2004). Physical activity in an Old Order Amish community. *Medicine & Science in Sports & Exercise,* 36, 79–85.

Berling, J. et al. (2006). The effect of handrail support on oxygen uptake during steady state treadmill exercise. *Journal of Cardiopulmonary Rehabilitation,* 26, 391–394.

Booth, F.W. & Roberts, C.K. (2008). Linking performance and chronic disease: Indices of physical performance are surrogates for health. *British Journal of Sports Medicine,* 42, 950–953.

Booth, F.W. et al. (2002). Waging war on physical inactivity: Using modern molecular ammunition against an ancient enemy. *Journal of Applied Physiology,* 93, 3–30.

Borg, G. (1998). *Borg's Perceived Exertion and Pain Scales.* Champaign, Ill.: Human Kinetics.

Cannon, C. et al. (2004). The talk test as a measure of exertional ischemia. *American Journal of Sports Medicine,* 6, 52–57.

Cordain, L., Gotshall, R.W., & Eaton, S.B. (1998). Physical activity, energy expenditure and fitness: An evolutionary perspective. *International Journal of Sports Medicine,* 19, 328–335.

Dehart, M. et al. (2000). Relationship between the talk test and ventilatory threshold. *Clinical Exercise Physiology,* 2, 34–38.

Esteve-Lanao, J. et al. (2007). Impact of training intensity distribution on performance in endurance athletes. *Journal of Strength and Conditioning Research,* 21, 943–949.

Esteve-Lanao, J. et al. (2005). How do endurance runners actually train? Relationship with competition performance. *Medicine & Science in Sports & Exercise,* 37, 496–504.

Foster, C. (1998). Monitoring training in athletes with reference to overtraining syndrome. *Medicine & Science in Sports & Exercise,* 30, 1164–1168.

Foster, C. & Cotter, H.M. (2006). Blood lactate, respiratory and heart rate markers on the capacity for sustained exercise. In: Maud, P.J. & Foster, C. (Eds.) *Physiological Assessment of Human Fitness* (2nd ed.). Champaign, Ill.: Human Kinetics.

Foster, C., Daniels, J., & Seiler, S. (1999). Perspectives on correct approaches to training. In: Lehmann, M. et al. (Eds.) *Overload, Performance Incompetence and Regeneration in Sport.* New York, Kluwer Academic/Plenum Publishers.

Foster, C., Porcari, J.P., & Lucia, A. (2008). Endurance training. In: Durstine, J.L. et al. (Eds.) *Pollock's Textbook of Cardiovascular Disease and Rehabilitation.* Philadelphia: Lippincott Williams & Wilkins.

Foster, C. et al. (2008). The risk of exercise training. *American Journal of Lifestyle Medicine,* 10, 279–284.

Foster, C. et al. (2007). Training in the aging athlete. *Current Sports Medicine Reports,* 6, 200–206.

Foster, C. et al. (2001a). Monitoring exercise training during non-steady state exercise. *Journal of Strength Conditioning Research,* 15, 109–115.

Foster, C. et al. (2001b). Differences in perceptions of training by coaches and athletes. *South African Journal of Sports Medicine,* 8, 3–7.

Foster, C. et al. (1996). Athletic performance in relation to training load. *Wisconsin Medical Journal,* 95, 370–374.

Foster, C. et al. (1995). Effects of specific vs. cross training on running performance. *European Journal of Applied Physiology,* 70, 367–372.

Fox III, S.M., Naughton, J.P., & Haskell, W.L. (1971). Physical activity and the prevention of coronary heart disease. *Annuals of Clinical Research,* 3, 404–432.

Gellish, R.L. et al. (2007). Longitudinal modeling of the relationship between age and maximal heart rate. *Medicine & Science in Sports & Exercise*, 39, 5, 822–829.

Gorostiaga, E.M. et al. (1991). Uniqueness of interval and continuous training at the same maintained exercise intensity. *European Journal of Applied Physiology,* 63, 101–107.

Hansen, A.K. et al. (2005). Skeletal muscle adaptation: Training twice every second day vs. training once daily. *Journal of Applied Physiology,* 98, 93–99.

Haskell, W.L. et al. (2007). Physical activity and public health: Updated recommendations of the American College of Sports Medicine and the American Heart Association. *Medicine & Science in Sports & Exercise,* 39, 1423–1434.

Herman, L. et al. (2006). Validity and reliability of the session RPE method for monitoring exercise training intensity. *South African Journal of Sports Medicine,* 18, 14–17.

Karvonen, M. et al. (1957). The effect of training on heart rate: A longitudinal study. *Annales Medicinae Experimentalis et Biologiae Fenniae,* 35, 307–315.

Katch, V. et al. (1978). Validity of the relative percent concept for equating training intensity. *European Journal of Applied Physiology,* 39, 219–227.

Laursen, P.B. et al. (2002). Interval training program optimization in highly trained endurance cyclists. *Medicine & Science in Sports & Exercise,* 34, 1801–1807.

Loy, S.F., Holland, G.J., & Mutton, D.K. (1993). Effects of stair climbing vs. run training on treadmill and track running. *Medicine & Science in Sports & Exercise,* 25, 1275–1278.

McConnell, T.R. et al. (1991). Prediction of functional capacity during treadmill testing: Effect of handrail support. *Journal of Cardiopulmonary Rehabilitation,* 11, 255–260.

Meeusen, R. et al. (2006). Prevention, diagnosis and treatment of overtraining syndrome. *European Journal of Sport Science,* 6, 1–14.

Meyer, T. et al. (2005). A conceptual framework for performance diagnosis and training prescription from submaximal parameters: Theory and application. *International Journal of Sports Medicine,* 26, 1–11.

Persinger, R. et al. (2004). Consistency of the talk test for exercise prescription. *Medicine & Science in Sports & Exercise,* 36, 1632–1636.

Porcari, J.P. et al. (2001). Prescribing exercise using the talk test. *Fitness Management,* 17, 9, 46–49.

Recalde, P.T. et al. (2002). The talk test as a simple marker of ventilatory threshold. *South African Journal of Sports Medicine,* 9, 5–8.

Seiler, K.S. & Kjerland, G.O. (2006). Quantifying training intensity distribution in elite athletes: Is there evidence for an 'optimal' distribution. *Scandinavian Journal of Medicine & Science in Sports,* 16, 49–56.

Sjodin, B. & Jacobs, I. (1981). Onset of blood lactate accumulation and marathon running performance. *International Journal of Sports Medicine,* 2, 23–26.

Sjodin, B. et al. (1982). Changes in onset of blood lactate accumulation (OBLA) and muscle enzymes after training at OBLA. *European Journal of Applied Physiology,* 49, 45–57.

Stepto, N.K. et al. (1998). Effect of different interval training programs on cycling time trial performance. *Medicine & Science in Sports & Exercise,* 31, 736–741.

Tabata, I. et al. (1996). Effects of moderate-intensity endurance and high-intensity intermittent training on anaerobic capacity and $\dot{V}O_2$max. *Medicine & Science in Sports & Exercise,* 28, 1327–1330.

Tanaka, H., Monahan, K.D., & Seals, D.R. (2001). Age-predicted maximal heart revisited. *Journal of the American College of Cardiology,* 37, 153–156.

U.S. Department of Health & Human Services (2008). *2008 Physical Activity Guidelines for Americans: Be Active, Healthy and Happy.* www.health.gov/paguidelines/pdf/paguide.pdf

Voelker, S.A. et al. (2002). Relationship between the talk test and ventilatory threshold in cardiac patients. *Clinical Exercise Physiology,* 4, 120–123.

Wilmore, J.H., Costill, D., & Kenney, W.L. (2008). *Physiology of Sport and Exercise* (4th ed.). Champaign, Ill.: Human Kinetics.

World Health Organization (1968). Exercise tests in relation to cardiovascular function: Report of a WHO meeting. *World Health Organization Technical Report Series,* 388, 1–30.

Suggested Reading

American College of Sports Medicine (2009). *ACSM's Resource Manual for Guidelines for Exercise Testing and Prescription* (6th ed.). Philadelphia: Lippincott Williams & Wilkins.

Daniels, J. (2005). *Daniels' Running Formula* (2nd ed.). Champaign, Ill.: Human Kinetics.

Edwards, S. (1993). *The Heart Rate Monitor Book.* Sacramento, Calif.: Fleet Feet Press.

Noakes, T. (2001). *The Lore of Running* (4th ed.). Champaign, Ill.: Human Kinetics.

Powers, S.K. & Howley, E.T. (2008). *Exercise Physiology: Theory and Application to Fitness and Performance* (7th ed.). New York: McGraw-Hill.

Wilmore, J.H., Costill, D.L., & Kenney, W.L. (2008). *Physiology of Sport and Exercise* (4th ed.). Champaign, Ill.: Human Kinetics.

IN THIS CHAPTER:

Case Study 1: Sharon

Functional Movement and Resistance Training—Phase 1: Stability and Mobility Training

Cardiorespiratory Training—Phase 1: Aerobic-base Training

Functional Movement and Resistance Training—Phase 2: Movement Training

Cardiorespiratory Training—Phase 2: Aerobic-efficiency Training

Functional Movement and Resistance Training—Phase 3: Load Training

Cardiorespiratory Training—Phase 2: Aerobic-efficiency Training (Progression)

Conclusion

Case Study 2: David

Functional Movement and Resistance Training—Phase 1: Stability and Mobility Training

Cardiorespiratory Training—Phase 2: Aerobic-efficiency Training

Functional Movement and Resistance Training—Phase 2: Movement Training

Cardiorespiratory Training—Phase 3: Anaerobic-endurance Training

Conclusion

Case Study 3: Jan

Functional Movement and Resistance Training—Phase 2: Movement Training

Functional Movement and Resistance Training—Phase 3: Load Training

Functional Movement and Resistance Training—Phase 4: Performance Training

Conclusion

Case Study 4: Stanley

Functional Movement and Resistance Training—Phase 1: Stability and Mobility Training

Cardiorespiratory Training—Phase 1: Aerobic-base Training

Functional Movement and Resistance Training—Phase 2: Movement Training

Cardiorespiratory Training—Phase 1: Aerobic-base Training (Progression)

Conclusion

Case Study 5: Meredith

Functional Movement and Resistance Training—Phase 2: Movement Training

Cardiorespiratory Training—Phase 2: Aerobic-efficiency Training

Functional Movement and Resistance Training—Phase 3: Load Training

Cardiorespiratory Training—Phase 2: Anaerobic-endurance Training (Progression)

Functional Movement and Resistance Training—Phase 4: Performance Training

Cardiorespiratory Training—Phase 2: Aerobic-efficiency Training (Progression)

Conclusion

Case Study 6: Kelly

Functional Movement and Resistance Training—Phase 2: Movement Training

Functional Movement and Resistance Training—Phase 3: Load Training

Conclusion

Summary

***PETE MCCALL, M.S.**, is an exercise physiologist with the American Council on Exercise (ACE), where he creates and delivers fitness education programs to uphold ACE's mission of enriching quality of life through safe and effective exercise and physical activity. Prior to working with ACE, McCall was a full-time personal trainer and group fitness instructor in Washington, D.C. He has a Master's of Science degree in exercise science and health promotion from California University of Pennsylvania and is an ACE-certified Personal Trainer.*

CHAPTER 12

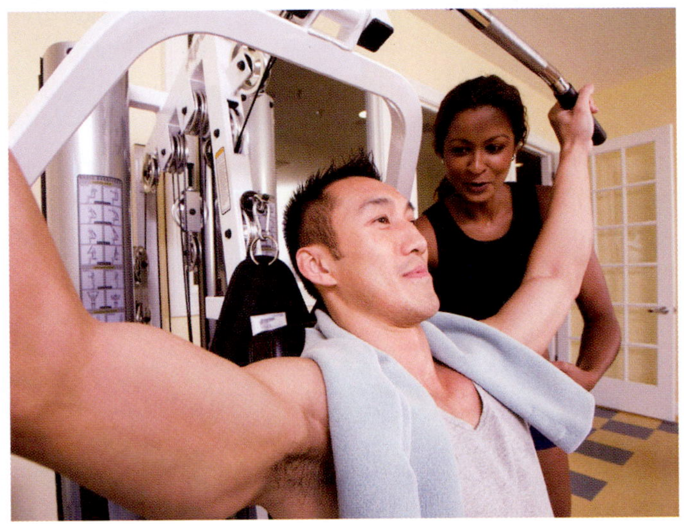

The ACE Integrated Fitness Training™ Model in Practice

Pete McCall

The purpose of this chapter is to provide practical examples that show how the ACE Integrated Fitness Training (ACE IFT™) Model can be applied to different types of clients that ACE-certified Personal Trainers might commonly encounter in the course of their professional careers. These case studies demonstrate how a personal trainer can utilize the ACE IFT Model to choose assessments and design exercise programs for a diverse selection of clientele based on each client's current stage of behavior change, health, fitness, and individual needs and goals. Each case study provides a scenario in which a personal trainer has to determine a client's current stage of behavior change, conduct the most effective assessments for the client, and design an exercise program based on the results of the assessments that will also meet the client's goals. These case studies are not meant to be the *only* solution for each client's needs and goals, but instead are designed to demonstrate potential solutions based on the application of the ACE IFT Model and how to successfully progress an exercise program if the client shows a favorable response.

> The aim of these case studies is to enable trainers to identify, design, and implement the various physiological stages of the ACE IFT Model to help clients attain their goals. To achieve this learning objective, the content intentionally deemphasizes discussion of the psychological and emotional components so that the reader can understand the physiological programming appropriate for each stage. In reality, however, trainers should always remember to include psychological or emotional strategies that will maximize opportunities for success and create a positive and memorable experience for each client (see Chapters 2 through 4).

For the purpose of these case studies, the health histories only include pertinent information; details not included would not make a significant impact on the client's program.

The assessments discussed in the case studies were covered in detail in Chapters 7 and 8. Please refer back as needed to better understand the goal and protocol for each assessment chosen.

Case Study 1: Sharon

Sharon is a 33-year-old female who works from home and has two children under the age of four. Prior to her pregnancies, Sharon was a recreational runner who ran two to three times a week to train for 5K and 10K races and played on a coed soccer team for fun on the weekends. Sharon also worked out in a health club doing group strength training and group indoor cycling classes to stay in shape for her activities, but rarely worked out on her own because she preferred the camaraderie of group activities. She was a high school and Division III college soccer player.

Sharon exercised during both pregnancies, continuing the group strength training classes, but replacing the running with prenatal **yoga** classes and walking. Now that both kids are a little older and can be left with a babysitter during her workouts (her youngest child is 12 months old), Sharon wants to work with a personal trainer to start working out regularly and get back in her pre-pregnancy shape.

Sharon has approached Mike, a trainer at her health club, about using his services. Mike led Sharon's introductory sessions when she joined the club three years ago, and he has continued to talk with her and ask about her family, so there is existing **rapport.** Sharon decides that she will invest in a package of 20 personal-training sessions in an effort to return to her pre-pregnancy fitness level. Mike sets the first appointment with Sharon so he can update her health-history information, measure her **blood pressure,** identify her specific training goals, and have her start on a basic exercise program. The health history reveals that other than her recent pregnancies and a knee sprain suffered while playing soccer in college, Sharon has no medical issues, but she does indicate that she has been experiencing mild soreness in her low back since the birth of her second child, though it has never been severe enough for her to seek the attention of a doctor (Table 12-1).

Table 12-1

Sharon: Health-risk Appraisal

Age	33
Height/weight	5'5"/150 lb (1.7 m/68 kg)
Exercise history	Previously a frequent exerciser. Played recreational sports, ran regularly, and participated in group exercise classes. Wants to get in pre-pregnancy shape and return to prior activities.
Medical history	Gave birth to two children in the past four years, the last was one year ago; no complications from the pregnancies Sprained knee 14 years ago, some recent mild low-back soreness No serious health issues Currently taking no medications except over-the-counter pain reliever for her back, as needed
Risk factors	Resting heart rate: 62 bpm Blood pressure: 118/74 mmHg No history of high cholesterol or fasting blood glucose Her uncle passed away from a heart attack at age 67

Note: bpm = Beats per minute

Sharon identifies her goals as returning to her pre-baby bodyweight and resuming her pre-pregnancy fitness activities, such as running and group strength training classes. Sharon is not concerned about her back, but is aware that she has lost core strength since her recent pregnancy and cites that as the cause of the soreness. In their discussion, Mike learns that the only concern Sharon has about her exercise program is that she will need to work around her childcare and work schedules and might not be able to make it to the club for every workout. Therefore, she wants a routine that she can do on her own with the stability ball, medicine ball, and dumbbells she has at home.

Based on the health-risk appraisal and the goal-setting discussion, Mike determines that Sharon is in the **preparation** stage of change because she is motivated to exercise regularly, but has yet to adopt a regular routine. Mike notes that she has the potential to move fairly quickly into the **action** stage because she is motivated to exercise, has been successful at following a regular exercise program in the past, and just needs structure for a proper training progression to achieve her goals. Upon the conclusion of the health history and blood-pressure assessments, Mike conducts a basic assessment of her posture to identify any major muscle imbalances and finds slight thoracic kyphosis and increased low-back lordosis. He decides to spend the last 20 minutes of the first session teaching Sharon basic core-activation exercises, including the birddog, plank, side-plank, and glute bridge exercises so that she can start working on her core **stability.**

Sharon is a highly motivated ex-athlete who wants to include running as a mode of exercise, but she has not been exercising regularly since before the birth of her second child. Mike will first implement a cardio-respiratory program that helps her rebuild her **aerobic** base. Once she can complete 20 to 30 minutes of steady-state moderate-intensity exercise in zone 1 [**ratings of perceived exertion (RPE)** of 3 to 4], he will have her perform a submaximal **talk test** to establish her heart rate at the **first ventilatory threshold (VT1).** He will then use her heart rate at VT1 to progress her cardiorespiratory program to help her work toward her running goals.

Mike determines that he will assess Sharon's lower-body **flexibility** and test the strength and endurance of her core muscles in an effort identify the cause of her low-back discomfort. During the second session, Mike will conduct the passive straight-leg raise assessment and the Thomas test, along with the trunk flexor, trunk lateral, and trunk extensor endurance tests, in an effort to identify any abnormal muscle tightness or weakness that can be addressed with the exercise program. Mike will use the results from these assessments to establish Sharon's baseline levels of flexibility and core strength for comparison with future assessments to determine program effectiveness. In their initial conversation, Sharon identifies her primary objective as weight loss and indicates that she is motivated by tracking her results, so Mike decides to take **body composition** and circumference measurements so they can track progress toward her goals. During the assessments, Sharon was able to complete all of the fitness tests without complications. Rather than compare her scores to "norms," Mike decides to simply record Sharon's scores to use as baseline values when measuring progress during future assessments, and to help with program design. Table 12-2 presents Mike's notes.

Functional Movement and Resistance Training—Phase 1: Stability and Mobility Training

Due to the imbalances in flexibility and muscular strength and endurance, Mike will start Sharon with a program focusing on stability and **mobility.** This phase will last until Sharon demonstrates effective strength of the core muscles and improved **range of motion (ROM)** of the hips. Mike estimates that Sharon will spend two to four weeks in this phase.

- *Frequency:* Sharon will train two times per week with Mike and once a week on her own.
- *Intensity:* These exercises focus on using bodyweight to create an overload, leading to enhanced conditioning and stability of the core muscles.
- *Type:* Based on her goals and the results of the assessments, Mike designs a program that will focus on exercises to

Table 12-2

Sharon: Trainer's Assessment Notes

Assessment	Results	Observations
Posture	Stands with slight kyphosis and lordosis posture	Will need to improve postural stability and mobility
Body composition	28% body fat	She has an athletic build but is still carrying weight from the second baby.
Circumference measurements	Waist: 27 inches (69 cm) Hips: 33 inches (84 cm) Waist: hip ratio: 0.82 (average)	She states that one of her prime goals is to fit back into her "skinny jeans" and wear her pre-pregnancy clothes.
Passive straight-leg raise test	Right: Approximately 90 degrees Left: Approximately 80 degrees	Right leg has more ROM than the left leg (the left knee was the one sprained in college).
Thomas test	Right: Right femur lies flat on the table, knee is in slight extension Left: Hip flexes slightly, does not stay flat along the table, knee maintains slight extension	She is tight in both quadriceps. Left hip flexors are tighter than the right—asymmetrical ROM in hips could be cause of back soreness. She needs to increase ROM of hip flexors.
Core function assessment	Demonstrates that she can activate her TVA successfully	
Trunk flexor endurance test	Held trunk flexion for 85 seconds	Has a flexor:extensor ratio of 1.4; needs to work on strength and endurance of core muscles
Trunk extensor test	Maintained trunk extension for only 60 seconds	
Trunk lateral endurance—right side	Held position for 34 seconds	Has a right-left side score differential of 0.27. Her right side is the dominant side, but she usually carries one of her kids in her left arm, so that side has more strength and endurance. Her ratio of lateral bridge to extension is more than 0.05 from 1.0, so she needs to balance her right- and left-side core strength.
Trunk lateral endurance—left side	Held position for 46 seconds	

Note: ROM = Range of motion; TVA = Transverse abdominis

help improve her core strength while also addressing the ROM of her hips.

- *Time:* Each workout should last approximately one hour, including a five-minute warm-up of walking on the treadmill and a 10-minute cool-down that includes stretching of the hip flexors, adductors, and extensors, as well as the back, chest, and calves.

Table 12-3 presents Sharon's initial functional-movement program, which is designed to improve core stability and mobility. She will start with two sets of each exercise, with rest intervals of 60 seconds. As Sharon adapts to the exercises and progresses through the training program, Mike will increase the volume to three sets of each exercise and minimize the rest intervals so that Sharon begins to do all of the exercises in a circuit format, moving from one exercise to the next and not resting until the end of the series of exercises. Mike will teach Sharon how to do a modified version of the workout with the equipment that she has available at home.

Once Sharon is able to complete the exercise circuit three to four times with good coordination and while maintaining a high work rate, Mike will change the exercise selection and progress the resistance-training workout into the movement-training phase (phase 2).

Table 12-3				
Sharon: Functional Movement and Resistance Training Phase 1—Stability and Mobility Training				
Exercise Selection	**Intensity**	**Repetitions**	**Rest Interval**	**Sets**
Exercise progression for core activation	<50% MVC	1	10–15 seconds	1–2
Birddog	Bodyweight	10–12	30–60 seconds	2–3
Dirty dog	Bodyweight	10–12	30–60 seconds	2–3
Plank	Bodyweight	1 (30–45 second hold)	30–60 seconds	2–3
Side plank	Bodyweight	1 (20–30 second hold)	30–60 seconds	2–3
Glute bridge	Bodyweight	12–15	30–60 seconds	2–3
Thoracic matrix in neutral stance (seated or kneeling); progress to standing, staggered-stance, and split stance	Bodyweight	15	30–60 seconds	2–3

Note: MVC = Maximum voluntary contraction

Cardiorespiratory Training—Phase 1: Aerobic-base Training

During this phase, Sharon will train at an aerobic level that falls below the "talk test" level. Since VT1 will not be assessed until the next phase, Mike will teach her how to gauge her intensity using the RPE scale (0 to 10 scale), and instruct her to exercise at an RPE of 3 to 4, with initial goals of performing regular cardiorespiratory exercise while focusing on increased duration. Mike will plan three aerobic-training sessions per week during this phase of training. Since Sharon wants to get back into running, Mike will start her with a program built on brisk walking and then introduce jogging into her cardiorespiratory training. This also meets her requirement of being able to exercise on her own by going outside for walks or runs when she does not have time to make it to the health club. Table 12-4 presents Sharon's aerobic-base training program.

Once Sharon is consistently performing 25 to 30 minutes of walking/jogging at an RPE of 4 and is ready to do more, Mike will have her perform a submaximal talk test to determine her HR at VT1 and then progress her program by introducing low–zone 2 intervals with intensities slightly above VT1.

Table 12-4		
Sharon: Cardiorespiratory Training Phase 1—Aerobic-base Training		
Warm-up	**Workout**	**Cool-down**
Fast walk for 5 minutes Dynamic stretches (e.g., bodyweight forward and side lunges)	Frequency: >3 days per week Intensity: Below the talk-test threshold, or at a perceived exertion that is "moderate" to "somewhat hard" (RPE = 3 to 4) Time: Work up to 30 minutes of continuous exercise	Walk for 5 minutes Static stretching of hip flexors, hip adductors, hamstrings, and calves
	Type: Walking, with jogging introduced as fitness improves	

Note: RPE = Ratings of perceived exertion

Functional Movement and Resistance Training—Phase 2: Movement Training

This phase will last until Sharon demonstrates effective and efficient control of the basic movement patterns: squatting, lunging, pushing, pulling, and rotational (see page 330 for more information on the five basic movement patterns). Mike estimates that Sharon will spend four to six weeks in this phase

- *Frequency:* Sharon will train twice per week with Mike and once a week on her own.
- *Intensity:* These exercises primarily use bodyweight as resistance, but Sharon

can progress to using external-resistance equipment like medicine balls and dumbbells as her movement patterns and strength improve.

- *Type:* The focus of the exercise selection is to retrain basic patterns of movement and work on integrated muscle coordination.
- *Time:* Each workout should last approximately one hour, including the warm-up and cool-down.

Table 12-5 presents Sharon's movement-training program.

Table 12-5

Sharon: Functional Movement and Resistance Training Phase 2—Movement Training

Exercise Selection	Intensity	Repetitions	Rest Interval	Sets
Dynamic warm–up • Plank • Side plank • Glute bridge • Crunches on ball	Bodyweight	12–15 (1 for planks; hold for 30–60 seconds each)	90 seconds (after all four exercises)	3
Hip hinge	Bodyweight; progress to 3-kg (~6.5-lb) medicine ball	12–15	30 seconds	2–3
Bodyweight squats	Bodyweight	12–15	30 seconds	2–3
Prone lies on stability ball with torso movements	Bodyweight	12–15	30 seconds	2–3
Half-kneeling wood chops (progress to full standing)	Bodyweight; progress to 3-kg (~6.5-lb) medicine ball	12–15	30–60 seconds	2–3
Half-kneeling hay bailers (progress to full standing)	Bodyweight; progress to 3-kg (~6.5-lb) medicine ball	12–15	30 seconds	2–3
Forward lunges, progress to include side, backward, and rotational lunges	Bodyweight	12–15	30 seconds	2–3
Supine and seated scapular packing exercise	Bodyweight	12– 15	30 seconds	2–3
Seated bilateral cable press	65% 1 RM	15	30 seconds	2–3
Modified (assisted) pull-ups	Bodyweight	15	30 seconds	2–3
Bilateral overhead dumbbell press	65% 1 RM	12–15	30 seconds	2–3

Note: 1 RM = One-repetition maximum

Cardiorespiratory Training—Phase 2: Aerobic-efficiency Training

Mike has Sharon perform a submaximal talk test and determines her HR at VT1 to be 140 bpm. Mike continues to recommend three zone 1 cardiorespiratory sessions per week during this phase of training, but will modify the workouts to all running that progresses to include zone 2 intervals that have Sharon exercising at, or just above, her HR at VT1 (approximately 140 to 150 bpm), with adequate recovery intervals to build aerobic efficiency. Sharon has been enjoying the workouts and has invested in a heart-rate monitor so she can track her intensity more efficiently. Table 12-6 presents Sharon's aerobic efficiency program.

Once Sharon demonstrates the proper coordination, strength, and control through the basic movement patterns, Mike can increase the intensity of her training so that she progresses to phase 3 (load training), at which point she can focus on training for muscular strength. Sharon has lost weight and is on the way to achieving her goal of regaining her pre-pregnancy fitness level. She now wants to work on increasing her strength so that she can do full-body pull-ups like she could in college. The next stage of program design will focus on helping Sharon gain the necessary strength to complete three full-body pull-ups while also emphasizing muscular definition.

Functional Movement and Resistance Training—Phase 3: Load Training

Sharon will continue in this phase until she reaches her goal of completing three bodyweight pull-ups. Once that goal is achieved, she and Mike will establish new goals.

- *Frequency:* Sharon is now working with Mike only once a week and is able to train twice a week on her own.
- *Intensity:* Mike sets the intensity to achieve strength and advises Sharon that she should fatigue by the twelfth repetition of each set. If not, she should increase the resistance.

Table 12-6

Sharon: Cardiorespiratory Training Phase 2—Aerobic-efficiency Training

Warm-up	Workout	Cool-down
Fast walk for 5 minutes Dynamic stretches (e.g.,bodyweight squats and lunges)	Frequency: 3 days per week Intensity: Warm-up, cool-down, steady state, and recovery intervals in zone 1 with HR below 140 bpm. Work intervals in zone 2 at an HR range of 140 to 150 bpm, which is at, or up to 10 bpm above, HR at VT1 (140 bpm) Time: 30 minutes per session, with time to increase as her schedule allows Type: Walking for zone 1 exercise and jogging for zone 2 intervals. Progress to all jogging for exercise in zones 1 and 2.	Walk for 5 minutes Static stretching of hip flexors, hip adductors, hamstrings, and calves

Note: HR = Heart rate; VT1 = First ventilatory threshold; bpm = Beats per minute

- *Type:* The focus of the exercise selection is on compound movements that create integrated, total-body strength.
- *Time:* Each workout should last approximately one hour, including the warm-up and cool-down.

Table 12-7 presents Sharon's load-training program.

Table 12-7

Sharon: Functional Movement and Resistance Training Phase 3—Load Training

Exercise Selection	Intensity	Repetitions	Rest Interval	Sets
Dynamic warm-up • Plank • Side plank • Glute bridge–feet on ball • Crunches on ball • Medicine ball wood chops	Bodyweight Medicine ball	12–15 (1 for planks; hold for 30–60 seconds each)	2 minutes after the circuit	2–3
Barbell deadlifts	70% 1 RM	10–12	30–60 seconds	2–3
Dumbbell incline chest flys	70% 1 RM	10–12	30–60 seconds	2–3
Dumbbell side lunges	70% 1 RM	10–12	30–60 seconds	2–3
Modified pull-ups	Bodyweight	To fatigue	30–60 seconds	2–3
Dumbbell squat to shoulder press	70% 1 RM	10–12	30–60 seconds	2–3
Bent-over barbell rows	70% 1 RM	10–12	30–60 seconds	2–3
Dumbbell biceps curls	70% 1 RM	10–12	30–60 seconds	2–3
Cable triceps push-downs	70% 1 RM	10–12	30–60 seconds	2–3

Note: 1 RM = One-repetition maximum

Cardiorespiratory Training—Phase 2: Aerobic-efficiency Training (Progression)

The goal of this phase of Sharon's program is to perform aerobic intervals for improving aerobic efficiency. In this phase, Sharon will progress her cardiorespiratory training to prepare for an upcoming 5K (3.1 mile) run. Mike will continue to recommend three runs per week during this phase of training, progressing to include intervals of different intensities. Mike reassesses Sharon's HR at VT1 by having her perform another submaximal talk test. Her new HR at VT1 is 144 bpm, which Mike uses as an intensity marker for her work intervals. Sharon has been enjoying the workouts and uses her heart-rate monitor to track her intensity and work rate. To reduce her risk of repetitive-stress injuries from running, Sharon plans on varying her cardiorespiratory workouts by replacing one day of running per week with an indoor cycling class. Sharon has consistently worn her heart-rate monitor during training and feels that it helps her track her progress and improves her consistency with following her exercise routine. Table 12-8 presents Sharon's new cardiorespiratory training program.

Table 12-8

Sharon: Cardiorespiratory Training Phase 2—Aerobic-efficiency Training (Progression)

Warm-up	Workout	Cool-down
Fast walk for 5 minutes Dynamic stretches (e.g., bodyweight squats and lunges)	Frequency: 3 days per week Intensity: Warm-up, cool-down, steady state, and recovery intervals in zone 1 with HR below 144 bpm. Work intervals in zone 2 at an HR range of 144 to 154 bpm, which is at, or up to 10 bpm above, HR at VT1 (140 bpm) Time: 30 minutes per session, with time to increase as her schedule allows Type: Running in zone 1 with work intervals in zone 2	Walk for 5 minutes Static stretching of hip flexors, hip adductors, hamstrings, and calves

Note: HR = Heart rate; VT1 = First ventilatory threshold; bpm = Beats per minute

Conclusion

This exercise program demonstrates a possible progression for a person who is self-motivated to exercise, but needs the guidance and structure from a personal trainer to help her achieve her specific goals. Based on Sharon's fitness level, assessments, goals, and available time to commit to training, Mike started her in the first phase for both training components. Because she was consistent with her workouts, he was able to progress the intensity so she could achieve the results she desired.

Case Study 2: David

David, a 57-year-old business executive, is an avid runner, cyclist, and golfer. David grew up playing baseball, football, and golf and is extremely competitive. He enjoys being active, but does not specifically train for his activities. Instead, he uses jogging, cycling, and golf as a means to stay in shape. During an ideal week, David will ride his bike three to four times, play golf twice, and run twice. His job requires travel that sometimes makes it difficult to maintain this schedule. David is a good golfer with a low handicap. He generally golfs with clients and colleagues, which includes entering corporate-sponsored tournaments, where he usually places near the top. A health club recently opened up in the same building as David's office and his company has arranged for employees to purchase discounted memberships. David has been experiencing back and knee soreness the last few times he went golfing and he has recently read numerous articles in golf publications about core exercise for golf, so he decides to take advantage of the new health club to begin an exercise program to enhance his golf game. In addition, David is planning to complete a century (100 mile) bike ride in four months with some friends and wants to aim for completing the event in under 6.5 hours (~15.4 mph average speed). David visits his doctor for annual check-ups and is in great health, with the exception of occasional muscle and joint soreness that he attributes to his active lifestyle. Before joining the health club, David checked with his doctor and received a full medical clearance for exercise.

Phyllis is an ACE-certified Personal Trainer at the new health club and conducts the complimentary fitness session that David receives as part of his membership. While reviewing his health-risk appraisal form, Phyllis asks David about his specific goals, which he identifies as getting in better shape for golf and cycling. Phyllis asks David how often he plays golf and when he feels the back soreness, and how often he rides and for what distances. David tells Phyllis about the knee and low-back soreness that he feels occasionally after running or after two consecutive days of playing golf, and indicates that he thinks some of the golf-specific strength-training workouts he has read about recently could improve his fitness for golf. He says that he generally rides three days most weeks—completing one- to three-hour rides on Saturday and Sunday, with a third ride mid-week that is generally one hour long. Phyllis tells David that she can help him improve his flexibility and core strength, which could have a direct impact on his golf game, in addition to helping him improve his strength and endurance for his cycling event. As a result of the conversation, David decides to invest in a series of 20 training sessions with Phyllis for the express purpose of improving his golf game and preparing for the 100-mile bike ride. They schedule the first training session, during which Phyllis plans to conduct some specific exercise assessments to determine David's current level of fitness. Table 12-9 presents David's health-risk appraisal data.

Table 12-9

David: Health-risk Appraisal

Age	57
Height/ weight	5'11"/172 lb (1.8 m/78 kg)
Exercise history	Has exercised on most days of the week, alternating between jogging, cycling, and playing golf, for 25 years. Tries to run when on business trips, but sometimes his schedule does not allow for it.
Medical history	Client is in good shape. Complains of occasional low-back and knee discomfort related to his activities, but it is not severe so he has not sought medical attention.
Risk factors	Resting heart rate: 54 bpm Blood pressure: 122/80 mmHg No history of high cholesterol or high blood pressure—client attributes his higher than normal blood pressure to the coffee he drank on the way to the session (the appointment was at 6:30 a.m.)

Note: bpm = Beats per minute

Training to improve his performance in golf is one of David's primary goals, so Phyllis decides to use a number of assessments to check David's flexibility and identify any possible muscle imbalances that she can address in his exercise program. Golf requires mobility in the hips, thoracic spine, and shoulders, as well as stability in the deep core muscles. Phyllis decides to use the assessments that will provide her with the most information about those areas. A postural assessment and modified hurdle step test will evaluate potential muscle imbalances and overall postural instability, while Apley's scratch test (shoulder flexion/extension, internal/external rotation), and the trunk rotation test will identify potential upper-extremity mobility issues. The passive straight-leg raise and the Thomas test will identify mobility issues in the lower body. Core endurance tests, along with the core function test, will assess David's core fitness. Finally, Phyllis will administer the submaximal talk test using a cycle ergometer (stationary bicycle) instead of a treadmill, to match David's training and goal specificity and determine his HR at VT1 for individualized training based on this metabolic marker. Table 12-10 presents Phyllis's notes.

Because David is competitive and active, he is extremely motivated to follow an exercise program, especially one that will enhance his performance for golf and prepare him for his 100-mile bike ride. Phyllis identifies that as a long-time regular exerciser, David is in the **maintenance** stage of change. She will start working with David two times a week to strengthen his core and improve his flexibility. The only barriers to David's **adherence** are his work and travel schedules. David admits that if he schedules the time for his exercise, he is extremely consistent about doing it, which is one reason why he wants to work with a trainer. He knows that if the appointment is in his schedule, he will follow through on the commitment. David did not identify weight loss as one of his goals, so Phyllis decides to focus on designing an exercise program that will increase his cardiorespiratory fitness level for cycling and enhance his golf-specific strength and flexibility.

Table 12-10
David: Trainer's Assessment Notes

Assessment	Results	Observations
Posture	Slight ankle pronation (both feet) Internal knee and hip rotation (both legs) Forward-rounded shoulders	Foot position creates instability and the potential internal rotation may exacerbate knee and hip issues during his golf swing, running, and possibly even his cycling. His rounded shoulders may alter healthy mechanics in the shoulder girdle.
Modified hurdle step test	Ankle pronation of the stance leg Slight torso sway during the leg movement Slight anterior pelvic tilting in the raised-leg position	Possible instability within his kinetic chain due to his inability to prevent pronation Possible core instability due to torso sway Possible tightness in his hip flexors preventing posterior rotation of the pelvis during the leg raise
Trunk rotation test	Good rotation to the left side, limited rotation to the right side	Rotation to the left side is good, but right-side rotation is limited, which could limit his golf backswing. Client needs to improve thoracic mobility.
Apley's scratch test Shoulder mobility test	Right shoulder: Can reach halfway down medial border of left scapula Left shoulder: Can barely reach the superior-medial border of the right scapulae	Client notices tightness in left shoulder when performing the assessment
Shoulder flexion test Shoulder extension test	Right arm can lie flat on the ground. Left shoulder cannot flex to 180 degrees.	When David tries to force his left shoulder flat, it causes his lumbar spine to go into extension. Both shoulders demonstrate adequate ROM during extension.
Shoulder internal rotation Shoulder external rotation	Right: The right shoulder demonstrates limitations in external rotation, but internal rotation is okay. Left: The left shoulder demonstrates less external rotation than the right shoulder; internal rotation is within normal limits.	The shoulder assessments identify that David needs to work on his shoulder mobility, because golf performance depends on flexibility through the thoracic spine and shoulders.
Core function assessment	Not successful at recruiting his TVA to reduce the pressure on the cuff.	Client needs to retrain the TVA and do core stabilization training.
Passive straight-leg raise test	Right: Flexibility limited to approximately 75 degrees Left: Flexibility limited to approximately 75 degrees.	Client notices tightness in both of his hamstrings as he attempts the assessments. As the client moves beyond 75 degrees with either leg, the lumbar spine moves into flexion.
Thomas test	Right: Femur stays in slight flexion Left: Femur stays in flexion, slightly more than right	Client cannot keep either femur flat on the table; when he tries to keep the femur on the table, the lumbar spine moves into extension.
Flexor endurance test	Maintained trunk flexion for 1 minute and 20 seconds	Client exhibits adequate flexor endurance
Back extensor test	Held trunk extension for 50 seconds	Has a flexor:extensor ratio of 1.6; noticed that his low back became sore at the end of the assessment
Lateral endurance—right side	Held right side bridge for 40 seconds	Is stronger on right side, but it was difficult to maintain the position for the duration of the test The right-side bridge:extension ratio is 0.8
Lateral endurance—left side	Held left side bridge for 25 seconds	Did not have good strength or endurance in the left-side core muscles The left-side bridge:extension ratio is 0.50 Needs to work on strength and endurance of oblique and core muscles
Submaximal talk test on cycle ergometer to find HR at VT1	Talk-test threshold was identified at an HR of 145 bpm, his HR at VT1	David demonstrated good cardiorespiratory fitness; will design a workout program to enhance aerobic efficiency

Note: TVA = Transverse abdominis; HR = Heart rate; VT1 = First ventilatory threshold; bpm = Beats per minute

Phyllis has identified that David will need to start in the first phase of program design for functional movement and resistance training—stability and mobility—to address his postural and core instability, and his flexibility issues. Because David has good cardiorespiratory fitness, Phyllis is going to design his program to emphasize aerobic efficiency (phase 2). In addition to the training sessions, she recommends that David try to include one indoor cycling class to incorporate additional cycling time into his training, and start taking beginner yoga to improve his flexibility. Phyllis teaches one of the cycling classes, so she can instruct him on the set up and use of an indoor cycling bike. David likes the fact that the club offers early-morning classes and that he can schedule specific times for his workouts based on the class schedule. He agrees to try to make the classes a part of his routine, and says that he will try to complete one strength-training workout per week on his own. David is health conscious and attempts to make healthful food choices, but is not always able to do so due to the demands of his schedule. He sometimes has to skip meals or eat late at night.

Functional Movement and Resistance Training—Phase 1: Stability and Mobility Training

Due to David's weak core musculature and ROM limitations in the hips and shoulders, Phyllis will start David with a phase 1 program focused on developing stability and mobility. Phyllis will train David in this phase until he demonstrates effective strength in his core muscles and improved ROM in the hips. Phyllis tells David that if he follows her suggestions, he will spend about four weeks in this phase and could start seeing improvements in his golf game sooner than that.

- *Frequency:* David will train twice per week with Phyllis and try to complete one workout per week on his own. He will also try to attend one beginner yoga class per week.
- *Intensity:* The first phase of the program will focus on using bodyweight and isometric contractions to enhance the strength and stability of the core muscles.
- *Type:* Based on his goals and assessment results, Phyllis advises David that his exercise program will focus on improving his core strength and muscular strength and endurance, while also addressing the flexibility of his hips, back, and shoulders.
- *Time:* Each workout should last approximately one hour, including a five-minute warm-up of cycling on a stationary bike and a 10-minute cool-down consisting of static stretching of the hip flexors, adductors, and extensors, as well as the back, chest, and calves.

Table 12-11 presents David's stability and mobility training program.

David will start with two sets of each exercise with rest intervals of 60 seconds. As David adapts to the exercises and progresses through the training program, Phyllis will increase the volume to three sets of each exercise and reduce the length of the rest intervals so that David begins to do all of the exercises in a circuit format, moving from one exercise to the next with only brief recovery periods until the end of the circuit. To improve David's adherence to the program, Phyllis will teach him how to do a modified version of the workout when he has to travel for work.

Cardiorespiratory Training—Phase 2: Aerobic-efficiency Training

David is a regular exerciser who already has a strong aerobic base. Since his goals are focused on achieving a strong performance (sub-6.5 hour ride) in a century ride that is four months away, his cardiorespiratory training will focus first on building aerobic efficiency and then progress to building **anaerobic** endurance to help him reach his goal. Phyllis introduces David to the three-zone training model and explains that he will begin with his training in zones 1 and 2, and will then progress in about six weeks to working in all three zones. Phyllis sets David's zone 1 training HR at 10 bpm below his HR at VT1, which was determined to be 145 bpm, giving him a zone 1 training HR range of 135 to 144

Table 12-11

David: Functional Movement and Resistance Training Phase 1—Stability and Mobility Training

Exercise Selection	Intensity	Repetitions	Rest Interval	Sets
Cat-camel	Bodyweight	10–12	30–60 seconds	2–3
Pelvic tilts, progress to supine bent-knee marches	Bodyweight	12–15	30–60 seconds	2–3
Birddog	Bodyweight	12	30–60 seconds	2–3
Plank	Bodyweight	1 (15–30 second hold)	30–60 seconds	2–3
Side plank	Bodyweight	1 per side (10–20 second hold)	30–60 seconds	2–3
Shoulder (glute) bridge with pelvic tilt	Bodyweight	12–15	30–60 seconds	2–3
Supine arm lifts in various positions (I, Y, W, O); progress to standing and then stability ball (progress to prone)	Bodyweight	2–4 per position	30–60 seconds	2–3
Thoracic spine mobilization exercises: spinal twists	Bodyweight	2–4 per side	30–60 seconds	2–3
Triplanar closed kinetic chain weight shifts (for scapulothoracic joint)	Bodyweight; progress hand positions	2–4 per plane	30–60 seconds	2–3
Hip flexor mobility progression: half-kneeling triplanar stretch	Bodyweight	1 in each plane (hold >15 seconds each)	30–60 seconds	2–3

Note: 1 RM = One-repetition maximum

bpm. Phyllis then sets David's initial zone 2 HR range at 10 bpm above HR at VT1, for a zone 2 training HR range of 145 to 155 bpm. To help David better gauge his efforts on the bike, Phyllis teaches him how to use RPE (0 to 10 scale) to gauge his intensity in zone 1, where his efforts should be "moderate" (RPE = 3) to "somewhat hard" (RPE = 4), and zone 2, where his efforts should be "hard" (RPE = 5 to 6). She also suggests that he invest in a heart-rate monitor to help him stay within the recommended heart-rate zones during his workouts, especially during indoor cycling classes. Table 12-12 presents David's aerobic-efficiency training program.

Table 12-12

David: Cardiorespiratory Training Phase 2—Aerobic Efficiency

Warm-up	Workout	Cool-down
Slow cycling for 8–10 minutes, gradually building the pace/intensity	Outdoor cycling: Ride at a steady-state in zone 1 with HR within 10 bpm of HR at VT1 (145 bpm): HR range = 135 to 144 bpm. Can also use perceived exertion of "moderate" to "somewhat hard" (RPE = 3 to 4) Indoor cycling classes: Cycle in zone 1 (HR range = 135 to 144 bpm) during the warm-up, cool-down, and all recovery intervals, and cycle in zone 2 during higher-intensity intervals with HR ranges up to 10 bpm above VT1 (HR range = 145 to 155 bpm). Can use perceived exertion of "hard" (RPE = 5 to 6) for all zone 2 intervals.	Gradually slow the pace of cycling to let the heart rate fall to <100 bpm Static stretching of hip flexors, hip adductors, hamstrings, and calves

Note: HR = Heart rate; bpm = Beats per minute; VT1 = First ventilatory threshold

Functional Movement and Resistance Training—Phase 2: Movement Training

David enjoys exercising in the morning with the group classes and likes working with Phyllis, but finds that he has a tough time making it to the club when he does not have a specific activity scheduled. David has made progress with his workouts and demonstrates improvements in both his core conditioning and flexibility, so Phyllis decides it is time to progress him to movement training (phase 2). Phyllis will keep David in this phase until he demonstrates effective and efficient control of the five basic movement patterns. Phyllis estimates that David will spend four to six weeks in this phase.

- *Frequency:* David wants to increase to training three times per week with Phyllis, since he has a hard time making it to the health club on his own. However, Phyllis's schedule is full at the times that David wants to train, so she enlists the help of one her colleagues, Darrell, who agrees to train David one time per week following Phyllis's program. David enjoys the beginner yoga class when he can fit it into his schedule. His flexibility is improving, but he will stay in the beginner class for now.
- *Intensity:* The intensity will increase through the introduction of movement-training exercises, with progressions that move from body weight training to the addition of light resistance (e.g., medicine balls, cables)
- *Type:* The focus of the exercise selection for the next phase of David's program is to integrate muscle coordination for the basic movement patterns, while improving his thoracic rotation and hip mobility for golf and enhancing his muscular strength and endurance for his cycling trip.
- *Time:* Each workout should last approximately one hour, including the warm-up and cool-down.

Table 12-13 presents David's movement-training program.

Table 12-13

David: Functional Movement and Resistance Training Phase 2—Movement Training

Exercise Selection	Intensity	Repetitions	Rest Interval	Sets
Dynamic warm-up • Cat-camel • Plank • Side plank • Single-leg shoulder (glute) bridge with knee to chest	Bodyweight	12–15 (1 for planks; hold for 30–60 seconds each)	90 seconds (after all four exercises)	2–3
Hip hinge (progress to a single-leg hip-hinge)	Bodyweight	12–15	30 seconds	2–3
Squats (neutral stance, then add foot variations)	Body weight; progress to medicine ball	12–15	30–60 seconds	2–3
Prone lies on stability ball with torso movements	Bodyweight	12–15	30 seconds	2–3
Supine and seated scapular packing exercise	Bodyweight	12–15	30 seconds	2–3
Half-kneeling wood chop; progress to cables	Bodyweight; progress to 65% 1 RM	12–15	30 seconds	2–3
Half-kneeling hay bailer; progress to cables	Bodyweight; progress to 65% 1 RM	12–15	30 seconds	2–3
Standing two-arm cable press	65% 1 RM	12–15	30–60 seconds	2–3
Standing two-arm cable rows	65% 1 RM	12–15	30–60 seconds	2–3
Lunges with arm drivers • Forward • Side • Rotational	Bodyweight	10 (each direction)	30–60 seconds (after circuit of all 3 lunges)	2–3
Dumbbell shoulder presses	65% 1 RM	12–15	30–60 seconds	2–3

Note: 1 RM = One-repetition maximum

Cardiorespiratory Training—Phase 3: Anaerobic-endurance Training

After working on his aerobic efficiency for six weeks, David has shown great progress and is now completing four sets of five-minute zone 2 intervals with a 1:1 work-to-recovery interval ratio one day per week. He has also progressed the time of his long ride to four hours and 30 minutes. He is now completing approximately eight to nine hours of cycling per week, including the indoor cycling class, and is ready to progress to the anaerobic-endurance training phase (phase 3), where exercise programming can utilize the three-zone cardiorespiratory-training model.

Phyllis has David perform another submaximal talk test to determine if his HR at VT1 has changed. She also has him perform the VT2 threshold test to determine his **second ventilatory threshold (VT2).** Both tests were conducted using the cycling ergometer that was used during his initial submaximal talk test. His HR at VT1 is determined to now be 147 bpm and his average HR during the final five minutes of the field test for VT2 is 168 bpm, which Phyllis multiplies by 0.95 to find his HR at VT2 (160 bpm). Phyllis then establishes new HR ranges for David to use when training in zone 1 (136 to 146 bpm), zone 2 (147 to 159 bpm), and zone 3 (≥160 bpm). Phyllis also explains that when performing intervals in zone 3, David should generally be at a perceived effort of "very hard" (RPE = 7) and occasionally "very, very hard" (RPE = 8).

David has 10 weeks until the century bike ride that he wants to complete in under 6.5 hours. The primary challenges related to this event will be feeling relatively strong during the entire ride, improving pacing to work toward a sub-6.5 hour effort for 100 miles, and improving David's ability to climb short hills and recover, as the ride is on a course with many hills that will take one to five minutes to climb. As such, Phyllis designs a 10-week program consisting of three **mesocycles,** each lasting three weeks, with weeks 1 and 2 focusing on increasing the total training volume and week 3 focusing on recovery from the previous two weeks. Each week will include one long ride, one zone 2 interval day focused on improving pacing between VT1 and VT2, and one zone 3 interval day focused on higher intensity, shorter (1- to 3-minute) intervals to improve anaerobic endurance and recovery between short anaerobic efforts. Due to David's travel schedule, interval sessions can be performed during indoor cycling classes to help him fit these important workouts into his routine. The total training volume during each week will be distributed among the three zones as follows:

- Zone 1 = 80% of total training volume
- Zone 2 = 10% of total training volume
- Zone 3 = 10% of total training volume

The total 10-week program will have increasing time and intensity during weeks 1 and 2, 4 and 5, and 7 and 8, with recovery weeks of decreased time and intensity during weeks 3, 6, and 9. Week 10 will be a taper week prior to the century ride. Coupled with the recovery during week 9, David should be very fit and recovered for this event. Table 12-14 presents David's anaerobic-endurance training program during weeks 4 through 7.

Conclusion

This exercise program demonstrates a possible progression for a client who is self-motivated to exercise and has specific goals, but has difficulty making time for exercise unless he has a scheduled appointment with a personal trainer. David had poor core stability and flexibility, so Phyllis started him at the stability and mobility phase for functional movement and resistance training. This program also demonstrates how the cardiorespiratory-training phases of the ACE IFT Model can be used to help an athlete—recreational or highly competitive—train for peak performance at a specific event.

Case Study 3: Jan

Jan is a 17-year-old female athlete who plays high school volleyball and basketball and is a member of a traveling volleyball club. Her positions are outside hitter (volleyball) and forward (basketball).

It is the spring of Jan's junior year in high school, just after the end of the high school volleyball season. She is still practicing and playing with her club volleyball team. Jan's high school coach is encouraging her to improve her strength and power so that she

Table 12-14

David: Cardiorespiratory Training Phase 3—Anaerobic Endurance

Training Parameter	Week 4—Increase Intensity	Week 5—Increase Intensity	Week 6—Recovery Week	Week 7—Increase Intensity
Training volume	Total time = 10 hours	Total time = 11 hours	Total time = 8 hours	Total time = 12 hours
Zone 1 (~80% of volume) 2–3 workouts per week plus warm-up, cool-down, and rest intervals (during zone 2 and 3 workouts)	1 time/week Long ride = 5 hours 1 time/week 60-minute ride (RPE = 4) 1 time/week (optional) 45-minute ride (RPE = 3)	1 time/week Long run = 5 hours 30 minutes 1 time/week 75-minute ride (RPE = 4) 1 time/week (optional) 60-minute ride (RPE = 3)	1 time/week Long run = 4 hours 1 time/week 60-minute ride (RPE = 4)	1 time/week Long run = 6 hours 1 time/week 90-minute ride (RPE = 4) 1 time/week (optional) 60-minute ride (RPE = 3)
Zone 2 (~10% of volume) 1 workout per week (can substitute indoor cycling class during travel weeks)	3 x 5-minute intervals 1:1½ work:rest ratio 50-minute workout with warm-up and cool-down	3 x 7-minute intervals 1:1½ work:rest ratio 65-minute workout with warm-up and cool-down	2 x 8-minute intervals 1:2 work:rest ratio 60-minute workout with warm-up and cool-down	3 x 8-minute intervals 1:1 work:rest ratio 65-minute workout with warm-up and cool-down
Zone 3 (~10% of volume) 1 workout per week (can substitute indoor cycling class during travel weeks)	2 sets: 3 x 90-second intervals 1:3 work:rest ratio 10 minutes between sets 60-minute workout with warm-up and cool-down	2 sets: 3 x 2-minute intervals 1:3 work:rest ratio 10 minutes between sets 70-minute workout with warm-up and cool-down	2 sets: 2 x 3-minute intervals 1:3 work:rest ratio 10 minutes between sets 60-minute workout with warm-up and cool-down	2 sets: 3 x 3-minute intervals 1:3 work:rest ratio 10 minutes between sets 80-minute workout with warm-up and cool-down
Strength training	Circuit training 2 days/week 1 hour/session	Circuit training 2 days/week 1 hour/session	Circuit training 1 day/week 1 hour/session	Circuit training 2 days/week 1 hour/session

will be a good candidate for college scholarships during her senior year. Jan's coach has told her that she needs to work specifically on her upper-body strength, vertical jump, and agility. Jan has experienced shoulder soreness, but has no chronic medical issues. The doctor has attributed Jan's shoulder soreness to overuse and recommended that she rest and strengthen her rotator cuff muscles to handle all of the volleyball she is playing. Jan is hesitant to take time off from playing, but agrees to take a month off from her club team to focus on strengthening her shoulders.

Even though Jan is a competitive athlete, she has a difficult time focusing on strength training because she finds it "boring." She is motivated to train to improve her chances at a scholarship, but has to work around her school schedule as well as the practice and competition schedule for her club volleyball team. The team practices twice each week and plays weekend tournaments twice a month.

Jan's parents put her in touch with Oscar, an ACE-certified Personal Trainer who works at their health club and specializes in strength and conditioning for sports, and has experience working with high school athletes. Oscar agrees to work with Jan twice a week in an effort to improve her volleyball performance. Jan will be attending a two-week volleyball camp beginning the third week in July and will be on a week-long family vacation during the second week of August. Jan's school starts again after Labor Day. Practice for her high school volleyball team will not start again until October, so she will be able to train with Oscar until then. Oscar schedules the first appointment with Jan and her mother to go through her health history and to determine her specific goals for training. Table 12-15 presents Jan's health history.

Table 12-15

Jan: Health-risk Appraisal

Age	17
Height/weight	5'9"/140 lb (1.75 m/64 kg)
Exercise history	A competitive two-sport athlete (high school and club leagues); has practice or competitions on most days of the week. Exercises to stay in shape for her sports.
Medical history	In very good shape. Complains of occasional shoulder discomfort related to the repetitive motion of hitting a volleyball. She has seen her doctor, who did not find any medical complications and recommended she strengthen her rotator cuff muscles.
Risk factors	Resting heart rate: 60 bpm Blood pressure: 114/70 mmHg No history of high cholesterol or high blood pressure—her father has type 1 diabetes and had a minor heart attack last year when he was 50

Note: bpm = Beats per minute

Jan tells Oscar what her coaches have told her that she needs to improve her jumping ability and upper-body strength to be more competitive for a scholarship. She indicates that she is motivated to train, especially if it will help her increase her chances of a scholarship, but is concerned that it will take away from her social life with her friends. Oscar knows that she is in the action stage of change as it relates to her volleyball seasons, and that her barriers include her school schedule and her social life. Oscar knows that to keep Jan focused on her program he will have to demonstrate that she is making progress. He plans on using regular testing and assessments as a way to keep her motivated.

Oscar will use a number of assessments to measure Jan's current fitness and skill levels so that he can track her ongoing progress. The schools that will be evaluating Jan want to see specific results in a variety of fitness categories, so Oscar will design a program to improve her overall conditioning level as well as prepare her for the fitness tests she will see as she prepares for college. The initial assessments will measure lower- and upper-body flexibility, lower-body strength using a free-weight leg press, power using the vertical jump test, core muscular endurance, upper-body strength on a free-weight chest press, anaerobic endurance with the 300-yard shuttle run, and the ability to change direction while running with the pro agility test. The results of the tests will be used to monitor the progress of the program and, since she is competitive, she will be reassessed once a month as a way to let her compete against her previous results.

Jan has not identified weight loss as one of her goals. Although she expresses concern about gaining weight and becoming too muscular, she is looking forward to developing more power and strength. Oscar is sensitive to the issues that female athletes face with body image, so he purposely does not take Jan's body composition or circumference measurements and will instead use the scores of her fitness assessments to measure her progress. Jan tells Oscar that she is conscious about what she eats, but admits to enjoying fast food while hanging out with her friends. Oscar does not want Jan to become fixated on her weight, so he explains the need to properly fuel for the workouts and reminds her that she should eat immediately after training so she can recover and prepare for the next session or competition. Table 12-16 presents Oscar's notes.

Jan's assessments show that she has very good core stabilization, strength, and, with the exception of some restriction in her

Table 12-16

Jan: Trainer's Assessment Notes

Assessment	Results	Observations
Trunk rotation	Slightly more than 45 degrees of rotation in both directions	Jan has good thoracic rotation, but has a tendency to sit and stand with a slouched posture.
Apley's scratch test Shoulder mobility	Right: Excellent ROM, can reach to the inferior-medial border of her left scapula (this is her dominant hitting arm for striking in volleyball). Left: Good ROM, not as much as the right, but can easily reach the medial border of her right scapula	Very good shoulder mobility when she maintains good posture, but her tendency to slouch can restrict her ROM
Shoulder flexion test Shoulder extension test	Both arms can easily lie flat on the floor while reaching overhead and demonstrate good ROM in extension, with the right shoulder having just a little more mobility.	Client displays good shoulder mobility
Shoulder internal rotation test Shoulder external rotation test	Both shoulders demonstrate good ROM for internal rotation. The right shoulder does not reach all the way to the ground in the external rotation test—possible tight internal rotators, which could be related to the shoulder soreness.	A combination of poor posture and tight internal rotators could be the cause of the soreness in the right shoulder. Will address these issues with stretching and strengthening in the exercise program.
Passive straight-leg raise test	Can easily move both legs past 90 degrees of hip flexion while maintaining a stable, neutral pelvis.	Client has good hip/hamstrings mobility
Thomas test	The femurs of both legs easily lie flat along the table, but the left knee does not drop straight down and maintains a position of slight extension.	Her left quadriceps is tighter than her right. She is a right-handed hitter, so she jumps more off of her left leg than her right.
Flexor endurance test	Able to hold a flexed position for 1 minute and 55 seconds	Flexor:extensor ratio of 0.88
Back extensor test	Able to hold the extended position for 2 minutes and 10 seconds	
Lateral endurance test—right side	Held right side position for 50 seconds	Said that her shoulder got sore from being in that position Right side bridge:extensor ratio of 0.38
Lateral endurance test—left side	Held left side position for 40 seconds	Differential of 0.20 between right and left sides. Her right side is dominant. She needs to balance core strength. Left side bridge:extensor ratio of 0.31 Due to strength-related conditioning for her two competitive sports, she has good core stabilization.
Leg press strength test	Warm-up: 95 lb (43 kg) for 2 sets of 12 repetitions with a 2-minute rest interval Test: 180 lb (82 kg) for 6 repetitions Her strength-to-weight ratio = 210 lb/140 lb = 1.5 Her score ranks her in the 60th percentile	180 lb (82 kg) x 6 repetitions = 210 lb (95 kg) maximum
Bench press strength test	Warm-up: 55 lb (25 kg) for 2 sets of 10 repetitions with a 2-minute rest interval Test: 85 lb (39 kg) for 4 repetitions Her strength-to-weight ratio = 95 lb/140 lb = 0.68 Her score ranks her in the 63rd percentile	85 lb (39 kg) x 4 repetitions = 95 lb (43 kg) maximum

Continued on next page

Table 12-16 *continued*

Jan: Trainer's Assessment Notes

Assessment	Results	Observations
Vertical jump test	Three trials: 15 inches (38 cm) 16 inches (41 cm) 16 inches (41 cm)	Squats into her knees when she jumps; does not generate power from her hips. Currently ranks in the 30th percentile in the vertical jump for NCAA women; she needs to get better to improve her chance of earning a scholarship.
300-yard shuttle run	Completed in 65.5 seconds	Her score puts her in the 50th percentile of NCAA women volleyball players. Decent for a high school junior, but increasing her speed, agility, and quickness will strengthen her chances for a scholarship.
Pro agility test (20-yard shuttle)	Three trials: 5.2 seconds 5.15 seconds 5.10 seconds	Jan had never run this test before, but got faster with each trial. Her score puts her in the 30th percentile for NCAA women volleyball players; it needs to improve.

Note: ROM = Range of motion; NCAA = National Collegiate Athletic Association

right shoulder, good flexibility. Jan needs to work on her strength, power, speed, agility, and quickness, all of which college teams will evaluate during the recruiting process. During her vertical jump test, Jan was performing the countermovement (downward movement prior to jumping) by flexing her knees (quad-dominant) before flexing her hips, so Oscar will start her strength-training program in the movement-training phase (phase 2) to teach her the proper movement mechanics of using the hips during squats and jumps. Volleyball is a sport that relies on the anaerobic energy system to develop speed and power, so Oscar will try to progress Jan to phase 4 (performance training), where her workouts will include a variety of speed, agility, and quickness drills and have Jan perform jump rope intervals when they are not training together in effort to work on her foot quickness. Jan scored relatively low in the vertical jump test, so Oscar will make sure to progress her program to include **plyometric** jump training.

Functional Movement and Resistance Training— Phase 2: Movement Training

Jan's program will begin in phase 2 to help her develop proper movement patterns prior to loading them with heavier external resistance. Oscar will keep Jan in this phase of training until she demonstrates that she can control the ROM and perform the five basic movements with coordination and strength. Oscar will focus on teaching Jan how to effectively use her hips to generate power for jumping and agility movements.

- *Frequency:* Jan is taking a month off from competing with her club team to focus on her strength training. She will work with Oscar three days per week, and will join her club for their conditioning practice one day a week.
- *Intensity:* The goal is to focus on strength and endurance for the basic movement patterns, so Jan will be using enough resistance for 12 to 20 repetitions.
- *Type:* The exercise selection will focus primarily on bodyweight exercises, but medicine balls, dumbbells, cables, and resistance tubing will be used when and where appropriate.
- *Time:* The workouts will last approximately one hour, including a five-minute warm-up of walking on a treadmill and a 10-minute cool-down consisting of static stretching of the shoulders, upper back, chest, hip flexors, hip adductors, hip extensors, and calves.

Table 12-17 presents Jan's movement-training program.

Table 12–17

Jan: Functional Movement and Resistance Training Phase 2—Movement Training

Exercise Selection	Intensity	Repetitions	Rest Interval	Sets
Dynamic warm-up • Plank • Side plank • Glute bridge; progress to single-leg glute bridge • Birddog • Single-leg balance with arm drivers	Bodyweight and medicine balls	10–12 (1 for planks; hold for 30–60 seconds each)	Circuit training with 90 seconds rest	2–3
Hip hinge	Bodyweight	12–15	30 seconds	1–2
Body weight squats; add arm drivers (triplanar)	Bodyweight	12–15	30 seconds	1–2
Prone arm lifts (I, Y, W, O); progress to stability ball	Bodyweight	2–4 per position	30–60 seconds	1–2
Wood chops (standing)	Bodyweight; progress to 3-kg (~6.5-lb) medicine ball	12–15	30 seconds	2–3
Hay bailers (standing)	Bodyweight; progress to 3-kg (~6.5-lb) medicine ball	12–15	30 seconds	2–3
Seated bilateral overhead dumbbell press; progress to unilateral	65% 1 RM	12–15	30–60 seconds	2–3
Push-ups with a plus	Bodyweight	To fatigue	30–60 seconds	2–3
Seated bilateral cable pull-downs, progress to unilateral	65% 1 RM	12–15	30–60 seconds	2–3
Triplanar lunges, progress with arm drivers	Bodyweight	12–15	30–60 seconds	2–3
Shoulder internal and external rotations with tubing	65% 1 RM	12–15	30–60 seconds	2–3

Note: 1 RM = One-repetition maximum

To help condition Jan's anaerobic energy system as the workout intensity increases, Oscar will reduce the time of the rest intervals and progress Jan to circuit training.

After four weeks of training, Oscar put Jan through the same fitness assessments that he conducted during their initial meeting. Jan demonstrates improvements in the following areas:

- Upper-body strength and flexibility
- Core strength and endurance
- Lower-body strength and power
- Agility
- 300-yard shuttle run

Jan is motivated by her progress and, now that she has improved her upper-body strength, will start playing with her club volleyball team again. Based on the results of her reassessments, Oscar progresses Jan to load training (phase 3).

Functional Movement and Resistance Training—Phase 3: Load Training

Oscar recommends that this phase last for at least eight weeks and plans on testing again in four weeks to measure Jan's progress and make any necessary adjustments to her program. Jan is scheduled to attend a volleyball skills camp in eight weeks, so the short-term goal is focused on helping her develop strength and mobility for the camp.

- *Frequency:* Jan has been doing conditioning drills with her club team once a week and will start practicing and playing with them again during this phase. Oscar will train Jan three times a week when she does not have a tournament on the weekend and will train her two times during the weeks when she does have a tournament.

- *Intensity:* Oscar will implement strength-training protocols and will estimate 75% of her **one-repetition maximum (1 RM)** by using loads that cause muscular fatigue by the tenth repetition. After the initial four weeks of this phase—and once reassessments have taken place—Oscar will increase the load so Jan fatigues by the sixth repetition.
- *Type:* The exercise selection will focus on integrated movements involving both upper- and lower-body muscles. Oscar selects exercises that will strengthen movement patterns specific to Jan's volleyball position and will add in plyometric exercises once she progresses to phase 4 (performance training).
- *Time:* Oscar teaches Jan a dynamic warm-up routine that she can do on her own so that they can focus on resistance training during their time together. Each session should last one hour, including 10 minutes of static stretching of the shoulders, upper back, chest, hip flexors, hip adductors, hip extensors, and calves. The exercises in the dynamic warm-up, which Jan will perform before her session with Oscar begins, will provide an adequate warm-up and will continue to facilitate proper movement patterns learned during movement training (phase 2).

Table 12-18 presents Jan's load-training program.

As Jan adapts to the workload and training volume of this phase, Oscar will again reduce the time of the rest intervals and incorporate more circuit training in an effort to help condition her anaerobic energy systems. Oscar is helping Jan improve her strength, but by structuring her workouts in a circuit-training format, he is also helping her improve her ability to perform at a high work rate and

Table 12-18

Jan: Functional Movement and Resistance Training Phase 3—Load Training

Exercise Selection	Intensity	Repetitions	Rest Interval	Sets
Dynamic warm–up • Plank • Side plank • Birddog • Bodyweight squats • Single-leg hip hinge • Medicine ball wood chops and hay bailers • Lunge matrix	Bodyweight Medicine balls	10–12 (1 for planks; hold for 30–60 seconds each)	Bodyweight exercises comprise one circuit with 90 seconds of rest between each circuit	2–3
Dumbbell raise in scapular plane	75% 1 RM	10–12	60–90 seconds	2–3
Single-leg step-ups with dumbbells	75% 1RM, 6-inch (15-cm) step	10–12	60–90 seconds	2–3
Front squat	75% 1 RM	10–12	60–90 seconds	2–3
Dumbbell incline press	75% 1 RM	10–12	60–90 seconds	2–3
Dumbbell pull-overs	75% 1 RM	10–12	60–90 seconds	2–3
Forward lunges	75% 1 RM	10–12	60–90 seconds	2–3
Side lunges	75% 1 RM	10–12	60–90 seconds	2–3
Reverse dumbbell flys	75% 1 RM	10–12	60–90 seconds	2–3
Chair dips	75% 1 RM	10–12	60–90 seconds	2–3

Note: 1 RM = One-repetition maximum

recover rapidly during the rest intervals, which should translate well to sport-specific fitness for volleyball and basketball.

Oscar conducts two different testing sessions with Jan during the load-training phase to monitor her progress. Jan again shows consistent improvements in:

- Upper-body strength and flexibility
- Core strength and endurance
- Lower-body strength and power
- 300-yard shuttle run

At the conclusion of the eight weeks of load training, Jan went to the skills camp, where she impressed the coaches and other players with her improved strength and power. Once Jan returns from her volleyball camp, Oscar will progress her training sessions to the performance-training phase (phase 4) to help her prepare for her senior season of volleyball.

Functional Movement and Resistance Training—Phase 4: Performance Training

Oscar plans the workouts to gradually progress intensity until one week prior to the start of the season. Jan will then have a week off for active recovery before she begins practice.

- *Frequency:* Oscar and Jan will continue the training schedule of three times on non-tournament weekends and two times during tournament weekends until the end of the club season. Once Jan's club volleyball season ends, she will train with Oscar three times a week and work out twice a week on her own, doing moderate-intensity cardiorespiratory exercise to enhance her aerobic base for improved endurance and recovery.
- *Intensity*: Jan's dynamic warm-up will begin with bodyweight and medicine-ball strength exercises and progress to agility drills and medicine-ball throws. The workout will focus on plyometric jumps (to improve her vertical jumping ability) and explosive exercises. The volume will start with three sets per exercise and progress to five sets per exercise as she becomes more efficient in the exercise movement patterns.
- *Type:* Exercise selection focuses on plyometric jumps and explosive lifts to enhance her activation of fast-twitch muscle fibers.
- *Time:* Jan will continue to start the dynamic warm-up on her own so she and Oscar can focus on the challenging jumps and lifts during the training sessions. Each session should last one hour, including 10 minutes of static stretching of the shoulders, upper back, chest, hip flexors, hip adductors, hip extensors, and calves. The exercises in the dynamic warm-up, which Jan will perform before her sessions with Oscar begin, will provide an adequate warm-up.

Table 12-19 presents Jan's performance-training program.

Table 12-19

Jan: Functional Movement and Resistance Training Phase 4—Performance Training

Exercise Selection	Intensity	Repetitions	Rest Interval	Sets
Dynamic warm-up • Medicine ball wood chops • Lunge with trunk rotation • Inchworms • Bear crawls • High-knees • Medicine-ball throw sequence • Skip sequence	Bodyweight Medicine balls	10–12 for chops 10-meter distance for agility drills 6–8 for throws	Circuit training with 90 seconds of rest	2–3
Jumps to box	Bodyweight 12-inch (30-cm) box	4–6	1 minute	2–3
Single-leg jumps to box	Bodyweight 6-inch (15-cm) box	4–6	1 minute	2–3
Depth jumps	Bodyweight 12-inch (30-cm) box	4–6	1 minute	2–3
Hang cleans	50% 1 RM	4–6	3 minutes	3–5
1-arm kettlebell snatches	50% 1 RM	4–6	3 minutes	3–5
Dumbbell push-jerks	50% 1 RM	4–6	3 minutes	3–5
Triceps press-downs	80% 1 RM	8	30–60 seconds	2–3

Note: 1 RM = One-repetition maximum

Conclusion

Thanks to Oscar's help, Jan enters the senior season of her high school volleyball career having greatly improved her agility, jumping power, and anaerobic fitness. Jan improved her vertical jump by 4.5 inches (11 cm), lowered her time in the agility test by half a second, and reduced her time in the 300-yard shuttle by six seconds, making her a much more attractive candidate for a college scholarship.

Case Study 4: Stanley

Stanley is a 28-year-old male who works as a software designer by day and enjoys playing interactive video games by night. The only activity that Stanley does is yard work and other chores around the house and the occasional walk around the neighborhood with his wife, who just found out she is pregnant with their first child. Otherwise, Stanley is **sedentary** and has no history of adhering to an exercise program as an adult. While growing up, Stanley considered himself to be non-athletic and consequently did not participate in many sports or unstructured play activities. Stanley's low self-efficacy toward exercise has carried over into his adulthood and is the reason why he has never made exercise a priority. Exercise makes him feel uncomfortable and brings back negative memories from his childhood. Now that his wife is pregnant with their first child, she is encouraging Stanley to stop smoking and become healthy so they can enjoy life with their child. At his recent physical, Stanley's doctor told him that he was at risk for the **metabolic syndrome** and strongly recommended that he begin an exercise program to improve his health. The combination of expecting his first child, the encouragement from his wife, and his current state of health is the motivation behind his interest in starting an exercise program. Stanley recently joined his wife's health club, where she takes **Pilates** and yoga classes on a regular basis. His goals are to lose weight and improve his health; he will also try to quit smoking, eat better, and develop more effective methods of managing his stress.

When joining the health club, Stanley took advantage of a special offer to buy a series of 20 personal-training sessions. The sales consultant wants to see Stanley achieve his goals, so she introduces him to Toby, an ACE-certified Personal Trainer who earned his certification and changed his career after losing 100 pounds (45 kg). Stanley likes the fact that he will be working with a trainer who has experience in losing a lot of weight, because it helps reduce the intimidation that he feels about going to a gym. Toby and Stanley schedule an initial appointment so that Toby can conduct a full health-risk assessment (Table 12-20), and have Stanley sign a liability waiver and informed consent.

Table 12-20
Stanley: Health-risk Appraisal

Age	28
Height/weight	5'10"/245 lb (1.8 m/111 kg)
Exercise history	Occasional walks with his wife or does chores around the house, but no consistent exercise program
Medical history	At a recent check-up, he was found to be at risk for the metabolic syndrome. His physician recommended that he begin an exercise program to lower his weight and improve his health and provided him with a prescription for exercise as tolerated with no contraindications for exercise listed.
Risk factors	Resting heart rate: 74 bpm Blood pressure: 138/82 mmHg BMI: 35 kg/m^2 Smoker: "about a pack a day" Sedentary

Note: bpm = Beats per minute; BMI = Body mass index

Upon reviewing Stanley's information, Toby thanks Stanley for bringing the physician's release and tells him that by losing weight he should be able to decrease his risk for metabolic syndrome. Toby recognizes that because Stanley has purchased a membership along with the accompanying training sessions, he has recently transitioned to the **preparation** stage of behavior change, and will need assistance to develop adherence to a regular exercise program. Because he prefers interactive gaming and junk food over exercise, Stanley readily acknowledges that he is **overweight** and out of shape. Toby decides not to subject him to fitness assessments that will only reaffirm his current lack of fitness and decides to have him start his exercise program right away (since he has provided the medical clearance to do so). Toby knows that since Stanley has not followed an exercise routine, it is more important to have him start on a low-to-moderate intensity exercise program to help him develop adherence and favorable behavior patterns than to put him through a barrage of assessments that will just reinforce the fact that he is in poor shape.

During their first training session together, Stanley admits to Toby that he might have a difficult time staying committed to the program because his work schedule is dictated by product launch timelines, which means that he often works nights and weekends.

When Toby asks Stanley about his nutritional choices, Stanley confesses that while his wife is relatively health-conscious and tries to keep healthy food in the house, he likes to drink sodas and snack while playing interactive video games and will buy these for himself. Stanley tells Toby that he will often skip the lunches she prepares for him in favor of what he considers better-tasting fast-food options. Toby explains that diet and proper nutrition play a major role in losing weight and maintaining a healthy weight for the long run. Toby does not recommend any specific diet, but educates him on portion size and provides strategies for food selection and preparation to help him adopt a more healthful diet. Toby admitted that he used to eat fast food for almost every meal and that one of the main factors behind his weight loss was taking the time to prepare his own meals and make healthful food choices. Toby tells Stanley that if he can lower his caloric intake and increase his energy expenditure by a combined 500 calories a day, he will be well on the way to losing weight at a rate of approximately 1 pound per week. Toby points out that a 20-ounce bottle of soda and a small bag of potato chips each have over 200 calories, so if Stanley could play video games without snacking and cut out at least three fast-food meals a week, then he would be making a very important change that will help him reach his weight-loss goal.

Functional Movement and Resistance Training—Phase 1: Stability and Mobility Training

Toby starts Stanley's exercise program with a focus on stability and mobility. Not only does Stanley need to work on his core strength and flexibility, but more importantly, Toby knows that he has to provide Stanley with easily achievable initial goals that can help him develop a sense of accomplishment. This will help Stanley develop long-term adherence to his exercise program. From his own experience, Toby is sensitive to the fact that Stanley needs exercises that he can do successfully and not ones that will "kick his butt," making him sore and only reinforcing his poor level of fitness. Toby recorded Stanley's blood pressure, **resting heart rate (RHR),** and bodyweight, but did not have him perform any physical assessments. Once Stanley shows the initial adherence and physical improvements, Toby will increase the intensity of his workouts.

- *Frequency:* Although he is serious about following through on the exercise program, Stanley has recently been placed on a project at work that will take up a lot of his time. Toby is sensitive to the time challenge, so he and Stanley agree to meet twice a week for 30-minute sessions. In addition, Toby provides Stanley with a copy of the program so he can make an effort to exercise twice a week on his own. The 30-minute sessions provide Toby enough time to coach Stanley through a basic core-stabilization routine with exercises that are challenging, but are not too much in terms of time commitment or level of difficulty. When Stanley demonstrates that he can adhere to the 30-minute exercise sessions and his schedule opens up, Toby will increase the intensity of the programs by progressing to one-hour training sessions and design a program that Stanley can complete on his own in 45 minutes or less.

- *Intensity:* Stanley's workouts feature bodyweight exercises that emphasize core stabilization.
- *Type:* The primary goal is to help Stanley feel comfortable with exercise so that he develops adherence to his program. Therefore, exercise selection focuses primarily on bodyweight.
- *Time:* The initial workouts with Toby are only 30 minutes in duration, so Stanley is encouraged to arrive early to perform five minutes of walking on the treadmill as a warm-up. Toby also teaches Stanley some stretches to do on his own at the conclusion of the workout. These static stretches focus on the shoulders, upper back, chest, hip flexors, hip adductors, hamstrings, and calves.

Table 12-21 presents Stanley's stability and mobility training program.

Cardiorespiratory Training—Phase 1: Aerobic-base Training

Toby recommends that Stanley try to walk at least three times per week with his wife for an initial duration of 10 to 15 minutes at a "moderate" intensity (RPE = 3). Toby tells Stanley that the goal of these walks is to develop a walking routine that they can enjoy together now, throughout his wife's pregnancy, and after their child is born.

The initial phase of the program is designed to be low intensity to help Stanley feel comfortable with exercise. Given that Stanley is a video game enthusiast, Toby suggests that Stanley invest in an interactive fitness video game bundle so he can combine exercise with his preferred hobby. Stanley thinks this is a good idea because it will give him an opportunity to exercise when he cannot make it to the health club, plus it will be an opportunity to do something active with his wife while still participating in his favorite hobby.

At the six-week point of the program, Toby points out to Stanley that he has cancelled almost a third of their scheduled training sessions and that if Stanley is serious about reaching his goals he needs to have more commitment to the program. Stanley has been trying to exercise in the evening after work, but given his workload and deadlines it is sometimes challenging to get out of work in time to make it to the health club. Stanley also admits to being tired at the end of the day and just wants to go home to have dinner, relax, and play video games.

Even with the sporadic adherence, Stanley has lost a couple of pounds and noticed an

Table 12-21

Stanley: Functional Movement and Resistance Training Phase 1—Stability and Mobility Training

Exercise Selection	Intensity	Repetitions	Rest Interval	Sets
Cat-camel	Bodyweight	10–12	20–30 seconds	1–2
Modified forearm planks	Bodyweight	3 (5–10 second hold)	20–30 seconds	1–2
Quadruped TVA contractions; progress to single-arm raises and single-leg raises	Bodyweight	10–12 per side	20–30 seconds	1–2
Glute bridges	Bodyweight	10–12	20–30 seconds	1–2
Pelvic tilts; progress to supine bent-knee marches	Bodyweight	10–12	20–30 seconds	1–2
Reverse flys with supine 90-90	Bodyweight	2–4	20–30 seconds	1–2
Thoracic spine mobilization: prisoner rotations	Bodyweight	2 per side	20–30 seconds	1–2

Note: TVA = Transverse abdominis

increase in both his strength and energy, so he tells Toby that he will make an effort to be more committed to the workouts. Toby points out that a major barrier to Stanley's adherence is his unpredictable work schedule, which makes going to the gym tough in the evening. Consequently, he makes the recommendation that Stanley consider switching his workouts to the morning so he can complete them before work. Stanley claims that it will be difficult waking up that early, but decides he will try the morning workouts. Stanley tells Toby he has been changing his dietary habits to include healthful snacks, which he admits take some getting used to, along with cutting back on his trips to fast-food restaurants. Toby congratulates Stanley on these changes, indicates that those could be the primary drivers for his initial weight loss and energy changes, and encourages him to keep up the good work.

Toby and Stanley agree to a morning schedule and stay with the 30-minute sessions to help Stanley make the transition to the earlier wake-up times. Three weeks after the switch to the morning schedule, Stanley has not missed one session and finds that he likes exercising in the morning. Toby decides to increase the duration of his program to one-hour sessions and progress to the next phase of training. Along with his gym workouts, Stanley has been using the fitness video games quite a bit and has found that he enjoys the games and the friendly competition with his wife.

Toby asks Stanley about his smoking. Stanley replies that he has been doing his best not to smoke, but admits to still having an occasional cigarette with a buddy at work. Stanley already feels better from the exercise program, his dietary changes, and reduced smoking, but admits that with all of the changes he has made to this point he occasionally finds himself craving a cigarette. Toby congratulates Stanley on the progress and acknowledges his accomplishments to date. He does not chastise Stanley about the smoking and instead encourages him to do his best to focus on his program and his goals. Toby wants to support and encourage the positive behavior rather than be punitive and focus on repercussions for smoking the occasional cigarette. This strategy helps Stanley focus on the positive benefits of following a consistent exercise program rather than the negative effects of non-adherence.

Functional Movement and Resistance Training— Phase 2: Movement Training

Toby will keep Stanley in this phase of training until he demonstrates that he can complete the basic movement patterns with control through the full ROM.

- *Frequency:* Stanley likes the progress he has made to date, so he invests in another 20 training sessions with Toby and stays with the morning schedule. In addition to his scheduled training sessions, Stanley will make an effort to make it to the gym at least one additional time during the week to work out on his own in addition to walking with his wife.
- *Intensity:* During the movement-training phase, Toby will teach Stanley how to control his own bodyweight through the basic movements of exercise. In addition to bodyweight exercises, Toby challenges Stanley with equipment such as medicine balls, dumbbells, and cable machines. The emphasis of this phase is on developing muscular strength and endurance through the movement patterns, so the intensity is enough to allow 12 to 15 repetitions.
- *Type:* Exercise selection focuses on the basic movements of exercise: squats, lunges, pushes (both in the horizontal plane and overhead), pulls, and rotational movements.
- *Time:* Now that Stanley's adherence has improved, he and Toby meet for one-hour training sessions, which include a warm-up of five to 10 minutes of treadmill walking and a cool-down consisting of static stretches for the shoulders, upper back, chest, hip flexors, hip adductors, hamstrings, and calves.

Stanley has lost 10 pounds (4.5 kg) and is interested in seeing how his fitness has improved. Before beginning the next phase of training, Toby schedules a session to conduct some assessments to track Stanley's ongoing progress. At the beginning of the program, Toby did not want to do any assessments because he did not want to embarrass or intimidate Stanley. After working with Toby for a while and experiencing some initial results, Stanley actually asks Toby to measure his **body fat** so he can learn what it is. In addition to the body-composition measurement, Toby selects the core muscular endurance test, push-up test, bodyweight squat test, and passive straight-leg raise. Toby will use the results of these assessments to measure the effects of Stanley's exercise program. Once Stanley can see how much he has improved in these categories, it will help him maintain long-term adherence to the program. Table 12-22 presents Stanley's movement-training program.

Cardiorespiratory Training—Phase 1: Aerobic-base Training (Progression)

Stanley has progressed to the action stage of behavior change and is making exercise a regular habit. Until now, the only cardiovascular exercise that Stanley has been doing is the warm-ups for his workouts, the frequent walks that he has been taking with his wife, and playing the Wii Fit®. Toby begins incorporating more cardiorespiratory exercise into Stanley's program by showing him how to use the elliptical machine, treadmill, and stationary bike. Toby adds 15 to 20 minutes of cardiorespiratory exercise on the machine of Stanley's choice to his cool-down following his training sessions. Stanley indicates that he is enjoying the walks with his wife, so Toby teaches him how to use the RPE scale so he can work on his aerobic-base training by working at a perceived effort that

Table 12-22

Stanley: Functional Movement and Resistance Training Phase 2—Movement Training

Exercise Selection	Intensity	Repetitions	Rest Interval	Sets
Birddog	Bodyweight	12	30 seconds	2–3
Plank	Bodyweight	One 15-second hold	30 seconds	2–3
Side plank	Bodyweight	One 10-second hold	30 seconds	2–3
Glute bridges; progress to single-leg with alternate knee to chest	Bodyweight	15	30 seconds	2–3
Single-leg balance with arm and leg drivers	Bodyweight	10–12	30 seconds	2–3
Hip hinges	Bodyweight	10–12	30 seconds	2–3
Bodyweight squats	Bodyweight	12–15	30 seconds	2–3
Seated bilateral chest press—selectorized machine	65% 1 RM	12–15	60 seconds	2–3
Seated bilateral pull-downs—selectorized machine	65% 1 RM	12–15	60 seconds	2–3
Step-ups	Bodyweight	10–12	60 seconds	2–3
Seated bilateral overhead press—selectorized machine	65% 1 RM	12–15	60 seconds	2–3
Kneeling wood chops and hay bailers; spiral pattern progressing to full pattern	Bodyweight, progressing to 3-kg (~6.5-lb) medicine ball	12–15	60 seconds	2–3

Note: 1 RM = One-repetition maximum

is "moderate" (RPE = 3) and progressing to "somewhat hard" (RPE = 4). Toby asks Stanley to begin increasing the time of his walks by two minutes each week until they are 25 to 30 minutes in length; then Toby can progress Stanley to phase 2 (aerobic-efficiency training).

Conclusion

This is an example of how to use the ACE IFT Model to develop a program to help a sedentary adult begin an exercise program. Stanley did not have a history of exercise or being active, but Toby was able to meet him at his current state of fitness and design a program that allowed him to be successful and slowly change his behavior to make regular exercise a habit.

Case Study 5: Meredith

Meredith is a 64-year-old grandmother who recently retired from a career in business. She is an active older adult who was the vice president of a large corporation. Meredith enjoys walking, aquatic exercise classes, and playing with her two grandchildren (five- and eight-year-old boys). Her hobbies also include playing golf and tennis. She is extremely competitive and has played in her club's tennis league for a long time, but has not done so recently due to a demanding pre-retirement work schedule and her sore knees. She enjoys exercise and used to work with a personal trainer twice a work for the purpose of staying in shape and being fit for her tennis matches. The trainer got married and moved away two years ago and, even though Meredith was referred to another trainer, she never followed up because she became too busy at work.

Meredith has gained approximately 15 pounds (6.8 kg) during the last two years, which she attributes to her busy schedule and her lack of regular workouts with a trainer. Now that she is retired from her fast-paced career, Meredith is ready to begin working with a new personal trainer. Recently, Meredith was diagnosed with **osteoarthritis** in her knees and hips. Her doctor has given her written clearance for exercise as tolerated and told her that if she lost the weight she has gained and resumed her former activity levels, it should reduce the effects of the arthritis. Meredith's goals are to reestablish a regular exercise program with a trainer to improve her health, lose weight, minimize the effects of the arthritis, and get back into shape so she can be competitive in the upcoming tennis season at her club.

When Meredith's trainer moved away two years ago, she referred Meredith to Dwight, an ACE-certified Personal Trainer at the health club. Meredith had intended to contact Dwight to begin working with him, but ended up getting too busy. Now that Meredith has retired, she wants to get herself back into shape and has contacted Dwight to begin a series of training sessions with him. Meredith appreciates the value of working with a personal trainer and has heard very good things about Dwight from her former trainer. She invests in a series of 30 sessions to jump-start her fitness program.

Dwight schedules an initial appointment with Meredith to conduct a health-risk appraisal and some basic fitness testing (Table 12-23). Dwight knows Meredith from the health club and knows her

Table 12-23

Meredith: Health-risk Appraisal

Age	64
Height/weight	5'5"/158 lb (1.65 m/84 kg)
Exercise history	Normally very active with golfing, cross-country skiing, tennis, water aerobics, weight training, and walking. Used to work with a personal trainer 2–3 times per week, but the trainer moved away and Meredith became busy at work, so she has not followed a consistent routine for approximately two years. For the last two years, she has been consistent with walking and water aerobics, but not any of her other exercise routines.
Medical history	Recently diagnosed with osteoarthritis, she is approximately 15 pounds (7 kg) overweight. She had surgery on her low back a number of years ago and recently it has been bothering her; not painful, just noticeable.
Risk factors	Resting heart rate: 66 bpm Blood pressure: 124/80 mmHg BMI: 26 kg/m^2

Note: bpm = Beats per minute; BMI = Body mass index

competitive reputation in tennis, so he wants to use the fitness assessments as a way to have Meredith compete against herself to help her adhere to her program. Meredith has exercised regularly for years, and while she did not have time for working with a trainer over the past two years, she was still fairly consistent with water aerobics and walking. Dwight identifies her stage of behavior change as preparation, because she is in the process of resuming her former regular exercise habits, but is yet to follow a regular program for any period of time. Her primary barrier to maintaining a regular exercise program is her schedule. Even though Meredith recently retired, she serves on the boards of two different charities and has an extensive social schedule. She also enjoys traveling, which she wants to do more of now that she has time.

The initial assessments were the upper- and lower-body flexibility tests, core muscular endurance test, and submaximal talk test to determine her HR at VT1, all of which are important components related to Meredith's goal of being a competitive tennis player. Table 12-24 presents Dwight's notes from the assessments.

Table 12-24

Meredith: Trainer's Assessment Notes

Assessment	Results	Observations
Trunk rotation	Had more motion rotating to the right than rotating to the left	Asymmetrical motion between right and left rotation
Apley's scratch test Shoulder mobility	Right hand could easily reach the top of the left scapula; left hand could barely reach the top of the right scapula	Asymmetrical motion between right and left shoulders
Shoulder flexion test Shoulder extension test	Both arms were able to lie flat on the floor. Each shoulder had a symmetrical ROM in the extension test.	There was a little movement in the lumbar spine as the arms reached full overhead flexion.
Core function assessment	Demonstrated effective core function	Indicated that her previous trainer had her do a lot of core work
Passive straight-leg raise test	Right leg barely made it to 90 degrees; the left leg easily made it slightly beyond 90 degrees	Asymmetrical flexibility in the hips
Thomas test	Both legs lay flat along the table, but the right knee stayed in a position of extension during the test.	Asymmetrical flexibility in the knee extensors
Flexor endurance test	Maintained position for 150 seconds	Performed well in back extensor test; mentioned that her back fatigues after a long day of golf Flexor:extensor ratio of 0.83 (150/180)
Back extensor test	Held back extensor position for 180 seconds	
Lateral endurance—right side	Maintained right-side balance (RSB) for 88 seconds	Has a RSB:LSB ratio of 0.96 (88/92), a differential score of only 0.04 from 1.00
Lateral endurance—left side	Maintained left-side balance (LSB) for 92 seconds	
Submaximal talk test to determine HR at VT1	Using a treadmill due to her consistent walking, determined HR at VT1 to be 134 bpm	Use this HR to set heart-rate ranges for exercise in zones 1 and 2.

Note: ROM = range of motion; VT1 = First ventilatory threshold; HR = Heart rate

Functional Movement and Resistance Training—Phase 2: Movement Training

Since Meredith exhibited good core stability and joint mobility during her initial assessments, Dwight decides to start her in the movement-training phase of functional movement and resistance training (phase 2). She will work in this phase until she demonstrates good strength and control through the movement patterns.

- *Frequency:* Meredith has the time to meet with Dwight two times a week. In addition to the training sessions, Meredith plans on doing one aquatic exercise class each week, walking two to four times per week with her neighbor for approximately 30 minutes, as well as playing tennis and golf at least one day per week each.
- *Intensity:* The emphasis of this phase is on developing muscular strength and endurance through the movement patterns, so the intensity will be enough to allow 12 to 15 repetitions. Meredith will use bodyweight, medicine balls, stability balls, tubing, and cable machines for the resistance-training exercises.
- *Type:* Exercise selection focuses on the basic movements of exercise: squats, lunges, pushes (both in the horizontal plane and overhead), pulls, and rotational movements. Meredith showed a couple of asymmetries during the assessments that will be addressed in the course of the training program.
- *Time:* Meredith and Dwight meet for two one-hour exercise sessions per week, during which the focus is on strength and flexibility training. Each one-hour session includes a warm-up circuit that focuses on core conditioning and a cool-down that features static stretches for the hips, calves, chest, back, and shoulders.

Table 12-25 presents Meredith's movement-training program.

Table 12-25

Meredith: Functional Movement and Resistance Training Phase 2—Movement Training

Exercise Selection	Intensity	Repetitions	Rest Interval	Sets
Dynamic warm-up: • Cat-camel • Glute (shoulder) bridges • Forearm planks • Side planks • Birddog	Bodyweight	10–12 (1 for planks; hold for 30–60 seconds each)	30 seconds	2–3
Triplanar dynamic movement patterns: single arm, single leg, and integrated arm/leg	Bodyweight	10–20 (per side)	30 seconds between sets	1–2
Step-up to balance	Bodyweight	10–12	30 seconds	2–3
Kneeling wood chops; progress to standing	Bodyweight	12–15	45–60 seconds	2–3
Kneeling hay bailers, progress to standing	Bodyweight	12–15	45–60 seconds	2–3
Hip hinge	Bodyweight	12–15	45–60 seconds	2–3
Seated bilateral cable chest press; progress to standing	60% 1 RM	12–15	45–60 seconds	2–3
Seated bilateral cable pull-downs; progress to standing	60% 1 RM	12–15	45–60 seconds	2–3
Prone arm lifts (W-I-T-Y); progress to standing with hip hinge	Bodyweight	2–4	45–60 seconds	2–3
Forward lunges; progress with arm drivers and then lateral and rotational lunges	Bodyweight	10–12 each direction	45–60 seconds	2–3

Note: 1 RM = One-repetition maximum

Cardiorespiratory Training—Phase 2: Aerobic-efficiency Training

Even though Meredith stopped working with a trainer and has not followed a regular weight-training routine for almost two years, she has maintained her aerobic fitness through walking and aquatic exercise. Therefore, Dwight will begin her cardiorespiratory-training program with aerobic-efficiency training (phase 2). To alleviate any potential discomfort with her knees, Dwight will have Meredith perform most of her cardiorespiratory training on an elliptical machine or stationary bicycle. Dwight performed Meredith's submaximal talk test on a treadmill due to her consistent walking exercise, and determined her HR at VT1 to be 134 bpm. Based on this result, Dwight sets her exercise heart rate range at 124 to 133 bpm for zone 1 training and 134 to 144 for exercise in zone 2.

Meredith will do the cardiovascular work on her own when she is not training with Dwight. Meredith's initial program focuses on increasing her aerobic efficiency, so Dwight wants her to maintain an average heart rate below 134 bpm for a majority of the training. Once she completes a five-minute warm-up, Meredith works at a steady-state intensity below an HR of 134 bpm, with short-duration intervals that take her to a perceived exertion of "hard" (RPE = 5 to 6) with her HR between 134 and 144 bpm to help her increase her aerobic efficiency. Meredith mentions that she finds using cardiovascular machines "boring," so Dwight recommends that Meredith complete 15 minutes of training on the elliptical machine and then 15 minutes of cycling on a stationary bicycle for variety.

Functional Movement and Resistance Training—Phase 3: Load Training

Once Meredith demonstrates that she can successfully complete the basic movements of exercise with skill and coordination, Dwight will progress her to the load-training phase. Another reason for the progression is to help Meredith develop the necessary muscular strength to be competitive in recreational tennis tournaments. Meredith does not like the fact that she did not play tennis regularly for two years, so she is focused on getting in shape to win. Increasing her muscular strength will help her achieve that goal. Dwight will have Meredith work in this phase until she has made significant gains and is ready to progress to the performance-training phase (phase 4).

- *Frequency:* Meredith continues seeing Dwight for two training sessions to prepare for the tennis season. She also starts playing tennis two or three times each week.
- *Intensity:* The emphasis of this phase is on developing muscular strength, so Dwight uses loads that fatigue Meredith in eight to 12 repetitions. The purpose of this phase is to enhance muscle-force production in preparation for increasing the velocity of force production as she progresses.
- *Type:* Exercise selection focuses on developing strength in the movement patterns most commonly used primarily for tennis, with a secondary focus on golf and cross-country skiing.
- *Time:* Meredith and Dwight meet for two one-hour exercise sessions, during which the focus is on increasing muscle-force production. Each one-hour session includes a dynamic warm-up circuit, as well as a cool-down consisting of static stretching of the hips, calves, shoulders, chest, and back.

Table 12-26 presents Meredith's load-training program.

Cardiorespiratory Training—Phase 2: Anaerobic-endurance Training (Progression)

Meredith has found that using two different pieces of cardiovascular equipment does keep her from getting bored, so when Dwight mentions that it is time to progress her program, she asks him to recommend another piece of equipment so she can do a mini-triathlon for her aerobic-fitness training. Dwight recommends that Meredith

Table 12-26
Meredith: Functional Movement and Resistance Training Phase 3—Load Training

Exercise Selection	Intensity	Repetitions	Rest Interval	Sets
Dynamic warm-up—Stability ball circuit: • Hip bridges • Crunches • Russian twists • Planks • Prone arm lifts (W-I-T-Y)	Bodyweight on stability ball	10–12 (1 for planks; hold for 30–60 seconds each) 2–4 for prone arm lifts	60–90 seconds after the circuit	2–3
Lunge matrix	Bodyweight	1 in each direction	45–60 seconds	2–3
Kneeling wood chops; progress to standing	2-kg (~4.5-lb) medicine ball	12–15	45–60 seconds	2–3
Kneeling hay bailers; progress to standing	2-kg (~4.5-lb) medicine ball	12–15	45–60 seconds	2–3
Dumbbell squat to 90-degree knee bend	70% 1 RM	8–12	2 minutes	3–4
Standing one-arm cable row	70% 1 RM	8–12	2 minutes	3–4
Step-ups with dumbbell onto 6-inch (15-cm) step	70% 1 RM	8–12 (each leg)	2 minutes	3–4
Rotational dumbbell shoulder presses	70% 1 RM	8–12	2 minutes	3–4
Modified (assisted) pull-ups	Bodyweight	8–12	2 minutes	3–4
Dumbbell bench press	70% 1 RM	8–12	2 minutes	3–4

Note: 1 RM = One-repetition maximum

start doing intervals with two-minute work intervals in zone 2 (HR = 134 to 144), followed by four-minute recovery intervals in zone 1 (HR <134). After working up to four of these intervals, Meredith progresses by first decreasing the recovery interval to three minutes; then decreasing the recovery interval to two minutes; and then increasing both the work and recovery intervals to three minutes for a set of four intervals. Dwight teaches Meredith how to use a Stepmill machine and recommends that she increase her training time to 45 minutes so that she can spend 15 minutes on each piece of equipment.

Functional Movement and Resistance Training—Phase 4: Performance Training

Meredith enjoys the challenge of the weight training. After seven weeks, she feels that she has her old fitness level back. At first, Meredith was concerned that weight training would increase her weight and size, but Dwight explained that women do not produce the amount of **testosterone** necessary for developing large amounts of muscle mass. Meredith enjoys the weight training and can feel the impact on the court, where her shots have a lot more power and she does not get tired as easily during a longer match.

There are only two months before the competitive tennis league begins at Meredith's club, so Dwight helps her prepare by progressing the intensity of the training to the performance-training phase. The prior phase improved Meredith's ability to generate muscular force, and the performance phase of functional movement and resistance training will help her prepare for the competition at her tennis club by increasing her velocity of muscular force production. Dwight will progress Meredith in this phase for the two months leading up to the start of competition and maintain the intensity for the duration of the season, which is usually three months long.

- *Frequency:* Meredith plays in the competitive tennis league once a week, plays with her friends once a week, and works with a coach every other week. Meredith trains with Dwight twice a week, unless she is scheduled to meet with her coach, in which case they only meet once a week.
- *Intensity:* The emphasis of this phase is on developing muscular power. The loads are bodyweight for jumps and light resistance for the lifts and throws, so Meredith can focus on the explosive muscle action.
- *Type:* Exercise selection focuses on movements consistent with tennis, with a special focus on rotational core exercises to enhance her swinging power and racquet speed.
- *Time:* Meredith performs one or two one-hour training sessions per week. She performs a warm-up (dynamic flexibility circuit) and cool-down (static stretching for the calves, hamstrings, quadriceps, hip flexors, chest, back, and shoulder muscles) on her own so she and Dwight can focus their entire hour on performance training.

Table 12-27 presents Meredith's performance-training program.

Cardiorespiratory Training—Phase 2: Aerobic-efficiency Training (Progression)

Meredith is beginning her recreational tennis season and will be getting plenty of exercise playing tennis, but Dwight has her continue with at least one day of

Table 12-27

Meredith: Functional Movement and Resistance Training Phase 4—Performance Training

Exercise Selection	Intensity	Repetitions	Rest Interval	Sets
Dynamic warm-up, medicine ball strength circuit • Wood chops • Rotational wood chops • Side lunge • Forward lunge with reach	2-kg (~4.5-lb) medicine ball	10–12	30 seconds	2–3
Jumps in place	Bodyweight	6–8	1 minute	2–3
Lateral hops	Bodyweight	6–8	1 minute	2–3
Agility drills • T drill • Hexagon drill	Fast	3–4 each drill	1 minute	1
Medicine ball throw circuit • Rotational passes/throws • Overhead throws • Throw-downs	2-kg medicine ball	6–8	1 minute	2–3
Stability ball core circuit • Hip bridges—single-leg • Crunches—with resistance • Russian twists —with resistance • Push-ups	Bodyweight, on stability ball 2-kg (~4.5-lb) medicine ball for exercises with resistance	8–10	45–60 seconds	2–3

aerobic-efficiency training to help maintain her cardiorespiratory fitness using the three different pieces of cardiorespiratory equipment for variety. Meredith is now working on speed, agility, quickness, and power with Dwight and her tennis coach, which helps her gain the tennis-specific fitness she needs to be successful in her matches.

Conclusion

Dwight's exercise program helped Meredith regain her previous fitness levels and lose the 15 pounds (6.8 kg) she had gained since reducing her activity level after her previous trainer moved away. The explosive strength and power Meredith developed as a result of Dwight's program helped her regain her form as a competitive tennis player. Meredith also has the energy and stamina to teach her two grandsons how to play tennis and enjoys the time interacting and playing with them.

Case Study 6: Kelly

Kelly is a 30-year-old professional woman preparing for her wedding. She is an active career woman who wants to get in shape and look great for her wedding day. She has not played sports since she was a kid and does not consider herself an athlete. She enjoys socializing with her friends and spending evenings out with her fiancé. Ever since she graduated from college almost eight years ago, she has been exercising sporadically and finds it easy to make excuses or do things other than go to a gym. Generally, Kelly is comfortable with her body. When she does exercise, it is primarily because she enjoys her social life and wants to be able to eat and drink without being too concerned about gaining weight. She has a health club membership and wants to work out more often, but usually lets other things like work and her social life interfere. She does enjoy being active in terms of walking, hiking, and dancing at nightclubs with her friends on the weekends, but she is concentrating on her corporate career and finds it challenging to maintain a consistent exercise schedule during the week. When Kelly does make it to the health club, she generally takes exercise classes like indoor cycling, Latin dance, step, yoga, or "ab training." She uses the cardiovascular equipment, but finds weights to be intimidating. She wants to exercise to lose weight and fears that strength training will only "bulk her up."

Kelly's wedding is four months away, and she wants to look great in her dress. Kelly has read articles in women's fitness magazines that identify weight training as an effective method for burning fat, which is her primary goal when it comes to preparing for her wedding. Kelly has approached Andy, an ACE-certified Personal Trainer and Group Fitness Instructor who teaches Kelly's favorite abs class, about hiring him to train her for her wedding. Kelly felt comfortable with Andy's personality, and since she always enjoys his group fitness classes, he was her first choice when considering hiring a personal trainer. Andy agrees to help Kelly prepare for her wedding. Kelly purchases a package of 20 personal-training sessions, and Andy schedules the initial health-risk appraisal and assessment (Table 12-28).

Table 12-28

Kelly: Health-risk Appraisal

Age	30
Height/weight	5'3"/148 lb (1.6 m/67 kg)
Exercise history	Participates in group fitness classes such as indoor cycling, Latin dance, step, yoga, and "ab training"
Medical history	Kelly has type 1 diabetes—she regularly monitors her insulin levels and knows not to exercise if her blood glucose is too low. She has a physician's release for exercise as tolerated, as long as she manages her blood glucose. The physician's note lists no other contraindications.
Risk factors	Resting heart rate: 68 bpm Blood pressure: 115/64 mmHg

Note: bpm = Beats per minute

Kelly's primary goals are weight loss and muscular development. The assessments Andy selects for Kelly include assessments for posture, core function, and hip mobility. He also measures her body composition and waist-to-hip ratio. Table 12-29 presents Andy's notes.

Table 12-29
Kelly: Trainer's Assessment Notes

Assessment	Results	Observations
Posture	Stands with lordosis posture	Lordosis appears to stem from anterior pelvic tilt
Body-composition assessment	28% body fat	She falls into the "average" category for body fat. Her percent fat will be useful in goal setting and to measure progress.
Waist circumference	28 inches	She falls into the low-risk category for the waist circumference. The measurement will be used to gauge progress.
Core function assessment	Change of >10 mmHg on the cuff	She possesses effective recruitment patterns of core muscles.
Passive straight-leg raise test	Both legs can move efficiently to 90 degrees.	She has symmetrical flexibility in the hip extensors.
Thomas test	Neither thigh is able to lie flat on the table; each hip stays in flexion—when they are pushed to the table it pulls her lumbar spine into extension.	She needs to improve the flexibility and extensibility of both of hip flexor muscles.

Kelly has four months to prepare for her wedding, so Andy divides her training into two distinct phases. He designs a program to address her total body strength, but with a special emphasis on the back, shoulders, and arms, because she will be a wearing an off-the-shoulder dress. Andy knows that Kelly has stayed away from resistance training because she does not want to gain weight, but he reaffirms what she has read in the magazines: that strength training is an effective component of a program for decreasing body fat. Since Kelly's primary goals are fat burning and weight loss, Andy focuses the training sessions on resistance training. Andy knows that Kelly likes the social aspect of group fitness, so he recommends that she use a combination of indoor cycling, Latin dance, and step training for her cardiorespiratory training. Early training sessions focus on teaching Kelly the basic movement patterns of exercise through movement training (phase 2).

Kelly has not always been consistent with exercise programs in the past, but she is focused on her goal of looking great for her wedding day. Therefore, Andy identifies that she is in the preparation stage of behavior change.

Functional Movement and Resistance Training—Phase 2: Movement Training

This phase of training will last six weeks, at which point Andy will progress Kelly to load training (phase 3) so she can focus on muscular development.

- *Frequency:* Kelly and Andy meet twice a week for training sessions that focus on movement training. Kelly is extremely motivated to look great for her wedding day, so in addition to the training sessions she trains on her own three to five times a week, taking a variety of group fitness classes.
- *Intensity:* The intensity focuses on Kelly's bodyweight and light resistance.
- *Type:* Kelly primarily does group fitness classes and uses the cardiovascular machines. Therefore, Andy starts her in the movement-training phase to teach her how to perform the basic movements of exercise both efficiently and effectively.
- *Time:* Andy and Kelly meet for two one-hour training sessions each week. Each session includes a warm-up of five to eight minutes of walking on a treadmill with a cool-down consisting of 10 to 15 minutes of static stretching focusing on the upper- and lower-back, chest, calf muscles, and the hip flexors, extensors, adductors, and abductors.

Table 12-30 presents Kelly's movement-training program.

Table 12-30

Kelly: Functional Movement and Resistance Training Phase 2—Movement Training

Exercise Selection	Intensity	Repetitions	Rest Interval	Sets
Glute bridges	Bodyweight	12–15	30–45 seconds	2–3
Plank	Bodyweight	One 25-second hold	30–45 seconds	2–3
Side plank	Bodyweight	One 15-second hold	30–45 seconds	2–3
Crunches	Bodyweight	12–15	30–45 seconds	2–3
Step-ups to balance	Bodyweight 6-inch (15-cm) step	10–12	30–45 seconds	2–3
Hip hinge	Bodyweight	10–12	30–45 seconds	2–3
Standing bilateral cable chest press	65% 1 RM	12–15	30–45 seconds	2–3
Prone arm lifts (W-I-T-Y); progress to incline on stability ball	Bodyweight	2-4	30–45 seconds	2–3
Side lunge	Bodyweight	12–15	30–45 seconds	2–3
Pull-ups on an assisted pull-up machine	Bodyweight	To fatigue, or a maximum of 15 repetitions	30–45 seconds	2–3
Seated bilateral dumbbell overhead press	65% 1 RM	12–15	30–45 seconds	2–3
Dumbbell biceps curls and overhead triceps extensions (superset)	65% 1 RM	15	45 seconds after both exercises	2–3

Note: 1 RM = One-repetition maximum

Kelly makes great progress and enjoys the results of the resistance training. She has found some group fitness classes that she really likes, so she has been consistent with both her resistance and cardiorespiratory exercise. When she has successfully completed four weeks of movement training, Andy progresses Kelly's workout to phase 3 of the functional movement and resistance training component so she can complete 12 weeks of load training prior to the wedding. Kelly will continue going to her favorite group fitness classes for her cardiorespiratory training. Therefore, she and Andy can specifically focus on strength training during their sessions.

Functional Movement and Resistance Training—Phase 3: Load Training

Kelly works in this phase throughout the rest of the program until her wedding.

- *Frequency:* Kelly is now working with Andy three times a week and takes group fitness classes three or four times a week to focus on aerobic calorie burning.
- *Intensity:* Load training is an effective method of enhancing lean mass and muscular appearance. Andy has Kelly progress to circuit training so that she is doing four or five exercises in a row before a rest interval. This ensures that she is not only increasing her lean muscle, but also maximizing caloric expenditure during each training session.
- *Type:* Kelly wants her shoulders and back to be the focus of her program, as they will be revealed by her wedding dress. The day after the wedding, the couple is leaving for a 10-day honeymoon. Therefore, in addition to preparing her to look great in her dress, Andy selects exercises that will help her look great on the beach.

- *Time:* Kelly will arrive early enough to perform a 10-minute general warm-up on cardiovascular equipment so that she and Andy can focus on strength training during their one-hour sessions. Each session also includes a cool down consisting of 10 to 15 minutes of static stretching focusing on the upper- and lower-back, chest, calf muscles, and the hip flexors, extensors, adductors, and abductors.

Table 12-31 presents Kelly's load-training program.

Conclusion

At the completion of the 12 weeks of load training, Kelly is looking lean and fit. She has lost 5% body fat, 2 inches (5.1 cm) off of her waist, and 3 inches (7.6 cm) off of her hips, and is feeling confident for her big day. This is an example of how the ACE IFT Model can be used to design a program for a client who has a specific goal related to muscular development and changes in body composition. It is also an example of how a trainer can provide focused functional movement and resistance training programming for a client who is highly motivated to do his or her own cardiorespiratory training through group exercise classes.

Summary

Each case study presented in this chapter provides an example of how the ACE IFT Model can be applied to real-life situations that a personal trainer might encounter during the course of his or her career. As mentioned previously, the information provided in each case study is not the only solution to that client's needs, but is instead an example of how a progressive model of exercise program design can be applied to help clients safely achieve meaningful results.

Table 12-31

Kelly: Functional Movement and Resistance Training Phase 3—Load Training

Exercise Selection	Intensity	Repetitions	Rest Interval	Sets
Dynamic warm-up—core training circuit • Plank • Side plank • Glute bridge on stability ball • Crunches on stability ball	Bodyweight and stability ball	12–15 (1 for planks; hold for 30–60 seconds each)	90 seconds after the circuit	3–4
Front squat	70% 1 RM	10–12	60 seconds	2–3
Standing squat-to-row on cable machine	70% 1 RM	10–12	30–45 seconds	2–3
Bent-over barbell rows	70% 1 RM	10–12	60 seconds	2–3
Dumbbell incline chest presses	70% 1 RM	10–12	60 seconds	2–3
Lunge circuit • Forward • Side • Rotational	Bodyweight	8 for each lunge	90 seconds after the circuit	2–3
Standing dumbbell overhead press	70% 1 RM	10–12	60 seconds	2–3
Dumbbell raise in scapular plane	70% 1 RM	10–12	60 seconds	2–3
Reverse dumbbell flys with hip hinge	70% 1 RM	10–12	60 seconds	2–3
Dumbbell biceps curl superset with dumbbell triceps extension	70% 1 RM	10–12	60 seconds after the superset	2–3

Note: 1 RM = One-repetition maximum

PART IV

Special Exercise Programming Topics

Chapter 13
Mind-body Exercise

Chapter 14
Exercise and Special Populations

IN THIS CHAPTER:

Neurobiological Foundations of Mind-body Exercise

Roots of Contemporary Mind-body Exercise Programs

Differentiating Characteristics of Mind-body Exercise

Research-supported Outcomes and Benefits of Mind-body Exercise

- Yoga Research
- Qigong and Tai Chi Research

Mind-body Exercise Modalities and Programs

- Yoga
- Qigong Exercise
- Tai Chi

Contemporary Mind-body Exercise Programs

- Pilates
- Alexander Technique
- Feldenkrais Method
- Nia
- Native American and Alaskan Spiritual Dancing

Assessing Outcomes

Indications for Mind-body Exercise

- Mind-body Exercise and Chronic Disease Management
- Mind-body Modalities and Acute Coronary Syndromes

Personal Trainers and Mind-body Exercise

Summary

RALPH LA FORGE, M.S., *is a clinical lipid specialist and managing director of the Duke Lipid Disorder Physician Education Program, Duke University Medical Center, Endocrine Division, Durham, N.C. He has worked for 30 years in clinical cardiology/endocrinology and as an instructor of exercise physiology at the University of California, San Diego. La Forge has authored more than 300 consumer and professional publications on cardiovascular disease management, applied exercise science, and preventive cardiology. He has helped organize and inaugurate cardiovascular disease risk reduction and preventive endocrinology programs for more than 450 healthcare institutions and medical groups throughout the United States, including the Department of Defense.*

CHAPTER 13

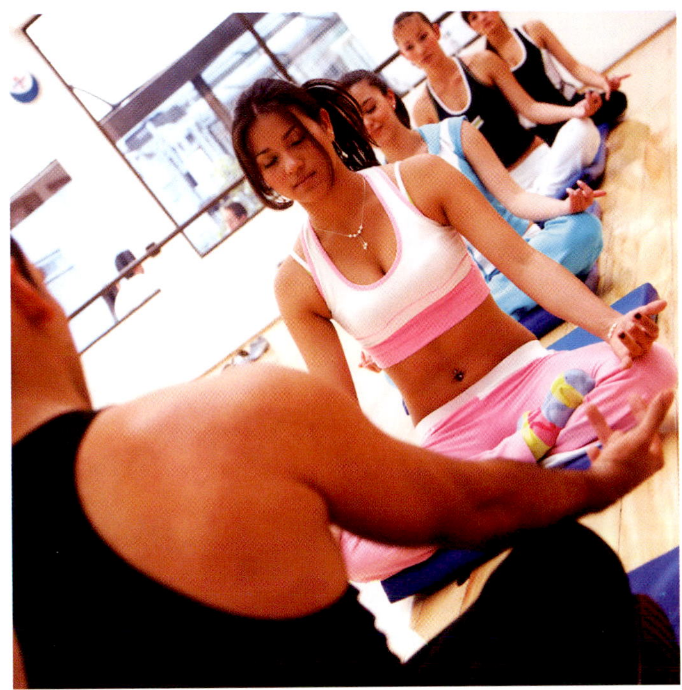

Mind-body Exercise

Ralph La Forge

Mind-body exercise programs continue to establish themselves as significant players in individual and group exercise programming. In its most unadulterated form, mind-body exercise is perhaps best characterized by low-to-moderate intensity physical activity performed with a meditative, proprioceptive, or sensory-awareness component. Clearly, any form or level of physical activity can be "mind-body," but less intense physical activity may provide a preferable platform for cognitive benefits. Mind-body exercise can also be described simply as physical exercise executed with a profound inward mental focus. This inwardly directed attention should be focused in a nonjudgmental fashion on self versus, for example, target heart rate zone or performance. Self-focus includes specific attention to breathing and **proprioception.** For example, from the viewpoint of someone who is unfamiliar with **yoga,** the popular cobra pose (see pose 7 of Figure 13-7 on page 461) may appear to be nothing more than a back extension exercise.

Nonetheless, the yogi's cognition is entirely and deeply entrained on the simple **kinesthesis** of the pose and breath-centering—nothing more and nothing less. Many clients will find these attributes beneficial in managing specific fitness and health concerns, including stress-related disorders, deterioration of musculoskeletal health, decreased **balance** control, **hypertension, depression,** and decreased self-confidence. Table 13-1 is a simple taxonomy of some of the mind-body forms of exercise that have gained considerable popularity in the West in recent years. For many, the calming/contemplative states experienced may confer health benefits, precluding the need for higher-intensity exercise for those who either cannot perform, or do not require, higher-intensity traditional exercise.

With mind-body exercise practice, the physical exercise itself can be executed with a specific choreographic movement pattern, such as in **tai chi,** or can be a free-form pattern as observed in ethnic spiritual dancing (e.g., Native American/Alaskan spiritual dancing). Regular participation in mind-body exercise has been associated with improved muscular strength, **flexibility,** balance, and coordination, but perhaps most importantly from a health promotion viewpoint, increased mental development and **self-efficacy.**

The purpose of this chapter is to briefly introduce the essential tenets of mind-body exercise, describe the more influential forms, and provide useful education, training, and research resources. It is not the intent of this chapter to disclose all that is necessary to fully appreciate or competently teach yoga, tai chi, or **qigong** exercise. Each modality addressed here requires hundreds of hours of personal exploration to attain reasonable kinesthetic proficiency and knowledge of that system's tradition. This discussion is limited to the classical and several contemporary forms of mind-body exercise.

Table 13-1

A Simple Taxonomy of Mindful Exercise Programs

Contemporary	Classical (>200-year heritage)
Feldenkrais Method	Tai chi chuan
Alexander Technique	Qigong exercise
Pilates	Hatha yoga
Laban Movement Analysis®	Spiritual and ethnic dance (e.g., Native American/Alaskan, capoeira, hula)
Integrative yoga programs (e.g., Integral yoga, Somatic yoga, Yogaflow, Viniyoga)	Some ancient martial arts (e.g., karate, judo, aikido)
Composite mind-body exercise programs (e.g., Nia, E-MOTION,® Gyrokinesis, Shatki Exercise, mind-body circuit programs, Brain Gym,® aqua tai chi, ChiBall Method,® ChiRunning,® Yogarobics)	
Tai chi chih	
Somatics	
Contemporary martial arts (e.g., tae kwon do)	
Meditation walking	
Native American yoga	

Neurobiological Foundations of Mind-body Exercise

There is intuitive neurobiological support for how and why mind-body therapies such as acupuncture, meditation, and mind-body exercise interact with important cognitive functions of the brain. The early pioneering work by such esteemed physiologists as Walter Canon (1914) and Hans Selye (1946) formed much of the foundation for understanding the neuroendocrine response to stress, which gave unprecedented clarity to brain-body interactions. This and other early investigational work became the biological template from which all mind-body and psychophysiological processes operate. However, it was not until 1972 when the scientific framework for understanding body-mind interactions was achieved when G.M. Goodwin, Ian McCloskey, and Peter Matthews carried out careful behavioral studies that demonstrated that **muscle afferents** have direct access to mechanisms of perception, and implied that there must be projections of the muscle afferent pathways to the cortex for this to occur (Goodwin, McCloskey, & Matthews, 1972). Subsequent studies have confirmed the presence of these pathways. Figure 13-1 illustrates some of the afferent muscle fiber–brain pathways that are involved in affective responses to muscular contraction dynamics (e.g., yoga **asanas**). Ascending muscle afferent pathways carry sensory information from the muscles and joints to a variety of thalamic, limbic, and cortical structures in the brain, thereby forming a body-mind conduit (i.e., affording direct access of muscular activity to the mechanisms of perception and cognition). Figure 13-2 depicts the fundamental neuroendocrine "mind-body" interactions involved with meditative and breathwork activities. Two key hormones of behavior [**corticotropin releasing hormone (CRH)** and **adrenocorticotropin hormone (ACTH)**] inextricably bond brain (hypothalamus and higher brain centers) and body (pituitary-adrenal glands) together and play an extensive role in mind-body visceral and cognitive responses. This hypothalamus–pituitary CRH interface is truly the consummate "mind-body connection."

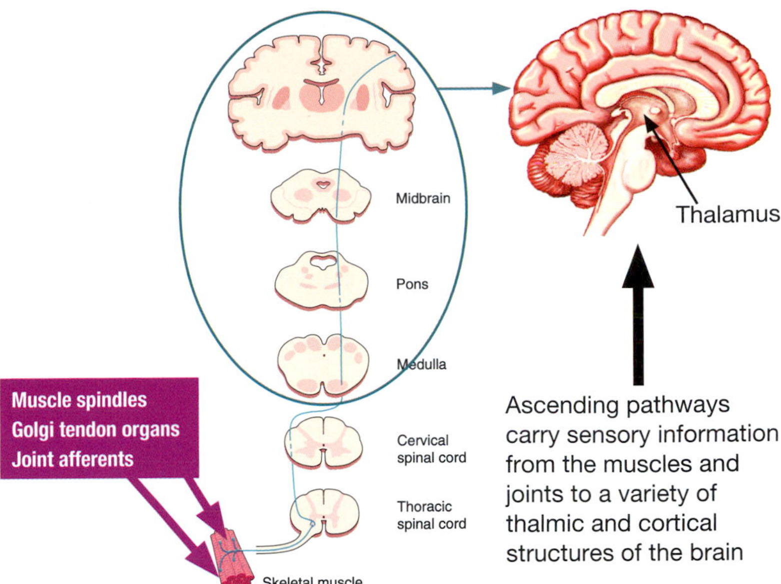

Figure 13-1
Muscle-brain pathways involved in muscle-mind responses

Source: LifeART image copyright 2008 Wolters Kluwer Health, Inc., Lippincott Williams & Wilkins. All rights reserved.

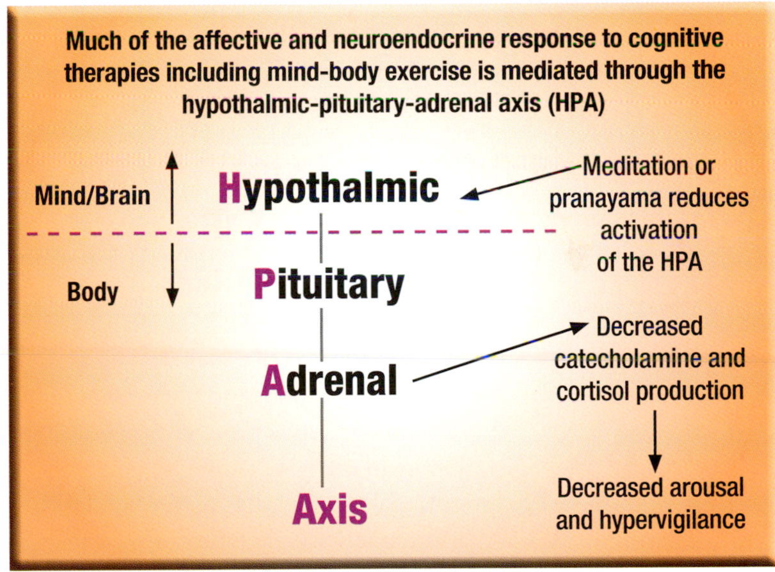

Figure 13-2
Neuroendocrine basis for mind-body responses

Roots of Contemporary Mind-body Exercise Programs

The Asian yoga and tai chi disciplines are at the root of most contemporary mind-body exercise programs taught today. These two ancient forms have intensively integrated mind and body along with an overt sense of spirituality and groundedness with nature. At the heart of all meditative practice in Asia is what Indians call yoga. Yoga is a complex system of physical and spiritual disciplines that is fundamental to a number of Asian religions (e.g., Hinduism and Buddhism). For example, classical yoga as described in the *Yoga Sutra,* an ancient text of yogic principles attributed to Patanjali, is composed of eight components, or "limbs": moral principles, observances, posture, breath control, withdrawal of the senses, concentration, meditation, and pure contemplation (Miller, 1998). Here, posture refers to yogic exercises, or asanas, that originally were used to prepare the individual for practicing breath control and meditation. In other words, yoga exercise was used as a means to an end—meditation and spiritual freedom. The physical arm of yoga, **hatha yoga,** when coupled with a meditative-contemplative component, is perhaps the most practiced form of mind-body exercise in the West today.

Tai chi has a nearly 4,000-year heritage and is derived from the practice of qigong (also called chi kung), which describes the entire tradition of spiritual, martial, and health exercises developed in China. Qigong is the primary Chinese methodology for activating the "medicine within," or the naturally occurring self-healing resource. This ancient practice is a combination of two ideas: *qi* is the vital energy of the body and *gong* is the skill of working with the qi (also called chi). Tai chi, the martial art derivative of qigong, is best described as a moving meditation. In some way, most contemporary mind-body exercise programs [e.g., **neuromuscular integrative action (Nia),** meditation walking, E-MOTION] are derived from early yoga and qigong practice.

Differentiating Characteristics of Mind-body Exercise

Mind-body exercise such as yoga and tai chi is attentive to the present moment and is process-oriented, in contrast to many, if not most, forms of conventional exercise that center on body or performance-oriented measures, such as fat-burning, body-sculpting, power output, or **target heart rate.** Mind-body exercise generally relies on self-monitoring of perceived effort, breathing, and nonjudgmental self-awareness rather than cueing entirely from an exercise leader as is experienced in conventional group exercise classes. Unquestionably, conventional aerobic and resistance-training programs can manifest each of these mind-body qualities; however, with mind-body exercise, these cognitive features are both the means and the outcome. Mind-body exercise, when taught appropriately and individually, can assist in the management of a number of chronic disease states, including **cardiovascular disease (CVD), diabetes,** and **arthritis.** Moreover, this form of activity can be readily executed at low-to-moderate exercise intensities adaptable to a wide range of functional capacities.

Research-supported Outcomes and Benefits of Mind-body Exercise

Mind-body exercise programs such as tai chi and hatha yoga generally require minimal equipment or exercise tools and can be performed in the home or outside of fitness facilities. Perhaps most importantly, they are relatively safe and provide a low-impact workout. Specific hatha yoga exercises are particularly helpful for arthritis, **asthma,** low-back pain, and postural problems, while tai chi is helpful in improving balance and motor coordination. Because of its slow contemplative nature, tai chi can help reduce **anxiety, blood pressure,** and symptoms of depression. There is a growing body of scientific evidence supporting various mind-body exercise modalities as significant means of improving a variety of health outcomes. Perhaps the most comprehensive meta-analytic review of mind-body practices, including mind-body exercise, was executed by Ospina and colleagues (2007). This review of more than 1,000 studies indicates that although many studies were inadequately designed and poorly controlled, there were clear trends in blood-pressure reduction, decreased stress-related outcomes, and reduced pain and disease symptomology. Qigong, tai chi, and yoga trials comprise approximately 95% of the research literature on mind-body exercise. Table 13-2 depicts some of the more significant research outcomes of mind-body practices, particularly hatha yoga, qigong, and tai chi, that have a reasonable volume of research support.

Table 13-2

Research-supported Outcomes and Benefits of Yoga and Tai Chi

Cardiorespiratory

- Decreased resting blood pressure
  (Yeh et al., 2008; Taylor-Piliae et al., 2006; Murugesan, Govindarajulu, & Bera, 2000; Selvamurthy et al., 1998; Channer et al., 1996)
- Increased pulmonary function
  (Malhotra et al., 2002; Birkel & Edgren, 2000; Joshi, Joshi, & Gokhale, 1992)
- Improved respiratory function in patients with asthma
  (Manocha et al., 2002; Khanam, 1996; Fluge, 1994; Jain & Talukdar, 1993)
- Increased parasympathetic tone, increased heart-rate variability
  (Vaananen et al., 2002; Bernardi et al., 2001 & 2002; Sakakibara, Tekeuchi, & Hayano, 1994)
- Improvement in baroreflex function/sensitivity
  (Bernardi et al., 2002; Selvamurthy et al., 1998; Bowman et al., 1997)
- Decreased blood lactate and resting oxygen consumption
  (Raju et al., 1994)
- Enhanced arterial endothelial function
  (Sivasankaran et al., 2006; Wang, Lan, & Wong, 2001)
- Increased maximum oxygen consumption and physical work capacity
  (Manchanda, 2000; Lan et al., 1998 & 1999; Lai et al., 1993)
- Regression of coronary artery disease
  (Yogendra et al., 2004; Manchanda, 2000; Ornish et al., 1990)
- Improved cardiovascular disease risk factor profile (e.g., blood lipids)
  (Yogendra et al., 2004; Manchanda, 2000; Mahajan et al., 1999; Schmidt, 1997)

Musculoskeletal

- Increased muscular strength and flexibility
  (Tran et al., 2001; Lan et al., 1996 & 1998; Wolfson et al., 1996)
- Increased balance control
  (Yang et al., 2007; Wong et al., 2001; Hong, Li, & Robinson, 2000; Schaller, 1996; Wolfson et al., 1996)
- Reduced knee arthritis symptoms
  (Chen et al., 2008)
- Improved posture
  (Wong et al., 2001)
- Decreased falls in seniors
  (Faber et al., 2006; Wolf et al., 1996; Province et al., 1995)
- Decreased low-back pain
  (Tekur et al., 2008; Donzelli et al., 2006; Rydeard et al., 2006)

Psychobiological

- Increased cognitive performance
  (Naveen et al., 1997; Jella & Shannahoff-Khalsa, 1993)
- Improved relaxation and psychological well-being
  (Telles et al., 2000; Schell, Allolio, & Schonecke, 1994; Wood, 1993; Berger & Owen, 1992)
- Decreased stress hormones (e.g., cortisol)
  (Kamei et al., 2000)
- Decreased anxiety and depression scores
  (Chen et al., 2009; Danhauer et al., 2008; Gupta et al., 2006; Ray et al., 2001; Sovik, 2000; Janakiramaiah et al., 2000)
- Reduction in frequency of panic episodes
  (Clark, Salkovskis, & Chalkley, 1985)
- Reduced symptoms of insomnia
  (Koch et al., 1998)
- Reduced physiological and psychological responses to threat or stress
  (Sakakibara & Hayano, 1996; Bera, 1995; Cappo & Holmes, 1984; McCaul, Solomon, & Holmes, 1979)
- Decreased symptoms associated with pain, angina, asthma, and chronic fatigue
  (Manchanda, 2000; Nespor, 1991)

Metabolic

- Increased glucose tolerance and insulin sensitivity
  (Innes & Vincent, 2007; Xin et al., 2007; Innes et al., 2005; Jain et al., 1993)
- Decreased HbA1c (glycosylated hemoglobin) and C-peptide levels in type 2 diabetes
  (Kerr et al., 2002; Monro et al., 1992)
- Decreased blood lactate levels
  (Sharma et al., 2003; Tsujiuchi et al., 2002)
- Improved blood lipid profile and lipid oxidation
  (Gordon et al., 2008)

Other

- Increased physical functioning in older persons
  (Faber et al., 2006; Li et al., 2001; Kutner et al., 1997)
- Decreased obsessive-compulsive disorder symptoms
  (Shannahoff-Khalsa & Beckett, 1996)
- Decreased osteoarthritis symptoms
  (Garfinkel et al., 1994)
- Decreased carpal-tunnel symptoms
  (Garfinkel et al., 1999)
- Decreased cancer symptoms and cancer therapy symptoms
  (Danhauer et al., 2008; Raghavendra et al., 2007)

Common Components of Mind-body Exercise Programs

For mind-body exercise to be optimally fulfilling, it requires more than merely adding a "cognitive component" to conventional physical activity. The criteria for what constitutes mind-body exercise continue to evolve as more definitive research is conducted and published and more programs are developed. The following criteria are recommended for mind-body exercise:

- *Meditative/contemplative:* This noncompetitive, present-moment, and nonjudgmental introspective component is process-centered versus strictly outcome- or goal-oriented.
- *Proprioceptive and kinesthetic body awareness:* Mind-body exercise is generally characterized by relatively low-level muscular activity coupled with mental focus on muscle and movement sense.
- *Breath-centering or breathwork:* The breath is frequently cited as the primary centering activity in mind-body exercise. There are many breath-centering techniques in yoga, tai chi, and qigong exercise.
- *Anatomic alignment or proper choreographic form:* Disciplining oneself to a particular movement pattern or spinal alignment is integral to many forms of mind-body exercise such as hatha yoga, Alexander Technique, Pilates, and tai chi. It is also important to note that not all mind-body exercise forms utilize a set choreography or disciplined anatomical alignment characteristics. Examples include Nia and expressive ethnic dance exercises such as Native American spiritual dancing or hula, which exhibit significant free-form movement.
- *Energycentric:* This component refers to the perceptive movement and flow of one's intrinsic energy, vital life force, chi, prana, or other positive energy commonly described in many classical mind-body exercise traditions.

Yoga Research

Approximately 1,600 studies on yoga are listed by Monroe, Ghosh, & Kalish (1989) and many more have been undertaken since that bibliography was published. Perhaps the most dedicated yoga research repository and publication is the *Yoga Mimamsa,* which is managed and published by the Kaivalyadhama Yoga Institute (www.kdham.com). The International Association of Yoga Therapy (www.iayt.org), periodically publishes original investigations on yoga in their *International Journal of Yoga Therapy*. Additionally, the National Center for Complimentary and Alternative Medicine (NCCAM), a division of the National Institutes of Health (NIH), maintains a somewhat limited repository of recently published and controlled yoga trials, as well as chi and meditation studies.

The majority of the published hatha yoga research still suffers from inadequate subject number, low statistical power, and subject selection bias, and/or is void of adequate controls. That said, the overall trend of reported results in most studies is statistically significant with or without controls. There is a growing number of adequately controlled yoga trials demonstrating reasonably clear outcomes (see Table 13-2). For example, research by Berger and Owen comparing hatha yoga to aerobic exercise demonstrated that exercise does not need to be aerobic to decrease anxiety and anger scores and improve mood (Berger & Owen, 1992). One of the most referenced studies in the West is the Lifestyle Heart Trial conducted by Dr. Dean Ornish and colleagues (Ornish et al., 1990). This study, however, did not isolate hatha yoga itself as a therapeutic agent. In this study, a blend of a healthy dietary cuisine (10 to 12% fat), social and group support, moderate aerobic exercise (walking), and regular hatha yoga (sequence of eight to 15 poses) demonstrated a modest regression of atherosclerotic disease in CVD patients as determined by quantitative coronary angiography. More recently, an investigational study by Manchanda demonstrated similar results (Manchanda, 2000). Manchanda evaluated the possible role of lifestyle modification, including hatha yoga, on retardation of **coronary atherosclerotic disease.** In this prospective, randomized, controlled trial, 42 men with angiographically proven **coronary artery disease (CAD)** were randomized to control (n = 21) and yoga intervention groups (n = 21) and followed for one year. The active yoga group was treated with a program consisting of hatha yoga, control of risk factors, diet control, and moderate aerobic exercise. The control group was managed by conventional methods (i.e., risk factor control, moderate exercise, and the American Heart Association's Step I diet, which allows a maximum of 30% of energy from fat and is high in carbohydrate).

At one year, the yoga group showed significant reduction in the number of anginal episodes per week, improved exercise capacity, and decreased body weight. Serum total cholesterol, **low-density lipoprotein (LDL)** cholesterol, and **triglyceride** levels also showed greater reductions as compared with the control group. Revascularization procedures (coronary angioplasty or bypass surgery) were less frequently required in the yoga group (one versus eight patients; relative risk = 5.45; p = 0.01). Coronary angiography repeated at one year showed that significantly more lesions regressed (20% versus 2%) and fewer lesions progressed (5% versus 37%) in the yoga group (p <0.0001). Compliance with the total program was excellent and no side effects were observed. One can conclude that the active yoga program was truly an integrated intervention program blending a low-fat diet with meditation and hatha yoga principles. More recently, Yogendra et al. (2004) replicated much of Manchanda's findings in 71 CAD patients undergoing intensive yogic lifestyle therapy.

In 2005, Kim Innes at the University of Virginia received a $375,000 grant award from the NCCAM and the Office of Women's Health to conduct a study about the effects of yoga on women's heart health. Her subjects are sedentary, overweight, and postmenopausal women—a population that has a higher risk of **cardiometabolic disease.** Participants in the study will be divided randomly into two groups. The study's control group will attend eight weeks of interactive group sessions where they will view and discuss films on women's issues, including menopause, aging, and heart disease. The experimental group will receive eight weeks of intensive instruction in Iyengar yoga because of its gentleness, slow pace, and use of props and supports. This is just one of 13 NCCAM-sponsored research trials investigating the role of yoga in disease management and prevention.

The Ornish, Manchanda, and Yogendra studies show that for a yoga program to either cause regression or at least slow the progression of coronary disease there must be a significant modification of blood **lipids** and **lipoproteins** (i.e., LDL cholesterol), primarily by dietary means. In the final analysis, yogic lifestyle intervention, rather than hatha yoga alone, is perhaps the necessary stimulus required for generating significant clinical outcomes as evidenced in these and other trials.

Qigong and Tai Chi Research

In the early 1980s, scientists in China began investigating the many potential benefits of qigong and tai chi. Since 1985, approximately 1,800 research papers have been published on qigong practice alone (the Qigong and Energy Medicine Database includes more than 4,000 research papers). Much of this research has involved qigong exercise and tai chi. A number of these research trials were well-controlled studies that reported statistically significant decreases in the incidence of **stroke** and stroke mortality, increases in bone mineral density, improved balance, improved lipid profile, decreased blood pressure, improved effectiveness of cancer therapy, and increased psychological well-being.

Despite all of the interest and perceived benefits of yoga and tai chi in the West, there still remains a great need for more peer-reviewed and adequately controlled research investigating the impact of yoga on chronic disease, musculoskeletal function, and behavioral outcomes. Although there is a considerable international body of research in terms of the total number of research citations—more than 5,000 papers published worldwide—the majority of these trials are statistically underpowered, lack adequate controls, and/or are fraught with selection bias. Still, there are a growing number of well-controlled experimental trials that support the many biological and psychological benefits associated with both classical and contemporary forms of mind-body exercise. To be sure, there are a number of well-controlled trials in progress evaluating low-back pain, aging, and multiple sclerosis. Vijay Vad at the Hospital for Special Surgery in Manhattan is studying 50 patients with herniated disks who are suffering from low-back pain and comparing a combination of yoga and Pilates (70% yoga, 30% Pilates exercise) to drug therapy. After three months, 80% of the patients in the yoga/Pilates group reported that their pain was reduced by at least 50% versus only 44% of the patients in the drug-treated group reporting reduced pain. The NIH is currently funding studies evaluating the effects of hatha yoga on insomnia, **insulin resistance,** and multiple sclerosis.

For more information, go to the NIH website (www.clinicaltrials.gov) and enter the search word "yoga." The quantity and quality of this level of research will surely escalate as Western graduate schools develop structured course work involving the psychobiology of mind-body exercise modalities and students pursue study and investigational projects in these promising forms of contemplative physical activity.

Mind-body Exercise Modalities and Programs

Hatha yoga, qigong, tai chi, and pranayama (yogic breathing), all classical forms of mind-body exercise, have been practiced by young and old alike for centuries and each has spawned numerous styles for a variety of age groups and functional capacities. More contemporary forms of mind-body exercise (e.g., Pilates, Nia, Somatics, E-MOTION, **Feldenkrais Method,** and **Alexander Technique**) have been largely inspired by these early forms and also deserve consideration in their own right.

Yoga

It is important for personal trainers to know the difference between "yoga" and what much of the fitness industry refers to as yoga exercise or hatha yoga. The word yoga originated from the ancient Sanskrit language spoken by the religious elite of India. Yoga literally means "union," or integration of mind and body disciplines. According to Patanjali's philosophical analyses contained in the *Yoga Sutra,* yoga historically refers to the complex system of physical and spiritual disciplines that are fundamental to Buddhist, Jain, and Hindu religious practice throughout Asia. It is important to differentiate a "yogic lifestyle" from participation in hatha yoga classes such as those offered in yoga studios and fitness centers in the United States (e.g., Iyengar yoga and power yoga classes). Those who live yogic lifestyles, while perhaps not in full compliance with the teachings of the *Yoga Sutra,* generally embark upon daily dietary, meditation, and spiritual centering and regular hatha yoga exercise, whereas the routine practice of hatha yoga poses may or may not include dietary or other lifestyle changes. This is an important point because some yoga research outcomes are based on following yogic lifestyle principles that clearly transcend the mere practice of yoga exercise.

All six branches of yoga (Inana, Karma, Mantra, Tantra, Raja, Hatha) attempt to accomplish the same final goal; however, hatha yoga will be the focus of this section, as it is perhaps the most relevant branch for personal trainers. Hatha yoga is the physical aspect of yogic disciplines and includes a vast repertoire of physical postures, or asanas, done seated, standing, or lying prone or supine on the floor, and, in some instances, inverted positions. Several basic movement patterns are involved in most asanas: backbends, twists, and forward bends.

The principal challenge of hatha yoga is to become proficient at handling increasingly greater amounts of "resistance" (i.e., complexity and the degree of difficulty) in the various postures and breathing patterns while maintaining a steady and comfortable equilibrium of mind and body. As a general rule, hatha yoga sessions start and end with a relaxation pose (a savasana, or corpse pose) and include a variety of asanas focusing on spinal, postural, and limb muscle groups so that the exerciser spends 30 seconds to one minute with each pose before transitioning to the next. Optimally, early stages of hatha yoga are taught individually, with a certified yoga teacher providing hands-on assessment and guidance through each pose. The use of props (e.g., blankets, blocks, neck and lumbar rolls, and bolsters) is very helpful in early stages of training to help the individual achieve safe and proper alignment, minimizing undue musculoskeletal stress. In virtually all forms of hatha yoga it is paramount that yogic breathing be executed in synchrony with each pose. There are countless yogic breathing techniques [see "Yogic Breathing Training (Pranayama)," page 463]. As a general rule, yogic breathing is combined with yoga exercise in a very logical way. Whenever a yoga movement or pose expands the chest or abdomen, the participant inhales. Conversely, when a movement contracts or compresses the chest or abdomen, the participant exhales.

The following sections present several methods of hatha yoga that are commonly practiced throughout the United States and Europe.

Restorative Yoga

This style of hatha yoga is a derivative of the Iyengar yoga tradition and is perhaps most appropriate for those who are just embarking on a yoga program because of the use of props and the elementary nature of the poses. Judith Lasater and others have introduced this form of Iyengar yoga. Restorative yoga is easier and more relaxing for those who are relatively weak, fatigued, or experiencing peak stressful periods in life. Some of the more popular poses in this form are legs-up-the-wall pose, supported half-dog pose, chair forward bend, and half-wall hang (Figures 13-3 through 13-6) (Lasater, 2003 & 1995).

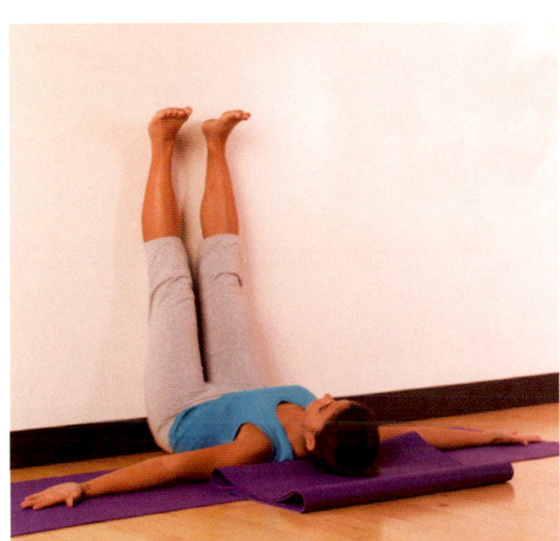

Figure 13-3
Legs-up-the-wall pose

Source: Adapted from Lasater, J. (1995). *Relax and Renew: Restful Yoga for Stressful Times.* Berkeley, Calif.: Rodmell Press.

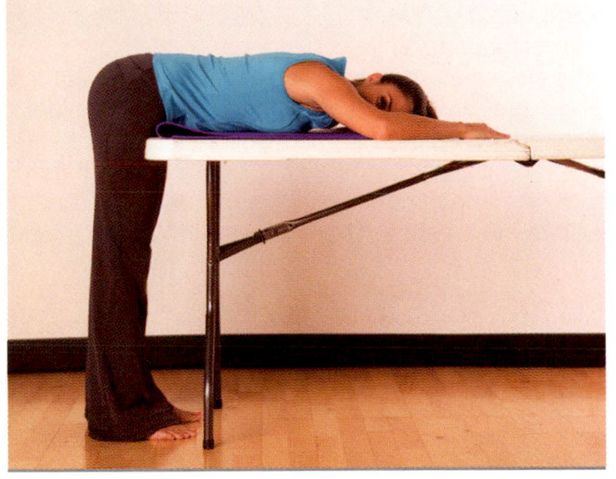

Figure 13-4
Supported half-dog pose

Source: Adapted from Lasater, J. (1995). *Relax and Renew: Restful Yoga for Stressful Times.* Berkeley, Calif.: Rodmell Press.

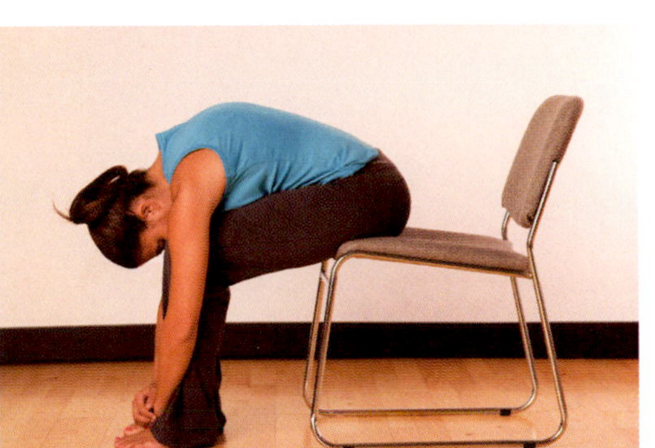

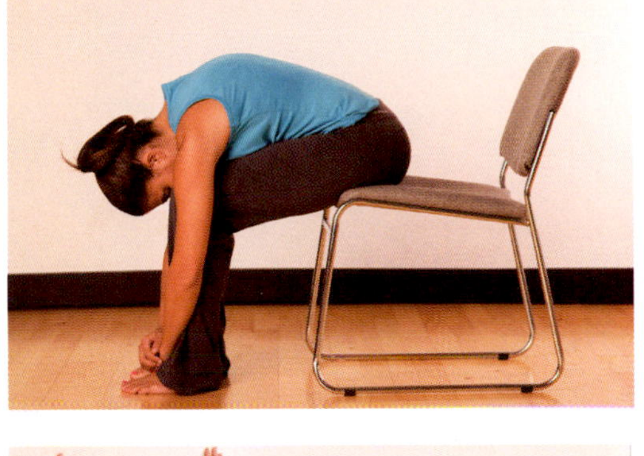

Figure 13-5
Chair forward bend

Source: Adapted from Lasater, J. (1995). *Relax and Renew: Restful Yoga for Stressful Times.* Berkeley, Calif.: Rodmell Press.

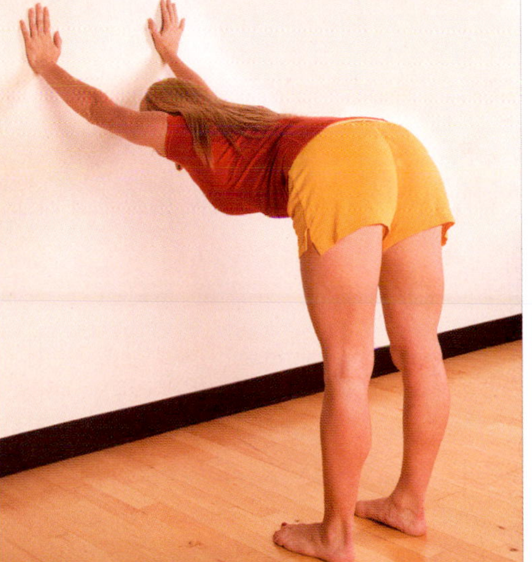

Figure 13-6
Half-wall hang

Source: Adapted from Lasater, J. (1995). *Relax and Renew: Restful Yoga for Stressful Times.* Berkeley, Calif.: Rodmell Press.

Sivananda Yoga

A style of classical yoga with traditional poses, breathing exercises, and relaxation, Sivananda teaches 12 postures comprising the Sun Salutation sequence and can be readily adapted to beginners or those who have low functional capacities (Figure 13-7). The Sivananda Yoga Vedanta Center (see Teacher Training Resources, page 477) has trained more than 10,000 yoga teachers worldwide and is widely respected for teaching authentic hatha yoga.

Figure 13-7
Sun salutation
The sun salutation was introduced to the West in the early 1950s and is one of the most popular hatha yoga sequences. This pose series is an excellent example of how breath is coordinated with yoga pose sequencing. Although this yoga series is for those who are reasonably healthy and fit (e.g., without significant back problems), it exemplifies a method that can improve posture by stretching the spine and strengthening the muscle groups that support it. Coordination and muscular endurance are two additional benefits. There are several styles of sun salutation, including Ashtanga and Shivandana styles.

The following sun salutation 12-step yoga sequence illustrates an intermediate level performance, in contrast to a full Ashtanga or Shivandana style, in which greater flexibility is exhibited. This sequence begins and ends with the standing position with the palms together (prayer pose).

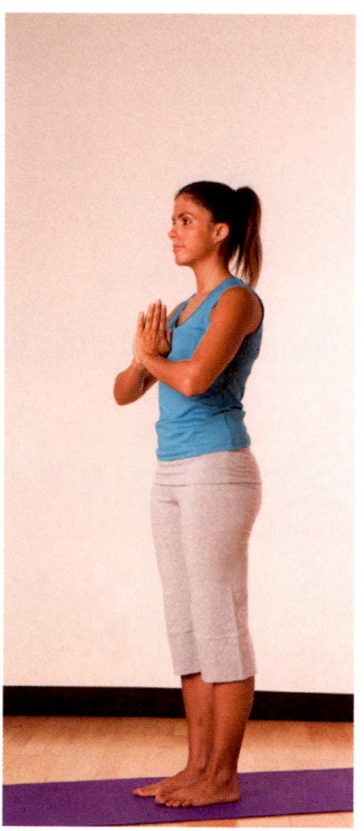

1. Normal relaxed respiration, standing in prayer pose

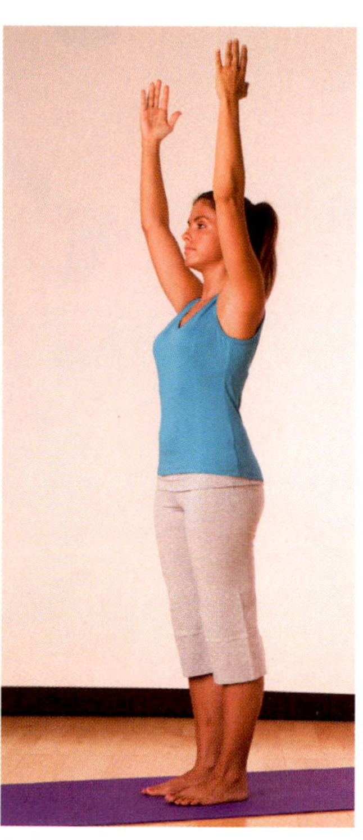

2. Breathe in, back slightly arched

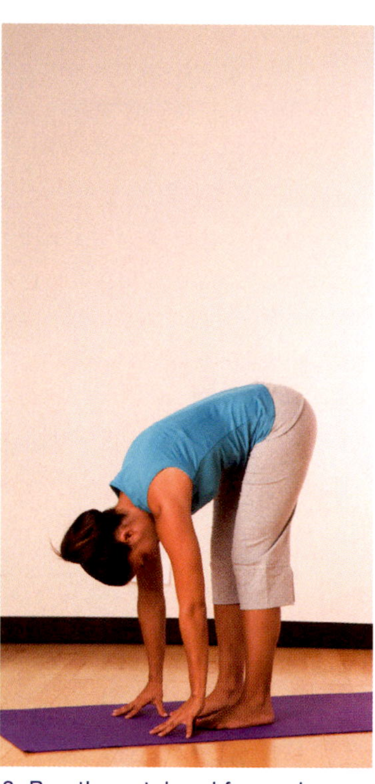

3. Breathe out, bend forward

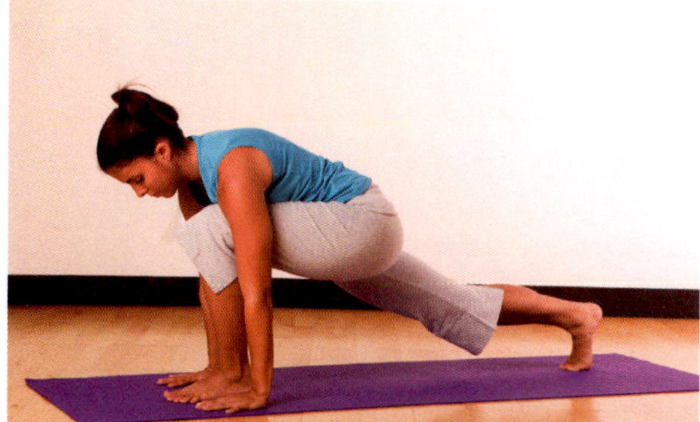

4. Breathe in, step back with the right leg

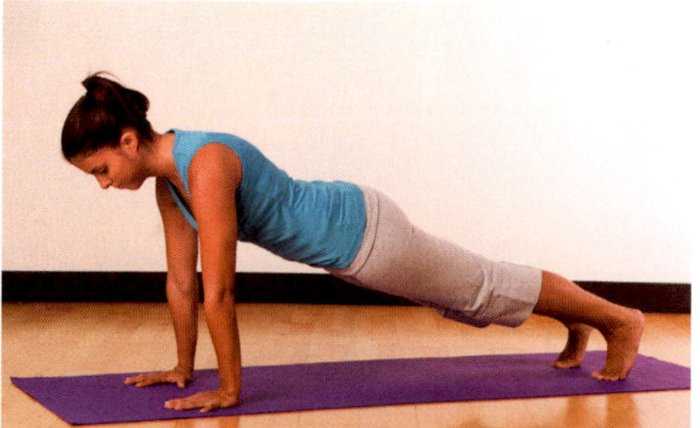

5. Breathe out, bring the left foot back with the right foot (press-up position)

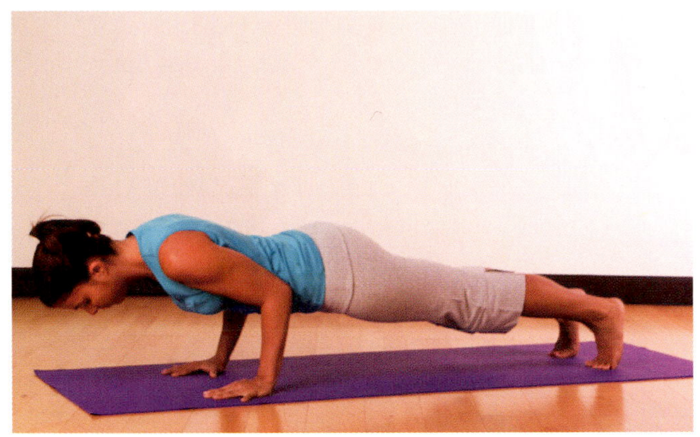
6. Lower your body slowly to the floor

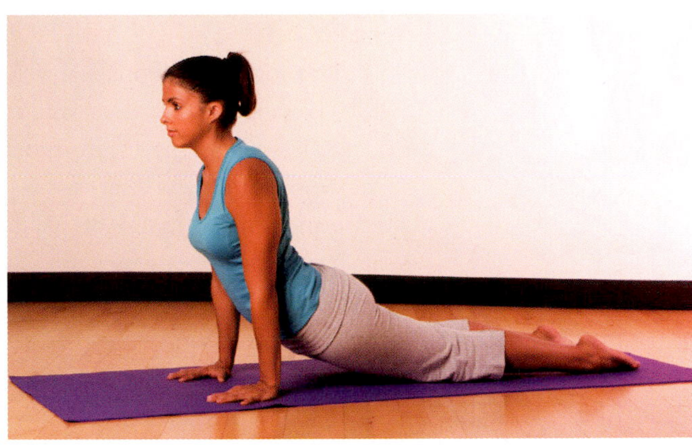
7. Breathe in, with upper body raised

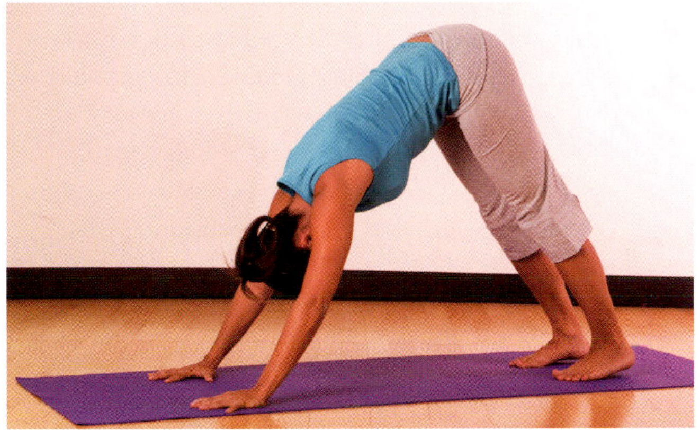
8. Breathe out, assume inverted V position

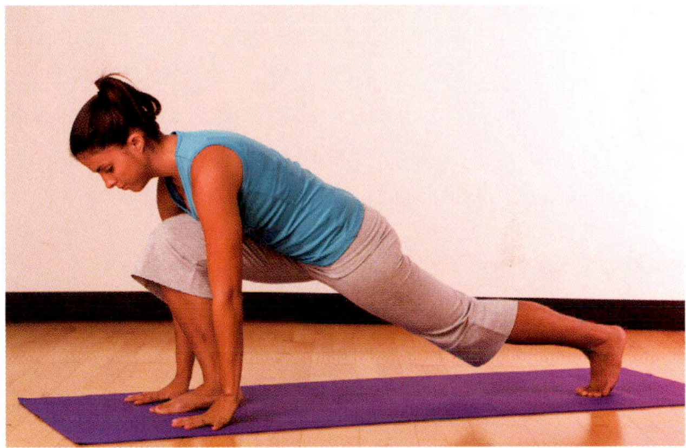
9. Breathe in, bend the right knee and step in between the hands

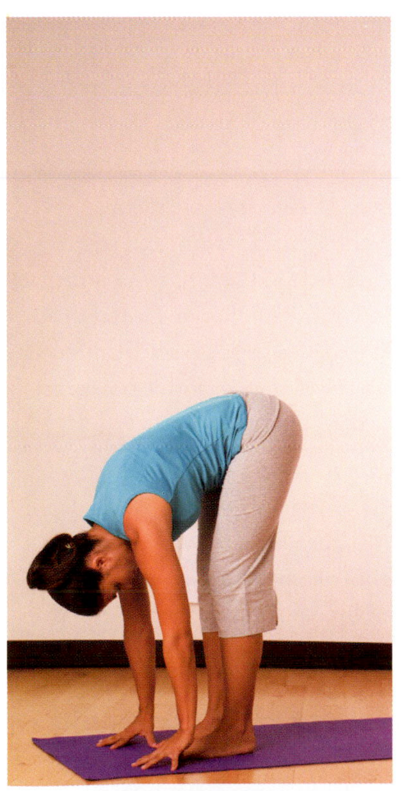
10. Breathe out, bring the left foot up to meet the right, bend forward

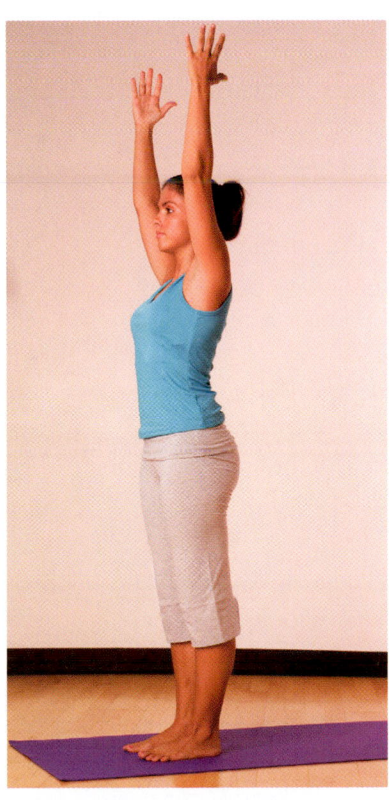
11. Breathe in, reassume pose #2 with back arched

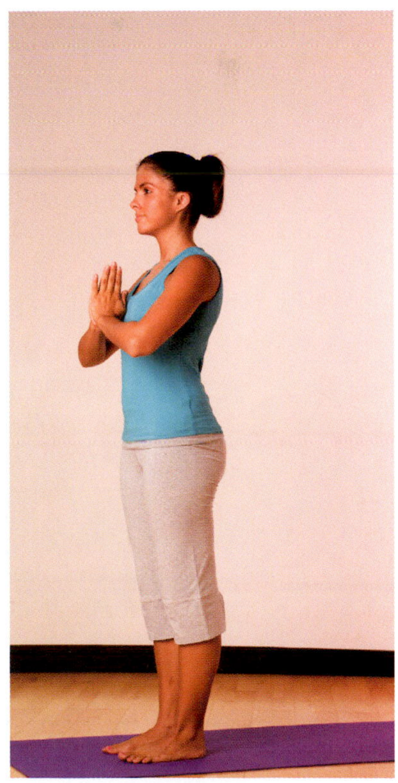
12. Finish by returning to a prayer pose

Iyengar Yoga

Iyengar yoga was originally developed by B.K.S. Iyengar, who systematized more than 200 classical asanas (poses) from very simple to very difficult. Much emphasis is placed on precise anatomical alignment, which over the years has refined the therapeutic aspects of yoga. One preferred form of Iyengar yoga uses standing poses in which the person assumes a stationary position using **isometric** contractions to attain precise body alignment. As with nearly all styles of hatha yoga, Iyengar places much emphasis on breathing (pranayama). The use of props to assist with attaining appropriate spinal alignment is one of the characteristics of Iyengar classes. Perhaps the most authoritative and detailed illustrated text on Iyengar yoga is B.K.S. Iyengar's *Light on Yoga.*

Ashtanga Yoga

This is the ancient system of hatha yoga currently taught by Pattabhi Jois. This method synchronizes a progressive series of postures with a specific breathing method (ujjayi pranayama). The asanas in Ashtanga yoga are sequenced in groups of poses that range from moderate to very difficult. The sequence pace and pose difficulty is what often characterizes Ashtanga as "power yoga." Ashtanga places equal emphasis on strength, flexibility, and mental and physical stamina.

Anusara Yoga

Founded by John Friend, this form of hatha yoga closely resembles Iyengar and stresses three focus points: attitude, alignment, and action.

Participants are taught to be cognizant of their "key power center" or focal point (i.e., the point at which most of the body weight or musculoskeletal force is placed).

Viniyoga

This is a softer and more individualized form of hatha yoga known for its therapeutic application of the classical asanas or poses. Emphasis is placed on breathing (pranayama) and coordination of breath and movement. Viniyoga is usually taught on a one-on-one basis. Kraftsow's *Yoga for Wellness: Healing with the Timeless Teachings of Viniyoga and Yoga for Transformation,* as well as Desikachar's *The Heart of Yoga* are consummate descriptive works on Viniyoga.

Kripalu Yoga

This is a three-level style of hatha yoga customized to the needs of Western students. Stage 1 teaches the basic mechanics of the postures, including body alignment and coordination of breath and movement. Stage 2 includes a prolonged holding of the poses as the student learns to practice a disciplined mental concentration. Stage 3 involves a spontaneous moving meditation set to the individual's internal awareness and energy. The Kripalu method of teaching and practicing yoga blends the physical postures of hatha yoga with the contemplative meditation of Raja yoga, the principal tenets of which extend well beyond those of hatha yoga and include moral discipline, self restraint, meditation, concentration, breath control, and physical postures.

Integral Yoga

Another yoga form that gently stretches, strengthens, and calms the body and mind, Integral yoga includes comfortable postures, deep relaxation, and breathing practices. This form of yoga emphasizes diet and is employed in Dr. Dean Ornish's heart disease reversal programs around the United States.

Bikram Yoga

Bikram yoga is a vigorous 90-minute, 26-pose series designed to warm and stretch muscles, ligaments, and tendons in a particular sequence. Since most studios are heated to 90 to 105° F (32 to 41° C), each participant needs to have a large towel, a washcloth (sometimes two), and a water bottle for class.

Kundalini Yoga

Also called the yoga of awareness, kundalini yoga's principal purpose is to awaken the serpent power (kundalini, or coiled-up energy) with postures, breath control, chanting, and meditation. Originated by Yogi Bhajan, a kundalini yoga class usually entails a spine and flexibility warm-up, specific asana sequences commensurate with one's "coiled up energy," and relaxation. Each asana is symbolic of life habits and emotion and a specific associated breath (e.g., long-deep breath, segmented breathing, breath of fire).

Somatic Yoga

Eleanor Criswell Hanna developed this moderate-intensity form of hatha yoga that shares many characteristics of the Alexander Technique and Feldenkrais Method (see pages 467–468). Somatic yoga sessions emphasize contracting particular muscle groups and then relaxing them. Each yoga pose is done slowly and is followed by one minute of deep breathing, self-awareness, and what Hanna refers to as "integration." Classes end with pranayama, guided relaxation (quieting of the senses), and meditation.

Yogic Breathing Training (Pranayama)

In the yogic and qigong traditions, breathing functions as an intermediary between the mind and body. Pranayama (the practice of voluntary breath control, consisting of conscious inhalation, retention, and exhalation) is often practiced in conjunction with meditation and yoga asanas but can stand by itself as an important mind-body exercise method. Breathwork studies have demonstrated it as an independent method of increasing relaxation, reducing anxiety, and improving mental alertness, focus, and overall psychological well-being (Bhatia et al., 2003; Janakiramaiah et al., 2000; Sakakibara & Hayano, 1996; Sakakibara, Tekeuchi, & Hayano, 1994). Yogic breathing also has been used as a therapeutic modality in managing chronic heart failure (Bernardi et al., 2002). Yogic breathwork can either be isolated as a training modality itself or function as a necessary component of mind-body exercise. The fundamental purpose of breathwork is to develop the ability to: (a) sustain relaxed attention to the flow of the breath, (b) refine and control respiratory movements, and (c) integrate awareness and breathing to reduce stress and enhance psychological functioning. Sovik (2000) characterizes optimal breathwork as:

- Diaphragmatic
- Nasal (inhalation and exhalation)
- Deep
- Smooth
- Even
- Quiet
- Free of pauses

General Precautions With Hatha Yoga Programs

Because many styles of hatha yoga involve acute dynamic changes in body position, it is important to understand the **hemodynamic** and cardiac ventricular responses to such exercise and how these may alter cardiac function in people diagnosed with CVD, including hypertension or diabetes. Inverted poses in which the head is below the heart (e.g., downward facing dog, headstands) and sequences in which a head-down position is alternated with a head-up pose should be avoided, at least in the early stages of a yoga program. In most cases, those who are initially deconditioned or have a chronic disease should: (a) minimize acute rapid changes in body position (e.g., changes in the limbs and trunk in relation to the heart) in early stages of hatha yoga training, and/or (b) use slower transitions from one yoga pose to the next.

Ashtanga, Iyengar, and Bikram yoga asanas and sequences require considerable muscular strength and mental concentration. Therefore, they may be more appropriate for higher functioning individuals (i.e., those with >11–12 **MET** exercise capacity). Some yoga poses may cause significant and rapid changes in blood pressure and may be inappropriate for those with stage 2 or higher hypertension (i.e., those with blood pressures equal to or greater than 160/100 mmHg). DiCarlo and colleagues (1995) demonstrated significantly greater **systolic** and **diastolic blood pressures** in yoga practitioners practicing Iyengar style yoga when compared to moderate treadmill walking (~4 miles per hour). This, however, does not contraindicate Iyengar-style yoga for reasonably conditioned adults with stable cardiovascular disease.

Because some yoga programs involve advanced breathing techniques (e.g., breath retentions and breath suspensions), caution must be used with those who have cardiovascular or pulmonary disease. Breath retentions are brief pauses (two to five or more seconds) taken at the end of a controlled inspiration. Breath suspensions are similar pauses taken at the end of controlled expirations. While very brief pauses appear to be relatively safe, those with cardiovascular disease, hypertension, obstructive pulmonary disease, or asthma should avoid retentions or suspensions of greater than four to five seconds and focus on the standard breathwork taught in most yoga programs.

Qigong Exercise

Qigong is a system of self-healing exercise and meditation that includes healing postures, movement, visualization, breathwork, and meditation. Qigong exercise, otherwise known as Chinese health exercise, has a heritage dating back more than 3,000 years. Qigong movements are executed at very low metabolic levels, usually between 2 and 4 METs, and include standing, seated, and supine positions. The ultimate goal of qigong is to improve the balance of the functions of the body. There are two general categories of qigong: active, or physical, qigong exercise (dong gong) and tranquil, or passive, qigong (jing gong). The active category is what is discussed here, as this is the most popular form of qigong in both China and in the West. There are perhaps many thousands of qigong exercise styles all based on balance, relaxation, breathing, and good posture.

Many qigong styles are named after animals whose movements they imitate, (e.g., dragon, crane, snake, wild goose, and animal frolics styles). According to qigong tradition, inhaling brings positive qi into the body and usually accompanies an "opening" movement (e.g., arms opening away from the body), while exhaling releases the negative qi and accompanies a "closing" movement (e.g., arms back to the body). One simple qigong series is Taiji qigong, which consists of only 18 movements taken from the tai chi and qigong forms (Tse, 1996). Figure 13-8 presents the four-movement Taiji qigong sequence called Pushing the Wave. Taiji qigong is ideal as a preparation for higher-intensity conditioning exercise or as a cool-down. It is recommended that this series be practiced once or twice a day for 15 to 20 minutes. There are numerous published studies, mostly with small subject numbers, demonstrating many health benefits of qigong exercise (e.g., reduced blood pressure, pain management, anxiety, and tension reduction) (see Table 13-2). Two resources that describe qigong exercise in good detail are Michael Tse's *Qigong for Health and Vitality* and Kenneth Cohen's *The Way of Qigong*.

Tai Chi

Tai chi (shorthand for tai chi chuan or taijiquan) is only one form of the more ancient practice of qigong. Tai chi chuan is a complex martial arts choreography of 108 flowing graceful movements that can be practiced for health, meditation, and self-defense. There are numerous forms or styles of tai chi chuan, including the original Chen, and the relatively more recent Yang, Chang, and Wu styles. Each form emphasizes a particular aspect, such as breathing, generating power, or relaxation. Some styles have a short form that may be more adaptable to those with disabilities or for seniors. In tai chi, students are taught to allow the practice to evolve into a free-flow exercise such that the movements and breathing become one unified energy flow. As with hatha yoga, it is important that the movements and breathing are coordinated so that the student may derive the energy-centric benefits (i.e., unobstructed flow of perceived positive energy). Another way of looking at tai chi is as a form of inner contemplation choreographed with movement. Students are first taught to be mindful of the postures and movements, then of the coordination of movement with breathing. Finally, students are taught to be "mindful not to be mindful" (i.e., not to become overly focused on the postures, movements, and breathing). **Tai chi chih,** developed by American Justin Stone, is a simpler form of tai chi chuan and consists of a series of 20 movements and one ending pose. Qigong exercise involves even

Figure 13-8
Qigong—pushing the wave
Pushing the wave is part of an 18-movement Taiji qigong sequence taught by Michael Tse (1996) and is choreographed to replicate other Taiji forms, dance, and daily life movements. The pushing the wave sequence is characterized by a straight front leg with slow but intentional arm and hand movements. The movement coordinates and connects various qi (energy) points throughout the body, particularly the upper extremities, lungs, and stomach. As with yoga's sun salutation (see Figure 13-7), the movements are coordinated with the breath.

1.
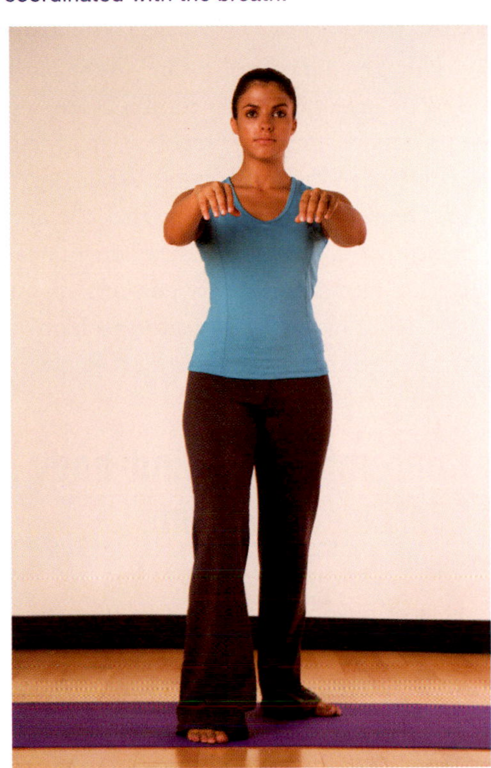

2.
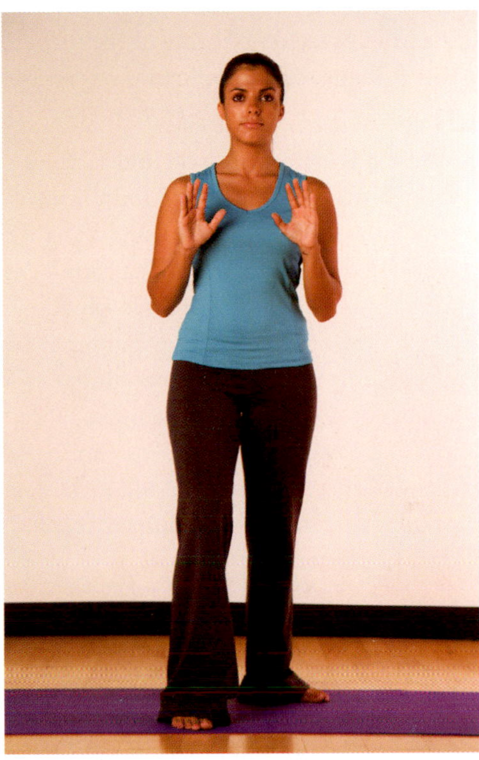

3.
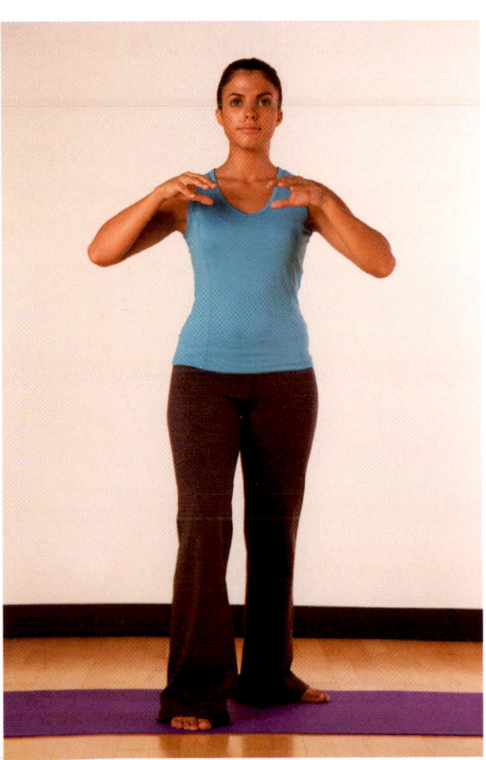

4.
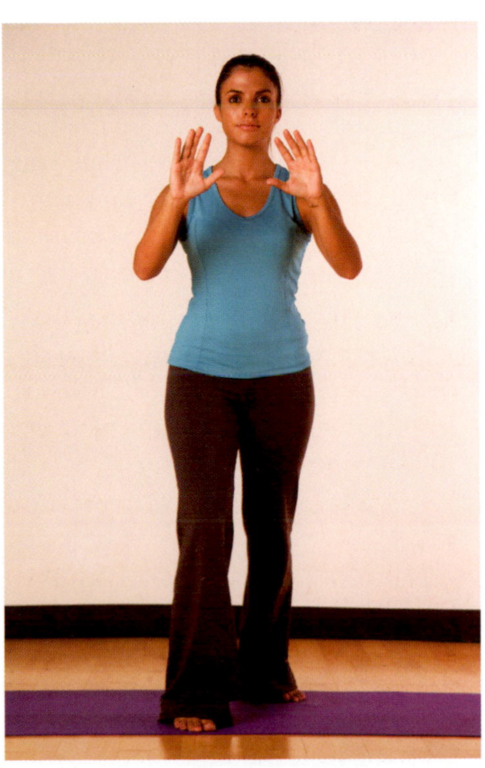

a simpler set of movements than its martial arts relative tai chi.

It is commonly accepted that all tai chi styles follow similar essential principles: deep synchronous breathing, profound mental concentration, and perceptive and intentional movement of chi. The following is a brief overview of some of the major distinguishable styles of tai chi.

Original Chen Style

The original Chen style (old form) is thought to be the template form from which the more recent Wu and Yang forms descended. The original Chen form contains motions including jumping, leaping, scurrying, bouncing, discharging, and other quick movements that may make it difficult for seniors or those with poor functional capacity. The newer Chen style has eliminated many of these movements and involves more circular choreography and is suitable for a broad range of fitness levels.

Yang Style

Originated by Yang Luchan in the 1800s, the Yang form is the most widely practiced form in the West today. The original Yang form consists of 108 movements (Yang Long Form); however, the Yang 24–Short Form is a popular modification practiced today. As with all styles of tai chi, Yang-style movements reflect the principle of opposites commonly called yin and yang, in which offensive and defensive movements unite to form a graceful flow of martial arts choreography and, more importantly, chi.

Chang Style

This is a relatively new style of tai chi developed by Chang Tung-sheng in the 1930s. Chang style consists of more than 100 movements and is based on modifications to the Yang Long Form.

Wu Style

This style of tai chi was developed by Master Wu Chien-chuan and is second in popularity only to Yang-style tai chi. Wu style is an easier form of tai chi, with smaller steps and movements that involve less twisting and impose less stress on the legs and knees. The condensed form of Wu style includes 36 postures, including grasping the sparrow's tail, slant flying, embrace tiger, and push mountain. Other versions of Wu style include 54 movements (e.g., 54 Forms by Master Wu Tai Sin and Sifu Eddie Wu).

Sun Style

Developed by Sun Lu-tang in the late 1800s, Sun-style tai chi combines elements of Wu and Yang-style tai chi. Sun style is characterized by lively steps. When one foot moves forward or backward, the other foot follows. Turns include an opening and closing movement, a very powerful qigong practice. This style also features a high stance, making it easy for older people to learn.

Contemporary Mind-body Exercise Programs

Over the past century, numerous mind-body exercise derivatives have grown from the classical traditions of qigong, tai chi, and yoga. Pilates, Alexander, Feldenkrais, and various modern hatha yoga styles have matured as respected mind-body exercise methods as their techniques have been largely standardized. There are many more contemporary mind-body exercise programs that combine attributes from several classical forms, including Nia, Chi Ball Method, E-MOTION, BrainGym, Yogarobics, Aqua Tai Chi, Yo Chi,® and many ethnic dance routines. The Asian martial arts (e.g., aikido, karate, tae kwon do, kempo, and judo) also clearly employ associative and disassociative cognitive methods to center their attention and direct their movements and strikes.

Pilates

The Pilates Method was developed by German immigrant Joseph H. Pilates in the early 20th century. Pilates is an orderly system of slow, controlled, distinct movements that demand a profound internal cognitive focus and attention to breathing. Fundamentally, this method is based on the idea that there is a core set of postural muscles that help to keep the body balanced and are essential to providing good support to the spine. This method is divided into two modalities, floor/mat work and work on a Reformer, a piece of resistance equipment originally developed by Pilates (Figure 13-9). With either modality, but especially with the Reformer, the principal goal is to achieve efficient functional movement and improved performance. There are several versions of Reformers, including lightweight consumer, rehabilitation, and professional models. Fundamentally, Pilates is a form of movement re-education in which the exerciser learns to overcome faulty compensatory movement patterns. These inefficient movement patterns are broken down into components by using springs for resistance (with a Reformer) and changing the body's orientation to gravity. Pilates exercises are designed to facilitate more efficient movement behavior by allowing the exerciser to be in a position that minimizes undesirable muscle activity, which can cause early fatigue and lead to injury. The Reformer is constructed to adapt to many human anatomic variations. For example, the springs, ropes, and foot bar of the clinical Reformer can be adjusted so that similar properties of movement sequencing can be applied to a variety of body types and limb/torso lengths. Pilates work involves considerable mental focus and coordinated breathwork, particularly during very slow concentric and eccentric muscular contractions. The Pilates method is utilized for rehabilitation, post-rehabilitation, and fitness.

There is some variation in technique among contemporary Pilates education and training programs, most of which assert many advantages and benefits of Pilates-style training when compared to conventional strength and muscle re-education training. Pilates is advantageous for those who desire low-impact exercise to improve posture, flexibility, core-strength, and functionality. For example, Hutchinson, Christiansen, and Beitzel (1998) demonstrated significant improvements in leap height, explosive power, and reaction time in six elite athletes after one month of Pilates training. More recently, a growing body of research has provided increased support for Pilates-based therapy, particularly in those with low-back pain (Donzelli et al., 2006; Rydeard et al., 2006). Those interested in exploring a reasonably detailed scientific introduction into Pilates-based exercise and rehabilitation are referred to Anderson and Spector's "Introduction to Pilates-Based Rehabilitation" (2000).

Alexander Technique

The Alexander Technique, as established by Frederick Alexander in the late 19th century, is a method that teaches the

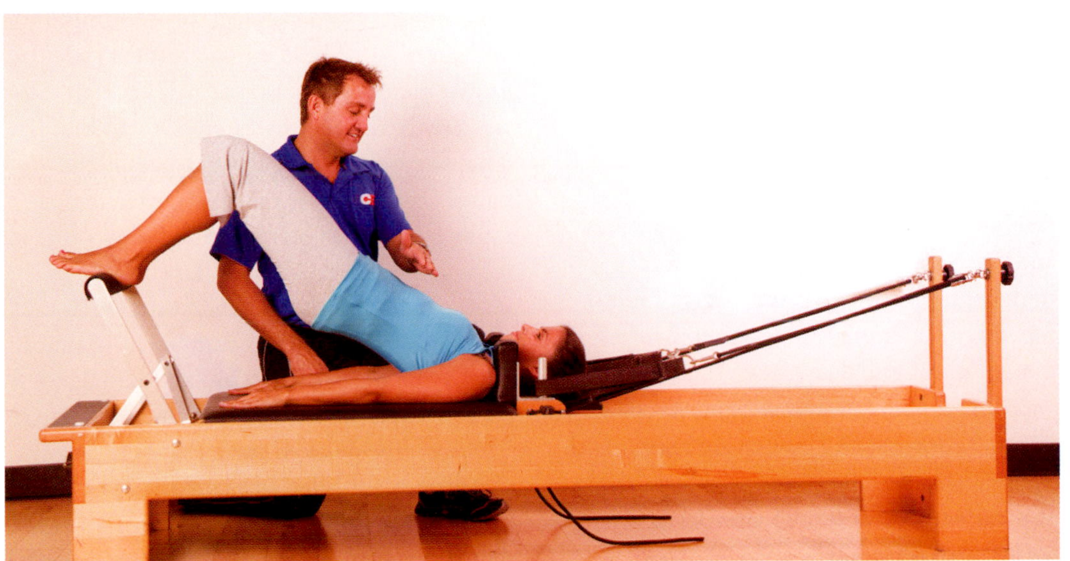

Figure 13-9
One of many styles of Pilates Reformers. The machine glides forward and backward on rollers, uses springs for resistance, and may include other attachments for a wide variety of movements and positions.

transformation of neuromuscular habits by helping an individual focus on sensory experiences. It corrects unconscious habits of posture and movement that may be precursors to injuries. This method is useful for individuals with disc trouble, sciatica, low-back pain, whiplash injury, shoulder/arm pain, neck pain, or arthritis, and athletes who wish to move with more ease and greater coordination. It is important to remember that this is not an exercise program per se, but rather a proprioceptive, postural, and movement technique that is applied to routine day-to-day domestic, recreational, and sports activities. The Alexander Technique is taught one-on-one or in small groups by an Alexander-certified teacher.

Feldenkrais Method

The Feldenkrais Method was developed by the Russian Moshe Feldenkrais in 1904 and consists of two interrelated, somatically based educational methods. The first method, Awareness Through Movement (ATM), is a verbally directed technique designed for group work. The second method, Functional Integration, is a nonverbal manual-contact technique designed for people desiring or requiring more individualized attention. The ATM method incorporates active movements, imagery, and other forms of directed attention. These are gentle, non-strenuous exercises designed to re-educate the nervous system, with the emphasis placed on learning from the individual's own kinesthetic feedback. A significant emphasis is placed on posture, breathing, somatically based imagery, and visualization that pertains to perception, cognition, and other aspects of motor function. Functional Integration involves directing and enhancing the efficiency, coordination, grace, and self-possession of a person's movement. Lessons are taught with the practitioner gently touching or moving the student in a variety of ways to facilitate awareness and vitality.

Nia

Nia, or what was originally known as the Neuromuscular Integrative Action technique, was created by Debbie and Carlos Rosas in 1983 and represents a composite of both Eastern and Western mind-body exercise influences and has grown in popularity in many health clubs and fitness centers throughout the United States. Nia classes blend movements and concepts from a variety of mind-body programs, including tai chi, yoga, martial arts, and ethnic and modern dance. Unlike other mind-body exercise programs, Nia also includes a moderate-level aerobic component to address cardiorespiratory endurance. The aerobic segment is designed to foster creativity and spontaneity rather than strict adherence to standard group movement patterns. Nia movements provide a wide variety in range of motion and numerous choreographed movement choices. Participants are taught to move with self-expression and couple movement tempo with their emotion. E-MOTION, developed by Laura Sachs, is somewhat similar to Nia and involves a sensory-directed warm-up that uses visualization and tai chi–like low-impact movements.

Native American and Alaskan Spiritual Dancing

Native American and Alaskan spiritual dancing share common features with many contemporary and classical forms of mind-body exercise. These unique forms have grown in popularity in recent years, particularly in the Southwestern United States. These expressive and artful dances blend nature, spirituality, and expressive choreography together as one meaningful movement form as evidenced by their dance names (e.g., sun, arrow, hoop deer, corn, eagle, rain, snake, and pipe). The mental focus is almost entirely on deeply respected and heritage-specific experience with natural phenomena. Much can be gleaned from these ethnic mind-body routines, but perhaps most important is the integration of nature (earth, animals, plants, cosmos) into the movement pattern, thereby instilling a genuine devotion to interconnectedness.

Assessing Outcomes

There are a variety of methods, other than muscular strength and flexibility measures, available to objectively measure the response to mind-body exercise, particularly for hatha yoga, tai chi, and qigong.

Quality of life: Quality-of-life measures, as assessed and scored on a variety of quality of life inventories such as QualityMetric's SF-8 and SF-12 self-report instruments, are reasonably well suited for characterizing the overall functional response (www.qmetric.com). The Centers for Disease Control and Prevention's (CDC) National Center for Chronic Disease Prevention and Health Promotion is one source of a simple measure of health-related quality of life (CDC, 2002).

Blood pressure: Baseline and serial resting blood pressure measurement is also an accepted outcome measure responsive to four to six weeks of mind-body exercise—especially if the participant has a resting blood pressure in the prehypertension or higher range (i.e., >120/80 mmHg).

Pulmonary function: Pulmonary function measures such as **FEV1** (maximum forced expiratory volume in one second) are valid indicators when baseline FEV1 is less than 80%. **Vital capacity** itself is not likely to change, but some studies have demonstrated increases in lung volumes and FEV1 with yoga programs that incorporate significant breathwork.

Balance control: Balance assessment (see Chapter 7) is appropriate for evaluating the response to tai chi and qigong exercise or other mind-body exercise programs in which balance control is a primary component.

Anxiety and tension: Anxiety measures may also be helpful in evaluating stress and tension. The Spielberger State Trait Anxiety Inventory (STAI) contains two 20-item self-report scales that assess anxiety-proneness (trait) and report the current level of anxiety (state). The STAI Computer Program (www.mhs.com) is an inexpensive administration and scoring program that is an alternative to paper-and-pencil versions and takes about 10 minutes to administer.

Spirituality: Although very few mind-body exercise studies objectively examine spirituality, it is an outcome measure worthy of consideration. There are a number of validated spirituality assessment tools that may be useful for evaluating a client's sense of spirituality before and after a period of mind-body exercise training. The following are three examples: the Brief Serenity Scale (Kreitzer et al., 2009), the Mindful Attention Awareness Scale (Brown & Ryan, 2003), and the Spirituality Index of Well-Being (Daaleman & Frey, 2004).

Indications for Mind-body Exercise

There are a number of indications for choosing mind-body exercise modalities for clients, including as a complement to conventional aerobic or resistance-training exercise when additional muscular fitness and stress-reduction benefits are desired. Mind-body exercise, particularly tai chi, qigong, restorative yoga, and Pilates, may also be appropriate for those with low functional capacity (e.g., deconditioned individuals, seniors, or those with chronic conditions). Many older adults seek better balance, and numerous studies have demonstrated improved balance and reduced falls in seniors who practice tai chi and qigong-type exercise on a regular basis. Mind-body exercise is also appropriate for clients with chronic disease (e.g., high-normal and stage 1 hypertension, **type 2 diabetes,** anxiety and depression disorders, arthritis, and poor functional capacity), as well as for stable individuals requiring cardiac and/or pulmonary rehabilitation, pain management, or anger management. The chosen mind-body exercise modality should follow accepted and current pre-exercise assessment and exercise-training guidelines for individuals with medical conditions (American College of Sports Medicine, 2010; Fletcher et al., 2001).

Mind-body Exercise and Chronic Disease Management

In recent years, mind-body exercise programs, particularly yoga, qigong, and tai chi, have played increasing roles in managing a number of chronic disease states. The major chronic disease states include cardiovascular disease (primarily heart disease and stroke), cancer, diabetes, and arthritis.

There are two key considerations when selecting mind-body exercise in chronic disease management:

- Clients should only use forms of mind-body exercise where the degree of difficulty and intensity of effort begins with very low physical effort (e.g., 2–3 METs) and can be graduated slowly.
- Only those with chronic disease states where the disease course is stable (i.e., no unstable symptoms) should consider mind-body exercise.

For clarification purposes, mind-body exercise here denotes low-to-moderate intensity physical exercise coupled with a significant meditative/contemplative and breathwork component.

Characteristics of mind-body exercise programs that are helpful for those with stable chronic disease include the following:

- Can be taught at a relatively low-intensity level (e.g., 2–4 METs) and can be individualized
- Decrease real-time cognitive arousal and stress hormone activation
- Enhance proprioception (muscle sense) and kinesthesis
- Can improve muscular strength, posture, and balance
- Can improve self-efficacy and confidence

In a review of 32 studies on yoga and chronic disease risk factors, Yang (2007) found that yoga interventions are generally effective in reducing body weight, blood pressure, glucose level, and high cholesterol. However, only a few studies examined long-term adherence.

Mind-body Modalities and Acute Coronary Syndromes

Employing yogic breathing and meditation therapy can help reduce the potential for triggering **acute coronary syndromes (ACS)** (i.e., heart attacks and acute chest pain episodes) in individuals who have coronary disease and are vulnerable to cholesterol plaque rupture. When skillfully taught, mind-body therapies can be used to reduce the emotional-cognitive triggers for ACS.

There are a variety of stimuli that can "trigger" ACS [e.g., stress/anger, tobacco use, sudden onset exercise, and acute dietary factors (ingestion of a high-fat meal, caffeine consumption, cigarette smoking on a full stomach)], and there are current medical therapies that can reduce those stimuli. Teaching clients mind-body behaviors to reduce acute stress, such as yogic breathwork, meditation, tai chi, qi gong, and restorative yoga, can help reduce these triggers by either replacing them and/or inducing a more relaxed psychological state. Such mind-body therapy can reduce the heart rate and blood pressure response to anxiety-provoking situations. Integrating medical and mind-body therapy can reduce the vulnerability of a coronary artery cholesterol plaque rupture, which often is the initial event before a heart attack **(myocardial infarction)** or other forms of ACS. Yogendra et al. (2004), among others (Manchanda, 2000), have also shown with coronary angiography and myocardial perfusion imaging that yogic lifestyle therapy (meditation, asanas, walking, and low-fat dietary therapy) can slow the progression of coronary artery disease and even induce regression of **atherosclerosis** in some coronary blood vessels.

Personal Trainers and Mind-body Exercise

Health-promotion and fitness professionals should become familiar with the basic tenets of at least the classical forms of mind-body exercise for two reasons. First, this knowledge will reduce the number of unfortunate misconceptions that many people have about yoga, tai chi chuan, or qigong. Most contemporary mind-body exercise methods were and continue to be developed on a platform of qigong, yoga, and/or Native American spiritual exercise. Second, by attaining a better grasp of the cultural, health, and fitness benefits of these unique forms of exercise, personal trainers can more confidently refer clients to qualified mind-body exercise teachers, perhaps even inspiring a personal interest and participation. Chinese health exercise (i.e., qigong and its countless forms) is practiced by millions of people world-wide, yet the majority of fitness professionals in the West would find it difficult to produce even a cursory definition of this time-honored activity. Until recently, these distinctive exercise methods have been ignored and underappreciated by the Western fitness culture. Very few contemporary exercise science texts even mention their existence despite a rather large and increasing body of published research. Moreover, personal trainers should avoid the temptation to overly critique, particularly the classical forms of mind-body exercise, from a Westernized **biomechanics** or target conditioning zone perspective. The central function of most of these methods is to enhance the individual's sense of self-empowerment and personal spirituality while being respectful of their existing faith. Mind-body exercise, when taught respectfully and skillfully, is an opportunity to improve health for those who wish to complement their existing fitness program or who are otherwise sedentary and are looking for some greater meaning in their daily exercise routine.

Practical Suggestions for Personal Trainers

Structured mind-body techniques can be incorporated into a host of personal-training settings, although it is important to understand that these techniques do not substitute for the many cognitive and health-related benefits of, for example, a restorative yoga or tai chi chuan class.

The following are several methods whereby one or more mind-body exercise characteristics can be integrated into a personal-training session:

- Before and during a resistance-training session, personal trainers can teach a client to use two mind-body techniques that are the focuses of nearly all stress-reduction programs: sustained attention to the present and internal awareness. The client should prioritize his or her mental focus on the kinesthesis of each muscle contraction as well as the breath—this focus is entirely nonjudgmental. This process is in contrast to thoughts generated by the actual physical load or effort, where there is some level of negative appraisal assigned to the difficulty of each exercise repetition.
- Meditation and yogic-breathing exercises can be integrated with existing warm-up and cool-down exercises. For example, begin the warm-up session with a three- to five-minute quiet contemplation or meditation session before progressing to low-level aerobic or flexibility exercise. One to two minutes of yogic breathing exercise can also be added here. The client can end the entire exercise session with a similar meditation component.
- Personal trainers can incorporate a mind-body component in the aerobic phase of an exercise session. This is optimally executed with low- to moderate-intensity aerobic or strength exercise (e.g., 30 to 60% of maximum effort level or aerobic capacity). Adding a mindful component to a flexibility exercise, low-level cycling, slow intentional muscular contractions during strength training, or walking can be quite rewarding. For example, during low-level cycling exercise (i.e., with minimal resistance on the pedal crank axis), clients can add a present-moment nonjudgmental focus on "muscle sense" while synchronizing slow abdominal breathing with every two or three pedal crank revolutions. ChiRunning is an excellent example of this kind of mind-body integration process (www.chirunning.com).
- Personal trainers can incorporate any of the select yoga poses described in the restorative or Iyengar tradition into the flexibility and strength-training components of the program. For example, inserting the seated or standing spinal twist pose, child's pose, or cobra pose between resistance-training exercises may increase flexibility and serve as a welcome period of relative rest and energy restoration. It is imperative that proper yogic breathing accompany these exercises.
- The popular tree pose can be included as part of a circuit of exercises to help stimulate balance control. Balance is seldom addressed by personal trainers, even when working with those clients who need

it most—older adults. The tree pose is attained by starting with a slow exhalation and assuming a single-leg stance on the right foot while bending the left knee and placing the sole of the left foot, toes pointing down, on the inside of the right leg between the knee and groin (Figure 13-10). While inhaling, the client brings the arms overhead and joins the palms together. He or she holds this pose for three to five breaths in the beginning sessions, and six to eight breaths in later sessions. He or she then repeats the pose while standing on the opposite leg. Using a nearby table or wall for support will be helpful in early stages of training for this pose.

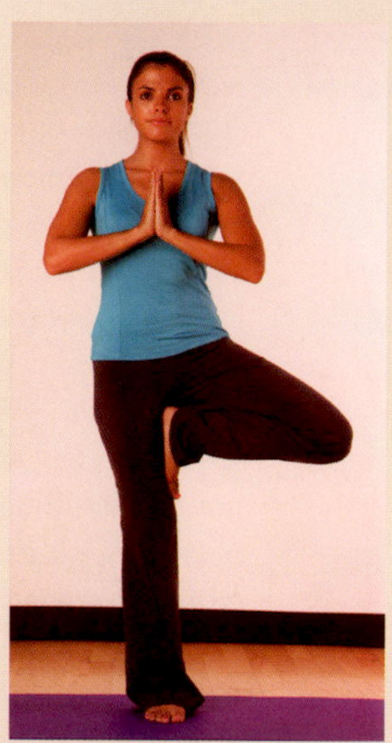

Figure 13-10
Tree pose

A Simple Breathwork Exercise

The following is a simple introductory breathing exercise (diaphragmatic breathing emphasis) that personal trainers can present to clients, many of whom will find it very therapeutic.

- Lie supine and place one hand on the chest and the other on the abdomen. Place a small pillow or folded blanket under the head (i.e., corpse pose or savasana).
- Take 10 to 15 slow, deep breaths. Expand the abdomen during inhalation and contract the abdomen during exhalation—while keeping the chest as still as possible.
- Pause for a couple of seconds between the inhalation and exhalation phase of each breath.

Summary

Mind-body exercise continues to emerge as an effective fitness and health-enhancement modality. There is scientific evidence that hypertension, insulin resistance, pain, cardiovascular disease, anxiety, and depression all respond favorably to regular participation in mind-body exercise such as tai chi, qigong, and hatha yoga. The core benefits from these programs include increased balance, strength, and flexibility, as well as relaxation and mental quiescence. Regular and self-regulated mind-body exercise may also be ideal for many clients because of its portability and relative low-intensity nature.

It is not beyond reason that in the near future the fitness and health-promotion industry will benefit from the inclusion of mind-body exercise guidelines and professional resources in respected exercise consensus publications that recommend the appropriate quality and quantity of exercise for primary and secondary disease prevention. The alliance of traditional health promotion programming with mind-body interventions should further reduce healthcare utilization and the unnecessary burden of degenerative diseases. Given the present mandate for implementing integrated disease prevention and disease-management programs to effectively reduce healthcare costs and inspire self-care in clients, mind-body exercise programs will be a necessary element.

References

American College of Sports Medicine (2010). *ACSM's Guidelines for Exercise Testing and Prescription* (8th ed.). Philadelphia, Pa.: Wolters Kluwer/Lippincott Williams & Wilkins.

Anderson, B.D. & Spector A. (2000). Introduction to pilates-based rehabilitation. *Orthopaedic Physical Therapy Clinics of North America,* 9, 395–410.

Bera, T.K. (1995). Recovery from stress in two different postures and in Shavasa yogic relaxation positions. *Indian Journal of Physiological Pharmacology,* 42, 473–478.

Berger, B. & Owen, D. (1992). Mood alteration with yoga and swimming: Aerobic exercise may not be necessary. *Perceptual and Motor Skills,* 75, 1331–1343.

Bernardi, L. et al. (2002). Slow breathing increases arterial baroreflex sensitivity in patients with chronic heart failure. *Circulation,* 105, 143–145.

Bernardi, L. et al. (2001). Beyond science? Effect of rosary prayer and yoga mantras on autonomic cardiovascular rhythms: Comparative study. *British Medical Journal,* 323, 1446–1449.

Bhatia, M. et al. (2003). Electrophysiologic evaluation of Sudarshan Kriya: An EEG, BAER, and P300 study. *Indian Journal of Physiology and Pharmacology*, 47, 157–163.

Birkel, D.A. & Edgren, L. (2000). Hatha yoga: Improved vital capacity in college students. *Alternative Therapies in Health and Medicine,* 6, 55–63.

Bowman, A.J. et al. (1997). Effects of aerobic exercise training and yoga on the baroreflex index in healthy elderly persons. *European Journal of Clinical Investigation,* 27, 443–449.

Brown, K.W. & Ryan, R.M. (2003). The benefits of being present: Mindfulness and its role in psychological well-being. *Journal of Personality and Social Psychology*, 84, 822–848.

Canon, W. (1914). Emotional stimulation of adrenal secretion. *American Journal of Physiology,* 33, 356–372.

Cappo, B.M. & Holmes, D.S. (1984). The utility of prolonged respiratory exhalation for reducing physiological and psychological arousal in non-threatening and threatening situations. *Journal of Psychosomatic Research*, 28, 265–273.

Centers for Disease Control and Prevention (2002). *Methods and Measures.* Atlanta, Ga.: National Center for Chronic Disease Prevention and Health Promotion. www.cdc.gov/hrqol/methods.htm

Channer, K.S. et al. (1996). Changes in hemodynamic parameters following tai chi chuan and aerobic exercise in patients recovering from myocardial infarction. *Postgraduate Medicine*, 72, 347–351.

Chen, K.M. et. al. (2009). Sleep quality, depression state, and health status of older adults after silver yoga exercises: Cluster randomized trial. *International Journal of Nursing Studies,* 46, 2, 154–163.

Chen, K.W. et al. (2008). Effects of external qigong therapy on osteoarthritis of the knee: A randomized controlled trial. *Clinical Rheumatology,* 27, 12, 1497–1505.

Clark, D.M., Salkovskis, P.M., & Chalkley, A.J. (1985). Respiratory control as a treatment for panic attacks. *Therapeutic and Experimental Psychiatry,* 16, 22–30.

Daaleman, T. & Frey, B. (2004). The Spirituality Index of Well-Being: A new instrument for health-related quality-of-life research. *Annals of Family Medicine,* 2, 499–503.

Danhauer, S.C. et al. (2008). Restorative yoga for women with ovarian or breast cancer: Findings from a pilot study. *Journal of the Society for Integrative Oncology,* 6, 47–58.

DiCarlo, L.J. et al. (1995). Cardiovascular, metabolic, and perceptual responses to hatha yoga standing poses. *Medicine, Exercise, Nutrition, and Health,* 4, 107–112.

Donzelli, S. et al. (2006). Two different techniques in the rehabilitation treatment of low back pain: A randomized controlled trial. *Europa Medicophysica*, 42, 205–210.

Faber, M.J. et al. (2006). Effects of exercise programs on falls and mobility in frail and pre-frail older adults: A multicenter randomized controlled trial. *Archives of Physical Medicine and Rehabilitation,* 87, 885–896.

Fletcher, G.A. et al. (2001). Exercise standards for testing and training: A statement for healthcare professionals from the American Heart Association. *Circulation,* 104, 1694–1740.

Fluge, T. (1994). Long-term effects of breathing exercises and yoga in patients with bronchial asthma. *Pneumologie,* 48, 484–490.

Garfinkel, M.S. et al. (1999). Yoga based intervention for carpal tunnel syndrome: A random trial. *Journal of the American Medical Association,* 281, 2087–2099.

Garfinkel, M.S. et al. (1994). Evaluation of a yoga-based regimen for treatment of osteoarthritis of the hands. *Journal of Rheumatology,* 21, 2341–2343.

Goodwin, G.M., McCloskey, I., & Matthews, P. (1972). The contribution of muscle afferents to kinesthesia shown by vibration-induced illusions of movement and by effects of paralyzing joint afferents. *Brain,* 95, 705.

Gordon L.A. et al. (2008). Effect of exercise therapy on lipid profile and oxidative stress indicators in patients with type 2 diabetes. *BMC Complementary and Alternative Medicine,* 8, 21.

Gupta, N. et al. (2006). Effect of yoga based lifestyle intervention on state and trait anxiety. *Indian Journal of Physiology and Pharmacology,* 50, 41–47.

Hong, Y., Li, J., & Robinson, P.D. (2000). Balance control, flexibility, and cardiorespiratory fitness among older tai chi practitioners. *British Journal of Sports Medicine,* 34, 29–34.

Hutchinson, M.R., Christiansen, T.L., & Beitzel, J. (1998). Improving leaping ability in elite rhythmic gymnasts. *Medicine & Science in Sports & Exercise,* 30, 1543–1547.

Innes, K.E. & Vincent, H.K. (2007). The influence of yoga-based programs on risk profiles in adults with type 2 diabetes mellitus: A systematic review. *Evidence-Based Complementary and Alternative Medicine,* 4, 469–486.

Innes, K.E. et al. (2005). Risk indices associated with the insulin resistance syndrome, cardiovascular disease and possible protection with yoga: A systematic review. *Journal of the American Board of Family Practice,* 18, 491–519.

Jain, S.C. & Talukdar, B. (1993). Evaluation of yoga therapy programme for patients with bronchial asthma. *Singapore Medical Journal,* 34, 306.

Jain, S.C. et al. (1993). A study of response pattern of non-insulin dependent diabetics to yoga therapy. *Diabetes Research and Clinical Practice,* 19, 69–74.

Janakiramaiah, N. et al. (2000). Antidepressant efficacy of Sudarshan Kriya Yoga (SKY) in melancholia: A randomized comparison with electroconvulsive therapy (ECT) and Imipramine. *Journal of Affective Disorders,* 57, 255–259.

Jella, S.A. & Shannahoff-Khalsa, D.S. (1993). The effects of unilateral forced nostril breathing on cognitive performance. *International Journal of Neuroscience,* 73, 61–68.

Joshi, L.N., Joshi, V.D., & Gokhale, L.V. (1992). Effect of short term pranayama practice on breathing rate and ventilatory functions of the lung. *Indian Journal of Physiological Pharmacology,* 36, 105–108.

Kamei, T. et al. (2000). Decrease in serum cortisol during yoga exercise is correlated with alpha wave activation. *Perceptual and Motor Skills*, 90 (Pt. 1), 1027–1032.

Kerr, D. et al. (2002). An Eastern art form for a Western disease: Randomised controlled trial of yoga in patients with poorly controlled insulin-treated diabetes. *Pract Diabetes Intern,* 19, 164–166.

Khanam, A.A. (1996). Study of pulmonary and autonomic functions of asthma patients after yoga training. *Indian Journal of Physiological Pharmacology*, 40, 318–324.

Koch, U. et al. (1998). Yoga treatment in psychophysiological insomnia. *Journal of Sleep Research,* 7 (suppl. 2), 137.

Kreitzer, M.J. et al. (2009) The brief serenity scale: A psychometric analysis of a measure of spirituality and well-being. *Journal of Holistic Nursing,* 27, 7–16

Kutner, N.G. et al. (1997). Self-report benefits of tai chi practice by older adults. *Journal of Gerontology, Biological Psychology and Social Sciences,* 52, 242–246.

Lai, J.S. et al. (1993). Cardiorespiratory responses of tai chi chuan practitioners and sedentary subjects during cycle ergometry. *Journal of the Formosa Medical Association,* 92, 894–899.

Lan, C. et al. (1999). The effect of tai chi on cardiorespiratory function in patients with coronary artery bypass surgery. *Medicine & Science in Sports & Exercise,* 31, 634–638.

Lan, C. et al. (1998). 12-month tai chi training in the elderly: Its effect on health fitness. *Medicine & Science in Sports & Exercise,* 30, 345–351.

Lan, C. et al. (1996). Cardiorespiratory function, flexibility, and body composition assessment of geriatric tai chi chuan practitioners. *Archives of Physical Medicine and Rehabilitation,* 77, 612.

Lasater, J. (2003). *30 Essential Yoga Poses for Beginning Students and Their Teachers.* Berkeley, Calif.: Rodmell Press.

Lasater, J. (1995). *Relax and Renew: Restful Yoga for Stressful Times.* Berkeley, Calif.: Rodmell Press.

Li, F. et al. (2001). An evaluation of the effects of tai chi exercise on physical function among older persons: A randomized controlled trial. *Annals of Behavioral Medicine*, 23, 139–146.

Mahajan, A.S. et al. (1999). Lipid profile of coronary risk subjects following yogic lifestyle intervention. *Indian Heart Journal,* 51, 37–40.

Malhotra, V. et.al. (2002). Study of yoga asanas in assessment of pulmonary function in NIDDM patients. *Indian Journal of Physiology and Pharmacology,* 46, 313–320.

Manchanda, S.C. (2000). Retardation of coronary atherosclerosis with yoga lifestyle intervention. *Journal of the Associated Physicians of India,* 48, 687.

Manocha, R. et al. (2002). Sahaja yoga in the management of moderate to severe asthma: Randomized controlled trial. *Thorax,* 57, 110–115.

McCaul, K.D., Solomon, S., & Holmes, D.S. (1979). Effects of paced respiration and expectation on the physiological and psychological responses to threat. *Journal of Personality and Social Psychology,* 37, 564–571.

Miller, B.S. (1998). *Yoga Discipline of Freedom: The Yoga Sutra.* New York: Bantam Books.

Monro, R. et al. (1992). Yoga therapy for NIDDM: A controlled trial. *Complement Med Research,* 6, 66–68.

Monroe, R., Ghosh, A.K., & Kalish, D. (1989). *Yoga Research Bibliography: Scientific Studies on Yoga and Meditation.* Cambridge, England: Yoga Biomedical Trust.

Murugesan, R., Govindarajulu, N., & Bera, T.K. (2000).

Effects of selected yoga practices on hypertension. *Indian Journal of Physiological Pharmacology,* 44, 207–210.

Naveen, K.V. et al. (1997). Yoga breathing through a particular nostril increases spatial memory scores without lateralized effects. *Psychology Reports,* 81, 555–561.

Nespor, K. (1991). Pain management and yoga. *International Journal of Psychosomatics,* 38, 76–81.

Ornish, D. et al. (1990). Lifestyle Heart Trial. *Lancet,* 336, 129–133.

Ospina, M.B. et al. (2007). Meditation practices for health: State of research. *Evidence Report: Technology Assessment (Full Rep),* 155, 1-263.

Province, M.A. et al. (1995). The effects of exercise on falls in elderly patients. A preplanned meta-analysis of the FICSIT Trials. Frailty and Injuries: Cooperative Studies of Intervention Techniques. *Journal of the American Medical Association,* 273, 1341–1347.

Raghavendra, R.M. et al. (2007). Effects of an integrated yoga programme on chemotherapy-induced nausea and emesis in breast cancer patients. *European Journal of Cancer Care,* 16, 462–474.

Raju, P.S. et al. (1994). Comparison of effects of yoga and physical exercise in athletes. *Indian Journal of Medical Research*, 100, 81–86.

Ray, U.S. et al. (2001). Effect of yogic exercises on physical and mental health of young fellowship course trainees. *Indian Journal of Physiological Pharmacology*, 45, 37–53.

Rydeard, R. et al. (2006). Pilates-based therapeutic exercise: Effect on subjects with nonspecific chronic low back pain and functional disability: A randomized controlled trial. *Journal of Orthopedic and Sports Physical Therapy,* 36, 472–484.

Sakakibara, M. & Hayano, J. (1996). Effect of slowed respiration on cardiac parasympathetic response to threat. *Psychosomatic Medicine,* 58, 32–37.

Sakakibara, M., Takeuchi, S., & Hayano, J. (1994). Effects of relaxation training on cardiac parasympathetic tone. *Psychophysiology,* 31, 223–228.

Schaller, K.J. (1996). Tai chi chih: An exercise for older adults. *Journal of Gerontological Nursing*, 22, 12–17.

Schell, F.J., Allolio, B., & Schonecke, O.W. (1994). Physiological and psychological effects of hatha-yoga exercise in healthy women. *International Journal of Psychosomatics,* 41, 46–52.

Schmidt, T. (1997). Changes in cardiovascular risk factors and hormones during a comprehensive residential three month kriya yoga training program and vegetarian nutrition. *Acta Physiologica Scandinavia Supplement*, 640, 158–162.

Selvamurthy, W. et al. (1998). A new physiological approach to control essential hypertension. *Indian Journal of Physiological Pharmacology,* 42, 205.

Selye, H. (1946). The general adaptation syndrome and the diseases of adaptation. *Journal of Clinical Endocrinology,* 6, 117–230.

Shannahoff-Khalsa, D.S. & Beckett, L.R. (1996). Clinical case report: Efficacy of yogic techniques in the treatment of obsessive compulsive disorder. *International Journal of Neuroscience,* 85, 1–17.

Sharma, H. et al. (2003). Sudarshan Kriya practitioners exhibit better antioxidant status and lower blood lactate levels. *Biological Psychology,* 63, 281–291.

Sivasankaran, S. et al. (2006). The effect of a six-week program of yoga and meditation on brachial artery reactivity: Do psychosocial interventions affect vascular tone? *Clinical Cardiology,* 29, 393–398.

Sovik, R. (2000). The science of breathing: The yogic view. In: Mayer, E.A. & Sayer, C.B. (Eds.). *Progress in Brain Research.* pp. 491–505. New York: Elsevier Science BV.

Taylor-Piliae, R.E. et al. (2006). Hemodynamic responses to a community-based tai chi exercise intervention in ethnic Chinese adults with cardiovascular disease. *European Journal of Cardiovascular Nursing,* 5, 165–174.

Tekur, P. et al. (2008). Effect of short-term intensive yoga program on pain, functional disability and spinal flexibility in chronic low back pain: A randomized control study. *Journal of Alternative Complementary Medicine,* 14, 637–644.

Telles, S. et al. (2000). Oxygen consumption and respiration following two yoga relaxation techniques. *Applied Psychophysiology and Biofeedback*, 25, 221.

Tran, M.D. (2001). Effects of hatha yoga practice on fitness parameters. *Preventive Cardiology,* 4, 165–170.

Tse, M. (1996). *Qigong for Health and Vitality.* New York: St. Martin's Griffin.

Tsujiuchi, T. et al. (2002). The effect of qigong relaxation exercise on the control of type 2 diabetes mellitus. *Diabetes Care*, 25, 241–242.

Vaananen, J. et al. (2002). Taichiquan acutely increases heart rate variability. *Clinical Physiology and Functional Imaging,* 22, 2–3.

Wang, J.S., Lan, C., & Wong, M.K. (2001). Tai chi chuan training to enhance microcirculatory function in healthy elderly subjects. *Archives of Physical Medicine and Rehabilitation,* 82, 1176–1180.

Wolf, S.L. et al. (1996). Reducing frailty and falls in older persons: An investigation of tai chi and computerized balance training. *Journal of the American Geriatric Society,* 44, 489–497.

Wolfson, L. et al. (1996). Balance and strength training in older adults: Intervention gains and tai chi maintenance. *Journal of the American Geriatric Society,* 44, 498–506.

Wong, A.M. et al. (2001). Coordination exercise and postural stability in elderly people: Effects of tai chi chuan. *Archives of Physical Medicine and Rehabilitation,* 82, 608–612.

Wood, C. (1993). Mood change and perceptions of vitality: A comparison of the effects of relaxation, visualization, and yoga. *Journal of the Royal Society of Medicine*, 86, 254.

Xin, L. et al. (2007). A qualitative review of the role of qigong in the management of diabetes. *Journal of Alternative Complementary Medicine,*13, 27–33.

Yang, K. (2007). A review of yoga programs for four leading risk factors of chronic diseases. *Evidence-based Complementary Alternative Medicine,* 4, 487–491.

Yang, Y. et al. (2007). Effect of combined taiji and qigong training on balance mechanisms: A randomized controlled trial of older adults. *Medical Science Monitor,* 13,CR339–348.

Yeh, G.Y. et al. (2008). The effect of tai chi exercise on blood pressure: A systematic review. *Preventive Cardiology,* 11, 82–89.

Yogendra, J. et al. (2004). Beneficial effects of yoga lifestyle on reversibility of ischaemic heart disease: Caring heart project of International Board of Yoga. *Journal of Association of Physicians of India,* 52, 283.

Suggested Reading

Chance, J. (1999). *Thorson's Principles of the Alexander Technique.* New York: Harper Collins.

Cohen, K.S. (1998). *The Way of Qigong*. New York: Ballantine Books.

Desikachar, T.K.V. (1999). *The Heart of Yoga.* Rochester, Vt.: Inner Traditions.

Dong, P. & Esser, A. (2008). *Chi Gong: The Ancient Chinese Way to Health.* New York: Marlowe & Co.

Feuerstein, G. & Payne, L. (2000). *Yoga For Dummies*. Indianapolis, Ind.: IDG Books.

Gallagher, S.P. & Kryzanowska, R. (1999). *The Pilates Method of Body Conditioning.* Philadelphia, Pa.: BainBridge Books.

Huang, A. (1993). *Complete Tai-Chi.* Tokyo: Tuttle Publishing.

Iyengar, B.K.S. (1977). *Light on Yoga: The Yoga Journey to Wholeness, Inner Peace, and Ultimate Freedom*. New York: Rodale Books.

Jahnke, R. (2002). *The Healing Promise of Qi: Creating Extraordinary Wellness Through Qigong and Tai Chi.* New York: McGraw-Hill.

Khalsa, S.K. (2001). *KISS Guide to Yoga.* New York: Dk Publications.

Kraftsow, G. (2002). *Yoga for Transformation.* New York: Penguin Compass.

Kraftsow, G. (1999). *Yoga for Wellness: Healing With The Timeless Teachings of Viniyoga.* New York: Penguin Books.

La Forge, R. (2008). Coronary artery disease. In: American Council on Exercise. *ACE Advanced Health & Fitness Specialist Manual.* San Diego, Calif.: American Council on Exercise.

Lasater, J. (2003). *30 Essential Yoga Poses for Beginning Students and Their Teachers.* Berkeley, Calif.: Rodmell Press.

Monro, R., Nagarathna, R., & Nagendra H.R. (2000). *Yoga for Common Ailments.* London: Gaia Books.

National Museum of the American Indian (Heth, C., Editor) (1993). *Native American Dance: Ceremonies and Social Traditions.* Golden, Colo.: Fulcrum Publishing.

Rosas D. & Rosas C. (2005). *The Nia Technique: The High-Powered Energizing Workout that Gives You a New Body and a New Life.* New York: Broadway Books.

Rywerant Y. (2003). *The Feldenkrais Method: Teaching by Handling.* Laguna Beach, Calif.: Basic Health Publications.

Shafarman, S. (1997). *Awareness Heals: The Feldenkrais Method for Dynamic Health*. New York: Da Capo Press.

Stone, J. (1995). *Tai Chi Chih: New Revised Edition.* Fort Yates, N.D.: Good Karma Publishing.

Tse, M. (1996). *Qigong for Health and Vitality.* New York: St. Martin's Griffin.

Wilson, S.D. (1997). *Qi Gong for Beginners: Eight Easy Movements for Vibrant Health.* Portland Ore.: Rudra Press.

Teacher Training Resources

There are many teacher training and certification programs for prospective tai chi, qigong, Pilates, Nia, and particularly yoga teachers. Many of these programs do not follow a common set of consensus guidelines that cover a core curriculum such as exercise and health assessment and evidenced-based applied exercise science specific to the method taught. This does not mean there are not many thoughtfully planned and professionally conducted yoga and tai chi teacher training programs; however, historically there have been no central practice guidelines or regulations governing core material in such programs. The Yoga Alliance, which is a nonprofit organization, maintains a national registry of yoga teachers and schools who meet the Alliance's recommended educational standards and strongly encourages the inclusion of core competencies.

Select Yoga, Tai Chi, Qigong, Nia, and Pilates Education and Training Resources

Balanced Body
www.pilates.com
Phone: 800-745-2837

East West Academy of
The Healing Arts (qigong) Way
www.eastwestqi.com
Phone: 415-285-9400

Inner IDEA (annual conference of
many mind-body exercise programs)
www.inneridea.com
800-462-1876

Integrative Yoga Therapy
www.iytyogatherapy.com
Phone: 800-750-9642

International Association of Yoga Therapists
www.iayt.org
Phone: 928-541-0004

Justin Stone's Tai Chi Chih
www.taichichih.org

Kripalu Center for Yoga and Health
www.kripalu.org
Phone: 866-200-5203

Mad Dogg Athletics (Peak Pilates)
www.spinning.com
Phone: 800-847-7746

National Qigong Association USA
www.nqa.org
Phone: 888-815-1893

Nia
www.nianow.com
Phone: (503) 245-9886

Pilates Method Alliance
www.pilatesmethodalliance.org
Phone: 866-573-4945

Polestar Pilates
www.polestarpilates.com
Phone: 305-666-0037

Qigong Association of America
www.qi.org
Phone: 541-752-6599

Qigong Institute
www.qigonginstitute.org

Relax and Renew® Restorative Yoga Teacher
Training with Judith Lasater
www.yogatreesf.com/teachertraining/
www.restorativeyogateachers.com/teach/

Sivananda Yoga Vedanta Center of New York
www.sivananda.org
Phone: 212-255-4560

Stott Pilates
www.stottpilates.com
Phone: 800-910-0001

Yoga Alliance
www.yogaalliance.org
Phone: 877-964-2255

YogaFit
www.yogafit.com
Phone: 888-786-3111

Yoga Research and Education Center
www.yrec.org

IN THIS CHAPTER:

Cardiovascular Disorders
- Exercise and Coronary Artery Disease
- Exercise Guidelines
- Sample Exercise Recommendation for Clients With Cardiovascular Disease

Hypertension
- Exercise and Hypertension
- Exercise Guidelines
- Sample Exercise Recommendation for Clients With Hypertension

Stroke
- Exercise and Stroke
- Exercise Guidelines
- Sample Exercise Recommendation for Clients With Stroke

Peripheral Vascular Disease
- Exercise and Peripheral Vascular Disease
- Exercise Guidelines
- Sample Exercise Recommendation for Clients With Peripheral Vascular Disease

Dyslipidemia
- Exercise and Dyslipidemia
- Exercise Guidelines
- Sample Exercise Recommendation for Clients With Dyslipidemia

Diabetes
- Diabetes Control
- Benefits of Exercise for Type 1 Diabetics
- Benefits of Exercise for Type 2 Diabetics
- Exercise Guidelines
- Exercise Training for Clients With Type 1 Diabetes
- Exercise Training for Clients With Type 2 Diabetes
- Precautions
- Sample Exercise Recommendation for Clients With Diabetes

Metabolic Syndrome
- Exercise and the Metabolic Syndrome
- Exercise Guidelines
- Sample Exercise Recommendation for Clients With the Metabolic Syndrome

Asthma
- Exercise and Asthma
- Exercise Guidelines
- Sample Exercise Recommendation for Clients With Asthma

Cancer
- Exercise and Cancer
- Exercise Guidelines
- Precautions
- Sample Exercise Recommendation for Clients With Cancer

Osteoporosis
- Exercise and Osteoporosis
- Exercise Guidelines
- Sample Exercise Recommendation for Clients With Osteoporosis

Arthritis
- Exercise and Arthritis
- Exercise Guidelines
- Sample Exercise Recommendation for Clients With Arthritis

Fibromyalgia
- Exercise and Fibromyalgia
- Exercise Guidelines
- Sample Exercise Recommendation for Clients With Fibromyalgia

Chronic Fatigue Syndrome
- Exercise and Chronic Fatigue Syndrome
- Exercise Guidelines
- Sample Exercise Recommendation for Clients With Chronic Fatigue Syndrome

Low-back Pain
- Exercise and Low-back Pain
- Exercise Guidelines
- Sample Exercise Recommendation for Clients With Low-back Pain

Weight Management
- Exercise and Weight Management
- Exercise Guidelines
- Sample Exercise Recommendation for Weight Management

Exercise and Older Adults
- Cardiovascular System
- Musculoskeletal System
- Sensory Systems
- Mental Health
- Exercise Guidelines
- Sample Exercise Recommendation for Older Adults

Exercise and Youth
- Exercise Guidelines
- Sample Exercise Recommendation for Youth

Pre- and Postnatal Exercise
- Exercise Guidelines for Pregnant Women
- Postnatal Exercise Guidelines
- Sample Exercise Recommendation for Pregnant Women

Summary

BRAD A. ROY, Ph.D., FACHE, FACSM, *is the administrator at The Summit Medical Fitness Center and is part of the executive team for Kalispell Regional Medical Center in Kalispell, Montana. Dr. Roy has more than 30 years experience in healthcare and the fitness industry. Dr. Roy oversees a nearly 115,000 square foot medical fitness center, in addition to managing community health promotion, cardiac and pulmonary rehabilitation, occupational medicine, employee health, home health, hospice care, private care, and the stroke program.*

CHAPTER 14

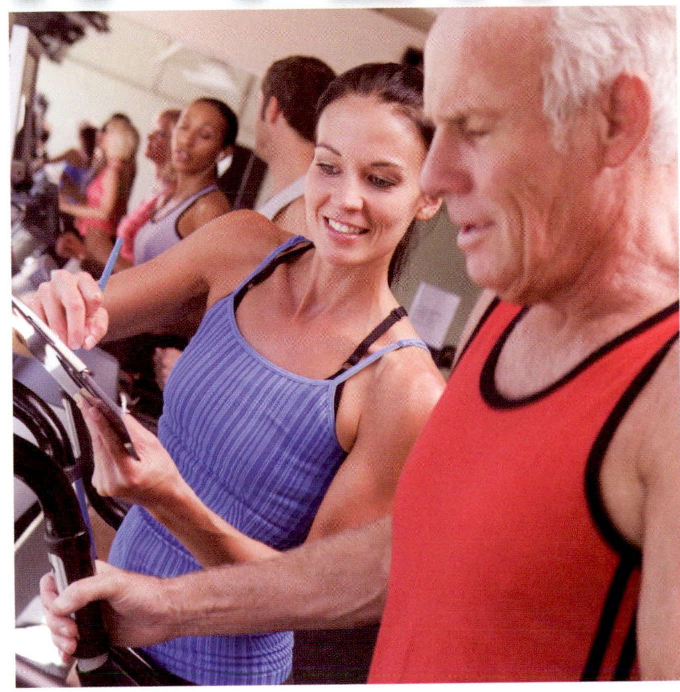

Exercise and Special Populations

Brad A. Roy

Personal trainers frequently encounter clients with special needs and health concerns. **Chronic diseases** such as cardiovascular disorders, cancer, **diabetes,** and the **metabolic syndrome** are the leading causes of death and disability in the United States. These health conditions are responsible for seven out of every 10 deaths in the U.S. and affect the quality of life of more than 130 million Americans. Frequently thought of as conditions seen in older adults, **obesity,** diabetes, and **hypertension** are becoming increasingly common in children and young adults. The U.S. Centers for Disease Control and Prevention (CDC) estimate that reducing three **risk factors**—poor diet, physical inactivity, and smoking—would dramatically reduce the incidence of chronic disease (CDC, 2008a).

Because of this rapid rise in chronic disease, it is important for a personal trainer to identify and address health conditions before working with a client. Such conditions may significantly influence exercise program development and should be identified as part of the initial screening portion of the client–trainer interaction. A personal trainer should regularly update client records to identify and effectively address changes in health status as they occur.

Once a client's medical and/or health conditions have been identified, the personal trainer must obtain physician approval before proceeding with exercise program development, testing, or training. Along with physician approval, the trainer should also request exercise guidelines and limitations from the client's physician. In many cases, a physician may choose to appoint another health professional to assist in providing exercise and educational guidelines. This may be, for example, a nurse, physical therapist, clinical exercise physiologist, diabetes educator, and/or a licensed dietitian. It is important that the personal trainer adheres to the guidelines and restrictions provided and maintains close communication with the health professional to have questions answered and to provide status reports at predetermined intervals.

Documentation of client encounters, health status, and progress is important for the trainer to appropriately adjust each client's program and prepare communication to the health provider. The **SOAP note** (an acronym for subjective, objective, assessment, and plan) is commonly used by healthcare providers to document patient progress. Content for each section of the SOAP note as used by fitness professionals is defined as follows:

- *Subjective:* Observations that include the client's own status report, a description of symptoms, challenges with the program, and progress made
- *Objective:* Measurements such as vital signs, height, weight, age, posture, exercise and other test results, as well as exercise and nutrition log information
- *Assessment:* A brief summary of the client's current status based on the subjective and objective observations and measures
- *Plan:* A description of the next steps in the program based on the assessment

Wording in each section of the SOAP note should be concise and accurately reflect the activities documented. The entire note could be written on an index card, depending on the size of one's writing. It is essential that every SOAP note is dated by the personal trainer. The SOAP note is an elegant and efficient way to communicate both what the client feels and what the personal trainer observes. Over time, SOAP notes document patterns of self-image versus actual performance, and can be useful tools when providing feedback to the client.

Typically, a client who has been released to take part in **independent activities of daily living** (including a limited exercise program) will also be cleared to work with a personal trainer who can provide additional guidance, motivation, and an appropriate rate of progression. An ACE-certified Personal Trainer is certified to work with clients that have health challenges only after they have been cleared by their personal physicians.

This chapter addresses basic guidelines for working with clients with the following health conditions and/or special needs:

- Coronary artery disease
- Hypertension
- Stroke
- Peripheral vascular disease
- Dyslipidemia
- Diabetes
- Metabolic syndrome
- Asthma
- Cancer
- Osteoporosis
- Arthritis
- Fibromyalgia
- Chronic fatigue syndrome
- Low-back pain
- Weight management
- Older adults
- Youth
- Pre- and postnatal

Generally speaking, clients with one or more of the above should follow a low- to moderate-intensity exercise program that progresses gradually. The exact nature of the program will depend on each person's current health status, physical condition, and other factors identified in the screening and referral process. The program must be individualized to the specific characteristics of the client, with appropriate modifications made to the activities that will enhance the safety and effectiveness of the exercise program. Many people with chronic health conditions have **comorbidities** (e.g., a person with heart disease and diabetes who is also **overweight**) that also impact the exercise program and further emphasize the importance of individualizing each program. A personal trainer who chooses to train clients with special needs has a responsibility to expand his or her knowledge and skills in this area through continuing education opportunities and close communication with healthcare professionals.

Cardiovascular Disorders

Cardiovascular disease (CVD) continues to be the leading cause of death in the developed world and for more than 100 years has caused more deaths in Americans than any other major cause. The American Heart Association (AHA) estimates that 80.7 million Americans have one or more types of cardiovascular disorders, including: **dyslipidemia, coronary artery disease (CAD), congestive heart failure (CHF),** hypertension, **stroke,** and **peripheral vascular disease.** Well-established risk factors that contribute to cardiovascular disease include family history, hypertension, smoking, diabetes, age, dyslipidemia, and lifestyle (i.e., poor diet and physical inactivity) (AHA, 2009a).

CAD, also called **atherosclerotic heart disease,** is characterized by a narrowing of the coronary arteries that supply the heart muscle with blood and oxygen. The narrowing is an inflammatory response within the arterial walls resulting from an initial injury (due to high blood pressure, elevated levels of **low-density lipoprotein (LDL)** cholesterol, elevated blood glucose, or other chemical agents such as those produced from cigarettes) and the deposition of lipid-rich plaque and calcified **cholesterol.** Heart attacks, or **myocardial infarctions (MI),** frequently result from the rupture of vulnerable plaques and the associated release of **thrombotic** (blood-clotting) substances that critically narrow or completely close the diameter of the artery.

Atherosclerosis is also the underlying cause of cerebral and peripheral vascular diseases. Manifestations of atherosclerosis include **angina,** heart attack, stroke, and intermittent **claudication.** Dyslipidemia (blood **lipid** disorder) significantly contributes to the development of atherosclerosis and associated disease conditions. It is estimated that 16.8 million Americans have CAD, 785,000 people will have an initial heart attack in 2009, and 445,687 will experience a recurrent event (AHA, 2009a).

Exercise and Coronary Artery Disease

Physical inactivity is a major independent risk factor for CAD in both men and women. People participating in moderate amounts of physical activity have a 20% lower risk, while those undertaking higher amounts of exercise have a 30% or more reduction in the risk of developing CAD (Haskell et al., 2008).

Exercise is also a critical part of the treatment regimen for people with CAD. For many years, heart attack patients were restricted to bed rest for six weeks or more. Unfortunately, this prolonged immobilization did not improve the healing process. In fact, it exposed the patient to additional risks of blood clots, lung infections, muscle wasting, and deconditioning. Since the early 1960s, many reports have been published documenting the benefits of progressive physical activity in reducing the **mortality** and **morbidity** among patients with CAD. Today, exercise training is an essential component of the therapeutic regimen for people with CAD. In almost all cases, an individual's recovery from a myocardial infarction, cardiac surgery, or other cardiac procedure (e.g., **angioplasty,** stenting) will benefit from an appropriately designed and monitored exercise program.

Clients with a history of CAD should be evaluated by their physicians, who should refer eligible candidates to supervised comprehensive cardiac rehabilitation programs before allowing them to start an exercise training program with a personal trainer. Most patients who have been released to take part in **activities of daily living (ADL)** will also have been given some basic activity guidelines. It is appropriate for the personal trainer to inform prospective clients that cardiac rehabilitation programs are available, and that clients should ask their physicians if participation is recommended. Unfortunately, many eligible patients are not referred to, or do not have access to, a cardiac rehabilitation program. In all cases, it is imperative that a client with two or more risk factors and/or active CAD is evaluated by his or her physician and obtains a physician release prior to starting an exercise program with a personal trainer (see Table 6-1, page 108).

Exercise Guidelines

All clients with documented CAD should have a physician-supervised **maximal graded exercise test** to determine their **functional capacity** and cardiovascular status to establish a safe exercise level. The physician or other designated health professional should then provide the personal trainer with basic exercise program parameters such as heart-rate limits, exercise limitations, and other program recommendations. These guidelines will usually be based on the exercise test results, medical history, clinical status, and symptoms. Additionally, there are published guidelines available to assist the personal trainer in working with CAD clients and interacting with their healthcare team [American College of Sports Medicine (ACSM), 2010; Wenger, 2008; Balady, 2007; American Association of Cardiovascular and Pulmonary Rehabilitation (AACVPR), 2004].

Exercise guidelines are based on the clinical status of the client, and it is most appropriate for personal trainers to work with low-risk CAD clients. Low-risk cardiac clients should have stable cardiovascular and physiological responses to exercise. The term low-risk is generally applied to clients who have all of the following characteristics (Roberts, 2003):

- An uncomplicated clinical course in the hospital
- No evidence of resting or exercise-induced **ischemia**
- Functional capacity greater than 7 **metabolic equivalents (METs)** three weeks following any medical event or treatment that required hospitalization (e.g., angina, heart attack, cardiac surgery)
- Normal ventricular function with an **ejection fraction** greater than 50%
- No significant resting or exercise-induced **arrhythmias** (abnormal heart rhythms)

Most low-risk clients with CAD can also benefit from the improvement of muscular strength and endurance that occurs with an appropriate resistance-training program. However, there are safety concerns that need to be considered by the personal trainer prior to implementing a resistance-training program with CAD clients, and physician clearance, recommendations, and limitations should be obtained before proceeding. Clients should be taught proper technique that includes breathing (avoiding a **Valsalva maneuver**) and moving through a full, pain-free **range of motion (ROM).** Begin with low-level exercises that use light weight (hand dumbbells can be a good starting point) and gradually progress to weight machines. Many low-risk, stable CAD clients that a personal trainer works with will have already undergone a course of cardiac rehabilitation that included resistance training, so the client may already be using weight machines. Other potential modes include bands/tubing, calisthenics, exercise balls, and, for a few clients, free weights. Generally, clients should perform one set of 12 to 15 repetitions using eight to 10 exercises that target the major muscle groups, twice a week. Heart rates should not exceed the training targets and/or **ratings of perceived exertion (RPE)** of 11 to 14 (6 to 20 scale). The client's physician or designated healthcare professional should provide initial guidelines for the client.

It is important for personal trainers to be knowledgeable about abnormal signs or symptoms that necessitate delaying or terminating the exercise session. Exercise should not continue if any abnormal signs or symptoms are observed, such as angina, **dyspnea,** lightheadedness or dizziness, pallor, or rapid heart rate above established targets. Personal trainers should question clients and observe them for such signs and symptoms before, during, and immediately following each exercise session. If symptoms occur and persist, the emergency medical system should be activated and the client's physician notified. It is also important to teach clients to recognize signs and symptoms that indicate they should stop exercising and to report such experiences to their healthcare providers.

Sample Exercise Recommendation for Clients With Cardiovascular Disease

Mode: For most clients, the initial mode should consist of low-intensity endurance exercise, such as low-impact aerobics, walking, swimming, stationary cycling, or other ergometer use. Clients can gradually be progressed to moderate-intensity exercise utilizing interval-type training. **Isometric** exercises should be avoided because they can dramatically raise blood pressure and the associated work of the heart. The resistance-training program should utilize one set of 12 to 15 repetitions of eight to 10 exercises.

Intensity: Low-risk, stable CAD clients initiating an exercise program should begin at an intensity of 40 to 50% of HRR or an RPE of 9 to 11 (6 to 20 scale) or at an HR 20 to 30 beats over **resting heart rate.** Low-risk, stable CAD clients who are already exercising may gradually be progressed to an intensity of 60 to 85% of HRR or an RPE of 11 to 14 (ACSM, 2010). The personal trainer should be aware that some clients might be on medications that alter (i.e., lower) the heart-rate response to exercise. In such cases, RPE and careful observation of the client should be utilized.

Duration: The total duration should be gradually increased to 30 minutes or more of continuous or **interval training,** plus additional time for warm-up and cool-down activities.

Frequency: Clients should perform three to five days per week of aerobic training and two days per week of resistance training.

Hypertension

Hypertension, sometimes referred to as the "silent killer," is one of the most prevalent chronic diseases in the United States. One in three U.S. adults have high blood pressure, defined as having **systolic blood pressure (SBP)** ≥140 mmHg or **diastolic blood pressure (DBP)** ≥90 mmHg or taking antihypertensive medication. Approximately 55,000 hypertension-related deaths occur in the U.S. each year. Additionally, just over 37% of the U.S. population aged 20 years or older has **prehypertension,** defined as an untreated SBP of 120 to 139 mmHg or an untreated DBP of 80 to 89 mmHg. Prehypertensive individuals have twice the risk of developing high blood pressure compared to those with normal values (AHA, 2009a).

Approximately 69% of people who have a first heart attack, 77% who have a first stroke, and 74% who have CHF have a blood pressure higher than 140/90 mmHg. It is estimated that each 20 mmHg rise in SBP or 10 mmHg rise in DBP doubles the risk of developing cardiovascular disease (Chobanian et al., 2003).

Exercise and Hypertension

Exercise, weight loss, sodium reduction, and reduced **fat** and alcohol intake are important lifestyle therapy components for controlling hypertension and, in some cases, augment a client's pharmacological intervention. The personal trainer should work closely with clinicians and dietitians to optimize lifestyle modifications with the pharmacotherapy regimen.

Regularly performing 150 minutes of exercise per week has consistently been shown to reduce SBP by an average of 2 to 6 mmHg (Kenney & Holowatz, 2008), with the greatest reductions occurring in hypertensive individuals. Exercise also has an **acute** post-exercise effect on both SBP and DBP. This post-exercise decrease in BP is related to reduced peripheral vascular resistance that is not compensated for by an increase in **cardiac output** and can persist for up to 22 hours. **Post-exercise hypotension (PEH)** can be of the magnitude of 15 and 4 mmHg for SBP and DBP, respectively, and emphasizes the potential benefits of daily activity.

Exercise Guidelines

Both prehypertensive and hypertensive individuals should participate in 30 minutes or more of regular exercise at least five days each week. Aerobic activities such as walking, cycling, swimming, and using ergometers are excellent modes and should be supplemented with resistance training. Trainers should avoid isometric exercise and teach and emphasize appropriate technique and breathing (i.e., avoiding the Valsalva maneuver). **Circuit training** utilizing low to moderate resistance and high repetitions, as opposed to heavy lifting, is an excellent resistance-training option.

Many hypertensive clients will be on pharmacologic therapy. The personal trainer should be aware of the client's medications and their potential impact on the exercise response. Some medications (e.g., **beta blockers, calcium channel blockers**) can alter heart-rate response and cause **orthostatic hypotension** and PEH. Clients should be taught to use RPE to monitor exercise intensity, change positions slowly, and follow each exercise session with a gradual and prolonged cool-down period. Many clients may also be taking **diuretic** medications and should be taught to pay careful attention to hydration, especially in warm environments. The personal trainer should ask for a list of current medications and recommendations from the client's physician when obtaining the exercise release and guidelines.

Exercise should be terminated if any abnormal signs or symptoms are observed before, during, or after exercise, and the client's physician should be notified. The exercise program should be discontinued until the client's physician gives clearance to resume. If symptoms persist, the personal trainer should activate the emergency medical system.

Both hypertensive and hypotensive responses are possible during and following exercise. The personal trainer should measure the client's pre- and post-exercise blood pressure. Physicians may instruct their hypertensive patients to record their resting and post-exercise blood pressure and the personal trainer should review their logs prior to each training session. It is important to carefully monitor each client's blood pressure during exercise initially, and possibly long-term, depending on the client's BP responses and physician recommendations. The exercise session should be discontinued if the SBP or DBP rise to 250 mmHg or 115 mmHg, respectively, or if the SBP fails to increase with increasing workload or drops ≥20 mmHg.

Other forms of exercise, such as **yoga** and **tai chi,** have been shown to be beneficial for clients with high blood pressure. These activities can be used to add variety to the exercise program and to promote relaxation, strength, and flexibility. The trainer should advise clients to avoid isometric muscle contractions and inverted positions (i.e., the head below the level of the heart) and make sure the dynamic movements associated with all recommended activities are within the current abilities of the client.

Sample Exercise Recommendation for Clients With Hypertension

Mode: The overall exercise training recommendations for individuals with mild-to-moderate hypertension are similar to those for healthy individuals. Endurance exercise, such as low-impact aerobics, walking, cycling, using ergometers, and swimming, should be the primary exercise mode. Exercises with a significant isometric component should be avoided. Weight training should feature low resistance and a high number of repetitions, as in a circuit-training program. Mind-body exercise such as yoga and tai chi can be used to provide additional variety and promote strength, flexibility, and relaxation.

Intensity: Exercise training performed at lower intensities appears to lower blood pressure as much as, if not more than, exercise at higher intensities (Pescatello et al., 2004). For most clients, an RPE of 9 to 13 (6 to 20 scale) will be the preferred exercise intensity, especially for those clients on heart rate–altering medications. When using heart rate, the target should be set at the lower end of the heart-rate range (40 to 65%).

Frequency: Personal trainers should encourage hypertensive clients to exercise four to seven days per week. Clients should ideally strive to exercise on a daily basis due to the acute hypotensive effect of exercise. Elderly clients or those with an initially low functional capacity may exercise daily for shorter durations.

Duration: Gradual warm-up and cool-down periods lasting longer than five minutes should be advised. Personal trainers can gradually increase total exercise duration to as much as 40 to 60 minutes per session, depending on the medical history and clinical status of the individual. The duration can be continuous or intermittent. However, if it is intermittent, each bout should last for a minimum of 10 minutes and total 30 to 60 minutes for the day.

Stroke

Stroke, or brain attack, affects 795,000 Americans each year, resulting in more than 150,000 deaths. Strokes occur when the blood supply to the brain is cut off (**ischemic stroke**) or when a blood vessel in the brain bursts (**hemorrhagic stroke**) (AHA, 2009a). Approximately 80% of strokes are ischemic, and many can be treated with the drug t-PA (tissue plasminogen activator) if the person seeks immediate help. The t-PA must be administered within the initial three hours of a stroke and can significantly reduce or eliminate the impairments that typically occur. The personal trainer should be aware of the warning signs of a stroke:

- Sudden numbness or weakness of the face, arms, or legs
- Sudden confusion or trouble speaking or understanding others
- Sudden trouble seeing in one or both eyes
- Sudden walking problems, dizziness, or loss of balance and coordination
- Sudden severe headache with no known cause

Many people survive strokes, but not without damage, making it the leading cause of chronic disability. Strokes can dramatically reduce a person's quality of life, robbing him or her of the ability to speak or utilize facial, arm, and leg muscles, and can cause other neurologic impairments. Additionally, people with stroke typically present in a severely deconditioned state, leading to a variety of metabolic disorders and significantly increased risk of recurrent stroke and myocardial infarction. The deconditioning and associated metabolic changes, such as impaired **glucose** tolerance and **type 2 diabetes** along with other risk factors, are typically worsened by physical inactivity resulting from stroke-related physical impairments. Risk factors for stroke include high blood pressure, smoking, heart disease, previous stroke, physical inactivity, and **transient ischemic attacks (TIA),** which are momentary reductions in oxygen delivery to the brain, possibly resulting in sudden headache, dizziness, blackout, and/or temporary neurologic dysfunction.

Exercise and Stroke

Rehabilitation following stroke typically focuses on optimizing **basic activities of daily living skills,** regaining balance, coordination, and functional independence, and preventing complications and stroke reoccurrence. Unfortunately, this low-level rehabilitation does not provide adequate aerobic stimulus to reverse the physical deconditioning, muscular **atrophy,** increased cardiovascular risk resulting from stroke, and associated neurologic impairment. A number of publications have demonstrated improved functional capacity resulting from a variety of exercise modalities, such as bicycle ergometer exercise, water exercise, and weight-supported treadmill exercise, as well as gait, balance, and coordination activities. Exercise has also been shown to impact CVD risk factors in stroke patients (e.g., SBP, lipid profiles, **insulin** sensitivity, glucose metabolism, and **body composition**), reducing the overall risk of CAD and recurrent stroke. Additionally, exercise has been shown to improve fibrinolytic activity, the system responsible for dissolving blood clots.

Exercise Guidelines

For many years, clinicians have considered the window for motor improvement following stroke to be within the first three to six months. However, increasing clinical and experimental data show that exercise has the potential to improve selected motor performance even years after a stroke. Therefore, people with stroke may gain additional benefit and improved quality of life by working with a personal trainer following release from a clinical rehabilitation program. Ideally, program guidelines for the personal trainer to utilize should come from the physical, occupational, and/or recreational therapist overseeing the clinical course of rehabilitation. Clients who are at risk for, or have experienced, a stroke, should follow the same guidelines and recommendations used for coronary artery disease and hypertension. Exercise activities may vary depending on the client's neurologic deficit profile, current functional capacity, and risk-factor status. Modalities such as using a cycle ergometer, walking/treadmill training, water exercise, and other exercise classes can be modified to accommodate stroke clients. Activities that improve balance and coordination can also be helpful and should be recommended by the client's physician and/or clinical therapist.

Sample Exercise Recommendation for Clients With Stroke

Mode: Appropriate modes of exercise include walking, stationary and recumbent bicycling, upper-extremity ergometers, and water exercise, depending on the client's condition and loss of function. Some individuals may have lost significant limb function, requiring that activities are adapted (e.g., strap one foot to the ergometer). Balance exercises and light resistance training should also be included when possible. As conditioning improves, the personal trainer can add a series of cognitive challenges as the client exercises.

Intensity: Intensity should be light to moderate depending on the client's condition and medical history.

Duration: Clients should begin with short bouts of activity—three to five minutes—and gradually build to 30 minutes over time. The personal trainer should also consider using intermittent exercise with rest periods as needed.

Frequency: Clients should preferably exercise five days per week, though many may need to begin with three days and gradually progress to five.

Peripheral Vascular Disease

Peripheral vascular disease (PVD) is caused by atherosclerotic lesions in one or more peripheral arterial and/or venous blood vessels and is an important medical concern because of the high risk of concomitant coronary and cerebral artery disease. Risk factors for PVD are similar to those of CAD and include **hyperlipidemia,** smoking, hypertension, diabetes, family predisposition, physical inactivity, obesity, and stress. The most prominent risk factors are smoking and diabetes. It is estimated that 90% of individuals with PVD are smokers and that PVD occurs 11 times more frequently in diabetic than non-diabetic individuals (AHA, 2009a; Barnard & Hall, 1989).

One of the most common forms of PVD is **peripheral artery occlusive disease (PAOD),** which results from atherosclerosis of the arteries of the lower extremities. The most common sites for lower-extremity lesions include the abdominal aorta and the iliac, femoral, popliteal, and tibial arteries. Consequently, blood flow distal to the lesion is reduced, significantly impacting ambulation.

Peripheral vascular occlusive disease (PVOD) is characterized by muscular pain caused by ischemia, or lack of blood flow to the muscle. This ischemic pain is usually the result of spasms or blockages and is referred to as claudication. Most claudication pain is brought on by physical activity, but some people with more severe cases can also have pain at rest. Pain associated with PVOD is frequently described as a dull, aching, cramping pain and is usually reproducible at a given exercise workload. Many individuals with PVOD can only walk a limited distance before needing to rest. Positional change is not required to bring symptomatic relief, and following a brief rest period the individual usually is able to walk another short distance before stopping again. A subjective rating of pain can be made with the four-point scale presented in Table 14-1.

Table 14-1

Subjective Grading Scale for Peripheral Vascular Disease

Grade I —	Definite discomfort or pain, but only of initial or modest levels
Grade II —	Moderate discomfort or pain from which the client's attention can be diverted, by conversation, for example
Grade III —	Intense pain (short of Grade IV) from which the client's attention cannot be diverted
Grade IV —	Excruciating and unbearable pain

Exercise and Peripheral Vascular Disease

Exercise consistently has been shown to be effective in improving ambulation distances in individuals with PVD. Improvement has been associated with changes in blood viscosity and capillary and mitochondrial density, along with increases in oxidative and glycolytic **enzymes,** all of which improve oxygen utilization. Additionally, improvement in walking mechanics and pain perception also significantly influence exercise performance. Since the risk factors for PVD are similar to those for CAD, one of the primary benefits of exercise is that it helps to lower overall CAD risk, in addition to improving blood flow and overall cardiovascular endurance.

Exercise Guidelines

Before starting an exercise program with a personal trainer, people with PVD should undergo a complete medical evaluation. The client's physician or designated healthcare provider should provide exercise clearance and basic exercise guidelines. The goals of the exercise program are to improve arterial flow, increase oxygen extraction, and improve walking mechanics that ultimately serve to decrease oxygen demand at a given workload. Additional goals include modifying underlying risk factors, such as smoking, and educating the client about PVD (e.g., symptoms, foot care, nutrition). Education is particularly important because of the anxiety associated with the pain that individuals with PVD experience.

Generally, walking is the exercise of choice because it uses the lower-leg muscles, effectively producing ischemia in the affected limb(s). This is important, as ischemia may be the primary stimulus for development of collateral circulation and other improvements in oxidative metabolism. To improve exercise capacity, it is important to encourage clients to walk to the point of intense pain (between Grades II and III) before stopping. The client should then rest until the pain subsides and then repeat the ambulatory activity once again. The process should initially be repeated for a total of 20 to 30 minutes with gradual progression to 30- to 60-minute sessions. The initial workload intensity should stimulate claudication pain within two to six minutes of walking. When eight to 12 minutes of continuous walking can be tolerated, consider increasing the walking pace or progressing the total activity time.

Selected clients may also benefit from supplementing the walking program with other low-intensity, non-weightbearing activities that further promote conditioning. Light upper-extremity resistance training may also be helpful. However, caution should be taken to ensure that clients are free of cardiovascular symptoms, stay within moderate intensities (e.g., RPE of 9 to 13 on the 6 to 20 scale), and are taught appropriate lifting techniques. It is important to obtain physician clearance before advancing clients with PVD to these more intense activities.

Personal trainers should be aware that people with PVD may also have underlying CAD. Some clients may develop CAD symptoms as walking distance and/or speed increases. In such cases, the exercise session should be discontinued until the client is evaluated by his or her physician and released back to activity. Additionally, proper foot care is essential. The personal trainer should pay close attention to the client's feet, especially if the client is diabetic, and encourage proper footwear. Clients with PVD should avoid exercising in cold air or water to reduce the risk of **vasoconstriction.**

Sample Exercise Recommendation for Clients With Peripheral Vascular Disease

Mode: For overall conditioning and risk reduction, use of non-impact endurance exercise such as swimming, cycling, and other ergometer use, may allow for longer-duration and higher-intensity exercise. Personal trainers can recommend weightbearing activities, such as walking, that are shorter in duration and lower in intensity with more frequent rest periods, to improve walking distance and delay pain onset.

Intensity: For aerobic exercise, clients should use low to moderate intensities, depending on the current medical status, conditioning, and physician or healthcare provider recommendations. Weightbearing activities such as walking should be carried out to the point of moderate to intense pain (Grade II to Grade III on the claudication pain scale; see Table 14-1). As functional capacity improves, it is okay to gradually increase intensity.

Duration: Longer and more gradual warm-up and cool-down periods (longer than 10 minutes) are recommended. It is important to gradually increase total exercise duration to 30 to 60 minutes, depending on the client's status and exercise progress.

Frequency: Daily exercise is recommended initially. As functional capacity improves, frequency can be reduced to four to five days a week.

Dyslipidemia

Elevated levels of total cholesterol and LDL cholesterol are well-recognized as lipid parameters with the highest correlation to CVD, along with suboptimal levels of **high-density lipoprotein (HDL)** cholesterol and elevated levels of **triglycerides.** Chronic elevation of triglyceride levels has been associated with endothelial dysfunction and is considered an independent risk factor for CVD [Grundy et al., 2004; National Cholesterol Education Program (NCEP), 2002].

The American Heart Association reports that 106.7 million Americans age 20 and older have total cholesterol levels >200 mg/dL, while more than 37.2 million are estimated to have total blood cholesterol levels >240 mg/dL (AHA, 2009b).

Cholesterol is a waxy, fat-like substance that is found in all cell membranes and is transported in the blood **plasma.** It is manufactured by the liver and found in certain foods such as dairy products, meat, and eggs. Cholesterol is an essential component of cell function and the production of **hormones,** vitamin D, and the bile acids that assist with fat digestion. However, while essential for life, high levels of cholesterol in circulation are strongly associated with atherosclerosis and the development of cardiovascular disorders.

Cholesterol travels through the body attached to a **protein,** referred to as a **lipoprotein.** The primary lipoproteins are classified as follows:

- *Low-density lipoprotein (LDL):* This is the major carrier of cholesterol in the circulation, containing 60 to 70% of the body's total serum cholesterol. LDL is frequently referred to as the "bad" cholesterol because of its role in **atherogenesis,** the early stages of atherosclerosis.
- *Very low-density lipoprotein (VLDL):* As the major carrier of triglyceride, VLDL contains 10 to 15% of the body's total serum cholesterol. Triglyceride is a major form of fat that tends to be associated with low levels of HDL and elevated levels of LDL.
- *High-density lipoprotein (HDL):* Often referred to as the "good" cholesterol, HDL is produced in the intestine and liver and normally contains 20 to 30% of the body's total cholesterol. HDL levels are inversely correlated to CAD, meaning that the higher the level of HDL, the lower the risk of developing CAD.
- *Non-HDL cholesterol (non-HDL):* Non-HDL is defined as total cholesterol minus HDL, or put another way, the sum of the LDL, VLDL, and **intermediate-density lipoprotein (IDL).** Non-HDL cholesterol is strongly associated with the development of CVD, and non-HDL levels appear to be equal or better than LDL levels at identifying atherogenic particles.

Table 14-2 presents the classification of LDL, total, and HDL cholesterol, while Table 14-3 shows the classification of triglycerides.

Treatment for elevated cholesterol and triglycerides and/or low HDL is based on a person's overall CVD risk profile and blood lipid levels. Treatment generally encompasses diet, exercise, and medications. NCEP (2002) guidelines recommend at least six months of non-pharmacologic therapy prior to initiating a medication regimen.

Table 14-2

ATP III Classification of LDL, Total Cholesterol, and HDL Cholesterol (mg/dL)

LDL Cholesterol	
Optimal	<100
Near optimal/above optimal	100–129
Borderline high	130–159
High	160–189
Very high	≥190
Total Cholesterol	
Desirable	<200
Borderline high	200–239
High	≥240
HDL Cholesterol	
Low	<40
High	≥60

Note: LDL = Low-density lipoprotein;
HDL = High-density lipoprotein

National Cholesterol Education Program (2002).Expert Panel on Detection, Evaluation and Treatment of High Blood Cholesterol in Adults: Summary of the second report of NCEP Expert Panel on Detection, Evaluation and Treatment of High Blood Cholesterol in Adults (Adult Treatment31 Panel III). NIH Publication No. 02-5213. *Journal of the American Medical Association*, 285, 2486–2497.

Table 14-3

Classification of Triglycerides (mg/dL)

Normal	<150
Borderline high	150–199
High	200–499
Very high	≥500

Exercise and Dyslipidemia

Exercise and dietary modification are considered to be effective in the management of high serum cholesterol and triglyceride levels, and are particularly effective in elevating low HDL levels. While there are limited randomized, controlled studies investigating the lipid response to exercise, studies that have been published indicate a benefit. Exercise appears to have the greatest affect on HDL levels, with increases ranging from 4 to 43% in various studies. However, the majority of studies suggest a more modest increase of 3 to 8%. Improving the HDL level is important in reducing the risk of cardiovascular morbidity and mortality. While lowering the LDL level by 1 mg/dL reduces CAD risk by 1%, raising the HDL level by 1 mg/dL results in a 2% risk reduction in men and a 3% reduction in women (Kodama et al., 2007; Kelley & Kelley, 2006; Leon & Sanchez, 2001; Maron, 2000).

Triglyceride levels are also responsive to exercise training, with reductions occurring 18 to 24 hours after exercise and persisting for 48 to 72 hours. The effect of exercise on LDL levels is less definitive, with most studies reporting zero to only moderate improvements. These results may be partly due to challenges with study design.

The impact of exercise on blood lipid profiles is most profound with corresponding decreases in body fat. Therefore, exercise, when combined with dietary changes that lower body weight, is an effective means of improving lipid profiles in many people.

Exercise Guidelines

Prior to beginning an exercise program with a personal trainer, an individual with one or more lipid disorders should see his or her physician and obtain exercise clearance. This is important, because many people with abnormal lipids also have other CVD risk factors (e.g., smoking, overweight, high blood pressure, diabetes, lack of physical activity) and are at increased risk for CAD. The physician should provide guidelines for exercise, including any restrictions or limitations that need to be considered. People at high CVD risk should undergo a graded exercise test to evaluate cardiovascular function and fitness along with exercise intensity parameters.

The exercise program for clients with known health conditions in addition to an abnormal lipid profile should be developed according to the specific guidelines for their medical condition and be modified according to physician recommendations. Exercise programming for clients who have abnormal lipid levels, but who are free of other health conditions, can be developed utilizing the general age-specific guidelines presented in the U.S. Department of Health & Human Service's *2008 Physical Activity Guidelines*.

Sample Exercise Recommendation for Clients With Dyslipidemia

Mode: Aerobic activities, such as walking, jogging, cycling, and swimming, are appropriate unless contraindicated by other health conditions. Resistance training twice a week using light to moderate weights at 10 to 12 repetitions may provide additional benefit.

Intensity: Clients should begin at a low to moderate intensity with a focus on duration, especially overweight clients. Some clients may be able to progress to short bouts of vigorous-intensity exercise, depending on medical history and overall condition.

Duration: Depending on client status, workouts should begin at 15 minutes and build to 30 to 60 minutes per day. The goal is to exercise for a total of 150 to 200 minutes each week.

Frequency: Five days per week is an appropriate frequency for this population.

Diabetes

Diabetes is a group of diseases characterized by high levels of blood glucose resulting from defects in insulin production, insulin action, or both. Diabetes causes abnormalities in the metabolism of **carbohydrate,** protein, and fat and, when left untreated or inadequately treated, results in a variety of chronic disorders and premature death. People with diabetes are at greater risk for developing chronic health problems, including heart disease, stroke, kidney failure, nerve disorders, and eye problems. Approximately 23.6 million children and adults (7.8% of the population) have diabetes, 17.9 million of whom have been officially diagnosed. Unfortunately, because symptoms associated with diabetes are not always present during the early stages of the disease, approximately 5.7 million people are unaware that they have diabetes [American Diabetes Association (ADA), 2009].

Healthcare providers use a fasting plasma glucose (FPG) test or an oral glucose tolerance test (OGTT) to diagnose diabetes. With the FPG test, a fasting blood glucose level ≥126 mg/dL indicates diabetes. An FPG between 100 and 125 mg/dL signals prediabetes, a condition that occurs when levels are higher than normal but not in the diagnostic range of diabetes. Approximately 57 million Americans have prediabetes, in addition to the 23.6 million with diabetes (ADA, 2009).

There are three primary types of diabetes. **Type 1 diabetes,** previously called **insulin-dependent diabetes mellitus (IDDM),** develops when the body's immune system destroys pancreatic **beta cells** that are responsible for producing insulin. While type 1 diabetes can occur at any age, it most frequently occurs in children and young adults. People with type 1 diabetes require regular insulin delivered by injections or a pump to regulate blood glucose levels. In adults, type 1 diabetes accounts for 5 to 10% of all diagnosed cases of diabetes.

The typical symptoms of type 1 diabetes are excessive thirst and hunger, frequent urination, weight loss, blurred vision, and recurrent infections. During periods of insulin deficiency, a higher-than-normal level of glucose remains in the blood, a result of reduced glucose uptake and storage. A portion of the excess glucose is excreted in the urine, leading to thirst, reduced appetite, and weight loss. A chronically elevated blood glucose level is a condition referred to as **hyperglycemia.**

Type 2 diabetes, previously referred to as **non-insulin dependent diabetes mellitus (NIDDM),** is the most common form of diabetes, accounting for 90 to 95% of all diagnosed cases. Typically, type 2 diabetes initially presents as **insulin resistance,** a disorder (affecting a third of adults aged 20 years or older) in which the cells do not use insulin properly. As the demand for insulin rises, the pancreas gradually loses its ability to produce it. The combination of insulin resistance and impaired insulin production leads to frequent states of hyperglycemia. Initial treatment usually includes weight loss, diet modification, and exercise. Approximately 75% of people with type 2 diabetes are obese or have a history of obesity, making weight loss an important objective that in some cases can reverse the condition. Many people with type 2 diabetes are placed on oral and, less frequently, injectable medications.

Gestational diabetes is a form of glucose intolerance that occurs during pregnancy and is present in approximately 7% of all pregnancies. It is more common among obese women, those with a history of gestational diabetes, African Americans, Hispanic/Latino Americans, and American Indians. Treatment is required to avoid complications in the infant. Women who have experienced gestational diabetes have a 40 to 60% chance of developing diabetes over the subsequent five to 10 years.

Diabetes Control

The primary treatment goal is twofold—to normalize glucose metabolism and to prevent diabetes-associated complications and disease progression. Proper management of diabetes requires a team approach that includes physicians, diabetes educators, dietitians, exercise specialists, and the diabetic person's self-management skills. The personal trainer can provide assistance to the team and the diabetic by motivating the client to safely and regularly participate in physical activity and by providing feedback to the team regarding the client's progress and responses.

Benefits of Exercise for Type 1 Diabetics

The role of exercise in controlling glucose levels in type 1 diabetes has not been well demonstrated. A number of studies have failed to show an independent effect of exercise training on improving glycemic control in people with type 1 diabetes. Even so, individuals with type 1 diabetes can improve their functional capacity, reduce their risk for CAD, and improve insulin-receptor sensitivity with a program of regular physical activity. Therefore, the reason for exercise has shifted from glucose control to the establishment of an important positive life behavior with multiple benefits.

Benefits of Exercise for Type 2 Diabetics

The benefits of exercise for the client with type 2 diabetes are substantial, including prevention of CAD, stroke, peripheral vascular disease, and other diabetes-related complications. Regular exercise has consistently been shown to improve lipid profiles and **hypertension fibrinolysis** and reduce elevated body weight, all of which can be present in type 2 diabetes. With excessive blood glucose elevation, blood fats rise to become the primary energy source for the body, putting people with diabetes at a greater risk for heart disease. The combination of weight loss and exercise can positively affect lipid levels, thereby lowering this risk.

Exercise Guidelines

It is important that individuals with diabetes are appropriately prepared for a safe and enjoyable exercise experience, including proper screening and education regarding precautions and self-management skills. Before beginning an exercise program, a client with diabetes should be screened thoroughly by his or her physician and clearance to exercise should be obtained. Additionally, the client should develop a program of diet, exercise, and medication with guidance from his or her physician and/or diabetes educator. Ideally, the client will have been referred to and completed a diabetes self-management course taught by a certified diabetes educator. Clients who have not participated in a diabetes self-management program should be encouraged to talk to their physicians about participating in a local program. Diabetes self-management programs focus on self-care behaviors such as healthy eating, physical activity, weight loss, blood sugar monitoring, and recognition of **hypoglycemia** and hyperglycemia signs and symptoms—skills that every person with diabetes should have.

Gradual warm-up and cool-down periods should be part of every exercise session. The warm-up should consist of five to 10 minutes of light aerobic activity and a period of gentle stretching. Following the activity session, the cool-down should last five to 10 minutes and gradually bring the heart rate down to its pre-exercise level.

The blood glucose level should be measured before and after each exercise session. The session should be delayed or postponed if the pre-exercise blood glucose level is below 100 mg/dL. With additional carbohydrate consumption, the blood glucose level should normalize and exercise may be allowed to take place. Exercise should also be curtailed if the pre-exercise blood glucose is greater than 300 mg/dL or greater than 250 mg/dL with the presence of **ketosis.** In the latter scenario, exercise should be postponed until the client's blood sugar is under control. Clients should follow specific guidelines from their healthcare providers should these situations arise.

Exercise Training for Clients With Type 1 Diabetes

The primary goals of exercise are better glucose regulation and reduced heart disease risk. Clients with type 1 diabetes should be encouraged to consistently exercise at least three to five times per week, if not every day. Exercise should be combined with a regular pattern of diet and insulin dosage on each exercise day to ensure consistent glucose control and exercise response. All levels of exercise, including leisure activities, recreational sports, and competitive sports, can be performed by people with type 1 diabetes who do not have complications or comorbidities and are in good blood glucose control. Most type 1 diabetes clients can comfortably exercise at an intensity between 55 and 75% of functional capacity or at an RPE of 11 to 14 (6 to 20 scale). RPE is preferred, especially as the disease progresses, due to potential inaccuracies in the heart-rate measurement as a result of complications such as **autonomic** and **peripheral neuropathy.** Long-duration and high-intensity exercise should be avoided, as long-duration activities increase the risk of hypoglycemia, and high-intensity exercise can increase the risk of hyperglycemia. Clients should build their activity session up to 30 minutes or more, depending on their medical profiles. Strength training should be included for individuals who are without complications.

Exercise Training for Clients With Type 2 Diabetes

The primary goals of exercise for most people with type 2 diabetes are better glucose regulation and weight loss, as 80% of this population is overweight. Weight loss through appropriate diet and exercise may allow the client, with physician direction, to reduce (and in some cases eliminate) the amount of oral insulin medication required. Generally, aerobic exercise at low to moderate intensities [e.g., 50 to 80% of HRR or an RPE of 11 to 16 (6 to 20 scale)] for 40 to 60 minutes, five or six days per week, is recommended, depending on the client's overall condition and risk profile. Individuals with type 2 diabetes may also derive benefit from low- to moderate-intensity resistance training consisting of eight to 12 repetitions of eight to 10 different exercises twice a week. In fact, a combined program of aerobic and resistance training may yield the best improvement in glycemic control and overall functional capability (Marcus et al., 2008).

Precautions

A personal trainer who chooses to work with a diabetic client should be aware of the potential complications associated with exercise and know how to appropriately respond should such complications occur. Table 14-4 presents preventive measures that should be taken to ensure a safe and effective exercise experience for diabetic clients.

Sample Exercise Recommendation for Clients With Diabetes

Mode: Appropriate exercises include walking, cycling, swimming, and recreational sports, depending on the client's age and condition. It is essential to utilize gradual warm-up and cool-down periods. Twice-a-week resistance training is appropriate and beneficial for clients who are without complications, using eight to 10 exercises at eight to 12 repetitions. Clients should monitor blood glucose before and after exercise.

Intensity: Clients should train at a moderate intensity, such as an RPE of 11 to 14 (6 to 20 scale) for type 1 diabetes and 11 to 16 for type 2 diabetes.

Duration: Clients with type 1 diabetes should gradually work up to 30 minutes or more per session, while 40 to 60 minutes is recommended for individuals with type 2 diabetes.

Frequency: Five to six days per week is an appropriate exercise frequency, though some clients may need to start out with several shorter daily sessions. The initial goal is to establish a "regular" pattern of physical activity and then gradually progress to higher levels of activity.

Table 14-4
Exercise Precautions for Clients With Diabetes
• Metabolic control before exercise ✓ Avoid exercise if fasting glucose levels are ≥250 mg/dL and ketosis is present or if blood glucose levels are >300 mg/dL and no ketosis is present. ✓ Ingest additional carbohydrate if glucose levels are <100 mg/dL.
• Blood glucose monitoring before and after exercise ✓ Identify when changes in insulin or food intake are necessary. ✓ Be aware of the glycemic response to different exercise conditions.
• Food intake ✓ Consume additional carbohydrate as needed to avoid hypoglycemia. ✓ Carbohydrate-based foods should be readily available during exercise.
• Avoid injecting insulin into the primary muscle groups that will be used during exercise, because it will be absorbed more quickly, potentially resulting in hypoglycemia.
• Avoid exercise during periods of peak insulin activity.
• Exercise at the same time each day with a regular pattern of diet, medication, and duration/intensity.
• Exercise with a partner and wear a medical identification tag.
• Proper hydration is extremely important. Drink water before, during, and following exercise to prevent dehydration. Be especially cautious on hot days, as blood glucose can be impacted by dehydration.
• Focus on careful foot hygiene and proper footwear. Cotton socks and correctly fitting athletic shoes are important. Regularly check feet for sores, blisters, irritation, cuts, and other injuries.
• Do not ignore pain. Discontinue exercise that results in unexpected pain.

Metabolic Syndrome

The metabolic syndrome (MetS) is a cluster of conditions that increases a person's risk for developing heart disease, type 2 diabetes, and stroke. Affecting more than 25% of the population, MetS is characterized by abdominal obesity, **atherogenic dyslipidemia,** elevated blood pressure, insulin resistance, prothrombotic state, and proinflammatory state. The prevalence is higher in certain ethnic groups, such as African Americans, Hispanics, and Native Americans.

The AHA and the National Heart, Lung, and Blood Institute (NHLBI) recommend that MetS be identified as the presence of three or more of the following components (AHA/NHLBI, 2005):

- Elevated waist circumference
  - ✓ Men ≥40 inches (102 cm)
  - ✓ Women ≥35 inches (88 cm)
- Elevated triglycerides
  - ✓ ≥150 mg/dL
- Reduced HDL cholesterol
  - ✓ Men <40 mg/dL
  - ✓ Women <50 mg/dL
- Elevated blood pressure
  - ✓ ≥130/85 mmHg
- Elevated fasting blood glucose
  - ✓ ≥100 mg/dL

The metabolic syndrome has been

associated with physical inactivity, excessive caloric intake, obesity, genetics, and aging. Excess **visceral** fat is of particular concern and typically is the result of physical inactivity and poor nutritional habits.

The primary treatment objective for MetS is to reduce the risk for developing cardiovascular disease and type 2 diabetes. Lifestyle interventions, such as weight loss, increased physical activity, healthy eating, and tobacco cessation are typically the initial strategies implemented. Some people with MetS are also placed on medications to treat hypertension and elevated lipids (high LDL cholesterol and/or triglycerides) and low HDL. Klein et al. (2004) studied the metabolic effects of removing abdominal tissue in obese individuals with liposuction. They concluded that removal of abdominal adipose tissue with liposuction does not appear to improve insulin resistance or risk factors for CAD. This suggests that the negative energy balance induced by diet and exercise are necessary for achieving the metabolic benefits of weight loss (Tortosa et al., 2007; Klein et al., 2004).

Exercise and the Metabolic Syndrome

A variety of studies have shown that MetS is inversely associated with physical activity, with more active individuals having a lower incidence of MetS (Yang et al., 2008). These results are not surprising, since physical inactivity has been shown to predispose people to a variety of health conditions, such as hypertension, insulin resistance, obesity, elevated lipids, and low HDL, among others. The level of cardiorespiratory fitness has also been shown to independently influence the risk of premature mortality in people with increased body weight and/or the presence of MetS (Katzmarzyk, 2005).

Individuals with MetS should be evaluated by their physicians and exercise clearance should be obtained prior to starting an exercise program with a personal trainer. Because the vast majority of people with MetS are obese, the exercise program should be designed around guidelines for the treatment of overweight and obese clients [**body mass index (BMI)** ≥25 kg/m^2 and ≥30 kg/m^2, respectively] (ACSM, 2009; AHA/NHBLI, 2005). However, additional factors such as underlying CAD, hypertension, dyslipidemia, and other risk factors should be evaluated and considered during program development.

Most studies on exercise and MetS have evaluated the effect of various aerobic modes of activity, such as walking, elliptical training and other similar ergometers, and stationary cycling. Some obese individuals may be better served by aquatic exercise or other forms of non-weightbearing activities. Additionally, resistance training has been shown to be inversely associated with the prevalence of MetS (Yang et al., 2008).

Exercise Guidelines

Individuals with MetS should be encouraged to develop an active lifestyle by looking for opportunities to expend energy throughout their daily routines. Simple strategies such as taking the stairs, parking farther away from a destination, periodically getting up and moving about, and performing a variety of recreational and leisure-time physical activities may produce significant benefits. ACSM recommends that overweight and obese individuals accumulate 200 to 300 minutes of physical activity per week (equivalent to ≥2,000 kilocalories per week) (ACSM, 2010).

Exercise intensity will vary depending on the client's weight status, overall conditioning, and medical profile. Deconditioned individuals should begin at a lower intensity and gradually progress to moderate levels (40 to 75% **$\dot{V}O_2$ reserve** or an RPE of 9 to 13 on the 6 to 20 scale). Because a primary goal is to burn calories and lose weight, a frequency of three to five times per week or more is recommended and can consist of both continuous and intermittent activity.

Sample Exercise Recommendation for Clients With the Metabolic Syndrome

Mode: Clients should begin with low-impact activities (e.g., walking, elliptical training, low-impact aerobics). Personal trainers should consider using non-weightbearing activities (e.g., water exercise, cycling) for obese clients and those with musculoskeletal challenges. Twice-a-week resistance training is appropriate and beneficial for clients who are without complications, using eight to 10 exercises at eight to 12 repetitions. It is also important to encourage a physically active lifestyle, incorporating stairs, gardening, household work, and a variety of recreational activities into the overall program.

Intensity: Clients should exercise at an RPE of fairly light to somewhat hard (11 to 13 on the 6 to 20 scale) or 30 to 75% of $\dot{V}O_2$ reserve. Clients should begin at a low intensity and gradually progress as conditioning improves and weight loss occurs. They should initially work on increasing duration rather than intensity to optimize caloric expenditure.

Duration: Clients should target a total weekly accumulation of 200 to 300 minutes using a gradual progression. Intermittent short exercise bouts (10 to 15 minutes) accumulated throughout the day may be easier and more beneficial for some individuals in maximizing weight loss.

Frequency: Clients should exercise at least three to five days per week, preferably daily.

Asthma

Asthma is a complex reactive airway disorder affecting more than 22 million Americans and is one of the most common childhood chronic diseases, affecting approximately 6 million children (NHLBI, 2007). Asthma is a chronic inflammatory disorder that is characterized by variable and recurring symptoms, such as shortness of breath, wheezing, coughing, and chest tightness. The inflammatory response and subsequent cascade of events are typically set off by environmental triggers, such as **allergens** (animal dander, dust mites, cockroaches, mold), irritants (cigarette smoke, air pollution, strong odors and sprays, pollens), viruses, stress, cold air, and exercise. These triggers can activate an inflammatory response that leads to airway hyper-responsiveness and airway obstruction due to constriction of smooth muscle around the airways, swelling of mucosal cells, and/or increased secretion of mucus.

Approximately 80% of people with asthma experience asthma attacks during and/or after physical activity, referred to as **exercise-induced asthma (EIA).** Exercise-induced asthma typically occurs after ventilation of large quantities of air, especially dry, cold air that contains environmental allergens and/or pollutants. The severity of the response is related to the intensity of exercise (ventilatory requirement) and the environmental conditions. EIA typically occurs during or shortly after vigorous activity, and can easily be brought on by sudden intense exercise in some individuals. Symptoms usually peak five to 10 minutes after the individual stops exercising and can last for 20 to 30 minutes. Some individuals will also develop a hacking cough two to 12 hours after exercise that can last for one to two days.

Approximately 50% of individuals incurring an EIA episode experience a relative refractory period, lasting for up to two hours, during which another exercise bout will not produce an EIA attack or will result in a less intense reaction. Late asthmatic responses, six to eight hours after the initial **bronchospasm,** also occur in approximately half the EIA population. These late responses are typically mild in nature.

Exercise and Asthma

While asthma is not a **contraindication** to exercise, people with asthma should receive medical clearance from their physicians before starting an exercise program. A physician can provide guidance regarding potential triggers, medication use, and what to do in case of an asthmatic episode during and/or following exercise. Many people with asthma are placed on medications that lessen or prevent the EIA response, such as bronchodilators, anti-inflammatory agents, and a variety of other medications. It is important that the client reviews the use of these medications with his or her physician, especially prophylactic treatment prior to exercise.

Most people with controlled asthma will benefit from regular exercise and can follow exercise guidelines for the general population. Exercise conditioning can help to reduce the ventilatory requirement for various tasks, making it easier for asthmatic individuals to participate in normal daily activities, recreational events, and competitive sports. There is also some evidence that regular exercise can reduce the number and severity of exercise-induced asthma attacks (ACSM, 2010).

Since EIA is brought on by hyperventilation, individuals with asthma should be encouraged to undertake gradual and prolonged warm-up and cool-down periods. The prolonged, gradual warm-up period will allow some people to utilize the refractory period to lessen the bronchospastic response during subsequent higher-intensity exercise.

Exercise Guidelines

As with all chronic conditions, a client with asthma should be cleared by his or her physician prior to beginning an exercise program. The physician should provide the client with a medication/treatment plan to prevent EIA attacks and a response plan to lessen the effects should an attack occur. Only people with stable asthma should exercise without medical supervision. The following general activity guidelines will assist the personal trainer in developing, monitoring, and progressing an exercise program for clients with asthma.

- Clients with asthma should have rescue medication with them at all times and be instructed on how to use it should symptoms occur. Some physicians will also instruct their patients to use a bronchodilating inhaler prior to beginning the exercise session.
- Clients should drink plenty of fluids before, during, and after exercise to prevent dehydration.
- Clients should avoid asthma triggers during exercise and consider moving indoors on extremely hot or cold days or when pollen counts and/or air pollution are high. Some individuals may benefit by wearing a face mask during exercise to help keep inhaled air warm and moist.
- Asthmatic clients should utilize gradual and prolonged warm-up and cool-down periods.
- It is important to keep the initial intensity low and gradually increase it over time. The peak exercise intensity should be determined by the client's state of conditioning and asthma severity. Clients should reduce the intensity if asthma symptoms begin to occur.
- Personal trainers should closely monitor the client for early signs of an asthma attack and respond immediately. Reduce intensity, and terminate the exercise session should symptoms worsen.
- If an asthma attack is not relieved by medication, the personal trainer should activate the emergency medical system.
- People with asthma often respond best to exercise in mid-to-late morning.
- Clients with well-controlled asthma can typically use the exercise guidelines for the general population for cardiovascular and strength training.

Sample Exercise Recommendation for Clients With Asthma

Mode: Walking, cycling, ergometer use, and swimming are good choices for clients with asthma. Younger, more highly conditioned individuals may also be able to jog and/or run. Swimming may be particularly beneficial because it allows people with asthma to inhale the moist air just above the surface of the water. For some clients, upper-body exercises such as arm cranking, rowing, and cross-country skiing may not be appropriate because of the higher ventilation demands.

Intensity: Personal trainers should recommend low- to moderate-intensity dynamic exercise based on the client's fitness status and limitations. Clients should begin easy and gradually increase intensity during the session.

Duration: Clients with asthma should gradually progress total exercise time to 30 minutes or more. Personal trainers should encourage longer, more gradual warm-up and cool-down periods (10 minutes or more).

Frequency: People with asthma should exercise at least three to five times per week. Some clients, especially those with initially low functional capacities and those who experience symptoms during prolonged exercise, may benefit from intermittent exercise (two or three 10-minute sessions, or interval training).

Cancer

Cancer, which is the second leading cause of death in the United States, is a general term for a group of diseases in which abnormal cells divide without control and are capable of invading other tissues through the blood and lymph systems. In 2008, there were more than 1.4 million new cases of cancer and an estimated 565,650 cancer-related deaths. These figures do not include the more than 1 million basal and squamous cell skin cancers. Cancer affects 11 million Americans and it is estimated that 40.35% of all men and women born today will be diagnosed with one or more types of cancer types in their lifetime [National Cancer Institute (NCI), 2008a].

Although cancer rates have been declining in recent years, decreasing by 0.8% per year for all cancers and both sexes combined from 1999 through 2005, it still represents a significant health challenge. With the aging population, continued population growth, and rapidly improving detection technology, cancer rates may dramatically increase over the next decade (Jemal et al., 2008; NCI, 2008b).

While prostate cancer and breast cancer are the most common forms of cancer in men and women, respectively, lung cancer continues to be the leading cause of cancer death for both genders. According to the NCI, the five-year survival rate for all cancers is currently estimated at 65%. African Americans have lower survival rates (58%) for all cancers compared to other groups (Horner et al., 2009).

Cancer is a group of more than 100 diseases that are characterized by uncontrolled growth and spread (**metastasis**) of cells within the body. Cancer begins at the cellular level (the cell is the body's basic unit of life). Normal cells grow and divide in an orderly, controlled fashion to produce new cells that replace old and/or damaged cells. Cancer cells develop when the **deoxyribonucleic acid (DNA)** of normal cells is damaged, producing mutations that affect the orderly, controlled process. The damaged DNA and associated mutations result in uncontrolled cell growth, formation of tissue masses called tumors, and in some cases metastasize to other areas of the body through the blood and lymph systems. Cancer tumors and metastasized cells can eventually interfere with organ and organ system function, possibly leading to death.

Malignant cells typically metastasize, while **benign** cells stay locally at the site of origin and do not spread throughout the body. However, like malignant cells, benign cells can still pose a challenge when tumors grow too large and compress and/or interfere with vital organs, organ systems, and their important bodily functions.

The cause of cancer is complex and linked to many factors, such as environmental exposures (e.g., pollutants, ultraviolet light, chemicals), lifestyle practices (e.g., smoking, physical inactivity, alcohol use, diet), medical interventions, viral infections, genetic traits, gender, and aging.

Exercise and Cancer

Studies have shown that physical activity can help protect active people from acquiring some cancers (i.e., colon, prostate, and breast cancer), either by balancing caloric intake with energy expenditure or by other means, including changes that positively affect the hormonal environments. An increased risk for developing cancer of the colon, prostate, endometrium, breast, and kidney has been linked to weight gain and obesity (Drouin & Pfalzer, 2008). While exercise has not been shown to be "preventative" for other forms of cancer, it does have a significant role in improving risk factors associated with cancer development. There is some evidence that physical activity improves immune function and that improvement may be an additional benefit of exercise in the prevention and treatment of some forms of cancer. However, research at this time is not conclusive.

Traditionally, people being treated for, or recovering from, cancer were told to rest and limit their physical activity. This reduction in activity and the resulting loss of strength, endurance, and mobility only served to intensify the deterioration of function and led to a worsening of signs and symptoms related to cancer and associated treatments. Research has shown that exercise is not only safe and possible during cancer treatment, but also serves to improve physical function, mental outlook, and quality of life (Temel et al., 2009; Hayes, Reul-Hirsche, & Turner, 2009; Klika, Callahan, & Golik, 2008; Schneider et al., 2007; Galvao & Newton, 2005; Knols et al., 2005; Stevinson, Lawlor, & Fox, 2004; Courneya, 2003). Exercise benefits include preservation of muscle mass and increase of muscular strength and endurance; improved balance and overall physical function; reductions in fatigue, nausea, **anxiety,** and **depression;** and decreased risk for heart disease, **osteoporosis,** and diabetes. In the case of breast cancer, studies have shown that walking at a brisk pace for three to five hours per week will decrease breast cancer relapse by 50%. Cardiorespiratory fitness has also been shown to be protective against the development of breast cancer and its progression after diagnosis (Peel et al., 2009; Matthews et al., 2007; Dallal et al., 2007; Slattery et al., 2007; Holmes et al., 2005).

The goal of exercise in the treatment of cancer is to maintain and improve cardiovascular conditioning, prevent musculoskeletal deterioration, reduce symptoms such as nausea and fatigue, and improve the client's mental health outlook and overall quality of life. For the breast cancer patient, adequate daily cardiorespiratory training will decrease the chance of a cancer relapse. The specific exercise program undertaken should be tailored to the client's needs, type of cancer, treatments he or she is undergoing, and current medical and physical-fitness status. Activity that may be low intensity for one cancer client may be high intensity for another of the same age and gender. The training protocol should center on aerobic activities, light strength training, and stretching, and be supplemented with recreational activities. People undergoing chemotherapy and/or radiation may be **anemic** and require reduced exercise intensity, while others may have compromised skeletal integrity that may prevent weightbearing activities.

Exercise Guidelines

- People with cancer should obtain physician clearance prior to starting an exercise program with a personal trainer. Some physicians may choose to refer the patient to a physical therapist and/or clinical exercise physiologist for initial program development and monitoring. Personal trainers should ask each client's physician and/or allied health professional for exercise recommendations and precautions.
- It is important that the client starts slowly and builds gradually, focusing on duration more than intensity. The personal trainer should consider intermittent activity with frequent rest breaks.
- Intensity should be light to moderate, depending on the client's condition and responses to treatment and activity. Intensity may vary day to day based on treatments and related fatigue.
- Clients with cancer that is in remission may be able to exercise at higher intensities with appropriate physician approval.
- Resistance training should utilize light weights with 10 to 15 repetitions. It is important to emphasize proper technique. *Note:* For the breast cancer patient who has undergone axillary (underarm) lymph node removal and who may be at risk for lymphedema, initial repetitions should be limited to 10 and a set of arm exercises should be alternated with exercises for another part of the body (abdominals, legs) to allow the arm time to fully recover.
- Personal trainers must emphasize the importance of proper warm-up and cool-down periods, and include light stretching to maintain range of motion.
- Clients that have numbness in the feet and/or balance challenges are at higher risk for falls. They should avoid uneven surfaces or any independent weightbearing exercise that could cause a fall and injury. Stationary equipment, such as upright or recumbent cycles, may be better than treadmill or outdoor walking. For these individuals, balance exercises are particularly important

and should be carefully monitored by the personal trainer.

- To avoid irritation, clients should not expose skin that has had radiation or recent surgical wounds to the chlorine in swimming pools. Additionally, clients with indwelling catheters should avoid swimming until the catheter is removed.
- Personal trainers should encourage clients to eat a balanced diet and drink plenty of fluids. Clients may benefit from counseling provided by a registered dietitian and should discuss this with their physicians.

Precautions

- Clients who are anemic should not exercise without physician clearance and may require reduced intensity levels.
- Clients with low white blood cell counts (neutropenia) and those taking medications that may reduce their ability to fight infection should consider avoiding public gyms and instead exercise at home. Exercise should be avoided if there is a fever above 100.4° F (38° C).
- Clients who have experienced frequent vomiting and/or diarrhea may be dehydrated and in mineral imbalance and should therefore be encouraged to drink a lot of fluids and check with their physicians before resuming exercise.
- Personal trainers should watch for swollen ankles, unexplained weight gain, and/or shortness of breath at rest or with limited exertion. These symptoms should be reported to the client's physician.
- Clients with low platelet counts **(thrombocytopenia)** and those taking blood thinners have an increased risk of bruising and bleeding and should avoid activities that raise the risk of falls and physical contact. Unusual bruising or symptoms such as nose bleeds should be reported to the client's physician.
- Clients should not exercise if they experience unrelieved pain, nausea or vomiting, or any other symptom of concern. Exercise should be postponed until physician clearance is obtained.
- Cancer clients that have a catheter should avoid aquatic exercise and other exposures that may cause infections. They should also avoid resistance training that incorporates exercises in the area of the catheter to avoid dislodging it. The client's physician should provide recommendations.
- People should not exercise within two hours of chemotherapy or radiation therapy, as increases in circulation may impact the effects of therapy.

Sample Exercise Recommendation for Clients With Cancer

Mode: Many cancer patients are at increased risk of developing osteoporosis due to treatment side effects combined with inactivity during treatment. Thus, weightbearing exercise, particularly walking, is an appropriate first step in the cardiovascular recovery phase for most cancer clients. Low-impact or non-weightbearing aerobic activities such as elliptical trainers, treadmills, and cycles are generally considered secondary options, although they may be more appropriate for some individuals. Aquatic exercise may be a good choice for a client with treatment-related hand and foot numbness, if the individual is not undergoing radiation treatments, does not have an indwelling catheter, and all surgical sites are healed.

Intensity: Light- to moderate-intensity exercise (RPE of 9 to 13 on the 6 to 20 scale) is recommended for most clients. Clients in remission and with good conditioning may be able to increase their exercise intensity levels. Intensity may need to be adjusted from session to session depending on client responses to treatment and exercise, and associated fatigue and symptoms. Personal trainers should focus more on duration and consistency than intensity.

Duration: Low-functioning clients may be required to begin with multiple short bouts of activity, three to five minutes in duration with frequent rest breaks. They should progress to 10-minute intermittent bouts and gradually build to 30 to 40 minutes of accumulated exercise.

Frequency: A cardiovascular, flexibility, and balance program can be performed on a daily basis. Strength training can be performed two to three times a week, with at least a full 24 hours of rest between sessions.

Osteoporosis

Osteoporosis, characterized by low bone mass and disrupted microarchitecture, is one of the most prevalent public health issues in America. Defined as a **bone mineral density (BMD)** that is 2.5 standard deviations (s.d.) or more below the mean for young adults, osteoporosis affects more women than men. An estimated 8 million women and 2 million men have BMD values 2.5 s.d. or more below the mean [National Osteoporosis Foundation (NOF), 2009].

Low BMD and associated deterioration in bone microarchitecture result in structural weakness and increased risk for fracture. An estimated 50% of all women and 25% of all men over the age of 50 will suffer an osteoporotic fracture within their lifetime. Women with a hip fracture have a fourfold risk of incurring another fracture. The most common fracture sites are the proximal femur (hip), vertebrae (spine), and distal forearm (wrist). The consequences of hip and spine fractures are significant, especially in older adults. Mortality in people over 50 years old during the first year following a hip fracture has been reported to be an average of 24% for both genders combined (NOF, 2009). The incidence of hip fractures increases exponentially with age due to bone density declines, loss of muscular strength, and poor balance. Falls are responsible for more than 90% of all hip fractures.

An additional 33.6 million Americans have a BMD between 1.0 and 2.5 s.d. below the mean, a condition referred to as **osteopenia** (NOF, 2009). Similar to prediabetes and pre-hypertension, osteopenia is seen as a possible precursor to osteoporosis. Individuals with osteopenia are at a greater risk for fracture and further bone deterioration to osteoporosis.

During the early growth years, the rate of **bone formation** is typically greater than the rate of **bone resorption,** resulting in an overall gain in bone mineral. This "remodeling" balance is disrupted as people age and the amount of bone formation no longer keeps pace with the amount of bone being resorbed. Lifestyle also plays an important role in bone health, as physical inactivity, poor nutrition, and other lifestyle factors (e.g., smoking) further impact bone density. Additional risk factors include genetics, age, gender, race, and certain hormones that control or influence calcium levels.

Exercise and Osteoporosis

Exercise is an important part of the prevention and treatment plan for osteoporosis, along with adequate nutrition (especially caloric intake, calcium, and vitamin D), pharmacologic intervention, and in some fracture cases, surgery. The primary goal of treatment is to prevent or retain bone mineral loss and to decrease the risk of falls and fractures. The personal trainer should encourage the client to meet with a registered dietitian for recommendations regarding vitamin supplementation and appropriate caloric intake.

Exercise Guidelines

While the optimal strategy for preserving bone health remains unclear, it is known that physical stress determines the strength of bone. Mechanical stress applied to bone results in a small deformation, or bending, of bone, referred to as strain. This response to bone loading stimulates bone deposition and associated gains in bone mass and strength. Forces that result in bone strain are easily induced via impact with the ground. For this reason, weightbearing exercises (such as jogging, hopping, skipping, jumping, and other **plyometric** exercises) are recommended and can be incorporated into a variety of games and activities. However, it is important to remember that the type of activity chosen will depend on the physical and medical condition of the individual client.

The intensity of the loading force is a key determinant of the bone response to exercise. Bone loading forces should be above those incurred with activities of daily living, as higher stress results in greater strain. Bone's response to strain is also dependent on the frequency of loading, with higher-intensity loads requiring less frequency than lower-intensity loads. Shorter, frequent loading cycles have been shown to be more effective in increasing bone strength than longer single sessions. Improvement has been demonstrated with loading cycles from five to 50 impacts per session. Therefore, frequent sessions of multiple, brief loading that are separated by a few hours of recovery may have the greatest impact on bone formation.

Resistance training is also an important component in the prevention of osteoporosis. Depending on the client's physical condition and medical profile, higher-intensity strength-training exercises [eight-repetition maximum (8 RM)] may derive the most benefit to bone. Additionally, improved strength will also assist in reducing the risk of falling. Since many individuals with osteoporosis are older, the personal trainer should refer such clients to their physicians for medical clearance prior to beginning an exercise program. Some activities may need to be modified or avoided, depending on the client's condition.

To prevent further injury and falls, some clients (e.g., those with spinal and other fractures) may need to avoid:

- Spinal flexion, crunches, and rowing machines
- Jumping and high-impact aerobics
- Trampolines and step aerobics
- Abducting or adducting the legs against resistance
- Pulling on the neck with hands behind the head

Sample Exercise Recommendation for Clients With Osteoporosis

Mode: Personal trainers should choose weightbearing exercises such as walking, group fitness classes, and resistance training, depending on the client's physical and medical condition and physician recommendations. If walking is performed as the primary exercise modality, it should be accompanied by high-intensity (8 RM) strength-training. It is important to supplement weightbearing activities with traditional aerobic exercise to stimulate cardiovascular conditioning. Activities that promote balance and coordination should also be included to reduce the risk of falling and associated fractures.

Intensity: Weightbearing activities are best performed at high intensities that promote high strain and stimulate bone adaptation. For cardiovascular activities, clients can follow the general exercise guidelines for children, adults, and older adults, excluding any jarring, high-impact activities such as running. Strength-training activities should be of higher intensity (8 RM) to stimulate bone changes. Personal trainers must be sure to obtain physician clearance prior to initiating a high-intensity program.

Duration: For prevention of osteoporosis, the actual number of strain impacts can be small (50 to 100), so the duration of loading activities can be short (five to 10 minutes), depending on the type of activity chosen. For cardiovascular exercise, clients with osteoporosis can follow the age-appropriate guidelines for the general public, excluding any jarring, high-impact activities such as running.

Frequency: Multiple bouts of bone-loading exercises are more effective than a single longer-duration session. It is important to provide for adequate rest between exercise bouts, depending on the number of strain cycles and the intensity. For cardiovascular exercise, clients can follow the age-appropriate guidelines for the general public, excluding any jarring, high-impact activities such as running.

Arthritis

More than 21% of American adults (over 46 million people) have arthritis or another diagnosed rheumatic condition (CDC, 2008b). Arthritis is a chronic condition that is characterized by inflammation and associated joint pain. Prevalence is higher in women, obese and overweight individuals, and physically inactive people. Prevalence also increases with age in both genders. The two primary forms of arthritis are **osteoarthritis,** a degenerative joint disease that leads to deterioration of cartilage and development of bone growth (spurs) at the edges of joints, and **rheumatoid arthritis,** a chronic and systemic inflammatory disease. Additionally, it is estimated that 294,000 children under age 18 have some form of arthritis or rheumatic condition (CDC, 2008b).

Rheumatoid arthritis, the most crippling form of arthritis, affected 1.3 million Americans in 2005, down from an estimated 2.1 million in 1990 (Helmick et al., 2008; Reva et al., 2008). Part of this change in incidence was related to a narrowing of the diagnostic criteria for rheumatoid arthritis. Rheumatoid arthritis affects three times more women than men and can strike at any age, but most commonly surfaces between the ages of 20 and 50 years. While rheumatoid arthritis is classified as an autoimmune disease, the exact cause, or **etiology,** remains unknown. Rheumatoid arthritis is characterized by joint pain, swelling, stiffness, and in more severe cases, **contractures.**

Osteoarthritis is the most common type of arthritis, affecting nearly 27 million Americans. It results from overuse, trauma, obesity, or the degeneration of the joint cartilage that takes place with age. While some individuals will develop osteoarthritis with no identifiable underlying cause, the majority of cases are secondary to trauma and/or obesity.

The treatment of arthritis can include medication, physical therapy, physiotherapy, occupational therapy, and surgery, depending on the type and severity of arthritis. Individuals with arthritis can be classified into four categories of functional capacity (Table 14-5).

Table 14-5

American College of Rheumatology Revised Criteria for Classification of Functional Status in Rheumatoid Arthritis

Class I	Completely able to perform usual activities of daily living (self-care, vocational, and avocational)
Class II	Able to perform usual self-care and vocational activities, but limited in avocational activities
Class III	Able to perform usual self-care activities, but limited in vocational and avocational activities
Class IV	Limited in ability to perform usual self-care, vocational, and avocational activities

Note: Usual self-care activities include dressing, feeding, bathing, grooming, and toileting. Avocational activities (recreational and/or leisure) and vocational (work, school, homemaking) activities are patient-desired and age- and sex-specific.

Hochberg, M.C. et al. (1992). The American College of Rheumatology 1991 revised criteria for the classification of global functioning status in rheumatoid arthritis. *Arthritis and Rheumatism,* 35, 5, 498–502.

Exercise and Arthritis

Exercise is also an important part of the therapy regimen and benefits people with arthritis in a number of ways. People experiencing chronic pain and inflammation typically shy away from physical activity, thereby causing their health to spiral downward. Physical inactivity causes significant deconditioning, which results in diminished endurance and muscular strength, as well as joint weakness, all of which accelerate the negative effect of arthritis and associated pain. Additionally, physical inactivity increases the risk for CAD, diabetes, and other chronic health conditions, while the decreased bone loading that occurs with physical inactivity increases the risk for osteoporosis.

A consistent exercise program that promotes cardiovascular fitness, improved muscular strength and endurance, and joint mobility will break this negative health cycle and significantly improve daily function and associated quality of life. Additional benefits include lower risk for cardiovascular disease, improved psychosocial well-being, decreased pain and stiffness, and improved neuromuscular coordination.

Exercise programs should be carefully designed in conjunction with a physician and/or physical therapist, and must be based on the functional status of the individual. The primary goals of the exercise program are to improve cardiovascular fitness and lower CAD risk, increase muscular endurance and strength, and maintain or, when indicated, improve range of motion and flexibility around the affected joint(s).

Exercise Guidelines

Clients with arthritis should undergo a complete medical evaluation and obtain physician consent before beginning an exercise program with a personal trainer. Some clients may have recently completed a physical-therapy program and the therapist can provide specific exercise guidelines for the client and personal trainer to follow.

Encourage clients to use a variety of low-impact aerobic activities to avoid overstressing the joints. Activities such as walking on soft surfaces, elliptical training, cycling, rowing, and aquatic exercise are excellent choices. Clients with hip and/or knee arthritis should avoid jarring exercises such as jogging, running, and stair climbing, while those with elbow symptoms should avoid rowing. Personal trainers should emphasize the importance of gradual and extended warm-up and cool-down periods. Other important guidelines include the following:

- Focus on duration rather than intensity, gradually lengthening the workout to 30 minutes, three to five days per week. Clients who are fairly deconditioned may benefit from short-duration (three to 10 minutes) intermittent activities at a low intensity. RPE initially may be in the 9 to 13 range (6 to 20 scale), gradually progressing to 11 to 15.
- Personal trainers must emphasize proper body alignment and proper exercise technique at all times. Poor posture combined with reduced joint mobility and strength significantly impacts movement patterns and results in more rapid fatigue and greater risk of injury. Special precautions must be taken when working with clients who have undergone a hip replacement (Table 14-6).
- Clients with arthritis should be encouraged to put all joints through their full range of motion at least once a day to maintain mobility.
- Strength training should focus on increasing the number of repetitions rather than increasing the weight being lifted. Clients can gradually increase repetitions from two or three to 10 to 12. Some clients may benefit from isometric exercises that strengthen the joint structures and surrounding muscle while placing less stress on the joint itself.
- Individuals with rheumatoid arthritis should not exercise during periods of inflammation, and regular rest periods should be stressed during exercise sessions.
- Personal trainers should modify the intensity and duration of exercise based on the client's response, changes in medication, and pain symptoms.
- It is important to encourage clients to take an extra day or two of rest if they continue to complain about pain during or following an exercise session. Clients who are still experiencing pain or joint discomfort more than two hours after a workout should have the exercise intensity reduced.
- If severe pain persists following exercise, clients should consult with their physicians.
- It is important to keep in mind that clients with arthritis may be more limited by joint pain than by cardiovascular function.

Table 14-6

Exercise Guidelines for Individuals With a Hip Replacement

• Lift knee no higher than hip level or 90° flexion
• Toes straight ahead, no "pigeon" or "duck" toes
• No adduction past midline
• Need leg/hip abduction and lateral movements and strengthening

Sample Exercise Recommendation for Clients With Arthritis

Mode: Non-weightbearing or non-impact activities such as elliptical training, cycling, warm-water aquatic exercise, and swimming are preferred because they reduce joint stress. For warm-water exercise, temperature should be in the 83 to 88° F range (28 to 31° C). Personal trainers should encourage recreational activities such as golf, gardening, table tennis, or bowling to supplement the exercise program.

Intensity: Personal trainers should emphasize low-intensity, low-impact dynamic exercise rather than high-intensity, high-impact activities. The exercise intensity should be based on the client's comfort level before, during, and after exercise. Generally, the intensity should be in the 9 to 15 RPE range (6 to 20 scale).

Duration: Personal trainers can stress the importance of prolonged and gradual warm-up and cool-down periods (greater than 10 minutes). Clients can begin initial exercise sessions at 10 to 15 minutes and gradually progress to 30 minutes. Some individuals may require intermittent exercise with shorter durations, at least initially.

Frequency: Three to five times per week is an appropriate exercise frequency.

Fibromyalgia

Fibromyalgia is classified as a **syndrome,** and it is characterized by long-lasting widespread pain and tenderness at specific points on the body. The term "fibromyalgia" comes from the Latin roots *fibro* (connective tissue fibers), *my* (muscle), *al* (pain), and *gia* (condition of), and the term syndrome refers to a group of signs and symptoms that occur together and characterize an abnormality. While not defining characteristics, sleep disturbances and fatigue are also integral symptoms of fibromyalgia.

Chronic pain syndromes such as fibromyalgia present some of the most challenging and frustrating therapeutic dilemmas that physicians and patients face. Fibromyalgia syndrome is not new. More than 2,000 years ago, Hippocrates described a condition he observed in patients with diffuse, musculoskeletal pain that resembled fibromyalgia, while in 1816, William Balfour, a surgeon at the University of Edinburgh, described similar symptomatology in his patients. In 1904, William Gowers labeled this collection of symptoms "fibrositis," a somewhat misleading term because fibromyalgia is not characterized by inflammation. In 1976, Dr. P. Kahler Hench coined the current term, "fibromyalgia syndrome" to better reflect the true nature of the condition.

While considered an arthritis-related condition, fibromyalgia is not truly a form of arthritis, as it does not cause inflammation or associated damage to the joints, muscles, and/or soft tissues. However, it is considered a rheumatic condition because it impairs the joints and/or soft tissues and causes chronic pain (Arthritis Foundation, 2009).

Fibromyalgia is more common in women than men and typically strikes between the ages of 30 and 50 years. It is estimated that 3 to 5% of adult women and 0.5% of adult men have a fibromyalgia diagnosis. While it has been hypothesized that fibromyalgia results when a genetically susceptible individual comes in contact with some environmental trigger that sets the symptoms in motion, the exact cause of fibromyalgia remains unclear. Many people with fibromyalgia attribute the onset to a stressor, such as an acute injury, illness, surgery, or long-term psychosocial stress.

The most common symptoms of fibromyalgia include the following:

- Aches and pains similar to flu-like exhaustion
- Multiple tender points
- Stiffness
- Decreased exercise endurance
- Fatigue
- Muscle spasms
- **Paresthesis**

Aches and pains are generally widespread and diffuse, fluctuate in intensity, and frequently are accompanied by marked stiffness. Other symptoms commonly described include excessive fatigue, disruptive sleep patterns, bowel and bladder irritability, anxiety, depression, cognitive difficulties, **temporomandibular joint syndrome (TMJ),** sensitivity to loud noises, and "allergic" symptoms such as nasal congestion and rhinitis.

Accurately diagnosing fibromyalgia is

challenging, as no definitive test or markers exist to make the diagnosis. Instead, the diagnosis is based on nonspecific, generalized symptoms such as pain, fatigue, and sleep disturbances. In 1990, the American College of Rheumatology developed criteria for the diagnosis of fibromyalgia (Wolfe et al., 1990). The criteria is characterized by a history of widespread pain occurring for longer than three months, in combination with pain on palpation of 11 of 18 tender point sites (Table 14-7).

Because the primary cause of fibromyalgia remains unknown, there is no one definitive treatment for it. Typical treatment modalities include the following:

- Treatment of any underlying sleep disorder
- Allergy testing and treatment
- Medications such as analgesics, **nonsteroidal anti-inflammatory drugs (NSAIDs)** including ibuprofen, **selective serotonin reuptake inhibitors (SSRI),** tricyclic antidepressants, muscle relaxants, and other medications
- Exercise
- Relaxation techniques
- Other complementary therapies

Table 14-7

American College of Rheumatology Diagnostic Criteria for Fibromyalgia

History of Widespread Pain
Pain is considered widespread when all of the following are present: • Pain in the left side of the body • Pain in the right side of the body • Pain above the waist • Pain below the waist
In addition, axial skeletal pain (in the cervical spine or anterior chest, or thoracic spine or low back) must be present. "Low-back" pain is considered lower-segment pain.
Pain on digital palpation in 11 of 18 tender-point sites: 1. Occiput: bilateral, at the suboccipital muscle insertions 2. Low cervical: bilateral, at the anterior aspects of the intertransverse spaces at C5-C7 3. Trapezius: bilateral, at the midpoint of the upper border 4. Supraspinatous: bilateral, at origins, above the scapular spine and near the medial border 5. Second rib: bilateral, at the second costochondral junctions, just lateral to the junctions on upper surfaces 6. Lateral epicondyle: bilateral, 2 cm (0.8 inches) distal to the epicondyles 7. Gluteal: bilateral, in upper, outer quadrants of the buttocks in the anterior fold of the muscle 8. Greater trochanter: bilateral, posterior to the trochanteric prominence 9. Knee: bilateral, at the medial fat pad proximal to the joint line

Wolfe, F. et al. (1990). The American College of Rheumatology 1990 Criteria for the Classification of Fibromyalgia: A report for the multicenter criteria committee. *Arthritis Rheumatology,* 33, 160–172.

Exercise and Fibromyalgia

People with fibromyalgia, like people with other chronic pain conditions, are typically deconditioned and tend to shy away from exercise due to fear of exacerbating symptoms and the level of fatigue. Unfortunately, this lack of physical activity becomes a downward spiral that produces further decreases in fitness and results in lower levels of exertion that bring on fatigue and pain. Studies have shown that exercise is beneficial for people with fibromyalgia, easing symptoms and preventing the development of other chronic conditions associated with physical inactivity (Abeles et al., 2008; Assis et al., 2006; Gusi et al., 2006; Burckhardt et al. 1994; McCain et al., 1988). Aerobic exercise has an analgesic and antidepressant effect that can significantly reduce the pain, depression, and anxiety frequently associated with fibromyalgia.

Exercise Guidelines

Individuals with fibromyalgia should discuss their exercise goals with their physicians and obtain medical clearance prior to starting an exercise program. Fibromyalgia clients should be encouraged to exercise on a regular basis. Gentle stretching should become part of the daily routine, with extra care being taken to avoid overstretching. Warm-water exercise can be especially beneficial for individuals with fibromyalgia, along with other low-impact activities (Abeles et al., 2008). Low- to moderate-intensity exercise is recommended, with a goal of developing consistent exercise patterns rather than intense workouts. Intensity and/or duration should be reduced during periods of flare-up and increased fatigue or pain resulting from previous activity. Personal trainers should encourage variety, rather than one particular type of activity, to reduce repetitive trauma and potential adverse symptoms.

Sample Exercise Recommendation for Clients With Fibromyalgia

People with fibromyalgia should avoid physical inactivity and develop a pattern of "regular" exercise with the type and amount matched to their abilities and the severity of their condition. They may require off days during intense flare-ups, but should avoid prolonged inactivity.

Mode: Walking and low-impact activities such as elliptical training, recumbent cycling, warm-water aquatic exercise, and swimming are excellent activities for a client with fibromyalgia. Personal trainers should include light stretching as part of the daily routine, along with resistance exercise activities utilizing resistance bands. Some individuals can use light weights and/or perform other functional strengthening activities.

Intensity: These clients should generally perform at a low to moderate intensity—RPE of 9 to 13 (6 to 20 scale)—depending on age and condition.

Duration: Gradually progress to a goal of 150 minutes or more per week of aerobic activity. Some people may need to begin with frequent short-duration sessions (10 minutes) and gradually build over time.

Frequency: The key is to establish a "regular" pattern of exercise three to five days per week.

Chronic Fatigue Syndrome

Chronic fatigue syndrome (CFS) is a debilitating and complex illness that is characterized by profound, incapacitating fatigue lasting at least six months that results in a substantial reduction in occupational, recreational, social, and educational activities. The fatigue does not improve with bed rest and may worsen with physical and/or mental activity. It is estimated that 1 million or more Americans have CFS and that less than 20% of Americans with CFS have been diagnosed. The female-to-male ratio of CFS is 4:1. CFS occurs most often in the 40 to 59 age group (Griffith & Zarruof, 2008).

Chronic fatigue syndrome is accompanied by characteristic symptoms, including problems with memory and concentration, unrefreshing sleep, muscle and joint pain without inflammation and redness, headaches, tender cervical or axillary lymph nodes, recurrent sore throat, and extreme exhaustion lasting more than 24 hours following physical or mental exercise. Some people with CFS also report additional symptoms such as abdominal pain, bloating, chest pain, chronic cough, diarrhea, dizziness, nausea, chills and night sweats, psychological problems (e.g., depression, irritability, anxiety, panic attacks), and visual disturbances.

There is considerable variation in the clinical course of CFS and the condition can remain active for years. Some people remain homebound and others improve to the point that they can resume work and other activities even though they still experience symptoms. Recovery rates from CFS are unclear. However, full recovery from CFS may be rare, with an average of only 5 to 10% sustaining total remission (CDC, 2008c).

The diagnosis of CFS is based on exclusion, as there are no diagnostic tests or laboratory markers for CFS, and its associated pathophysiology is unknown. Diagnosis can be challenging, as many of the signs and symptoms of CFS also occur with other diseases and health conditions (Table 14-8). People with CFS must be carefully evaluated by their physicians to rule out common conditions that may mimic CFS (e.g., mononucleosis, Lyme disease, various cancers).

Despite extensive research, no clear cause of CFS has been identified. Current research has focused on the role of the immune, endocrine, and nervous systems as possible mechanisms. Genetic and environmental factors may also play a role in both the development and course of CFS. It appears that CFS is not caused by depression, although the two illnesses often coexist.

Table 14-8

Chronic Fatigue Syndrome Criteria

• Unexplained, persistent fatigue that is not due to ongoing exertion, is not substantially relieved by rest, is of new onset (not lifelong), and results in a significant reduction in previous levels of activity
AND
• Four or more of the following symptoms present for six months or more: ✓ Impaired memory or concentration ✓ Post-exertional malaise (extreme, prolonged exhaustion and exacerbation of symptoms following physical or mental exertion) ✓ Unrefreshing sleep ✓ Muscle pain ✓ Multijoint pain without swelling or redness ✓ Headaches of a new type or severity ✓ Sore throat that is frequent or recurring ✓ Tender cervical or axillary lymph nodes

Sources: Griffith, J.P. & F.A. Zarruof (2008). A systematic review of chronic fatigue syndrome: Don't assume it's depression. Primary Care Companion. *Journal of Clinical Psychiatry*, 10, 2, 120–128; Centers for Disease Control and Prevention (2006a). *Toolkit for Healthcare Professionals: Chronic Fatigue Syndrome.* www.cdc.gov/cfs

Managing CFS is as complex as the illness itself, as no single therapy exists that helps all people with CFS. Treatment is generally aimed at providing symptom relief and improving function. There are currently no prescription drugs that have been developed specifically for CFS. The treatment regimen may include the following (adapted from Mayo Clinic, 2009):

- *Moderating daily activity:* Patients are frequently encouraged to slow down and avoid excessive physical and psychological stress. However, too much rest can be detrimental and worsen long-term symptoms. Thus, the goal is moderation of activity, not total cessation.
- *Gradually progressing exercise:* Patients may be referred to a physical therapist or ACE-certified Advanced Health & Fitness Specialist for guidance in beginning an exercise program that gradually progresses from lower levels to higher levels of effort. Research has shown that exercise, when progressed gradually, can improve symptoms associated with CFS.
- *Cognitive behavior therapy:* Often used in association with graduated exercise, cognitive behavior therapy helps individuals identify negative beliefs and behaviors that might adversely impact recovery and replace them with healthy, positive ones.
- *Treatment of depression:* Depression is common in people with CFS and is frequently treated with low-level physical activity, counseling, and medications.
- *Treatment of existing pain:* Acetaminophen and NSAIDs such as aspirin and ibuprofen are frequently recommended to reduce pain and fever.
- *Treatment of allergy-like symptoms:* Antihistamines and decongestants are often prescribed to relieve allergy-like symptoms such as runny nose.

There are also a variety of other therapies, both experimental and non-experimental, that are used for treatment of certain individuals, based on their individual profile and symptomatology.

Exercise and Chronic Fatigue Syndrome

Most people with CFS cannot tolerate traditional exercise routines that are aimed at optimizing **aerobic capacity** and building muscular strength and endurance. Instead of helping people with CFS, these moderate- to vigorous-intensity activities can cause an exacerbation in fatigue and other symptoms associated with CFS. Even worse, these types of activities can precipitate a full-scale relapse that lasts for days or weeks. However, activity with appropriate rest has been shown to decrease psychological stress and improve fatigue, functional capacity, and fitness (Griffith & Zarruof, 2008).

Exercise Guidelines

The primary objective of exercise for people with CFS is to create a balance that allows the client to avoid post-activity malaise, while also preventing deconditioning so they can achieve better function and improved quality of life. The key is to avoid the extremes of activity (i.e., no exercise or vigorous exertion) and develop an exercise program that is well-balanced and consistent. Appropriate rest is an important element of the activity program and clients must learn to stop activity before illness and fatigue are worsened. The following guidelines apply to people with CFS (Griffith & Zarruof, 2008; CDC, 2006a):

- Personal trainers should teach clients with CFS that all exercise should be followed by a rest period at a 1:3 ratio (i.e., resting for three minutes for each minute of exercise). Some individuals can exercise for only remarkably short periods, just two to five minutes, without risking a relapse.
- Deconditioned clients should limit themselves to the basic activities of daily living until their symptoms are stabilized. Several daily sessions of brief, low-impact activity can slowly be added, such as a few minutes of stretching, strength exercises, or light activity like walking or cycling. These sessions are increased by one to five minutes a week as tolerance develops.
- Should exercise worsen symptoms, clients should be encouraged to return to the most recent manageable level of activity that did not result in increased symptoms. Daily exercise may be divided into two or more sessions to avoid symptom flare-ups.
- Clients should start with simple stretching and strengthening exercise, using only body weight for resistance. They can gradually add activities such as wall push-ups, modified chair dips, and toe raises to the routine. Repetitions should be increased gradually, beginning with two to four repetitions and building to a maximum of eight.
- These clients can add resistance exercise as strength improves by using exercise bands or light weights.
- Some clients may not tolerate an upright position and may benefit by swimming or using a recumbent bicycle.

Sample Exercise Recommendation for Clients With Chronic Fatigue Syndrome

Mode: Activities of daily living and walking or low-impact activities such as cycling are recommended. Light stretching and light resistance training using resistance bands are also recommended. Other forms of resistance may be appropriate for higher conditioned clients.

Intensity: Low-intensity exercise is recommended. The goal is to develop a "regular" pattern of activity that does not result in post-activity malaise.

Frequency: Three to five days per week is generally recommended.

Duration: Clients can begin with multiple two- to five-minute exercise periods followed by six- to 15-minute rest breaks (i.e., 1:3 ratio). Gradually build to 30 minutes of total activity.

Low-back Pain

Low-back pain (LBP) is an extremely common and significant source of medical costs and disability. Affecting almost every person at some point, LBP interferes with work, routine activities of daily living, and recreation. It is estimated that Americans spend more than $50 billion each year on LBP, which is the leading contributor to job-related disability. Back strain/sprain is the most common type of workers' compensation claim, accounting for 25% of all claims (higher in some vocations) and significantly affecting an individual's productivity. People with LBP are more likely to report symptoms of depression, anxiety, and sleep disruption than those without it. LBP is the number-one disability for people under the age of 45 and it is estimated that 1.2 million adults are disabled as a result of their LBP at any given time (Wong & Transfeltd, 2007). Approximately 5% of people with acute back pain will go on to develop chronic LBP, which accounts for 10% of all chronic health conditions in the U.S. and 25% of lost work days. There is little wonder why reducing low-back injuries is a major focus of most employers.

Acute, or short-term, LBP typically lasts from a few days to a few weeks and is usually mechanical in nature. There are many ideas about what causes LBP, but no single explanation can be applied to everyone. Typical causes are trauma (e.g., sports injury; lifting, bending, or reaching; sudden jolt as in a car accident), certain disorders such as arthritis, and aging. Symptoms vary, ranging from muscle ache to shooting or stabbing pain. While symptoms can be severe for a few days, they often improve significantly within two to four weeks.

Chronic back pain is generally defined as pain that persists for more than three months. It is usually progressive and the exact cause can be challenging to determine. In some people, the spine becomes overly strained or compressed, resulting in a disc rupture or outward bulge that places pressure on one of the more than 50 nerves rooted to the spinal cord. Other causes include conditions such as **spinal stenosis,** osteoporosis and associated fractures, spinal degeneration, and spinal irregularities (such as **scoliosis, kyphosis,** and **lordosis**).

While LBP most frequently occurs between the ages of 30 and 50, it can affect people of all ages. A number of lifestyle-related factors, such as physical inactivity, being overweight or obese, inappropriate posture, poor sleeping position, stress, and smoking are associated with the development of LBP. Additionally, the incidence of LBP in pre-teen children has increased, in part due to overloaded school backpacks and improper lifting techniques.

Exercise and Low-back Pain

Exercise is one of the cornerstones of both the prevention and treatment of LBP. In fact, many physicians feel that the major cause of LBP is physical deconditioning, especially in large muscle groups such as the back extensors (Dugan, 2006). Aerobic training and exercises for the lower back should be performed on a regular basis and proper technique for each exercise should be taught and practiced. Maintaining and improving muscular balance across the joints is particularly important for people with skeletal irregularities.

Exercise Guidelines

Clients with LBP should be cleared by their physicians prior to beginning an exercise program with a personal trainer. Many clients will be referred to, or have just completed, a program with a physical therapist, so the personal trainer will be able to work with the client on reinforcing the skills and training exercises the therapist implemented. Those who have not been evaluated by a physical therapist should be encouraged to speak to their physicians regarding a physical-therapy program. There is no one single exercise program that fits all people with low-back pain and it is important that the program be individualized based on each client's profile. What is helpful for some clients may exacerbate symptoms for another.

Cardiorespiratory training, resistance training, and basic core exercises should be the primary components of the training program. Clients should not be encouraged to "work through the pain," as pain is an indication of improper technique and/or the wrong exercise being performed. Generally, people with LBP should avoid the following:

- Unsupported forward flexion
- Twisting at the waist with turned feet, especially when carrying a load
- Lifting both legs simultaneously when in a prone or supine position
- Rapid movements, such as twisting, forward flexion, or hyperextension

Therapeutic aquatic exercise may be beneficial for some clients with LBP, particularly pregnancy-related LBP (Waller, Lambeck, & Daly, 2009).

Muscular endurance—as opposed to muscular strength—has been shown to have the strongest positive association with low-back health. Therefore, the training program should focus on building muscular endurance, utilizing higher repetitions and lower resistance and emphasizing proper technique at all times. The program should also be composed of specific low-back core exercises and supplemented with aerobic exercise to improve cardiovascular health.

The personal trainer should share the following guidelines with clients with LBP:

- Clients with LBP, or a history of chronic LBP, should consult with a physician and get specific recommendations for exercise. Clients with active LBP who have not had a course of physical therapy should be encouraged to ask their physicians about a referral.

- Adequately warm up and cool down before and after each workout session.
- Always be aware of proper form and alignment.
- Do not try to work through pain.
- Always maintain neutral pelvic alignment and an erect torso during any exercise movements.
- Avoid head-forward positions in which the chin is tilted up.
- When leaning forward or lifting or lowering an object, always bend the knees. Do not lift objects that are too heavy, do not twist when lifting, and keep objects close to the body.
- Avoid hyperextending the spine in an unsupported position.
- If applicable, quit smoking. Smoking reduces blood flow to the lower spine and has been associated with spinal disc degeneration.
- If experiencing LBP following exercise, sit or lie down in a comfortable position and apply ice to the affected area. Take a few days off from exercise if experiencing a mild back strain.
- Focus on the importance of good posture. Do not slouch while standing or sitting and keep weight balanced on the feet. Work surfaces should be at a comfortable height that will promote good posture.

Dr. Stuart McGill (2007), a prominent expert on low-back health and injury prevention, recommends that clients with low-back pain keep the following guidelines in mind:

- While there is a common belief that exercise sessions should be performed at least three times per week, it appears that low-back exercises have the most beneficial effect when performed daily.
- The "no pain, no gain" axiom does not apply when exercising the low back in pained individuals, particularly when applied to weight training.
- General exercise programs that combine cardiovascular components (like walking) with specific low-back exercises have been shown to be more effective in both rehabilitation and for injury prevention.
- Diurnal variation in the fluid level of the intervertebral discs (discs are more hydrated in the morning after rising from bed) changes the stresses on the discs throughout the day. Specifically, these stresses are highest following bed rest and diminish over the subsequent few hours. It would be very unwise to perform full-range spine motion while under load shortly after rising from bed.
- Low-back exercises performed for maintenance of health need not emphasize strength; rather, more repetitions of less-demanding exercises will assist in the enhancement of endurance and strength. There is no doubt that back injury can occur during seemingly low-level demands (such as picking up a pencil) and that injury due to a motor-control error can occur. While it appears that the chance of motor-control errors, which can result in inappropriate muscle forces, increases with fatigue, there is also evidence documenting the changes in passive tissue loading with fatiguing lifting. Given that endurance has more protective value than strength, strength gains should not be overemphasized at the expense of endurance.
- There is no such thing as an ideal set of exercises for all individuals. An individual's training objectives must be identified (e.g., rehabilitation specifically to reduce the risk of injury, optimize general health and fitness, or maximize athletic performance), and the most appropriate exercises chosen. While science cannot evaluate the optimal exercises for each situation, the combination of science and clinical experiential "wisdom" must be utilized to enhance low-back health.
- Encourage clients to be patient and stick with the program. Increased function and pain reduction may not occur for three months.

Daily Routine for Enhancing Low-back Health

The following exercises will spare the spine, enhance the muscle challenge, and enhance the motor control system to ensure that spine stability is maintained in all other activities. Keep in mind that these are only examples of well-designed exercises and may not be for everyone—the initial challenge may or may not be appropriate for every individual, nor will the graded progression be the same for all clients. These are simply examples to challenge the muscles of the torso.

Cat-Camel

The routine should begin with the cat-camel motion exercise (spine flexion-extension cycles) to reduce spine viscosity (internal resistance and friction) and "floss" the nerve roots as they outlet at each lumbar level. Note that the cat-camel is intended as a motion exercise—not a stretch—so the emphasis is on motion rather than "pushing" at the end ranges of flexion and extension. Five to eight cycles have shown to be sufficient to reduce most viscous-frictional stresses.

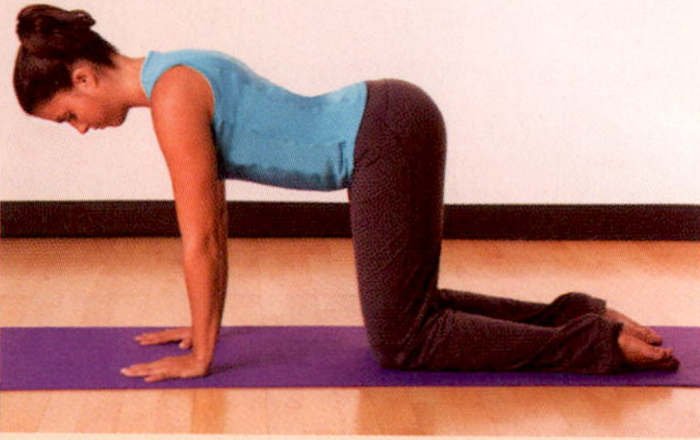

Camel position

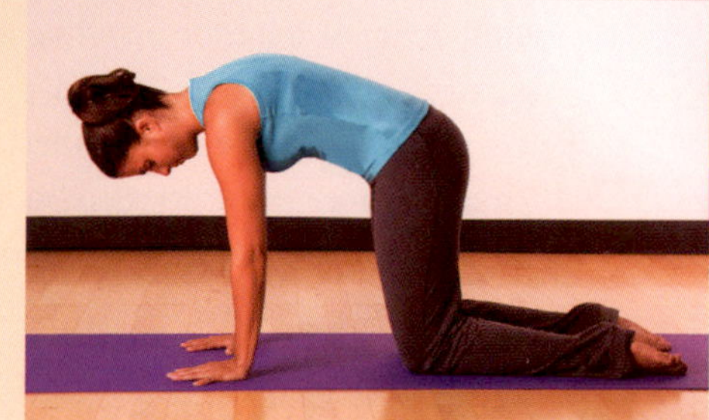

Cat position

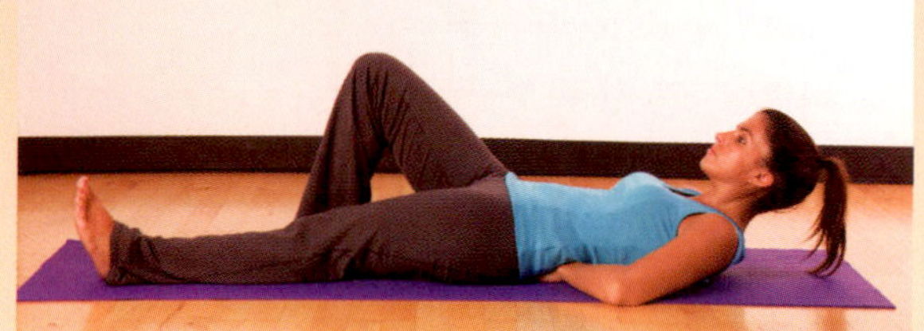

Modified Curl-up

The cat-camel motion exercise is followed by anterior abdominal exercises, in this case the curl-up. The hands or a rolled towel are placed under the lumbar spine to preserve a neutral spine posture. Do not allow the client to flatten the back to the floor, as doing so flexes the lumbar spine, violates the neutral spine principle, and increases the loads on the discs and ligaments. One knee is flexed but the other leg is straight to lock the pelvis–lumbar spine and minimize the loss of a neutral lumbar posture. Have clients alternate the bent leg (right to left) midway through the repetitions.

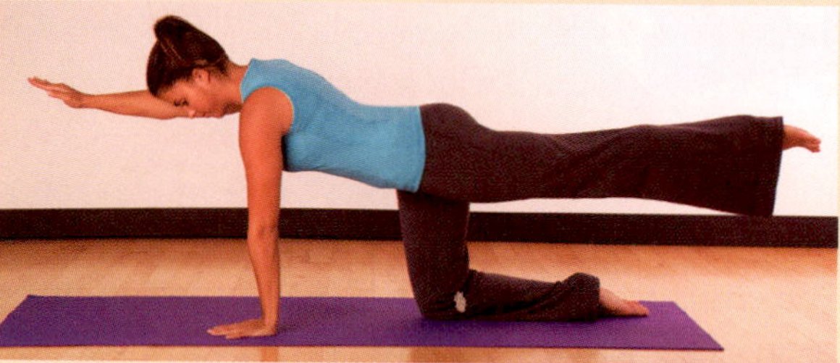

Birddog

The extensor program consists of leg extensions and the "birddog." In general, these isometric holds should last no longer than seven to eight seconds given evidence from near infrared spectroscopy indicating rapid loss of available oxygen in the torso muscles when contracting at these levels; short relaxation of the muscle restores oxygen. The evidence supports building endurance with increased repetitions rather than extending "hold time."

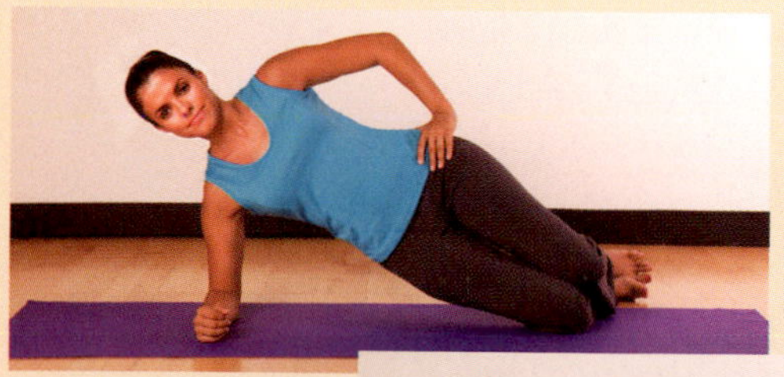

Side Bridge

The lateral muscles of the torso (i.e., quadratus lumborum and abdominal obliques) are important for optimal stability, and are targeted with the side bridge exercise. The beginner level of this exercise involves bridging the torso between the elbow and the knees. Once this is mastered and well-tolerated, the challenge is increased by bridging using the elbow and the feet. It is important when performing the side bridge exercise to maintain a neutral neck and spine position and not let the hips rotate forward.

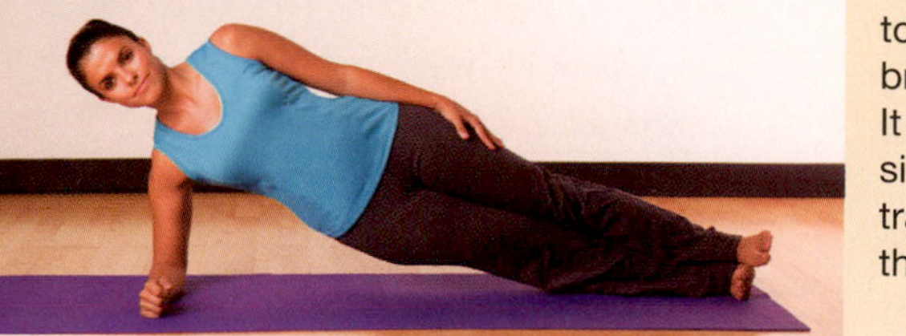

Sample Exercise Recommendation for Clients With Low-back Pain

Mode: Walking, stationary biking, and swimming are generally recommended depending on the client's condition and his or her health professional's recommendations. Some activities may exacerbate symptoms and should be avoided (e.g., prolonged sitting while cycling). Variety is good. Core strengthening exercises, light resistance training, and stretching may also be included; the client's healthcare professional can provide specific guidelines for these activities.

Intensity: Light to moderate intensity is recommended initially. As conditioning improves and symptoms dissipate, some individuals may be able to progress to moderate to vigorous activity.

Frequency: Three to five days per week is recommended, with a goal of establishing a regular pattern of activity.

Duration: Gradually build to 30 to 60 minutes per session. Some individuals may need to begin with multiple short (10-minute) bouts of activity.

Weight Management

Overweight and obesity has become a public health crisis in the United States. Adult obesity rates have doubled from 15 to 30% since 1980, and two-thirds of American adults are now overweight or obese (Vinter et al., 2008). More than 20% of adults are obese in every state except for Colorado, where the rate is at 18.3%. Additionally, the incidence of childhood obesity has nearly tripled since 1980, from 6.5% to 16.3% (Vinter et al., 2008).

Rising obesity rates have significant health consequences, contributing to more than 20 chronic diseases, including type 2 diabetes, hypertension, CAD, some cancers, arthritis, **Alzheimer's disease,** and **dementia.** Furthermore, obese children and teenagers are developing diseases that were formerly seen only in adults. Approximately 176,500 youth under the age of 20 years have type 2 diabetes and 2 million adolescents age 12 to 19 years have prediabetes (CDC, 2005).

Obesity is defined as an excessive amount of adipose tissue or body fat in relation to **lean body mass.** The most common measure used to define overweight and obesity is the body mass index (BMI), which is calculated using the following formula:

$$\text{BMI} = \text{Weight (kg)}/\text{Height}^2\text{ (m)}$$

Adults with a BMI of 25.0 to 29.9 are considered overweight, while those with a BMI ≥30 are considered obese (see Tables 8-7 and 8-8 on pages 185 and 186). While BMI measurement is not without controversy (e.g., BMI does not distinguish between fat and muscle; certain ethnic groups may have greater amounts of lean tissue and, thus, higher baseline BMIs), it is currently accepted as the primary tool for diagnosing overweight and obesity. BMI levels are simple to measure and quick to produce information. Other measures may enhance the BMI categorization, such as waist size and **waist-to-hip ratio.**

The diagnosis and treatment of obesity can be challenging and frustrating for the healthcare professional. Detailed medical, physical-activity, and dietary histories are necessary before a physician can begin to determine the cause(s) of obesity in patients. Although caloric consumption and physical inactivity are directly related to obesity, they are not the only causes. In many cases, obesity is caused by complex psychosocial issues that may require referral to a psychologist or professional counselor. However, many lifestyle habits and cultural changes contribute to weight gain and obesity, including the following (Vinter et al., 2008):

- Caloric intake increased by 300 calories per day from 1985 to 2002. Overeating is often related to stress, portion size and value perceptions, and high caloric-density foods.
- The proliferation of microwaveable and ready-to-eat high-fat foods has worsened the average diet.
- People do less in-home cooking and eat out and on-the-go more frequently.
- Marketing entices people to choose foods that are higher in calories and fat.

- Sixty percent of Americans do not meet the recommended amount of physical activity and 22% report no physical activity. This is compounded by the fact that many communities are not designed for safe and effective physical activity.
- People spend excessive amounts of time doing sedentary activities, such as computer-based work and play, video games, and television viewing.
- Jobs have become more sedentary in nature and many worksites offer limited or no opportunity for physical activity during the workday. In addition, many worksite cafeterias and lunch options offer a variety of unhealthy food choices.
- Many people no longer walk and/or bike to work and school, but instead spend a significant amount of time driving. This is especially problematic in areas of heavy traffic and long commutes.

Exercise and Weight Management

Exercise plays an important role in the reduction of excess body weight and in achieving weight stability. Studies have shown a strong dose-response relationship between the volume (frequency, intensity, and duration) of endurance and/or resistance exercise, the training duration, and the amount of total and regional fat loss (Haskell et al., 2008). In the absence of concurrent caloric restriction, aerobic exercise in the range of 150 minutes per week has been associated with modest weight loss [4.4 to 6.6 lb (2 to 3 kg)], while 225 to 420 minutes per week results in a 11 to 16.5 lb loss (5 to 7.5 kg) in studies with durations ranging from 12 to 18 weeks (ACSM, 2009). Individuals seeking weight loss should include exercise as a key component of their programs, and overweight and obese adults should accumulate more than 150 minutes of moderate-intensity exercise each week, and when possible, more than 225 minutes per week (ACSM, 2009).

While it is generally accepted that people can lose weight, most cannot maintain significant weight loss over time. The exact amount of physical activity required to reduce or maintain weight remains unclear due to design flaws in many of the published studies. However, evidence suggests that "more is better" and that increased levels of physical activity are necessary to promote weight loss and weight stability. Stevens and colleagues (2006) defined weight stability as less than a 3% change in body weight, and a change of 5% or more is considered clinically significant. For example, a 5% change for a 200-pound person would equate to a 10-pound weight loss. While the exact amount of physical activity required to maintain weight remains uncertain, research suggests that the gross energy expenditure required to achieve weight maintenance following substantial weight loss is approximately 4.4 kcal/kg/day (e.g., walking at 3 mph for 80 minutes per day, walking at 4 mph for 54 minutes, or jogging at 6 mph for 26 minutes) (Haskell et al., 2008). However, the literature is not consistent and the amount may significantly vary among individuals. Because of these limitations, ACSM states that weight maintenance (weight fluctuation <3%) is likely to be associated with ~60 minutes of physical activity (~4 to 5 miles of walking per day) at a moderate intensity (ACSM, 2009).

Exercise Guidelines

The combination of exercise and a sensible eating plan produces the best long-term weight-loss and weight-maintenance results. Individuals undertaking non-medically supervised weight-loss initiatives should reduce energy intake by 500 to 1,000 kcal per day to elicit a weight loss of approximately 1 to 2 pounds (0.5 to 0.9 kg) per week (ACSM, 2009). However, the key to successful, long-term weight stability is the adoption of life-long physical activity and sensible eating habits.

One of the benefits of exercise is its impact on **resting metabolic rate** and **fat-free mass.** Both strength training and aerobic exercise have been shown to make the greatest contribution to a weight-management program when the caloric intake does not go below 1,200 kcal per day. Regular exercise also helps control appetite and improve psychological outlook when a person is trying to lose weight.

Sample Exercise Recommendation for Weight Management

Mode: Walking is a highly effective form of exercise for weight loss and control, as are cycling and group exercise classes such as aerobics. Aquatic exercise and swimming may be appropriate activities for some overweight individuals. The key is to find safe, effective, and enjoyable activities that promote consistent physical activity. Resistance exercise may derive additional benefits for overweight and obese individuals.

Intensity: The intensity level should be low to moderate. These clients should begin at low intensity and gradually progress to higher levels as conditioning improves. The RPE scale is an excellent tool for monitoring exercise intensity. Personal trainers should be aware of signs that the client is working too hard, such as excessive sweating, shortness of breath, or fatigue, or an inability to complete the exercise session—and modify intensity as required.

Duration: Exercise duration is a critical component of the exercise program. Clients should be encouraged to accumulate 150 to 200 or more minutes of exercise each week.

Frequency: Overweight and obese clients should exercise five to six days per week to maximize caloric expenditure. Initially, some clients may need to start out with two to three days per week.

Exercise and Older Adults

Regular physical activity is essential for older adults (≥65 years) who wish to maintain independence and quality of life. It is no secret that the United States population is aging, and by 2030 it is estimated that one in five Americans, or 71 million individuals, will be 65 years or older. The most rapidly growing age group in America is those 85 years and older, due in part to healthcare advances and health-promotion activities (CDC, 2009). However, while the health of America's aging population is improving, many older people suffer from one or more chronic conditions that limit activity and reduce quality of life. For some, activities of daily living become strenuous due to chronic conditions and the associated loss of physical function, resulting in a loss of independence. As people age, being physically active, eating right, and not smoking become even more important.

Older adults are a varied group. Many, but not all, have one or more chronic conditions that vary in type and severity. All have experienced a loss of physical fitness with age, some more than others. The typical signs of aging are familiar to everyone, and include graying and loss of hair, loss of height, reduced lean body mass, loss of skin elasticity and associated wrinkles, thickening of nails, changes in eyesight, and reduced coordination. Additionally, there are noticeable changes in the cardiovascular, endocrine, respiratory, and musculoskeletal systems. The extent that these changes may be affected by exercise is not completely understood.

Cardiovascular System

Maximum heart rate declines with age, and in many cases is affected by medication, thus diminishing the accuracy of estimating training intensity based on heart rate. Other intensity-monitoring methods, such as the RPE or the **talk test** may be more effective. Cardiac output (the amount of blood pumped out by the heart each minute) is typically lower in older individuals, and resting cardiac output declines by approximately 1% per year upon reaching adulthood. Resting **stroke volume** declines approximately 30% from the age of 25 to age 85 and, when combined with the decrease in maximum heart rate, leads to a drop in cardiac output of 30 to 60%. While the heart rate decline with age does not appear to be impacted by exercise training, stroke volume has been shown to increase or be maintained in healthy older subjects who exercise, thereby counteracting the impact of reduced heart rate on cardiac output.

Associated with the decrease in heart rate and stroke volume is a reduction in **maximal**

oxygen uptake ($\dot{V}O_2$max). This decline is estimated to be 8 to 10% per decade after age 30 and is impacted by decreased oxygen extraction by working muscles. There is clear evidence that aerobic capacity can be improved via exercise training at any age.

Musculoskeletal System

Muscle mass declines with age, resulting in reduced muscular strength and endurance. For each decade after the age of 25, 3 to 5% of muscle mass is lost. This is primarily attributed to changes in lifestyle (i.e., less physical activity) and decreased use of the neuromuscular system. Studies have consistently shown muscular strength and endurance gains following exercise training in older adults. The aging process also affects bones, as they become more fragile and porous with advancing years, placing older adults at a greater risk of fractures. Debilitating fractures become more common and many older individuals that sustain a hip fracture will die of related complications. With age, loss of calcium results in decreased bone mass, but weightbearing and resistance-training exercises have been shown to help maintain bone mass.

As lean body mass declines with age, body fat typically increases. These changes in body composition are primarily due to decreased muscle mass, **basal metabolic rate,** and reduced, or lack of, physical activity. On average, there is a 10% reduction in basal metabolic rate between early adulthood and retirement age, and a further 10% decline after that time. Regular physical activity helps to stimulate protein synthesis, preserve lean body mass, and decrease fat stores.

Sensory Systems

As people age, balance and coordination tend to decline, increasing the risk of falls and fall-associated injury. This is due to the loss of muscle mass and associated strength and a decline in sensory systems that provide the **central nervous system** with information regarding the body's position in space. The **visual, vestibular,** and **somatosensory systems** provide essential information to the central nervous system to maintain balance. Each of these systems is affected by aging. People rely heavily on visual input for balance. Vision typically declines as people age, and the resulting poor visual acuity distorts information that is sent to the central nervous system, impacting balance. It is not unusual to see older people hunched over as they walk, partly due to poor vision. Declines in the functioning of the vestibular system, which provides information regarding the position of the head in space, and the somatosensory system (e.g., muscle and joint proprioceptors, cutaneous and pressure receptors) also significantly impact balance and coordination. Physical activity has been shown to improve balance and coordination in older adults, especially activities that focus on the mind-body connection, such as tai chi, yoga, and **Pilates.**

Mental Health

Cognitive decline has been associated with aging and there is some evidence that physical activity prevents or delays cognitive impairment and disability and improves sleep (Nelson et al., 2007). As people age, depression and anxiety disorders increase, though physical activity has been shown to be beneficial in preventing these disorders. Additionally, people tend to have fewer friends and acquaintances as they age, and this loss of social stimulation can lead to depression. Physical activity provides a mechanism for older adults to have regular social interaction.

Exercise Guidelines

Before starting an exercise program, older adults should first see their physicians for a pre-exercise evaluation that may include a medical history review, physical, and exercise test. Physical-activity recommendations for older adults include the following (Nelson et al., 2007):

- Older adults should perform moderate-intensity aerobic physical activity for a minimum of 30 minutes five days each week, or vigorous-intensity aerobic activity for a minimum of 20 minutes, three days each week. Moderate-intensity aerobic activity involves a moderate level of effort relative to an individual's aerobic fitness. On a 10-point scale, where sitting is 0 and all-out effort is 10, moderate activity is a 5 or 6 and should produce noticeable increases in heart rate and breathing. On the same scale, vigorous-intensity activity is a 7 or 8 and produces large increases in heart rate and breathing rate. Combinations of moderate- and vigorous-intensity activity can be performed to meet this recommendation.

- At least twice each week, older adults should perform muscle-strengthening activities that maintain or increase muscular strength and endurance using the major muscles of the body. It is recommended that eight to 10 exercises be performed on at least two non-consecutive days per week using a resistance that allows 10 to 15 repetitions for each exercise.
- Because of the dose-response relationship between physical activity and health, older persons who wish to further improve their personal fitness, reduce their risk for chronic diseases and disabilities, or prevent unhealthy weight gain will likely benefit from exceeding the minimum recommended amount of physical activity.
- To maintain the flexibility necessary for regular physical activity and daily life, older adults should perform activities that help maintain or increase flexibility at least twice each week for at least 10 minutes each day.
- To reduce the risk of injury from falls, community-dwelling older adults with a substantial risk of falling should perform exercises that maintain or improve balance.
- Older adults with one or more medical conditions for which physical activity is therapeutic should perform physical activity in a manner that effectively and safely treats the condition.
- Older adults should have a plan for obtaining sufficient physical activity that addresses each recommended type of activity. Those with chronic conditions for which activity is therapeutic should have a single plan that integrates prevention and treatment. For older adults who are not active at recommended levels, plans should include a gradual (or stepwise) approach to increase physical activity over time. Many months of activity at less than recommended levels is appropriate for some older adults (e.g., those with low fitness) as they increase activity in a stepwise manner. Older adults should also be encouraged to self-monitor their physical activity on a regular basis and to reevaluate plans as their abilities improve or as their health status changes.

Sample Exercise Recommendation for Older Adults

Mode: Endurance exercise, such as low-impact aerobics, walking, using cardiovascular equipment such as elliptical trainers and cycles, and swimming, should be the primary exercise mode for most older adults. Personal trainers should recommend a program of weight training that features low resistance and high repetitions (at least initially) and include exercises that maintain or improve balance, such as backward walking, sideways walking, heel walking, toe walking, standing from a sitting position, and tai chi, always being certain to teach appropriate technique and monitor for safety. It is important to encourage an active lifestyle and participation in recreational activities (e.g., tennis, dancing) as appropriate.

Intensity: Depending on the level of physical conditioning, current state of health, and age, exercise intensity will range from low to moderate, with relatively few individuals performing vigorous exercise. Most older adults should be encouraged to exercise at a moderate level (RPE of 11 to 13 on the 6 to 20 scale).

Duration: Older clients should perform longer and more gradual warm-up and cool-down periods. Clients can gradually increase exercise duration to 30 to 60 minutes per session, depending on their medical history and clinical status.

Frequency: Older clients should exercise at least five days each week. Daily exercise of shorter duration may be appropriate for some individuals with an initially low functional capacity.

Exercise and Youth

Regular physical activity in children and adolescents is essential to promote health and fitness. Unfortunately, millions of American youths do not get the recommended amount of physical activity and are at risk for developing degenerative diseases in their adult years. Additionally, lack of physical activity and poor nutritional habits have resulted in an exponential increase in overweight and obese children and adolescents, placing them at risk for premature death. Youth have been negatively impacted by the decline in physical-activity requirements in schools and sedentary pursuits such as surfing the Internet, computer gaming, and television viewing. On average, young people between the ages of 2 and 18 spend an astounding four to five hours per day using electronic media. Couple that with the time spent sitting in a classroom and the lack of school-based physical education and the result is a generation of young people that spend the majority—and in extreme cases all—of their waking time in sedentary activities.

The negative health consequences of physical inactivity, poor dietary habits, and associated weight gain include hypertension, type 2 diabetes, osteoporosis, and the development of atherosclerosis. Furthermore, behaviors established at a young age have a high probability of persisting into adulthood, making it likely that physically inactive youth will remain sedentary as adults, placing them at risk for premature death.

Youth can achieve substantial health benefits by doing moderate- and vigorous-intensity physical activity for periods of time that add up to 60 minutes or more each day (U.S. Department of Health & Human Services, 2008). This activity should include aerobic activities as well as age-appropriate muscle- and bone-strengthening exercises. As with adults, it appears that the total amount of physical activity accumulated each week is more important for achieving health benefits than is any one component (frequency, intensity, or duration). However, bone-strengthening activities are especially critical for children and young adolescents, because the greatest gains in bone mass occur during the period just before and during puberty.

Exercise Guidelines

The primary exercise activities for children and adolescents are aerobic conditioning, muscle strengthening, and bone strengthening. Most of the 60-plus minutes of physical activity each day should be either moderate- or vigorous-intensity aerobic exercise, and should include vigorous-intensity physical activity performed at least three days per week. Activities such as running, hopping, skipping, jumping rope, swimming, and bicycling should be encouraged. Recreational and competitive sports are excellent ways to improve fitness and should provide an element of fun.

Muscle-strengthening activities are an important part of the activity program and should be included on at least three days of the week. Muscle-strengthening activities do not have to be structured (e.g., weight training), but can be incorporated into play and games (climbing trees, tug-of-war, jumping).

Although there are fewer resistance-training studies involving children than adults, the evidence that demonstrates increases in strength following structured resistance training in children is mounting (ACSM, 2010; Faigenbaum & Westcott, 2009). These studies indicate that strength increases in children are similar to those observed in older age groups. Furthermore, the safety and efficacy of resistance-training programs for prepubescent children has been well-documented.

The risk of injuries to children participating in resistance-training programs is low. However, injuries can occur in any sport or strenuous physical activity. To minimize the risk of injury during resistance training, personal trainers should adhere to the following guidelines:

- Obtain medical clearance or instructions regarding physical needs.
- Children should be properly supervised and use proper exercise technique at all times.

- Do not allow children to exercise unless the weight-training facility is safe for them.
- Never have children perform single maximal lifts, sudden explosive movements, or try to compete with other children.
- Teach children how to breathe properly during exercise movements.
- Never allow children to use any equipment that is broken or damaged, or that they do not fit on properly.
- Children should rest for approximately one to two minutes between each exercise, and for longer if necessary. In addition, they should have scheduled rest days between each training day.
- Encourage children to drink plenty of fluids before, during, and after exercise.
- Tell children that they need to communicate with their coach, parent, or teacher when they feel tired or fatigued, or when they have been injured.

Bone-strengthening is stimulated by activities that produce a force on the bones, such as running, jumping rope, hopping, skipping, and playing basketball, tennis, or hopscotch. Table 14-9 shows examples of moderate- and vigorous-intensity aerobic activities, as well

Table 14-9

Examples of Moderate- and Vigorous-intensity Aerobic Activities and Muscle- and Bone-strengthening Activities for Children and Adolescents

Type of Physical Activity	Children	Adolescents
Moderate-intensity aerobic	• Active recreation, such as hiking, skateboarding, and rollerblading • Bicycle riding • Brisk walking	• Active recreation, such as canoeing, hiking, skateboarding, and rollerblading • Brisk walking • Bicycle riding (stationary or road bike) • Housework or yard work, such as sweeping or pushing a lawn mower • Games that require catching and throwing, such as baseball and softball
Vigorous-intensity aerobic	• Active games involving running and chasing, such as tag • Bicycle riding • Jumping rope • Martial arts, such as karate • Running • Sports such as soccer, ice or field hockey, basketball, swimming, and tennis • Cross-country skiing	• Active games involving running and chasing, such as flag football • Bicycle riding • Jumping rope • Martial arts, such as karate • Running • Sports such as soccer, ice or field hockey, basketball, swimming, and tennis • Vigorous dancing • Cross-country skiing
Muscle strengthening	• Games such as tug-of-war • Modified push-ups (with knees on the floor) • Resistance exercises using body weight or resistance bands • Rope or tree climbing • Sit-ups (curl-ups or crunches) • Swinging on playground equipment/bars	• Games such as tug-of-war • Push-ups and pull-ups • Resistance exercises with exercise bands, weight machines, and hand-held weights • Climbing wall • Sit-ups (curl-ups or crunches)
Bone strengthening	• Games such as hopscotch • Hopping, skipping, and jumping • Jumping rope • Running • Sports such as gymnastics, basketball, volleyball, and tennis	• Hopping, skipping, and jumping • Jumping rope • Running • Sports such as gymnastics, basketball, volleyball, and tennis

Note: Some activities, such as bicycling, can be moderate or vigorous intensity, depending upon level of effort.

U.S. Department of Health & Human Services (2008). *2008 Physical Activity Guidelines for Americans: Be Active, Healthy and Happy.* www.health.gov/paguidelines/pdf/paguide.pdf

as examples of activities that promote the strengthening of bone and muscle.

Children and adolescents with disabilities and health conditions such as asthma and diabetes are less likely to be active than youth without these conditions. Youth with health challenges should work with their healthcare providers to understand the types and amounts of physical activity that are appropriate for them.

Children exercising in extremely cold temperatures are at increased risk of dehydration and **hypothermia.** Careful attention should be given to ensure proper hydration and layering of clothing when exercising in cold conditions. In extremely cold conditions, trainers should consider moving activities indoors.

Hot environments present a challenge as well, and concern has existed that children may be at greater risk of heat-related illnesses than adults due to their:

- Higher ratio of body surface area to mass
- Lower exercise economy
- Diminished sweating capacity
- Lower cardiac output at a similar workload

Research suggests that children and adults are similar in terms of their risk for heat-related illness and that no maturational differences exist in thermal balance or endurance performance during exercise in the heat (Rowland, 2008; Naughton & Carlson, 2008; Rowland et al., 2008; Falke & Dotan, 2008). Therefore, the following precautions are applicable for children as well as adults (CDC, 2006b):

- Reduce the intensity of exercise when it is very hot, humid, or sunny.
- Cancel activity or move indoors to an air conditioned environment during periods of very hot and especially humid conditions.
- Maintain hydration; encourage children to drink every 15 to 30 minutes when exercising, even if they do not "feel" thirsty.
- Encourage frequent breaks/rest periods in the shade, and have children drink fluids during these breaks.
- Encourage lightweight, light-colored, loose-fitting clothing, as well as the use of sunscreen.
- To prevent hyponatremia, it is important to replace both lost water and salt, either with a sports drink or a meal. Use of salt supplements is not recommended.

Over the past few years, the volume of overuse injuries and sports-related traumatic injuries has been steadily increasing in children and adolescents. It is important to remember that children are not just small versions of adults and that training activities must be age-appropriate. Far too many children participating in competitive sports are being pushed too hard in an effort to "win," resulting in injury, loss of the fun element of sport, and ultimately a decline in participation. Vigorous exercise is good for youth. However, it must be age-appropriate and not of the magnitude that it increases injury risk. The following guidelines are important to keep in mind when working with children and adolescents (U.S. Department of Health & Human Services, 2008):

- Children and adolescents who do not currently meet the recommended physical-activity guidelines for youth (e.g., 60 or more minutes of daily physical activity) should slowly increase their activity levels in small steps and in ways that they enjoy. A gradual increase in the number of days and time spent being active will help reduce the risk of injury.
- Children and adolescents who do meet the guidelines should continue being active on a daily basis and, if appropriate, become even more active. Evidence suggests that performing more than 60 minutes of daily activity may provide additional health benefits.
- Children and adolescents who exceed the guidelines should maintain their activity levels and vary the kinds of activities they do to reduce the risk of overtraining or injury.

Sample Exercise Recommendation for Youth

Mode: Personal trainers should encourage children and adolescents to participate in sustained activities that use large muscle groups (e.g., swimming, running, jogging, aerobics). It is important to incorporate fun activities, such as recreational sports that develop other components of fitness (speed, power, flexibility, muscular endurance, agility, and coordination). Personal trainers should also encourage children and adolescents to include muscle-strengthening and bone-strengthening exercise as part of their physical activity at least three days per week and to live active lifestyles by walking to school and playing outdoors whenever possible.

Intensity: Children and adolescents who have not been active should start with low-intensity activity and gradually progress. As conditioning progresses, children and adolescents should be encouraged to participate in moderate- and vigorous-intensity activity. Activities that encompass all three intensity zones are an excellent choice.

Duration: Children and adolescents should accumulate 60 minutes or more of daily physical activity.

Frequency: Children and adolescents should be encouraged to exercise daily. Daily sessions do not have to be heavily structured, but should include a variety of play and recreational activities.

Pre- and Postnatal Exercise

For many years, the medical community encouraged pregnant women to reduce their physical-activity levels and refrain from starting vigorous exercise programs, due to concerns that exercise might harm the fetus. Since the mid-1990s, an increasing amount of research on exercise during pregnancy has shown that pregnant women can exercise safely without harming the fetus. ACSM developed a Roundtable Consensus Statement in 2006 that provides evidence in support of the safety of exercise and physical activity during pregnancy and the postpartum period (ACSM, 2006b). The expert panel concluded that exercise during pregnancy and the postpartum period:

- Reduces the risk of preeclampsia
- Treats or prevents gestational diabetes
- Helps manage or alleviate pregnancy-related musculoskeletal issues such as low-back pain, pregnancy-related incontinence, abdominal muscle disturbances, and joint and muscle injuries
- Positively affects mood and mental health. Many women experience mood changes during pregnancy and the postpartum period. Exercise has been shown to improve mood, increase vigor, improve self-concept, and reduce fatigue, stress, anxiety, and depression.
- Is safe and does not harm offspring health or development

Women undergo a variety of physical changes during pregnancy that can limit the ability to exercise. On average, pregnant women gain 25 to 40 pounds (11 to 18 kg), placing additional stress on joints of the back, pelvis, hips, and legs. As the fetus grows and weight gain occurs, the **center of gravity (COG)** moves upward and out. The changes in weight and COG often result in low-back discomfort and affect balance and coordination. Many women are more flexible during pregnancy due to hormone-related joint laxity (**relaxin**).

Cardiac reserve, or the difference between resting and maximum cardiac function, is reduced in pregnant women. During the early months of pregnancy, hormonal signals stimulate increases in heart rate, blood volume, stroke volume, and cardiac output. As pregnancy progresses, these cardiovascular changes can make increased physical demands more difficult than normal, especially in the supine position. This is why pregnant women should be discouraged from exercising at high intensity levels or participating in activities that require sudden bursts of movement.

The thermoregulatory system is also affected by pregnancy, resulting in a slight improvement in women's ability to dissipate heat. This may be due to increased blood flow to the skin and increases in tidal volume. However, it is critical that the pregnant exerciser is aware of the **ambient temperature** prior to each workout. Exercise increases body temperature, and increased ambient temperature and/or humidity may significantly affect the woman's ability to dissipate heat and could result in **hyperthermia** and potentially harm the fetus. However, there have been no reports that hyperthermia associated with exercise causes malformations of the embryo or fetus.

Exercise Guidelines for Pregnant Women

A review of current research supports the recommendation that a moderate level of exercise on a regular basis during a low-risk pregnancy has minimal risk for the fetus and beneficial metabolic and cardiorespiratory effects for the exercising woman. Recommendations from ACSM, the Canadian Academy of Sport Medicine (CASM), the American College of Obstetricians and Gynecologists (ACOG), the Society of Obstetricians and Gynaecologists of Canada (SOGC), the Royal College of Obstetricians and Gynaecologists (RCOG), and others, have concluded that physician-guided exercise is beneficial during and following pregnancy (CASM/ACSM, 2008; ACMS, 2006b; RCOG, 2006; SOGC, 2003; ACOG, 2002).

Pregnant women should obtain physician clearance and guidelines for exercise before initiating an exercise program. The physician will ensure that there are no health conditions present that would limit activity. Pregnant women with the following health conditions should not exercise:

- Risk factors for pre-term labor
- Vaginal bleeding
- Premature rupture of membranes

Generally, pregnant women should adhere to the following guidelines:

- Do not begin a vigorous exercise program shortly before or during pregnancy.
- Women who have been previously active may continue their exercise programs during the first trimester to a maximum of 30 to 40 minutes at a frequency of three to four days per week, as tolerated.
- Women who have not previously been active should begin slowly, with 15 minutes of low-intensity exercise and a gradual increase to 30 minutes. Some women may need to begin with even shorter durations and/or perform intermittent activity.
- Gradually reduce the intensity, duration, and frequency of exercise during the second and third trimesters. For example, a woman who walks or runs an average of 40 minutes per session might reduce her time to 30 minutes during the first trimester and then further reduce duration and/or exercise intensity in the second and third trimesters.
- Use the RPE scale rather than heart rate to monitor exercise intensity. Choose an intensity that is comfortable (e.g., RPE of 9 to 13 on the 6 to 20 scale). A pounding heart rate, breathlessness, and dizziness are indicators that intensity should be reduced.
- Avoid the following exercises:
  - ✓ Activities that require extensive jumping, hopping, skipping, bouncing, or running
  - ✓ Deep knee bends, full sit-ups, double-leg raises, and straight-leg toe touches
  - ✓ Contact sports such as softball, football, basketball, and volleyball
  - ✓ Bouncing while stretching
  - ✓ Activities where falling is likely (e.g., downhill or cross-country skiing, horseback riding)
- After the first trimester, prolonged exercise in the supine position (greater than five minutes) should be discouraged due to the potential for fetal hypoxia.
- Avoid long periods of standing and instead keep moving or sit and rest.
- Exercise should be avoided when the temperature and/or humidity is high.
- Body temperature, which should not exceed 100° F (38° C), should be taken immediately after exercise. If body temperature exceeds 100° F (38° C), exercise intensity and duration should be modified and the client should be encouraged to exercise during cooler parts of the day or indoors.

- Focus on proper fluid intake to balance loss of fluids from exercise and prevent dehydration.
- Utilize extended warm-up and cool-down periods and incorporate some stretching.
- Avoid skiing, contact sports, scuba diving, jumping/jarring motions, and quick changes in movement.
- Walking and running should occur on flat, even surfaces to reduce the likelihood of falls.
- Wear supportive shoes while walking or running.
- Wear a bra that fits well and gives lots of support to help protect the breasts.
- Some pregnant women may benefit from a small snack prior to exercise to help avoid hypoglycemia. Pregnant women should consume the required extra daily calories needed during pregnancy.

Exercise during pregnancy is not without risk and it is important that personal trainers and their pregnant clients are aware of the following warning signs. Should any of these occur, the exercise session should be postponed and the client should discuss the condition with her physician prior to resuming exercise training (ACOG, 2002).

- Vaginal bleeding
- Dizziness or feeling faint
- Increased shortness of breath
- Chest pain
- Headache
- Muscle weakness
- Calf pain or swelling
- Uterine contractions
- Decreased fetal movement
- Fluid leaking from the vagina

Sample Exercise Recommendation for Pregnant Women

Mode: Aerobic and strength-conditioning exercises such as brisk walking, elliptical training, stationary cycling, cross-country skiing (no downhill), and swimming are recommended. Pregnant women should avoid jumping and jarring activities and contact sports.

Intensity: Light- to moderate-intensity exercise is recommended. The talk test or RPE scale can be used to monitor intensity (e.g., 9 to 13 on the 6 to 20 scale).

Duration: Pregnant women should begin with 15 minutes of continuous exercise and gradually build to 30-minute sessions. Women who are already exercising may be able to start at 30 to 40 minutes.

Frequency: Three times per week is the general recommendation, though some women may be able to progress to four to five times per week.

Postnatal Exercise Guidelines

Following delivery, women require some recovery time to regain strength. Taking care of a newborn—and coping with the associated sleep interruption—can easily lead to a fatigued state. Generally, the goal during the initial six weeks following delivery is to gradually increase physical activity as a means of relaxation, personal time, and a regaining of the sense of control, rather than improving physical fitness. Women who have had a Caesarean delivery may require additional recovery time. After the initial two months, the goal of exercise is to gradually improve the fitness level. After delivery, women should adhere to the following general guidelines:

- Obtain physician clearance and guidelines prior to resuming or starting an exercise program.
- Begin slowly, and gradually increase duration and then intensity. The goal is to develop consistency, not to see how hard one can work.
- Start with walking several times per week.
- Avoid excessive fatigue and dehydration.
- Wear a supportive bra.
- Stop the exercise session if unusual pain is experienced.
- Stop the exercise session and seek medical evaluation if bright red vaginal bleeding occurs that is heavier than a normal menstrual period.
- Drink plenty of water and eat appropriately.

Summary

Trends show that Americans continue to be sedentary and gain weight, resulting in numerous chronic health conditions. Personal trainers may be asked to work with one or more clients who have a chronic health condition. It is important that the personal trainer work closely with the client's physician and/or healthcare professional to establish a safe and effective exercise program. Training people with health challenges and seeing them progress can be quite rewarding, especially when programs are appropriately designed, implemented, and monitored.

The aging of America and the rapid rise in chronic health conditions provide a challenge for personal trainers, as the likelihood of working with one or more "special population" clients is high. The personal trainer is encouraged to become a student of clients' health conditions by researching and reading about them, and by communicating with healthcare professionals. The personal trainer must be careful not to step beyond the defined **scope of practice** and always obtain physician clearance and program recommendations prior to working with clients who have special health conditions.

Personal trainers can advance their careers by participating in a variety of continuing education opportunities and by seeking advanced certifications. The American Council on Exercise offers the Advanced Health & Fitness Specialist certification, which is an advanced certification that focuses on special populations. There are a number of annual national and regional conferences that provide exceptional continuing education and networking opportunities. Many of these conferences focus on specific diseases or disorders, and offer targeted educational opportunities. Online continuing education options (see www.acefitness.org/continuingeducation) and peer-reviewed journals are also available to assist personal trainers in advancing their knowledge bases. A number of medical fitness facilities also offer clinical internship opportunities, and additional education and professional degrees in exercise science are available at universities and colleges across the world.

References

Abeles, M. et al. (2008). Update on fibromyalgia therapy. *American Journal of Medicine,* 121, 555–561.

American Association of Cardiovascular and Pulmonary Rehabilitation (2004). *Guidelines for Cardiac Rehabilitation and Secondary Prevention Programs* (4th ed.). Champaign, Ill.: Human Kinetics.

American College of Obstetricians and Gynecologists (2002). ACOG Committee Opinion No. 267: Exercise during pregnancy and the postpartum period. *Clinical Obstetrics and Gynecology,* 99, 171–173.

American College of Sports Medicine (2010). *ACSM's Guidelines for Exercise Testing and Prescription* (8th ed.). Philadelphia: Wolters Kluwer/Lippincott Williams & Wilkins.

American College of Sports Medicine (2010). *ACSM's Resource Manual for Exercise Testing and Prescription* (6th ed.). Philadelphia: Lippincott Williams & Wilkins.

American College of Sports Medicine (2009). Position stand: Appropriate physical activity intervention strategies for weight loss and prevention of weight regain for adults. *Medicine & Science in Sports & Exercise,* 41, 2, 459–471.

American College of Sports Medicine (2006b). *American College of Sports Medicine Offers Guidance on Physical Activity During Pregnancy and the Postpartum Period.* www.acsm.org/AM/PrinterTemplate.cfm?Section=Chinese1&CONTENTID=5334&TEMPLATE=/CM/ContentDisplay.cfm

American Diabetes Association (2009). Total Prevalence of Diabetes and Pre-diabetes. www.diabetes.org/diabetes-statistics/prevalence.jsp. Retrieved January 22, 2009.

American Heart Association (2009a). *Statistical Fact Sheet: Risk Factors, 2008 Update. High Blood Cholesterol and Other Lipids: Statistics.* www.americanheart.org/downloadable/heart/1197995624080FS13CHO8.pdf

American Heart Association (2009b). Heart disease and stroke statistics 2009 update: A report from the American Heart Association Statistics Committee and Stroke Statistics Subcommittee. *Circulation,* 119, e21–e181.

American Heart Association/National Heart, Lung, and Blood Institute (2005). Scientific statement: Diagnosis and management of the metabolic syndrome. *Circulation,* 112, e285–e290.

Arthritis Foundation (2009). *Fibromyalgia (FMS).* www.arthritis.org/disease-center.php?disease_id=10. Retrieved January 22, 2009.

Assis, M.R. et al. (2006). A randomized controlled trial of deep water running: Clinical effectiveness of aquatic exercise to treat fibromyalgia. *Arthritis & Rheumatism,* 55, 1, 57–65.

Balady, G.J. (2007). Core components of cardiac rehabilitation. *Circulation,* 115, 2675–2682.

Barnard, R.J. & Hall, J.A. (1989). Patients with peripheral vascular disease. In: Franklin, B.A. (Ed.) *Exercise in Modern Medicine.* Baltimore: Williams & Wilkins.

Burckhardt, C.S. et al. (1994). A randomized, controlled clinical trial of education and physical training for women with fibromyalgia. *Journal of Rheumatology,* 21, 4, 714–720.

Canadian Academy of Sport Medicine/American College of Sports Medicine (2008). *Position Statement: Exercise and Pregnancy.* www.sirc.ca/newsletters/may08/documents/PregnancyDiscussionPaper.pdf

Centers for Disease Control and Prevention (2009). *Healthy Aging for Older Adults.* www.cdc.gov/aging/. Retrieved April 8, 2009.

Centers for Disease Control and Prevention (2008a). *Chronic Disease Prevention and Health Promotion.* www.cdc.gov/nccdphp/. Retrieved January 25, 2009.

Centers for Disease Control and Prevention (2008b). *Arthritis.* www.cdc.gov/arthritis. Retrieved January 26, 2009.

Centers for Disease Control and Prevention (2008c). *CFS Basic Facts.* www.cdc.gov/cfs/cfsbasicfacts.htm. Retrieved January 22, 2009.

Centers for Disease Control and Prevention (2006a). *Toolkit for Healthcare Professionals: Chronic Fatigue Syndrome.* www.cdc.gov/cfs. Retrieved January 26, 2009.

Centers for Disease Control and Prevention (2006b). *Extreme Heat: A Prevention Guide to Promote Your Personal Health and Safety.* www.bt.cdc.gov/disasters/extremeheat/heat_guide.asp. Retrieved April 8, 2009.

Centers for Disease Control and Prevention (2005). National Diabetes Fact Sheet. www.cdc.gov/diabetes/pubs/factsheet05.htm

Chobanian, A.V. et al. (2003). *JNC 7 Express: The Seventh Report of the Joint National Committee on Prevention, Detection, Evaluation, and Treatment of High Blood Pressure. NIH Publication No. 03-5233.* Washington D.C.: National Institutes of Health and National Heart, Lung, and Blood Institute.

Courneya, K.S. (2003). Exercise in cancer survivors: An overview of research. *Medicine & Science in Sports & Exercise,* 35, 11, 1846–1852.

Dallal, C.M. et al. (2007). Long-term recreational physical activity and risk of invasive and in situ breast cancer: The California teachers study. *Archives of Internal Medicine,* 167, 408–415.

Drouin, J. & Pfalzer, L. (2008). *Cancer and Exercise.* www.ncpad.org/disability/fact_sheet.php?sheet=195&PHPSESSID=1885bf557db02b163c17febef9239406. Retrieved January 18, 2009.

Dugan, S.A. (2006). Role of exercise in prevention and management of acute low back pain. *Clinics in Occupational and Environmental Medicine,* 5, 3, 615–632.

Falke, B. & Dotan, R. (2008). Children's thermoregulation. *Applied Physiology, Nutrition, and Metabolism,* 33, 2, 420–427.

Faigenbaum, A.D. & Westcott, W.L. (2009). *Youth Strength Training.* Champaign, Ill: Human Kinetics.

Galvao, D.A. & Newton, R.V. (2005). Review of exercise intervention studies in cancer patients. *Journal of Clinical Oncology,* 23, 899–909.

Griffith, J.P. & Zarruof, F.A. (2008). A systematic review of chronic fatigue syndrome: Don't assume it's depression. Primary Care Companion. *Journal of Clinical Psychiatry,* 10, 2, 120–128.

Grundy, S.M. et al. (2004). Implication of recent clinical trials for the National Cholesterol Education Program Adult Treatment Panel III Guidelines. *Circulation*, 110, 227–239.

Gusi, N. et al. (2006). Exercise in waist-high warm water decreases pain and improves health-related quality of life and strength in the lower extremities in women with fibromyalgia. *Arthritis & Rheumatism,* 55, 1, 66–73.

Haskell, W.L. et al. (2008). *Physical Activity Guidelines Advisory Committee Report.* www.health.gov/paguidelines/Report/

Hayes, S.C., Reul-Hirsche, H., & Turner, J. (2009). Exercise and secondary lymphedema: Safety, potential benefits, and research issues. *Medicine & Science in Sports & Exercise,* 41, 3, 483–489.

Helmick, C.G. et al. (2008). Estimates of the prevalence of arthritis and other rheumatic conditions in the United States: Part I. *Arthritis and Rheumatism,* 58, 1, 15–25.

Hochberg, M.C. et al. (1992). The American College of Rheumatology 1991 revised criteria for the classification of global functioning status in rheumatoid arthritis. *Arthritis and Rheumatism,* 35, 5, 498–502.

Holmes, M.D. et al. (2005). Physical activity and survival after breast cancer diagnosis. *Journal of the American Medical Association,* 293, 2479–2486.

Horner, M.J. et al. (Eds.) (2009). *SEER Cancer Statistics Review,* 1975–2006. Bethesda, Md.: National Cancer Institute. www.seer.cancer.gov

Jemal, A. et al. (2008). Annual Report to the Nation on the Status of Cancer, 1975–2005, Featuring trends in lung cancer, tobacco use, and tobacco control. *Journal of the National Cancer Institute,* 100, 23, 1672–1694.

Katzmarzyk, P.T. (2005). Metabolic syndrome, obesity, and mortality: Impact of cardiorespiratory fitness. *Diabetes Care,* 28, 2.

Kenney, W. & Holowatz, L.A. (2008). Hypertension. In: American Council on Exercise. *ACE Advanced Health & Fitness Specialist Manual*. San Diego, Calif.: American Council on Exercise.

Kelley, G.A. & Kelley, K.S. (2006). Aerobic exercise and lipids and lipoproteins in men: A meta-analysis of randomized controlled trials. *Journal of Men's Health and Gender,* 3, 1, 61–70.

Klein, S. et al. (2004). Absence of an effect of liposuction on insulin action and risk factors for coronary heart disease. *New England Journal of Medicine,* 350, 25, 2549–2557.

Klika, R.J., Callahan, K.E., & Golik, S.K. (2008). Exercise capacity of a breast cancer survivor: A case study. *Medicine & Science in Sports & Exercise,* 40, 10, 1711–1716.

Knols, R. et al. (2005). Physical exercise in cancer patients during and after medical treatment: A systematic review of randomized and controlled clinical trials. *Journal of Clinical Oncology,* 23, 3830–3842.

Kodama, S. et al. (2007). Effect of aerobic exercise training on serum levels of high-density lipoprotein cholesterol: A meta-analysis. *Archives of Internal Medicine,* 167, 999–1008.

Leon, A.S. & Sanchez, O.A. (2001). Response of blood lipids to exercise training alone or combined with dietary intervention. *Medicine & Science in Sports & Exercise,* 33, 6 Suppl., s502–s515.

Marcus, R.L. et al. (2008). Comparison of combined aerobic and high-force eccentric resistance exercise with aerobic exercise only for people with type 2 diabetes mellitus. *Physical Therapy,* 88, 11, 1345–1354.

Maron, D.J. (2000). The epidemiology of low levels of high-density lipoprotein cholesterol in patients with and without coronary artery disease. *American Journal of Cardiology,* 86, 12A, 11L–14L.

Matthews, C.E. et al. (2007). Evaluation of a 12-week home-based walking intervention for breast cancer survivors. *Support Care Cancer,* 15, 203–211.

Mayo Clinic (2009). *Chronic Fatigue Syndrome.* www.mayoclinic.com/health/chronic-fatigue-syndrome/DS00395. Retrieved January 18, 2009.

McCain, G.A. et al. (1988). A controlled study of the effects of a supervised cardiovascular fitness training program on the manifestations of primary fibromyalgia. *Arthritis & Rheumatism,* 37, 9, 1135–1141.

McGill, S.M. (2007). *Low Back Disorders* (2nd ed.). Champaign, Ill.: Human Kinetics.

National Cancer Institute (2008a). *Cancer Topics.* www.cancer.gov/cancertopics. Retrieved January 14, 2009.

National Cancer Institute (2008b). Annual report to the nation finds declines in cancer incidence and death rates: Special feature reveals wide variations in lung cancer trends across states. www.cancer.

gov/newscenter/pressreleases'ReportNation2008/Release. Retrieved January 12, 2009.

National Cholesterol Education Program (2002). Expert Panel on Detection, Evaluation and Treatment of High Blood Cholesterol in Adults: Summary of the second report of NCEP Expert Panel on Detection, Evaluation and Treatment of High Blood Cholesterol in Adults (Adult Treatment Panel III). NIH Publication No. 02-5213. *Journal of the American Medical Association,* 285, 2486–2497.

National Heart, Lung, and Blood Institute (2007). *National Asthma Education and Prevention Program Expert Panel Report 3: Guidelines for the Diagnosis and Management of Asthma.* NIH Publication Number 08-5846. Washington, D.C.: U.S. Department of Health & Human Services.

National Osteoporosis Foundation (2009). *Fast Facts on Osteoporosis.* www.nof.org/osteoporosis/diseasefacts.htm. Retrieved January 19, 2009.

Naughton, G.A. & Carlson, J.S. (2008). Reducing the risk of heat-related decrements to physical activity in young people. *Journal of Science and Medicine in Sport,* 11, 1, 58–65.

Nelson, M.E. et al. (2007). Physical activity and public health in older adults: Recommendation from the American College of Sports Medicine and the American Heart Association. *Medicine & Science in Sports & Exercise,* 39, 8, 1435–1445.

Peel, J.B. et al. (2009). A prospective study of cardiorespiratory fitness and breast cancer mortality. *Medicine & Science in Sports & Exercise,* 41, 4, 742–748.

Pescatello, L.S. et al. (2004). American College of Sports Medicine position stand: Exercise and hypertension. *Medicine & Science in Sports & Exercise,* 36, 533–553.

Reva, L.C. et al. (2008). Estimates of the prevelance of arthritis and other rheumatic conditions in the United States: Part II. *Arthritis and Rheumatism,* 58, 1, 26–35.

Roberts, S. (2003). Special populations and health concerns. In: American Council on Exercise. *ACE Personal Trainer Manual* (3rd ed.). San Diego, Calif.: American Council on Exercise.

Rowland, T. (2008). Thermoregulation during exercise in the heat in children: Old concepts revisited. *Journal of Applied Physiology,*105, 2, 718–724.

Rowland, T. et al. (2008). Exercise tolerance and thermoregulatory responses during cycling in boys and men. *Medicine & Science in Sports & Exercise,* 40, 2, 282–287.

Royal College of Obstetricians and Gynaecologists (2006). *RCOG Statement No.4: Exercise in Pregnancy.* www.rcog.org.uk/index.asp?PageID=1366

Schneider, C.M. et al. (2007). Cancer treatment-induced alterations in muscular fitness and quality of life: The role of exercise training. *Annals of Oncology,* 18, 12, 1957–1962.

Slattery, M.L. et al. (2007). Physical activity and breast cancer risk among women in the southwestern United States. *Annals of Epidemiology,* 17, 342–353.

Society of Obstetricians and Gynaecologists of Canada (2003). Exercise in pregnancy and the postpartum period. *Journal of Obstetrics and Gynaecology Canada,* 25, 6, 516–522.

Stevens, J. et al. (2006). The definition of weight maintenance. *International Journal of Obesity,* 30, 3, 391–399.

Stevinson, C., Lawlor, D.A., & Fox, K.R. (2004). Exercise interventions for cancer patients: A systematic review of controlled trials. *Cancer Causes & Control,* 15, 1035–1056.

Temel, J.S. et al. (2009). A structured exercise program for patients with advanced non-small cell lung cancer. *Journal of Thoracic Oncology,* 4, 5.

Tortosa, A. et al. (2007). Mediterranean diet inversely associated with the incidence of metabolic syndrome: The SUN prospective cohort. *Diabetes Care,* 30, 2957.

U.S. Department of Health & Human Services (2008). *2008 Physical Activity Guidelines for Americans: Be Active, Healthy and Happy*. www.health.gov/paguidelines/pdf/paguide.pdf

Vinter, S. et al. (2008). F as in fat: How obesity policies are failing America, 2008: Trust for America's Health. Robert Wood Johnson Foundation. www.healthyamericans.org/reports/obesity2008/. Retrieved January 23, 2009.

Waller, B., Lambeck, S., & Daly, D. (2009). Therapeutic aquatic exercise in the treatment of low back pain: A systematic review. *Clinical Rehabilitation,* 23, 1, 3–14.

Wenger, N.K. (2008). Current status of cardiac rehabilitation. *Journal of the American College of Cardiology,* 51, 17, 1619–1631.

Wolfe, F. et al. (1990). The American College of Rheumatology 1990 Criteria for the Classification of Fibromyalgia: A report for the multicenter criteria committee. *Arthritis Rheumatology,* 33, 160–172.

Wong, D. & Transfeltd, E. (2007). *Macnab's Backache* (4th ed.). Philadelphia: Lippincott Williams & Wilkins.

Yang, X. et al. (2008). The longitudinal effects of physical activity history on metabolic syndrome. *Medicine & Science in Sports & Exercise,* 40, 8, 1424–1431.

Suggested Reading

American College of Sports Medicine (2009). *ACSM's Exercise Management for Persons with Chronic Diseases and Disabilities* (3rd ed.). Champaign, Ill.: Human Kinetics.

American College of Sports Medicine and American Diabetes Association (1997). Diabetes mellitus and exercise: A joint position statement of the American College of Sports Medicine and the American Diabetes Association. *Medicine & Science in Sports & Exercise,* 29, i-vi.

American Council on Exercise (2009). *ACE Fit Fact: Managing Cholesterol With Exercise*. San Diego, Calif.: American Council on Exercise.

American Council on Exercise (2005). *Exercise for Older Adults* (2nd ed.). San Diego, Calif.: American Council on Exercise.

American Council on Exercise (2008). *ACE Advanced Health & Fitness Specialist Manual.* San Diego, Calif.: American Council on Exercise.

Anthony, L. (2002). *Pre- and Post-Natal Fitness.* San Diego, Calif.: American Council on Exercise

Barry, D.W. & Kohrt, W.M. (2008). Exercise and the preservation of bone health. *Journal of Cardiopulmonary Rehabilitation and Prevention.* 28, 3, 153–162.

Chu, D., Faigenbaum, A., & Falkel, J. (2006). *Progressive Plyometrics for Kids.* Monterey, Calif.: Healthy Learning.

Churilla, J.R. (2009). The metabolic syndrome: The crucial role of exercise prescription and diet. *ACSM's Health and Fitness Journal,* 13, 1, 20–25.

Cohen, D. & Townsend, R.R. (2007). Yoga and hypertension. *Journal of Clinical Hypertension,* 9, 800–801.

Franklin, B.A. & Gordon, N.F. (2005). *Contemporary Diagnosis and Management in Cardiovascular Exercise.* Newtown, Penn.: Handbooks in Healthcare Company.

Frederick, M.I., Hafer-Macko, C.E., & Macko, R.F. (2008). Exercise training for cardiometabolic adaptation after stroke. *Journal of Cardiopulmonary Rehabilitation and Prevention,* 28, 2–11.

Hassink, S.G. (2006). *A Clinical Guide to Pediatric Weight Management and Obesity.* Philadelphia: Lippincott Williams & Wilkins.

Janiszewski, P.M., Saunders, T.J., & Ross, R. (2008). Lifestyle treatment of the metabolic syndrome. *American Journal of Lifestyle Medicine,* 2, 2, 99.

Kaelin, C.M. et al. (2007). *The Breast Cancer Survivor's Fitness Plan.* New York: McGraw-Hill.

Kraemer W. & Fleck, S. (2004). *Strength Training for Young Athletes* (2nd ed.). Champaign, Ill.: Human Kinetics.

Kraus, W.E. & Levine, B.D. (2007). Exercise training for diabetes: The "strength" of the evidence. *Annals of Internal Medicine,* 147, 6, 423–424.

Lavie, C.J. & Milani, R.V. (2005). Cardiac rehabilitation and exercise training in metabolic syndrome and diabetes. *Journal of Cardiopulmonary Rehabilitation,* 25, 2, 59–66.

Mediate, P. & Faigenbaum, A. (2007). *Medicine Ball for All Kids.* Monterey, Calif.: Healthy Learning.

Pate, R. et al. (2006). Promoting physical activity in children and youth. *Circulation,* 114, 1214–1224.

Pescatello, L.S. et al. (2004). Position stand: Exercise and hypertension. *Medicine & Science in Sports & Exercise,* 36, 3, 533–553.

Rippe, J.M. (1999). *Lifestyle Medicine.* Malden, Mass.: Blackwell Science.

Ruderman N. et al. (Eds.) (2002). *Handbook of Exercise in Diabetes* (2nd ed.). Alexandria, Va.: American Diabetes Association.

Schairer, J.R. & Keteyian, S.J. (2006). Exercise training in patients with cardiovascular disease. In: Kaminsky, L.A. (Ed.) *ACSM's Resource Manual for Guidelines for Exercise Testing and Prescription* (5th ed.). Philadelphia: Lippincott Williams & Wilkins.

Tipton, C.M. (1991). Exercise training and hypertension: An update. *Exercise and Sport Sciences Reviews,* 19, 447–505.

U.S. Department of Health & Human Services (1996). *Physical Activity and Health: A Report of the Surgeon General.* Atlanta, Ga.: U.S. Department of Health & Human Services, Centers for Disease Control and Prevention, National Center for Chronic Disease Prevention and Health Promotion.

Van Baar, M.E. et al. (1999). Effectiveness of exercise therapy in patients with osteoarthritis of the hip or knee: A systematic review of randomized clinical trials. *Arthritis and Rheumatism,* 42, 7, 1361–1369.

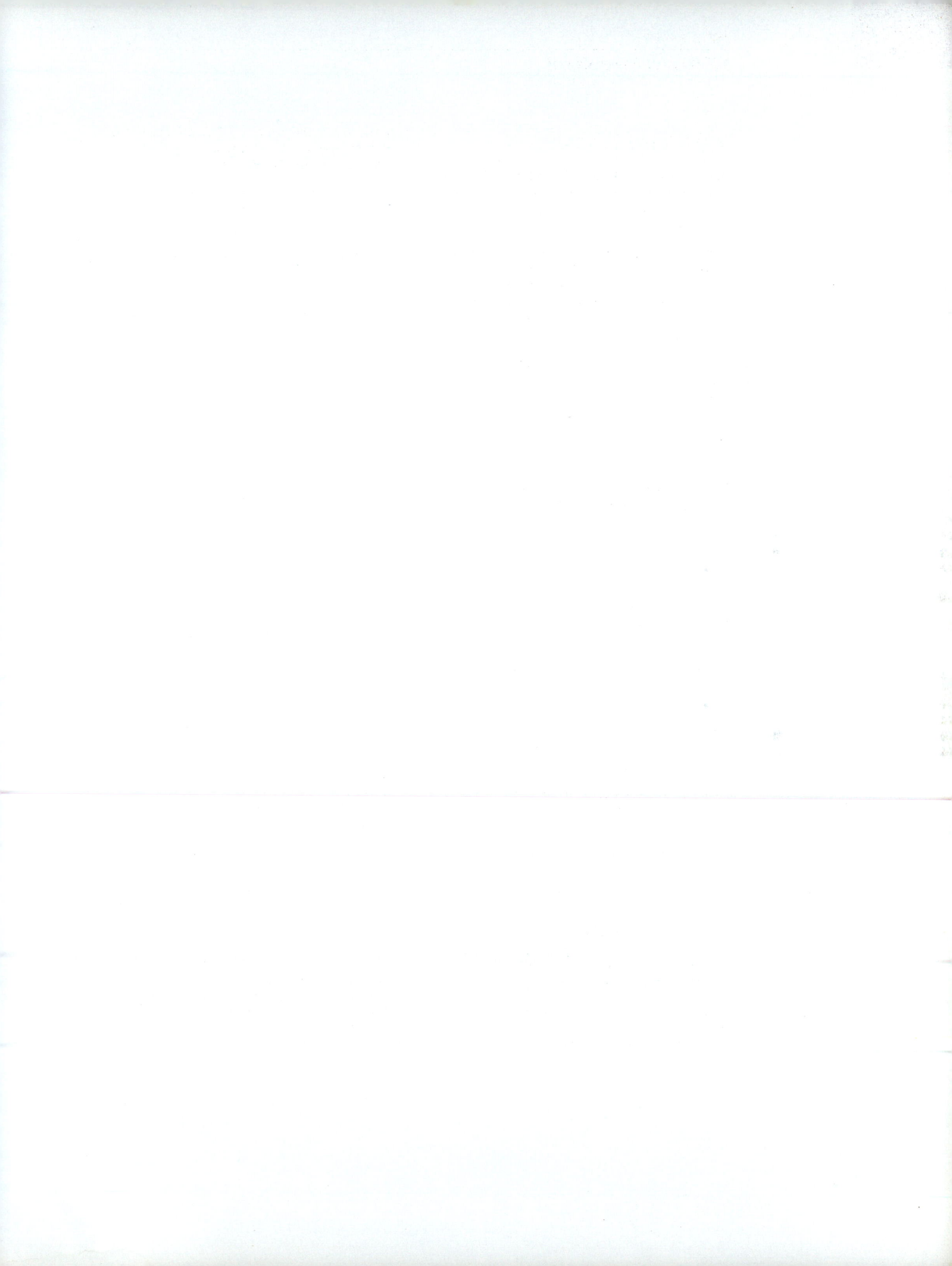

PART V
Injury Prevention and First Aid

Chapter 15

Common Musculoskeletal Injuries and Implications for Exercise

Chapter 16

Emergency Procedures

IN THIS CHAPTER:

Types of Tissue and Common Tissue Injuries
- Muscle Strains and Tendinitis
- Ligament Sprains
- Overuse Conditions
- Cartilage Damage
- Bone Fractures

Tissue Reaction to Healing
- Signs and Symptoms of Inflammation

Managing Musculoskeletal Injuries
- Pre-existing Injuries
- Program Modification
- Acute Injury Management

Flexibility and Musculoskeletal Injuries

Upper-extremity Injuries
- Shoulder Strain/Sprain
- Rotator Cuff Injuries
- Elbow Tendinitis
- Carpal Tunnel Syndrome

Low-back Pain
- Causes of Low-back Pain

Lower-extremity Injuries
- Greater Trochanteric Bursitis
- Iliotibial Band Syndrome
- Patellofemoral Pain Syndrome
- Infrapatellar Tendinitis
- Shin Splints
- Ankle Sprains
- Achilles Tendinitis
- Plantar Fasciitis

Record Keeping
- Medical History
- Exercise Record
- Incident Report
- Correspondence

Summary

SCOTT CHEATHAM, DPT, OCS, ATC, CSCS, PES, *is owner of Bodymechanix Sports Medicine & PT. He previously taught at Chapman University and is currently a national presenter. He has authored various manuscripts and has served on the exam committee for the National PT Board Exam and the National Athletic Training Certification Exam. Dr. Cheatham is currently a reviewer for the* Journal of Athletic Training *and* NSCA Strength & Conditioning Journal, *and is on the editorial board for NSCA's* Performance Training Journal.

CHAPTER 15

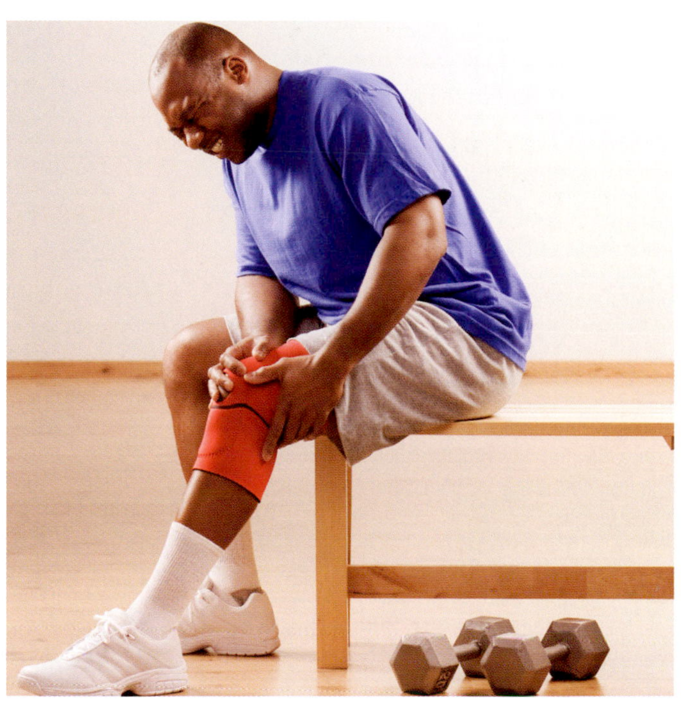

Common Musculoskeletal Injuries and Implications for Exercise

Scott Cheatham

When there is an injury to the human body, a variety of structures can be damaged, including bone, **cartilage, ligaments,** and muscle. Additionally, it is common for damage to the skin, nerves, blood vessels, and **viscera** to occur at the same time. Thus, having a basic understanding of common musculoskeletal injuries will help a personal trainer provide safe and effective exercise programming and make appropriate referrals to the healthcare team when warranted.

Types of Tissue and Common Tissue Injuries

Muscle Strains and Tendinitis

Muscle **strains** are injuries in which the muscle works beyond its capacity, resulting in microscopic tears of the muscle fibers. In mild strains, the client may report tightness or tension.

In more severe cases, the client may report feeling a sudden "tear" or "pop" that leads to immediate pain and weakness in the muscle. In addition, swelling, discoloration (**ecchymosis**), and loss of function often occur after the injury (Anderson, Hall, & Martin, 2008). Strains are frequent in the lower extremity and primarily occur in major muscle groups such as the hamstrings, groin, and calf (i.e., the gastrocnemius and soleus). Table 15-1 provides a description of the grades of muscle strains.

Table 15-1

Grading System for Muscle Strains

Grade	Description
Grade I strain	This is a mild strain; a few muscle fibers are stretched or torn. The injured muscle is tender and painful but has normal strength.
Grade II strain	This is a moderate strain; a large number of fibers are injured and there is more severe muscle pain and tenderness. Mild swelling is present, with a noticeable loss of strength and possible bruising.
Grade III strain	This is a complete tear. Sometimes a "tear" or "pop" sensation is felt as the muscle tears. Grade III strains result in complete loss of muscle function, severe pain, swelling, tenderness, and discoloration.

Adapted from Anderson, M.K., Hall, S.J., & Martin, M. (2008). *Foundations of Athletic Training: Prevention, Assessment, and Management* (4th ed.). Baltimore, Md.: Lippincott Williams & Wilkins.

Muscle strains of the hamstrings group are often caused by a severe stretch or a rapid, forceful contraction (e.g., sprinting). The hamstrings have the highest frequency of strains in the body, with the injury being especially common among athletes in running and jumping sports (Anderson, Hall, & Martin, 2008). Risk factors include poor **flexibility,** poor posture, muscle imbalance, improper warm-up, and training errors (Anderson, Hall, & Martin, 2008).

Muscle strains of the hip (e.g., adductor strains) are common in sports such as ice hockey and figure skating that require explosive acceleration, deceleration, and change of direction with a **lateral** movement component. With injury, the client may report an initial "pull" of the muscles inside the thigh, followed by intense pain and loss of function. Muscle imbalance between the hip adductors and abductors is the most prevalent risk factor for this injury (Anderson, Hall, & Martin, 2008).

Muscle strains in the calf are common among athletes in most running and jumping sports. Risk factors include muscle fatigue, fluid and **electrolyte** depletion, forced knee extension while the foot is dorsiflexed, and forced **dorsiflexion** while the knee is extended (Anderson, Hall, & Martin, 2008).

Ligament Sprains

Ligament **sprains** often, but not always, occur with trauma, such as a fall, or during contact sports. The most common joints for sprains include the ankle, knee, thumb/finger, and shoulder. If a sprain occurs, the client may report hearing a "popping" sound followed by immediate pain, swelling, instability, decreased **range of motion (ROM),** and a loss of function (Anderson, Hall, & Martin, 2008). Table 15-2 provides a general grading system for ligament sprains. Of particular medical significance are injuries to the anterior cruciate ligament (ACL) and the medial collateral ligament (MCL) of the knee.

ACL injuries are the most common *sports-related* injury of the knee, with 70 to 80% of ACL injuries occurring without contact (Figure 15-1) (Boden & Garrett, 1996; Griffin, 2000). These injuries often occur in relatively young athletic individuals 15 to 45 years of age (Mankse, 2006). The ACL's primary role

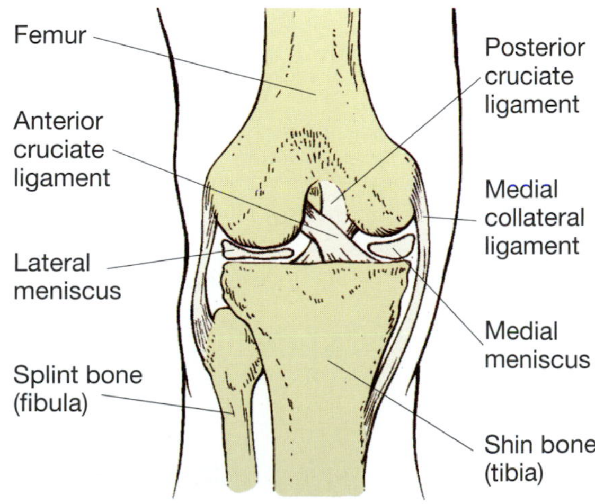

Figure 15-1
Knee joint anatomy depicting the anterior cruciate ligament (ACL), the medial collateral ligament (MCL), the posterior cruciate ligament, and the medial and lateral menisci

Table 15-2

Grading System for Ligament Sprains

Severity	Physical Examination Findings	Impairment	Pathophysiology	Typical Treatment
Grade I	Minimal tenderness Minimal swelling	Minimal	Microscopic tearing of collagen fibers	Weightbearing as tolerated No splinting/casting Isometric exercises Full ROM Stretching/strengthening exercises as tolerated
Grade II	Moderated tenderness Moderate swelling Decreased ROM Possible instability	Moderate	Complete tears of some, but not all, collagen fibers in the ligament	Immobilization with air splint Physical therapy ROM, stretching Strengthening exercises
Grade III	Significant swelling Significant tenderness Instability	Severe	Complete tear/rupture of ligament	Immobilization Physical therapy over a longer period Possible surgical reconstruction

Note: ROM = Range of motion

Adapted from Anderson, M.K., Hall, S.J., & Martin, M. (2008). *Foundations of Athletic Training: Prevention, Assessment, and Management* (4th ed.). Baltimore, Md.: Lippincott Williams & Wilkins.

is to prevent anterior glide of the tibia away from the femur. The mechanism of injury often involves deceleration of the body (e.g., a sudden stopping or cutting motion), combined with a maneuver of twisting, pivoting, or side-stepping (Griffin, 2000). When an ACL injury occurs, it is often traumatic and typically requires immediate medical care (Maxey & Magnusson, 2001).

It is common for individuals to injure the MCL at the same time as the ACL. However, injuries to the MCL are less common, but are often associated with complex knee injuries in which more than one tissue disruption occurs. The primary role of the MCL ligament is to prevent **medial** bending (**valgus**) on the knee. The mechanism of injury for isolated MCL trauma often involves an impact to the outer knee with no twisting involved. MCL damage is most often associated with a significant injury such as ACL or medial meniscal injuries (Anderson, Hall, & Martin, 2008). The signs and symptoms of an isolated MCL injury closely follow the grading scale presented in Table 15-2. The "Lower-extremity Injuries" section on page 543 provides a more in-depth discussion of knee sprains.

Overuse Conditions

When the body is put through excessive demands during activity, it often results in overuse conditions such as **tendinitis, bursitis,** and **fasciitis.** Tendinitis (i.e., inflammation of the **tendon**) is commonly diagnosed in the shoulders, elbows, knees, and ankles. Typically, clients begin new activities or exercise programs too quickly and the tendon cannot handle this new level of demand, resulting in an irritation that triggers an inflammatory response. Bursitis is an inflammation of the bursa sac due to **acute** trauma, repetitive stress, muscle imbalance, or muscle tightness on top of the **bursa.** Bursitis commonly affects the shoulders, hips, and knees. Lastly, fasciitis is inflammation of the connective tissue called **fascia** (Anderson, Hall, & Martin, 2008). It most commonly occurs in the bottom and back of the foot and has been linked to various intrinsic and extrinsic factors. "Upper-extremity Injuries" (page 538) and "Lower-extremity Injuries" (page 543) offer more in-depth discussions of these specific conditions.

Cartilage Damage

In addition to ligaments, the knee also consists of cartilage, another important type of tissue. Damage to the joint surface of the knee often involves damage to both the hyaline cartilage (which covers the bone) and the menisci cartilage (which act as shock absorbers).

The most commonly reported knee injury is damage to the menisci. The menisci have an important role within the knee due to their multiple functions—shock absorption, **stability,** joint congruency, lubrication, and **proprioception** (see Figure 15-1) (Manske, 2006). Meniscal injuries predominantly occur from trauma or degeneration. When meniscal injuries are the result of trauma, they are usually associated with a combination of loading and twisting of the joint or occur in conjunction with traumatic injuries such as ACL tears (i.e., lateral meniscus) or MCL injuries (i.e., medial meniscus) (Manske, 2006). Older individuals with degenerative joints are more predisposed to less acute meniscal tears (Goldstein & Zuckerman, 2000).

Regardless of their degree of acuity, when a client has a meniscal tear, he or she may complain of signs such as stiffness, clicking or popping with weightbearing activities, giving way, catching, and locking (in more severe tears). Symptoms may include joint pain, swelling, and muscle weakness (e.g., in the quadriceps) (Manske, 2006).

The cartilage under the patella (i.e., the knee cap) can also become damaged, resulting in **chondromalacia**. Chondromalacia is a softening or wearing away of the cartilage behind the patella, resulting in inflammation and pain. This is caused by the posterior surface of the patella not properly tracking in the femoral groove. Chondromalacia is commonly associated with improper training methods (e.g., overtraining, poor running style), sudden changes in training surface (e.g., from grass to concrete), lower-extremity muscle weakness and/or tightness, and even foot overpronation (i.e., flat feet). The affected knee may appear swollen and warm, and pain often occurs behind the patella during activity (Anderson, Hall, & Martin, 2008).

Bone Fractures

The causes of bone fractures are classified as either low or high impact. Low-impact trauma, such as a short fall on a level surface or repeated microtrauma to a bone region, can result in a minor fracture or a **stress fracture,** respectively. Stress fractures often occur in distance runners, track athletes, and court sport athletes (e.g., volleyball, basketball) (Figure 15-2). It is important not to confuse stress fractures with shin splints (refer to "Shin Splints" on page 548). Stress fractures have the following specific signs and symptoms (Cosca & Navazio, 2007):

- Progressive pain that is worse with weightbearing activity
- Focal pain
- Pain at rest in some cases
- Local swelling

High-impact trauma often occurs in motor vehicle accidents or during high-impact sports such as football. These injuries are often

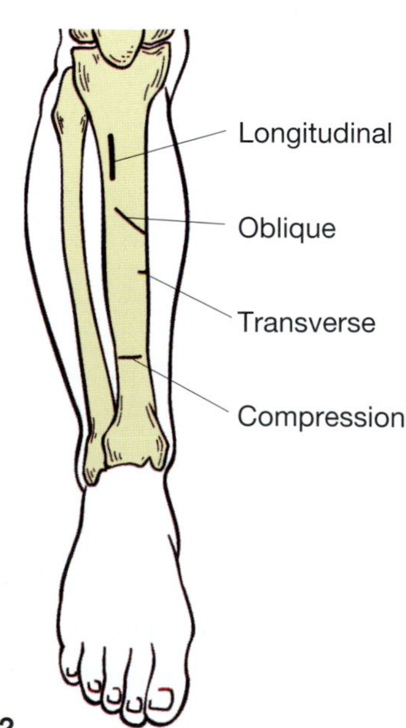

Figure 15-2
Types of stress fractures

disabling and require immediate medical attention. Other medical conditions such as infection, cancer, or **osteoporosis** can weaken bone and increase the risks for fracture (Cosca & Navazio, 2007). Such fractures are commonly called pathological fractures given their association with disease.

Tissue Reaction to Healing

When an injury occurs, the healing process begins immediately. The body goes through a systematic process with three distinct phases. These phases must be understood if a personal trainer is going to be able to design safe fitness programs for their clients following injury.

The first phase is the inflammatory phase, which can typically last for up to six days, depending on the severity of the injury. The focus of this phase is to immobilize the injured area and begin the healing process. Increased blood flow occurs to bring in oxygen and nutrients to rebuild the damaged tissue.

The second phase is the fibroblastic/proliferation phase, which begins approximately at day 3 and lasts approximately until day 21. This phase begins with the wound filling with **collagen** and other cells, which will eventually form a scar. Within two to three weeks, the wound can resist normal stresses, but wound strength continues to build for several months (Anderson, Hall, & Martin, 2008).

The third phase, the maturation/remodeling phase, begins approximately at day 21, and can last up to two years. This phase begins the remodeling of the scar, rebuilding of bone, and/or restrengthening of tissue into a more organized structure (Anderson, Hall, & Martin, 2008). Exercise progression must always be cautious when working with individuals recovering from a musculoskeletal injury.

Signs and Symptoms of Inflammation

When the tissues of the body (e.g., muscles, tendons, and ligaments) become inflamed, they will elicit specific signs and symptoms of which the fitness professional needs to be aware. This is particularly important for clients who are post-injury or post-surgery. The goal is to give these individuals a challenging exercise program that will not cause further damage to the injured area. The signs and symptoms of tissue inflammation are as follows (Magee, 2007):

- Pain
- Redness
- Swelling
- Warmth
- Loss of function

Managing Musculoskeletal Injuries

Pre-existing Injuries

If a client suffers from a pre-existing injury, proper management is essential. Clients will often approach a fitness professional seeking advice for present or past injuries. A personal trainer must respect the defined **scope of practice** and refrain from diagnosing the injury. A thorough medical history and assessment will help a personal trainer make appropriate decisions regarding the client's exercise programming. It is important to be able to answer the most important question: "Is the client appropriate for exercise or should he or she be cleared by a medical professional?" This will ensure client safety and provide the personal trainer with guidelines to follow. However, with local injuries (e.g., ankle sprains), the client should be able to participate in a modified exercise program using the non-injured parts of the body. For example, he or she can still exercise the upper body or do seated exercises that do not load the ankle. After obtaining medical clearance and guidelines, the personal trainer can proceed with a program that incorporates the injured region.

Program Modification

If a client has a pre-existing condition, his or her exercise program may need to be modified. The client should be monitored for any changes in symptoms, including pain. The following are some commonly reported symptoms of post-injury/post-surgery overtraining (Brotzman & Wilk, 2003):

- Soreness that lasts for more than 24 hours
- Pain when sleeping or increased pain when sleeping
- Soreness or pain that occurs earlier or is increased from the prior session
- Increased stiffness or decreased ROM over several sessions
- Swelling, redness, or warmth in healing tissue
- Progressive weakness over several sessions
- Decreased functional usage

Acute Injury Management

Acute injuries need to be handled quickly, but with caution. Client safety is paramount. A personal trainer needs to refer the client to an appropriate medical professional when an injury is serious enough (e.g., a client who is unable to walk after twisting an ankle during agility exercises or who feels sudden shoulder pain and weakness after swinging a kettlebell).

If an acute injury occurs, early intervention often includes medical management. The acronym P.R.I.C.E. (protection, rest or restricted activity, ice, compression, and elevation) describes a safe early-intervention strategy for an acute injury. In the following example, an ankle injury has taken place.

- *Protection* includes protecting the injured ankle with the use of crutches and appropriate ankle bracing.
- *Rest or restricted activity,* especially weightbearing activity, is advised until cleared by the physician.
- *Ice* should be applied every hour for 10 to 20 minutes until the tendency for swelling has passed.
- *Compression* involves placing a compression wrap on the area to minimize local swelling.
- *Elevation* of the ankle 6 to 10 inches above the level of the heart will also help control swelling. This is done to reduce hemorrhage, inflammation, swelling, and pain (Anderson, Hall, & Martin, 2008).

Flexibility and Musculoskeletal Injuries

Decreased flexibility has been associated with various musculoskeletal injuries, including muscle strains and the overuse conditions described previously. When a muscle becomes shortened and inflexible, it cannot lengthen appropriately or generate adequate force. This inflexible and weakened state often leads to injury.

To address this inflexibility and help prevent further injury, fitness professionals commonly develop stretching programs for their clients. A thorough flexibility assessment should be done prior to beginning any stretching program. A more in-depth discussion on this topic is presented in Chapter 7.

The following are **relative contraindications** to stretching that need to be considered to prevent injury (Kisner & Colby, 2007):

- Pain in the affected area
- Restrictions from the client's doctor
- Prolonged immobilization of muscles and connective tissue
- Joint swelling (**effusion**) from trauma or disease
- Presence of osteoporosis or **rheumatoid arthritis**
- A history of prolonged **corticosteroid** use

There are also **absolute contraindications** to stretching (Kisner & Colby, 2007):

- A fracture site that is healing
- Acute soft-tissue injury
- Post-surgical conditions
- Joint hypermobility
- An area of infection

If a client presents with any type of contraindication, the personal trainer should get further clearance from a medical professional prior to beginning a stretching routine.

Upper-extremity Injuries

Shoulder Strain/Sprain

Shoulder strain/sprain occurs when the soft-tissue structures (e.g., bursa, rotator cuff tendons) get abnormally stretched or compressed. Strains most often involve a tendon, while sprains usually involve a ligament. Additionally, shoulder strains/sprains can result from an impingement secondary to the compression and end up as tendinitis. These injuries can eventually lead to rotator cuff tears if they are not managed properly (Anderson, Hall, & Martin, 2008). Impingement is particularly common in young individuals who participate in overhead activities such as tennis, baseball, and swimming. Middle-aged adults can also be at risk from doing repetitive overhead activities such as painting or lifting objects (Anderson, Hall, & Martin, 2008). In general, strains/sprains are common in the shoulder as a result of this joint's significant mobility and its sacrifice of stability to achieve it.

Signs and Symptoms

Clients who suffer from shoulder strains/sprains often complain of local pain at the shoulder that radiates down the arm. Aggravating activities may include lifting objects and reaching overhead or across the body or any movements that stretch the strained/sprained tissues. There may be swelling and tenderness in the shoulder that causes pain and stiffness with movement (Anderson, Hall, & Martin, 2008).

Management

The conservative management of common musculoskeletal injuries is presented in Table 15-3. In the case of shoulder sprain/strain, aggravating activities or movements that should be avoided include overhead and across-the-body movements, as well as any movements that involve placing the hand behind the back.

Table 15-3

Conservative Management of Common Musculoskeletal Injuries

- Avoiding aggravating activities or movements
- Physical therapy
- Modalities (e.g., ice, heat)
- Oral anti-inflammatory medication
- Cortisone injections

Adapted from Brotzman, B. & Wilk, K. (2003). *Clinical Orthopedic Rehabilitation* (2nd ed.). St. Louis, Mo.: Mosby.

Exercise Programming

The personal trainer should educate the client on avoiding aggravating activities and improving posture and body positioning. The exercise program should emphasize regaining strength and flexibility of the shoulder complex. More specifically, strengthening the scapular stabilizers (e.g., rhomboids, middle trapezius, serratus anterior) and rotator cuff muscles will help restore proper scapulohumeral motion. The client should focus on stretching the major muscle groups around the shoulder to restore proper length to these muscles. In the presence of injury, exercise modifications may be needed to prevent further injury. With shoulder injuries, overhead activities often need to be modified. The overhead press exercise can be modified so that the exerciser only moves through a portion of the ROM. For example, the client can be instructed to not fully extend the arms. The shoulders should be positioned more toward the front of the body (i.e., in the scapular plane, where the shoulder is positioned 30 degrees between the **sagittal** and **frontal planes**) (Figure 15-3). This shoulder position helps prevent pinching of shoulder structures.

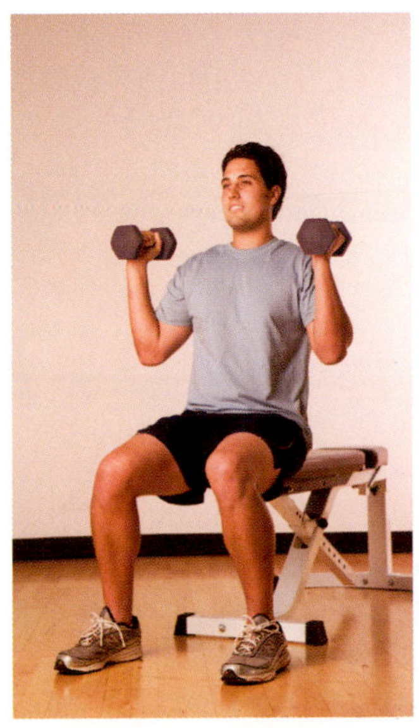
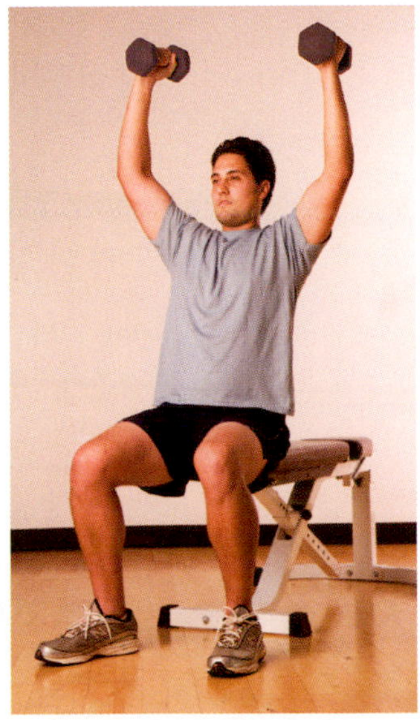

Figure 15-3
Shoulder press in the scapular plane

Rotator Cuff Injuries

Injuries to the rotator cuff are common among individuals who engage in activities involving overhead movements, as well as among middle-aged individuals. A tear may result from an acute injury or begin with a sprain/strain that eventually progresses to a rotator cuff tear. Rotator cuff injury can be classified into two main categories: acute and **chronic.** Acute injuries are often related to some type of trauma, such as falling on the shoulder or raising the arm against overwhelming resistance. These types of injuries commonly occur in individuals younger than 30 years old and are often accompanied by severe loss of function (Malanga, 2009; Cioppa-Mosca et al., 2006). Consequently, chronic tears present as a gradual worsening of pain and weakness. Often, these tears are a result of a degenerative process in individuals over the age of 40, with the dominant arm being most affected. Males are more susceptible to this injury than females (Malanga 2009; Cioppa-Mosca et al., 2006).

Signs and Symptoms

If an acute rotator cuff tear occurs, the client will likely complain of feeling a sudden "tearing" sensation followed by immediate pain and loss of motion. The client will typically have trouble lifting his or her arm above the head. Chronic tears show a gradual worsening, with increased pain at night or after increased activity. Reaching overhead or behind the back is painful. Basic tasks such as putting on a shirt or grabbing an object from a high shelf become difficult to impossible to perform (Malanga, 2009; Manske, 2006).

Management

A rotator cuff tear is typically traumatic in nature and results in loss of function. If a tear is suspected (either acute or chronic) the client should see a physician for proper diagnosis and management. Initially, the client may be referred to physical therapy for treatment while the physician orders other imaging [e.g., **magnetic resonance imaging (MRI)**] to obtain a more extensive diagnosis. It is common for other structures within the shoulder complex to be damaged, including the glenoid labrum or biceps tendon. These structures may have been affected by the trauma or degenerative process. The client is typically restricted from performing overhead activities and lifting heavy objects. If there is no progress with physical therapy or the tear is too severe, surgery is indicated to repair the torn muscle (Cioppa-Mosca et al., 2006).

Exercise Programming

The client is typically immobilized for six to eight weeks to allow the repair to heal. During this time, he or she will be limited to only passive range of motion (PROM), because actively contracting the repaired muscle could cause it to re-tear. The client may be cleared for gym activity after approximately 16 weeks, at which point the client may be transitioning from physical therapy (Cioppa-Mosca et al., 2006). This is a crucial time, when the personal trainer must obtain specific exercise guidelines from the physical therapist and, if applicable, the surgeon. The goal should be to continue what has been done in physical therapy in a safe, progressive manner. Ultimately, the personal trainer should obtain specific guidelines for what "should" and "should not" be done during gym activity. With a rotator cuff repair, exercise modifications may be needed to prevent further injury. In general, the personal trainer should be cautious with specific shoulder positions during activity. For example, performing overhead activities or keeping the arm straight during exercise should be limited due to the strain these actions will cause in the healing tissue. Exercises with the elbows bent will create less torque on the healing muscles (Figure 15-4).

Elbow Tendinitis

Tendinitis of both the flexor and extensor muscle tendons of the elbow and wrist can occur with overuse of the upper extremity. Two of the most common injuries are **lateral** and **medial epicondylitis.**

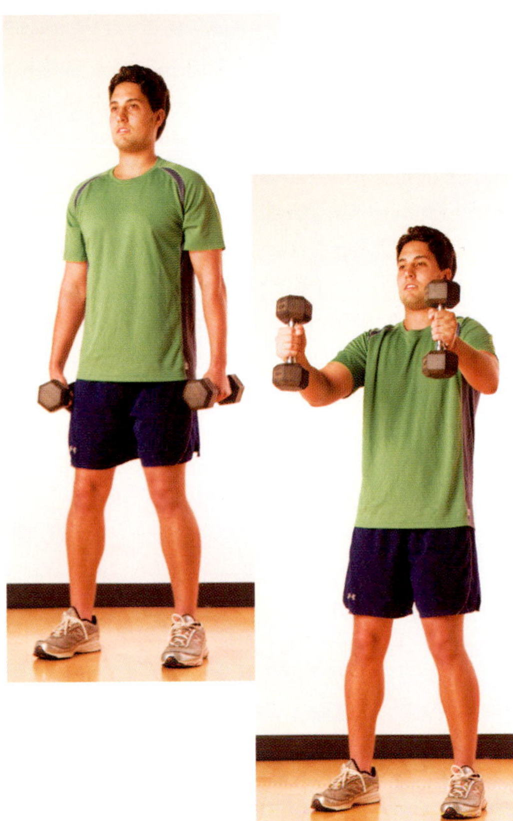

Figure 15-4
Front raise with elbows bent

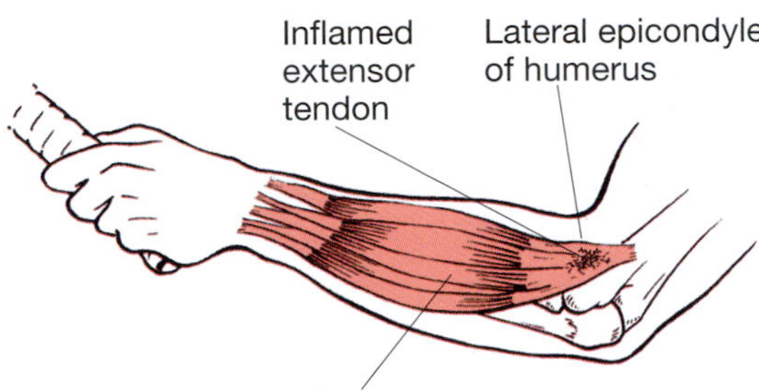

Figure 15-5
Lateral epicondylitis, or "tennis elbow"

Lateral epicondylitis, which is commonly called "tennis elbow," is defined as an overuse or repetitive-trauma injury of the wrist extensor muscle tendons near their origin on the lateral epicondyle of the humerus (Figure 15-5). Medial epicondylitis, which is sometimes called "golfer's elbow," is an overuse or repetitive-trauma injury of the wrist flexor muscle tendons near their origin on the medial epicondyle. These conditions are common in adults 30 to 55 years old (Anderson, Hall, & Martin, 2008; Brotzman & Wilk, 2003).

Signs and Symptoms

Clients will often complain of nagging elbow pain at the lateral epicondyle or medial epicondyle during aggravating activities (e.g. shaking hands, turning door knobs, lifting/carrying loads, cooking). Pain will diminish with rest, but tends to get worse over time if not addressed properly.

Management

The conservative management of common musculoskeletal injuries is presented in Table 15-3 (page 539). In the case of elbow tendinitis, aggravating activities or movements that should be avoided include repetitive elbow and wrist flexion/extension activities.

Exercise Programming

The exercise program should emphasize educating the client on avoiding aggravating activities and improving posture and body positioning. Regaining strength and flexibility of the flexor/pronator and extensor/supinator muscle groups of the wrist and elbow is important. The client may be prescribed a wrist or elbow splint to wear during activity, and the personal trainer should monitor for increased symptoms (Anderson, Hall, & Martin, 2008; Brotzman & Wilk, 2003). In the presence of injury, exercise modifications may be needed to prevent further injury. Clients with elbow tendinitis should avoid high-repetition activity (e.g., 15 to 20 repetitions) at the elbow and wrist. Exercises such as dumbbell biceps and wrist curls should begin with low weight and repetitions. Also, full elbow extension (i.e., locking the elbow) when performing shoulder exercises such as dumbbell front raises should be done with caution, since this can cause excessive loading of the muscle.

Carpal Tunnel Syndrome

Carpal tunnel syndrome is the most frequently occurring compression syndrome of the wrist. Repetitive wrist and finger flexion when the flexor tendons are strained results in a narrowing of the carpal tunnel due to inflammation, which eventually compresses the median nerve (Figure 15-6). Women are three times more likely than men to develop the syndrome and the dominant hand is

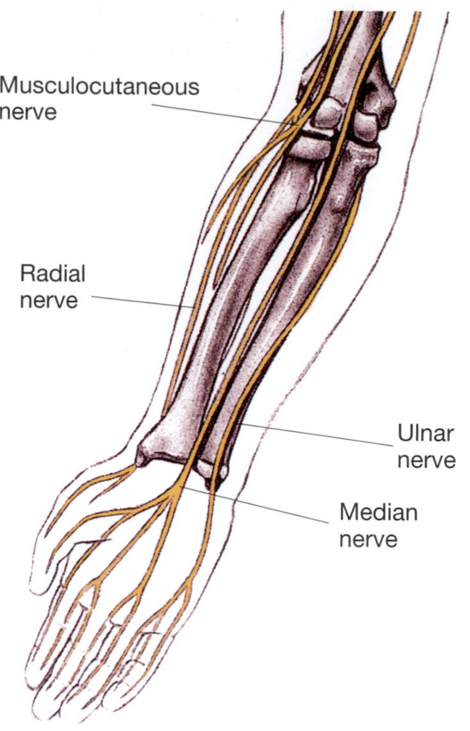

Figure 15-6
The nerves of the wrist, highlighting the median nerve

Source: Human Anatomy, 3rd ed., by Martini, F.H., Timmons, M.J., & McKinley, M.P. Copyright 2008. Reprinted by permission of Pearson Education.

usually affected first (Prentice, 1994; Calliet, 1978). Anything that narrows the carpal tunnel can result in this syndrome.

Signs and Symptoms

Carpal tunnel syndrome usually starts gradually with pain, weakness, or numbness in the radial three-and-a-half digits of the hand and the palmar aspect of the thumb. As the condition progresses, more specific symptoms begin to appear (Prentice, 1994; Calliet, 1978):

- Night or early-morning pain or burning
- Loss of grip strength and dropping of objects
- Numbness or tingling in the palm, thumb, index, and middle fingers

Long-standing affects may include atrophy of the thumb side of the hand, loss of sensations, and **paresthesias.**

Management

The conservative management approach presented in Table 15-3 (page 539), with the exception of cortisone injections, is often prescribed by physicians before surgical options are considered (Prentice, 1994; Calliet, 1978). In addition, individuals with carpal tunnel syndrome may be prescribed wrist splints to wear during activity.

Exercise Programming

The personal trainer should provide education on avoiding aggravating activities and improving posture and body positioning. The exercise program should emphasize regaining strength and flexibility of the elbow, wrist, and finger flexors and extensors. The client should wear the prescribed wrist splint during activity and the personal trainer should monitor for increased symptoms and adjust accordingly. In the presence of injury, exercise modifications may be needed to prevent further injury. With carpel tunnel syndrome, the client should avoid movements that involve full wrist flexion or extension. These end-range positions can further compress the carpel tunnel, which can increase symptoms. Exercise should focus on the mid-range of these motions.

Low-back Pain

The prevalence of low-back pain has reached nearly epidemic levels in America. Low-back pain equally affects men and women and most often occurs in individuals between 30 and 50 years of age. In fact, approximately two-thirds of adults will suffer from low-back pain at some time in their lives (Deyo & Weinstein, 2001). Common risk factors associated with low-back pain include, but are not limited to, the following (Pai & Sundaram, 2004; Maetzel & Li, 2002; Deyo & Weinstein, 2001):

- Heavy lifting, pushing, and pulling with twisting of the spine
- Prolonged static postures
- **Obesity**
- Stress or depression
- Poor physical fitness
- Inherited diseases (e.g., disc disease)
- Smoking
- Pregnancy
- Other diseases: **osteoarthritis,** rheumatoid arthritis, **ankylosing spondylitis,** and cancer

Causes of Low-back Pain

It is important for a personal trainer to understand the **etiology** of a client's low-back pain. This information will allow for safe and accurate exercise program development. The most frequently cited causes are mechanical back pain, **degenerative disc disease (DDD),** and **sciatica.**

Mechanical Pain

Mechanical low-back pain can simply be described as pain that is produced with movement of specific anatomical structures. This pain originates from abnormalities or deviations in the vertebrae, intervertebral discs, or facet joints. Pain is elicited when these injured structures are repeatedly stressed through movement (Hills, 2006).The weakened back is vulnerable to re-injury due to the lack of support from the injured structures. Poor muscular strength and flexibility are often present due to a decrease in activity secondary to pain. Other causes include muscle spasms, muscle tension, and myofascial restrictions (Hills, 2006; Deyo & Weinstein, 2001).

Degenerative Disc Disease and Sciatica

DDD commonly occurs in individuals between the ages of 30 and 50 years. It is typically due to an aging process, where the intervertebral disc gradually gets worn down and eventually degenerates. Along with DDD, disc herniations and bulging discs occur between the fourth and fifth lumbar vertebrae or between the fifth lumbar vertebra and the first sacroiliac joint 95% of the time (Cioppa-Mosca et al., 2006; Deyo & Weinstein, 2001). In both DDD and disc herniations, if the nerves coming out of the spinal cord at these levels get "pinched" due to a narrowing of the outlet holes called **foramina** (i.e., stenosis), the client may develop signs of sciatica or other nerve **radiculopathy,** which is a broad term used to describe nerve involvement at these levels. A client will often report a clear path of pain, numbness, and tingling along the affected nerve. Additionally, there may be accompanying weakness in the affected extremity (Cioppa-Mosca et al., 2006; Deyo & Weinstein, 2001). Precautions should be taken when working with individuals with low-back pain to protect the spine. These clients should avoid repeated bending and twisting due to the high stress caused in the spinal structures. The clients should learn how to stabilize the trunk with a moderate **lordosis** or "neutral" position and also use back support during overhead activities.

Lower-extremity Injuries

Greater Trochanteric Bursitis

Greater trochanteric bursitis is characterized by painful inflammation of the greater trochanteric bursa between the greater trochanter of the femur and the gluteus medius tendon/proximal **iliotibial (IT) band** complex (Bierma-Zeinstra et al., 1999). This condition is more common in female runners, cross-country skiers, and ballet dancers (Anderson, Hall, & Martin, 2008; Lievense, Bierma-Zeinstra, & Schouten, 2005). Inflammation of the bursa may be due to an acute incident or repetitive (cumulative) trauma to the area. Acute incidents may include trauma from falls, contact sports (e.g., football), and other sources of impact. Repetitive trauma may be due to excessive friction from prolonged running, cycling, or even kickboxing, or increases or changes in activity (Foye & Stitik, 2006).

Signs and Symptoms

Trochanteric pain and/or parasthesias (i.e., tingling, prickling, and numbness) often radiate from the greater trochanter to the posterior lateral hip, down the iliotibial tract, to the lateral knee (Little, 1979). Symptoms are most often related to an increase in activity or repetitive overuse, which irritates the bursa and causes irritation. The client may walk with a limp (e.g., **Trendelenberg gait** or sign) due to pain and weakness. This often results in decreased muscle length (e.g., quadriceps, hamstrings), myofascial tightness (e.g., in the iliotibial band complex), and decreased muscular strength.

Management

Conservative management of greater trochanteric bursitis is consistent with Table 15-3 (page 539). In addition, individuals with this condition should utilize an assistive device such as a cane as needed (Foye & Stitik, 2006).

Exercise Programming

When the client is ready to return to gym activity, a written clearance from his or her physician may be necessary. The client should slowly return to activity with an emphasis on proper training techniques, proper equipment (e.g., footwear), and early injury recognition. The exercise program should focus on regaining flexibility and strength at the hip.

Stretching of the iliotibial band complex, hamstrings, and quadriceps should be the focus to ensure proper lower-extremity mobility. Strengthening the gluteals and deeper hip rotator muscles is important to maintain adequate strength. Proper **gait** techniques in walking and running should be a priority.

In the presence of injury, exercise modifications may be needed to prevent further injury. These clients should avoid side-lying positions that compress the lateral hip, as they may still have tenderness over the affected area. Higher-loading activity such as squats or lunges may not be immediately tolerated. These clients may benefit from aquatic exercise, because the buoyancy of the water can unload the hips and help provide a gradual return to land-based exercises.

Educating Clients on Proper Footwear

Proper footwear is mentioned several times in this chapter as a point of emphasis when working with clients following lower-extremity injuries. Personal trainers can offer some basic guidelines to help their clients purchase appropriate footwear for their activities.

When shopping for athletic shoes, the first step is deciding what type is needed. If a client engages in a specific activity two or three times each week, such as running, walking, tennis, basketball, or aerobics, he or she will want a shoe designed specifically for that sport. Multipurpose shoes such as cross trainers may be a good alternative for clients who participate in several sports or activities, such as cardiovascular and weight training, in a single workout. Ideally, clients should look for a specialty athletic shoe store with a good reputation in the community. Their sales staffs are more likely to be knowledgeable about selecting appropriate shoes for the individual, considering his or her activity level and specific foot type.

General recommendations include the following:

- Get fitted for footwear toward the end of the day. It is not unusual for an individual's foot to increase by half a shoe size during the course of a single day. However, if an individual plans to exercise consistently at a specific time, he or she should consider getting fitted at that exact time.
- Allow a space up to the width of the index finger between the end of the longest toe and the end of the shoe. This space will accommodate foot size increases, a variety of socks, and foot movement within the shoe without hurting the toes.
- The ball of the foot should match the widest part of the shoe, and the client should have plenty of room for the toes to wiggle without experiencing slippage in the heel.
- Shoes should not rub or pinch any area of the foot or ankle. The client should rotate the ankles when trying on shoes, and pay attention to the sides of the feet and the top of the toes, common areas for blisters.
- The client should wear the same weight of socks that he or she intends to use during activity. Clients should look for socks that are made with synthetic fibers such as acrylic, polyester, or Coolmax® for better blister prevention.

It is also important to be aware of when shoes need to be replaced. If they are no longer absorbing the pounding and jarring action, the client is more likely to sustain ankle, shin, and knee injuries. Athletic shoes will lose their cushioning after three to six months of regular use [or 350 to 500 miles (~560 to 800 km) of running]. However, clients should look at the wear patterns as a good indicator for replacement. Any time the shoe appears to be wearing down unevenly, especially at the heel, it is time to replace the shoes. Additionally, if the traction on the soles of the shoes is worn flat, it is time for new shoes.

Iliotibial Band Syndrome

Iliotibial band syndrome (ITBS) is a repetitive overuse condition that occurs when the distal portion of the iliotibial band rubs against the lateral femoral epicondyle (Anderson, Hall, & Martin, 2008; Brotzman & Wilk, 2003). ITBS is common among active individuals 15 to 50 years of age and is primarily caused by training errors in runners, cyclists, volleyball players, and weight lifters (Anderson, Hall, & Martin, 2008; Martinez & Honsik, 2006). Risk factors may include the following (Anderson, Hall, & Martin, 2008; Martinez & Honsik, 2006):

- Overtraining (e.g., increased speed, distance, or frequency)
- Improper footwear or equipment use
- Changes in running surface
- Muscle imbalance (e.g., weakness or tightness)
- Structural abnormalities (pes planus, knee valgus, and leg-length discrepancy)
- Failure to stretch correctly

Signs and Symptoms

Clients often report a gradual onset of tightness, burning, or pain at the lateral aspect of the knee during activity. The pain may be localized, but generally radiates to the outside of the knee and/or up the outside of the thigh. The pain may appear as a sharp "stabbing" pain along the lower outside of the knee. Snapping, popping, or pain may be felt at the lateral knee when it is flexed and extended (Anderson, Hall, & Martin, 2008; Martinez & Honsik, 2006; Brotzman & Wilk, 2003). Aggravating factors may include any repetitive activity such as running (especially downhill) or cycling. Symptoms are often resolved with rest, but can increase in intensity and frequency if not properly treated.

Management

Conservative management of ITBS is consistent with Table 15-3 (page 539). In addition, individuals with ITBS may be prescribed an assistive device such as a cane if needed (Foye & Stitik, 2006).

Exercise Programming

The client may present with weakness in the hip abductors, iliotibial band shortening, and tenderness throughout the iliotibial band complex (Martinez & Honsik, 2006; Brotzman & Wilk, 2003). As in trochanteric bursitis, this can cause a limp due to pain. A slow return to activity is recommended with an emphasis on proper training techniques, proper equipment (e.g., shoe wear), and early injury recognition. The exercise program should focus on regaining flexibility (Figure 15-7) and strength at the hip and lateral thigh.

In the presence of injury, exercise modifications may be needed to prevent further injury. Clients with ITBS may not tolerate higher-loading activities such as lunges or squats. These activities should be introduced at a slower pace. Lunges and squats limited to 45 degrees of knee flexion can be introduced with a progression to 90 degrees and beyond, if tolerated. Aquatic exercise may also be beneficial if these clients have pain with activity.

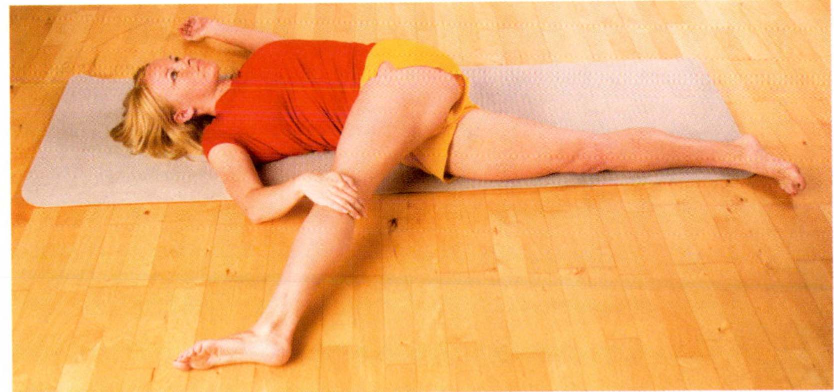

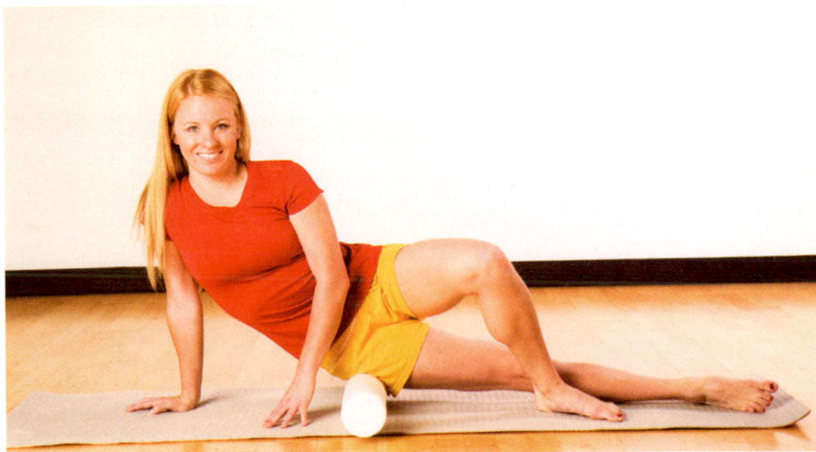

Figure 15-7
Iliotibial band range-of-motion exercises

Is Softer Always Safer?

A common misconception is that softer running surfaces are gentler on the lower extremities and therefore safer. While it is true that running on soft surfaces can be easy on the joints of the lower body because of a dampening of the ground-reaction forces, running on too soft of a surface (e.g., sand or plush grass) can introduce a level of instability that may actually increase injury potential. These uneven surfaces appear to place an excessive challenge on the foot and ankle to maintain whole-body balance while running. Some research has shown an increased risk of Achilles tendon issues when running on sand surfaces compared to running on asphalt, which was deemed safer (Knobloch, Yoon, & Vogt, 2008). The following tips can help protect individuals' lower extremities when they run on soft, uneven surfaces:

- Wear an athletic shoe with good motion control.
- Supplement running workouts with exercises that dynamically strengthen the foot and ankle joints (e.g., calf raises performed on a wobble board or a BOSU™).
- Avoid soft/uneven surfaces if clients have a history of lower-extremity problems, especially involving the ankle joint.

Patellofemoral Pain Syndrome

Patellofemoral pain syndrome (PFPS) is often called "anterior knee pain" or "runner's knee" and is often confused with chondromalacia. This syndrome has been found to have the highest prevalence among runners. In fact, PFPS makes up 16 to 25% of all running injuries (Dixit et al., 2007). The cause of PFPS is often considered multifactorial and can be classified into three primary categories: overuse, biomechanical, and muscle dysfunction.

Overuse

PFPS can occur when repetitive loading activities cause abnormal stress to the knee joint, leading to pain and dysfunction. The excessive loading exceeds the body's physiological balance, which leads to tissue trauma, injury, and pain (Dixit et al., 2007). Recent changes in intensity, frequency, duration, and training environment (e.g., surface) may contribute to this condition.

Biomechanical

Biomechanical abnormalities can alter tracking of the patella and/or increase patellofemoral joint stress (Dixit et al., 2007). Pes planus (i.e., flat foot) has been associated with PFPS, because it alters the alignment of the knee. Loss of the medial arch flattens the foot, causing a compensatory internal rotation of the tibia or femur that alters the dynamics of the patellofemoral joint (Dixit et al., 2007). Conversely, **pes cavus** (i.e., high arches) provides less cushioning than a normal foot. This leads to excessive stress to the patellofemoral joint, particularly with loading activities such as running (Dixit et al., 2007).

Muscle Dysfunction

Muscle tightness and length deficits have been associated with PFPS. Tightness in the IT band complex (e.g., gluteals) causes an excessive lateral force to the patella via its fascial connection. Tightness in the hamstrings can cause a posterior force to the knee, leading to increased contact between the patella and femur. Also, tightness in the gastrocnemius/soleus complex can lead to compensatory pronation during walking and excessive posterior force that results in increased patellofemoral contact pressure (Brotzman & Wilk, 2003; Juhn, 1999). Muscle weakness in the quadriceps and hip musculature has been associated with PFPS. In fact, research has shown that hip abductor and external rotator weakness can be present in individuals with PFPS (Boling, Padua, & Creighton, 2009; Souza & Powers, 2009). This weakness can cause femoral internal rotation and abnormal knee valgus during activity, which can cause abnormal patellofemoral tracking (Boling, Padua, & Creighton, 2009).

Signs and Symptoms

Commonly reported symptoms include pain with running, ascending or descending stairs, squatting, or prolonged sitting (i.e., "theater sign"). The client will typically describe a gradual "achy" pain that occurs behind or underneath the patella, but may be immediate if trauma has occurred (Dixit et al., 2007). Clients may also report knee stiffness, giving way, clicking, or a popping sensation during movement (Juhn, 1999).

Management

Management of PFPS includes the following (Dixit et al., 2007; Brotzman & Wilk, 2003):

- Avoiding aggravating activities [e.g., prolonged sitting, deep squats, running (particularly downhill running)]
- Modifying training variables (e.g., frequency, intensity, duration)
- Proper footwear
- Physical therapy
- Patellar taping
- Knee bracing
- Foot orthotics
- Client education
- Oral anti-inflammatory medication
- Modalities (e.g., ice, heat)

Exercise Programming

The focus of the exercise program is to progress what has been done in the early stages of physical therapy. The personal trainer must remember that restoring proper flexibility and strength is the key with PFPS. Addressing tightness in the IT band complex through stretching and **myofascial release** (e.g., on a foam roller) can have a major impact on the dynamics of the patellofemoral joint. Stretching of the hamstrings and calves will also help to restore muscle-length balance across the knee joint. Clients with PFPS may have tightness in these muscle groups from compensatory patterns that developed in response to pain. Exercise should focus on restoring proper strength throughout the hip, knee, and ankle. Exercises for the hip and ankle complex should be included due to their effects on the knee joint. For example, improving femoral control through strengthening of the hip muscles will help control the forces imposed on the knee joint. Closed-chain exercises such as squats and lunges may be beneficial. Caution should be taken with open-chain knee exercises due to the abnormal stress it can impose on the patella. The muscles that control the ankle complex may need to be strengthened to establish stability distally to allow the knee to function properly. Resistance band exercises for the ankle are commonly used to build strength.

In the presence of injury, exercise modifications may be needed to prevent further injury. With these clients, exercising in the mid-range (i.e., 45 degrees) of closed-chain activities may provide the most comfort. As mentioned above, open-chain knee activity such as leg extensions should be done with caution. One alternative is having the client do a straight-leg raise in a sitting or supine position, which is a great way to challenge the quadriceps group without imposing extra stress to the patella (Figure 15-8).

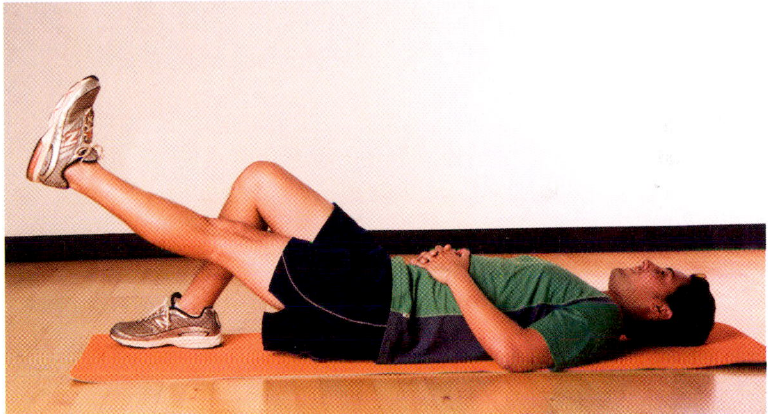

Figure 15-8
Straight-leg raise in a supine position

Infrapatellar Tendinitis

Infrapatellar tendinitis or "jumper's knee," is an overuse syndrome characterized by inflammation of the patellar tendon at the insertion into the distal part of the patella and the proximal tibia. This injury is common in sports such as basketball, volleyball, and track and field due to the jumping aspects producing significant strain in the tendinous tissues in this area. Potential causes include improper training methods (e.g., poor running style, overtraining), sudden change in training surface, lower-extremity inflexibility, and muscle imbalance (Brotzman & Wilk, 2003).

Signs and Symptoms

Commonly reported symptoms include pain at the distal kneecap into the infrapatellar tendon. Pain has also been reported with running, walking stairs, squatting, or prolonged sitting (i.e., "theater sign") (Anderson, Hall, & Martin, 2008).

Management

Management of infrapatellar tendinitis includes the following (Anderson, Hall, & Martin, 2008; Dixit et al., 2007):

- Avoiding aggravating activities (e.g., **plyometrics,** prolonged sitting, deep squats, running)
- Modifying training variables (e.g., frequency, intensity, duration)
- Proper footwear
- Physical therapy
- Patellar taping
- Knee bracing
- Arch supports
- Foot orthotics
- Client education
- Oral anti-inflammatory medication
- Modalities (e.g., ice, heat)

Exercise Programming

As with PFPS, the focus when training a client with infrapatellar tendinitis should be to restore proper flexibility and strength in the lower extremity. Addressing tightness in the quadriceps through stretching and myofascial release (e.g., on a foam roller) can have a major impact on the dynamics of the infrapatellar tendon. Stretching and self–myofascial release of the IT band, hamstrings, and calves will also help restore muscle-length balance across the knee joint. Exercise should focus on restoring strength throughout the hip, knee, and ankle. Exercises for the hip and ankle complex should be included due to their effects on the knee joint. The muscles that control the ankle complex may need to be strengthened to establish stability distally to allow the knee to function properly.

In the presence of injury, exercise modifications may be needed to prevent further injury. Clients with patellar tendinitis may not immediately tolerate high-impact activities such as running or plyometrics. A slow return to loading activity is recommended to further reduce the chances of re-injury. For example, having the client jog on a trampoline before progressing to grass and eventually to a court or other playing surface may allow him or her to progress safely.

Shin Splints

"Shin splints" is a general term used to describe exertional leg pain (Anderson, Hall, & Martin, 2008). Shin splints are typically classified as one of two specific conditions: **medial tibial stress syndrome (MTSS),** which is also called posterior shin splints, and **anterior shin splints** (Figure 15-9).

MTSS, an overuse injury that occurs in the active population, is an exercise-induced condition that is often triggered by a sudden change in activity and has been associated with pes planus (Anderson, Hall, & Martin, 2008; Brotzman & Wilk, 2003). MTSS is actually **periostitis,** or inflammation of the **periosteum** (connective tissue covering the bone). MTSS is the most frequently diagnosed injury in runners and is common in dancers and military personnel (Anderson, Hall, & Martin, 2008).

Anterior shin splints are also common in the active population, and pain often occurs in the anterior compartment of the leg. The etiology of anterior shin splints is not completely known, but is often associated with exertional activity (Brotzman & Wilk, 2003). The anterior compartment muscles of the leg (i.e., tibialis anterior, extensor digitorum longus, and extensor hallucis longus), fascia, and periosteal lining are most commonly affected. Anterior shin splints are also common in runners and military personnel (Anderson, Hall, & Martin, 2008).

Signs and Symptoms

Clients with MTSS commonly complain of a "dull ache" along the distal two-thirds of the posterior medial tibia, while those with anterior shin splints complain of the same type of pain along the distal anterior shin (Brotzman & Wilk, 2003). The pain is elicited by initial activity, but diminishes as activity continues. Typically, the pain then returns hours after activity. If the condition progresses, the pain becomes constant and tends to restrict performance (Anderson, Hall, & Martin, 2008).

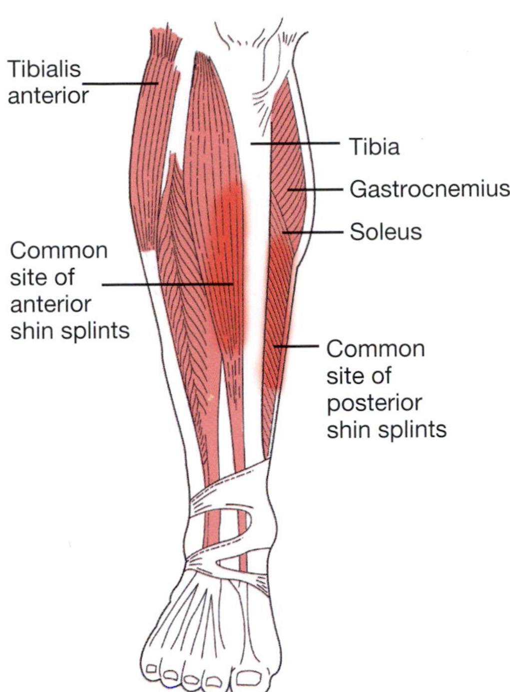

Figure 15-9
Site of pain for anterior and posterior shin splints

Management

Management of both types of shin splints includes modifying training with lower-impact/lower-mileage conditioning and cross-training (e.g., aquatic exercise). However, the best intervention may just be to rest. Modalities (e.g., ice, ultrasound), oral anti-inflammatory medication, cortisone injections, heel pads, and bracing may also be beneficial to relieve symptoms (Anderson, Hall, & Martin, 2008). The client may be referred to physical therapy to address these issues through modalities, stretching, therapeutic exercise, and other soft-tissue mobilizations.

Exercise Programming

The client may be restricted with activity or limited due to pain. The role of the personal trainer is to slowly introduce the client back to full unrestricted activity without exacerbating the symptoms. Cross-training to maintain adequate levels of fitness is indicated in the early stages. For both conditions, stretching and strengthening have been shown to be beneficial. Pain-free stretching of the calf muscles, especially the soleus, has been shown to be effective in relieving symptoms related to MTSS. Stretching the anterior compartment has been shown to help relieve symptoms associated with anterior shin splints (Anderson, Hall, & Martin, 2008; Brotzman & Wilk, 2003).

A general lower-body stretching program should accompany more specific stretching to address any secondary muscle-length deficits that may affect the foot and ankle. Rest and modified activity are the primary interventions for symptom relief. However, there may be some residual strength deficits and imbalances in the muscles that control the ankle. Targeting these muscles is the goal, especially the calf and anterior leg muscles.

In the presence of injury, exercise modifications may be needed to prevent further injury. These clients may be sensitive to a rapid return to activity or an extreme change in surfaces. For example, an immediate return to full activity or having the client run on different surfaces such as sand could further stress the healing region. Logically, clients who are post-injury are often deconditioned (e.g., decreased muscular strength and endurance) and will require a gradual return to activity. This often allows time for the body and healing tissues to re-adapt to the demands of the activity or sport.

Ankle Sprains

Ankle sprains are very common in the athletic population. They account for 10 to 30% of sports-related injuries in young athletes (Pearl, 1993). Ankle sprains are most common in basketball, volleyball, soccer, and ice skating (Ivins, 2006). There is a lack of data regarding risk factors for ankle sprains, other than a history of ankle sprains, foot type (e.g., overpronators), general laxity, and gender (i.e., males are more susceptible), which have all been linked to incidents of ankle sprains (Ivins, 2006).

Types of Ankle Sprains

Lateral, or inversion, ankle sprains are the most common type (Figure 15-10). In fact, most ankle sprains (approximately 85%) are to the lateral structures of the ankle (Garrick, 1982; Balduini & Tetzlaff, 1982). The mechanism of injury is typically

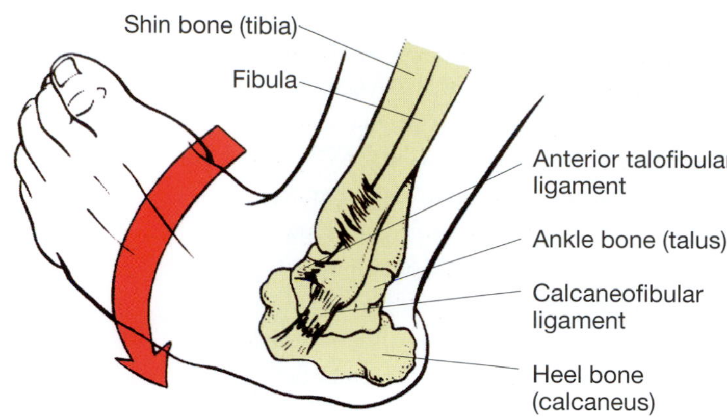

Figure 15-10
Lateral ankle sprain

inversion with a plantarflexed foot. The lateral ankle ligaments, which include the anterior talofibular ligament (ATFL), calcaneofibular ligament (CFL), and posterior talofibular ligament (PTFL), are the most common structures involved.

Medial, or **eversion,** ankle sprains are relatively rare and result from forced dorsiflexion and eversion of the ankle. The medial deltoid ligament is the most common structure involved, and injury often requires further examination to rule out a fracture (Anderson, Hall, & Martin, 2008).

Signs and Symptoms

With lateral ankle sprains, the individual can often recall the mechanism of injury and may report hearing a "pop" or "tearing" sound. Specific signs and symptoms for ligament sprains are described in Table 15-2 (page 535). Medial ankle sprains rarely happen in isolation. The individual is often unable to recall the specific mechanism of injury, but can reproduce discomfort by dorsiflexing and everting the ankle. There may be medial swelling with tenderness over the deltoid ligament (Anderson, Hall, & Martin, 2008).

Management

Individuals with lateral and medial ankle sprains are sometimes referred to their medical doctors for further diagnosis and treatment. Grade I and II lateral sprains are often immobilized with an ankle brace for several days. Grade III lateral sprains are often immobilized with a removable cast boot for up to three weeks (Brotzman & Wilk, 2003).

Early intervention can begin one to three weeks after injury unless a severe ankle sprain has occurred, which may require further immobilization (Brotzman & Wilk, 2003). The client may be sent to physical therapy to improve strength, flexibility, proprioception, and endurance, and to control swelling.

Exercise Programming

A personal trainer may begin to see the client for exercise activity as soon as one or two weeks after a Grade I sprain, two to three weeks after a Grade II sprain, and three to six weeks after a Grade III sprain (Brotzman & Wilk, 2003). During this time, the client may still be in physical therapy and be ready to transition to gym activity. Remember, the client can return to exercise for non-injured regions, such as the upper body. The injured area should always be protected during activity to avoid re-injury.

Restoring proper proprioception, flexibility, and strength is the key with these types of injuries. Clients who have suffered ankle sprains may also have deficits in balance. The ligaments and joints they stabilize are major sources of proprioceptive feedback for balance and joint position sense (Brotzman & Wilk, 2003). Stretching of the gastrocnemius and soleus muscles may be beneficial if the client has tightness in these muscles and decreased length in the Achilles tendon after immobilization. In addition, general stretches for the lower extremity should be included to maintain adequate lower-extremity flexibility. Strengthening the lower leg will also be beneficial, with particular emphasis on the muscles that control the foot and ankle. Targeting the peroneal muscle group for inversion ankle sprains is important for prevention of re-injury. For example, exercises such as side stepping with a band or ankle eversion with resistive bands can challenge the peroneal muscle group. Clients with eversion ankle sprains may have more global deficits due to the fact that eversion ankle sprains are rarely seen in isolation; they often follow other trauma, such as a fracture. Strengthening programs for these injuries are often individual and are determined by the injury.

In the presence of injury, exercise modifications may be needed to prevent further injury. These clients often lack stability with side-to-side and multidirectional motions. It is often recommended that personal trainers progress these individuals first with straight-plane motions such as forward running, then side-to-side motions such as sidestepping, and then multidirectional motions such as carioca (Figure 15-11).

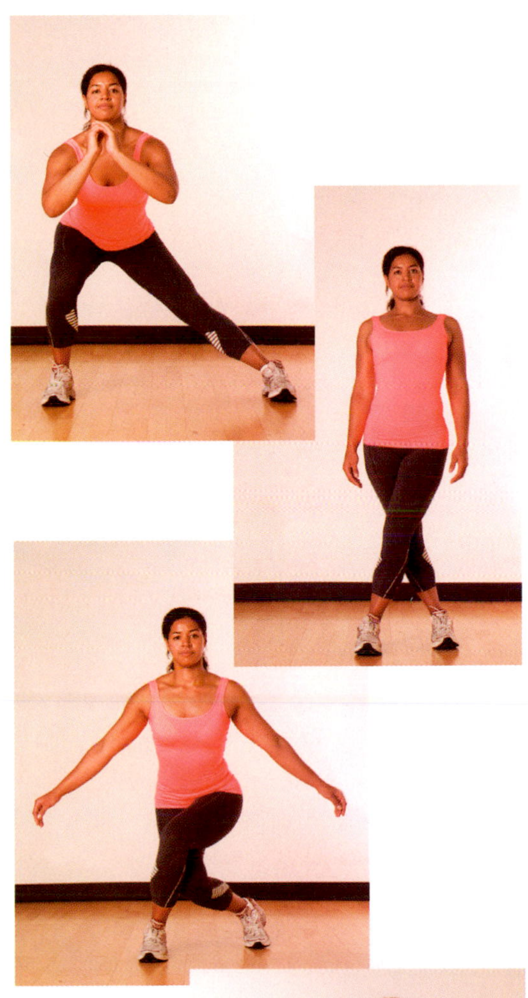

Figure 15-11
Carioca

Achilles Tendinitis

Injury to the Achilles tendon is common in athletes as well as the active population. The condition is most common in runners, gymnasts, and dancers. Other sports where it is common include track and field, volleyball, and soccer. Typically, older individuals are more affected by Achilles tendinitis than teens or children (Mazzone, 2002). This condition can eventually lead to a partial tear or complete tear (i.e., rupture) of the Achilles tendon if not addressed appropriately.

There are various intrinsic and extrinsic factors that are associated with this condition. Intrinsic factors include the following (Paavola et al., 2002; Kader et al., 2002; Mazzone, 2002):

- Age
- Pes cavus
- Pes planus
- Leg-length discrepancies
- Lateral ankle instability

Extrinsic factors include the following (Paavola et al., 2002; Kader et al., 2002; Mazzone, 2002):

- Errors in training
- Prior injuries
- Poor footwear
- Muscle weakness
- Poor flexibility

The extrinsic factors are typically responsible for acute tendon trauma. Overuse and chronic injuries are often multifactorial and include a combination of intrinsic and extrinsic factors (Paavola et al., 2002).

Signs and Symptoms

Individuals often complain about pain that is 2 to 6 cm (0.8 to 2.3 inches) above the tendon insertion into the calcaneus (i.e., heel). The typical pattern is initial morning pain that is "sharp" or "burning" and increases with more vigorous activity. Rest will often alleviate the pain, but as the condition worsens the pain becomes more constant and begins to interfere with **activities of daily living (ADL)** (Mazzone, 2002).

Management

Management includes controlling pain and

inflammation by using modalities (e.g., ice), rest, and oral anti-inflammatory medication (Mazzone, 2002). Proper training techniques, losing weight, proper footwear, orthotics, strengthening, and stretching can help alleviate pain and prevent progression of the condition (Paavola et al., 2002; Mazzone, 2002). It is important for the personal trainer to monitor a client's symptoms as he or she returns to activity. It is common for clients to exercise in the presence of discomfort and put themselves at risk for an Achilles rupture. Individuals aged 45 and older are at higher risk for Achilles ruptures (Kettunen et al., 2006). Personal trainers must teach these clients that Achilles tendinitis can progress to a rupture if not managed properly. If a client is in physical therapy, it would be good to work with the physical therapist on educating the client about the risks.

Exercise Programming

The client may be cleared to exercise immediately to tolerance or may have some activity restrictions. A gradual, pain-free return to activity is indicated for this condition. Modifications in training techniques and environment should be addressed with an emphasis on client education. The objective is to design a program that helps to meet a client's overall goals but does not exacerbate the condition.

Restoring proper length to the calf muscles can reduce strain to the musculotendinous unit and decrease symptoms (Kader et al., 2002). The client should be cautioned to stretch to tolerance and avoid overexertion. Overstretching of the Achilles tendon can cause irritation to the musculotendinous unit and should be avoided.

Controlled eccentric strengthening of the calf complex has been shown in the literature to be beneficial for relieving symptoms. Eccentric exercise may reduce pain and improve strength in the presence of Achilles tendinitis (Wasielewski & Kotsko, 2007). Progressively loading the Achilles tendon carefully with eccentric activity can benefit the client, but may be even more beneficial when combined with other interventions.

In the presence of injury, exercise modifications may be needed to prevent further injury. Regaining calf flexibility is a key component of managing this problem. In particular, when stretching the calf in a standing position, the client should wear supportive shoes. The client should be taught to properly position the back foot to point straight ahead, which will ensure that the target muscle will be stretched (Figure 15-12). Figure 15-13 shows alternative stretches for the calf.

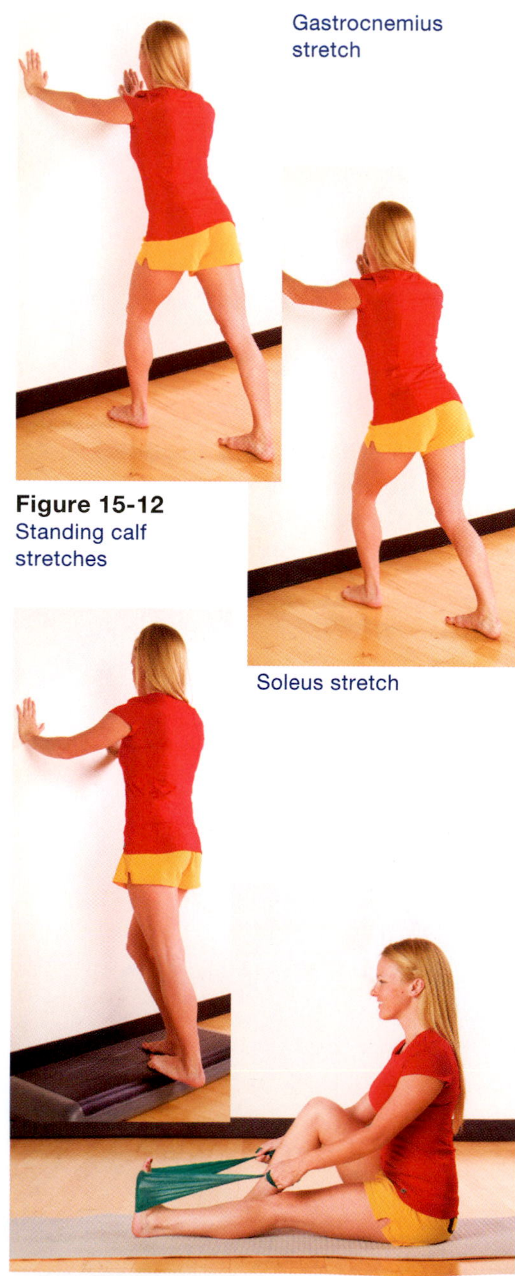

Figure 15-12
Standing calf stretches

Figure 15-13
Calf stretch modifications

Plantar Fasciitis

Plantar fasciitis is an inflammatory condition of the plantar aponeurosis (i.e., fascia) of the foot. This condition has been reported to be the most common cause of heel pain and heel spur formation, and accounts for 10% of running pain (Buchbinder, 2004). Plantar fasciitis is more common in obese individuals and people who are on their feet for long periods of time (Cole, Seto, & Gazewood, 2005).

There have been several intrinsic and extrinsic risk factors associated with this condition. Intrinsic factors include (Buchbinder, 2004):

- Pes planus
- Pes cavus

Extrinsic factors include (Buchbinder, 2004):

- Overtraining
- Improper footwear
- Obesity
- Unyielding surfaces

Signs and Symptoms

Typically, individuals report pain on the plantar, medial heel at its calcaneal attachment that worsens after rest but improves after 10 to 15 minutes of activity (Buchbinder, 2004). In particular, clients will commonly report excessive pain during the first few steps in the morning. It is important to keep in mind that plantar fasciitis can be seen throughout the plantar surface of the foot.

Management

Conservative management of this condition may include the following:

- Modalities (e.g., ice)
- Oral anti-inflammatory medication
- Heel pad or plantar arch
- Stretching
- Strengthening exercises

A medical doctor may prescribe physical therapy, a night splint, or orthotics, or inject the area with cortisone (Cole, Seto, & Gazewood, 2005; Buchbinder, 2004).

Exercise Programming

A client with plantar fasciitis may be cleared to exercise immediately to tolerance, but most often with restrictions from his or her medical professional. The goal is to design a program that challenges the client but does not excessively load the foot. Integrating specific foot exercises into the client's general fitness program often provides the best results. This allows the client to work toward his or her fitness goals as well as address the foot problems.

Stretching of the gastrocnemius, soleus, and plantar fascia is beneficial and has been shown to help relieve symptoms. Self–myofascial release techniques, which include rolling the foot over a baseball, golf ball, or dumbbell, may help to break up myofascial adhesion in the plantar fascia.

Strengthening the foot's intrinsic muscles (i.e., the muscles that have their bellies and tendons completely in the foot) may help to improve arch stability and help decrease the stresses imposed across the plantar fascia. Strengthening of the gastrocnemius, soleus, peroneals, tibialis anterior, and tibialis posterior muscles may be needed to help improve strength at the ankle.

In the presence of injury, exercise modifications may be needed to prevent further injury. The calf stretches shown in Figures 15-12 and 15-13 should be included in the stretching program for clients with plantar fasciitis. Another alternative stretch for these clients is to bend the toes with the hands or against the wall, which helps to isolate the plantar fascia for a more effective stretch (Figure 15-14).

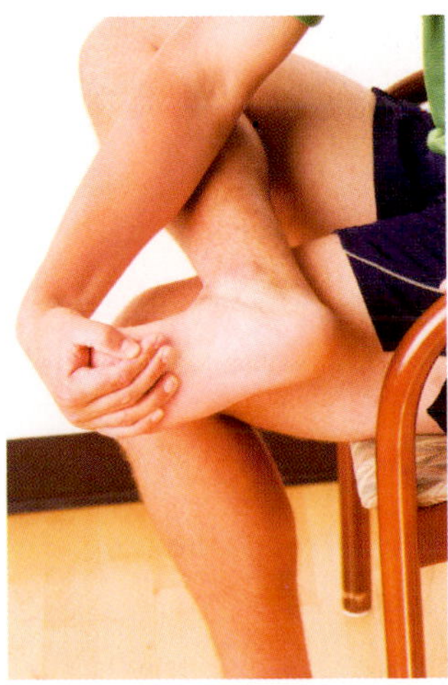
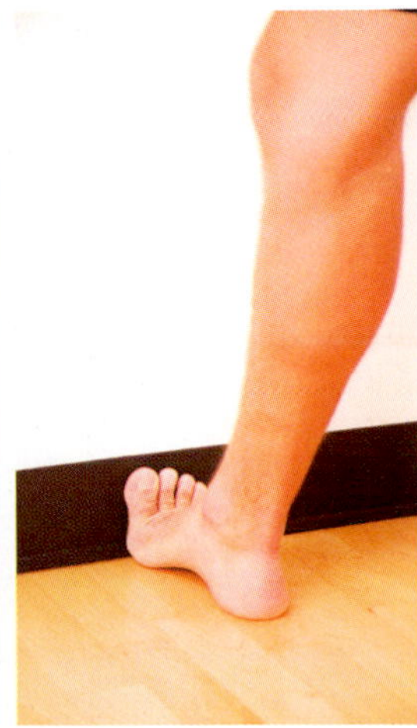

Figure 15-14
Plantar fascia stretches

Record Keeping

Keeping current and accurate records for every client is essential for a personal trainer. The important principle to remember is that if information is not written down, then it did not occur and it does not exist.

Medical History

A personal trainer must maintain current records of each client's medical conditions. This includes present and past medical conditions and current medications. It is advisable for the trainer to update each client's records every three months, including medical clearances. Additionally, a trainer should document details of clients' present conditions, especially their condition prior to beginning any exercise programs. This will provide the trainer with a baseline to compare to in the future. Positive changes from this baseline can be used for motivation and goal development.

Exercise Record

A client's exercise record needs to stay current with specific notations for any changes, such as a new onset of "pain." This will provide the personal trainer with an accurate record of any program changes when the incident occurred. A good practice is to write down some important details of every single session.

Incident Report

If an injury does occur during a workout session, it needs to be handled appropriately. First, the client's injury will need immediate medical attention. This may include minor first aid or activation of EMS. Client safety is the number-one priority. Second, after the client is safe, a formal written account of the incident needs to be documented. Most organizations will have a specific "incident" report that is filled out after an accident has occurred. Third, the personal trainer needs to keep his or her own account of what occurred and maintain any pertinent documentation. This will ensure an accurate account of the incident. Chapter 17 provides a more in-depth discussion of the legal responsibilities of the personal trainer.

Correspondence

Due to the 1996 **Health Insurance Portability and Accountability Act (HIPAA),** all medical records that the personal trainer has on each client are confidential, which means that he or she must obtain written permission prior to discussing this information with an outside party. If outside consultation is necessary, obtaining a written clearance from the client is a must. The goal is to keep the client information private. The personal trainer should document all conversations and sharing of information. This will ensure protection of the client's personal information. Refer to Appendix A for the ACE Code of Ethics.

Summary

All personal trainers work with clients who have sustained, or will sustain, musculoskeletal injuries in the course of their activities. The key when working with such clients is avoiding exercises that aggravate pre-existing conditions. An understanding of how the body reacts to injury and resulting repair will help clients plan an appropriate program. Recognizing the signs and symptoms of inflammation and knowing the proper steps in acute injury care can allow the trainer to help the injured client recover more quickly.

It is also important for trainers to know the common injuries associated with physical activity. The ability to design a program for a client that will avoid injury is critical to the success of the program.

All trainers should receive as much training as is available in first aid and injury recognition. Doing so will increase one's confidence in dealing with clients in these types of situations.

References

Anderson, M.K., Hall, S.J., & Martin, M. (2008). *Foundations of Athletic Training: Prevention, Assessment, and Management* (4th ed.). Baltimore, Md.: Lippincott Williams & Wilkins.

Balduini, F.C. & Tetzlaff, J. (1982). Historical perspectives on injuries of the ligaments of the ankle. *Clinical Sports Medicine,* 1, 1, 3–12.

Bierma-Zeinstra, S. et al. (1999). Validity of American College of Rheumatology criteria for diagnosing hip osteoarthritis in primary care research. *Journal of Rheumatology,* 26, 1129–1133.

Boden, B.P. & Garrett, W.E. (1996). Mechanism of injuries to the anterior cruciate ligament. *Medicine & Science Sports & Exercise,* 28, 5s, 156–168.

Boling, M.C., Padua, D.A., & Creighton, R. (2009). Concentric and eccentric torque of the hip musculature in individuals with and without patellofemoral pain. *Journal of Athletic Training,* 44, 1, 7–13.

Brotzman, B. & Wilk, K. (2003). *Clinical Orthopedic Rehabilitation* (2nd ed.). St. Louis, Mo.: Mosby.

Buchbinder, R. (2004). Plantar fasciitis. *New England Journal of Medicine*, 350, 21, 2159–2167.

Calliet, R. (1978). *Rehabilitation of the Hand.* St. Louis, Mo.: Mosby.

Cioppa-Mosca, J.M. et al. (2006). *Postsurgical Rehabilitation Guidelines for the Orthopedic Clinician*. St. Louis, Mo.: Mosby.

Cole, C., Seto, C., & Gazewood, J. (2005). Plantar fasciitis: Evidence-based review of diagnosis and therapy. *American Family Physician*, 72, 11, 2237–2243.

Cosca, D. & Navazio, F. (2007). Common problems in endurance athletes: Meniscal tears. *American Family Physician,* 76, 2, 237–244.

Deyo, R.A. & Weinstein, J. (2001). Low-back pain. *New England Journal of Medicine,* 344, 5, 363–371.

Dixit, S. et al. (2007). Management of patellofemoral pain syndrome. *American Family Physician,* 75, 194–204.

Foye, P.M. & Stitik, T.P. (2006). Trochantaric bursitis. *E-Medicine Online Journal* (Web MD), Dec 21, 1–14.

Garrick, J.G. (1982). Epidemiologic perspective. *Clinical Sports Medicine,* 1, 1, 13–21.

Goldstein, J. & Zuckerman, J.D. (2000). Selected orthopedic problems in the elderly. *Rheumatic Disease Clinics of North America,* 26, 3, 593–616.

Griffin, L.Y. (2000). Non-contact anterior cruciate ligament injuries: Risk factors and prevention strategies. *Journal of American Academy of Orthopedic Surgeons,* 8, 141–150.

Hills, E.C. (2006). Mechanical low-back pain. *E-Medicine Online Journal* (Web MD). June, 1–14.

Ivins, D. (2006). Acute ankle sprains: An update. *American Family Physician,* 74, 1714–1720.

Juhn, M. (1999). Patellofemoral pain syndrome: A review and guidelines for treatment. *American Family Physician,* 60, 2012–2022.

Kader, D. et al. (2002). Achilles tendinopathy: Some aspects of basic science and clinical management. *British Journal of Sports Medicine,* 36, 4, 239–250.

Kettunen, J.A. et al. (2006). Health of master track and field athletes: A 16-year follow-up study. *Clinical Journal of Sports Medicine,* 16, 2, 142–148.

Kisner, C. & Colby, L. (2007). *Therapeutic Exercise: Foundations and Techniques* (5th ed.). Philadelphia, Pa.: F.A. Davis Company.

Knobloch, K., Yoon, U., & Vogt, P.M. (2008). Acute and overuse injuries correlated to hours of training in master running athletes. *Foot & Ankle International,* 29, 7, 671–676.

Lievense, A., Bierma-Zeinstra, S., & Schouten, B. (2005). Prognosis of trochantaric pain in primary care. *British Journal of General Practice,* 55, 512, 199–204.

Little, H. (1979). Trochanteric bursitis: A common cause of pelvic girdle pain. *Canadian Medical Association Journal,* 120, 456–458.

Maetzel, A. & Li, L. (2002). The economic burden of low-back pain: A review of studies published between 1996 and 2001. *Best Practice Research of Clinical Rheumatology,* 16, 23–30.

Magee, D.J. (2007). *Orthopedic Physical Assessment* (5th ed.). Philadelphia: WB Saunders.

Malanga, G.A. (2009). Rotator cuff injury. www.emedicine.medscape.com. Retrieved April 20, 2009.

Manske, R.C. (2006). *Postsurgical Orthopedic Sports Rehabilitation: Knee and Shoulder*. St. Louis, Mo.: Mosby.

Martinez, J.M. & Honsik, K. (2006). Iliotibial band syndrome. *E-Medicine Online Journal* (Web MD). Dec 6, 1–14.

Martini, F.H., Timmons, M.J., & McKinley, M.P. (2008). *Human Anatomy* (3rd ed.). Upper Saddle River, N.J.: Pearson Education.

Maxey, L & Magnusson, J. (2006). *Rehabilitation for the Post Surgical Orthopedic Patient* (2nd ed.). St. Louis, Mo: Mosby.

Mazzone, M. (2002). Common conditions of the Achilles tendon. *American Family Physician,* 65, 1805–1810.

Paavola, M. et al. (2002). Current concepts review: Achilles tendinopathy. *Journal of Bone & Joint Surgery,* 84-A, 11, 2062–2076.

Pai, S. & Sundaram, L.J. (2004). Low-back pain: An economic assessment in the United States. *Orthopedic Clinics of North America,* 35, 1–5.

Pearl, A.J. (1993). *The Athletic Female.* Champaign, Ill.: Human Kinetics.

Prentice, W. (1994). *Rehabilitation Techniques in Sports Medicine* (3rd ed.). St. Louis, Mo.: Mosby.

Souza, R.B. & Powers, C.M. (2009). Differences in hip kinematics, muscle strength, and muscle activation between subjects with and without patellofemoral pain. *Journal of Orthopaedic and Sports Physical Therapy,* 39, 1, 12–19.

Wasielewski, N.J. & Kotsko, K.M. (2007). Does eccentric exercise reduce pain and improve strength in physically active adults with symptomatic lower extremity tendinosis? A systematic review. *Journal of Athletic Training,* 42, 3, 409–422.

Suggested Reading

Anderson, M.K., Hall, S.J., & Martin, M. (2008). *Foundations of Athletic Training: Prevention, Assessment, and Management* (4th ed.). Baltimore, Md.: Lippincott Williams & Wilkins.

Brotzman, B. & Wilk, K. (2003). *Clinical Orthopedic Rehabilitation* (2nd ed.). St Louis Mo.: Mosby.

Kisner, C. & Colby, L. (2007). *Therapeutic Exercise: Foundations and Techniques* (5th ed.). Philadelphia, Pa.: F.A. Davis Company.

IN THIS CHAPTER:

Personal Protective Equipment

Scene Safety

Emergency Policies and Procedures for Fitness Facilities

Record Keeping and Confidentiality

Emergency Assessment
- Primary Assessment
- Secondary Assessment

Activating EMS
- When to Call 9-1-1
- Land Lines vs. Cell Phones
- Emergency Call Centers

Initial Response
- Cardiopulmonary Resuscitation
- Automated External Defibrillation

Common Medical Emergencies and Injuries
- Dyspnea
- Choking
- Asthma
- Cardiovascular Disease, Chest Pain, and Heart Attack
- Syncope
- Stroke
- Diabetes and Insulin Reaction (Hypoglycemia)
- Heat Illness
- Cold Illness
- Seizures
- Soft-tissue Injuries
- Fractures
- Head Injuries
- Neck and Back Injuries
- Shock

Universal Precautions and Protection Against Bloodborne Pathogens

Summary

__JULIA VALENTOUR, M.S., EMT-B,__ is the program coordinator for live workshops for the American Council on Exercise, an American Heart Association (AHA) Training Center Coordinator, and an instructor for Basic Life Support and Heartsaver courses. She is an ACE-certified Personal Trainer and holds a health and fitness specialist certification from the American College of Sports Medicine. Valentour has developed content for ACE webinars and has contributed material for the AHA's Start! Walking Program. She is an assistant professor of kinesiology for California State University San Marcos. Valentour spent several years working for the U.S. Navy, where she served as the Afloat Fitness Director aboard the aircraft carrier USS NIMITZ (CVN-68), including an eight-month deployment to the Persian Gulf in 2003 for Operation Iraqi Freedom.

CHAPTER 16

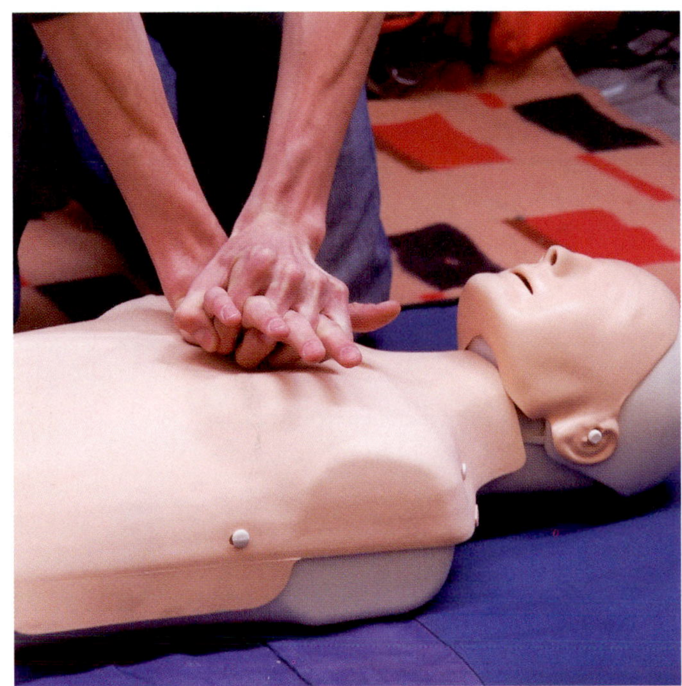

Emergency Procedures

Julia Valentour

Over the long term, exercise can greatly improve health and wellness and play an important role in enhancing overall public health. However, there are inherent risks involved with exercise due to the physical demands placed on the body. During exercise, the risk of heart attack and sudden death are increased, even in athletic individuals. The likelihood of injuries also increases. Therefore, fitness professionals work in an environment where they might be called upon to react to an emergency as a first responder.

Handling emergency situations requires quick, decisive action. The person who takes charge should be capable of assessing the victim and managing the scene. Because this person's demeanor will affect how others react, it is important for him or her to stay in control and remain calm. Emergencies can vary widely, including such minor incidents as when a basketball player **sprains** his ankle or when a woman with **diabetes** starts to become hypoglycemic while weight training.

Although rare, some situations are much more serious, and can involve a person who is bleeding heavily or who is unconscious with impaired breathing or circulation. Having a systematic approach for handling any of these situations, no matter how severe, requires training and practice.

Personal Protective Equipment

Dealing with emergencies begins with protecting one's own safety as well as the safety of others and the victim. When administering first aid, a personal trainer should start by wearing personal protective equipment (PPE). Gloves are a universal standard and should be worn in all cases, but other equipment, such as eye protection and a mask, may also be necessary to avoid the possible transfer of **pathogens** (microorganisms that cause disease) (Mistovich & Karren, 2008). **Human immunodeficiency virus (HIV)** and **hepatitis** are the bloodborne diseases of most concern to a personal trainer. Universal precautions state that everyone is to be treated as if he or she is infected, and first responders should always avoid contact with a victim's bodily fluids [American Heart Association (AHA), 2006] (see "Universal Precautions and Protection Against Bloodborne Pathogens" on page 585 for more information).

Scene Safety

Scene safety requires knowing when it is safe to approach a victim and when it is not. For example, people are sometimes struck and killed on the road while trying to help at the scene of an accident. Other dangerous situations might involve a smoke-filled building, downed power lines, hazardous materials, a crime in progress, or unstable surfaces such as a car on its side. If in doubt, a potential rescuer should wait for trained help to arrive, as he or she can make the situation much worse by becoming another victim. For personal trainers, scene safety requires situational awareness, whether training clients in the gym or in their homes (Mistovich & Karren, 2008). What are the potential hazards? Is there a first-aid kit or an **automated external defibrillator (AED)** on the premises? Where is the nearest phone, or is there cell phone coverage in the area? Where is the nearest hospital? Are there others nearby who can help in case of an emergency?

Maintaining a First-aid Kit

A first-aid kit should be systematically maintained and stocked with the following supplies:

For airway management:
- CPR microshield or pocket mask with one-way valve for protected mouth-to-mouth ventilations (Figure 16-1)

For assessing circulation:
- Sphygmomanometer (blood pressure cuff)
- Stethoscope
- Penlight or flashlight

For general wound management:
- Personal protective equipment, including latex gloves, mask, and eye protection
- Sterile gauze dressings (medium and larger sizes)
- Adhesive tape (1- and 2-inch sizes)
- Bandage scissors
- Liquid soap or hand sanitizer (if soap is unavailable in the workplace)

For suspected sprains or fractures:
- Splinting materials
- Chemical cold pack, or ice and plastic bag
- Compression wrap

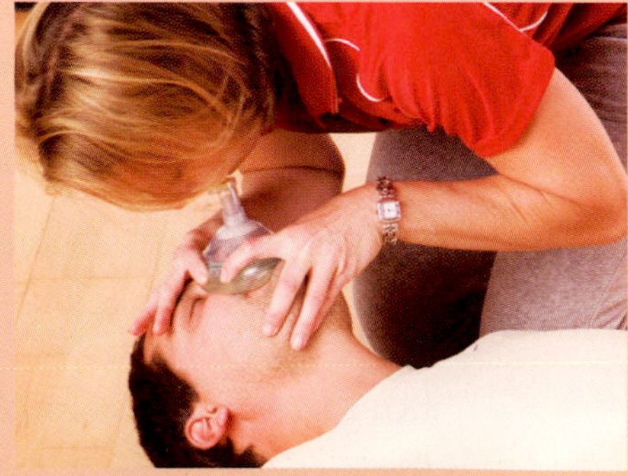

Figure 16-1
Mouth-to-mask ventilations: A mask with a one-way valve prevents contact with a victim's face during mouth-to-mouth resuscitation. Small pocket masks are also effective, inexpensive, and convenient.

Emergency Policies and Procedures for Fitness Facilities

While some emergency situations are unavoidable, the best approach is to be prepared. The AHA and American College of Sports Medicine (ACSM) published guidelines for fitness facilities in 1998 that involve pre-screening members, having adequate staffing, and establishing emergency policies. A fitness facility can take the following steps to minimize the risk of injuries (Balady et al., 1998):

- All employees should be trained in first aid, **cardiopulmonary resuscitation (CPR),** and AED usage. CPR and AED training is required by ACE. Also, many states now have laws that require health clubs to have at least one AED on the premises, as well as staff members who are trained to use them.
- Fitness staff should hold current accredited certifications in their specialty areas (e.g., personal training, group fitness instruction, lifeguarding). If a staff member works with a special population such as seniors, youth, or pre- or postnatal women, additional training for working safely and effectively with that population is recommended (Canadian Fitness Matters, 2004).

Facilities should screen new members to identify those at high risk for cardiovascular events by using a simple screening questionnaire such as the **Physical Activity Readiness Questionnaire (PAR-Q)** (see Chapter 6). People with cardiac disease are 10 times more likely to have a cardiovascular event during exercise than those who are apparently healthy. The PAR-Q can help to identify high-risk individuals who need medical referral or require modifications to their exercise programs. This tool can also help identify the need for additional qualified staff members if there are a number of high-risk clients (Canadian Fitness Matters, 2004; Balady et al., 1998).

Fitness facilities should establish a method of notifying participants about the risk of injury with exercise, such as having new members sign **informed consent** forms. Personal trainers should also follow these guidelines by having clients complete medical screening forms and obtain medical clearance when necessary, as determined by the client's risk stratification (Canadian Fitness Matters, 2004; Balady et al., 1998).

The club should take responsibility for minimizing any additional risks by ensuring the following (Canadian Fitness Matters, 2004; Balady et al., 1998):

- Adequate staffing and supervision
- Cleanliness and clear walkways
- Adequate lighting
- Nonslip surfaces around showers and pools
- Caution signs for wet floors and other hazards (for example, "No Diving" signs at the shallow end of the pool)
- Regular maintenance and repair of equipment
- A clean drinking water supply
- Fire/smoke alarms installed
- Limiting the number of people in the building and in group fitness classes to avoid overcrowding
- First-aid kits that are kept in convenient locations and assigned to someone to restock on a regular basis
- Phones that can be easily accessed with emergency numbers posted nearby

Having the right equipment available is not enough—training and practice are also vital to effectively handle emergencies. Each club should have an emergency action plan taught to all employees and practiced quarterly. Documentation should be kept noting when this training took place and who was involved. The plan should include instructions on how to handle the types of emergencies that are more likely to occur when people are exercising, such as hypoglycemic events, cardiac events, **strokes,** heat illnesses, and orthopedic injuries. Handling other events such as fires should also be rehearsed. The personnel involved should understand the roles of first, second, and third responders. Staff members should know the location of emergency equipment, such as first-aid kits, AEDs, phones, emergency exits, and the most accessible route for emergency personnel. Someone at the club should be identified as the facility's coordinator for ensuring the facility is capable of handling an emergency. Local medical professionals can help the facility's management team create this emergency response plan (ACSM, 2007).

For emergencies with a single victim, staff members should *not* move a victim with head or neck injuries unless there is danger of further injury if the victim is not moved. When trained help is needed, one staff member should stay with the victim while another goes to call and wait outside for **emergency medical services (EMS)**. This person can guide rescuers by using the shortest route available to the scene of the incident. A third staff member (if available) can get a first-aid kit and AED. When rescuers arrive, staff members should be ready to assist as needed.

Record Keeping and Confidentiality

After an incident, complete documentation of the event should be done by the staff member who was the most directly involved. Each facility may have its own type of medical emergency response report, but all should include the name of the victim, the date and time of the incident, what happened, and what was done to care for the victim and by whom. The names, addresses, and phone numbers of witnesses should also be documented.

This form should be filled out immediately after the event with as much detail as possible and kept on file for several years, depending on company policy and state law. If no form exists, the personal trainer should write everything down exactly as it occurred and keep that on record. If the victim or the victim's family decides to take legal action, this report is vital to the facility's defense, as well as that of the rescuer.

Other than sharing the incident report with the medical director and/or facility general manager, rescuers need to keep the information about the incident and the victim confidential. The **Health Insurance Portability and Accountability Act (HIPAA)** of 1996 is a federal law that ensures the victim's privacy by putting him or her in control of who has access to personal health information. This means that the event should not be discussed with anyone who has not received appropriate permission to view such information. The records of the event should be stored in a locked file drawer or cabinet or a secure, password-protected electronic file.

Emergency Assessment

Primary Assessment

Some emergencies are easily recognizable as life-threatening, while others may not be. To make that determination, check the most vital indicators: **a**irway, **b**reathing, **c**irculation, and **s**evere bleeding (the ABCs). First check to see if the victim is conscious and able to speak. Tap the victim's shoulder and ask "Are you okay?" With a conscious victim, the rescuer should introduce him- or herself, ask what the problem is, and ask if he or she can provide any help. (Consent to receive help must be given verbally if the victim is conscious and alert.) If the victim is able to speak, that means there is a patent (open) airway and the person is breathing, conscious, and has a pulse. This quick assessment is valuable in determining the cause of the emergency (Mistovich & Karren, 2008). If there is no reply, the trainer should call EMS or, preferably, stay with the victim and send another person to call. In situations where the victim is unresponsive or disoriented, implied consent can be assumed (meaning that the victim agrees to treatment). Check for the ABCs. If there is no sign of trauma to the spine, perform a head tilt–chin lift (a technique for opening the airway) (Figure 16-2). This will remove the tongue from resting on the back of the throat, which could block the airway. If there is evidence of a fall or other signs of trauma to the face, neck, or head, open the airway by the jaw thrust method instead (Figure 16-3). (These techniques are learned and practiced in a CPR/AED course.)

To assess respirations (breathing), the rescuer should have an ear close to the victim's mouth to feel for breath on the rescuer's cheek and listen for air movement while watching to see if the chest rises and falls. This should be done for five to 10 seconds. If no breath is felt or heard and the chest does not visibly rise, or if breaths are gasping or irregular, the rescuer should give two breaths into the mouth of the victim while pinching the nose. (Having a pocket mask available in a first-aid kit will provide a protective barrier for mouth-to-mouth contact.) After delivering two breaths that cause the victim's lungs to expand, the third step is checking for a pulse (circulation). The carotid artery is located beside the trachea in the front of the neck. Pressing gently with two fingers, the rescuer should check for a pulse—or the absence of one—in 10 seconds or less. Without a pulse, the victim will need immediate CPR, starting with chest compressions. If others are available to help, it may be necessary to simultaneously control severe bleeding with gauze pads and direct pressure. This is secondary to performing CPR and is not urgent unless there is major blood loss, making the situation life-threatening.

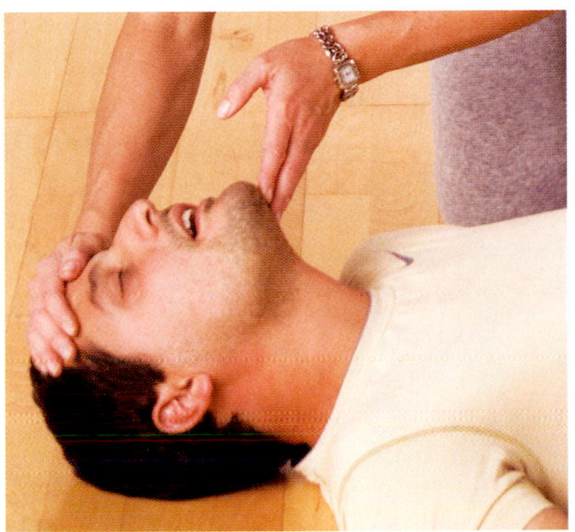

Figure 16-2
The head tilt–chin lift maneuver: Tilt the head back and lift the chin to move the tongue away from the back of the throat. Check for breathing by looking at the chest and listening and feeling for breath.

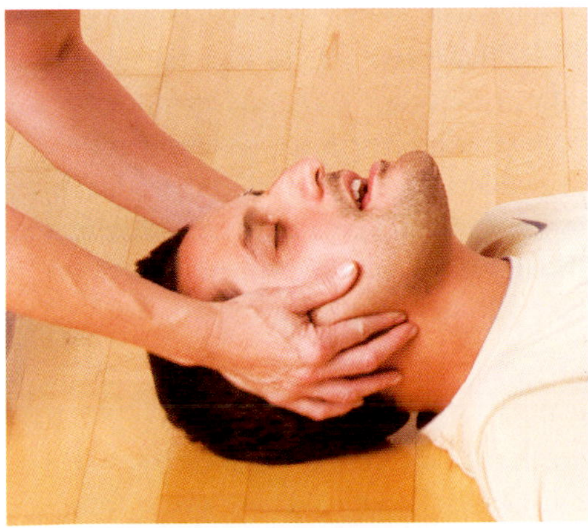

Figure 16-3
The jaw thrust method: Place the fingers on the angles of the jaw, and lift the jaw to move it forward. This moves the tongue away from the back of the throat and opens the airway.

Secondary Assessment

Once a person is conscious and speaking, or unconscious but with stable ABCs, a **secondary assessment** can be completed to address any issues that are not immediately life-threatening. If the cause of injury is not known, there could be something life-threatening that is not being recognized and treated, such as internal bleeding, heat stress, and shock. For a victim of trauma or someone who is unconscious, a head-to-toe assessment might be done to look for additional injuries, such as deformities, abrasions, tenderness, or swelling. This is also a good time to check for medical alert jewelry. Vital signs should be taken, such as pulse and **blood pressure,** and it is important to check skin color and temperature. Skin color can provide information about a person's general health. Skin that is warm and has a pinkish tone indicates adequate blood flow and oxygenation, whereas grayish, pale skin may indicate poor circulation (American Academy of Orthopedic Surgeons, 2006). A conscious victim might also be asked about his or her signs and symptoms, any known allergies, what medications he or she has been taking, pertinent medical history, the type and location of the pain, and any events that led up to the incident. The victim should be monitored closely, and if the person can talk, the rescuer should keep the conversation going to reassure him or her, let the person know what is happening, and keep monitoring the airway (Mistovich & Karren, 2008; Anderson, Hall, & Martin, 2000).

Activating EMS

Determining the likely cause of the emergency helps the 9-1-1 operator know what agency to call for help and what the responders should be prepared to handle.

When to Call 9-1-1

It is appropriate to call EMS when there is a life-threatening situation or anything that requires immediate medical attention, such as a person who is not breathing, has an open wound to the chest, or is bleeding profusely (Mistovich & Karren, 2008).

A personal trainer should phone the company's emergency response number (or 9-1-1) whenever someone is seriously ill or when unsure of what to do. For example, a personal trainer should call EMS when a victim (AHA, 2006):

- Does not respond to voice or touch
- Has chest pain or chest discomfort
- Has signs of stroke (see "Stroke," page 570)
- Has a problem breathing
- Has a severe injury or burn
- Has a seizure
- Suddenly cannot move a part of the body
- Has received an electric shock
- Has been exposed to a poison
- Tries to commit suicide or is assaulted, regardless of the victim's condition

Other situations that require EMS include:

- Crimes in progress
- First witnesses of a fire, traffic accident, or chemical spill
- When fire, smoke, or carbon monoxide alarms sound in a building
- Electrical hazards, such as sparking of a power line

It is appropriate for a personal trainer to call in any other emergency if he or she is unsure. However, a personal trainer should not call if there is *not* a true emergency, as doing so can delay response time to true emergencies. For non-emergencies, call the appropriate agency. For example, call the emergency contact listed in the client's file or another individual as requested by the client if he or she trips and appears to have a broken bone. While a broken bone requires immediate attention from a healthcare professional, it typically does not require the activation of EMS. Also, people should not call to inquire about the status of an emergency or fire. Instead, call 2-1-1 or listen to local news (San Diego Fire-Rescue Department, 2008).

Land Lines vs. Cell Phones

If the personal trainer has a choice, it is always better to call EMS from a land line than from a cellular phone. A call from a cell phone may have to be routed to different places depending on whether it is a police, fire, or medical emergency. Unlike with a land line, it is difficult to determine the caller's exact location when using a cell phone (depending on the technology in the phone and at the dispatch center), and even if a location is found it may be an area as large as three football fields. The caller may also need to provide the phone number, which would not be necessary if calling from a land line. Having to provide the additional information such as the address and phone number takes precious time away from responders. Cell phone callers who are driving should pull over so it is less likely that the signal will get dropped and it is easier for EMS to locate them.

Emergency Call Centers

Public Safety Answering Points (PSAPs) are the dispatch centers that receive 9-1-1 calls. They do not have the same technology as the callers. For example, they do not receive text messages—which may be a more desirable means of communication during times of disaster when the system is overloaded. A bill passed by Congress (The NET 911 Improvement Act of 2008) calls for the creation of a plan that will improve the 9-1-1 system from analog to digital to match newer technology, primarily by incorporating Internet protocol (IP) network technology into the emergency system. This will allow better connections and faster communication between PSAPs, responders, and emergency warning systems. Video, text, and data transmission could be used for calls, in addition to voice. This would help service those who are deaf and hearing impaired, although the 9-1-1 centers currently can take calls from TTYs (text telephones used by the deaf, hard of hearing, and speech impaired). This new directive would also help pinpoint the location where the call was made, which currently is more difficult for those in high-rise buildings or rural areas. However, how and when the implementation will occur has not yet been determined (Moore, 2008).

When calling 9-1-1, it is important to stay calm and try to give the dispatcher the exact location of the emergency. Stay on the line—the dispatcher will ask questions regarding the emergency to make sure rescuers are ready to respond to the exact situation when they arrive. Callers should give the number of victims in case it is necessary for the dispatcher to send multiple units to the scene. The dispatcher may give directions on providing immediate care for the victim, such as performing CPR and controlling bleeding. It is essential to have someone wait outside for EMS to direct rescuers to the exact location as quickly as possible. Remember, there may be locked doors or access codes to gated communities, and addresses may not be clearly marked. Also, it is important to secure any pets that may endanger the safety of rescuers. Finally, if the victim is taking medications, collect them in a bag for the rescuers to take along. This can give valuable information regarding the person's medical history, and the person may need them while hospitalized (Mistovich & Karren, 2008).

Calling 9-1-1

When a person phones the company's emergency response number (or 9-1-1), he or she should be prepared to answer some questions about the emergency. An emergency dispatcher might ask some or all of the following questions:

- "What is the emergency?"
- "Where is your emergency and what number are you calling from?"
- "What is your name?"
- "Is the victim conscious?"
- "Is the victim breathing normally?"
- "Are you able to assist with CPR?"
- "Do you have access to an AED?"

It is essential that the caller not hang up until the dispatcher tells him or her to do so (AHA, 2006).

Initial Response

It takes EMS an average of seven to 10 minutes to reach a victim, but brain death can occur in only four to six minutes (Gonzales & Lino, 2008). What can be done to help the person survive?

Cardiopulmonary Resuscitation

Sudden **cardiac arrest** (also called sudden cardiac death) is one of the leading causes of death in the United States, claiming about 250,000 lives every year (Aufderheide et al., 2006). Most of these deaths occur outside of hospitals, so it is important to be trained and ready to respond whenever this situation might occur. Cardiac arrest is the cessation of heart function, when the person loses consciousness, has no pulse, and stops breathing. The person may be gasping, snorting, or gurgling, but this is not breathing and should not deter someone from starting CPR. In this circumstance, the chance of survival is remote without an intervention. To educate the public about what to do, the American Heart Association has developed the Chain of Survival, which includes four steps or "links" to increase the likelihood of survival (Aufderheide et al., 2006):

- Early access
- Early CPR
- Early defibrillation
- Early advanced care

As previously mentioned, early access involves early recognition of the emergency and immediate activation of EMS. The second step, early CPR, is important to help the body maintain **perfusion** (blood flow and oxygen delivery to body tissues). CPR, a combination of breaths and compressions for a person who is in a state of cardiac arrest, should ideally begin within two minutes of the onset of cardiac arrest (Mistovich & Karren, 2008). Without treatment, the person's chance of survival declines by about 10% every minute.

Because EMS takes an average of seven to 10 minutes to arrive, CPR should be started by a bystander—a friend, family member, employee, or stranger (Mistovich & Karren, 2008). However, most victims of out-of-hospital cardiac arrest do not receive treatment. In fact, only 27% of out-of-hospital victims receive bystander CPR (Nichol et al., 1999), despite the fact that bystander CPR can more than double the chance of survival (Herlitz et al., 2005).

Interviews with people who witnessed a cardiac arrest have found that the major reason bystanders do not attempt to perform CPR is because they panic. Although more than half of the interviewees had CPR training at some time in their lives, many reported that they were afraid to cause harm or afraid they would not perform well. The fear of disease was not a factor because most were family members of the victim (Swor et al., 2006). In 2007, several AHA studies found that in some instances, CPR could be simplified to performing chest compressions only, which is referred to as "hands-only CPR" (Nagao et al., 2007; Bohm et al., 2007; Iwami et al., 2007). In this type of CPR, a bystander only needs to remember to push hard and fast on the center of the victim's chest until trained help arrives. This is effective for victims who are adults and who have been witnessed going into cardiac arrest. When the collapse is witnessed and CPR begins immediately, the victim's blood still contains oxygen, and oxygen remains in the lungs. By pumping the chest, this oxygenated blood can be distributed to the body. Because of its simplicity, hands-only CPR will hopefully encourage bystanders to do *something*—and any CPR is better than none for a victim of cardiac arrest (Sayre et al., 2008).

Although it is just as effective in some circumstances, hands-only CPR does not replace traditional CPR in situations where oxygen is needed. When an adult is found unconscious (and when the blood is no longer oxygenated), and in emergencies involving infants or children, drug overdoses, drowning victims, or any adult who collapses due to a respiratory problem, a combination of breaths and compressions is needed. It is absolutely essential that fitness professionals keep their CPR provider cards current (Sayre et al., 2008). *Note:* Current CPR certification is required for all ACE-certified Fitness Professionals.

Automated External Defibrillation

While CPR alone cannot change an abnormal heart rhythm, it is important to buy time before defibrillation. During cardiac arrest, the heart is beating erratically and ineffectively. The most common rhythm during cardiac arrest is **ventricular fibrillation (VF),** which is a spasmodic quivering of the heart that is too fast to allow the heart chambers to adequately fill and empty, so little or no blood is pushed out to the body or lungs. An AED is used to convert VF back to a normal rhythm by delivering an electric shock to the heart through two adhesive electrode pads on the person's chest. By keeping the tissues perfused with oxygenated blood, CPR preserves the heart and brain and can prevent VF from deteriorating into an unshockable rhythm while waiting for an AED to arrive.

The AED should be used as soon as it becomes available, ideally within the first three to five minutes. When a shock is provided within the first minute of cardiac arrest, victims with VF have survival rates as high as 90%. The number of AEDs in a fitness facility should depend on the size of the building and the time it takes to get the AED to any location in the facility. If a building has multiple floors, having one per floor is recommended. Defibrillation cannot treat all heart rhythms, and an AED will not shock a victim when a normal heart rhythm is found. The machine will first analyze the patient to determine if a shock is appropriate. When a shock is delivered, the heart's pacemaker (i.e., the **sinoatrial node**) is able to restart.

When an AED is used on a child between one and eight years old, a child key or switch—or a smaller set of electrode pads that delivers a lower shock dose—should be used. If the child pads are not available, use adult pads for a child from age one to eight and give an adult shock dose. Always use the adult pads and adult shock dose for a child eight and older. An AED should not be used on an infant under one year old—there is not yet conclusive data for using an AED in this situation, as most infant cardiac arrests are due to a respiratory problem. An AED must never be used on a person who is conscious, breathing, or has a pulse (Mistovich & Karren, 2008).

Many states, including Arkansas, California, Illinois, Indiana, Louisiana, Massachusetts, Michigan, New Jersey, New York, Oregon, and Rhode Island, as well as the District of Columbia, have passed laws that require at least one AED in health clubs, and several other states are considering adopting this legislation. Good Samaritan laws exist in most states that offer liability protection to the person who administers the AED. The federal government also passed the Cardiac Arrest Survival Act in 2000, which granted Good Samaritan protection for anyone in the U.S. who acquired an AED or who uses an AED in a medical emergency, except in cases of wanton misconduct or recklessness. This federal law does not override state policies, but fills in the gaps for those states without these laws. This legal protection should allay any fears of liability for those organizations that want to offer a public-access defibrillation program, as well as the first responders who use them.

Common Medical Emergencies and Injuries

The following sections present common medical emergencies and injuries, the signs and symptoms of each, and recommended treatments. It is a good idea for a trainer to have a general knowledge about these situations in case they occur sometime during his or her personal-training career.

Dyspnea

Dyspnea (difficult and labored breathing) can be a common occurrence, such as when an unconditioned person attempts to exercise vigorously. In some cases, however, dyspnea can come on suddenly and be a very uncomfortable and distressing situation for the client, and it can even become life-threatening. A trauma such as a blow to the chest in boxing or a barbell dropped on the chest during a bench press could cause air to escape the lungs and move into the pleural space. The high pressure this causes outside of the lungs reduces lung volume and the person can experience severe breathing difficulty (Mistovich & Karren, 2008). Other causes of dyspnea include emotional stress, **asthma,** and airway obstruction. Heart problems can also cause dyspnea when the heart is not pumping enough blood to properly oxygenate the tissues. How the trainer should react to the situation is determined by the severity of the breathing difficulty, the cause, and how suddenly the onset occurred.

Dyspnea Scale

The dyspnea scale is a subjective score that reflects the relative difficulty of breathing as perceived by the client during physical activity.

+1 Mild, noticeable to the exerciser, but not to an observer
+2 Mild, some difficulty that is noticeable to an observer
+3 Moderate difficulty, client can continue to exercise
+4 Severe difficulty, client must stop exercising

Breathing adequately involves both an appropriate rate and depth of inhalation. The respiratory rate for adults averages between 12 and 20 breaths per minute. A rate that is too fast may be just as bad as one that is too slow. When breathing is too fast, such as during **anxiety** or panic attacks, the lungs do not have time to fill between breaths, so oxygen exchange is insufficient. Inappropriate depth (i.e., shallow breathing) indicates an inadequate **tidal volume,** or too little air inhaled with each breath. This can be due to many causes depending on whether the onset was sudden or it is a chronic problem.

The outward signs of respiratory distress are poor movement of the chest wall, flaring of the nostrils, straining of the neck muscles, and poor air exchange from the mouth and nose. Pale, diaphoretic (sweaty) skin can be an early sign of respiratory distress. **Cyanosis,** a bluish color, can develop around the lips, nose, fingernails, and inner lining of the eyes as a late sign of respiratory distress. Because the brain is not receiving enough oxygen, the person can become restless, agitated, confused, and unresponsive.

To assess breathing in an unconscious person, a personal trainer can feel for air flow on his or her own cheek while looking for chest rise and fall, although chest rise and fall alone may not mean that the air flow is adequate. It is also important to listen for unusual sounds that may indicate a partial airway blockage such as snoring, gurgling, or high pitched "crowing" sounds caused by swelling of the larynx. If there is no chest movement or no sounds indicating air movement around the mouth and nose, the personal trainer should give breaths. If there is no pulse, CPR should be initiated.

A client with a severe breathing difficulty or who is not breathing (**apneic**) is considered a priority for EMS rescuers, so it is important to call for help and convey that information. Ambulances are equipped with tanks of 100% pure oxygen to use in a wide variety of situations (Mistovich & Karren, 2008). A conscious person should be placed in a position of comfort to wait for emergency personnel to arrive. In many cases, this may mean sitting up or a "tripod" position (i.e., sitting up, leaning forward, and using the hands for support). Lying down may increase the difficulty of breathing (Schenck, 2005).

Choking

A person who is choking will have a blocked airway, and this can be mild or severe. If the blockage is mild, the airway is not completely blocked, allowing some air to get through. An individual with a mild airway blockage can still cough or make sounds. No assistance is necessary in this situation unless the object cannot be dislodged and the person becomes **hypoxic** (oxygen deficient). The personal trainer (or someone else nearby) should call EMS immediately if this happens.

If the person cannot breathe, make sounds, or has a very quiet cough, or if a child cannot cry, the blockage is severe. A person in this situation may make the universal choking sign (holding the neck with one or both hands). The rescuer should stand behind the victim with both arms wrapped around the victim's waist, make a fist with one hand, and put the thumb side just above the victim's belly button. The other hand should grab the fist, and several upward thrusts should be done to compress the diaphragm and force the object out of the victim's airway. If the victim is much smaller than the rescuer, the rescuer can kneel. If the victim is larger, the rescuer can ask the victim to kneel. If the victim is very large or in the late stages of pregnancy, the rescuer can wrap his or her arms around the victim's breastbone instead of the abdomen. If the thrusts (i.e., the **Heimlich maneuver**) do not succeed in dislodging the object, the victim may become unconscious. If this occurs, the personal trainer should have someone call for help and start the steps of CPR (AHA, 2006).

Asthma

Asthma is chronic inflammation of the airway with symptoms such as wheezing, shortness of breath, tightness in the chest, and coughing. This could be caused by **allergens** (such as dust, animal dander, and pollen) or irritants (such as smoke or pollution). Viruses, exercise, and cold air may also trigger symptoms, which can range from intermittent and mild to persistent and severe. Depending on severity, different types of treatment exist (Miller et al., 2005).

Treatment for asthma should include avoiding allergens that trigger an attack. For severe asthma, medications to prevent symptoms (controller medications) are taken daily. They can be taken orally, by injection, or inhaled. For less severe cases, reliever medications are taken once symptoms appear. These medications dilate the bronchiole muscles and reduce inflammation. Some asthmatics might have medication in the form of a metered-dose inhaler that they carry with them (Miller et al., 2005). If a client has an asthma exacerbation during exercise, the trainer should reduce the intensity and allow the client to take his or her rescue medication. If necessary, the trainer should seek medical treatment if the client's breathing does not improve or gets worse (Saglimbeni, 2007).

Exercise-induced asthma (EIA), or **exercise-induced bronchospasm (EIB),** can develop during exercise at 80% or more of maximum workload (Parsons & Mastronarde, 2005). During exercise, smooth muscles of the bronchioles constrict and mucous production increases (Mellion et al., 2003). EIA is thought to be due to the loss of water, heat, or both from the small airways during exercise (especially when participating in endurance events in cold, dry air) (Parsons & Mastronarde, 2005; Miller et al., 2005). Symptoms such as coughing, shortness of breath, wheezing, and chest tightness start in the first five to eight minutes during exercise and resolve about 30 to 60 minutes after (Parsons & Mastronarde, 2005; Mellion et al., 2003). Factors that affect EIA are the type and intensity of exercise, air quality, temperature, humidity, and the existence of allergens and viral infections (Miller et al., 2005). To avoid EIA symptoms, clients may find that breathing through the nose or through a scarf helps to warm and humidify the air. It can also help to prolong the warm-up and cool-down, to reduce the intensity of aerobic training, or to do short bouts of exercise followed by periods of rest instead of continuous exercise. If necessary, a non-aerobic activity could be substituted (Miller et al., 2005).

Cardiovascular Disease, Chest Pain, and Heart Attack

The number-one cause of death in the U.S. is cardiovascular disease, averaging one death every 37 seconds (AHA, 2008a). Plaque is a substance made up of **fat, cholesterol,** calcium, and other substances found in the blood that can stick to artery walls and narrow or completely obstruct the vessels (Schenck, 2005). This condition is called **coronary artery disease** or **atherosclerosis,** and many of its risk factors are preventable, including the following:

- Smoking
- **Hypertension**
- High cholesterol
- Diabetes
- **Overweight** or **obesity**
- Physical inactivity

Unlike sudden cardiac death, which is an electrical abnormality that disrupts the heart rhythm, a heart attack is due to an obstruction in the vessel that prevents part of the heart muscle from getting oxygen. When plaque builds up in the arteries and prevents proper blood flow to the heart, chest pain called **angina pectoris** can occur. Angina pectoris is described as chest pressure or a squeezing feeling, which may be mistaken for heart burn. This pain can also travel to one or both arms (typically the left arm, as the heart is on the left side of the chest), the neck, jaw, shoulder, or stomach. The back may also be affected. Shortness of breath may accompany these symptoms, and they may even take place without any chest pain. Nausea, a cold sweat, and lightheadedness may also occur. For women, the most common symptom is also chest pain, but women are more likely than men to experience nausea, shortness of breath, and back or jaw pain. Most heart attack warning signs are not sudden and intense—most have such a gradual onset that the person experiencing the symptoms does not realize what is happening. This delay in getting treatment can be fatal. If sudden cardiac death follows a heart attack, it is most likely to occur during the first four hours (AHA, 2008a). Trainers should be able to recognize signs of heart attack even if the victim is in denial.

The best way to react if someone is suffering from a possible heart attack is to immediately call 9-1-1. Rescuers can administer treatment such as oxygen and nitroglycerine on the scene and while traveling to the hospital. Early treatment can make the difference between life and death. People who are alone and experience these symptoms should not drive themselves to the hospital unless it is absolutely necessary.

Although news of "cough CPR" (coughing forcefully when feeling the symptoms of a heart attack) has become widespread on the Internet, the AHA does not endorse it. It is always best for someone suffering a heart attack to get trained help to the scene instead of trying to save oneself.

Physical activity is an important step in preventing cardiovascular disease. Performing physical activity regularly not only eliminates the risk factor of being **sedentary,** but it also can positively influence other risk factors such as hypertension, diabetes, and obesity. As stated earlier, the long-term benefits of exercise heavily outweigh the risks involved. However, there are dangers to performing exercise. During exercise, the likelihood of a cardiac event is temporarily increased, especially for those who are sedentary and at risk for **coronary heart disease.** Trainers should be alert to the onset of any signs and symptoms in their clients and take the conservative approach to get treatment if there is a chance that it may be necessary.

Syncope

Syncope, or fainting, is a temporary loss of consciousness due to a lack of blood flow to the brain. There are many different causes, including emotional stress, severe pain, **dehydration**/heavy sweating, overheating, and exhaustion. Syncope may also be caused by sudden postural changes after blood has pooled in the legs, such as squatting for a period of time and then standing up. Violent coughing spells, especially in men, may cause syncope due to a rapid change in blood pressure. Neurologic, metabolic, or psychiatric disorders can also cause syncope, as well as problems with the heart and lungs. Syncope is also a side effect of some medications. Although syncope is usually benign, some cases may signal life-threatening situations. Syncope is considered to be serious when it occurs with exercise, is associated with palpitations or an irregular heartbeat, or there is a family history of syncope associated with sudden cardiac death. A careful physical examination can determine whether or not a person is at risk.

Before a person faints, he or she may feel a warm sensation, nausea, or lightheadedness. Sweaty palms and a visual "grayout" may also occur. When these warning signs happen, have the person sit or lie down. To avoid fainting, the person should drink plenty of fluids to keep blood volume at adequate levels. Some people may need to be treated with medication.

Stroke

Stroke is the third leading cause of death in the U.S. and the number-one cause of disability. Like a heart attack, an **ischemic stroke** results from a blockage in a vessel—but instead of the heart, it occurs in the brain. Ischemic strokes account for approximately 80% of all strokes and are usually caused by a fatty deposit in the lining of the vessel (atherosclerosis).

The second type of stroke—**hemorrhagic stroke**—is caused by the rupture of a blood vessel. Hemorrhagic strokes account for roughly 20% of all cases, and are the result of a weakened vessel rupturing and bleeding out into the surrounding tissue. An **aneurysm** is a balloon-type bubble in the vessel at a weak spot that can rupture if left untreated. A malformation of blood vessels can also lead to a hemorrhagic stroke.

The Stroke Collaborative (2008) lists the following warning signs:

- Walk: Is the victim's balance off?
- Talk: Is the victim's speech slurred or face droopy?
- Reach: Is one side weak or numb?
- See: Is the victim's vision all or partially lost?
- Feel: Is the victim's headache severe?

The brain controls various body functions, so symptoms of a stroke depend on what area of the brain is affected. If the right hemisphere of the brain is affected, the signs and symptoms will appear on the right side of the face but the left side of the body due to the crossover of cranial nerves. This can cause a facial droop on the right side, weakness or paralysis on the left side of the body, vision problems, memory loss, and a quick, inquisitive type of behavior. If the left hemisphere of the brain is affected, it can cause a facial droop on the left side, weakness or paralysis on the right side of the body, memory loss and speech or language problems, and a slow, cautious type of behavior. If the back of the brain is affected, it can impair vision.

Getting medical care quickly is important with a stroke, so the personal trainer should call EMS immediately. The FDA has approved a clot-busting medication called **tissue plasminogen activator (tPA)** that can reduce the severity and speed recovery from a stroke. However, tPA must be administered within the first three hours of the onset of symptoms, so make sure to note the time when symptoms began.

A **transient ischemic attack (TIA)** can mimic the symptoms of a stroke but causes only temporary disability. Symptoms usually last less than one hour and may be relieved within 10 or 15 minutes. If a person has a TIA, he or she may be just as frightened as someone who has a stroke and should receive medical treatment to determine the cause. One-third of people who have a TIA will later have a stroke, many within the next month.

Diabetes and Insulin Reaction (Hypoglycemia)

Diabetes is a condition in which the body does not produce enough **insulin** or becomes insensitive to it (unresponsive). Insulin, a **hormone** secreted by the pancreas, is necessary after a meal to extract **glucose** out of the blood and into the muscles for use as energy and stored energy in the form of **glycogen.** There are two principal types of diabetes, **type 1 diabetes** [also called **insulin-dependent diabetes mellitus (IDDM)**] and **type 2 diabetes** [also called **non-insulin-dependent diabetes mellitus (NIDDM)**]. In type 1 diabetes, the islet cells of the pancreas do not produce a sufficient amount of insulin and, therefore, insulin must be administered regularly (Gulve, 2008). The initial symptoms usually appear in childhood and include weight loss, fatigue, excessive thirst, and excessive urination (AHA, 2008b). An absolute lack of insulin production in type 1 diabetes requires exogenous insulin administration (e.g., injections, pump, or inhalation) to maintain normal glucose levels, minimize complications, and prevent excessive use of fatty acids for energy, resulting in **ketoacidosis.** Because a limited amount of insulin might be sufficient to prevent ketoacidosis, type 1 diabetes can sometimes go undiagnosed for years. For others, ketoacidosis might occur within hours of insulin withdrawal [American Diabetes Association (ADA), 2004]. People with type 2 diabetes usually develop the disease after age 30 and approximately 80% or more are obese (Dixon & O'Brien, 2002). With type 2 diabetes, a normal amount of insulin may be secreted, but the body becomes resistant to it (AHA, 2008b).

Without enough insulin, blood sugar becomes too high (**hyperglycemia**) and glucose is passed into the kidneys, where it is excreted with a lot of water and **electrolytes,** leaving the person weak, thirsty, and fatigued (ADA, 2004). A more common occurrence in the fitness setting is **hypoglycemia,** or low blood sugar. If the client has vomited, injected too much insulin, or has done physical activity without eating enough food, he or she may show signs of low blood sugar. The onset may be rapid and can be displayed as headache, hunger, weakness, sweating, or fatigue. This can happen during exercise because of the increased uptake of glucose to fuel working muscles, and mild symptoms can also occur in a non-diabetic person who exercises heavily without consuming enough food beforehand. A hypoglycemic event could still occur after a workout due to the continued metabolic effects of an acute exercise bout. In a more severe hypoglycemic reaction, a person could display personality changes, neurological impairment, seizures, and coma (ADA, 2003).

Personal trainers should know their clients' medical backgrounds and be able to quickly recognize the signs of hypoglycemia, especially when working with a client who is known to have diabetes. At the first suspicion of hypoglycemia, the personal trainer should discontinue exercise and help the client sit down to avoid falling. If the client is conscious and can swallow, he or she should consume 20 to 30 grams of **carbohydrates** such as a sugary drink (juice or regular soda) or a packet of sugar or honey to raise the blood sugar back to a normal level. It is important to not give foods with little sugar, such as chocolate, diet soda, or artificial sweeteners (AHA, 2006). Usually, the person will feel better in a short time and can resume activity 15 minutes after the symptoms are gone (Lillegard, Butcher, & Rucker, 1999). *Note:* It is wise to have diabetic clients check their blood glucose levels to see if they are at least 100 mg/dL before resuming activity. If the person still is not feeling better after a few minutes, the personal trainer should activate EMS.

During severe hypoglycemia, a person may become unresponsive or unconscious. If the person cannot sit up or swallow or is unresponsive, the personal trainer should not try to make him or her eat or drink and instead call EMS immediately. A personal trainer must never try to give anything (e.g., sugar) by mouth to an unconscious person, as doing so could cause aspiration of the substance and airway or respiratory compromise. If the victim vomits, turn the victim onto his or her side to prevent aspiration (Figure 16-4). The personal trainer must be aware of a possible seizure and be ready to start CPR if necessary (AHA, 2006). The person should have a medical evaluation before resuming an exercise program (Lillegard, Butcher, & Rucker, 1999).

Because of the daily variations of **growth hormone** and **cortisol,** the best time to exercise to avoid hypoglycemia is usually in the morning, one to three hours after a meal (Gulve, 2008; Mellion et al., 2003). Prior to exercise, people with diabetes should check their blood glucose levels. If they are below 100 mg/dL, a pre-exercise snack should be eaten that is high in **complex carbohydrates** and low in fat. Those with blood glucose between 100 and 250 mg/dL can exercise, but extra calories may need to be consumed during or after exercise (depending on the duration). Sports drinks can be sipped throughout the exercise session to maintain blood sugar. If a person has a blood sugar level above 250 mg/dL and there is a presence of **ketones** in the urine (or if blood sugar is above 300 mg/dL without ketones), exercise should not be done until blood sugar is better controlled. Ketone bodies, the end products of fat metabolism, signify that the body is burning fat for energy rather than glucose because of a lack of insulin (Gulve, 2008). Ketones are acidic and lower the pH of the body, which could lead to adverse side effects, including confusion, lethargy, sleepiness, and even diabetic coma. Although this is rare in individuals who exercise, those who display this type of behavior should be given glucose. Even if glucose levels are high, giving extra glucose will be insignificant and unlikely to cause harm. If improvement is not immediate, EMS should be called (Schenck, 2005).

Individuals with diabetes should be encouraged to talk to their physicians before starting new exercise programs. It is common to have the insulin prescription significantly decreased, especially prior to exercise sessions (Gulve, 2008). They may also need to eat more prior to training sessions, or keep candy or a carbohydrate drink on hand. Long-term treatment for type 2 diabetes includes medication, diet modification, weight loss, and exercise. Exercise,

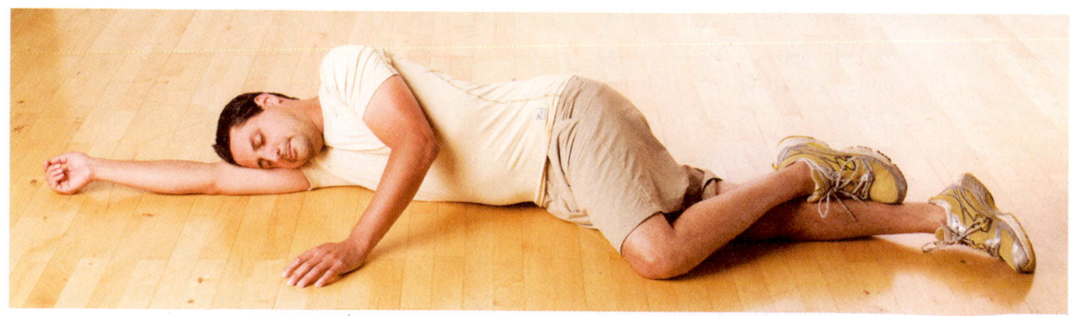

Figure 16-4
Side position for unconscious victim: Placing the victim on his or her side prevents airway blockage in case vomiting occurs. This position allows fluids to drain from the nose and mouth.

both aerobic and resistance training, helps to reduce fat weight and increase lean body mass, which together will lower the body's resistance to insulin (Gulve, 2008). Studies have shown that physical activity helps protect those at risk for developing type 2 diabetes, especially those with significant risk factors [high **body mass index (BMI)**, hypertension, and a family history of diabetes] (Helmrich et al., 1994; 1991).

Because exercise decreases blood sugar and increases insulin sensitivity, trainers should monitor their diabetic clients closely during exercise, especially when starting a new program. Increases in the intensity of the training program should be done slower and more conservatively (Gulve, 2008). A client with **peripheral neuropathy** due to diabetes may need to have a modified program to keep from damaging his or her feet. For example, non-weightbearing activities like biking and swimming are recommended, while running and jumping may need to be avoided. In addition, close attention should be paid to foot care, such as making sure the client wears properly fitting shoes and adequately cushioned socks. Any injuries should be immediately addressed (Mellion et al., 2003). However, when the problems are managed correctly, people with diabetes can function at very high levels.

Heat Illness

Exercise can raise body temperature by 4.5° F (Lillegard, Butcher, & Rucker, 1999). Blood that becomes heated flows to the skin, where **vasodilation** occurs and sweating begins. In the heat, normal body temperature is primarily maintained through the evaporation of sweat. Heat, high humidity, and some medications such as **diuretics,** antidepressants, and antihistamines place stress on the body's thermoregulatory system (Caris, Ramirez, & Van Durme, 2004). Profuse sweating resulting in fluid loss means there is less blood to carry nutrients and oxygen to working muscles. Clients are more likely to be at risk for heat illness during the summer months, particularly in geographic areas with high heat and humidity, in fitness facilities without air conditioning, and during high-intensity training in the heat. Those who are deconditioned are also at higher risk (Mellion et al., 2003).

There are several types of heat syndromes that range widely in their severity. Heat **edema** is a temporary swelling of the extremities, usually in people not acclimated to the elevated temperature. Swelling may affect the hands, feet, and ankles, but typically only for a few days. No treatment is necessary, although wearing support stockings may help (Mellion et al., 2003).

Heat cramps are spasms that affect the arms, legs, and abdominal muscles due to a loss of fluid and electrolytes, thereby causing cell size to decrease and affecting cell metabolism. Heat cramps can occur in individuals who sweat profusely, especially if they are not acclimated to heat. Treatment for heat cramps includes rest, direct pressure to cramp and release, gentle massage, replacing fluids and electrolytes, and passive stretching of the affected areas (Caris, Ramirez, & Van Durme, 2004). Activity can be resumed one or two days after symptoms have resolved. With more severe heat cramps that cause nausea and vomiting, medical attention may be needed to replace fluids intravenously (Lillegard, Butcher, & Rucker, 1999). Heat cramps can lead to more serious problems, such as **heat exhaustion** and **heat stroke** (Mellion et al., 2003) (Table 16-1).

Immediately after exercise, **heat syncope** can occur due to blood pooling in the legs and not enough blood reaching the brain (Mellion et al., 2003). This can also occur during exercise in a hot environment, as blood pressure falls rapidly when the higher body temperature causes blood to flow to the skin and limbs. There is a decrease in **stroke volume, cardiac output,** and blood pressure. To treat heat syncope, have the person drink fluids and rest with his or her feet raised. To avoid this situation, clients should avoid standing for prolonged periods in a hot environment. Exercise can resume the next day if the person is asymptomatic. However, if the person is lightheaded, or has abnormally low blood pressure, he or she should seek medical attention (Lillegard, Butcher, & Rucker, 1999).

Table 16-1

Heat Exhaustion and Heat Stroke

	Signs and Symptoms	Treatment
Heat Exhaustion	Weak, rapid pulse Low blood pressure Fatigue Headache Dizziness General weakness Paleness Cold, clammy skin Profuse sweating Elevated body core temperature (≤104° F or 40° C)	Stop exercising Move to a cool, well-ventilated area Lay down and elevate feet 12–18 inches (30–46 cm) Give fluids Monitor temperature
Heat Stroke	Hot, dry skin Bright red skin color Rapid, strong pulse Change in mental status (e.g., irritability, aggressiveness, anxiety) Labored breathing Elevated body core temperature (≥105° F or 41° C)	Stop exercising Remove as much clothing as feasible Try to cool the body immediately in any way possible (wet towels, ice packs/baths, fan) Give fluids Transport to emergency room immediately

Severe dehydration may cause uncoordinated movement and altered consciousness. To treat someone with severe dehydration, give fluids and cool the person by placing cool wet towels on the victim's body. Severe dehydration requires medical evaluation and one or more days of rest before returning to exercise (Lillegard, Butcher, & Rucker, 1999).

Individuals who are deconditioned or have been recovering from illness are at risk for heat exhaustion (Schenck, 2005). This condition is marked by the inability to continue exercise due to an elevated core temperature [but usually under 104° F (40° C)] (Mellion et al., 2003). Heat exhaustion occurs when the blood volume is inadequate to meet the demands for increased flow to the skin and working muscles (Caris, Ramirez, & Van Durme, 2004). Signs and symptoms include fatigue, general weakness, uncoordinated movement, lightheadedness, dizziness, and headache (Mellion et al., 2003). Dehydration (either fluid dehydration or salt depletion) can increase the risk of heat exhaustion. Salt depletion results in a loss of extracellular fluid, plasma volume, cardiac output, and blood pressure. A person experiencing salt depletion may not feel thirsty. Water depletion is more common and easier to treat because thirst is the main symptom (Lillegard, Butcher, & Rucker, 1999). The treatment for heat exhaustion includes moving the exerciser to a cool, well-ventilated area, rehydration, and having the person lie still and cool down while monitoring vital signs. It may be necessary to call EMS for a client who is vomiting, as he or she will need intravenous fluids to rehydrate (Caris, Ramirez, & Van Durme, 2004).

Heat stroke is a life-threatening failure of the body's cooling mechanisms. The victim's core body temperature reaches 105° F (41° C) or greater. This can suddenly occur after heat exhaustion. Even in cool to moderate outdoor temperatures, heat stroke can occur (Caris, Ramirez, & Van Durme, 2004). The signs and symptoms of heat stroke include a change in mental status, such as irritability and aggressiveness, which may progress to apathy, confusion, unresponsiveness, or even coma. An assessment of vital signs will indicate that the blood pressure is very low and the pulse is rapid and strong (Schenck, 2005). In some cases sweating may stop, but victims of exertional heat stroke are usually still sweating. Heat stroke is dangerous because all major organs and body systems can be affected (Mellion et al., 2003).

To care for a victim of heat stroke, call EMS if the person displays any abnormal signs, such as confusion, vomiting, inability to drink, red hot and dry skin due to an inability to sweat, shallow breathing, seizures, or unresponsiveness. Mild signs could get worse if the person does not receive treatment (AHA, 2006). Cool the victim immediately—do not wait for EMS to arrive. Get the person into a shady area, remove any tight or restrictive clothing, and apply ice packs to areas of high blood flow such as the groin, axilla (armpit), and neck or submerge the victim in a tub of ice water (Mellion et al., 2003). If the person can swallow, it is safe to give him or her cool fluids to drink, but not if the person is vomiting, is confused or unresponsive, or has had a seizure. Monitor the ABCs and core temperature. Once the person's behavior is back to normal, stop the cooling so that a state of **hypothermia** does not develop (AHA, 2006).

There are several factors that can help clients avoid heat illness:

- Clients should exercise during cooler times of day such as morning or evening.
- More water breaks should be taken on very hot and humid days.
- Clients should avoid exercise in extremely hot and humid conditions [**wet bulb globe temperature (WBGT)** above 82° F (28° C)]. WGBT combines temperature, humidity, and radiant heat. Heat index tables provide this information in an easy-to-read format (Table 16-2) (Mellion et al., 2003).

Table 16-2

Heat Index

	Actual Thermometer Reading (°F) (°C given in parentheses)										
	70 (21)	75 (24)	80 (27)	85 (29)	90 (32)	95 (35)	100 (38)	105 (41)	110 (43)	115 (46)	120 (49)
Relative Humidity	Equivalent or Effective Temperature* (°F) (°C given in parentheses)										
0	64 (18)	69 (21)	73 (23)	78 (26)	83 (28)	87 (31)	91 (33)	95 (35)	99 (37)	103 (39)	107 (42)
10	65 (18)	70 (21)	75 (24)	80 (27)	85 (29)	90 (32)	95 (35)	100 (38)	105 (41)	111 (44)	116 (47)
20	66 (19)	72 (22)	77 (25)	82 (28)	87 (31)	93 (34)	99 (37)	105 (41)	112 (44)	120 (49)	130 (54)
30	67 (19)	73 (23)	78 (26)	84 (29)	90 (32)	96 (36)	104 (40)	113 (45)	123 (51)	135 (57)	148 (64)
40	68 (20)	74 (23)	79 (26)	86 (30)	93 (34)	101 (38)	110 (43)	123 (51)	137 (58)	151 (66)	
50	69 (21)	75 (24)	81 (27)	88 (31)	96 (36)	107 (42)	120 (49)	135 (57)	150 (66)		
60	70 (21)	76 (24)	82 (28)	90 (32)	100 (38)	114 (46)	132 (56)	149 (65)			
70	70 (21)	77 (25)	85 (29)	93 (34)	106 (41)	124 (51)	144 (62)				
80	71 (22)	78 (26)	86 (30)	97 (36)	113 (45)	136 (58)					
90	71 (22)	79 (26)	88 (31)	102 (39)	122 (50)						
100	72 (22)	80 (27)	91 (33)	108 (42)							

*Combined index of heat and humidity and what it feels like to the body

How to Use Heat Index

1. Locate temperature across top
2. Locate relative humidity down left side
3. Follow across and down to find Apparent Temperature
4. Determine Heat Stress Risk on chart at right

Note: This Heat Index chart is designed to provide general guidelines for assessing the potential severity of heat stress. Individual reactions to heat will vary. In addition, studies indicate that susceptibility to heat disorders tends to increase among children and older adults. Exposure to full sunshine can increase Heat Index values by up to 15° F.

Apparent Temperature	Heat Stress Risk with Physical Activity and/or Prolonged Exposure
90–105 (32–41)	Heat cramps or heat exhaustion *possible*
106–130 (41–54)	Heat cramps or heat exhaustion *likely* Heat stroke *possible*
131–151 (54–66)	Heat stroke *highly likely*

- Becoming acclimatized, or getting physiologically adjusted to the heat, takes about 10 to 14 days. For the first few days, reduce intensity and take more rest breaks. Use **target heart rate** to identify the appropriate intensity (Mellion et al., 2003). While some researchers say that full **acclimatization** takes months, others say only 10 to 14 days is necessary. Once acclimatization occurs, it can be maintained with minimal exposure for several weeks (Schenck, 2005).
- Clients should always drink plenty of fluids before, during, and after exercise (Table 16-3). Drinking a slightly diluted sports drink is best. While water alone will quench thirst, athletes may not drink as much as when drinking flavored beverages. Flavored sports drinks are more likely to encourage intake as well as replenish electrolytes and carbohydrates to working muscles (Schenck, 2005).

Table 16-3

Fluid-intake Recommendations During Exercise

Fluid-intake Recommendations During Exercise
2 hours prior to exercise, drink 500–600 mL (17–20 oz)
Every 10–20 minutes during exercise, drink 200–300 mL (7–10 oz) or, preferably, drink based on sweat losses
Following exercise, drink 450–675 mL for every 0.5 kg body weight lost (or 16–24 oz for every pound)

Adapted with permission from Casa, D.J. et al. (2000). National Athletic Trainers' Association: Position statement: Fluid replacement for athletes. *Journal of Athletic Training*, 35, 212–224.

- Dress appropriately. Clothing that is lightweight, breathable, and light colored is best, and the skin should be exposed for maximal sweat evaporation. Sunscreen of at least SPF 15 will protect the skin from ultraviolet rays [American Cancer Society, 2008; Centers for Disease Control and Prevention (CDC), 2006].
- Be alert to early warning signs such as fatigue and cramping to avoid serious incidents.
- Individuals who are in good physical condition and well hydrated are less likely to be affected by the heat. Anyone with signs of heat illness should not participate in exercise for at least 24 hours (Schenck, 2005).

Cold Illness

Although "normal" body temperature is 98.6° F (37° C), the body can survive with core temperatures between 75 and 106° F (23.9 to 41° C). The core of the body (the brain heart, lungs, and abdominal organs) and the periphery of the body (the skin, muscles, and extremities) are affected differently by low temperatures. In a cold environment, the periphery of the body decreases its circulation to slow heat loss. Because of increased exposure, the hands, feet, ears, and face are often affected by the cold. Cells are made up mostly of water, which can actually freeze and damage the cells, also injuring nearby blood vessels and skin. The amount of damage can be more severe with high winds, lower temperatures, and longer exposure. Some examples of when cold illness might occur are during a cross-country ski trip, marathon training in winter months, hiking at a high altitude, ocean swimming, or any exercise in wet conditions (Schenck, 2005).

In cold temperatures, receptors in the skin signal the hypothalamus to begin shivering to increase core body temperature. Some of the signs and symptoms of mild hypothermia are confusion, **dysarthria** (difficulty speaking), fatigue, dizziness, amnesia, and apathy. When hypothermia goes from mild to moderate, victims can become lethargic, hallucinate, and even become unconscious. Shivering stops if the body temperature drops below 88 to 90° F (31 to 32° C). Victims of severe hypothermia may even appear dead, unresponsive to painful stimuli, and have fixed, dilated pupils (Mellion et al., 2003). In fact, medical professionals need to warm these victims before pronouncing them dead, as they may be in a coma (Mellion et al., 2003).

If a trainer needs to care for a victim of hypothermia, he or she should take the person to the nearest warm shelter and remove all wet clothing, pat the person dry, and dress him or her in warm clothing and blankets. Call for medical help immediately and keep the person lying down to prevent a drop in blood pressure (**orthostatic hypotension**). It is important to monitor the person to make sure he or she stays conscious. If there is an AED nearby, it should always be ready in the event of cardiac arrest. Arrhythmias may occur from hypothermia, and VF is common (AHA, 2006; Mellion et al., 2003).

Frostbite occurs when parts of the body are exposed to extreme cold. Tissues on the hands, face (especially the nose), feet, and ears may freeze and die. At first, the areas become numb and painful. The skin becomes grayish-white or yellow and has a waxy appearance that is hard to the touch. Frostbite is worsened by altitude, wind, exposure for long periods, and contact with cold objects that serve as conductors (e.g., sleeping on a cold ground). Those with diabetes and atherosclerosis are at higher risk for frostbite because circulation is already impaired (AHA, 2006; Mellion et al., 2003).

If there is not a chance of refreezing or if a medical facility is nearby, the personal trainer should warm the victim and remove any tight jewelry or clothing. Refreezing can cause more tissue damage than if the area had stayed frozen. Massaging the frostbitten area is not recommended, nor is warming with a heating pad, stove, or fire. As frostbitten areas are warmed, there may be a throbbing pain and swelling in the affected areas. Within 24 hours, blisters may form containing yellow or clear liquid. After one to two weeks, **eschars** may form (i.e., scabs that may give the appearance of having been burned). After three to six weeks, the skin may turn dark and eventually the scabs will fall off (Mellion et al., 2003; AHA, 2006). The skin may be painful for weeks—red, throbbing, and burning (Schenck, 2005).

To avoid overexposure, proper preparation is necessary. Clothing should be layered, as warm air trapped between layers helps maintain body temperature. The inner layer should be designed to wick moisture away. Some synthetic fabrics (lightweight polyester or polypropylene) are made for this purpose. The middle layer should be for insulation, and fabrics like fleece and wool are recommended. The outer layer should be a protective coating from elements such as wind and rain, but still allow moisture to evaporate (e.g., have mesh in areas such as the armpits). This layer can be removed when weather is clear and dry and it may only be necessary during rest periods. Hats, headbands, scarves, and gloves can help prevent frostbite in exposed areas. By increasing body heat and minimizing heat loss, the body can stay warm. However, overdressing is not recommended—when a person is not exercising, he or she should be somewhat chilly (Mellion et al., 2003).

Fluid loss via sweating occurs during cold-temperature exercise just as in warm weather, although thirst is not as noticeable. Frequent eating and drinking helps maintain blood volume and glycogen levels, and raises body heat through metabolism (Mellion et al., 2003).

Seizures

A seizure occurs when there is abnormal and excessive electrical activity in the brain. While 10% of the population may have a seizure at some point in their lives, only 1% of all seizures occur due to epilepsy (Schenck, 2005). Some seizures are caused by head injuries, low blood sugar, heat injuries, or poisons (AHA, 2006).

Seizures are either general or partial. The most common and well-known type of general seizure is the **tonic clonic seizure** or **grand mal seizure.** It usually starts with an "aura"—the person experiences a smell or sound that indicates a seizure is about to occur. When the seizure starts, the victim experiences a loss of consciousness and whole-body jerking movements (i.e., tonic clonic movements), where the muscles contract and relax, the jaw is clenched, and bowel or bladder control might be lost. This could last one or more minutes, and is followed by a state of exhaustion called the **postictal state.** The victim may still be unconscious in this state for 10 to 30 minutes (Schenck, 2005).

The emergency procedures for a generalized tonic clonic (grand mal) seizure are as follows (AHA, 2006):

- Clear the area so the victim will not hit his or her head on nearby furniture or objects.
- Place a towel under the victim's head to help protect it from injury.
- Never restrain the victim or place anything in the victim's mouth.
- Have someone phone EMS.

After the seizure, check to make sure the victim is breathing, and if not, start CPR. With a victim who is not suspected of having a head, neck, or spinal injury, roll him or her into the recovery position (on his or her side) to prevent vomit or mucus from obstructing the airway. The victim may be confused and very tired after a seizure, so it is important to stay nearby and reassure him or her upon awakening.

During a seizure, the person stops breathing. However, **hypoxia** is rarely a problem unless the seizure is prolonged—normal breathing resumes in the postictal state. It is important to make sure the airway is clear. If the seizure lasts more than five minutes, or multiple seizures occur without the person regaining consciousness in between, the personal trainer should call EMS immediately (Epilepsy Foundation, 2009).

Epileptic seizures are chronic and have no known cause (Schenck, 2005). They are actually less likely to occur during exercise than during rest, and exercise may be helpful in controlling them. If seizures are associated with exercise, they occur during prolonged exercise such as triathlons or marathons, when other metabolic states might act as contributing factors (such as **hyponatremia,** a sodium deficiency). Contact sports, even those involving head trauma, are unlikely to increase the prevalence of seizures (Mellion et al., 2003).

Interestingly, epilepsy is very controllable. Studies with children have found high remission rates after a child has remained seizure-free for two to four years on medication—even once the medication has been discontinued (Mellion et al., 2003).

Soft-tissue Injuries

Because the skin is the outer covering of the body, it is frequently injured. Blisters are caused by **shear force** in one or more directions, which causes fluid to go to the injury site and settle between the dermis and epidermis of the skin. Bruises occur when a compressive blow to the skin damages **capillaries** below the surface. The area fills with blood to cause bruising (**ecchymosis**). **Contusions** are similar to bruises in that they are caused by blunt trauma that does not break the surface of the skin, but contusions also feature swelling and the formation of a **hematoma,** a hard, localized mass of blood and dead tissue that could restrict movement or cause pain or even temporary paralysis due to nerve compression (Anderson, Hall, & Martin, 2000).

There are several types of breaks that can occur in the skin (Anderson, Hall, & Martin, 2000):

- **Abrasion**—A scraping of tissue from a fall against a rough surface, usually in one direction
- **Incision**—A clean cut to the skin from a tensile force, likely from a sharp edge
- **Laceration**—A jagged tear of the skin caused by both shear and tensile forces
- **Avulsion**—A severe laceration, with skin torn away from the tissue below
- **Puncture**—A penetration of the skin by an object

Treatment for these injuries is to clean the area thoroughly and irrigate with plenty of water, and then apply a dry dressing. Applying direct pressure over the injury site can help control bleeding (Figure 16-5). If the gauze gets soaked through, the personal trainer can apply more gauze pads without removing the first ones so as not to rip off any scab that starts to form. It is necessary to seek medical attention for large wounds where bleeding cannot be

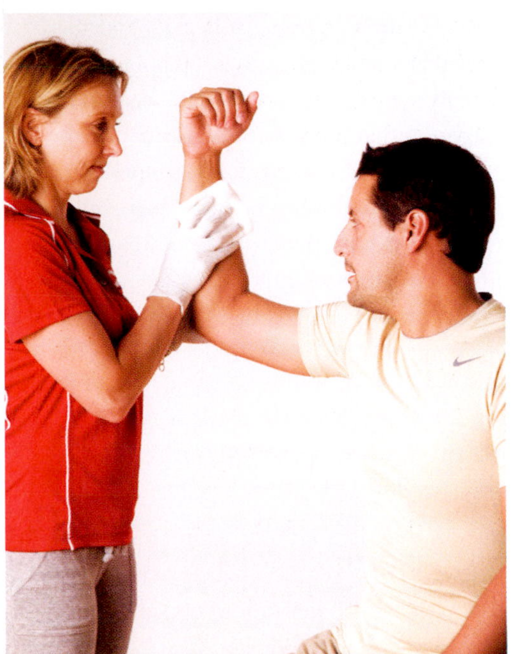

Figure 16-5
Direct pressure for hemorrhage control

controlled, or if the person begins to feel dizzy, confused, or agitated, and is pale, cold, and clammy—these may be signs of shock (Mellion et al., 2003). For any broken skin, the patient may be required to update his or her tetanus shot (Lillegard, Butcher, & Rucker, 1999). See "Universal Precautions and Protection Against Bloodborne Pathogens" on page 585 for more information on handling situations in which a personal trainer may come in contact with a client's blood or other bodily fluid.

Tendons and **ligaments** are formed primarily from **collagen** tissue. Collagen is a **protein** with fibers arranged in a wavy pattern, giving it a slight amount of stretch when under tension. However, injuries occur when tendons and ligaments are overstretched. A sprain is an acute trauma to a ligament, which connects bone to bone. Sprains are classified as first, second, or third degree, depending on the number of fibers torn and the amount of joint instability. Ligaments tear when bones become displaced, such as with an ankle sprain or shoulder dislocation. Although immediate stabilization and immobilization are necessary, healthcare professionals may not immobilize the joint for long, as doing so may cause **atrophy** and strength loss. Ligaments and tendons grow stronger as controlled stress is placed on them, so long periods of immobilization are detrimental to healing. Decreased blood flow in tendons and ligaments means slow healing times, even up to one year (Anderson, Hall, & Martin, 2000). See Chapter 15 for more information on sprains.

A **strain** involves injury to a tendon, which connects muscle to bone. Since tendons are stronger than the muscles they attach to, most strains are actually an injury to the muscle fibers and are commonly called pulled muscles. Strains can also be first, second, or third degree depending on the number of muscle fibers involved and the ability to contract the injured muscle (Mellion et al., 2003). Tendons are stronger than the muscles they attach to, so tendons usually do not tear (Anderson, Hall, & Martin, 2000). See Chapter 15 for more information on strains.

General primary treatment for soft-tissue injuries is RICE (rest or restricted activity, ice, compression, and elevation) or PRICES, which also includes protection and support. Rest or restricted activity is necessary to allow the body to heal. Ice should be applied for approximately 20 minutes to relieve swelling and pain. Although different theories exist, ice (not heat) is usually used in the first 24 hours. Ice massage is also a technique used to decrease pain and swelling. Water is frozen in a Styrofoam™ or paper cup, which is torn back about an inch from the top so that the ice can be rubbed on the injured area. Do this for approximately 20 minutes, depending on the type of cold pack applied, the area of injury, and sensitivity of the person (Holcomb, 2005). Ice gets colder than gel packs, so if the ice pack is held stationary on the skin, the personal trainer may want to place a towel under the ice pack so the tissue does not sustain damage. Compression bandages help prevent swelling and should be applied distally and wrapped proximally. Elevating the injury above the level of the heart can help further reduce swelling (Mellion et al., 2003).

Secondary treatment involves medical care and may include corticosteroid shots, physical therapy, something to brace the area, such as a cast or splint, and **non-steroidal**

anti-inflammatory drugs (NSAIDs), such as aspirin, ibuprofen, or naproxen, which relieve pain, fever, and inflammation. Heat is used to increase blood flow to muscle tissue to increase temperature, elasticity, and healing. Superficial heat such as hot packs or hot whirlpools is used to relieve muscle spasms and stiffness and to reduce pain (Mellion et al., 2003). Ultrasound is a deep heating modality used in athletic training and physical therapy settings to increase circulation to an area and decrease inflammation. Ultrasound delivers heat to tissues below the surface by using high- or low-frequency sound waves.

Remember that the diagnosis and treatment of injuries is outside the **scope of practice** of a personal trainer. If a client asks about an injury, the personal trainer should refer him or her to an appropriate healthcare provider and contact the provider to obtain guidelines and **contra-indications** related to fitness training and the injured area.

Fractures

A fracture is a disruption or break in bone continuity. The type of fracture depends on bone health, age, and the stress that caused it (Anderson, Hall, & Martin, 2000). The term "closed fracture" is used to describe a fracture where there is no break in the surface of the skin. With "open fractures," there is an open wound that may or may not have the end of the broken bone protruding through it. A trainer should suspect a broken bone when any of the following are present (Mistovich & Karren, 2008):

- Deformity or angulation—a difference in size or abnormal position
- Pain and tenderness
- Grating, **crepitus**—the sound of bone fragments grinding against each other
- Swelling
- Disfigurement
- Severe weakness and loss of function
- Bruising
- Exposed bone ends
- A joint locked in position

Stress injuries occur where there in an imbalance in **bone formation** and **bone resorption.** Stress fractures often occur in the tibia when abnormal stress is placed on the bone. The primary symptom is usually pain when bearing weight on that limb. Active individuals who are susceptible to stress fractures are typically those participating in high-repetition, high-intensity, or high-impact activities (e.g., endurance running, jumping, sprinting). An adequate intake of calcium and vitamin D is essential for optimal bone health, as are sufficient estrogen levels for women. Proper progression in an exercise program and supportive footwear can also help prevent stress fractures. Management involves resting the injured area and exercising only at levels that do not cause symptoms. Non-weightbearing exercises such as swimming or stationary biking are recommended during the healing process (Mellion et al., 2003). See Chapter 15 for more information on fractures.

A fracture is a serious injury not only because the bone is broken, but also because of the potential injury to the surrounding soft tissue. Tendons, ligaments, muscles, nerves, and blood vessels may be damaged, with a threat of permanent disability. Fractures may result from a direct blow or more indirect cause, such as a fall. The following are signs of possible bone fracture:

- Audible snap at the time of injury
- Abnormal motion or position of the injured limb
- Inability to bear weight on the limb (stand or walk)
- Swelling
- Deformity
- Discoloration
- Pain or tenderness to the touch

Immediate care for a victim with a suspected fracture involves controlling hemorrhage, preventing further injury to the bone and soft tissue, and providing first aid for shock, if necessary. If a personal trainer suspects a fracture, he or she should take the following steps:

- Keep the victim quiet; do not allow him or her to move the injured part or attempt to put weight on it
- Remove or cut away clothing that covers the injury. This step allows more

thorough assessment and prevents contamination of an open fracture.

- Cover an open fracture with a sterile gauze dressing or clean cloth to prevent further contamination. Activate the EMS system immediately and keep the victim lying down if there is significant bleeding to improve circulation to the heart and brain until help arrives. Apply gentle pressure to slow or stop the bleeding, using care not to disturb the fractured site.
- Leave the protruding ends of bone where they are. Attempting to push them back in place will increase risk of infection and further injury to soft tissues
- If the victim must be transported, splint the limb to immobilize it. However, if the extremity is grossly deformed and splinting may be difficult, merely prevent the injured limb from moving until medical help arrives. An untrained person's attempt to move a fractured limb can convert a closed fracture into an open one, or cause nerve and vascular injury in an uncomplicated fracture.

Splinting or immobilizing a fractured limb protects it against further injury during transportation, reduces pain, and prevents bone fragments from injuring arteries or other tissues. Many household objects or pieces of equipment in a health club may be converted to emergency splints—any object that provides support or prevents movement can serve this purpose. Some examples include heavy cardboard, newspapers, rolled blankets or towels, exercise mats, and straight sticks. The splint should simply be long enough to extend past the joints above and below the suspected fracture and should be padded to prevent pressure injuries due to contact with hard surfaces or sharp edges. A first-aid course will provide guidance in how to splint an extremity.

Figures 16-6 and 16-7 illustrate properly applied splints of the forearm and ankle, using materials commonly found in a home or fitness facility.

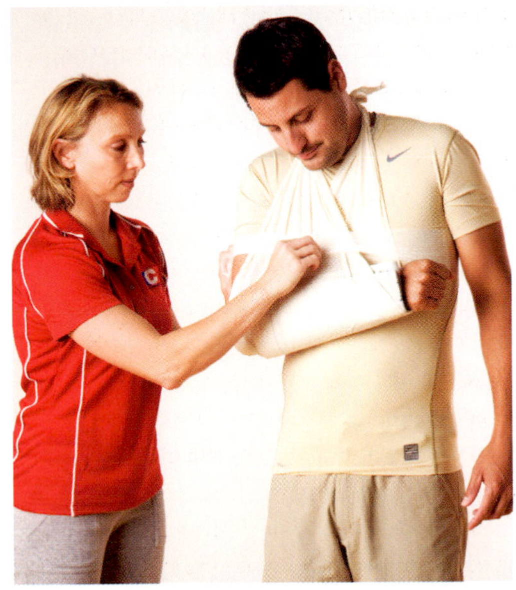

Figure 16-6
Splinting the forearm: The bone has been immobilized by newspaper that has been rolled up, padded with a towel, and tied with strips of material to hold the splint in place. Using a sling in combination with the splint will immobilize the joints below the fracture (wrist) and above the fracture (elbow). The sling also elevates the hand slightly above the elbow to minimize swelling.

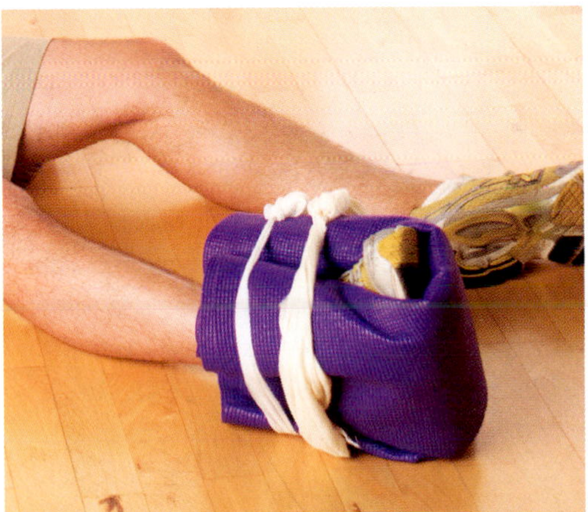

Figure 16-7
Splinting the ankle: Check circulation and sensation. Splint the ankle using a rolled blanket, towel, or exercise mat, applying it around the ankle and sole of the foot and tying it into place with cloth strips.

Head Injuries

The head has a natural protection from injury—the skull—which forms a bony covering around the brain and contains many cranial and facial bones. Three layers of protective covering called the **meninges** lie beneath the surface of the skull. Besides offering protection to the brain and spinal cord, the meninges also allow venous drainage through vessels that flow in between them and through the middle layer of the three meninges, the arachnoid mater—so named because of the spider-like web of vessels it contains. Just below the arachnoid mater is a space that contains cerebrospinal fluid that cushions the brain by distributing blunt forces over a larger area. When the skull is fractured, this clear fluid may be seen on bandages forming a "halo" or ring of clear wet liquid around the blood. It may also leak from ear canals due to a fracture at the base of the skull or through the nose if the fracture was in the anterior cranial area (Schenck, 2005).

A concussion is a brain injury that causes a change in mental status. Concussions can occur during contact sports, as the result of falls or blows to the head (such as in football or martial arts training). There may be an accompanying temporary loss of consciousness. The first signs of a concussion are often confusion and disorientation. The person may not be able to explain what happened and may experience memory loss that causes him or her to ask the same question repeatedly. Speech may be slow or slurred, and the person may be uncoordinated and have a headache or nausea. Following a concussion, the brain cells are in a vulnerable state and a second injury could be debilitating, so rest is absolutely necessary.

It is sometimes difficult to recognize a concussion, as the initial signs can be subtle. Personal trainers should be aware of the following warning signs:

- Amnesia
- Confusion
- Memory loss
- Headache
- Drowsiness
- Loss of consciousness
- Impaired speech
- **Tinnitus**
- Unequal pupil size
- Nausea
- Vomiting
- Balance problems or dizziness
- Blurry or double vision
- Sensitivity to light or noise
- Any change in the individual's behavior, thinking, or physical functioning

A common and sometimes dangerous misconception exists that a loss of consciousness always accompanies a concussion. It is important that personal trainers diligently watch for other symptoms after a possible brain injury, such as a vacant stare, delayed verbal or motor responses, increased sensitivity to light or sound, irritability, **depression,** poor coordination, fatigue, sleep disturbances, and loss of sense of taste or smell. Another disturbing misconception is the notion that if loss of consciousness does not occur, the concussion is minor and the athlete or client can safely return to the activity. It is essential that trainers understand that no concussion is ever minor.

For days or weeks after a concussion, there might be a number of symptoms still present, such as a mild headache and the inability to focus or concentrate (Mellion et al., 2003). Individuals who experience any concussion symptoms should be kept from activity until given permission to return by a healthcare professional with experience in evaluating for concussion. A repeat concussion that occurs before the brain recovers from the first can slow recovery or increase the likelihood of having long-term problems.

For any head trauma, the personal trainer should check the ABCs and start CPR if necessary. It is always prudent to assume there is a spinal injury until it can be ruled out, so the personal trainer must not try to move the victim. If the person can talk, check his or her level of consciousness by asking questions such as the victim's name, where he or she is, and what happened. Look for unequal pupil size, as that might indicate a serious head trauma.

Depending on how the head trauma occurred, individuals who suffer concussions may need to get additional medical attention for other possible injuries (Lillegard, Butcher, & Rucker, 1999):

- For any injury close to the eye area, it is essential that the victim get an evaluation from an ophthalmologist.

- For nasal injuries, the victim should be checked for damage to the nasal septum.
- If a tooth becomes avulsed (i.e., knocked out), the trainer should keep it clean and place it in milk or salt water, or have the victim keep the tooth in the cheek area and see a dentist immediately to re-implant it. A root canal might be required two to three weeks afterward.

Neck and Back Injuries

The most common neck injuries are cervical strains and sprains. A cervical strain is due to overstretching of the neck musculature, such as the paraspinals, upper trapezeius, and sternocleidomastoids. Similarly, cervical sprains can happen when ligaments are stretched beyond their capacities (Lillegard, Butcher, & Rucker, 1999). Although they may be more severe than strains, sprains have similar causes and symptoms (Anderson, Hall, & Martin, 2000). They can range from grade I (mild) to grade III (severe), depending on ligament laxity. Pain and stiffness are the usual symptoms, along with a decreased **range of motion.** To relieve spasm, ice massage for eight to 10 minutes is recommended. Symptoms may take a few days to a week to disappear. For these injuries, exercise is not recommended unless there is a pain-free range of motion and clearance to exercise has been provided by a doctor. Medical treatment might require the person to wear a cervical collar for six to 12 weeks if necessary (Lillegard, Butcher, & Rucker, 1999).

A "stinger" is a sharp burning pain down the arm after a head or shoulder injury. Short-term loss of arm function might accompany this injury. Symptoms usually last for five to 15 minutes. If they last any longer, medical treatment is recommended (Vaccaro, 2003).

Spine Injuries

The uppermost part of the spinal column, the cervical spine, is located in the neck and made up of seven cervical vertebrae (Figure 16-8). This part of the spinal cord is the most mobile and delicate, and the most likely to become injured. Some situations where a neck injury might occur are when a person falls from a height or sustains trauma to the face or head, such as in a diving or sports-related accident (Mistovich & Karren, 2008).

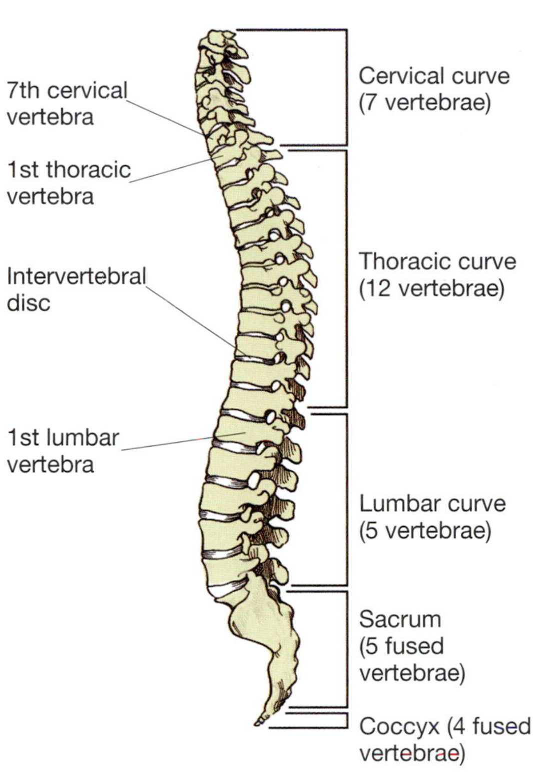

Figure 16-8
Vertebral column (lateral view)

When a neck injury is suspected, it is important that further damage is prevented. The victim should not be moved and the head must be immobilized until EMS professionals arrive. The personal trainer can check the ABCs. In an unconscious victim, open the airway with the jaw thrust method instead of the head tilt–chin lift (see Figures 16-2 and 16-3). If the person can talk, the trainer should instruct him or her to look straight ahead and *not* try to follow the trainer with his or her eyes when talking to keep the head as still as possible (Vaccaro, 2003). Damage to the spinal cord may interfere with the phrenic nerve's signals to the diaphragm, which interferes with breathing, so the personal trainer must be aware of possible respiratory distress or failure. Manual in-line stabilization (holding the head still as shown in Figure 16-9) should be done until EMS rescuers can strap the person to a backboard (Mistovich & Karren, 2008). The personal trainer should continue monitoring the victim until help arrives.

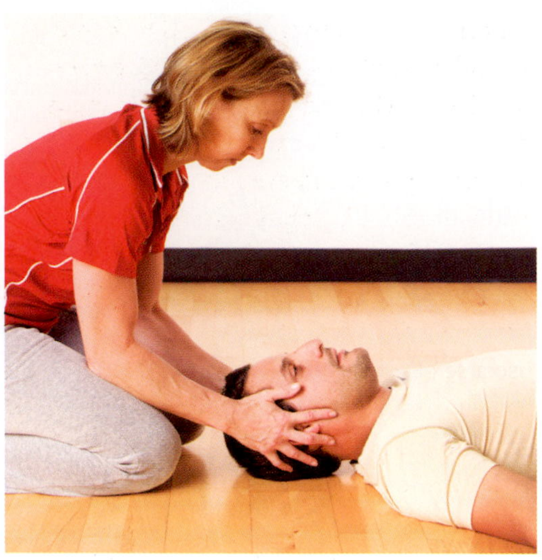

Figure 16-9
Immobilization of the head and neck: Kneel at the victim's head, placing the hands on either side of the head and neck, and hold them firmly in place. Keep the victim quiet and prevent movement of the head. Do not try to reposition the victim.

The middle part of the spinal column, the thoracic spine, is made up of 12 vertebrae of the upper back that allow **flexion, extension,** and **rotation** (see Figure 16-8). There are four normal curves of the spine (cervical, thoracic, lumbar, and sacral). The curve of the thoracic spine is **kyphotic,** which means that it curves posteriorly as a rounding of the upper back. An increase of this curvature has been called "swimmer's back" because swimming (especially the butterfly stroke) can cause this curve to become exaggerated due to the development of tight pectoral muscles. Similarly, weight trainers who overtrain the pectorals and do not adequately train the back muscles can develop this postural deviation (Anderson, Hall, & Martin, 2000).

The lower back, or lumbar spine, is made up of five vertebrae that allow flexion, extension, and side bending (see Figure 16-8). The **lordotic** curve of the lumbar spine curves anteriorly, making the low back curve into **hyperextension.** An example of an exaggerated lumbar curve can be seen in many gymnasts, for whom movements often require hyperextension of the back. Weak abdominal muscles and poor posture can also contribute to this excessive curvature, as does as a forward pelvic tilt. Altering any of these natural curves of the spine can interfere with load transfer between the upper and lower extremities and cause injury or low-back pain. A herniated disk, or a bulging of the fibrocartilaginous sac in between vertebrae, can cause burning pain, weakness, numbness, and tingling due to nerve compression. These commonly occur in the lumbar spine, most often between the fourth and fifth lumbar vertebrae (L4 and L5) or the fifth lumbar and first sacral vertebrae (L5 and S1). Treatment is determined by the severity of the injury (Anderson, Hall, & Martin, 2000; Lillegard, Butcher, & Rucker, 1999).

Low-back pain is estimated to affect 80% of the adult population at some point in their lives and is one of the leading causes of disability and missed work time (Lillegard, Butcher, & Rucker, 1999). Runners are likely to suffer from low-back pain because of their tendency to have tight hip flexors and hamstrings. These both act to tilt the pelvis anteriorly and to increase the lordotic curve of the lumbar spine. To reduce the likelihood of low-back pain, runners (and personal trainers) should be sure to include flexibility exercises for the hip flexors and hamstrings and be conservative when increasing distance and speed. Tension develops in the muscles surrounding the lumbar spine to counteract the body's tendency to lean forward, especially when running. Runners also might experience another type of lumbar injury—low-back muscle strain. This injury can occur when the runner overstrides, making this area susceptible to hyperextension (Lillegard, Butcher, & Rucker, 1999).

Personal trainers should teach their clients proper lifting technique to avoid low-back strains: keeping objects close to the body, bending at the knees while keeping the back straight, and contracting the abdominal and leg muscles to assist with the lift. It is a good idea to avoid simultaneous bending and twisting movements while lifting heavy weight and to exhale during the lift. Lifting weights with a slow, controlled motion is best to lower the compression and shear force on the spine and decrease the tension in the paraspinal muscles. Finally, good posture should be maintained when doing all **activities of daily living (ADL),** including sitting, standing, and walking, to avoid chronic strains or sprains (Anderson, Hall, & Martin, 2000).

Shock

Shock, also known as **hypoperfusion,** occurs when blood is not adequately distributed in the body and tissues do not receive the oxygen and nutrients needed for proper function and survival. There are four major types of shock: hypovolemic, obstructive, distributive, and cardiogenic. Hypovolemic shock occurs when fluid, such as blood, is lost as a result of severe dehydration or from severe internal or external bleeding. This should be suspected in any trauma victim who may be internally bleeding or when a person has lost a lot of blood from an open wound. Obstructive shock occurs when a blood clot or other mechanical obstruction does not allow blood to reach the heart. Distributive shock occurs when vessels are dilated and not allowing normal blood distribution. This can be due to a spinal or head injury, an allergy such as a bee sting or food allergy, or toxins from a severe infection. Cardiogenic shock is the inadequate function of the heart resulting from heart attack or coronary artery disease (Mistovich & Karren, 2008).

The signs and symptoms of shock are restlessness; anxiety; altered mental status; pale, cool, and clammy skin; fast and weak pulse; irregular breathing; nausea; and thirst. Shock is a serious condition that requires immediate medical attention. The personal trainer should check the ABCs and control severe bleeding. If there is no trauma to the lower body, it is important to elevate the victim's legs 8 to 12 inches (20 to 30 cm). It is also a good idea to cover the victim with a blanket, because shock decreases the ability to regulate body temperature, and the person may feel cold (Mistovich & Karren, 2008).

Universal Precautions and Protection Against Bloodborne Pathogens

Due to the threat of communicable disease, it is necessary to take universal precautions when dealing with another other person's blood or body fluids. The bloodborne pathogens of the most concern are **hepatitis B** and HIV. Rescuers should wear gloves, use a protective barrier device when performing CPR, and, if there is potential for blood to splash on the rescuer, a gown and eye protection should also be worn. To dispose of anything that touched blood or body fluid, use biohazard bags if they are available and be sure to properly seal them. If they are not available, use a sealable plastic bag. Do not toss these bags in the trash. Instead, dispose of them according to company policy or give them to trained emergency personnel. Make sure that all first-aid kits include latex gloves. All rescuers should wash their hands with soap and warm water for at least 10 to 15 seconds afterward, whether or not gloves were worn. Hand washing is the best way to prevent the spread of disease (AHA, 2006).

Hepatitis B and C are transmitted more easily than HIV. Hepatitis can be transmitted by drug injection, contact with mucous membranes or broken (non-intact) areas of skin, or possibly by casual contact such as living in close quarters with someone who is a hepatitis B carrier (Mellion et al., 2003).

HIV Infection and Exercise

Those infected with HIV are encouraged to be active and even participate in sports. There is very low risk to the other participants. As long as the infected person is healthy and asymptomatic, the disease can be managed better when he or she stays active, and the individual will have better overall health and quality of life. Some research has even found that exercise can slow the progression of the disease (Mustafa et al., 1999). Infected individuals should not exercise to a point of exhaustion and should discontinue competition when CD4 counts are below 500. CD4 cells, also known as T4 or T-Helper cells, are a type of white blood cell that fight infection. Normal ranges for healthy individuals are usually 500 to 1500. As HIV progresses, CD4 counts decrease, and with treatment the number increases. At a CD4 count of less than 200, a person infected with HIV is considered to have **acquired immunodeficiency syndrome (AIDS)** (American Association of Clinical Chemistry, 2005). When AIDS is diagnosed, the person can continue to stay active but should exercise only as symptoms allow (Mellion et al., 2003).

According to the CDC, there are no documented cases of HIV being transmitted during participation in sports. The very low risk of transmission during sports participation would involve sports with direct body contact in which bleeding might be expected to occur. Because most transmissions occur with deep hollow-bore needle sticks, transmission is very unlikely to occur during exercise (Mellion et al., 2003) and sweat has not been found to contain HIV (CDC, 2007). Universal precautions do not apply to sweat, tears, saliva, urine, and nasal sputum unless blood is visible (CDC, 1996). If someone is bleeding, his or her participation in the sport should be interrupted until the wound stops bleeding and is both antiseptically cleaned and securely bandaged. According to the CDC, there is no risk of HIV transmission through sports activities where bleeding does not occur.

Summary

Fitness facilities can better serve their members and avoid possible emergency situations by having a risk-management plan and maintaining a well-stocked first-aid kit. Although the diagnosis and treatment of injuries is outside of the scope of practice of a personal trainer, all personal trainers should have a knowledge and understanding of possible medical emergencies that can arise during the course of a career in the fitness industry. Personal trainers should learn to recognize medical emergencies and know when it is necessary to activate EMS. By staying current in first aid, CPR, and AED, a personal trainer just may save a person's life.

References

American Academy of Orthopedic Surgeons (2006). *First Aid and CPR* (5th ed.). Sudbury, Mass.: Jones and Bartlett.

American Association of Clinical Chemistry (2005). *CD4 Count.* www.labtestsonline.org/understanding/analytes/cd4/sample.html

American Cancer Society (2008). *Cancer Facts and Figures 2008.* Atlanta, Ga.: American Cancer Society.

American College of Sports Medicine (2007). *ACSM's Health/Fitness Facility Standards and Guidelines* (3rd ed.). Champaign, Ill.: Human Kinetics.

American Diabetes Association (2004). Hyperglycemic crises in diabetes. *Diabetes Care,* 27 (suppl. 1), s94–s102.

American Diabetes Association (2003). Hypoglycemia in diabetes. *Diabetes Care,* 26, 6, 1902–1912.

American Heart Association (2008a). *Heart Disease and Stroke Statistics—2008 Update.* Dallas, Tex.: American Heart Association.

American Heart Association (2008b). *About Diabetes.* www.americanheart.org/print_presenter.jhtml?identifier=3044757

American Heart Association (2006). *Heartsaver First Aid with CPR and AED Student Workbook.* Dallas, Tex.: American Heart Association.

Anderson, M., Hall, S.J., & Martin, M. (2000). *Sports Injury Management* (2nd ed.). Media, Pa.: Williams & Wilkins.

Aufderheide, T. et al. (2006). Community lay rescuer automated external defibrillator programs. *Circulation,* 113, 1260–1270.

Balady, G.J. et al. (1998). AHA/ACSM Scientific Statement: Recommendations for cardiovascular screening, staffing, and emergency policies at health/fitness facilities. *Circulation,* 97, 2283–2293.

Bohm K. et al. (2007). Survival is similar after standard treatment and chest compression only in out-of-hospital bystander cardiopulmonary resuscitation. *Circulation,* 116, 25, 2908–2912.

Canadian Fitness Matters (2004). *Canadian Fitness Safety Standards.* www.canadianfitnessmatters.ca/cf_standards.aro

Caris, E.E., Ramirez, A.M., & Van Durme, D.J. (2004). Heat illness in athletes: The dangerous combination of heat, humidity, and exercise. *Sports Medicine,* 34, 1, 9–16.

Casa, D.J. et al. (2000). National Athletic Trainers' Association: Position statement: Fluid replacement for athletes. *Journal of Athletic Training,* 35, 212–224.

Centers for Disease Control and Prevention (2007). *HIV and Its Transmission.* www.cdc.gov/hiv/resources/factsheets/transmission.htm

Centers for Disease Control and Prevention (2006). *Skin Cancer Questions and Answers.* www.cdc.gov/cancer/skin/chooseyourcover/qanda.htm#how

Centers for Disease Control and Prevention (1996). *Universal Precautions for Prevention of Transmission of HIV and Other Bloodborne Infections.* www.cdc.gov/ncidod/dhqp/bp_universal_precautions.html

Dixon, J.B. & O'Brien, P.E. (2002). Health outcomes of severely obese type 2 diabetic subjects 1 year after laparoscopic adjustable gastric banding. *Diabetes Care,* 25, 358–363.

Epilepsy Foundation (2009). *About Epilepsy.* www.epilepsyfoundation.org/about/firstaid/

Gonzales, L. & Lino, K. (2008). Workplace teamwork saves lives. *Currents in Cardiovascular Care,* Winter, 3.

Gulve, E.A. (2008). Exercise and glycemic control in diabetes: Benefits, challenges, and adjustment to pharmacotherapy. *Physical Therapy,* 88, 11, 1297–1321.

Helmrich, S.P. et al. (1994). Prevention of non-insulin-dependent diabetes mellitus with physical activity. *Medicine & Science in Sports & Exercise,* 26, 7, 824–830.

Helmrich, S.P. et al. (1991). Physical activity and reduced occurrence of non-insulin-dependent diabetes mellitus. *New England Journal of Medicine,* 325, 147–152.

Herlitz, J. et al. (2005). Efficacy of bystander CPR: Intervention by lay people and health care professionals. *Resuscitation,* 66, 3, 291–295.

Holcomb, W.R. (2005). Duration of cryotherapy application. *Athletic Therapy Today,* 10, 1, 60–62.

Iwami T. et al. (2007). Effectiveness of bystander-initiated cardiac-only resuscitation for patients with out-of-hospital cardiac arrest. *Circulation,* 116, 25, 2900–2907.

Lillegard, W.A., Butcher, J.D., & Rucker, K.S. (1999). *Handbook of Sports Medicine: A Symptom-Oriented Approach.* Stoneham, Ma.: Butterworth-Heinemann.

Mellion, M.B. et al. (2003). *Sports Medicine Secrets* (3rd ed.). Philadelphia, Pa.: Hanley and Belfus.

Miller, M.G. et al (2005). National Athletic Trainer's Association Position Statement: Management of asthma in athletes. *Journal of Athletic Training,* 40, 3, 224–245.

Mistovich, J.J. & Karren, K.J. (2008). *Prehospital Emergency Care* (8th ed.). Upper Saddle River, N.J.: Pearson Education.

Moore, L.K. (2008). *Emergency Communications: The Future of 911.* CRS Report for Congress.

Mustafa, T. et al. (1999). Association between exercise and HIV disease progression in a cohort of homosexual men. *Annals of Epidemiology,* 9, 2, 127–131.

Nagao K. et al. (2007). Cardiopulmonary resuscitation by bystanders with chest compression only (SOS-KANTO): An observational study. *Lancet,* 369, 920–926.

Nichol, G. et al. (1999). A cumulative meta-analysis of the effectiveness of defibrillator-capable emergency medical services for victims of out-of-hospital cardiac arrest. *Annals of Emergency Medicine,* 34, 517–525.

Parsons, J.P. & Mastronarde, J.G. (2005). Exercise-induced bronchioconstriction in athletes. *Chest,* 128, 6, 3966–3974.

Saglimbeni, A.J. (2007). *Exercise-induced Asthma: Treatment & Medication.* www.emedicine.medscape.com/article/88849-treatment

San Diego Fire-Rescue Department (2008). *What is 9-1-1?* The City of San Diego. www.sandiego.gov/fire-andems/911/whatis911.shtml

Sayre, M.R. et al. (2008). Hands-only (compression-only) cardiopulmonary resuscitation: A call to action for bystander response to adults who experience out-of-hospital sudden cardiac arrest: A science advisory for the public from the American Heart Association Emergency Cardiovascular Care Committee. *Circulation,* 117, 2162–2167.

Schenck, R.C. (Ed.). (2005). *Athletic Training and Sports Medicine* (4th ed.). Rosemont, Ill.: American Academy of Orthopedic Surgeons.

The Stroke Collaborative (2008). *Give Me Five for Stroke*. www.giveme5forstroke.org

Swor, R. et al. (2006). CPR training and CPR performance: Do CPR-trained bystanders perform CPR? *Academy of Emergency Medicine,* 13, 6, 596–601.

Vaccaro, A.R. (2003). Acute cervical spine injuries in the athlete: Diagnosis, management, and return-to-play. *International Sports Medicine Journal,* 4, 1, 1–9.

Suggested Reading

American Academy of Orthopedic Surgeons (2009). *Sports First Aid and Injury Prevention*. Sudbury, Mass.: Jones and Bartlett.

American Council on Exercise (2010). *ACE's Essentials of Exercise Science for Fitness Professionals.* San Diego, Calif.: American Council on Exercise.

American Council on Exercise (2009). *ACE Advanced Health and Fitness Specialist Manual*. San Diego, Calif.: American Council on Exercise.

Bahr, R. & Maehlum, S. (2004). *Clinical Guide to Sports Injuries,* Champaign, Ill.: Human Kinetics.

Carline, J.D. et al. (2004). *Mountaineering First Aid: A Guide to Accident Response and First Aid Care.* Seattle, Wash.: The Mountaineers Books.

Flegel, M.J. (1997). *Sport First Aid.* Champaign Ill.: Human Kinetics.

Wilmore, J.H., Costill, D., & Kenney, W.L. (2008). *Physiology of Sport and Exercise* (4th ed.). Champaign, Ill.: Human Kinetics.

PART IV

Professional and Legal Responsibilities and Business Strategies

Chapter 17
Legal Guidelines and Professional Responsibilities

Chapter 18
Personal-training Business Fundamentals

IN THIS CHAPTER:

Business Structure
- Sole Proprietorships
- Partnerships
- Corporations

Independent Contractors versus Employees

Contracts

Negligence

Vicarious Liability

Agreements to Participate, Informed Consent, and Waivers
- Agreement to Participate
- Informed Consent
- Inherent Risks
- Procedures

Legal Responsibilities
- Facilities
- Equipment
- Supervision
- Instruction
- Safety Guidelines

Scope of Practice

Liability Insurance
- Employees and Independent Contractors

Other Business Concerns With Legal Implications
- Marketing Activities
- Intellectual Property
- Transportation
- Financing

Risk Management

Summary

MARK S. NAGEL, ED.D., *teaches in the Sport and Entertainment Management Department at the University of South Carolina. Dr. Nagel has published extensively in a variety of areas of sport management, including law, finance, and marketing. Prior to becoming a professor, Dr. Nagel worked in campus recreation and intercollegiate athletics.*

CHAPTER 17

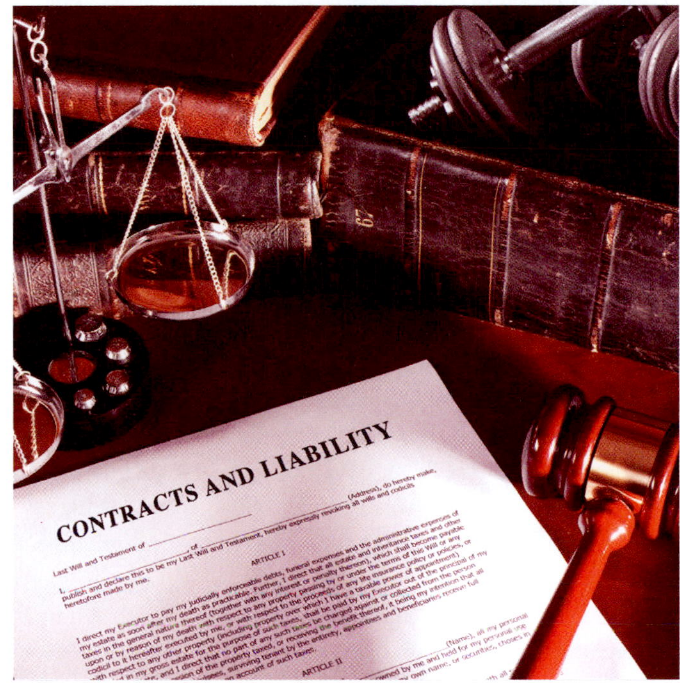

Legal Guidelines and Professional Responsibilities

Mark S. Nagel

Personal trainers typically do not need to be reminded of the importance of studying the latest research related to strength training, flexibility enhancement, cardiovascular fitness, and nutrition. Most personal trainers know that it is essential to spend considerable time and energy developing exercise programs to help clients achieve their goals. However, the majority of personal trainers often neglect the legal issues pertinent to operating a fitness business. Far too often, filed lawsuits are the first indication that a personal trainer has not adhered to established legal guidelines. In the vast majority of these cases, a simple understanding of the law and a trainer's responsibilities could have prevented the lawsuit or mitigated the potential damages.

This chapter addresses many of the standard legal and business concerns that personal trainers may have regarding business structure, employment status, **contracts,** insurance, and **risk management.** It also describes the **scope of practice** in personal training and summarizes legal responsibilities. The guidelines offered, while based on sport law and the experience of fitness professionals, are not intended as legal advice, but rather as guidance. Every personal trainer should utilize these principles when conferring with attorneys who specialize in the appropriate areas. As a personal trainer's knowledge of the law increases, the ability to anticipate potential legal concerns is heightened, which not only helps to decrease potential litigation, but also provides a better environment for clients, vendors, and **employees.** Ideally, personal trainers will regularly consult with an attorney who is aware of the unique laws governing the trainer's city, county, and state to remain abreast of recent legal developments. In addition, personal trainers should diligently read publications and attend conference presentations that address legal issues, as the **standards of care** and accepted business practices can be altered through legislation or case law.

Business Structure

Much of the personal-training industry is made up of entrepreneurs—individuals who undertake new financial ventures. Many personal trainers start their careers as an offshoot of their own physical training. New personal trainers often begin by working with close friends and family members before expanding their businesses to a greater assortment of clients. Most personal trainers, like many entrepreneurs in other industries, do not realize that the moment they begin providing advice in exchange for financial considerations they have created a business. Every business "owner," even one who is working part-time in a "hobby," should understand the ramifications of business structure.

Each personal trainer must decide the type of business structure under which he or she will operate. Each type retains certain legal and financial advantages and disadvantages. The size and scope of the business—both in the short- and long-term—will be important factors in the initial selection of the business entity. The business can be altered if conditions warrant, but personal trainers must understand that legal issues arising at a time when one structure was utilized cannot simply be mitigated by then switching to a different structure. The business entity employed at the time of the incident will usually be utilized by the courts in the event of a lawsuit. Typically, for-profit businesses* operate under one of the following structures: **sole proprietorship, partnership,** or **corporation.**

Sole Proprietorships

The vast majority of for-profit businesses in the United States operate as sole proprietorships. As the name implies, a sole proprietorship is a business owned and operated by one person. Since the individual owner operates the business, extensive meetings to determine strategy and company direction are not necessary, as the owner can simply make decisions. Creating a sole proprietorship does not require any formal paperwork, and there is minimal ongoing paperwork necessary (compared to other business types) to sustain the business. It exists as long as the owner operates the business, and profits from the business belong to the owner. However, financial losses and liabilities are also the sole responsibility of the owner. In a sole proprietorship there is no **corporate veil** that shields the actions of the business from the personal responsibility of the owner, even if the owner conducts business under a different company name. Delinquent debts and successful lawsuits against the business

*Though this chapter primarily focuses on for-profit businesses, there are government-operated businesses as well as non-profit organizations that operate with different legal and financial constraints. Even though a personal trainer may be training a client at a government-operated business (e.g., a community recreation center) or a non-profit organization (e.g., a YMCA fitness center), the personal trainer may retain a different business structure for liability purposes. Personal trainers should consult legal counsel prior to training any client.

can result in the owner being required to sell personal assets to pay the judgment. Personal training involves extensive physical movement, which often results in injuries even when proper techniques are utilized. The likelihood of injuries results in a greater opportunity for clients to potentially seek financial remuneration. One successful lawsuit against a sole proprietor could not only financially destroy the business, but also the owner's personal finances, as courts have often required sole proprietors to sell assets, including their homes, to pay for incurred debts.

There are other potential drawbacks to operating a personal-training business as a sole proprietorship. Since the business is owned by one individual, it can be more difficult to raise capital. In addition, though sole proprietorships may certainly hire employees, often the business cannot effectively function without the presence of the owner. Most personal trainers individually work with all of their clients, so if the owner takes a vacation, incoming revenue is potentially decreased. In addition, newly established personal trainers often maintain consistent contact with their clients to ensure that they do not have any reason to seek other potential trainers. This can create difficulties if the personal trainer is sick or has to attend to an emergency.

Partnerships

Two or more people who agree to operate a business and share profits and losses may form a partnership. Two personal trainers, for example, could form a company, or a trainer could become part owner of a fitness facility. Although partnerships may be created without filing paperwork, *any* partnership should have legal documents that establish the rules of operation. This agreement should clearly define and explain the structure for authority, the partners' rights, expected performance and contributions from each partner, buy-out clauses, income distribution, and responsibility for debts. Operating a partnership without a partnership agreement—even when it involves family members or close personal friends—is asking for potential disaster. Even partnerships that begin based on strong relationships can become strained as the business develops. Furthermore, even if the partners maintain a solid personal or professional relationship, other non-business-related occurrences can cause tremendous stress on the company. If one partner becomes divorced or deceased, other family members may become involved in the ownership and operation of the partnership. In extreme cases, the lack of a partnership agreement can result in the courts requiring the business to be dissolved to settle financial disputes. Partnership paperwork should be designed to address any eventuality, including the death or incapacity of one of the partners.

As potential partners plan and design their business, the type of partnership utilized should be identified. **General partnerships** are merely the joining of two or more individuals to own and operate a business. A general-partnership agreement could divide ownership equally or unequally. Most attorneys will advise against operating a business as a 50-50 partnership, even if it involves owners from the same family. A 50-50 partnership can result in a stalemate, because neither partner can institute policy without the permission of the other, since business decisions must be approved by a majority (50.1%) of the owners. However, disproportionate ownership positions in partnerships can also present problems for the **minority partner** or partners. If a two-person partnership is owned with a 60-40 split, the minority partner is only entitled to 40% of the profits and retains only 40% input regarding company decisions. That particular partner could be out-voted on any organizational issue. Some investors in partnerships who will take a minority position are not as likely to invest as much money as they would if they received operating control.

General partnerships can be established either formally or informally. An **express partnership** can be created by a contract between the parties. However, an **implied partnership** can be created and recognized by the judicial system if individuals act as partners (such as by sharing a company checking account or jointly signing for a business loan). It is critical that owners understand the consequences of their actions when operating a business, as the courts will likely examine the activities of the owners when determining potential liabilities if there is no clearly defined partnership agreement.

A partnership retains the same potential detriments as a sole proprietorship. Personal **liability** for company losses or judgments is retained by the partners. In some cases, minority partners may be personally liable for a greater share of the companies' liabilities than their percentage of ownership. If a partner who owns 55% of a business files for bankruptcy, a judgment against the business may result in the minority partner being required to cover the financial obligation of the insolvent general partner, even though the minority partner owns only 45% of the company. For this reason, some partnerships involve **limited partners.** While a general partner typically retains personal liability, limited partners are only liable for their direct financial contribution. However, in exchange for this limited liability, limited partners do not retain any formal managerial input regarding the operation of the business. Limited partners must also remember that the general partner or partners still retain personal liability and they should ensure that a judgment or other financial loss will not bankrupt the general partners, and hence the overall company. It is important to note that limited partners may retain more than 50% of the ownership in the company. For example, a limited partner who owns 70% of the organization still does not have any formal input into the companies' operation, but is entitled to 70% of the companies' profits.

At some point in a personal trainer's career, decisions regarding partnerships are likely to be contemplated. As personal trainers expand their client base, it may become difficult to organize a time for individual face-to-face interaction with each client. The trainer could elect to hire an employee or find a partner who could alleviate some concerns if multiple clients desire to work out at the same time. Personal training also involves marketing and advertising, as well as scheduling clients. Some personal trainers have entered into partnership agreements where one partner does the "hands-on" training while the other coordinates the "office" activities. These particular types of partnerships are especially prone to problems, as one partner may not understand or fully appreciate the importance of the other partner's duties and activities. Ultimately, any potential partnership can become contentious and should not be entered into without considerable contemplation, and only after seeking individualized legal advice.

A partnership ends when a partner dies or becomes bankrupt, or its partners engage in any illegal activity. A partnership could also be discontinued by the courts if one of the partners is deemed to be mentally incapacitated. One difficulty that sometimes arises when terminating partnerships is if the business is not making any money. Ultimately, if the business cannot make any money, the partnership will be dissolved. However, in some cases, one or more partners may have differing opinions about the future financial viability of the company. If one or more partners wish to continue the business, but one or more other partners do not, a resolution must occur. In many cases, these split decisions regarding continuing the business will require court intervention to dissolve the partnership or to determine how, and at what compensation, one or more partners may exit.

Though sole proprietorships and partnerships offer potential problems due to personal liability for the business' actions, they usually provide potential benefits from **flow-through taxation.** Typically, profits are taxed at lower personal rates rather than higher corporate rates. In addition, yearly losses can flow-through to be used by the owner to offset profits from other income. Potential investors, who will be providing money rather than day-to-day labor, will often desire to take a position as a limited partner in a business. The limited partnership protects them from personal liability (beyond their initial investment), but allows them to have a low tax rate on profits if the business is successful, or to use the losses during poorly performing periods to offset income from other investments.

Corporations

Corporations are designed to create a "separate" entity from the investors and operators of a business. Regulated by state and federal (and in some cases international) laws, corporations exist as distinct legal entities. Investors own shares of the corporation, which limits the investors' personal liability. As long as the corporation and the investors maintain "separate" existences, the corporate veil protects investors from personal liability. It is critical that investors in a corporation do not "act" as the corporation, or the corporate veil may be pierced. For example, if an investor mixes his personal checking account with that of the corporation, he or she may be deemed by the courts to be acting as the corporation and therefore be personally liable for potential corporate debts and judgments.

Forming and maintaining a corporation is much more burdensome than a sole proprietorship or partnership. Corporations are formed and registered in the office of the secretary of state (typically in the state where the business operates). Different states have various requirements, so a corporation that will operate in multiple states must determine the "best" state for short- and long-term operation. A person forming a corporation must select a name that has not previously been registered in that state. The appropriate notice of incorporation forms must be completed, fees must be paid, and a registered agent must be identified. The registered agent is the contact person in the event a lawsuit is filed against the corporation. Typically, it is one of the corporation's founders or it may be an attorney who represents the corporation. It is important that the person "registered" as the agent for the corporation be readily accessible. After being notified of a lawsuit, the registered agent must notify personnel to take appropriate action. In some cases, the registered agent must be a resident of the state in which the corporation operates. The secretary of state's office can help individuals complete the appropriate paperwork, but some entrepreneurs seek legal guidance to diminish the time and potential aggravation of incorporating.

Once the incorporation is complete, the corporation is recognized as a distinct legal entity. The shareholders will elect a board of directors who in turn will hire the executive management team. In cases where there are few shareholders in the corporation, such as when the corporation is first created, investors may fill all of the corporate positions. Once established, the company must annually complete and file operational paperwork with the state, and it also must file tax returns with appropriate local, state, and federal governments.

There are a variety of corporate structures and potential types of shareholders (e.g., preferred, common), and any personal trainer who is considering forming a corporation should seek legal advice to ensure that the proper corporate entity is created for both short- and long-term plans. Corporations can change their form, but this can require considerable time and may involve extensive (and costly) paperwork. In general, some of the main corporate structures include **subchapter S-corporations**, **limited liability corporations (LLCs)**, **limited liability partnerships (LLPs)**, and **C-corporations**, as well as franchise operation business models.

Subchapter S-Corporations

The main financial advantage of subchapter S-corporations (often called sub-S corps or simply S-corps) is that profits flow through the business to the shareholders and are taxed as ordinary income. S-corps are the most "typical" type of corporation used by personal-training businesses that do not operate as a sole proprietorship or partnership.

Shareholders in S-corps are shielded from personal liability—beyond their investment—by the corporate veil. S-corps can own subsidiaries that operate independently (from a legal standpoint), which enables the S-corp to be shielded from liability. S-corps do have some significant drawbacks, particularly if the business is going to grow and seek a wide variety of investors. S-corps must be based in the United States, can only have up to 100 total investors, and all of the investors must be from the United States. An S-corp can only issue one form of stock, meaning that every share must have the same voting rights and dividend allotments. Many businesses that do not anticipate having a large diversified ownership structure or operating in other countries choose to be incorporated as S-corps.

Limited Liability Corporations and Limited Liability Partnerships

Forming and operating a subchapter S-corporation requires extensive paperwork and attention to detail. For this reason, many small business owners have chosen to operate as LLCs or LLPs. An LLC or LLP operates in many ways like a subchapter S-corporation. Profits flow through to the investors and are taxed as ordinary income. The LLC and LLP also provide a corporate veil against personal liability. However, LLCs and LLPs typically can be established by filing simple paperwork in the state where the LLC/LLP will initially operate. Forms for taxes are also much easier to fill out and file than those for a subchapter S-corporation. However, unlike S-corps, which have been in existence for many decades, there are not any national standards regarding the operation of LLCs or LLPs, which are relatively new business entities. Individual states govern LLCs/LLPs in a variety of ways. In some states, the rules regarding LLCs/LLPs have been determined through legislative or judicial action. However, rules and operating procedures have not been firmly established in all states. In addition, some states have different laws regarding taxes owed by the owners of LLCs/LLPs. It is critical that investors seek financial and legal advice regarding the formation and operation of LLCs/LLPs. As consistent guidelines regarding LLCs and LLPs are established, they will likely become the preferred operating structures for personal trainers, as they combine the limited liability and flow-through taxation of the S-corp with easier creation and operation requirements.

C-Corporations

It is highly unlikely that most personal trainers will ever create a subchapter C-corporation (often called C-corporations or C-corps). Many, though not all, of the 500 largest companies in the United States operate as C-corps. The primary reason is that C-corps are structured in a manner that allows the company to seek investors and conduct business activities around the world. A company wishing to operate as a C-corp must annually file extensive paperwork in their home state and in countries where they conduct business. Companies classified as C-corps retain the corporate veil that protects investors from company liability. However, unlike an S-corp, C-corps are taxed as a company first and then any profits that are remaining may be provided to shareholders. Since the shareholders must then pay taxes on their dividends, C-corps are said to provide **double taxation.** For example, owners of an S-corp that profited $100,000 would have that money flow-through to their personal taxes. If their individual tax rate were 35%, then they would pay a total tax of $35,000. However, if the company were operated as a C-corp, then the company would first pay taxes on the $100,000 profit. In this case, if the corporate tax rate is also 35%, then the corporation first pays $35,000 in tax, leaving $65,000. If the company were to then issue a dividend of the entire $65,000 to the owners, the owners would then be required to pay 35% tax on the $65,000 (or $22,750 in taxes). The owners would have a remaining profit of $42,250 ($65,000 – $22,750).

Companies organized as C-corps do not have limits on the number of potential shareholders. In addition, different classifications of stock may be issued, and stock can be sold to foreign nationals and institutional investors. In many cases, profitable companies operated as partnerships, LLCs, or S-corps may elect to change their classification to a C-corp. “Going public” enables the owner or owners to potentially generate a tremendous amount of money, but it also allows other investors to take a significant stake in the operation of the company. In some cases, prominent founders of companies have been “forced out” of their management position by other shareholders. The decision regarding the direction of the company is ultimately retained by the majority of shareholders. If one person (or group of people) holds 50.1% of the stock, then he or she has the power to set policies. In most cases, when a company goes public, no one owner retains more than 50.1% of the stock. Factions of stockholders must vote together to establish or alter company policies.

Personal trainers must contemplate the advantages and disadvantages of their business structure (Table 17-1). In most cases, consultation with an attorney who specializes in this area can assist not only in reducing potential liability, but also in mitigating potential tax payments. In addition, the proper business structure will enable the personal trainer to properly prepare to expand the business if necessary.

Franchise Operation Business Models

Personal-training studio franchise opportunities are another option for trainers looking to open their own fitness businesses. Owning and operating a franchise provides some of the advantages of both an independent operation and a multiple-facility operation. The franchising model is based on the principle that local business owners will have greater success connecting their facilities to the local communities and more commitment to making them successful if they have an ownership stake in the business. A franchisee (the owner of a franchise) has the right to use an established brand name, trademark, logo, and business model. These individuals benefit from being associated with a recognized brand and a central franchising organization that provides operational and marketing assistance. A franchisee can purchase a specific location or the rights to open a number of locations for a specific market. The expectation is that the franchisee will meet certain financial requirements to make an investment in an individual franchise. Most franchise operations charge an individual franchisee an upfront fee that can range up to $25,000 and annual fees of a percentage of revenue earned from the business. There are other costs associated with owning a franchise, including the cost of purchasing operational and retail products through the franchiser's business structure.

The advantages of owning and operating a franchise include:

- Obtaining the rights to a recognized brand name that will assist the personal trainer in creating a strong presence in a specific market
- Access to the business and operating systems created by the franchiser, such as floor plans, equipment layouts, discounts on equipment purchases, operating plans, and marketing information
- Access to national advertising programs and the ability to share costs associated with marketing and brand identity with other franchise owners

Table 17-1

Advantages and Disadvantages of Various Business Structures

Type	Advantages	Disadvantages
Sole proprietorship	Easily created and managed Flow-through taxation	Personal liability Raising capital
Partnership	Easily created Flow-through taxation	Potential management disputes Personal liability (except limited partners)
S-corps	Flow-through taxation Limited liability	Limited number of potential investors Costs of formation and operation
LLC/LLP	Flow-through taxation Limited liability	Undefined operating standards in states
C-corps	Limited liability Unlimited number of investors	Cost of formation and operation Double taxation

- The ability to control the business, as long as the needs and requirements of the parent franchise company are met
- Franchisers that will provide training and advice on all aspects of marketing and operating the business, since it is in their best interest for each individual franchisee to be successful

The disadvantages of owning and operating a franchise include:

- The upfront costs for the franchise fee and the ongoing costs to maintain the association with the parent brand of the franchise
- The annual costs of maintaining the franchise, which include making necessary purchases through the franchise system
- An association with a particular brand, which could be a drawback if other franchisees within the network perform badly or conduct unethical business practices
- The fact that the franchisee agrees to follow the franchise's operating model, which could limit the franchisee's ability to adapt to changing market forces

Independent Contractors versus Employees

Once the business structure has been identified and implemented, personal trainers need to address other legal concerns. Of particular note for the personal-training industry is the definition of an employee versus an **independent contractor.** Employees "regularly" work for their employer, while independent contractors typically are hired on a short-term basis to perform a specific task or series of tasks. Once the specific identified tasks are complete, the independent contractor is compensated and then is no longer needed. A classic example of an independent contractor occurs when a homeowner has a leaking sink. The homeowner identifies the problem, hires a plumber, and pays the plumber once the leak is fixed. The plumber does not have an *expectation* of consistent work. Alternatively, an employer–employee relationship is created when a business hires a plumber full-time to address ongoing problems. In this case, the plumber would report to work daily, take direction from the employer regarding tasks, and be compensated on a regular basis (weekly, biweekly, monthly) rather than at the completion of each job.

The classification of a worker as an independent contractor versus an employee has numerous ramifications. In most cases, employers are responsible to train and supervise their employees and to maintain records regarding their employees' work. Employers usually must also withhold and match the employees' FICA (Federal Insurance Contributions Act) taxes for Social Security and Medicare. The employer usually offers and pays for unemployment coverage, workers' compensation coverage, and medical benefits. These requirements typically consume a tremendous amount of time and financial resources. In addition, employers often must provide justification for firing an employee. Conversely, someone hiring an independent contractor simply negotiates the job and the final compensation, and the independent contractor completes the work. If the independent contractor does not complete the work to the payer's satisfaction, the independent contractor will likely not be rehired in the future.

Certainly, most businesses would like to operate by limiting the number of employees and maximizing the number of independent contractors they retain. The time and expense necessary to adhere to laws regarding employer–employee relationships has caused some businesses to attempt to utilize *only* independent contractors. However, simply *designating* someone an independent contractor does not necessarily mean that an individual is *acting* as an independent contractor. Some companies have been penalized by the government for improperly classifying an employee as an independent contractor to avoid their financial and administrative duties. Companies should ensure that they are properly classifying and utilizing independent contractors at all times.

The main criteria the judicial system will utilize when addressing a potential complaint regarding independent contractor status is "control." In most cases, if the hiring authority maintains control over the worker, an employer–employee relationship has likely been established. Court cases have investigated control in the following areas:

- *Work details:* Creating schedules, requiring specific materials to be utilized, and overseeing procedures typically indicate an employment relationship.
- *Payment:* Regularly scheduled payments typically indicate employment, while payment by the "job" indicates an independent-contractor relationship.
- *Length of relationship:* People hired for short periods of time (a few weeks or less) are typically independent contractors.
- *Training and retraining:* An independent contractor will typically require no initial or ongoing training from the hiring agency.
- *Equipment:* Independent contractors typically provide their own equipment.
- *Number of clients:* Employees typically work for only one employer. An independent contractor usually services multiple clients.
- *Nature of the work:* If the work provided is integral to the core function of the business, the person is more likely to be deemed an employee. In addition, if the work is *typically* performed by independent contractors, then the courts will usually utilize that in their determination.
- *Intention of the parties:* The intent of the parties is a factor, though certainly not the only or deciding factor, in the eventual classification.

It is important to note that each of these areas in and of itself will typically not be the sole criteria utilized by the courts when adjudicating a potential status dispute. The courts will examine the entire relationship and the extent to which the potential employer "control' is present.

There are multiple issues that personal trainers and business owners must consider regarding the classification or status of employees. In most cases, personal trainers act as independent contractors. Personal trainers typically do not have long-term commitments to their clients to perform services beyond the immediate future. In addition, personal trainers provide the expertise during the workout, with the client utilizing the trainer's guidance. However, since the majority of trainers will work with clients at an established fitness center, the relationship between the center and the trainer needs to be clearly defined. Unlike a plumber who brings tools to complete a job, personal trainers who work with clients at fitness centers typically do not provide their own equipment (unless they own the center). Another potential concern is the solicitation of clients. A personal trainer who brings clients to a fitness center is operating in a different environment than one who arrives at the center and trains whoever has signed up that day.

Even though a personal trainer who is an independent contractor will adhere to the fitness center's general rules, he or she should be able to:

- Choose when and where to work
- Charge variable fees for different situations
- Begin working without extensive guidance
- Maintain autonomy in training decisions

By comparison, a fitness center employee will adhere to the general and specific guidelines of the employer when providing services. In many cases, a personal trainer who operates as an independent contractor retains greater personal and financial risk, while an employee exchanges the potential risks and rewards for the security of being an employee.

Both independent contractors and employees must be certain that every detail of their agreement is clear from the beginning of their professional relationship with a fitness facility. Often, the legal nature of the relationship is ambiguous, and trainers have filed lawsuits attempting to collect worker's compensation or unemployment insurance from clubs that consider them independent contractors. Other trainers who assumed that they were employees have been forced to pay back taxes and penalties for neglected FICA responsibilities once they were identified by the government as independent contractors. Ultimately, it is the responsibility of all parties to clearly define the relationship and ensure that the actions of the fitness center and the personal trainer adhere to guidelines that govern the actions of independent contractors or employees.

Contracts

Contracts are the best method to ensure that all aspects of a relationship are properly established. Whether a trainer works as an independent contractor or an employee, the basic tenets of contract law should be understood. The following elements are necessary to create a binding contract:

- An offer and acceptance with a mutual agreement of terms
- Consideration (an exchange of valuable items, such as money for services)
- Legality (acceptable form under the law)
- Ability of the parties to enter into a contract with respect to legal age and mental capacity

For example, a personal trainer may talk to a prospective client and mention potential services, such as designing individualized exercise sessions. The trainer and client may agree on dates and times for specific workouts. This negotiation constitutes an offer and an acceptance. Stating a fee of $50 per hour for services establishes an exchange of consideration (i.e., training services for money). Once these negotiations are settled, the trainer should prepare a written contract by filling out a basic contract form or by having one specifically written for each agreement. Regardless of the type of form, legal counsel should be consulted to ensure that the written form is valid under contract law before it is utilized. This document becomes a valid contract when signed by both the trainer and the client, assuming both parties are of legal age to enter into contracts. Certainly, difficulty can arise if a minor seeks to retain a personal trainer's services. Since minors may not legally sign a contract, the trainer is retaining some risk in this situation. Having the parents sign the contract to perform services may mitigate, but not completely solve, this potential problem.

Some personal trainers who are starting a business may feel that written contracts are unnecessary and that a brief chat and a handshake are sufficient when negotiating agreements. In the case of scheduling clients, that is often the standard practice. However, a potential miscommunication or misunderstanding may result in some difficulties, as any oral contract is subject to misinterpretation by the involved parties, and therefore is potentially dangerous. In the event of an oral contract dispute necessitating legal intervention, conflicting stories may be settled in a courtroom without sufficient evidence to support the trainer's account of what transpired.

In addition to scheduling, written contracts should be utilized to establish payment terms before any session occurs. There should also be considerations for issues such as rescheduling, bounced checks, agreements to follow instructions and adhere to proper techniques, confidentiality, termination of the agreement, and other aspects critical to the session. Typically, a **waiver** (Figure 17-1) will be signed as a component of the initial contract. Refer to "Vicarious Liability" on page 604 for more information on the purpose and proper use of waivers.

Personal trainers should insist upon a written contract not only with clients, but also with fitness centers, vendors, and any other entities with which they conduct business. In any case in which the agreement involves real estate or goods or services worth $500 or more, or requires more than one year to complete, the **statute of frauds** requires that there be a written contract if the agreement is to be valid. The courts will not intervene in a potential oral contract dispute if the contract violates the statute of frauds—it will simply invalidate the agreement.

Using valid contracts can save businesses money and mitigate a tremendous amount of time and stress. Far too often, personal trainers neglect to understand the importance of operating with valid contracts. In addition, they often fail to thoroughly read and understand the contracts presented to them by fitness centers and other vendors. A visit to

I, ________________________________, through the purchase of training sessions, have agreed to voluntarily participate in an exercise program, including, but not limited to, strength training, flexibility development, and aerobic exercise, under the guidance of [name of personal trainer and/or business]. I hereby stipulate and agree that I am physically and mentally sound and currently have no physical conditions that would be aggravated by my involvement in an exercise program. I have provided verification from a licensed physician that I am able to undertake a general fitness-training program.

I understand and am aware that physical-fitness activities, including the use of equipment, are potentially hazardous activities. I am aware that participating in these types of activities, even when completed properly, can be dangerous. I agree to follow the verbal instructions issued by the trainer. I am aware that potential risks associated with these types of activities include, but are not limited to: death, fainting, disorders in heartbeat, serious neck and spinal injuries that may result in complete or partial paralysis or brain damage, serious injury to virtually all bones, joints, ligaments, muscles, tendons, and other aspects of the musculoskeletal system, and serious injury or impairment to other aspects of my body, general health, and well-being.

I understand that I am responsible for my own medical insurance and will maintain that insurance throughout my entire period of participation with [name of personal trainer and/or business]. I will assume any additional expenses incurred that go beyond my health coverage. I will notify the [name of personal trainer and/or business] of any significant injury that requires medical attention (such as emergency care, hospitalization, etc.).

[name of personal trainer or business] or I will provide the equipment to be used in connection with workouts, including, but not limited to, benches, dumbbells, barbells, and similar items. I represent and warrant any and all equipment I provide for training sessions is for personal use only. [name of personal trainer or business] has not inspected my equipment and has no knowledge of its condition. I understand that I take sole responsibility for my equipment. I acknowledge that although [name of personal trainer and/or business] takes precautions to maintain the equipment, any equipment may malfunction and/or cause potential injuries. I take sole responsibility to inspect any and all of my or the [name of personal trainer and/or business]'s equipment prior to use.

Although [name of personal trainer and/or business] will take precautions to ensure my safety, I expressly assume and accept sole responsibility for my safety and for any and all injuries that may occur. In consideration of the acceptance of this entry, I, for myself and for my executors, administrators, and assigns, waive and release any and all claims against [name of personal trainer and/or business] and any of their staffs, officers, officials, volunteers, sponsors, agents, representatives, successors, or assigns and agree to hold them harmless from any claims or losses, including but not limited to claims for negligence for any injuries or expenses that I may incur while exercising or while traveling to and from training sessions. These exculpatory clauses are intended to apply to any and all activities occurring during the time for which I have contracted with [name of personal trainer and/or company].

I represent and warrant I am signing this agreement freely and willfully and not under fraud or duress.

HAVING READ THE ABOVE TERMS AND INTENDING TO BE LEGALLY BOUND HEREBY AND UNDERSTANDING THIS DOCUMENT TO BE A COMPLETE WAIVER AND DISCLAIMER IN FAVOR OF [name of personal trainer and/or business], I HEREBY AFFIX MY SIGNATURE HERETO.

____
Client's name (please print clearly)

______________________________ Date: ______________
Client's signature

____
Client's address

______________________________ Date: ______________
Parent/guardian signature (if applicable)

______________________________ Date: ______________
Trainer's signature

Figure 17-1

Sample waiver

Note: This document has been prepared to serve as a guide to improve understanding. Personal trainers should not assume that this form will provide adequate protection in the event of a lawsuit. Please see an attorney before creating, distributing, and collecting any agreements to participate, informed consent forms, or waivers.

an attorney's office is advisable before signing any contract, but it is particularly important in cases where an employer–employee relationship is established or an ongoing time or financial commitment is created. Long-term contracts should be examined with particular scrutiny, since much can change over time.

Negligence

One of the most important aspects of personal training is the adherence to established professional guidelines. Failing to perform as a reasonable and prudent person would under similar circumstances is considered **negligence.** In the case of personal trainers, a reasonable and prudent person is someone who adheres to the established **standard of care.** Attainment of ACE **certification** indicates that the personal trainer has demonstrated an acceptable level of competence and understanding of the established standards. Since standards of care can and do change, it is critical that personal trainers stay abreast of new guidelines. (*Note:* This is the role of continuing education.) A negligent act can occur if a trainer fails to act (act of omission) or acts inappropriately (act of commission). For example, a trainer could be successfully sued for neglecting to spot a client during a free-weight bench press (omission), or for programming straight-leg sit-ups for a client with known lower-back problems (commission). These actions would likely be found inappropriate as compared to what a reasonable and prudent professional would do in a similar situation.

To substantiate a charge of negligence in court, the plaintiff must establish four elements:

- The defendant had a duty to protect the plaintiff from injury.
- The defendant failed to uphold the standard of care necessary to perform that duty.
- Damage or injury to the plaintiff occurred.
- This damage or injury was caused by the defendant's breach of duty (proximate causation).

Negligence in personal training could occur, for example, if a trainer agreed to provide instruction and supervision for a weight-lifting regimen. The agreement between the trainer and the client establishes a legal duty that would not be present if both parties were simply working out at a fitness center at the same time. (Certainly there may be a moral duty to help a fellow patron in need, but there is not a legal duty to do so absent a special relationship such as parent–child.) If the trainer does not provide proper spotting during an exercise, the trainer has breached his or her duty to his client. If the client is injured as a direct result of the breach—which often happens when heavy weights are lifted without proper spotting—then the client will likely have a successful lawsuit for negligence against the personal trainer. The courts would examine the situation, the expected standard of care, the extent of the injury, and the result of the injury (e.g., medical bills, lost time at work) when assessing potential damages.

Vicarious Liability

Personal trainers who hire employees need to understand the concept of **vicarious liability** (also known as **respondeat superior**). Employers are responsible for the employment actions of their employees. If an employee is negligent while working within the normal scope of employment, it is likely that the injured party will sue not only the employee who breached the duty to cause injury, but also the employer or employers. Since employees often do not have the financial resources of employers, courts have typically upheld the right of the injured party to seek damages from the employer's "deep pockets." In most cases, litigants name every possible entity linked to the employee when negligence occurs.

The use of waivers is critical in personal training, as a properly worded **exculpatory clause** bars the injured from potential recovery (see Figure 17-1). There are some potential issues that every personal trainer must investigate with an attorney prior to crafting a waiver. Each state has slightly different rules regarding the validity of waivers, meaning that a waiver that is valid in one state may not be valid in another. In addition, confusion and litigation can arise when a fitness club utilizes personal trainers who are not employees. Consider the following court case, which addressed the situation in which a member of a health club signed a supplemental contract for personal-training services in the club setting. When the client was injured in a session with the personal trainer, she contended that the waiver signed with her membership contract did not extend and cover the services of the personal trainer. The court disagreed and ruled that the services of the personal trainer were part of the activities and benefits offered at the club and were therefore covered by the original waiver (Cotten, 2000a). Despite the outcome of this case, personal trainers should utilize their own waivers in addition to the ones potentially already signed when the client joined the fitness center or club.

Waivers also must detail the types of activities and potential risks of injury that would be barred from recovery. A client must knowingly understand the nature of the activities and the potential risks before he or she can waive the right to potentially sue for injuries occurring during participation. Waivers also typically do not protect the personal trainer from injuries directly caused by **gross negligence**—an action that demonstrates recklessness or a willful disregard for the safety of others. As a general rule, gross negligence occurs when someone deliberately acts in a manner that extends beyond the scope of employment or fails to meet the accepted standard of care. For example, a correctly worded waiver would likely not protect a personal trainer who did not properly spot a client completing a military press, as spotting would likely be considered part of the normal activities conducted during the course of personal training. However, if the personal trainer intentionally removed a safety screw from the seat prior to the client's arrival, the waiver would likely not apply, because removal of safety equipment is something that should *never* occur during the normal course of a personal trainer's activities. Ultimately, the use of proper waivers protects the personal trainer from lawsuits that arise not only from injuries that typically occur during exercises, but also from injuries that might occur due to mistakes the trainer may make while interacting with clients. Hopefully, mistakes are mitigated, injuries are limited, and potential lawsuits are completely avoided.

Even if a waiver is not utilized properly, a personal trainer may successfully defend against a negligence lawsuit in certain situations, even if he or she is partially at fault. Courts will typically examine every aspect of the scenario to determine who was at fault. In some cases, the client may have contributed to the potential injury. In certain states, **contributory negligence** laws prevent a plaintiff in a lawsuit who has played some role in the injury from receiving *any* remuneration. For example, if a client failed to notify a trainer that the soles of one of his shoes had been slipping, he would be partially to blame if his foot slipped while conducting a squat lift, even if the trainer did not properly spot the client. The clients' improper actions bar him from recovering any money, even though the trainer was partially at fault.

The majority of states do not use the contributory negligence standard, instead utilizing **comparative negligence** when deciding negligence cases. When multiple parties may have caused injuries, the court will apportion guilt and any subsequent award for damages. For instance, in the earlier example the client may be deemed to be 40% at fault for the injury (for failing to inform the personal trainer of the issue with his shoes) and the trainer 60% at fault (for failing to spot the client during the lift). If the court were to normally award $100,000 in damages, the award would be lowered to $60,000 (i.e., 60% of the damages). There are a variety of state standards regarding comparative negligence and its potential impact upon monetary awards.

Agreements to Participate, Informed Consent, and Waivers

There are a variety of potential contracts that personal trainers may utilize in their day-to-day operations. Of particular importance are contracts detailing the relationship between the trainer and the client as they pertain to the potential rigors and injuries associated with physical activity. Personal trainers should understand the concept and use of **agreements to participate**, **informed consent,** and waivers, as they can be important defenses to litigation for negligence. Ideally, each of these forms should be printed (avoid handwritten agreements) and signed by all clients *before* beginning the first exercise session.

Before a personal trainer begins using any of these documents, it is critical that legal counsel specializing in health and fitness in the personal trainer's state be consulted.

Agreement to Participate

An agreement to participate is designed to protect the personal trainer from a client claiming to be unaware of the potential risks of physical activity (Figure 17-2). An agreement to participate is not typically considered a formal contract, but rather serves to demonstrate that the client was made aware of the "normal" outcomes of certain types of physical activity and willingly assumed the risks of participation. Typically, the agreement to participate is utilized for "class" settings (e.g., step training, aquatic exercise) rather than for individualized personal-training situations. The agreement to participate should detail the nature of the activity, the potential risks to be encountered, and the expected behaviors of the participant (Cotten & Cotten, 2004). This last consideration is important, as the participant recognizes that he or she may need to follow instructions while participating.

Personal trainers should have a process to formally warn their clients about the potential dangers of exercise.

Typically, agreements to participate are incorporated into other documents, such as informed consent forms and waivers. One potential consideration for each of these documents is a general request, or in some cases a requirement, that participants consult with a doctor prior to beginning any exercise routine. Some attorneys may advise personal trainers not to train anyone unless that person has verified that, at the very least, a basic health examination has been performed by a medical doctor within the past six months. Though most personal trainers know to "start slowly" with new clients, personal trainers cannot evaluate the overall health of a client in the same manner as a medical doctor. Some agreements to participate also ask that health insurance information be provided. This not only lets the personal trainer know that the client has coverage, but also enables the trainer to provide that information if a client were in need of medical attention.

Informed Consent

An informed consent form can be utilized by a personal trainer to demonstrate that a client acknowledges that he or she has been specifically informed about the risks associated with the activity in which he or she is about to engage (Figure 17-3). Informed consent allows the client to have something done to him or her (e.g., strength test, flexibility regimen, measurement of **$\dot{V}O_2$max**) by the personal trainer, and therefore can differ slightly from an agreement to participate. It is primarily intended to communicate the potential benefits and dangers of the program or exercise testing procedures to the client. Informed consent forms should detail the possible discomforts involved and potential alternatives. Personal trainers should remember that many potential clients will be unaccustomed to straining their bodies through physical exertion. The informed consent form, combined with oral communication, prepares the client for the positive and negative effects of certain types of exercise.

The documents presented in this chapter have been prepared to serve as a guide to improve understanding. Personal trainers should not assume that they will provide adequate protection in the event of a lawsuit. Please see an attorney before creating, distributing, and collecting any agreements to participate, informed consent forms, or waivers.

"I, _________, have enrolled in a program of strenuous physical activity including, but not limited to, traditional aerobics, weight training, stationary bicycling, and the use of various aerobic-conditioning machinery offered by [name of personal trainer and/or business]. I am aware that participating in these types of activities, even when completed properly, can be dangerous. I agree to follow the verbal instructions issued by the trainer. I am aware that potential risks associated with these types of activities include, but are not limited to, death, serious neck and spinal injuries that may result in complete or partial paralysis or brain damage, serious injury to virtually all bones, joints, ligaments, muscles, tendons, and other aspects of the musculoskeletal system, and serious injury or impairment to other aspects of my body, general health, and well-being.

Because of the dangers of participating, I recognize the importance of following the personal trainer's instructions regarding proper techniques and training, as well as other organization rules.

I am in good health and have provided verification from a licensed physician that I am able to undertake a general fitness-training program. I hereby consent to first aid, emergency medical care, and admission to an accredited hospital or an emergency care center when necessary for executing such care and for treatment of injuries that I may sustain while participating in a fitness-training program.

I understand that I am responsible for my own medical insurance and will maintain that insurance throughout my entire period of participation with [name of personal trainer and/or business]. I will assume any additional expenses incurred that go beyond my health coverage. I will notify [name of personal trainer and/or business] of any significant injury that requires medical attention (such as emergency care, hospitalization, etc.).

Signed____

Printed Name_______________________ Phone Number_______________________

Address____

Emergency Contact_______________________ Contact Phone Number_______________________

Insurance Company____

Policy #_______________________ Effective Date _______________________

Name of Policy Holder____

Figure 17-2
Sample agreement to participate

Note: This document has been prepared to serve as a guide to improve understanding. Personal trainers should not assume that this form will provide adequate protection in the event of a lawsuit. Please see an attorney before creating, distributing, and collecting any agreements to participate, informed consent forms, or waivers.

Inherent Risks

Agreements to participate and informed consent forms, though potentially important in the defense against a lawsuit, primarily cover the **inherent risks** of participation in an activity. For instance, even if proper stretching and lifting techniques are utilized, injuries can occur to ligaments, tendons, muscles, and other parts of the body. An agreement to participate and an informed consent form would help to protect the personal trainer in the event that a lawsuit is filed by an injured client. However, it is often difficult to determine an inherent risk of participation and what might have been caused, in whole or in part, by the actions of the personal trainer. A client may claim that a personal trainer did not provide proper spotting during an exercise and that this action specifically caused an injury. The trainer might counter that an injury was unfortunate, but part of the normal, safe lifting process. This dispute would likely be settled in court. To potentially avoid this type of a scenario, personal trainers should have all clients sign a waiver prior to beginning any exercise routine. The waiver (sometimes called a release) will typically incorporate similar language included in an agreement to participate and an

Figure 17-3
Sample informed consent form

Note: This document has been prepared to serve as a guide to improve understanding. Personal trainers should not assume that this form will provide adequate protection in the event of a lawsuit. Please see an attorney before creating, distributing, and collecting any agreements to participate, informed consent forms, or waivers.

Circulatory and Respiratory Fitness Test

Informed Consent for Exercise Testing of Apparently Healthy Adults (without known heart disease)

Name____

1. Purpose and Explanation of Test

I hereby consent to voluntarily engage in an exercise test to determine my circulatory and respiratory fitness. I also consent to the taking of samples of my exhaled air during exercise to properly measure my oxygen consumption. I also consent, if necessary, to have a small blood sample drawn by needle from my arm for blood chemistry analysis and to the performance of lung function and body fat (skinfold pinch) tests. It is my understanding that the information obtained will help me evaluate future physical activities and sports activities in which I may engage.

Before I undergo the test, I certify that I am in good health and have had a physical examination conducted by a licensed medical physician within the last __________ months. Further, I hereby represent and inform the facility that I have accurately completed the pre-test history interview presented to me by the facility staff and have provided correct responses to the questions as indicated on the history form or as supplied to the interviewer. It is my understanding that I will be interviewed by a physician or other person prior to my undergoing the test who will in the course of interviewing me determine if there are any reasons that would make it undesirable or unsafe for me to take the test. Consequently, I understand that it is important that I provide complete and accurate responses to the interviewer and recognize that my failure to do so could lead to possible unnecessary injury to myself during the test.

The test that I will undergo will be performed on a motor-driven treadmill or bicycle ergometer with the amount of effort gradually increasing. As I understand it, this increase in effort will continue until I feel and verbally report to the operator any symptoms such as fatigue, shortness of breath, or chest discomfort that may appear. It is my understanding and I have been clearly advised that it is my right to request that a test be stopped at any point if I feel unusual discomfort or fatigue. I have been advised that I should, immediately upon experiencing any such symptoms or if I so choose, inform the operator that I wish to stop the test at that or any other point. My wishes in this regard shall be absolutely carried out.

It is further my understanding that prior to beginning the test, I will be connected by electrodes and cables to an electrocardiographic recorder that will enable the facility personnel to monitor my cardiac (heart) activity. During the test itself, it is my understanding that a trained observer will monitor my responses continuously and take frequent readings of blood pressure, the electrocardiogram, and my expressed feelings of effort. I realize that a true determination of my exercise capacity depends on progressing the test to the point of fatigue.

Once the test has been completed, but before I am released from the test area, I will be given special instructions about showering and recognition of certain symptoms that may appear within the first 24 hours after the test. I agree to follow these instructions and promptly contact the facility personnel or medical providers if such symptoms develop.

2. Risks

It is my understanding and I have been informed that there exists the possibility of adverse changes during the actual test. I have been informed that these changes could include abnormal blood pressure, fainting, disorders of heart rhythm, stroke, and very rare instances of heart attack or even death. Every effort, I have been told, will be made to minimize these

Initial: _____

occurrences by preliminary examination and by precautions and observations taken during the test. I have also been informed that emergency equipment and personnel are readily available to deal with these unusual situations should they occur. I understand that there is a risk of injury, heart attack, stroke, or even death as a result of my performance of this test, but knowing those risks, it is my desire to proceed to take the test as herein indicated.

3. Benefits to Be Expected and Alternatives Available to the Exercise Testing Procedure

The results of this test may or may not benefit me. Potential benefits relate mainly to my personal motives for taking the test (e.g., knowing my exercise capacity in relation to the general population, understanding my fitness for certain sports and recreational activities, planning my physical conditioning program, or evaluating the effects of my recent physical habits). Although my fitness might also be evaluated by alternative means (e.g., a bench step test or an outdoor running test), such tests do not provide as accurate a fitness assessment as the treadmill or bike test, nor do those options allow equally effective monitoring of my responses.

4. Confidentiality and Use of Information

I have been informed that the information that is obtained from this exercise test will be treated as privileged and confidential and will consequently not be released or revealed to any person without my express written consent or as required by law. I do, however, agree to the use of any information for research or statistical purposes so long as same does not provide facts that could lead to the identification of my person. Any other information obtained, however, will be used only by the facility staff to evaluate my exercise status or needs.

5. Inquiries and Freedom of Consent

I have been given an opportunity to ask questions about the procedure. Generally, these requests, which have been noted by the testing staff, and their responses are as follows:

____

____

____

I further understand that there are also other remote risks that may be associated with this procedure. Despite the fact that a complete accounting of all remote risks is not entirely possible, I am satisfied with the review of these risks, which was provided to me, and it is still my desire to proceed with the test.

I acknowledge that I have read this document in its entirety or that it has been read to me if I have been unable to read same.

I consent to the rendition of all services and procedures as explained herein by all facility personnel.

Date____________________

____

Client's Signature

____

Witness' Signature

____

Test Supervisor's Signature

Reprinted with permission from Herbert, D.L. & Herbert, W.G. (2002). *Legal Aspects of Preventive and Rehabilitative Exercise Programs* (4th ed.). Canton, Oh.: PRC Publishing. All rights reserved.

informed consent form, but will also include an exculpatory clause that bars the clients from seeking damages for injuries caused by the inherent risk of activities and by the ordinary negligence of the personal trainer and his or her employees and agents (see Figure 17-1).

Procedures

Valid agreements to participate, informed consent forms, and waivers must be administered properly to clients. There should not be any underhanded attempt to hide the true nature of these agreements prior to a client signing the document. Though some states permit **group waivers** that have a list of spaces for multiple patrons to sign below the waiver, it is advisable to have a stand-alone document for each client. Often, personal trainers properly insist that a new client sign a waiver prior to the first session, but then fail to allow sufficient time for the new client to read, understand, and ask questions about the document. Requiring a client to rush when reviewing a waiver can result in a court invalidating an otherwise properly crafted waiver. In addition, though courts have typically found that participants who cannot read English retain the responsibility to have someone translate the waiver prior to signing, it is a good practice to have someone available to assist with the translation if needed (Cotten & Cotten, 2004). If the document is multiple pages, a space for the client to initial the bottom of each page should be provided (see Figure 17-3 as an example).

Minors cannot legally sign a contract, so in most cases a waiver signed by a child will be invalidated by the courts. However, some states do allow parents to sign paperwork that may provide limited protection for the personal trainer. An attorney specializing in this area should be consulted if children will be utilizing a personal trainer's services. Personal trainers should remember to have every member of a family sign an individual waiver. A waiver signed by one spouse may not cover the other spouse (Cotten, 2000b). Once agreements to participate, informed consent forms, and waivers have been signed, the personal trainer should retain the paperwork on file at least until the **statute of limitations**—the time allotted to sue for damages—has elapsed. Some attorneys even recommend retaining records past the statute of limitations to ensure that a sudden change in the law does not negatively impact the ability of a service provider to defend against potential litigation.

Ultimately, the goal of any personal trainer should be to eliminate all client injuries. However, even in the safest conditions, physical activity will likely result in some physical injuries, even when proper care is provided. Personal trainers should utilize paperwork to notify new clients of *all* risks and potential dangers. This creates a situation in which the client knows and assumes the risks of participation. Personal trainers should then also utilize waivers to protect against costly lawsuits that arise both from the normal physical injuries associated with physical activity and from mistakes that may occur during personal-training sessions.

Legal Responsibilities

The use of proper paperwork prior to working with clients can mitigate some of the potential for litigation against the personal trainer. But even if clients waive their right to potentially sue, the personal trainer should still prepare for each training session with safety as the first priority. Not only is this a professional requirement, but it also provides a better experience for the client and increases the likelihood that the client will continue to utilize the trainer's services. One of the most important things a personal trainer can do is establish plans to regularly inspect facilities and equipment and review protocols regarding supervision and instruction.

Facilities

Personal trainers have an obligation to ensure that the facilities used are free from unreasonable hazards. At the very least, the physical environment should be inspected each day prior to beginning any training session, especially when the training area has been used by other patrons after the personal trainer last was present. Inspecting the facilities can be a problem if training sessions are conducted outdoors or in a client's home. Trainers should allocate sufficient time—which should *not* be charged to the client—to inspect the environment prior to the workout. In some cases, clients will recognize these inspections of the facility as a genuine concern for their well-being, which can have a positive impact on client retention and may generate new clients through referrals. The inspection should consider the following issues:

- Different floor surfaces are designed for different activities. Trainers should ensure that floor surfaces will cushion the feet, knees, and legs from excessive stress.
- There should be sufficient free space available to protect the client from other patrons and from hurting him- or herself on equipment.
- Functional lighting must be sufficient for chosen exercises.
- There must be functional heating and air conditioning systems.
- Proximity to drinking fountains and bathrooms is important for some clients.

Because a trainer's primary responsibility is the client's safety, regular inspection using a safety checklist is recommended. If an unsafe condition is noticed, the trainer should notify the facility's management and avoid that area until it has been addressed. If a fitness club owner does not repair the problem and the client is injured, the personal trainer can still be held partially liable. Though juries have often looked favorably on independent contractors or employees who have tried unsuccessfully to persuade management to correct dangerous conditions, there is always a potential risk when training in an unsafe environment. For this reason, personal trainers should develop relationships with reputable fitness centers that focus on safety. In addition, personal trainers should develop contingency plans (outside of cancelling the session and losing potential revenue) for unsafe facilities.

Working with clients in their homes can pose potential safety problems as well. Often, the client may be reluctant to alter the environment or change the overall décor. Though this type of situation may shift some or all of the responsibility for safety from the trainer to the client, an attorney should always be consulted in these instances.

Another consideration for training is the use of public spaces, especially the outdoors. For many trainers and clients, it is much more enjoyable to run on a trail than on a treadmill in a fitness center. However, in some jurisdictions it is illegal to train clients on public beaches, parks, or trails. It is the trainer's responsibility to know the local laws prior to using these areas. Once a "legal" outdoor area has been identified and selected for a training session, the trainer should be sure to understand the potential dangers of the area before meeting the client. Outdoor areas pose specific risks. Running on a public street may involve evading oncoming vehicular traffic, while running on a mountain trail could involve dodging loose rocks or tree roots. Training outdoors certainly can be an enjoyable experience, but it is the trainer's responsibility to ensure that the activities will not pose a significant risk for clients.

While most courts recognize that outdoor activities pose certain risks that a typical person would assume (such as loose dirt or rocks on a hiking trail), the trainer should inspect the area to identify any particularly unusual dangers. In addition, certain aspects of the environment may impact the choice to utilize it for a training session. If a client has never run on a specific outdoor trail, it is advisable to walk the trail with the client the first time rather than expecting an all-out initial effort. The safety of outdoor activities is also impacted by the weather. The courts often will remove a person's potential liability for **acts of God** (e.g., earthquakes, mudslides), but if the weather forecast indicates heightened dangers, the trainer should not engage in the activity. For example, though earthquakes and lightning storms are both acts of God, in many cases a lightning storm can be predicted. Courts might be willing to absolve trainers of potential liability from injuries caused by an earthquake, but they are less likely to rule in favor of a personal trainer if he or she knew, or should have known, that a lightning storm was in the area. In all outdoor training situations, extreme weather conditions such as freezing cold or excessive heat and humidity should be avoided. Acceptable exercise routines in 75° F (24° C) weather may not be acceptable in 95° F (35° C) or 35° F (2° C) weather conditions.

Some trainers use fitness centers without informing the management that there will be a training session. This is certainly not an ethical business practice, and in many areas is a violation of the law. In addition to adhering to the law and using good ethical behavior, developing a formal relationship with the fitness facility may eventually result in an expanded client base from fitness center referrals. An attorney should be consulted prior to establishing any formal relationship with a fitness center.

Equipment

Fitness programs may utilize a variety of equipment, and injuries from the use of exercise equipment are often a source of litigation in the fitness industry. All equipment should meet the highest safety and design standards and should be purchased from a reputable manufacturer. In most cases, the use of homemade equipment should be avoided, since designing and manufacturing are not considered part of the "normal" duties of a personal trainer. Equipment must be regularly inspected and properly maintained. Of particular concern is the protocol utilized when broken equipment is discovered. Once something is deemed unsafe, the personal trainer should immediately remove the equipment from the training area. If quick removal is not feasible, the equipment should be disabled to prevent further use until repaired. Unfortunately, broken equipment is often only marked with a sign that says "do not use." Far too often, these signs easily fall off and unsuspecting patrons may be injured when trying to use the broken equipment. Manufacturers typically provide maintenance schedules for equipment that personal trainers and club operators should follow. Regular maintenance should be logged and records retained for future referral in the event of a lawsuit.

The use of equipment owned by a client may create a conflict between professional practice and legal protection. A conservative legal stance would be to avoid any contact with the client's equipment, but most personal trainers accept some liability by using their expertise to adjust a client's equipment or recommend maintenance. For example, a personal trainer may arrive at a client's home for an initial fitness session and find a leg extension machine with a frayed cable. The trainer should inform the client that the equipment needs repairs, suggest that he or she call the company to order a replacement part, and then conduct sessions without using this equipment until it has been repaired.

Personal trainers should also understand the importance of non-exercise equipment when working with clients. Trainers should require that proper clothing and shoes be worn by their clients during sessions. Failure to stop a client from exercising with improper shoes may be deemed an endorsement of a bad practice. If the training sessions will be conducted outdoors, the trainer should provide water in containers that will be sufficient for the time, intensity, and temperature during the workout.

The use of safety equipment, such as **automated external defibrillators (AEDs),** has gained considerable attention in recent years. These devices can be found in many places of public assembly (e.g., airports, shopping malls, amusement parks) and are rapidly becoming standard emergency equipment in health and fitness facilities, not only because they can save lives, but also because they are legally *required* for fitness centers in many states (Agoglia, 2005). Even in states where AEDs are not required in fitness centers, courts can rule in favor of plaintiffs and change the standard of care (*Fowler v. Bally Total Fitness,* 2008).

Personal trainers will familiarize themselves with AEDs through **cardiopulmonary resuscitation (CPR)** and first aid courses, which are required prior to certification.

(Please visit www.acefitness.org for more information regarding AED training in your area.) Though usually not required, trainers may want to consider purchasing an AED for use in their own studios or when working with clients in their homes. It is likely that future legislation will establish AEDs as a standard piece of equipment for personal trainers working with clients in *all* settings (Wolohan, 2008). Every trainer should consult with his or her attorney to understand the local laws that may apply to a specific situation.

Supervision

General supervision involves overseeing a group of people, such as when a group fitness instructor leads a large class. **Specific supervision** occurs when an individual is supervised while performing a specific activity, such as what typically occurs during a personal-training session. When working with clients, trainers need to remember that most personal-training activities require specific supervision for safety purposes. A trainer should never leave a client when there is a potential for injury (such as when a spotter is needed on a bench press). Trainers who work with two or more clients during the same session should design the workouts to alternate between activities requiring general and specific supervision. For example, while the trainer provides specific supervision to one client (e.g., spotting), the other client should briefly rest or work on an activity that requires only general supervision (e.g., stretching or cardiovascular exercises). Trainers should eliminate any time that a client is not in their direct view, as this is when injuries can quickly occur. A trainer should never leave a client during a session.

Before beginning any session, the trainer must adequately plan for any emergencies that may arise. A client's emergency medical information should be immediately available in the event of an accident. This will eliminate the need to search for critical information about the client (such as emergency contact numbers) in the event of an emergency. If training is to occur in a remote area, cell phone coverage should be checked prior to the exercise session to ensure that 911 may be reached if necessary.

Proper supervision involves not only clients, but also employees. Personal trainers need to be aware of the actions of their employees. This awareness includes properly screening potential employees prior to hiring them. It is the responsibility of an employer to determine if the potential employee would pose a specific danger to clients due to his or her past history. Each employee should be trained regarding the unique aspects of the employer's operation and then supervised and retrained at regular intervals. Employers should conduct written performance evaluations with each of their employees and should retain those files even after an employee has stopped working for the employer.

Instruction

Personal trainers should utilize instructional techniques that are consistent with current professional practices. If one fails to demonstrate a movement or give proper instructions regarding how to use a piece of equipment and the client is injured, the trainer may be found negligent. Legal standards require that clients be given "adequate and proper" instruction before and during an activity. In a courtroom, an expert witness could be asked to assess "proper" or factually correct instruction. Adequate and proper instruction also means avoiding high-risk exercises, or those not recommended by professional peers. Advocating dangerous or controversial exercises puts the trainer at risk for a successful lawsuit if a client is injured. In one case (*Corrigan v. Musclemakers, Inc.*, 1999), a personal trainer put his client on a treadmill, but failed to appropriately adjust the speed for this first-time user or explain how to adjust the speed or stop the belt. The client could not keep pace, and she was catapulted backward and fractured her ankle in the ensuing fall.

Proper instruction also means individualizing workout routines for each client. An exercise may be appropriate for one client but completely inappropriate for another due to a variety of circumstances. In a reported case in the media, a personal trainer was sued for causing injuries to his client. The personal trainer, as is sometimes common, admitted to using the same workout routine with all of his clients. The injured woman was 42 years old and was not in proper physical condition to perform the same exercises as the trainer's other clients, who were much younger, healthier, and more advanced in their exercise training. After only her second workout, she was admitted to a hospital for nearly two weeks.

Personal trainers should insist on proper use of equipment and correct completion of activities at all times. Many personal trainers remember to properly demonstrate how to operate equipment the first time a client uses it, but if the client becomes sloppy in the future, trainers often become lax in terms of maintaining proper standards of performance. Personal trainers should demonstrate proper instruction by always using good technique during their own workouts. If a client is not corrected when using bad form or sees a trainer "bending the rules," the client may be more likely to exercise improperly, which can increase the likelihood of injury.

A relatively new aspect of instructional liability concerns the physical touching of clients. Trainers should avoid touching clients unless it is essential for proper instruction. Clients should be informed about the purpose of potential touching before it occurs. If a client objects, an alternative exercise should be utilized. Charges of sexual assault, even if groundless, can have disastrous consequences for a personal trainer's career.

Safety Guidelines

In reference to the above-mentioned areas of responsibility, personal trainers should adhere to the following safety guidelines in the conduct of their activities:

- Be sure that all sessions are well-planned, appropriate, and documented.
- Communicate and enforce all safety rules for equipment use.
- Ensure that equipment meets or exceeds all industry standards.
- Inspect all equipment prior to use and document adherence to maintenance schedules.
- Never allow unsupervised activity by the client.
- Limit participation to those under contract (i.e., no friends or family members).
- Clearly warn clients about the specific risks of planned activities.
- Only select activities within the defined scope of practice and appropriate areas of expertise.
- Ensure that clients wear any necessary protective equipment (e.g., athletic supporter or sports bra).
- Review the emergency plan [access to a phone and 911 for emergency medical services (EMS)].
- Stay up-to-date with certifications and education in the field.

Scope of Practice

One of the biggest difficulties for a personal trainer—particularly one who constantly spends time seeking to learn new information—is to remember the extent of one's professional qualifications (see Table 1-2, page 8). An ACE certification signifies the attainment of a specific level of knowledge, but it is narrowly focused in certain areas. Certainly, the more one learns, the greater the ability to help clients, but there is a danger that personal trainers may extend their service offerings beyond their area of established expertise or scope of practice. Many states allow exercise "prescriptions" to be developed only by a licensed doctor. Therefore, it is important that trainers provide exercise programs, not exercise prescriptions. Although the difference between these terms may sound like a technicality, it could become an important issue in a courtroom. Personal trainers should attempt to develop a network of doctors and other healthcare professionals, such as dietitians and physical therapists, who can provide meaningful information and services to their clients. Clients who need the specialized services of these healthcare professionals should be referred for treatment and counseling. In turn, these professionals may refer clients to the personal trainer.

In addition to having new clients seek

a physical exam from a doctor prior to beginning an exercise regimen with a trainer, it is also important for the trainer to have a completed health-history form. However, these documents should be utilized for the determination of an individual's level of fitness, rather than for the purpose of providing or recommending treatment for specific medical conditions.

Personal trainers should use the health-history form to screen the client for appropriate placement in a fitness program. In cases where any significant risk factors are indicated, the client should be referred to a physician for clearance before the program begins. If personal trainers were to use the health-history form to recommend treatment, they could be accused of practicing medicine without a license. Ideally, clients will have a physician sign a health clearance form and produce a letter on the doctor's letterhead prior to beginning exercise. However, if a client fakes a physician's signature to obtain acceptance to a fitness program, the trainer probably would not be held liable, unless, possibly, the trainer had knowledge of the forgery prior to the client's participation.

Trainers must understand how to use the information collected on the health-history form, asking only those questions that they can interpret and apply. Trainers must read and fully understand the answers the client provides. The forms are designed to alert the trainer to any potential problems that could occur; therefore, the trainer should not just see the completed form as an item to "cross off the checklist." Trainers should incorporate the information on the forms into the fitness programs they design for their clients.

Trainers should know and follow the exercise program guidelines recommended by leading professional organizations such as the American Council on Exercise (ACE), the National Strength and Conditioning Association (NSCA), the American College of Obstetricians and Gynecologists (ACOG), the American College of Sports Medicine (ACSM), and the American Heart Association (AHA). Trainers also should be familiar with the position statements (papers) for specific populations developed by these and other allied healthcare organizations. The NSCA has produced a position paper on weight training for prepubescent youth; ACOG has produced resource material on pregnant women and exercise; and ACSM has published numerous position statements regarding various aspects of exercise, fitness, and health.

Trainers may administer fitness assessments if the tests are recognized by a professional organization as appropriate for the intended use and are within the scope of the trainers' qualifications and training. For example, ACSM has established protocols for assessing a client's **cardiovascular disease (CVD)** risk to determine appropriate assessments and medical supervision needs during cardiorespiratory fitness assessments, and ACE has published established protocols for assessing posture, movement, flexibility, cardiorespiratory fitness, and muscular endurance, strength, and power (see Chapters 5 through 12). Trainers should carefully follow these risk-factor stratification and fitness assessment procedures and should never attempt to administer a test without proper training. In some cases, a qualified physician or other trained medical personnel must be present. It is important for trainers to only operate within their areas of expertise, particularly when exercise testing is conducted.

Most personal trainers can easily recognize certain situations in which they do not have the needed expertise. For example, most personal trainers would know immediately that a client who asked to have a sample of his or her blood drawn and analyzed would likely need to see a physician. However, in other situations, trainers may not recognize that they are providing advice beyond their qualifications. The unique, close personal relationship that often develops between personal trainers and their clients can cause potential areas of concern. Many clients view their personal trainer not only as their fitness advisor, but also as their physical therapist, dietitian, marriage counselor, or psychologist. When these types of perceived relationships develop, the trainer must pay particular attention to comments that may be construed as qualified professional advice. It is important for personal trainers to always stay within their scope of practice when providing professional advice or providing a personal opinion that could be taken as professional advice. Though trainers would never purposely hurt their clients, careless or misunderstood comments and actions can cause considerable pain, both physical and psychological.

When clients seek recommendations about exercise equipment, clothing, or shoes, it is important for trainers to remain cautious when responding, particularly when they may have a pre-existing endorsement arrangement with a service provider. Before giving advice, trainers should become knowledgeable about the products and equipment available, as well as their advantages and disadvantages. Another option would be to limit potential liability by referring clients to their choice of retail sporting goods stores. Advice based solely on personal experience should be given with that express qualification.

Though the choice of shoes and other equipment is important, of far greater concern and consequence is the solicitation of advice regarding nutrition and supplements (refer to Appendix C for ACE's Position Stand on Nutritional Supplements). One of the most noteworthy cases in this area concerned a personal trainer who suggested dietary supplements for a client in writing (*Capati v. Crunch Fitness*, 2002). The client died from a brain hemorrhage due to complications from an adverse interaction between the supplements and other medication she was taking. Unless personal trainers have received specific medical or nutritional training and have earned appropriate professional licenses, credentials, or certifications (e.g., M.D., R.D.), they should not provide advice in these areas. Most personal trainers know and understand this potential area of concern, but they often unwittingly provide advice to their clients. For example, there is a distinct difference between telling a client that a certain food, beverage, or supplement contains a high amount of **vitamins** and **minerals** and specifically telling a client to eat more of a particular food, beverage, or supplement. When a client is told to do something, it creates a potential liability for the personal trainer.

Personal trainers should also learn to recognize physical problems that their clients may be having. Unfortunately, impulsive behaviors regarding diet and exercise can lead some clients to engage in potentially destructive behaviors. It is important to learn to recognize dietary problems such as **anorexia**, **bulimia,** and **binge eating disorder.** In addition, despite various potential side effects, the use and overuse of supplements, steroids, and **growth hormone** has become more common. Personal trainers should never state, or even intimate, that they support their client's use of these products. When personal trainers recognize potential problems in their clients, they should have a plan to address the situation. Personal trainers should seek the advice of experts in the field when developing these protocols and should seek legal counsel when necessary.

Though a client–trainer relationship does not legally require the same standards for confidentiality as a physician–patient or attorney–client relationship, personal trainers should maintain that same level of expectation. It is inappropriate for trainers to discuss their client's workout regimens, strength and flexibility achievements, and weight loss with others. Violating a client's privacy is not only unethical, but can lead to significant negative repercussions (refer to Appendix A for the ACE Code of Ethics).

Liability Insurance

Even after taking precautions, it is important for personal trainers to be aware of the importance of insurance. The recent rise in litigation throughout the healthcare industry has caused nearly every personal trainer to seek some sort of insurance. The need for insurance is always present, but as personal trainers and their businesses become more financially successful, the importance of insurance also increases. Unfortunately, potential plaintiffs and their lawyers often "target" successful businesses, since there is a greater likelihood of "winning" a substantial financial reward. Though most trial attorneys will agree to work on a contingency fee basis, some unscrupulous attorneys will take meritless cases simply with the hope that they will be "successful" in convincing a judge or jury that their client deserves compensation. Judgments for millions of dollars are not uncommon, and few individuals or businesses could survive such a substantial financial loss. Insurance protection provides some peace of mind, as trainers can be secure in the knowledge that if someone were to be injured as a result of their actions or if a meritless lawsuit were to occur, insurance coverage would be adequate to recompense that individual for his or her losses. There are a variety of important insurance aspects to understand.

Generally, an insurance policy is a contract designed to protect trainers and their assets from litigation. There is, however, some truth to the saying that insurance companies are in the business of collecting premiums and denying claims. It is important to understand the basic components of insurance coverage before soliciting guidance from an insurance agent. Agents are in the business of selling policies, which means some agents will focus more on the potential sale than on providing accurate advice. Though it is important to never be "underinsured," personal trainers can purchase too much insurance given their unique situation. Talking with established personal trainers or seeking information from trusted industry organizations such as ACE can be a great way to be referred to a successful insurance agent who understands the unique aspects of the fitness industry. Not all insurance carriers are equal in their experience, acumen, and financial resources. The most reputable insurance carriers have a national affiliation, are licensed, have strong financial backing, have a reinsurer (corporate policy to ensure that policy holders' claims will be met even if their business collapses), and have not had any claims filed against them by the Better Business Bureau. It is the personal trainer's responsibility to investigate insurance carriers and coverage prior to beginning training sessions.

In general, personal trainers should not assume that any of their typically established personal insurance (e.g., auto, home) extends to their professional activities. For example, most homeowner's insurance has general liability to cover slips, trips, and falls that may occur while guests are visiting a person's home. This type of coverage would likely not cover a client who fell while being trained, since the training would be considered a business activity.

Personal trainers need to secure **professional liability insurance** that is specifically designed to cover the health and fitness industry. The selected liability insurance policy should cover personal injuries that can occur as a result of a training session. Injured clients may sue not only for medical expenses, but also for a variety of other compensation, such as lost wages from being unable to work, pain and suffering, and loss of consortium. ACE recommends retaining at least $1 million in coverage, as medical expenses can easily cost hundreds of thousands of dollars. In some instances, a higher liability coverage amount may be advisable.

> The American Council on Exercise has established relationships with reputable insurance carriers who specialize in the fitness industry. Visit www.acefitness.org/pdfs/personal-trainer-insurance.pdf for more information.

Personal trainers must understand the specific insurance needs that may arise given the location of the training activities. Home-based training has become popular, as many clients prefer to work with trainers in their own residence. In addition, some trainers would rather use their homes for training activities than maintain a formal relationship with a fitness center. General liability policies may not cover a personal trainer who works with clients in a private residence. Owners who will use their own home or a client's home should ensure that a specific insurance **rider**—a special addition to typical policy provisions—will cover those activities. In addition, specific language should provide liability protection for trainers who utilize outdoor settings for their training activities. In cases where personal trainers will work outside of a fitness center, it is imperative that the insurance carrier is aware of the professional activities that will occur. In most cases, home-based or outdoor training will require insurance (typically at higher rates) that specifically covers the trainer for these locations. For trainers who own their own fitness clubs, insurance should be retained that covers potential problems with the facility as well as the instruction and supervision of the trainer.

Most insurance agents now recommend that all professionals purchase an **umbrella liability policy.** The umbrella policy provides added coverage for all of the other insurance (e.g, auto, home, professional liability) that a person may have in place. For example, if a personal trainer was sued and the judgment exceeded his or her professional liability coverage, the umbrella policy would cover the insurance shortfall. When purchasing an umbrella policy, personal trainers should be sure that it covers professional activities associated with personal training. In addition, every liability policy should be examined to ensure that it covers the trainer while working in various locations (e.g., fitness center, personal home, client's home, outdoors).

Trainers who sell products may need to secure **product liability insurance** in the event a product fails to perform properly. This is particularly important for personal trainers who own and operate fitness centers. Though the manufacturer of a product retains most of the liability for design flaws, manufacturing defects, and product malfunctions, there have been cases where the "middleman" was also successfully sued.

Personal trainers who form partnerships or corporations may wish to investigate the purchase of **keyman insurance.** A keyman insurance policy is designed to compensate the business for the loss of a person who performs a unique and valuable function. If a business will experience significant financial trouble if one person has an extended illness or dies, keyman insurance should be purchased. Keyman insurance pays a specified amount to assist the business in its recovery from losing a critical human resource.

Employees and Independent Contractors

Many health and fitness industry employers now require their employees to demonstrate proof of liability insurance when they are hired, even though they will be potentially covered under the fitness center's insurance. Employers should ensure that employees renew and verify their policies annually. Potential employees may wish to verify that the fitness center has adequate coverage and that the employer's insurance will assist them in defending a potential lawsuit. It is *critical* that independent contractors working for fitness clubs or other facilities maintain adequate insurance, as the facility's legal representatives would likely seek to separate the facility itself from the actions of the personal trainer if a lawsuit occurs. The employment or independent contractor contract between the fitness center and the personal trainer should contain language detailing insurance requirements and responsibilities.

One important aspect of insurance is to obligate the insurance carrier to pay in the event of a loss. The following statement, or some version of it, should be included in any basic agreement:

> *We agree to pay those sums that the insured becomes legally obligated to pay as damages because of bodily injury or property damage to which this insurance applies, and these will include damages arising out of any negligent act, error, or omission in rendering or failing to render professional services described in this policy.*

One of the key provisions is that the insurance company will pay even if the trainer fails to provide a service. For example, if an injured person needed first-aid attention and the trainer did not provide it, the policy should still provide protection. If "failure to render" or "omission" is not specified, the policy covers the trainer only if the services provided were inadequate or improper.

A critical component of an insurance policy is related to coverage of legal fees, settlements, and defense charges. Trainers should look for the following type of clause in their policy:

> *We will have the right and duty to defend any suit seeking damages under this policy, even if the allegations are groundless, false, or fraudulent and may, at our discretion, make such investigation and settlement of any claim or suit deemed expedient.*

The best policies cover the cost of a legal defense *and* any claims awarded. Policies that only cover an amount equal to awarded damages are not recommended, as the trainer will be covered for the final judgment, but all of the trial expenses incurred will be the trainer's responsibility. One of the realities of insurance litigation is that the insurance company may make a strategic decision to settle rather than fight the case in court. It is important to have a policy that covers the cost of litigation, but the trainer should not necessarily be disappointed if the insurance company elects to settle a lawsuit out of court.

While it is important to identify and understand what is covered in the insurance policy, it is also critical to know what is not covered. Most policies delineate specific exclusions. The following liabilities are often excluded in fitness professional policies: abuse, molestation, cancer (resulting from tanning), libel, and slander. Trainers should also inquire whether bodily insurance coverage will cover lawsuits alleging mental stress. Most policies differentiate between the two, and a standard bodily injury clause does not necessarily include mental injuries. A client filing a suit might claim that the trainer was overly critical and, as a result, mental injuries were suffered. Mental injuries are difficult to define and determine. The courts are split on the issue of inclusion. For example, litigation in New York found that bodily injury included mental distress, while a California court said it did not.

Most policies exclude coverage for acts committed before the policy was purchased. Coverage also might be excluded for claims that occurred during the policy period but are filed after the coverage has been terminated. These issues are related to the"claims-made basis" of a policy. Though they can be expensive, trainers can purchase "prior acts coverage" from most insurance carriers for an additional cost if they have already begun training without insurance coverage. An "extended reporting endorsement" will ensure that claims made in the future for injuries during the policy period will be covered even if the policy is cancelled. Ideally, insurance coverage should be maintained until after the statute of limitations has expired for anyone who has been a client of a personal trainer.

Understanding insurance policies initially can be difficult. Proper research of potential insurance agents is critical. Once an insurance carrier has been indentified, the personal trainer should maintain an open line of communication with his or her agent. Ultimately, the agent and the insurance company work for the personal trainer, but it is the trainer's responsibility to maintain open communication. Any changes in business activity should be immediately relayed to the insurance company so that appropriate changes in the policy can be made. Adequate levels of insurance can change as a personal trainer's client list, employees, and income increase.

Other Business Concerns With Legal Implications

In addition to the legal responsibilities in the areas of business structure, scope of practice, facilities, equipment, testing, instruction, and supervision, personal trainers must be aware of the implications of certain other potential legal issues.

Marketing Activities

Identifying and procuring clients is the lifeblood of any business. Though many personal trainers maintain high ethical standards, some health clubs and fitness centers have relatively little concern for ethical behavior. Unfortunately, it has become common for some fitness centers to utilize improper marketing tactics and long-term contracts that contain devious language to attract and retain clients. In some extreme cases, fitness centers have even misused direct deposit agreements to commit fraud. Personal trainers should understand the marketing and operating activities that their fitness centers may utilize. If a fitness center is behaving unethically or illegally, the personal trainer may be "associated" with those practices, even if he or she had no direct involvement in the improper behavior. The widespread use of the Internet has enabled customer complaints to be relayed to current and potential clients, as well as to the Better Business Bureau. Since a significant portion of a personal trainer's business is related to reputation, it is important to only associate with fitness facilities that maintain high legal and ethical standards.

Intellectual Property

Music recordings sold commercially are intended strictly for the private, noncommercial use of the purchaser. In addition, there are rules regarding the use of television programming as a key component of any non-food or beverage service business. This means that in many cases copyright violations occur when a fitness center utilizes music or television broadcasts as a key component of its business. Although two groups, the **American Society of Composers, Authors, and Publishers (ASCAP)** and **Broadcast Music, Inc. (BMI)**, will issue licenses for the commercial use of broadcasts and recordings, their fees may be prohibitive in many situations. A good option is to purchase recordings produced specifically for use in fitness facilities. When training clients in their homes, personal trainers can have clients provide the music for each session. In effect, the clients are then using these recording for their own private, non-commercial enjoyment during exercise.

Some trainers may seek copyright or trademark protection for their own creative works. Trainers who develop specific routines or who write books or other materials may wish to profit from their creativity. For example, a book or instruction manual can be copyrighted so that any future sales provide a **royalty** to the author. Trainers who develop a company name or slogan may seek trademark protection so that other individuals or businesses cannot utilize that name or slogan without permission.

Proper Use of the ACE Name and Logo

The ACE-certified logo may be used by ACE-certified Professionals only and is a mark of excellence. ACE encourages its certified professionals to use this mark to promote themselves; however, it is important that ACE and its professionals work together to protect the American Council on Exercise name. The ACE logo and *ACE Logo Usage Guidelines* document are available for download by all ACE-certified Professionals at www.acefitness.org. This document provides complete details regarding proper and improper usage of both the ACE name and logo.

ACE-certified Professionals can use the ACE-certified logo mark to promote their credentials to clients. Examples include business cards, stationery, advertisements, or brochures marketing any ACE certifications earned and actively maintained, as well as the fitness services provided to consumers. ACE-certified Professionals may also use the ACE-certified logo on their professional websites or apparel.

To ensure the ACE name and logo are protected, please also note where usage would violate the ACE Code of Ethics and trademark laws. ACE-certified Professionals must not use the American Council on Exercise name or ACE-certified logo on any materials that promote their services as a trainer or instructor of other fitness professionals, such as continuing education courses, seminars, or basic training, unless it is contained within their personal biographical material. In additional, ACE-certified Professionals must not use the American Council on Exercise name or ACE-certified logo in conjunction with any other product or merchandise that they sell, such as videos or clothing.

Transportation

In most cases, personal trainers will meet their clients at a fitness center or some other location. However, there may be a situation where the personal trainer provides transportation for the client to or from a training session. Trainers should be aware that many "standard" automobile insurance policies may not cover injuries sustained by clients riding in the trainer's vehicle. If the trainer is going to provide a ride to a client, the trainer should check with his or her auto insurance company to ensure that potential injuries from accidents are covered.

Financing

As personal trainers create and expand their businesses, they may need to seek financing for certain activities. Even if the personal trainer is operating as an LLC/LLP or S-corp, banks and other lenders usually will only loan money if it is personally guaranteed by an individual. Unfortunately, many companies have advertised "business loans" that are in fact personal loans. Personal trainers who thought that only their businesses were liable for the financial obligation later learned that the lender was able to pursue the trainer for unpaid debts. Trainers should read and understand the "fine print" of any loan (or, better yet, hire an attorney to review the documents) prior to signing.

Risk Management

One of the most important aspects of any business is **risk management**. There are risks to any activity, but exercise programs carry certain special risks due to the physical movement and exertion often required. Personal trainers should constantly search for methods to make the environment safer for their clients. Periodically reviewing programs, facilities, and equipment to evaluate potential dangers allows the personal trainer to decide the best way to reduce potentially costly injuries in each situation.

Most authorities recommend a risk-management protocol that consists of the following five steps:

- *Risk identification:* This step involves the specification of all risks that may be encountered in the areas of instruction, supervision, facilities, equipment, contracts, and business structure.
- *Risk evaluation:* The personal trainer must review each risk, with consideration given to the probability that the risk could occur and, if so, what would be the conceivable severity. Table 17-2 can be used to assess the identified risks.

Table 17-2

Evaluating Risk Based on Frequency and Severity

	Frequency of Occurrence		
Severity of Injury or Financial Impact	High or often	Medium or infrequent	Low or seldom
High or vital	Avoid	Avoid or transfer	Transfer
Medium or significant	Avoid or transfer	Transfer, reduce, or retain	Transfer, reduce, or retain
Low or insignificant	Retain	Retain	Retain

- *Selection of an approach for managing each risk:* Several approaches are available to the personal trainer for managing and reducing the identified risks:
  - ✓ *Avoidance:* Remove the possibility of danger and injury by eliminating the activity.
  - ✓ *Transfer:* Move the risk to others through waivers, insurance policies, etc.
  - ✓ *Reduction:* Modify the risks by removing part of the activity.
  - ✓ *Retention:* Often there are risks that will be retained, especially if the removal of the risk would eliminate a potential benefit (e.g., no risks will occur if exercise is eliminated, but then no health benefits can be accrued).

The recommended approach for extreme risks is to avoid the activity completely. Risks that fall into one of the high categories can be managed either through insurance or viable actions to reduce the likelihood of occurrence or severity of outcome. Reduction is also the preferred method for addressing risks in the medium category, while risks with low impact can be retained (see Table 17-2).

- *Implementation:* Institute the plan
- *Evaluation:* Continually assess the outcome of risk-management endeavors. The standard of care regarding some risks may change over time. Therefore, risk-management approaches may need to be altered.

Personal trainers can also manage risk by examining procedures and policies and developing conduct and safety guidelines for clients' use of equipment. Strict safety guidelines for each activity, accompanied by procedures for emergencies, are particularly important. Trainers must not only develop these policies, but also become thoroughly familiar with them by mentally practicing emergency plans. Several lawsuits have resulted in substantial judgments against fitness professionals who failed to respond to the emergency medical needs of clients. In some cases, the initial injury was not a major concern, but the failure to adequately address the initial problem was the focus of the litigation. When an incident occurs, the personal trainer should first ensure the safety of all individuals involved. Once the immediate concern for safety has passed, the personal trainer should complete an incident report. The trainer should note any facts related to the incident and should solicit information from any witnesses. When collecting information from witnesses, it is critical to get phone numbers, physical addresses, email addresses, and signatures for future verification and follow-up. This information should be retained in a secure location for future reference in a lawsuit or when reviewing past performance and emergency-management procedures.

Summary

Although often overlooked when considering the technical aspects of providing quality personalized fitness instruction, legal and business concerns are of paramount importance. Personal trainers must always be aware of their scope of practice and the expected standard of care that should be provided. This chapter provided an introduction to the legal and professional responsibilities of personal trainers. In every instance, personal trainers should seek the guidance of qualified attorneys who specialize in the fitness industry. Personal trainers should establish their business in the proper structure, understand and utilize contracts, know the changing nature of their legal responsibilities, secure proper insurance, and implement a comprehensive risk-management plan. Ultimately, it is the personal trainer's responsibility to not only continually educate him- or herself regarding the "science" of personal training, but also to thoroughly understand the legal guidelines that must be followed to create a safe and enjoyable environment for clients.

References

Agoglia, J. (2005). *The AED Agenda.* www.fitnessbusinesspro.com/mag/fitness_aed_agenda/

Capati v. Crunch Fitness International, Inc. et al. (N.Y. App. 2002). 295 A.D.2d 181.

Corrigan v. Musclemakers, Inc. (1999). 686 N.Y.S. 2d 143.

Cotten, D.J. (2000a). Carefully worded liability waiver protects Bally's from liability for personal trainer negligence. *Exercise Standards and Malpractice Reporter*, 14, 5, 65.

Cotten, D.J. (2000b). Non-signing spouses: Are they bound by a waiver signed by the other spouse? *Exercise Standards and Malpractice Reporter*, 14, 2, 18.

Cotten, D.J. & Cotten, M.B. (2004). *Waivers & Releases of Liability.* Statesboro, Ga.: Sport Risk Consulting.

Fowler v. Bally Total Fitness (2008). Maryland Case No. 07 L 12258.

Herbert, D.L. & Herbert, W.G. (2002). *Legal Aspects of Preventive and Rehabilitative Exercise Programs* (4th ed.). Canton, Ohio: PRC Publishing.

Wolohan, J.T. (2008). Aftershocks. *Athletic Business*. www.athleticbusiness.com/articles/article.aspx?articleid=1758&zoneid=45

Suggested Reading

Broadcast Music, Inc. (2009). *Business Using Music: Fitness Clubs.* www.bmi.com/licensing/entry/C1299/pdf533620_1/

Herbert, D.L. & Herbert, W.G. (2002) *Legal Aspects of Preventive, Rehabilitative and Recreational Exercise Programs* (4th ed.). Canton, Ohio: PRC Publishing.

National Conference of State Legislatures (2008). *State Laws on Heart Attacks, Cardiac Arrest & Defibrillators.* www.ncsl.org/programs/health/aed.htm

Peragine, J.N. (2008). *How to Open and Operate a Financially Successful Personal Training Business*. Ocala, Fla.: Atlantic Publishing Group.

Reents, S. (2007). *Personal Trainers Should not Offer Nutritional Advice.* www.athleteinme.com/ArticleView.aspx?id=264

IN THIS CHAPTER:

The Direct-employee Model

The Independent-contractor Model

Starting a Career

Business Planning

- Executive Summary
- Business Description
- Marketing Plan
- Operational Plan
- Risk Analysis
- Decision-making Criteria

Creating a Brand

Communicating the Benefits

Marketing for Client Retention

Marketing Through General Communication

Choosing a Business Structure

Professional Services for Starting a Business

- Attorney
- Accountant
- Web Developer/Graphic Designer
- Insurance Broker
- Real Estate Broker
- Contractors

Financial Plan

Time Management

How to Sell Personal Training

- Selling Training Programs

Summary

PETE McCALL, M.S., *is an exercise physiologist with the American Council on Exercise (ACE), where he creates and delivers fitness education programs to uphold ACE's mission of enriching quality of life through safe and effective exercise and physical activity. Prior to working with ACE, McCall was a full-time personal trainer and group fitness instructor in Washington, D.C. He has a Master's of Science degree in exercise science and health promotion from California University of Pennsylvania and is an ACE-certified Personal Trainer.*

CHAPTER 18

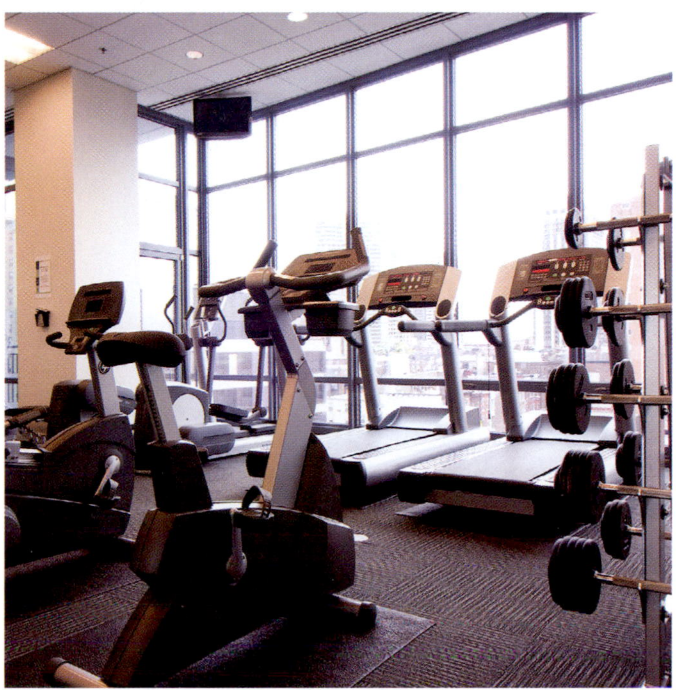

Personal-training Business Fundamentals

Pete McCall

When a person makes the decision to become an ACE-certified Personal Trainer, it is usually because he or she enjoys exercise, lives an active and healthy lifestyle, and wants to make a living helping others do the same. However, along with knowledge about anatomy, physiology, and exercise program design, a successful career as a personal trainer requires the ability to successfully run a business. Whether working with clients in their homes or for a major health club operator, a personal trainer needs to know how to properly manage and operate a business.

The fundamental purpose of a business is to generate profit by delivering a product or service to customers. Operating a successful personal-training business involves creating a budget, which is used to establish revenue (or income) goals and expense targets, developing a marketing plan, and having the ability to sell training sessions—which means asking people for money, something that many trainers (especially new ones) have difficulty doing.

A successful business needs customers that can use the goods or services being sold. Service businesses do not offer tangible products, but instead offer the knowledge, skill, and expertise to provide assistance to individuals with a specific need. Service companies build their businesses through interpersonal relationships (Beckwith, 1997). Once a person becomes an ACE-certified Personal Trainer, he or she possesses the level of education and professional skill necessary to provide a service by helping people who want to enjoy the benefits of exercise, such as weight loss, health improvement, improved appearance, or enhanced performance in a particular sport or activity. A personal trainer needs to be able to match his or her desire for helping clients improve their lives through exercise with the ability to quickly establish **rapport** with them. This combination will provide a strong foundation for a personal-training business.

A thriving business is based on delivering a product or service with honesty and integrity. The following is a brief overview of the different business environments that a personal trainer might encounter, with some considerations for a personal trainer's overall career development. The purpose of this overview is to provide an objective comparison of the differences among the many types of facilities and businesses in the fitness industry. Each option has very specific features, advantages, disadvantages, and benefits for fitness professionals. Prior to starting a career in the industry, a personal trainer should take the time to identify the type of business that would be most suitable for his or her needs.

The most important decision regarding employment options is whether to work directly for an employer, or independently by being a contractor to a fitness facility or training studio or working directly with clients in their own homes. A final option is to be an entrepreneur and start a training business, which opens up a much larger discussion.

The Direct-employee Model

In the direct-employee model, a trainer is usually paid one rate when working a scheduled shift on the fitness floor and a higher fee when working with a client as a personal trainer. The pay rate for delivering a personal-training session can range anywhere from 40 to 70% of what the client pays the club or training studio. In addition to the pay rates for hourly work and training sessions, many companies will reward trainers with bonuses if they meet certain performance objectives.

The decision to work for an employer in the direct-employee model requires further decisions, such as whether to work for a large health-club chain, a non-profit center like a YMCA or Jewish Community Center (JCC), a community or university recreation center, a corporate fitness facility, an independent health club with only one or two locations, or a personal-training studio. There is no decision that is right for everyone, but there are many factors to consider prior to making a commitment to an employer:

- The first consideration is to determine whether the facility attracts the type of clientele the trainer is interested in working with and if those potential clients have the disposable income to pay for personal-training services. If a trainer is interested in working with athletes, he or she should probably look for a suburban club with a large population of youth who play sports. However, if a trainer wants a consistent stream of clients who can afford to pay for training services, working in a club located in an affluent area that caters to a demographic with a high level of disposable income might be the best decision.
- The facility should be conveniently located for commuting. A personal trainer must be realistic about the costs and time associated with making a daily commute, especially if he or she is planning on training clients very early in the morning. In terms of providing quality

customer service, there is nothing worse than a client waiting for a trainer who is consistently late because he or she was stuck in traffic.

- The facility should be located in an area that gets steady traffic throughout the day. A suburban facility will generally have members coming in before work, stay-at-home parents or retirees who visit during the day, youth in the afternoon, and people who exercise in the evening before heading home, while an urban location will experience the highest number of visits in the morning before work, during lunch time, and right after work—with extremely slow periods in between. A personal trainer should identify the busiest times of day for a prospective employer and plan on being available to work with clients at those times.
- A personal trainer must do a little research to determine the reputation of a company for which he or she is considering working. As an employee, the trainer represents the organization, but it is important to keep in mind that the employer also represents the trainer. It is a wise for a personal trainer to determine if a prospective employer represents values that are consistent with his or her own. The facility should run a quality operation that caters to the needs of its members, and not simply focus on signing people up for a membership without providing the necessary back-end customer service. A good employer will run a business that receives favorable reviews from members. Taking the time to run a prospective employer through a few Internet search engines should provide some customer reviews from current or former members. A facility that does not treat its customers with a high level of service will probably not treat its employees that well either.
- It is important to determine the requirements for employment. Does the facility require specific education or a specific personal-training certification? Find out if the company provides any education or training on how to be a successful trainer. Finally, learn if the organization expects the trainer to follow a standardized method, or protocol, for exercise program design, which can be severely limiting and does not represent truly individualized programming and service.
- It is also important to identify the production expectations and whether the company provides any sales training. If an employee is expected to meet a certain sales quota in a specific time period, then the company should provide training on how to meet those expectations.
- Before beginning work at a facility, the personal trainer should ask the employer if they offer other revenue-making options for the trainer, such as teaching group exercise classes, conducting small-group training sessions that allow trainers to earn more money per hour, or conducting in-house workshops for the other fitness staff (some employers will pay trainers a set rate for educating other members of the staff).
- It is essential that ACE-certified Personal Trainers find out if a potential employer requires its employees to sell dietary supplements or any questionable fitness or nutritional products. Selling such products may place the trainer in legal jeopardy and in violation of the ACE Code of Ethics (see Appendix A). Refer to Appendix C for ACE's Position Statement on Nutritional Supplements.

Clearly, there are a lot of things to consider before making a commitment to an employer. Personal trainers must take the time to carefully think through these factors to identify the most effective place to start or advance their fitness careers.

The advantages of the direct-employee model include the following:

- The employer pays the cost of marketing to new facility members, all of whom are prospective clients for personal-training services.

- The employer pays for equipment and all expenses related to the repair and maintenance of the facility.
- Many employers will provide benefits, such as healthcare, paid vacation, or contributions to retirement accounts for employees who meet certain criteria.
- Some employers will provide uniforms and offer continuing education opportunities (which are required to maintain any ACE certification) at no charge to their employees.
- Working as a direct employee means that the employer is required to submit taxes on behalf of the trainer and issue an annual W-2 form indicating the amount of federal, state, and local taxes paid on the employee's behalf. This is beneficial when applying for car and home loans, filling out an application to rent an apartment, or preparing annual income tax documents.
- Before ordering equipment or changing the layout of a fitness floor, an employer will often check with the trainers (the people who use the floor the most) and let them take part in the decision-making process.
- Employers offer opportunities for promotion. Many health-club chains have a tiered system that rewards trainers with more experience by paying a higher per-session rate. A trainer may also be able to progress into management or leadership roles within the organization.
- Staying at the same location throughout the day means that clients will travel to see their trainer at a club or facility, as opposed to the trainer having to travel to see each client, thereby eliminating the cost of travel and additional commuting time.
- Many facilities offer group exercise classes for members. If a trainer earns a group fitness instructor (GFI) certification, this is an excellent way to meet many members. The facility will pay the trainer to teach a group fitness class, so he or she is able to get paid as an instructor while at the same time engaging a captive audience of potential personal-training clients.
- Many health clubs or studios provide opportunities for trainers to deliver small-group training sessions. This means that a trainer can see between two and six people at a time, allowing him or her to maximize the amount of money earned per hour (while providing a discount to each individual client). Refer to "Communicating the Benefits" on page 635 for more on group fitness instruction and small-group training.

The disadvantages of the direct-employee model include the following:

- As an employee, a trainer has to conform to the uniform and professional grooming standards of the employer.
- While many employers offer competitive per-session training fees, they are often lower than what the trainer could make working independently. However, it is important to keep in mind that to qualify for a car loan or a mortgage, an individual has to be able to demonstrate that he or she has a job with a consistent, steady stream of income.
- Many employers have requirements for the minimum number of hours to work and will terminate an employee if he or she fails to meet these requirements.
- When starting out in a fitness facility, a new trainer has to work hard to develop relationships and market his or her services to clients. In addition, many employers establish sales goals for their personal trainers, which can create a high-pressure sales environment. Some people thrive in this situation, while others are uncomfortable asking potential clients for their money.

In the direct-employee model, personal trainers should still act as if they are running their own businesses, because in a sense they are. In most facilities, personal trainers are expected to market their services directly to members in an effort to gain clients. The fitness industry is similar to the real estate industry in that a real estate license allows an agent to work for a firm, but the agent is responsible for generating all of his or her own business. If a personal trainer is unsure of whether he or she has the skills required to manage a business, working for an employer that requires the trainer to develop the skills to market for clients, handle all client paperwork, and manage business operations is often a good learning experience.

The Independent-contractor Model

Another option for employment is the independent-contractor model, in which the personal trainer contracts his or her services to a health club or training studio. In a contractor relationship, a trainer will pay either a per-client or monthly fee to a health club or training studio in return for being able to use that location with clients. The main difference is that rather than receiving a paycheck and other benefits, such as healthcare, paid time off, or a retirement account from an employer, the trainer will pay a fee to rent space from the club or studio. In this model, the trainer is responsible for paying all of his or her own operational costs, such as a fee to use the facility, marketing costs to attract new clients, and benefits such as healthcare or time off.

The independent-contractor model requires the trainer to make a decision about how much money to charge for his or her services. When just starting out, personal trainers will probably want to price themselves slightly lower than some of the competition (only 5% or so) to make the fees more attractive to the consumer. But once a trainer gains some experience, he or she can raise these rates accordingly. When setting their fees, trainers must remember that taxes are paid on any earned income. A personal trainer should not simply set a rate that sounds inexpensive. Instead, he or she must do the research to determine if the rate can indeed cover all of the required expenses of being in business for one's self. Just as when making a decision to work directly for an employer, there are many things to consider before making a decision to work as an **independent contractor:**

- What facility will be used? What arrangements will be made to use the facility? As an independent contractor, a personal trainer has to identify a facility that he or she can use with clients. Before renting space from a facility, a trainer should conduct the same research and level of due diligence that he or she would before agreeing to work for an employer. Prior to making a contractual obligation, a trainer needs to ensure that the facility he or she is renting space from does not conduct any unethical business practices that could have a negative impact on the personal-training business and/or the trainer's professional reputation.
- If the plan is to work in clients' homes, then the trainer should take the time to do the research on the local market to see if it has the demographic to support the fees for a private trainer. Another thing to think about is location. Specifically, do people live in close enough proximity to allow a trainer to easily travel from one client to the next?
- What type of marketing expenses will be required to advertise for new clients?
- What health-screening forms and liability waivers will be used to protect financial assets against litigation in the event that a client decides to sue (see Chapter 17)?
- What assistance will the trainer need from an accountant or lawyer in setting up a business plan or appropriate financial and tax records?

Training "Under the Table"

The personal trainer must keep in mind that some fitness facilities will prosecute trainers for shoplifting or trespassing if they are caught training "under the table"—taking money directly from a client without properly paying the facility operator for using the space. Because this practice is illegal and unethical, it violates the ACE Code of Ethics (see Appendix A) and could lead to the loss of the ACE credential. Training under the table might seem like a tempting option for a beginning or struggling trainer, but there are serious potential consequences.

The advantages of the independent-contractor model include the following:

- The personal trainer is able to establish the fees for training services based on experience and what the market will pay.
- Many personal trainers appreciate the opportunity to move around and work out of different facilities, such as apartment complex fitness centers, clients' homes, or facilities that allow independent trainers to rent space.
- The personal trainer is able to develop his or her own financial goals, while many employers will establish production goals for employees that they expect the trainer to achieve while working for their facilities.

The disadvantages of the independent-contractor model include the following:

- The personal trainer has to maintain business records and pay quarterly taxes. While it might be tempting to just take cash and not declare any income while working as a personal trainer, an individual needs to demonstrate a steady, documented source of income to qualify for a car loan, a rental application, or a mortgage. In addition, the Internal Revenue Service (IRS) issues stiff financial penalties and possible jail time to people who fail to declare income or pay taxes on earned income.
- The trainer is responsible for all of his or her own marketing costs.
- If a trainer is renting space (i.e., paying a fee to use a health club or training studio), the trainer does not have any control over the operations of the facility and will not have any input regarding the facility's hours of operation, equipment purchases, or floor-plan layouts.
- If training clients in their homes, the personal trainer will have to travel between different locations throughout the day. This requires budgeting time for traveling from one location to the other, which is not paid time. Also, traffic could cause the trainer to be late, thereby harming the client–trainer relationship. Other drawbacks include the expense of gas and additional mileage on the personal trainer's car.

Starting a Career

Considering all of the costs and planning involved in opening a fitness business, the best way to get started as a personal trainer and learn about the industry without taking any financial risks would be to work for an employer, such as a health club or other fitness facility. These facilities are always adding new members, so they provide a steady stream of potential training clients, and as discussed earlier, will give a personal trainer some of the experience needed to operate a fitness business without investing the time and money to start one and have to learn it from scratch. A good employer will train its personal trainers to market their skills and make sales, which can provide valuable experience before opening a business. Another benefit to working for health clubs is that they are often involved in community projects that can provide experience working with the public, thereby raising the community's awareness of the personal trainer. Some facilities will even have media opportunities that allow their trainers to be featured in the newspaper or on local television and radio shows talking about fitness-related topics. Beginning as a personal trainer working in the direct-employee model can establish the foundation for a long and rewarding career in the fitness industry.

Business Planning

When first working with a client, a personal trainer should take the time to conduct an assessment to evaluate the client's health risk factors and have the client perform some standardized tests to determine his or her current level of fitness. This information is then used to develop an exercise program specifically designed to meet the client's unique needs and wants. To have a successful career, a personal trainer should take the time to perform a similar assessment of his or her own financial fitness and use that information to develop a business plan. The result of this organizational exercise will be a detailed plan of how to operate a successful business.

No one starting a business plans to fail; they simply fail to develop a systematic plan for running a business. To run a successful fitness business, a personal trainer should take the time to create a detailed business plan that establishes definitive goals and a structure for achieving those goals. Any of the direct-employee, independent-contractor, or business-owner operating models (see Chapter 17) will require a detailed business plan. A comprehensive business plan will serve as an operating guide for achieving specific objectives, such as yearly income and the number of clients needed to achieve that income, as well as a marketing plan for attracting new clients. The components of a business plan are as follows:

- Executive summary
- Business description
- Marketing plan
- Operational plan
- Risk analysis
- Decision-making criteria

Executive Summary

The executive summary is a brief outline of the business and an overview of how the business fills a need within the marketplace. This should be a succinct synopsis of the business, with the rest of the business plan providing the exact specifications in greater detail. A well-written executive summary is one page and includes the following information:

- *Business concept:* A description of the business, the service it provides, the market for that service, and why this particular business holds a competitive advantage. A personal trainer interested in opening a studio would need to specify how his or her skills are different from what exists in the current marketplace.
- *Financial information:* The key financial points for the business, specifically the start-up costs for the first year of operation, the source of capital for the initial expenses, and the potential for sales revenue and profits, with an emphasis on the expected **return on investment (ROI)**
- *Current business position:* Relevant information about the owners of the business, their experiences in the industry, and the specific legal structure of the business. This section should highlight the trainer's experience in the field and identify the number of clients who plan on following the trainer to the new location.
- *Major achievements:* Any awards received, or clients who have given written permission for their names to be used in marketing materials. This section should identify a specific protocol for exercise program design that is different from competitors, such as sport-specific training, or list any local or national celebrities who will provide an endorsement of the trainer's work.

Business Description

This section of the business plan provides the details for the business as outlined in the executive summary, including the mission statement, business model, current status of the market, how the business fills a need within the market, and the management team. It is important to develop a succinct mission statement that describes the benefit of using this particular personal-training service. When describing the business, the personal trainer should:

- Identify the operating model and how it is different or unique when compared to other training studios in the area
- Describe the fitness industry specific to the local market, including the present financial situation and the outlook for future growth
- Provide details such as the number and location of competitors, how many employees they have, and the number of clients to whom they provide services
- List the members of the management team, highlighting their knowledge, skills, and experience

The purpose of this section of the plan is

to provide information about the structure of the business, the market it will serve, and the people who will run it. Potential lenders or investors will want to see all of this information before making a decision about providing capital.

Marketing Plan

This section of the business plan specifies how prospective clients become paying clients. Whether working as an employee or as an independent contractor, a trainer will need to develop a comprehensive marketing plan to communicate with prospective clients. Marketing is the process of promoting a service by communicating the features, advantages, and benefits to potential clients. Marketing tools for a service such as personal training should tell a story about how that service can enhance a person's life. All marketing pieces should communicate the benefits of working with an ACE-certified Personal Trainer, specifically showing how the trainer can help potential clients meet their health and fitness goals.

An effective marketing campaign will communicate how a specific product or service meets the needs of a potential client. Unfortunately, many people enter the fitness industry with the misperception that all they need to do is show off their athletic physiques to get clients—when nothing could be further from the truth. The marketing plan should list the details on the demographics for the area around the training business, the demand for personal-training services, the specific type or brand of training services being offered, and the plan for communicating the benefits of personal training to potential customers.

To develop a full schedule, a trainer should take the time to first identify a target audience that can benefit from his or her personal-training services. For example, if a trainer is working in a health club in a suburban location where a large percentage of the members are stay-at-home parents or retirees, the trainer needs to develop a plan to communicate with those specific audiences. Similarly, a trainer who is working in an urban location where a number of the facility's members are working professionals should identify the times of day that potential clients are available to train and should develop a plan to market his or her services to that audience to schedule those open timeslots.

Operational Plan

This portion of a business plan describes the structure for how a business will operate, including an organizational chart that identifies key decision makers and the employees responsible for executing those decisions. A business plan for a personal trainer will not need a lengthy operational plan if the trainer is working directly for an employer. However, if a personal trainer decides to follow the independent-contractor model, then he or she can make a decision about which operational model to use to create a business structure (see Chapter 17).

Risk Analysis

There are a number of risks involved in owning and operating a business. Risks can be categorized into one of the following general areas:

- Barriers to entry: The costs associated with starting a business, such as rental fees, equipment, employees, and marketing
- Financial: The access to the capital required to start or expand a business
- Competitive: Other players in the market who are competing for the same pool of customers
- Staffing: Issues associated with managing employees and budgeting for a consistent payroll

For personal trainers who decide to work as direct employees, most of the financial risks are covered by the employer. A personal trainer working as an employee in a health club or similar facility will experience limited risk, such as competition for clients from other trainers in the facility, or from other facilities that open nearby.

Independent personal trainers will need to conduct an analysis to identify competitors and categorize the risks of competing in a specific marketplace. A simple tool for conducting a risk assessment is the **SWOT analysis,** which stands for strengths, weaknesses, opportunities, and threats (Figure 18-1). A basic SWOT analysis is easy to perform. Begin by dividing a piece of paper into four squares. The upper-left square should be labeled "strengths"—under this heading list all of the strengths and competitive advantages of the business. Examples of strengths might include location, the brand name of the fitness facility, or the education of the particular personal trainer.

The upper-right square should be labeled "weaknesses"—under this heading identify all of the weaknesses of the business. Examples of weaknesses might include the limited visibility of a location, an inability to work with a variety of clients such as special populations or people released from physical therapy (post-rehabilitation clients), or lack of industry experience. It is important to be as honest and objective as possible about weaknesses, as this exercise will help turn any perceived weaknesses into new business opportunities.

The lower-left square should be labeled "opportunities"—under this heading list all of the opportunities for attracting new clients or expanding the business. As mentioned earlier, weaknesses can be turned into opportunities for new business. For example, if limited location visibility is a weakness, then it is also an opportunity to develop new signage or create a new marketing campaign. Another example is a lack of education in a specific area of exercise science, which could be turned into an opportunity to take a continuing education course or workshop to gain the necessary training.

Finally, the lower-right square should be labeled "threats"—under this heading list all of the threats that might impact the business. Examples of threats are the general economic climate, adverse weather that might impact clients' abilities to make it to their appointments, or competitors who plan on entering or expanding in the marketplace.

Decision-making Criteria

This component of the business plan includes a detailed cost-benefit analysis that demonstrates that the expenses for operating the business are worth the financial risks involved with establishing operations. The trainer should highlight the specifics about the business plan that prove that it will be a successful business venture. A well-written plan will present all of the components of the business in such a way that the final section is simply a conclusion summarizing how the business will be a profitable venture.

More time spent in the early planning stages detailing how the business will run to allow a business owner to focus his or her efforts on implementing the plan, attracting the clients, and providing the service once the business starts operating.

Figure 18-1
Sample SWOT analysis

Strengths	Weaknesses
Four-year degree in kinesiology ACE certification Like to help clients with lifestyle and weight-management issues; successful at helping clients adhere to exercise programs	Not confident when asking clients for money Need to learn more about marketing and sales Space to train clients when the club is crowded
Opportunities	**Threats**
Participate in a personal-training sales workshop Develop a talk on lifestyle and weight management Work for the largest health facility in town, which attracts 100-plus new members per month	Competition from other trainers in the club and the four other facilities and training studios in the immediate area Consumer confidence in the current economic climate

Creating a Brand

By definition, personal training is about establishing a "personal" connection with clients, and the trainer has to live up to that expectation if he or she is going to deliver results and create satisfied customers. A trainer should use the business-planning process to develop a brand identity for his or her training service. A brand represents what a service or product stands for and is an easy way to communicate its value to potential customers and clients. Creating a brand to define the quality of personal-training service that a client can expect is an important step in establishing an almost immediate emotional connection with a client. If a trainer invests the time to develop a specific brand for his or her service, it will help prepare the client for what to expect during the personal-training experience.

A brand establishes an instantly recognizable value for the product or service being sold. The benefit of developing a distinct brand of personal-training services is the establishment of a unique identity that effectively communicates the benefits of working with an ACE-certified Personal Trainer.

Think of some specific brands. What does the brand name communicate about the value of the product or service? When given the choice, which will people select—a known brand name that defines a specific level of quality or a brand that is unknown and has no unique qualities? Does the product that is more appealing have a higher level of quality, or does it have a higher *perceived* level of quality? This is where a distinct brand identity becomes valuable. Many people choose a specific brand because of a certain image the brand projects. That is the value of a strong brand identity.

When making the decision about whether to work in the direct-employee model or the independent-contractor model, a personal trainer should take the time to conduct some market research about whether the potential work environments provide access to the clients who will need his or her services. It is especially important to identify who would be the most interested and able to afford the expense of working with a personal trainer. This becomes the target demographic, or prospective customer base, of the training business. To build a brand of training that supports the chosen employment model, a trainer must identify some specific fitness goals that appeal to prospective clients. Examples might include training to help clients lose weight, post-rehabilitation strength training, functional training to improve movement skills, resistance training for muscular development, or sports conditioning for performance enhancement. Keep in mind that there might be an expectation to deliver a specific brand of training when working for a health club or studio, though a successful personal trainer will still be able to keep his or her unique personality and develop a singular identity.

The following list provides a few examples of the types of clients who might be interested in working with a personal trainer. A trainer can use these demographics to begin building a brand identity.

- New health club members who want to learn the basics of exercise training
- Brides preparing for their wedding days
- Over-50 adults looking to improve quality of life
- New mothers wanting to lose pregnancy weight
- People preparing for an adventure vacation, such as a ski trip or bicycle tour
- Competitive amateur athletes such as runners, cyclists, triathletes, tennis players, or golfers looking for sport-specific training
- High school athletes seeking performance enhancement for a particular sport

When building a brand and identifying a target demographic, a personal trainer should take a few minutes to answer the following questions:

- What can be done to create and communicate a unique brand identity that will attract the target demographic?
- Who is the ideal target customer?
- Where is this target customer located?
- What time of day will this customer be interested in working with a trainer?

- What marketing efforts can be used to reach the potential customer to convert him or her into an actual paying client?

One way a personal trainer can create a brand identity is to combine his or her strengths (as identified in the SWOT analysis) with research about the target demographic in his or her area to create a vision statement for the type of service he or she can provide. For example, a personal trainer who works in a downtown urban market has identified the following demographics at her health club during her daily (Monday–Friday) shift:

- Most members are urban professionals in the 25- to 45-year-old age bracket. The other members are retirees who still live in the city and enjoy active urban lifestyles.
- The trainer opens the club and works until 2:00 p.m. During those hours, the breakdown of people in the club is as follows:
    - ✓ 5:30 to 9:30 a.m.: Professionals exercising before work
    - ✓ 9:30 to 11:30 a.m.: Active older adults who either take a class or exercise using the cardiovascular and strength equipment
    - ✓ 11:30 a.m. to 2:00 p.m.: Professionals exercising during their lunch breaks
- A number of the members who the trainer has spoken with during these times either run or cycle for recreation and exercise, and might compete in a few running races a year, usually in the 10-kilometer to marathon distance.
- The older adults the trainer has spoken with indicate that they like to exercise to maintain active and healthy lifestyles. Some of the older adult members have told the trainer that they choose to exercise in an effort to alleviate chronic muscle and joint aches.

The trainer herself is a former runner and has taken the ACE Functional Training and Assessment Workshop, so she has an understanding of how to perform postural and movement assessments. The trainer has a four-year degree in exercise science and spent two semesters working an internship in the college's strength and conditioning program, so she has a strong background in sports conditioning and performance-enhancement training. In her SWOT analysis, the trainer identified the following traits as some of her strengths:

- The ability to design exercise programs for a number of different sports, but with a special emphasis on running
- An understanding of anatomy and the ability to conduct basic postural assessments and movement screens
- An interest in helping people train for specific goals like running a race or achieving certain muscular-fitness objectives

Based on her research and her work identifying her strengths, the trainer decides to create the following as her personal vision statement: "*High-performance Training for Life and Sport.*" This vision statement clearly identifies her brand of training as one that focuses on performance enhancement and sports conditioning that suits the wide variety of goals that the members who frequent her club during her shift might establish for themselves. The simplicity of this statement is that it could appeal to both recreational runners looking to boost their performance and active older adults who want to maintain their health and an active lifestyle. The trick to creating a vision statement or a brand is that it should be simple and clearly communicate what the intended customer can expect to receive from the service.

Communicating the Benefits

Once a brand of training has been created and the target demographic identified, the next step is to create a strategy to communicate the benefits of using the specific brand of training. There are a number of different ways to market to prospective clients, so it is important to identify the most cost-effective method that will have the greatest reach.

A personal trainer who is just starting a business could deliver a complimentary training session for new clients and be available to conduct as many complimentary fitness assessments to facility members as possible. Every new-member fitness assessment is an opportunity to demonstrate the benefits of working with a personal trainer, which include better results in a shorter period of time. The complimentary session or initial fitness assessment allows a potential client to experience some of the benefits of training services before making a commitment by investing in a package of sessions. During the initial session or complimentary assessment, it is important to be honest with new or potential clients and let them know that they will not see results immediately, but if they follow a consistent exercise program they can see results in a reasonable amount of time. Trainers should keep the conversation and questioning focused on the prospective clients' needs and interests. The initial session needs to accomplish two basic goals:

- Collect information about the client to screen for health risks and design an exercise program for his or her specific needs and abilities. The client will have some specific goals, but a good program should provide what he or she needs—for example, addressing muscular imbalances or inefficient movement patterns that were revealed during initial assessments—along with what he or she wants (i.e., goals).
- Give the potential client an opportunity to experience a specific brand of training so he or she can understand how working with a trainer will help him or her safely achieve fitness goals.

Personal trainers should also use the time working on the fitness floor to build as many relationships with club members as possible. The more people a trainer can meet during a work shift, the more familiar members will become with that trainer—and all health club members are prospective clients. The familiarity will lead to a rapport based on trust and communication, which can lead to new clients. When meeting a member on the fitness floor, a personal trainer should keep the interaction short and simple. Simply making an introduction and asking the member's name, and then using it whenever the client is on the floor, can go a long way. Once rapport is established, the trainer can ask about the member's interests, fitness goals, and personal stories related to exercise. Potential clients need to establish a familiarity and comfort level with a personal trainer before developing trust and investing in sessions. The process of developing clients becomes a numbers game. A trainer should set a goal to meet as many new people per day (or work shift) as possible, to increase the available pool of potential clients. Personal training is not an "impulse buy"—people do not decide in a few moments about whether they want to invest in training. It takes time to develop a relationship with the potential client so that he or she can develop trust and understand that benefits from exercise do not happen overnight and require a long-term commitment. The more personal the training experience, the greater the value added, leading to long-term clients who will reward the trainer's service and attention to detail by referring their friends and family members.

It is a good idea to make business cards and distribute them to as many people as possible. In the direct-employee model, many clubs will provide trainers with business cards, but independent contractors will have to design and purchase their own cards. It is important to keep the card simple, with name, title, contact information including phone number, email address, and website (if applicable), and perhaps one line describing the brand of training. Personal trainers should avoid putting their pictures on business cards, as doing so might be intimidating or attract the wrong type of attention. It is a good idea to make the business card also serve as a schedule reminder, so that a trainer can write down an appointment for a client, keeping the trainer at the forefront of the client's mind.

Personal trainers can also create a testimonial book or have testimonials from current and former clients on a web page. Nothing markets services as effectively as satisfied clients. A client who achieved his or her goal can become a strong advocate for a trainer and will speak to friends and family about the positive experience. Be sure to get a client's permission in writing before using his or her name, photos, or stories in any marketing or advertising materials, as failing to secure written permission would constitute a breach of confidentiality (see Appendix A). The following items can also be included in the testimonial book:

- A personal biography that tells a story about who the trainer is as a fitness professional and as a person
- Success stories from satisfied clients
- Pictures of clients in their wedding dresses, tuxedos, or athletic uniforms after working with the trainer
- Descriptions and photos of clients who the trainer has helped to achieve goals, such as running a marathon or entering a fitness competition
- Before and after pictures of clients

Once a prospective client becomes an actual paying client, the trainer can show his or her appreciation by hand writing a personalized thank you note, which is a great way to show how much the client's business is valued. Be sure to follow these guidelines when writing the note:

- Have an upbeat and positive tone.
- Mention the client's goals and explain that those goals are the basis of the program.
- Stay professional and use appropriate language, remembering that a client–trainer relationship is a professional business relationship. The note should simply thank the client for his or her business.

In the direct-employee model, trainers should make an effort to work with clients in a visible area of the facility so that other members can see the personal-training experience. Some members might have a misperception that personal training is too hard or is run like a military boot camp, so the idea is to make training sessions appear challenging yet fun so that others can witness the benefits of working with a trainer.

Independent contractors can create signage for their cars, so that when traveling or parked in front of a client's home, as many people as possible can be exposed to the trainer's name and contact information.

Trainers can make T-shirts for clients with the trainer's name and logo. This is a good idea for rewarding clients when they meet certain goals or when they buy a new series or program of personal training. The client will enjoy getting a free item, and people who see the shirt might ask about the trainer and the client's experience working with that trainer.

The Internet is a powerful and efficient tool for promoting personal-training services.

- *Create a website:* There are many services on the Internet that people can utilize to design professional websites without too much effort or financial expense. A website is a good tool for communicating with current clients by posting relevant fitness articles or featuring specific exercises of the week or month. It is important to regularly update the website as the trainer and business evolve.
- *Start writing a fitness blog:* It is relatively simple to start a blog, which can address specific issues related to training and exercise. There are a number of resources that teach how to start a blog and how to market it on the Internet. The more people who read the blog, the more prospective clients and potential colleagues and networking resources a trainer can reach.
- *Maintain a social networking account:* This allows trainers to market their services and provides an easy template for uploading new exercise videos showing people how to exercise safely and effectively.

Personal trainers can also expand their reach by becoming ACE-certified Group Fitness Instructors. People who take the time to attend a group exercise class have already demonstrated a commitment to fitness, so this is a way to reach facility members who are true prospective clients. Another benefit is that being in front of a room of people establishes expertise, leadership, and knowledge about exercise. Teaching group exercise classes creates familiarity with members, allowing participants to get to know the instructor and feel more comfortable asking for his or her services as a trainer. Finally, group fitness instructors are paid for each class they teach, so having a schedule of classes is a smart way to maintain a consistent income stream during slow periods of the year, like the Christmas holiday season or breaks from school, when many clients might travel out of town, taking their business with them.

Creating an **adherence** program is another great way for personal trainers to market their services. A personal trainer can set up a system whereby a client who does not cancel any sessions during the training package/program becomes eligible for an additional session at no charge, or receives a free item with the trainer's brand such as a T-shirt. This is a great advertising opportunity for independent trainers.

Personal trainers can also create an orientation program for new members. Trainers can establish specific times to take groups of new members around the club to provide a brief overview of how the club operates and how to use the exercise equipment. Trainers can also create an education program that covers specific aspects of exercise programming. This type of program creates "touches" with prospective clients. The more prospective clients a trainer can "touch," the more clients he or she will gain. Some possible education program topics include the following:

- A 30-minute education seminar on how to start a safe running program
- A 30-minute education seminar on techniques for exercising while traveling

It is also vital that personal trainers develop complementary relationships with other services related to health and wellness or with other employees of the fitness facility. Examples include the following:

- In a health club, the trainer can work with the membership office, front desk, and group fitness instructors.
- Outside the club, trainers can work with other health and wellness service providers, including massage therapists, athletic trainers, sports coaches, wellness centers, **registered dietitians,** and bicycle shops.
- Trainers can offer to run a conditioning program for local fundraising runs or walks.

Trainers should remember that it will take some time to develop rapport and trust with prospective clients before earning their business. In the direct-employee model, every interaction with a club member is an interaction with a potential client. The trainer needs to be able to communicate with the client and educate him or her about how a personal trainer can help the client reach his or her fitness goals.

Small-group Training

In recent years, the one-on-one concept of personal training has expanded to include a trainer servicing two or more clients during the same session. This concept, called small-group personal training or semiprivate training, is becoming more commonplace as personal trainers develop their group-teaching skills and become more concerned about effective time management. The benefits of small-group personal training extend to both the trainer and the client. From the trainer's perspective, semiprivate training provides advantages in the areas of finance, time management, and referrals. For the client, benefits include a lower cost per session, enhanced camaraderie among workout partners, and an opportunity to receive instruction in a small-group setting from a fitness professional.

Financial Benefits

Personal trainers who offer small-group training services increase their hourly earning power while giving each client a reduced cost of training. For example, a trainer who typically charges $60 per session can reduce the cost to $45 for each client, thereby increasing his or her hourly income to $90 for two participants. A lower cost per session helps clients extend the money they spend on personal training to cover more sessions, potentially achieving a more successful result and, in turn, better long-term program adherence.

Social Benefits

People who exercise in a group or with a friend are more likely to feel engaged in the activity and have an increased sense of personal commitment to continue. Social support during exercise can enhance program adherence in at least three ways:

- Dissociation, wherein an exerciser's attentional focus is diverted away from the unpleasant sensations related to exercise by engaging with others during the physical effort
- Enhanced self-efficacy through receiving compliments and support from others in the group who have similar goals
- Stimulus control through reminders from the group participants and the trainer to attend a scheduled session

Given the social benefit of group exercise, personal trainers might observe a reduced attrition rate among clients who participate in small-group training sessions.

Referrals

Another benefit of small-group personal training is the potential to develop a larger referral network simply because the number of clients trained per session is greater than in the traditional one-on-one setting. Having more clients in each session equates to more individuals who are exposed to the trainer's services and who can spread the word about the benefits of what he or she has to offer. Additionally, offering small-group training at a reduced session cost motivates interested clients to recruit others to join them in their training, which instantly increases a trainer's client base without the process of actively pursuing new clients.

Building the Program

There are two basic markets from which a trainer can attract small-group clients: current clientele and potential new clients. Each market holds limitless opportunity for building small-group training programs.

- *Referrals from current clientele:* Service-oriented businesses, such as personal training, typically attribute a majority of new client interest from word-of-mouth referrals. Satisfied clients can be a wellspring of enthusiasm and promotion for a personal-training business. To take advantage of this potential referral gold mine, trainers should entice clients to refer people to their business. One option is to reward current clients for bringing in new clients. An example of an enticing reward is to offer one complimentary private- or small-group training session for each referral that becomes a new client. Satisfied clients are the absolute best marketing tools a personal trainer can find. A periodic reminder to current clients about a new-client referral reward policy via email newsletters, brochures, and flyers can go a long way toward building a trainer's small-group and private training programs.
- *Attracting new clients*: One standard tenet of promoting any type of program is to define the customer who will be using the services. An excellent way to attract a specific type of customer is to develop a program that addresses a specific need among a group of people. In the case of small-group personal training, an easy way for a trainer to do this is to offer a limited-term program (lasting four to six weeks) that targets a certain aspect of fitness within his or her area of expertise. Examples include "Low-back Health," "Get Golf-ready," "Core Performance Blast," "Beginning Strength Training for Women," "Bone Builders," and "Strength for Seniors." Promoting these programs to existing and past clients through email newsletters or direct mail, and enticing current clients to refer new participants to these programs, are sound methods for building a new small-group training program.

Limitations

While small-group personal training can be advantageous to trainers and clients alike, there are several limitations that should be addressed when implementing this service. The following situations could negatively affect small-group training sessions:

- Clients who are dissimilar in their conditioning levels
- Clients who require constant individual attention
- Scheduling conflicts

One responsibility of a fitness professional is to ensure that each client receives proper instruction and supervision during exercise, which means that in some cases, small-group training might not be the best option for certain individuals. Strategies to circumvent these problems along with other information on how to create effective small-group programs can be found in ACE's Small-group Training Online Education Program (www.acefitness.org/continuingeducation).

Marketing for Client Retention

Once a prospective client becomes a paying client, it is important to have a retention plan. The challenge with marketing and selling a service like personal training is that it does take some time for the client to see the results of a training program. To retain a client for the long-term, a personal trainer should develop a long-term exercise plan for the client based on the concept of **periodization** (see Chapters 10 and 11).

Applying the science of periodized training allows the personal trainer to demonstrate to the client the benefits of working with a trainer on an ongoing basis. Most clients expect a personal trainer to provide a challenging workout, but a trainer who designs a long-term exercise program for his or her client based on the concept of periodization creates an added value to the personal-training experience. The ACE Integrated Fitness Training™ (ACE IFT™) Model presented in Chapters 5 through 12 uses periodization as a long-term, science-based plan for exercise program design that is aimed at meeting individual client needs, while also providing the personal trainer with a marketing strategy for client retention.

The trainer should identify the specific goals of the client, including the time of year in which the client wants to "peak" in terms of physical fitness. The workout plan should then be broken into phases of varying intensity so that the client is progressing to the next level of intensity as his or her existing series of training sessions is getting ready to expire. The client benefits because he or she receives a structured long-term program based on the understanding of how the body adapts to the physical stresses of exercise. The trainer benefits because it creates a scientifically based method of client retention.

For example, a new client invests in 20 training sessions (10 weeks x two sessions per week) at the beginning of January with the general goal of "losing weight and toning up." Early in the client–trainer relationship, when rapport is first being established, the trainer discovers that the client's family owns a beach house and the client is motivated to change her body to look great for bathing-suit season, which begins Memorial Day weekend. The trainer discovers that this client has tried numerous exercise programs before, but has quit because they have always gotten too hard or it was too difficult to find the time to make it to the gym. At the beginning of January, the trainer has the time to structure a 20-week exercise plan that will help the client achieve her desired beach body by the end of May.

The 20 sessions that the client has purchased will last until early March. In this example, the trainer could structure an exercise program to focus on the client's posture and base level of aerobic fitness during the first 16 workouts (i.e., eight weeks). Starting with a lower level of intensity in the stability and mobility phase (phase 1) will allow the client to gradually adapt to the stresses of exercise while improving the tonic muscles responsible for controlling posture and respiration, which will keep her from trying to do too much too quickly, a potential cause of injury. This method of allowing the client to adapt to the physical stresses of exercise over a structured period of time will help her avoid the overuse injuries she has experienced in the past and develop a positive, long-term relationship with exercise. As the client progresses in her workout program, her posture and base level of cardiorespiratory fitness will improve, allowing her to feel better and have more energy throughout the day, creating a tangible result from the exercise program. As the client comes to a point where she has only three or four training sessions left in the initial package, the trainer should transition the program to the movement-training phase (phase 2) and more challenging cardiovascular exercise. Since the client has made the adaptations to the exercises performed to enhance her posture, the trainer can change the variables of the exercise program, specifically exercise selection, intensity, repetitions, sets, and rest intervals, and the client can experience the difference made by the increased intensity.

The first phase of training over the course of 16 training sessions focused on helping the client progress from the **contemplation** phase to the **action** phase of the **transtheoretical model of behavioral change** by making exercise a regular habit (see Chapter 4). At this point, the client has made progress because the trainer has controlled the intensity of the exercise program. After the initial phase of training, the trainer can start increasing the intensity, since the client's body will be prepared for the more demanding workload. Once the client experiences four sessions of the new movement-training phase and can feel the results from the increased work rate and physical demand, she will likely want to continue working with the trainer and purchase another 10-week package (20 training sessions), which would last until Memorial Day weekend. The client has by then progressed fully into the movement-training phase, including the increased intensity in the cardiovascular exercise program (i.e., phase 2, the aerobic-efficiency phase).

Once the client demonstrates improved movement skills and neural recruitment for enhanced motor coordination, it will be time to progress her to the next stage of training: load training (phase 3). During the load-training phase, the client will perform exercises with external resistance using equipment such as free weights or machines and the trainer will apply the variables of program design in an effort to help the client achieve her original goal. As the client improves her muscular definition and physical appearance, the trainer and client can set more specific goals in an effort to help the client maintain adherence to the program. This will help the trainer retain the client once the current series of sessions nears its end. Applying the science of how the body adapts to exercise will allow the client to make the physiological adaptations to the imposed demands of the training program, while at the same time providing a science-based client-retention tool.

Marketing Through General Communication

Personal trainers must remember that the most common form of communication with potential clients on the gym floor occurs through visual means, since members in a fitness facility are always watching personal trainers as they work with clients. The members will base their perceptions of a trainer's skills and value on what they see as the trainer works with existing clients. New trainers need to be aware that having a neat appearance and conducting business in a professional but fun manner will help to establish effective nonverbal communication with prospective clients. For personal trainers, communication begins with a professional appearance. If a trainer looks professional, potential clients will likely treat the trainer like a professional, while a trainer who looks unkempt or is wearing clothing that is too revealing will send the wrong message to members who are prospective clients.

Every interaction should leave a positive impression. Time is an extremely valuable resource, arguably more valuable than money. Remember, clients hire trainers to maximize the efficiency of the time spent exercising. Marketing efforts should focus on why a potential client should invest money and time on a trainer and the value that working with a trainer will provide. A trainer should focus his or her communication efforts on helping prospective clients maximize their return on training time to achieve specific fitness results. New trainers should realize that it will take approximately three to six months of work to develop a full client schedule.

Choosing a Business Structure

Deciding whether to start a business requires the personal trainer to think about all aspects of starting, owning, and operating that business. Considerations for starting a business include how to structure the business, whether to work with partners, and whether to establish a corporate structure to create an additional layer of **liability** protection. Factors to consider when starting a personal-training business include the following:

- *The level of experience that the potential business owner has in the fitness industry:* If the personal trainer is newly certified and new to the fitness industry, then it might be a good idea to work for someone else for a period of time to learn about the fitness business before venturing out on one's own.
- *The level of self-motivation:* Personal trainers need to possess the ability to approach people they do not know to solicit their business, which includes making sales presentations and asking for money. If a person does not have a high level of self-motivation and the ability to be a salesperson, taking the steps to start a business might not be a good idea.
- *The ability to create and execute a business plan:* Success, whether in sports or business, does not "just happen." There has to be a well-structured plan that defines the steps to take to achieve established goals.
- *The size of the proposed business:* Will it be a single-person operation or will there be other people to help with the workload and provide service to clients?
- *The location of the proposed business:* Will the business provide services in clients' homes or will it have a specific location for seeing clients?
- *The cost of running the proposed business:* How much capital is required to start the business? The start-up costs for a personal-training business can run from hundreds of dollars for starting an in-home training business to tens of thousands of dollars for owning and operating a small studio.
- *The structure of the proposed business:* Will there be partners to help fund and run the business? If so, this requires consideration of what type of business structure to operate.

If a personal trainer is considering opening a personal-training business, he or she must keep in mind that there several different operating structures available, including those described in Chapter 17.

Professional Services for Starting a Business

Just as a person new to exercise should hire an ACE-certified Personal Trainer for guidance on how to safely structure and follow an exercise program to meet his or her goals, a personal trainer interested in opening a business needs to work with other professionals to get help in establishing that business. The following professional services are an important part of the process, and must be accounted for when calculating the costs associated with starting a business.

Attorney

Getting the right legal advice is critical when structuring the necessary articles of incorporation or partnership. The right attorney can be extremely helpful in providing advice and guidance for structuring an effective business that adheres to all state and local regulations. Though an attorney may seem like a large investment, trainers should think about the costs associated with a lawsuit if someone gets injured and the facility owner's assets are not protected with the appropriate corporate structure (see Chapter 17).

Accountant

While many off-the-shelf accounting software programs are available, consulting with an accountant can be extremely helpful for structuring the best cash-flow and financial-management system for the needs of a business. If a trainer is operating as a sole proprietor, an accountant is critical for learning what expenses and costs can be deducted as part of normal business operations.

Web Developer/Graphic Designer

One of the most important aspects of starting and operating a business is creating a brand and establishing a unique brand identity, a large proportion of which is accomplished through a logo and the right online presence. Like accounting software, many websites are available that help people create their own web pages, but having the right presence and the ability to collect personal-training fees and other revenue online requires the advice of a professional with that specific skill set. Taking the time to work with a graphic designer will also help a trainer create a unique and appealing logo that represents the business and can become instantly identifiable to prospective clients.

Insurance Broker

It is important to have the right insurance coverage for any and all potential losses or damages before starting a business. This will help protect any assets such as a house or retirement savings from being lost in the event of unfavorable litigation. Working with an insurance broker will be the most effective way to develop and structure a portfolio that will provide the necessary levels of protection.

Real Estate Broker

A commercial real estate specialist can help a personal trainer find the optimal location for a successful personal-training studio or fitness center. A real estate broker can help determine which neighborhoods have the highest disposable income and find the proper space for the needs of a studio, which include parking for clients and showers for people when they complete their workouts. In addition, a real estate broker can help negotiate the most favorable lease terms, including having the landlord properly prepare and build out the spaces for the needs of the potential business.

Contractors

When opening and operating a facility, it will be important to have good relationships with a variety of tradesmen, including electricians, plumbers, interior designers, landscapers, and commercial janitorial services. Nothing turns off customers faster than a facility with ongoing repair and maintenance issues. Having a network of the right professionals who can address any situation is critical for keeping a business open, operational, and profitable.

Financial Plan

To be successful, trainers should establish budget and revenue goals for themselves. This is especially true for any trainer interested in starting his or her own business. Once expenses have been identified, this information is used to determine the amount of money to charge per session as an independent trainer or the number of sessions to conduct if working as a direct employee. If a personal trainer is not able to set a monthly revenue budget based on his or her minimum expenses while working for an employer, it is not likely that he or she will be successful running a business while maintaining a budget that includes rent, repairs and maintenance on the facility, and any overhead costs such as salary and compensation for employees. One of the great things about the personal-training business is that the earning potential is limited only by the amount of time a trainer wants to work.

The first step to take when establishing a personal budget is to list monthly expenses. The trainer should identify all categories of fixed costs, such as rent, transportation, and utilities, as well as variable costs such as food, entertainment, and professional development (Figure 18-2). A trainer planning to work in the independent-contractor model and rent training space from a facility should include the monthly fee for the use of the facility. The total of these expenses must not exceed the trainer's total earnings.

Once the expenses are identified and totaled, the next step is to determine the number of training sessions required to achieve the revenue to cover these expenses if the trainer is going to work as a direct employee (Figure 18-3). A trainer working in the independent-contractor model should use the monthly expenses as a starting point for establishing his or her session rate, as well as when setting a goal for the number of sessions to deliver.

Another exercise is to start with a yearly income goal and then identify the amount of work needed to make that income. The personal trainer begins by setting a specific and attainable goal for the amount of yearly income desired as a new trainer in the fitness industry. This number then becomes a defined goal that can be used to gauge success (Figure 18-4).

Note that many health clubs will pay a bonus for training a certain number of sessions per pay period, month, or quarter (a fiscal year is divided into four three-month quarters).

The SMART acronym (see Chapter 3) is not only helpful for working with clients to establish their fitness goals, but is also extremely useful when applied to establishing financial goals for operating a personal-training business.

Figure 18-2
Personal expense worksheet

Expense	Weekly	Monthly
Rent		
Food		
Phone		
Internet/cable TV		
Transportation Gas Car payment Insurance		
Health insurance		
Clothing		
Entertainment/dining out		
Education/professional development (20 hours of education is required during every two-year period to maintain an ACE certification)		
Savings		
Retirement		
Taxes (if working as an independent contractor or sole proprietor, the IRS expects quarterly tax payments)		
Other		
Totals		

- *Direct-employee model:* List the compensation for each session performed: ______
- *Independent-contractor model:* List the amount that a client will pay for a training session: ______
- Divide the total monthly expenses (see Figure 18-2) by the amount earned for delivering a training session. This will identify the number of sessions to deliver to meet monthly expenses:
- ______ (monthly expenses)/______ (session fee/pay rate) = ______ (number of sessions required to meet monthly expenses)
    - ✓ At the current rate of pay, this is the number of sessions the trainer needs to deliver each month.
- Divide this number by four to determine the number of sessions needed to deliver per week:
- _____/4 = ______ (weekly session goal)
- Divide the weekly session goal by five (or the number of working days per week) to determine daily session goal:
- _____ (weekly session goal)/5 (number of days per week to work) = _____
    - ✓ This is the number of sessions that must be performed each day to achieve the monthly revenue goals.
- Multiply the minimum number of sessions to be conducted each month by 12 to determine the number of sessions that must be conducted in a year to meet *minimum* expenses. Then multiply this number by the compensation earned per session to determine *minimum* annual income (which will equal 12 times the monthly personal expenses calculated in Figure 18-2):
- _____ (number of sessions per month) x 12 x ____ (compensation per session) = ______ (minimum annual income)
    - ✓ An accurate calculation of annual income is necessary when filling out applications for things like renting an apartment or applying for a loan.

Figure 18-3
Calculating the number of sessions required to meet expenses

Example: How many sessions are needed to meet an annual income goal of $50,000, assuming the personal trainer earns a net of $40 per session?

- Yearly income goal: $50,000
- Weekly income: $50,000/50 weeks* = $1000

Weekly training session goal: $1000/$40 net per session = 25 sessions/week

* The number 50 is used instead of 52 to provide the trainer with two weeks of paid vacation per year.

Figure 18-4
Calculating the number of sessions needed to reach an income goal

- *Specific:* Once a trainer determines how many sessions are needed per week to make a specific income, he or she can determine how many prospective clients he or she needs to communicate with to successfully market the services. If a trainer speaks with five potential clients for every one paying client he or she recruits, then he or she has a **closing ratio** of 20%. The closing ratio can be used to set a specific goal for the number of prospective clients to speak with per week or per shift. For the trainer in this example to earn four new paying clients, he or she will need to set a goal to speak with 20 prospective clients each week, or four prospective clients per day during a five-day work week.
- *Measurable:* Using quantitative metrics such as the number of sessions rendered per month, week, or day or the amount of income earned per week, month, or quarter will help a trainer identify his or her level of success and whether he or she is on track to achieve the established goals.
- *Attainable:* A personal trainer must establish realistic goals for income and the number of sessions to deliver to achieve that income. If trainers work too many hours or too many days in a week, there is a high likelihood that they will not make time for their own exercise programs or possibly experience burnout

and leave the industry altogether. When establishing financial goals, a trainer must make sure they are realistically attainable and remember to make time for personal development as well as professional success.

- *Relevant:* A personal trainer must establish income and career goals that are relevant to the work environment. Not only is it rewarding to help clients improve their lives through exercise, but many health clubs also have compensation plans that allow trainers to earn a very good living. It is possible to earn a six-figure income as a personal trainer. However, it takes time to establish the business and develop a steady client base. For example, if a trainer has a pay rate of $45/session (not uncommon for trainers with two or three years of experience in an urban fitness facility), then he or she would need to conduct 35 training sessions per week, 50 weeks per year to make $78,750—and that does not include any bonuses he or she might receive for achieving production goals. If a trainer is only interested in working part-time, then he or she should set goals to reflect the amount of time he or she can commit to the employer and/or clients.
- *Time-bound:* Breaking down the number of sessions a personal trainer needs to deliver to meet certain revenue or income goals will help to establish the number of hours to work per day, the number of days to work per week, and finally the number of weeks to work in a year. If a trainer is working for him- or herself and wants to have a paid vacation, he or she will need to factor this time in when establishing SMART professional goals.

The financial plan provides the specific details for how a business will generate cash flow and produce a profit, which is the primary goal of a business. When developing the financial plan, a personal trainer must be as specific as possible to complete the proper level of due diligence. Investing the time to consider all of the issues related to cash flow in the planning process will allow a business owner to focus his or her time on the operation once the business is open.

Time Management

As a personal trainer takes on more clients, there will be many demands for his or her time. It is important for trainers to develop a schedule that accommodates all of their needs. It is not uncommon for a new trainer to try to be accommodating to all possible clients, getting to work early to see the morning clients and staying late to see evening clients. Being available at all hours might seem essential when starting a training business, but keep in mind that it is important to set strict guidelines for hours of availability and adhere to them.

A positive aspect of establishing a set schedule of hours is that it makes the trainer's time more valuable and creates the perception of demand; this is the "velvet rope" principle, which states that creating a sense that certain places or services are more scarce makes people perceive those things as even more attractive or valuable. A trainer who carefully manages his or her time and makes specific hours available to clients creates demand by giving the perception that this limited time is indeed extremely valuable. A second benefit is that clients will appreciate their timeslots and be more likely to show up for appointments.

If a prospective client is not able to adjust his or her schedule to fit into the time that a trainer has available, that client should be referred to another trainer who has availability at that time. For example, some trainers might prefer working early mornings and are willing to see clients at 5:00 or 6:00 a.m. If a client wants to work with one of these trainers at night, the trainer might be better off referring that client to a colleague who sees most of his or her clients in the evening. Likewise, the trainers that see clients at night might not be able to see a client at 5:30 a.m., so they will refer those clients to the early-morning trainers. Developing these relationships and the confidence to refer business away to other trainers will help a trainer establish a professional image. A prospective client will understand that a trainer might not be available at a certain time and will appreciate being referred to another qualified trainer. Having a reliable network of fitness professionals who refer clients back and forth will enhance everyone's business.

The schedule for a personal trainer should include time for all of the following activities:

- *Working with clients:* A trainer should establish the hours when he or she is available to see clients and consistently adhere to this schedule. Trainers should adhere to scheduled session times so that one client's session does not run into the next. A client has to understand that he or she is paying for an hour of time; if the client is late, the session should still end on time and not run into the next session. Everyone will appreciate the ability to establish and maintain a consistent schedule.

  A successful trainer will communicate the value of his or her time to clients, as this helps them appreciate the professionalism of a trainer and should reduce the number of clients who do not show up for an appointment or who continually arrive late or cancel their scheduled sessions. It is important to have a written cancellation policy that is clearly communicated to clients. A client should understand the penalty for not showing up or canceling an appointment at the last minute. If a client cancels with sufficient notice (the industry standard is a 24-hour cancellation window), the trainer is usually able to schedule another client in that timeslot. However, if a client cancels at the last minute or does not show up at all, he or she should be held accountable and charged for that session. Many fitness facilities have a policy of charging a client for a late cancellation, though this charge may be waived in the event of extenuating circumstances.
- *Client management:* Client management includes doing all necessary paperwork, such as preparing invoices or paperwork and collecting payments; developing or updating exercise programs; making follow-up phone calls, emails, or text messages to schedule and confirm appointments; and any other communication related to working with existing clients. Managing communications takes time, but clients appreciate the "extra touch" of an email or text message to remind them of an appointment. This practice also helps reduce the amount of no-shows a trainer might experience. If a client receives a reminder message the day before a session or on the morning of a scheduled appointment, it will serve as an opportunity for the client to provide notice to the trainer that the client's schedule has changed so that the trainer can adjust his or her own schedule accordingly.
- *Prospecting for new clients:* This is the time that a trainer might spend in the health club circulating on a fitness floor to meet members, provide assistance, and recruit new clients.
- *Developing marketing or advertising materials:* This includes the time to develop marketing pieces such as a flyer or a postcard for distribution, business cards, or a website. Many trainers use the Internet to market their services, communicate with clients or potential clients, and even collect payments. Creating successful marketing pieces is an effective method to build a business, but it does take time to develop and manage the ongoing communication, so a trainer must plan for it.
- *Other job duties:* In the direct-employee model, the employer might require the trainer to work an assigned shift during which the expectation is that the trainer is not working with private clients but instead providing assistance to all members. In the business-ownership

model, owning and operating a personal-training studio or other fitness facility will take a lot of time. If a trainer is working in clients' homes, he or she must schedule and plan for the time that will be required to travel from one location to the next.

- *Exercise:* An important part of being a personal trainer is maintaining a healthy lifestyle and serving as a role model, which includes following an exercise program. It is not uncommon for new trainers to become so busy with clients that they fail to make time for their own workouts. Personal trainers should not let this happen and should adhere to their personal workout schedules.
- *Personal time/home life:* To avoid burnout or fatigue, it is important for personal trainers to keep time in their schedules for family, friends, and things not related to work—so all trainers should schedule some time for having fun and recharging their batteries.

The biggest challenge when scheduling clients is that there are only a few specific times of day when most clients have the free time available to meet with a personal trainer. Most people generally have time in the morning before work, during their lunch hour, and after work, so those are the times when they are available to meet with personal trainers. The most popular times for clients to work with personal trainers are from 5:00 to 9:00 a.m., 12:00 noon to 2:00 p.m., and 4:00 to 8:00 p.m. There are always exceptions, but these are consistently the most popular timeslots. From 5:00 a.m. to 8:00 p.m. is a period of 15 hours, with 10 of those hours being the most popular among clients.

It might seem as if a trainer has to be available all of the time, which is why it is important to set aside specific times for working with clients. One option is to be a trainer who sees people mainly in the morning, which means being available at the crack of dawn, while another option is to sleep in and see clients mainly in the evening. There is no "best" way, as it all depends on the times of day that a trainer feels most comfortable working and being available to see clients. The unfortunate fact is that while a new trainer is developing a consistent and regular schedule of clients, he or she might have to be flexible to working at all hours of the day. In the long run, a successful personal trainer will have to adjust his or her schedule to be available for clients at peak times, while still maintaining a sense of balance and making time for his or her own quality of life.

How to Sell Personal Training

When a person makes the decision to purchase a health-club membership, he or she is primarily interested in achieving meaningful results. It is widely recognized that personal trainers play a critical role in the success of a fitness facility, as they come in direct contact with members on a daily basis and have the ability to help them achieve the results they desire. The harsh reality of the fitness industry is that for a personal trainer to have a successful career, he or she needs to be comfortable asking potential clients to make a commitment by spending money on the purchase of training sessions—and this requires the ability to be a sales professional.

"Sales" is not a four-letter word. Many personal trainers enter the profession because they sincerely want to help people, not because they want to be salespeople. A salesperson is just someone who sees a customer as a dollar sign, while a sales *professional* will help a consumer make an informed decision to meet a need. A sales professional is a problem solver and educator who can identify the problem that the consumer wants solved and then educate the consumer on the different options for a solution and how he or she will benefit from a product or service. People who are interested in becoming personal trainers enjoy exercise as part of a healthy and active lifestyle and want to make a living helping others improve their lives through exercise. Jeffrey Gitomer, sales expert and author of *The*

Sales Bible, states that "the best salespeople are the ones with the best attitude and product knowledge who give the best customer service" (Gitomer, 2003). ACE-certified Personal Trainers have the knowledge to design safe and effective exercise programs (the product), but they also need the positive attitude and ability to provide a high level of customer service to make the transition to sales professional.

The term "salesperson" often carries a negative connotation, but the sales process is based on helping others. When a person joins a health club or a potential client inquires about training services, he or she is really looking for the advice and guidance of an expert who can help him or her achieve specific results through exercise. Selling is the process of educating a potential client about how an exercise program can do just that. The sales process requires asking someone—a prospective client—to make a commitment to his or her personal fitness goals by investing in the personal trainer through the purchase of training sessions.

Sales professionals are also leaders who help clients make the best decisions for their needs by investing in a product or service. A leader can be defined as one who "changes people's attitudes and behaviors" (Carnegie, 1981). This is exactly what an ACE-certified Personal Trainer should do for his or her clients—lead them on a path to change their personal attitudes and behaviors toward exercise and healthy living.

If marketing is defined as the process of educating a prospective customer about *how* a product or service meets his or her needs, then selling involves helping that customer make the decision that a specific product or service meets those needs—and then making a purchase. Marketing fitness services involves effectively communicating how the knowledge and skills of a personal trainer can meet or exceed the needs of the potential client. Selling personal training is based on a model of helping clients. Personal trainers are able to help, but they need a commitment from the prospective client. It is not a "hard sell," but it involves developing the relationship so that the customer trusts that the trainer can help him or her achieve meaningful results. Selling is a win-win process, especially when it relates to personal training. When a trainer sells a package of training sessions to a client, the client "wins" because he or she is purchasing a needed and valuable service, and the trainer "wins" because he or she has gained a new client and a new source of revenue. While it can take a number of years to develop effective sales techniques, there are two basic components to being a successful sales professional:

- Marketing the personal-training service to potential clients
- Asking for the sale

While there are thousands of ways to sell, the most important involves taking the time to gain prospective clients' trust and discover what they need, and then educating them on how they will meet that need while working with a personal trainer. The following are seven basic rules for selling (Gitomer, 2003):

- Say it (make the presentation) in terms the customer wants, needs, and understands.
- Gather personal information and learn how to use it.
- Build friendships.
- Build a relationship "shield" that no competitor can pierce.
- Establish common ground.
- Gain confidence.
- Have fun and be funny.

While these rules were written for salespeople in general, they are applicable to the profession of personal training, especially the ones regarding building friendships and having fun. Think about what exercise represents to a client: For most of the day, clients have to be at work, school, or home taking care of the family or other essential responsibilities. The time spent in a health club or fitness studio is the client's personal time, so the exercise session has to be fun as well as productive. A client will look forward to working with a personal trainer if the trainer makes the session enjoyable and does not spend his or her time reprimanding the client for having too many snacks or talking to the client in dry, clinical, hard-to-understand language. If a client does experience a setback, the personal trainer should try to encourage the client by letting him or her know that occasional missteps are common and do not equal failure. A client should look forward to seeing his or her trainer, because it is the client's "play time." Trainers who can follow these basic rules and establish this type of relationship with clients will be rewarded with clients who will continue training after the initial package of sessions expires. If clients have fun with a trainer while working hard, they will be more likely to show up for training sessions and refer friends and family to enjoy the same positive experience. The best source of new clients is referrals from existing clients, so it literally pays to create a fun, engaging experience for clients.

Buying decisions are emotionally driven, meaning that prospective clients will think with logic, but act on emotion. **Empathy** is the ability to understand the thoughts and feelings of another person. Exercise deals with body image and feelings of self-confidence. As a result, the selling of a fitness service requires a personal trainer to make an emotional connection with a prospective client and have empathy for him or her. Keep in mind that having empathy for someone requires an understanding of how that person feels, but does *not* require the trainer to feel the same way. Try to imagine how a person feels the first time he or she steps into a health club or a training studio; it can be an extremely intimidating environment, especially if the person does not consider him- or herself to be athletic or in good shape. Empathy is one of the most important traits that a personal trainer can have when interacting with a prospective client. Other important traits for establishing a successful relationship with a prospective client are honesty and integrity. Selling personal training requires being able to sell one's self and create friendships with almost anyone. In the book *How to Win Friends & Influence People,* author Dale Carnegie (1981) identifies six ways to earn someone's immediate respect and trust:

- Become genuinely interested in other people.
- Smile.
- Remember that a person's name is to that person the sweetest and most important sound in any language.
- Be a good listener. Encourage others to talk about themselves.
- Talk in terms of the other person's interests.
- Make the other person feel important—and do it sincerely.

Although these principles were first drafted back in the 1930s, they accurately reflect the steps required to establish an almost instant rapport with a prospective personal-training client. The more solid the foundation of the prospective client–trainer relationship, the more likely it will progress to a client–trainer relationship.

A trainer needs to be able to identify the emotional needs behind the decision to start an exercise program, and work with the client to accommodate those needs. If a personal trainer can understand the motivation behind a client's decision-making process, then all subsequent conversations can be directed to achieving the desired results.

For example, a personal trainer might say: "I understand how difficult it has been to stay committed to an exercise program. You have expressed a feeling of frustration at not achieving your goals and I can relate to that. However, if we work together, I think you will find that having someone encourage you and hold you accountable for your goals will help you adhere to your program." A successful sales professional understands the buying experience from the customer's perspective, and every personal trainer should be able to understand and relate to the difficulty of finding time in a busy schedule to maintain consistent exercise participation. Sensitivity to another person's feelings, needs, and interests is required to be a successful personal trainer, and is a prerequisite for being a successful sales professional.

When a personal trainer meets with a potential client for the first time, it is important to keep in mind that no matter what, a sale *will* happen. Either the prospective client will be sold on the fact that working with the trainer will be worth the investment of time and money, or the client will sell the trainer on the fact that he or she is not actually committed to achieving results. It is important to note that research indicates that working with a trainer is more effective and will provide greater results than exercising on one's own (Faigenbaum et al., 2008). It is the trainer's responsibility to convince a prospective client of this reality.

At the first meeting, the trainer should congratulate the client for taking the steps to change his or her life and commend him or her for making the decision to join that particular fitness facility. Making this positive affirmation will validate the client's decision to take the first step, helping him or her feel more comfortable about meeting with a personal trainer. Trainers should be aware that if a client is over the age of 40 and deconditioned, he or she might be intimidated about being in the presence of a personal trainer, especially if the trainer is 15 to 20 years younger and in excellent shape. A sincere, positive affirmation of taking the step to join a club or meet with a trainer will serve to reinforce the client's decision-making process, making it more likely that he or she will be motivated to purchase a package of training sessions.

There are four basic questions that are required to move from presenting the information about personal training to closing the sale and turning a prospective client into an actual paying client. These questions should be asked once the prospective client has experienced the first full workout session with a trainer, especially if it was a complimentary session that the prospective client received when joining a health club.

- Did you enjoy the workout?
- Would you like to continue to experience the benefits of working with a trainer?
- Do you have the ability to invest in yourself by purchasing a package of training sessions?
- When would you like to schedule our next appointment?

When a conversation about personal training occurs, it is an opportunity for the trainer to make a sales presentation to the prospective client. The trainer should ask the prospective client both directive and non-directive questions. Directive questions can be answered with a simple "yes" or "no," while non-directive questions require a thoughtful, detailed answer from the client. The conversation should cover the client's fitness goals and expectations and how they are related to joining a fitness facility or starting an exercise program. The trainer should then focus the conversation on how the client's expectations can be met by working one-on-one with a personal trainer.

An effective method to close a sale and earn a new client is to ask a series of questions that relate back to the client's goals. For example, "You have explained that these are your goals, and that they are important to you. Can you see yourself when you have achieved these goals? What do you look like? How does that make you feel? If you invest in yourself with the purchase of personal-training sessions, you will be on the way to achieving your goals. Would you like to take that action now? Aren't you worth the investment?"

The conversation should focus on what the client needs and wants, as well as on how the trainer can help. The following questions focus on the needs of the client:

- You have told me your goals. How long have you had these goals?
- Why is it so important that you achieve these goals?
- What has kept you from achieving these goals in the past?
- From what you have told me, I think I can help you work toward meeting these goals. Would you like that?

Personal trainers can use questions to relate to the potential client and get the client feeling positively about the personal-training experience. By asking a series of directive questions, the trainer can *direct* the conversation so that the client continues to say "yes." This puts the client in a positive frame of mind, where he or she realizes that the clear solution for achieving his or her fitness goals is to work with a personal trainer.

The business of personal training is about changing people's lives, and a successful trainer will focus the conversation on how he or she is able to help change a prospective client's life. This is where the desire to help people meets the practical need to earn a living. If a trainer is sincere in his or her interest in providing a high level of service to change a person's life, no selling is involved. The sales process simply becomes a process of discovering what the client needs and then educating the client on the benefits of personal training. A prospective client wants to understand how his or her needs, wants, and desires are going to be satisfied. If a trainer can provide that information, the only decision left to make is when to schedule the next appointment.

Applying the transtheoretical model of behavioral change to the personal training sales process reveals that when a prospective client is inquiring about buying personal training, he or she is making the transition from the **preparation** to the action stage of change. The personal trainer should focus on helping the prospective client take the necessary steps to make exercise an integral part of his or her regular routine. The important thing about conversations at this level is to avoid overwhelming the client with how much work is involved in meeting a goal, and instead discussing how structuring a well-designed exercise program and focusing on doing a little exercise each day will help him or her achieve long-term goals.

Many fitness facilities provide new members with one or more complimentary sessions with a trainer. The primary purpose of the initial session is to conduct a health screening for the new member, but the session also represents an opportunity to learn more about the new member and for the personal trainer to introduce the member to the benefits of working with a trainer. The more a trainer can learn about the new member—and prospective client—during the screening process, the more information the trainer has to help sell his or her services. In addition, the exercise program can be personalized to meet the needs of the client and his or her readiness to change.

When working with new clients, a personal trainer should remember that clients want to know how much a trainer cares about them and their results. Take the time to learn about each client—his or her exercise history, injuries, the amount of time he or she can commit to a program, and his or her ability to adhere to an exercise program. The more detailed the information gathered, the more specific the exercise program that can be developed to produce the desired results. Keep in mind that clients want trainers who are enthusiastic, caring, empathetic, motivating, and genuinely interested in them. Displaying those traits honestly and with integrity is the quickest way to success.

Selling Training Programs

Rather than selling packages of one-hour sessions, personal trainers can offer their services through specific, defined training programs. A session package is a series of individual sessions. The client is purchasing a specific amount of the trainer's time, but the actual outcome of the training sessions is undefined and it is up to the trainer and client to identify specific goals through the intake and assessment process. The challenge with marketing and selling training sessions is that there is not a defined product or service being offered. It can be difficult for a personal trainer to market his or her services to a prospective client when the client does not have a clear expectation of the outcome. Consider the following situation from the client's point of view: The client understands that he or she can benefit from working with a personal trainer, but might not be interested in actually hiring and working with a trainer because he or she does not know what to expect from the experience.

Training programs, in contrast to session packages, clearly communicate a defined outcome so that the client knows what he or she is investing in when making the decision to work with a trainer. A training program is different than a series or package of individual personal-training sessions, because it is designed to progress each individual workout toward a predetermined goal. Selling "personal training" does not define an expected outcome. Marketing a specific outcome package (weight loss or physique/bodybuilding) defines the outcome and establishes the expectation for the client's experience with a trainer. An additional benefit of a defined-outcome training program is that it can help the client adhere to an exercise routine, because he or she is able to begin the program with a specific end in mind. If the client knows what to expect at the end of the program, then it will help him or her stay focused on the workouts to achieve the desired results. A series of training sessions marketed as a program should begin and end with the same specific assessment, test, or movement screen. This will allow the trainer to objectively quantify the results of the program for the client.

Marketing for training programs can be targeted toward specific audiences within a facility or community. During the spring wedding season, personal trainers can market programs designed to help brides and grooms look great on their big day, or they can market programs to prepare for specific seasonal activities such as training for a running race or conditioning for winter sports. The types of programs to offer might include the following:

- *Performance enhancement:* Tests that can be used to demonstrate progress in a performance-enhancement program include movement screens, the vertical jump, or the pro agility test (see Chapter 8).
- *Weight loss:* Assessments to demonstrate client progress include assessing the client's **body composition,** taking circumference measurements, or taking individual skinfold measurements (see Chapter 8).
- *Event preparation (e.g., wedding, trip, reunion):* When helping a client prepare for a specific event, personal trainers should determine the tests or assessments most relevant to the activity or event and use those as a way to measure progress.
- *Post-rehabilitation:* Movement screens are an effective way of measuring improvement from a personal-training program for clients who have been released from physical therapy.

Summary

Earning an ACE certification and starting a career as a personal trainer can be rewarding personally, professionally, and financially. However, earning the ACE certification is just the beginning. A successful career as a personal trainer requires forethought on the part of the trainer to develop a plan to attract clients and operate the business. Once a newly certified personal trainer makes a decision about which employment model to follow, he or she can take the critical steps to plan the business, just as he or she would take the time to plan a client's exercise program.

Even if the ultimate goal is to open a training studio or similar business, it is a good idea to start a fitness career in a relatively risk-free environment of a health club or similar facility. Working for an employer is an invaluable way to learn how a fitness business operates from the ground up without assuming the financial risk of starting a business. Once a personal trainer has learned the trade and developed a specific brand of fitness, it might be time for him or her to make the leap to opening a business, but only with a prudent plan to guide the way.

References

Beckwith, H. (1997). *Selling the Invisible: A Field Guide to Modern Marketing.* New York: Warner Books.

Carnegie, D. (1981). *How to Win Friends & Influence People* (revised edition). New York: Simon & Schuster.

Faigenbaum, A. et al. (2008). Self-selected resistance training intensity in healthy women: The influence of a personal trainer. *Journal of Strength and Conditioning Research,* 22, 1, 103–111.

Gitomer, J. (2003). *The Sales Bible* (revised edition). Hoboken, N.J.: John Wiley & Sons.

Suggested Reading

Covey, S. (2004). *The Seven Habits of Highly Effective People.* New York: Simon and Schuster.

Peterson, J. & Tharrett, S. (2008). *Fitness Management* (2nd ed.) Monterey, Calif.: Healthy Learning.

Ries, A. & Ries, L. (2004). *The Origin of Brands.* New York: Harper Business.

Ziglar, Z. (2003). *Secrets of Closing the Sale* (updated edition). Grand Rapids, Mich.: Fleming H. Revell.

Appendices

Appendix A
ACE Code of Ethics

Appendix B
Exam Content Outline

Appendix C
ACE Position Statement on Nutritional Supplements

APPENDIX A

ACE Code of Ethics

ACE-certified Professionals are guided by the following principles of conduct as they interact with clients/participants, the public, and other health and fitness professionals.

ACE-certified Professionals will endeavor to:

- ✔ Provide safe and effective instruction
- ✔ Provide equal and fair treatment to all clients
- ✔ Stay up-to-date on the latest health and fitness research and understand its practical application
- ✔ Maintain current CPR certification and knowledge of first-aid services
- ✔ Comply with all applicable business, employment, and intellectual property laws
- ✔ Maintain the confidentiality of all client information
- ✔ Refer clients to more qualified health or medical professionals when appropriate
- ✔ Uphold and enhance public appreciation and trust for the health and fitness industry
- ✔ Establish and maintain clear professional boundaries

Provide Safe and Effective Instruction

Providing safe and effective instruction involves a variety of responsibilities for ACE-certified Professionals. Safe means that the instruction will not result in physical, mental, or financial harm to the client/participant. Effective means that the instruction has a purposeful, intended, and desired effect toward the client's/participant's goal. Great effort and care must be taken in carrying out the responsibilities that are essential in creating a positive exercise experience for all clients/participants.

Screening

ACE-certified Professionals should have all potential clients/participants complete an industry-recognized health-screening tool to ensure safe exercise participation. If significant risk factors or signs and symptoms suggestive of chronic disease are identified, refer the client/participant to a physician or primary healthcare practitioner for medical clearance and guidance regarding which types of assessments, activities, or exercises are indicated, contraindicated, or deemed high risk. If an individual does not want to obtain medical clearance, have that individual sign a legally prepared document that releases you and the facility in which you work from any liability related to any injury that may result from exercise participation or assessment. Once the client/participant has been cleared for exercise and you have a full understanding of the client's/participant's health status and medical history, including his or her current use of medications, a formal risk-management plan for potential emergencies must be prepared and reviewed periodically.

Assessment

The main objective of a health assessment is to establish the client's/participant's baseline fitness level in order to design an appropriate exercise program. Explain the risks and benefits of each assessment and provide the client/participant with any pertinent instructions. Prior to conducting any type of assessment, the client/participant must be given an opportunity to ask questions and read and sign an informed consent. The types and order of assessments are dictated by the client's/participant's health status, fitness level, symptoms, and/or use of medications. Remember that each assessment has specific protocols and only those within your scope of practice should be administered. Once the assessments are completed, evaluate and discuss the results objectively as they relate to the client's/participant's health condition and goals. Educate the client/participant and emphasize how an exercise program will benefit the client/participant.

Program Design

You must not prescribe exercise, diet, or treatment, as doing so is outside your scope of practice and implies ordering or advising a medicine or treatment. Instead, it is appropriate for you to design exercise programs that improve components of physical fitness and wellness while adhering to the limitations of a previous injury or condition as determined by a certified, registered, or licensed allied health professional. Because nutritional laws and the practice of dietetics vary in each state, province, and country, understand what type of basic nutritional information is appropriate and legal for you to disseminate to your client/participant. The client's/participant's preferences, and short- and long-term goals as well as current industry standards and guidelines must be taken into consideration as you develop a formal yet realistic exercise and weight-management program. Provide as much detail for all exercise parameters such as mode, intensity, type of exercise, duration, progression, and termination points.

Program Implementation

Do not underestimate your ability to influence the client/participant to become active for a lifetime. Be sure that each class or session is well-planned, sequential, and documented. Instruct the client/participant how to safely and properly perform the appropriate exercises and communicate this in a manner that the client/participant will understand

and retain. Each client/participant has a different learning curve that will require different levels of attention, learning aids, and repetition. Supervise the client/participant closely, especially when spotting or cueing is needed. If supervising a group of two or more, ensure that you can supervise and provide the appropriate amount of attention to each individual at all times. Ideally, the group will have similar goals and will be performing similar exercises or activities. Position yourself so that you do not have to turn your back to any client/participant performing an exercise.

Facilities

Although the condition of a facility may not always be within your control, you are still obligated to ensure a hazard-free environment to maximize safety. If you notice potential hazards in the health club, communicate these hazards to the client and the facility management. For example, if you notice that the clamps that keep the weights on the barbells are getting rusty and loose, it would be prudent of you to remove them from the training area and alert the facility that immediate repair is required.

Equipment

Obtain equipment that meets or exceeds industry standards and utilize the equipment only for its intended use. Arrange exercise equipment and stations so that adequate space exists between equipment, participants, and foot traffic. Schedule regular maintenance and inspect equipment prior to use to ensure it is in proper working condition. Avoid the use of homemade equipment, as your liability is greater if it causes injury to a person exercising under your supervision.

Provide Equal and Fair Treatment to All Clients/Participants

ACE-certified Professionals are obligated to provide fair and equal treatment for each client/participant without bias, preference, or discrimination against gender, ethnic background, age, national origin, basis of religion, or physical disability.

The Americans with Disabilities Act protects individuals with disabilities against any type of unlawful discrimination. A disability can be either physical or mental, such as epilepsy, paralysis, HIV infection, AIDS, a significant hearing or visual impairment, mental retardation, or a specific learning disability. ACE-certified Professionals should, at a minimum, provide reasonable accommodations to each individual with a disability. Reasonable simply means that you are able to provide accommodations that do not cause you any undue hardship that requires additional or significant expense or difficulty. Making an existing facility accessible by modifying equipment or devices, assessments, or training materials are a few examples of providing reasonable accommodations. However, providing the use of personal items or providing items at your own expense may not be considered reasonable.

This ethical consideration of providing fair and equal treatment is not limited to behavioral interactions with clients, but also extends to exercise programming and other business-related services such as communication, scheduling, billing, cancellation policies, and dispute resolution.

Stay Up-to-Date on the Latest Health and Fitness Research and Understand Its Practical Application

Obtaining ACE-certification required you to have broad-based knowledge of many disciplines; however, this credential should not be viewed as the end of your professional development and education. Instead, it should be viewed as the beginning or foundation. The dynamic nature of the health and fitness industry requires you to maintain an understanding of the latest research and professional standards and guidelines, and of their impact on the design and implementation of exercise programming. To stay informed, make time to review a variety of industry resources such as professional journals, position statements, trade and lay periodicals, and correspondence courses, as well as to attend professional meetings, conferences, and educational workshops.

An additional benefit of staying up-to-date is that it also fulfills your certification renewal requirements for continuing education credit (CEC). To maintain your ACE-certification status, you must obtain an established amount of CECs every two years. CECs are granted for structured learning that takes place within the educational portion of a course related to the profession and presented by a qualified health and fitness professional.

Maintain Current CPR Certification and Knowledge of First-aid Services

ACE-certified Professionals must be prepared to recognize and respond to heart attacks and other life-threatening emergencies. Emergency response is enhanced by training and maintaining skills in CPR, first aid, and using automated external defibrillators (AEDs), which have become more widely available. An AED is a portable electronic device used to restore normal heart rhythm in a person experiencing a cardiac arrest and can reduce the time to defibrillation before EMS personnel arrive. For each minute that defibrillation is delayed, the victim's chance of survival is reduced by 7 to 10%. Thus, survival from cardiac arrest is improved dramatically when CPR and defibrillation are started early.

Comply With All Applicable Business, Employment, and Intellectual Property Laws

As an ACE-certified Professional, you are expected to maintain a high level of integrity by complying with all applicable business, employment, and copyright laws. Be truthful and forthcoming with communication to clients/participants, coworkers, and other health and fitness professionals in advertising, marketing, and business practices. Do not create false or misleading impressions of credentials, claims, or sponsorships, or perform services outside of your scope of practice that are illegal, deceptive, or fraudulent.

All information regarding your business must be clear, accurate, and easy to understand for all potential clients/participants. Provide disclosure about the name of your business, physical address, and contact information, and maintain a working phone number and email address. So that clients/ participants can make an informed choice about paying for your services, provide detailed information regarding schedules, prices, payment terms, time limits, and conditions. Cancellation, refund, and rescheduling information must also be clearly stated and easy to understand. Allow the client/participant an opportunity to ask questions and review this information before formally agreeing to your services and terms.

Because employment laws vary in each city, state, province, and country, familiarize yourself with the applicable employment regulations and standards to which your business must conform. Examples of this may include conforming to specific building codes and zoning ordinances or making sure that your place of business is accessible to individuals with a disability.

The understanding of intellectual property law and the proper use of copyrighted materials is an important legal issue for all ACE-certified Professionals. Intellectual property laws protect the creations of authors, artists, software programmers, and others with copyrighted materials. The most common infringement of intellectual property law in the fitness industry is the use of music in an exercise class. When commercial music is played in a for-profit exercise class, without a performance or blanket license, it is considered a public performance and a violation of intellectual property law. Therefore, make sure that any music, handouts, or educational materials are either exempt from intellectual property law or permissible under laws by reason of fair use, or obtain express written consent from the copyright holder for distribution, adaptation, or use. When in doubt, obtain permission first or consult with a qualified legal professional who has intellectual property law expertise.

Maintain the Confidentiality of All Client/Participant Information

Every client/participant has the right to expect that all personal data and discussions with an ACE-certified Professional will be safeguarded and not disclosed without the client's/participant's express written consent or acknowledgement. Therefore, protect the confidentiality of all client/participant information such as contact data, medical records, health history, progress notes, and meeting details. Even when confidentiality is not required by law, continue to preserve the confidentiality of such information.

Any breach of confidentiality, intentional or unintentional, potentially harms the productivity and trust of your client/participant and undermines your effectiveness as a fitness professional. This also puts you at risk for potential litigation and puts your client/class participant at risk for public embarrassment and fraudulent activity such as identity theft.

Most breaches of confidentiality are unintentional and occur because of carelessness and lack of awareness. The most common breach of confidentiality is exposing or storing personal data in a location that is not secure. This occurs when a client's/participant's file or information is left on a desk, or filed in a cabinet that has no lock or is accessible to others. Breaches of confidentiality may also occur when you have conversations regarding a client's/participant's performance or medical/health history with staff or others and the client's/participant's first name or other identifying details are used.

Post and adhere to a privacy policy that communicates how client/participant information will be used and secured and how a client's/participant's preference regarding unsolicited mail and email will be respected. When a client/participant provides you with any personal data, new or updated, make it a habit to immediately secure this information and ensure that only you and/or the appropriate individuals have access to it. Also, the client's/participant's files must only be accessed and used for purposes related to health and fitness services. If client/participant information is stored on a personal computer, restrict access by using a protected password. Should you receive any inquiries from family members or other individuals regarding the progress of a client/participant or other personal information, state that you cannot provide any information without the client's/participant's permission. If and when a client/participant permits you to release confidential information to an authorized individual or party, utilize secure methods of communication such as certified mail, sending and receiving information on a dedicated private fax line, or email with encryption.

Refer Clients/Participants to More Qualified Health or Medical Professionals When Appropriate

A fitness certification is not a professional license. Therefore, it is vitally important that ACE-certified Professionals who do not also have a professional license (i.e., physician, physical therapist, dietitian, psychologist, and attorney) refer their clients/participants to a more qualified professional when warranted. Doing so not only benefits your clients/participants by making sure that they receive the appropriate attention and care, but also enhances your credibility and reduces liability by defining your scope of practice and clarifying what services you can and cannot reasonably provide.

Knowing when to refer a client/participant is, however, as important as choosing to which professional to refer. For instance, just because a client/participant complains of symptoms of muscle soreness or discomfort or exhibits signs of fatigue or lack of energy is not an absolute indication to refer your client/participant to a physician. Because continual referrals such as this are not practical, familiarize and educate yourself on expected signs and symptoms, taking into consideration the client's/participant's fitness level, health status, chronic disease, disability, and/or background as they are screened and as they begin and progress with an exercise program. This helps you better discern between emergent and non-emergent situations and know when to refuse to offer your services, continue to monitor, and/or make an immediate referral.

It is important that you know the scope of practice for various health professionals and which types of referrals are appropriate. For example, some states require that a referring physician first approve visits to a physical therapist, while other states allow individuals to see a physical therapist directly. Only registered or licensed dietitians or physicians may provide specific dietary recommendations or diet plans; however, a client/participant who is suspected of an eating disorder should be referred to an eating disorders specialist. Refer clients/participants to a clinical psychologist if they wish to discuss family or marital problems or exhibit addictive behaviors such as substance abuse.

Network and develop rapport with potential allied health professionals in your area before you refer clients/participants to them. This demonstrates good will and respect for their expertise and will most likely result in reciprocal referrals for your services and fitness expertise.

Uphold and Enhance Public Appreciation and Trust for the Health and Fitness Industry

The best way for ACE-certified Professionals to uphold and enhance public appreciation and trust for the health and fitness industry is to represent themselves in a dignified and professional manner. As the public is inundated with misinformation and false claims about fitness products and services, your expertise must be utilized to dispel myths and half-truths about current trends and fads that are potentially harmful to the public.

When appropriate, mentor and dispense knowledge and training to less-experienced fitness professionals. Novice fitness professionals can benefit from your experience and skill as you assist them in establishing a foundation based on exercise science, from both theoretical and practical standpoints. Therefore, it is a disservice if you fail to provide helpful or corrective information—especially when an individual, the public, or other fitness professionals are at risk for injury or increased liability. For example, if you observe an individual using momentum to perform a strength-training exercise, the prudent course of action would be to suggest a modification. Likewise, if you observe a fitness professional in your workplace consistently failing to obtain informed consents before clients/participants undergo fitness testing or begin an exercise program, recommend that he or she consider implementing these forms to minimize liability.

Finally, do not represent yourself in an overly commercial or misleading manner. Consider the fitness professional who places an advertisement in a local newspaper stating: Lose 10 pounds in 10 days or your money back! It is inappropriate to lend credibility to or endorse a product, service, or program founded upon unsubstantiated or misleading claims; thus a solicitation such as this must be avoided, as it undermines the public's trust of health and fitness professionals.

Establish and Maintain Clear Professional Boundaries

Working in the fitness profession requires you to come in contact with many different people. It is imperative that a professional distance be maintained in relationships with all clients/participants. Fitness professionals are responsible for setting and monitoring the boundaries between a working relationship and friendship with their clients/participants. To that end, ACE-certified Professionals should:

- Never initiate or encourage discussion of a sexual nature
- Avoid touching clients/participants unless it is essential to instruction

- Inform clients/participants about the purpose of touching and find an alternative if the client/participant objects
- Discontinue all touching if it appears to make the client/participant uncomfortable
- Take all reasonable steps to ensure that any personal and social contacts between themselves and their clients/participants do not have an adverse impact on the trainer–client or instructor–participant relationship.

If you find yourself unable to maintain appropriate professional boundaries with a client/participant (whether due to your attitudes and actions or those of the client/participant), the prudent course of action is to terminate the relationship and, perhaps, refer the client/participant to another professional. Keep in mind that charges of sexual harassment or assault, even if groundless, can have disastrous effects on your career.

For the most up-to-date version of the Exam Content Outline please go to www.acefitness.org/PTexamcontent and download a free PDF.

Attention Exam Candidates!

When preparing for an ACE certification exam, be aware that the material presented in this manual, or any text, may become outdated due to the evolving nature of the fitness industry, as well as new developments in current and ongoing research. These exams are based on an in-depth job analysis and an industry-wide validation survey. By design, these exams assess a candidate's knowledge and application of the most current scientifically based professional standards and guidelines. The dynamic nature of this field requires that ACE certification exams be regularly updated to ensure that they reflect the latest industry findings and research. Therefore, the knowledge and skills required to pass these exams are not solely represented in this or any industry text. In addition to learning the material presented in this manual, ACE strongly encourages all exam candidates and fitness professionals to keep abreast of new developments, guidelines, and standards from a variety of valid industry sources.

APPENDIX B

Exam Content Outline

Purpose

In July 2005, the American Council on Exercise® (ACE®) and CASTLE Worldwide, Inc., conducted a role delineation study to identify the primary tasks performed by personal trainers. The fundamental purpose of this study was to establish and validate appropriate content areas for the ACE Personal Trainer Certification Examination. The result of this process includes this exam content outline, which sets forth the tasks, knowledge, and skills necessary for a personal trainer to perform job responsibilities at a minimum professional level. It is the position of ACE that the recommendations outlined here are not exhaustive to the qualifications of a personal trainer, but represent a minimum level of proficiency and theoretical knowledge. Please note that not all knowledge and skill statements listed in the exam content outline will be addressed on each exam administration.

Description

An ACE-certified Personal Trainer works in a health/fitness facility or in another appropriate setting administering individualized physical-activity programs to asymptomatic individuals or those who have been cleared by a physician. ACE-certified Personal Trainers will be competent to assess a client's health/medical/fitness status effectively; design safe and effective physical-activity programs utilizing goal setting, exercise science principles, and safety guidelines; implement the exercise program safely and effectively; modify the program as necessary to achieve reasonable goals; and adhere to all codes, laws, and procedures applicable within the recognized scope of practice for personal trainers. The ACE Personal Trainer Certification will be granted to those candidates who possess current adult CPR, are at least 18 years of age, and obtain the minimum passing score on an entry-level examination measuring ACE-identified competencies. This certification is appropriate for individuals working one-on-one, with small groups, or as floor staff, etc. The certification will be valid for a two-year period, at which time it may be renewed. Requirements for renewal will be obtaining a predetermined number of continuing education credits (CECs) and paying the applicable fee.

The ACE Personal Trainer Exam includes a Written Simulation portion that is designed to test the decision-making ability of the candidate. The problems in the exam are intended to simulate, as closely as possible, the types of situations that an actual certified personal trainer may encounter in a professional setting. Please visit www.acefitness.org to learn more.

The Examination Content Outline is essentially a blueprint for the exam. All exam questions are based on this outline.

Domains, Tasks, and Knowledge and Skill Statements

A Role Delineation Study completed for the Personal Trainer certification first identified the major categories of responsibility for the professional. These categories are defined as Domains and it was determined that the profession could be divided into four Performance Domains, or major areas of responsibility. These Performance Domains are:

- **Domain I: Client Interview and Assessment**
- **Domain II: Program Design and Implementation**
- **Domain III: Program Progression, Modification and Maintenance**
- **Domain IV: Professional Role and Responsibility**

The Personal Trainer, in performing his or her job, draws upon knowledge from four foundational sciences called Content Domains. The Content Domains include all exercise science topics important to the competence of the Personal Trainer in fulfilling the Performance Domains. These foundational sciences are:

- Anatomy and Biomechanics
- Physiology
- Nutrition
- Psychology

Within each Performance Domain are Task Statements that detail the job-related functions under the specific Domain. Each Task Statement is further divided into Knowledge and Skill Statements to further detail the scope of information required and how that information is applied in a practical setting for each Task Statement.

The Domains are presented in two dimensions:

- Performance Domains are listed vertically: client interview and assessment; program design and implementation; program progression, modification and maintenance; and professional role and responsibility
- Content domains tare listed horizontally: anatomy and biomechanics; physiology; nutrition; and psychology

Table 1
Exam Content Outline: Personal Trainer Certification

Applied Exercise Science					
Performance Domain	Total Items	Anatomy and Biomechanics (40)	Physiology (33)	Nutrition (20)	Psychology (22)
Client Interview and Assessment	40	14	11	7	8
Program Design and Implementation	41	14	12	7	8
Program Progression, Modification, and Maintenance	34	12	10	6	6
Professional Role and Responsibility	10	0	0	0	0
Total:	125	40	33	20	22

Domain I – Client Interview and Assessment 32%

Task 1 - Establish rapport and program value using effective communication and listening techniques to build trust, confidence, and enthusiasm and to maximize program participation.

Knowledge of:

Psychology

1. Communication techniques (e.g., active listening, appropriate eye contact, reflecting and other attending behaviors, nonverbal and verbal communication)
2. Effective interviewing techniques (e.g., open-ended questioning, clarifying, paraphrasing, probing, summarizing)
3. Factors that build and enhance rapport (e.g., empathy, genuineness, nonjudgmental responses, client confidentiality)
4. Cultural, ethnic, and personal differences as they affect communication, lifestyle, dietary habits, and personal and interpersonal behavior (e.g., common assumptions, misconceptions, complicating factors)
5. Environmental factors that affect communication (e.g., location, noise, temperature, distractions, sense of privacy)
6. Psychological factors that influence an individual's self-image and their impact on the communication process
7. Each interaction as an opportunity to enhance or improve an individual's lifestyle
8. Communication technology (e.g., software, email, website, telephone)

Skill in:

Psychology

1. Selecting an appropriate environment for consultation sessions
2. Applying interviewing and communication techniques (e.g., active listening)
3. Respecting the client's personal characteristics (e.g., gender, age, cultural/ethnic background) in all communication
4. Building rapport
5. Avoiding behaviors that are detrimental to building rapport (e.g., prejudicial statements, negative body language, and unproductive assumptions with regard to the client's body size, eating habits, past successes/failures with weight management)
6. Interpreting body language and recognizing incongruities between verbal and nonverbal behaviors
7. Identifying stage of behavioral change
8. Enhancing the perceived value of lifestyle modification for the client
9. Using technology as a communication tool

Task 2 - Assess client attitudes, preferences, motivations, and readiness for behavior change using questionnaires and interviews to set appropriate program goals and to identify potential barriers and unrealistic expectations.

Knowledge of:

Nutrition

1. Cultural, ethnic, and personal differences as they affect dietary habits
2. Potential barriers to healthful dietary choices and weight management

Psychology

1. Communication techniques (e.g., active listening, appropriate eye contact, reflecting and other attending behaviors, nonverbal and verbal communication)
2. Effective interviewing techniques (e.g., open-ended questioning, clarifying, paraphrasing, probing, summarizing)
3. Factors that build and enhance rapport (e.g., empathy, genuineness, nonjudgmental responses, client confidentiality)
4. Cultural, ethnic, and personal differences as they affect communication, lifestyle, dietary habits, and personal and interpersonal behavior (e.g., common assumptions, misconceptions, complicating factors)
5. Environmental factors that affect communication (e.g., location, noise,

temperature, distractions, sense of privacy)

6. Psychological factors that influence an individual's self-image and their impact on the communication process
7. Factors that indicate a client's readiness to change
8. Appropriate forms and assessment tools

Skill in:

Nutrition

1. Identifying potential barriers to healthful dietary choices and weight management

Psychology

2. Applying interviewing and communication techniques (e.g., active listening, empathy)
3. Respecting the client's personal characteristics (e.g., gender, age, cultural/ethnic background) in all communication
4. Interpreting body language and recognizing incongruities between verbal and nonverbal behaviors
5. Avoiding behaviors that are detrimental to building trust (e.g., prejudicial statements, body language, assumptions with regard to body size, eating habits, past successes and failures with weight management, activity history, and ability)
6. Identifying stage of behavioral change
7. Using stage-specific strategies for facilitating behavior change
8. Administering appropriate forms and assessment tools

Task 3 - Obtain health and exercise history and lifestyle information (e.g., nutrition habits, activity) using questionnaires, interviews, and available documents to determine risk stratification, to identify the need for medical clearance and referrals, and to facilitate program design

Knowledge of:

Anatomy and Biomechanics

1. General anatomy (e.g., neuromuscular, musculoskeletal, cardiovascular, respiratory)
2. Anatomical position, muscle actions, functional movements, and planes of motion
3. Normal joint range of motion
4. Physical laws of motion (e.g., inertia, acceleration, momentum, impact and reaction forces, lever classes, muscle and force production)
5. Static postural assessment and movement analysis (e.g., postural and muscle imbalances)
6. Static and dynamic balance (e.g., center of gravity, base of support, proprioception)

Physiology

1. General physiology (e.g., neuromuscular, musculoskeletal, cardiorespiratory, cardiovascular, endocrine)
2. General physiology of cardiorespiratory, metabolic, and musculoskeletal diseases and conditions (e.g., diabetes, osteoporosis, cardiovascular disease)
3. Population-specific considerations (e.g., youth, older adults, pregnancy)
4. Cardiovascular risk factors, risk stratification, and industry guidelines
5. Appropriate precautions with respect to prescription and nonprescription drugs

Nutrition

1. Appropriate allied health professionals to use as referrals (e.g., registered dietitians, physicians)
2. Physical and psychological signs and symptoms that might indicate the need for referral

Psychology

1. Communication techniques (e.g., active listening, appropriate eye contact, reflecting and other attending behaviors, nonverbal and verbal communication)
2. Effective interviewing techniques (e.g., open-ended questioning, clarifying, paraphrasing, probing, , summarizing)
3. Factors that build and enhance rapport (e.g., empathy, genuineness, nonjudgmental responses, client confidentiality)

4. Cultural, ethnic, and personal differences as they affect communication, lifestyle, dietary habits, and personal and interpersonal behavior (e.g., common assumptions, misconceptions, complicating factors)
5. Environmental factors that affect communication (e.g., location, noise, temperature, distractions, sense of privacy)
6. Psychological factors that influence an individual's self esteem and body image (e.g., anorexia, bulimia, body dysmorphia) and their impact on the communication process
7. Appropriate data-collection forms

Skill in:

Anatomy and Biomechanics

1. Applying knowledge of anatomy and biomechanics to the interpretation of health-history data

Physiology

1. Identifying and taking appropriate precautions with respect to prescription and nonprescription drugs
2. Identifying conditions based on observation and those addressed on the health-history and lifestyle questionnaires
3. Stratifying risk and identifying the need for referral

Nutrition

1. Recognizing physical and psychological conditions that might indicate the need for referral
2. Recognizing the need to refer clients to appropriate allied health professionals

Psychology

1. Applying interviewing and communication techniques (e.g., active listening)
2. Respecting the client's personal characteristics (e.g., gender, age, cultural/ethnic background) in all communication
3. Avoiding behaviors that are detrimental to building trust (e.g., prejudicial statements, body language, assumptions with regard to body size, eating habits, past successes and failures with weight management, activity history, and ability)
4. Identifying stage of behavioral change
5. Managing time during the interview and data-collection processes

Task 4 - Conduct appropriate baseline assessments (e.g., posture, function, cardiorespiratory fitness, muscular strength and endurance, flexibility, body composition, heart rate, blood pressure, diet, lifestyle) based on the client interview, questionnaire information, and standardized protocols to establish a safe, effective exercise program and to track changes over time.

Knowledge of:

Anatomy and Biomechanics

1. General anatomy (e.g., neuromuscular, musculoskeletal, cardiovascular, respiratory)
2. Anatomical position, muscle actions, functional movements, and planes of motion
3. Normal joint range of motion
4. Physical laws of motion (e.g., inertia, acceleration, momentum, impact and reaction forces, lever classes, muscle and force production)
5. Static postural assessment and movement analysis (e.g., postural and muscle imbalances)
6. Static and dynamic balance (e.g., center of gravity, base of support, proprioception)

Physiology

1. General physiology (e.g., neuromuscular, musculoskeletal, cardiorespiratory, cardiovascular, endocrine)
2. General physiology of cardiorespiratory, metabolic, and musculoskeletal diseases and conditions (e.g., diabetes, osteoporosis, cardiovascular disease)
3. Population-specific considerations (e.g., youth, older adults, pregnancy)
4. Acute physiological responses to exercise testing with consideration for individual differences (e.g., age, gender, disease, environmental conditions)

5. Normal and abnormal responses during physiological assessment
6. Effects of medications on physiological responses during testing
7. Factors that affect body composition
8. Standardized testing protocols, their intended use, and limitations
9. Signs indicating the need for test termination

Nutrition

1. Appropriate dietary assessment protocols and their uses (e.g., 24-hour diet recall, food logs, food frequency questionnaires)
2. Limitations of dietary data (e.g., inaccurate reporting, inaccurate recording)

Psychology

1. Communication techniques (e.g., active listening, appropriate eye contact, reflecting and other attending behaviors, nonverbal and verbal communication)
2. Factors that build and enhance rapport (e.g., empathy, genuineness, nonjudgmental responses, client confidentiality)
3. Cultural, ethnic, and personal differences as they affect communication, lifestyle, dietary habits, and personal and interpersonal behavior (e.g., common assumptions, misconceptions, complicating factors)
4. Motivating and demotivating factors of fitness testing

Skill in:

Anatomy and Biomechanics

1. Assessing posture and movement
2. Assessing static and dynamic balance
3. Monitoring movement patterns during fitness testing

Physiology

1. Selecting and administering a variety of physiological assessments (e.g., cardiorespiratory, muscular strength and endurance, body composition, flexibility)
2. Monitoring client responses during test administration (e.g., blood pressure, heart rate, RPE)
3. Measuring and recording exercise testing data accurately
4. Recognizing responses that indicate the need for test termination
5. Terminating exercise tests safely

Nutrition

1. Administering appropriate dietary assessment protocols
2. Collecting nutrition data

Psychology

1. Empathizing with the client's lack of experience, knowledge, or expertise in exercise methods and techniques
2. Modifying communication style and content appropriate to the client (e.g., learning style, sensory limitations, educational background, primary language)

DOMAIN II - PROGRAM DESIGN AND IMPLEMENTATION 33%

Task 1 - Interpret the results of the client interview and assessment by evaluating responses and data to facilitate goal setting and the design of a safe and effective exercise and lifestyle program.

Knowledge of:

Anatomy and Biomechanics

1. General anatomy (e.g., neuromuscular, musculoskeletal, cardiovascular, respiratory)
2. Anatomical position, muscle actions, functional movements, and planes of motion
3. Normal joint range of motion
4. Physical laws of motion (e.g., inertia, acceleration, momentum, impact and reaction forces, lever classes, muscle and force production)
5. Static postural assessment and movement analysis (e.g., postural and muscle imbalances)

6. Static and dynamic balance (e.g., center of gravity, base of support, proprioception)

Physiology

1. General physiology (e.g., neuromuscular, musculoskeletal, cardiorespiratory, cardiovascular, endocrine)
2. General physiology of cardiorespiratory, metabolic, and musculoskeletal diseases and conditions (e.g., diabetes, osteoporosis, cardiovascular disease)
3. Population-specific considerations (e.g., youth, older adults, pregnancy)
4. Data interpretation using standardized norms
5. Relationship between BMI, waist-to-hip ratio, and circumference measures and body weight, and determination of appropriate body weight

Nutrition

1. Methods for interpreting client assessment data in relation to established guidelines
2. Limitations of dietary assessment data
3. Applicable guidelines and standards published by accepted organizations (e.g., American Dietetic Association, U.S. Department of Agriculture, American Heart Association)

Psychology

1. Factors that indicate a client's readiness to change
2. Underlying motives that initiate program participation

Skill in:

Anatomy and Biomechanics

1. Evaluating musculoskeletal assessment data

Physiology

1. Interpreting physiological data relative to standardized norms

Nutrition

1. Evaluating the client's diet history, interview, and observations relative to accepted guidelines
2. Applying relevant standards and guidelines published by accepted organizations
3. Accounting for the limitations of dietary data

Psychology

1. Identifying stage of behavioral change
2. Identifying client goals, perceived and unperceived needs, and expectations for change
3. Helping the client to clarify and refine needs and motivations

Task 2 - Establish specific client goals using the interpretation of interview and assessment results and current standards to provide program direction.

Knowledge of:

Anatomy and Biomechanics

1. General anatomy (e.g., neuromuscular, musculoskeletal, cardiovascular, respiratory)
2. Anatomical position, muscle actions, functional movements, and planes of motion
3. Normal joint range of motion
4. Physical laws of motion (e.g., inertia, acceleration, momentum, impact and reaction forces, lever classes, muscle and force production)
5. Static postural assessment and movement analysis (e.g., postural and muscle imbalances)
6. Static and dynamic balance (e.g., center of gravity, base of support, proprioception)

Physiology

1. General physiology (e.g., neuromuscular, musculoskeletal, cardiorespiratory, cardiovascular, endocrine)
2. General physiology of cardiorespiratory, metabolic, and musculoskeletal diseases and conditions (e.g., diabetes, osteoporosis, cardiovascular disease)
3. Population-specific considerations (e.g., youth, older adults, pregnancy)
4. Expected physiological adaptations to exercise

Nutrition

1. Principles of nutrition and weight management for goal setting

Psychology

1. Principles of goal setting
2. Potential obstacles and challenges that may interfere with goal setting and goal attainment
3. Psychological and social factors that impact goal setting in the development of safe and effective programs
4. Communication styles and presentation techniques that assure collaborative goal setting based on the client's needs, preferences, and expectations
5. Behavior-change principles in goal setting

Skill in:

Anatomy and Biomechanics

1. Using musculoskeletal assessment results for goal setting and reinforcement

Physiology

1. Setting appropriate timeframes for goal attainment in accordance with industry standards

Nutrition

1. Applying the principles of nutrition and weight management to goal setting

Psychology

1. Assisting the client in setting personal goals based on the SMART framework
2. Guiding the goal-setting process to address short- and long-term goals
3. Helping the client identify potential barriers to goal attainment
4. Using communication styles and presentation techniques that assure collaborative goal setting based on the client's needs, preferences, and expectations

Task 3 - Apply appropriate exercise principles (e.g., frequency, intensity, duration, type) for cardiorespiratory fitness, muscular strength and endurance, and flexibility using current standards and appropriate techniques to develop a safe and effective exercise program.

Knowledge of:

Anatomy and Biomechanics

1. General anatomy (e.g., neuromuscular, musculoskeletal, cardiovascular, respiratory)
2. Anatomical position, muscle actions, functional movements, and planes of motion
3. Normal joint range of motion
4. Physical laws of motion (e.g., inertia, acceleration, momentum, impact and reaction forces, lever classes, muscle and force production)
5. Static postural assessment and movement analysis (e.g., postural and muscle imbalances)
6. Static and dynamic balance (e.g., center of gravity, base of support, proprioception)

Physiology

1. General physiology (e.g., neuromuscular, musculoskeletal, cardiorespiratory, cardiovascular, endocrine)
2. General physiology of cardiorespiratory, metabolic, and musculoskeletal diseases and conditions (e.g., diabetes, osteoporosis, cardiovascular disease)
3. Population-specific considerations (e.g., youth, older adults, pregnancy)
4. ACSM guidelines for frequency, intensity, duration, and type for cardiorespiratory, muscular strength and endurance, and flexibility programs
5. Principles of fitness (e.g., overload, specificity, diminishing returns, recovery, progression)
6. Techniques for measuring and monitoring cardiorespiratory intensity
7. Techniques for developing resistance-training programs (e.g., periodization, progression)
8. Techniques for aerobic and anaerobic training programs (e.g., intervals, steady state, tempo, low-intensity long-duration programs)

Skill in:

Anatomy and Biomechanics

1. Recognizing muscle functions, weaknesses, and imbalances

Physiology

1. Designing individualized programs in accordance with clients' goals for aerobic and anaerobic fitness, muscular strength and endurance, flexibility, and posture consistent with recognized standards (e.g., ACSM, ACE, NSCA)
2. Applying principles of fitness to individualized exercise programs
3. Measuring intensity and calculating target training zones for cardiorespiratory fitness

Task 4 - Implement appropriate lifestyle-modification strategies (e.g., stress management, nutrition, smoking cessation) using industry standards and best practices to improve quality of life and goal attainment.

Knowledge of:

Physiology

1. General physiology (e.g., neuromuscular, musculoskeletal, cardiorespiratory, cardiovascular, endocrine)
2. General physiology of cardiorespiratory, metabolic, and musculoskeletal diseases and conditions (e.g., diabetes, osteoporosis, cardiovascular disease)
3. Population-specific considerations (e.g., youth, older adults, pregnancy)
4. Physiology of cardiorespiratory and digestive systems
5. Physiological responses to lifestyle changes
6. Physiological changes with age

Nutrition

1. Appropriate application, safety, and effectiveness of various weight-management techniques
2. Safe and effective weight-loss methods and quantities
3. Different approaches to weight loss

Psychology

1. Communication techniques (e.g., active listening, appropriate eye contact, reflecting and other attending behaviors, nonverbal and verbal communication)
2. Factors that build and enhance rapport (e.g., empathy, genuineness, nonjudgmental responses, client confidentiality)
3. Cultural, ethnic, and personal differences as they affect communication, lifestyle, dietary habits, and personal and interpersonal behavior (e.g., common assumptions, misconceptions, complicating factors)
4. Motivating and demotivating factors of exercise and exercise environments
5. Stress-management techniques

Skill in:

Physiology

1. Educating and communicating about physiological improvements with lifestyle changes

Psychology

1. Helping clients identify sources of stress
2. Helping clients identify their reactions to stress
3. Recognizing the motivating and demotivating factors of exercise and exercise environments

Task 5 - Incorporate functional exercise (e.g., balance, agility, and core) in accordance with scientific research to improve movement efficiency, activities of daily living, and overall physical performance.

Knowledge of:

Anatomy and Biomechanics

1. General anatomy (e.g., neuromuscular, musculoskeletal, cardiovascular, respiratory)
2. Anatomical position, muscle actions, functional movements, and planes of motion
3. Normal joint range of motion
4. Physical laws of motion (e.g., inertia, acceleration, momentum, impact and reaction forces, lever classes, muscle and force production)

5. Posture and movement (e.g., postural and muscle imbalances)
6. Static and dynamic balance (e.g., center of gravity, base of support, proprioception)

Physiology

1. General physiology (e.g., neuromuscular, musculoskeletal, cardiorespiratory, cardiovascular, endocrine)
2. General physiology of cardiorespiratory, metabolic, and musculoskeletal diseases and conditions (e.g., diabetes, osteoporosis, cardiovascular disease)
3. Population-specific considerations (e.g., youth, older adults, pregnancy)
4. Neuromuscular adaptations to functional exercise
5. Physiological demands of activities of daily living
6. Differences in neuromuscular adaptations to functional training across the lifespan and in chronic disease

Skill in:

Anatomy and Biomechanics

1. Selecting and integrating appropriate methods for functional exercise (e.g., balance, agility, core) based on the client's needs
2. Implementing safe and effective exercise programs to address muscle weakness and imbalance

Physiology

1. Adapting functional exercises to the individual based on current neuromuscular ability and/or limitations

Task 6 - Teach safe and effective techniques using a variety of methods and resources to attain desired results and to promote lifestyle modification.

Knowledge of:

Anatomy and Biomechanics

1. General anatomy (e.g., neuromuscular, musculoskeletal, cardiovascular, respiratory)
2. Anatomical position, muscle actions, functional movements, and planes of motion
3. Normal joint range of motion
4. Physical laws of motion (e.g., inertia, acceleration, momentum, impact and reaction forces, lever classes, muscle and force production)
5. Posture and movement (e.g., postural and muscle imbalances)
6. Static and dynamic balance (e.g., center of gravity, base of support, proprioception)

Physiology

1. General physiology (e.g., neuromuscular, musculoskeletal, cardiorespiratory, cardiovascular, endocrine)
2. General physiology of cardiorespiratory, metabolic, and musculoskeletal diseases and conditions (e.g., diabetes, osteoporosis, cardiovascular disease)
3. Population-specific considerations (e.g., youth, older adults, pregnancy)
4. Musculoskeletal injury prevention
5. Physiological effects of overtraining and undertraining
6. Reliable resources to promote desired results and promote lifestyle modification (e.g., authoritative websites, training manuals from respected organizations, textbooks)
7. Physiological effects of lifestyle modification (e.g., smoking cessation, stress management, nutritious eating plan)

Nutrition

1. Healthful food and beverage selections at home, in restaurants, and at the grocery store based on food guidelines, food labels, methods of preparation, and key words on menus
2. Nutritional requirements during physical activity (e.g., hydration, energy needs)
3. Supplements, weight-loss products, and fad diets and the associated risks of each
4. Concepts of energy balance, including dietary intake and expenditure

5. Different approaches to weight management and/or body-composition change
6. Dietary guidelines emphasizing balance, variety, and moderation

Psychology

1. Learning styles (e.g., visual, verbal, kinesthetic)
2. Verbal and nonverbal communication
3. Learning theories

Skill in:

Anatomy and Biomechanics

1. Teaching proper use of a variety of equipment and offering appropriate feedback
2. Teaching safe and effective exercise techniques and offering appropriate feedback

Physiology

1. Designing safe and effective exercise and lifestyle-modification programs that improve physiological systems

Nutrition

2. Approximating caloric intake and expenditure
3. Explaining concepts related to nutrition and weight management
4. Selecting healthful foods and beverages at home, in restaurants, and at the grocery store based on food guidelines, food labels, methods of preparation, and key words on menus
5. Implementing appropriate nutritional strategies during physical activity (e.g., hydration, energy needs)
6. Educating clients to supplements, weight-loss products, and fad diets and the associated risks of each
7. Applying the concepts of energy balance, including dietary intake and expenditure
8. Applying dietary guidelines emphasizing balance, variety, and moderation

Psychology

1. Empathizing with the client's lack of experience, knowledge, or expertise in exercise methods and techniques
2. Modifying teaching style and content appropriate to the client's personal characteristics

Task 7 - Promote program adherence by applying the principles of motivation to maintain interest in physical activity and achievement of program goals.

Knowledge of:

Physiology

1. General physiology (e.g., neuromuscular, musculoskeletal, cardiorespiratory, cardiovascular, endocrine)
2. General physiology of cardiorespiratory, metabolic, and musculoskeletal diseases and conditions (e.g., diabetes, osteoporosis, cardiovascular disease)
3. Population-specific considerations (e.g., youth, older adults, pregnancy)
4. Client education about physiology as a tool for motivating clients to work at appropriate levels

Psychology

1. Self-efficacy as it relates to exercise participation
2. Common barriers to program compliance (e.g., time, energy, money)
3. Psychological effect of exercise program participation
4. Locus of control as it relates to program adherence and motivation
5. Principles of reinforcement and punishment

Nutrition

1. Accepted industry standards and weight-management planning to educate and motivate clients

Skill in:

Physiology

1. Educating clients on the response of physiological systems to various levels of training

Nutrition

1. Using accepted industry standards and weight-management planning to educate and motivate clients

Psychology

1. Recognizing the client's needs, expectations, and fears
2. Identifying barriers that influence program adherence
3. Manipulating factors to maximize adherence
4. Recognizing the personal trainer's influence on the client's adherence
5. Providing appropriate reinforcement

DOMAIN III - PROGRAM PROGRESSION, MODIFICATION, AND MAINTENANCE 27%

Task 1 - Evaluate ongoing progress using assessments, current standards, observation, and client feedback and performance to provide program direction and to optimize program adherence.

Knowledge of:

Anatomy and Biomechanics

1. General anatomy (e.g., neuromuscular, musculoskeletal, cardiovascular, respiratory)
2. Anatomical position, muscle actions, functional movements, and planes of motion
3. Normal joint range of motion
4. Physical laws of motion (e.g., inertia, acceleration, momentum, impact and reaction forces, lever classes, muscle and force production)
5. Static postural assessment and movement analysis (e.g., postural and muscle imbalances)
6. Static and dynamic balance (e.g., center of gravity, base of support, proprioception)

Physiology

1. General physiology (e.g., neuromuscular, musculoskeletal, cardiorespiratory, cardiovascular, endocrine)
2. General physiology of cardiorespiratory, metabolic, and musculoskeletal diseases and conditions (e.g., diabetes, osteoporosis, cardiovascular disease)
3. Population-specific considerations (e.g., youth, older adults, pregnancy)
4. Physiological responses to chronic training
5. Principles of progression as it relates to cardiorespiratory, muscular fitness, and flexibility training programs
6. Appropriate frequency for reassessment
7. Standardized testing protocols, their intended use, and limitations
8. Signs indicating the need for test termination
9. Current standards for training progression and weight loss

Nutrition

1. Appropriate dietary assessment protocols, purposes, inherent risks, and benefits (e.g., 24-hour diet recall, food logs, food frequency questionnaires)
2. Methods for interpreting client assessment data as it relates to established guidelines
3. Applicable guidelines and standards published by accepted organizations (e.g., ADA, USDA, AHA, Institute of Medicine)
4. Relationship between BMI, waist-to-hip ratio, and circumference measures and body weight, and determination of appropriate body weight

Psychology

1. Self-efficacy and locus of control as they relate to program adherence
2. Communication and listening techniques

Skill in:

Anatomy and Biomechanics

1. Assessing posture and movement in comparison to baseline data
2. Assessing static and dynamic balance in comparison to baseline data
3. Determining appropriate tests for reassessment to compare with baseline results
4. Evaluating data from musculoskeletal reassessment

Physiology

1. Identifying physiological responses based on observation and feedback during exercise
2. Selecting and administering a variety of physiological assessments (e.g., cardiorespiratory, muscular strength and endurance, body composition, flexibility)
3. Monitoring client responses during test administration (e.g., blood pressure, heart rate, RPE)
4. Measuring and recording exercise testing data accurately
5. Recognizing responses that indicate the need for test termination
6. Terminating exercise tests safely
7. Determining whether rate of progress is appropriate for the individual based on the expected physiological responses and current standards

Nutrition

1. Administering appropriate dietary assessment protocols
2. Interviewing and collecting nutrition data
3. Processing the client's diet history, evaluations, and observations, relative to accepted guidelines
4. Gathering, applying, and interpreting applicable standards and guidelines published by accepted organizations

Psychology

1. Recognizing the personal trainer's influence on the client's adherence
2. Recognizing client misconceptions about program progress
3. Communicating the results of the reassessments to effectively promote adherence
4. Managing time in the data-collection process

Task 2 - Identify lapses and barriers to success by reassessing baseline measures and evaluating compliance to redefine goals and to modify the program.

Knowledge of:

Anatomy and Biomechanics

1. General anatomy (e.g., neuromuscular, musculoskeletal, cardiovascular, respiratory)
2. Anatomical position, muscle actions, functional movements, and planes of motion
3. Normal joint range of motion
4. Physical laws of motion (e.g., inertia, acceleration, momentum, impact and reaction forces, lever classes, muscle and force production)
5. Posture and movement
6. Static and dynamic balance (e.g., center of gravity, base of support, proprioception)

Physiology

1. General physiology (e.g., neuromuscular, musculoskeletal, cardiorespiratory, cardiovascular, endocrine)
2. General physiology of cardiorespiratory, metabolic, and musculoskeletal diseases and conditions (e.g., diabetes, osteoporosis, cardiovascular disease)
3. Population-specific considerations (e.g., youth, older adults, pregnancy)
4. Principles of fitness (e.g., overload, specificity, diminishing returns, recovery, reversibility, progression)
5. How to modify the program based on changes in fitness and health status

Nutrition

1. Cultural, ethnic, and personal differences as they affect dietary habits
2. Potential barriers to healthful dietary choices and weight management
3. Accepted industry standards and weight-management planning

Psychology

1. Common barriers to program compliance (e.g., time, energy, money)
2. Self-efficacy and locus of control as they relate to program participation and adherence

Skill in:

Anatomy and Biomechanics

1. Identifying inappropriate movement patterns that may impede progress or adherence

2. Modifying exercise techniques as needed

Physiology

1. Modifying program components to accommodate fitness and/or health status

Nutrition

1. Using accepted industry standards and weight-management planning
2. Avoiding prejudicial statements and negative and/or unproductive assumptions with regard to client body size, eating habits, and past successes and failures with weight management.
3. Identifying potential barriers to healthful dietary choices and weight management

Psychology

1. Identifying barriers and enhancers that influence program adherence
2. Recognizing the client's needs, desires, expectations, and fears
3. Recognizing the personal trainer's influence on the client's adherence
4. Providing appropriate reinforcement

Task 3 - Modify program goals using appropriate educational and motivational techniques to improve compliance and awareness of the benefits of physical activity and a healthful lifestyle.

Knowledge of:

Anatomy and Biomechanics

1. General anatomy (e.g., neuromuscular, musculoskeletal, cardiovascular, respiratory)
2. Anatomical position, muscle actions, functional movements, and planes of motion
3. Normal joint range of motion
4. Physical laws of motion (e.g., inertia, acceleration, momentum, impact and reaction forces, lever classes, muscle and force production)
5. Posture and movement
6. Static and dynamic balance (e.g., center of gravity, base of support, proprioception)

Physiology

1. General physiology (e.g., neuromuscular, musculoskeletal, cardiorespiratory, cardiovascular, endocrine)
2. General physiology of cardiorespiratory, metabolic, and musculoskeletal diseases and conditions (e.g., diabetes, osteoporosis, cardiovascular disease)
3. Population-specific considerations (e.g., youth, older adults, pregnancy)
4. Physiological plateaus in cardiorespiratory, resistance, and weight-loss programs

Nutrition

1. Complexity of issues related to obesity, body size, eating disorders, and related lifestyle factors
2. Safe and effective weight loss and lifestyle change in regard to nutrition
3. Role of nutrition, supplements, weight-loss products, and fad diets, their effect on weight management and performance, and the associated risks

Psychology

1. Strategies that facilitate behavior change
2. Self-efficacy and locus of control as they relate to exercise participation
3. Principles of reinforcement and punishment
4. Principles of goal setting
5. Potential obstacles and challenges that may interfere with goal setting and attainment
6. Biological, psychological, and social factors that impact program compliance

Skill in:

Anatomy and Biomechanics

1. Modifying exercise techniques to promote goal attainment

Physiology

1. Identifying program components that can be modified to promote a positive training effect

2. Educating clients about the physiological benefits of continued training

Nutrition

1. Communicating the benefits of healthful nutrition to weight management and performance
2. Applying principles of nutrition to redefine short- and long-term goals

Psychology

1. Assisting the client in reevaluating and modifying goals
2. Helping the client recognize potential and actual barriers to adherence
3. Assisting the client in developing coping strategies to overcome barriers
4. Enhancing the client's self-efficacy through challenging yet manageable tasks

Task 4 - Implement progressions to the client's program as appropriate using established methods and techniques to facilitate goal achievement and long-term compliance.

Knowledge of:

Anatomy and Biomechanics

1. General anatomy (e.g., neuromuscular, musculoskeletal, cardiovascular, respiratory)
2. Anatomical position, muscle actions, functional movements, and planes of motion
3. Normal joint range of motion
4. Physical laws of motion (e.g., inertia, acceleration, momentum, impact and reaction forces, lever classes, muscle and force production)
5. Posture and movement
6. Static and dynamic balance (e.g., center of gravity, base of support, proprioception)

Physiology

1. General physiology (e.g., neuromuscular, musculoskeletal, cardiorespiratory, cardiovascular, endocrine)
2. General physiology of cardiorespiratory, metabolic, and musculoskeletal diseases and conditions (e.g., diabetes, osteoporosis, cardiovascular disease)
3. Population-specific considerations (e.g., youth, older adults, pregnancy)
4. Appropriate rate of progression according to established methods and guidelines
5. Various methods of progression for aerobic, anaerobic, muscular strength and endurance, and flexibility training

Skill in:

Anatomy and Biomechanics

1. Implementing appropriate exercise technique progressions

Physiology

1. Implementing appropriate exercise progressions to facilitate long-term success

DOMAIN IV - PROFESSIONAL ROLE AND RESPONSIBILITIES 8%

Task 1 - Maintain a professional client–trainer relationship by adhering to legal requirements, professional boundaries, and standards of care and by operating within the scope of practice, as defined in the ACE Code of Ethics, to protect the client and to limit liability.

Knowledge of:

1. Professional boundaries pertaining to the client-trainer relationship
2. American Council on Exercise Code of Ethics
3. Accepted standards of care
4. Liability issues associated with acting outside the appropriate standard of care, scope of practice, and the American Council on Exercise Code of Ethics
5. Scope of practice
6. Professional ethics regarding technology and communication

Skill in:

1. Assessing areas of risk (e.g., client, facilities, use of technology)

2. Identifying professional boundaries based on professional and ethical obligations

Task 2 - Treat all individuals with respect, empathy, and equality regardless of weight, appearance, ethnicity, nationality, sexual orientation, gender, age, disability, religion, marital status, socioeconomic status, and health status to maintain integrity in all professional relationships.

Knowledge of:

1. Abilities and limitations of various disabilities
2. Cultural differences related to professional relationships
3. Acceptable and unacceptable behavior related to individual differences
4. Personal issues and biases
5. Qualities of respect, empathy, and equality

Skill in:

1. Demonstrating compassion, empathy, and respect for all individuals
2. Maintaining appropriate behavior patterns regardless of personal issues and biases

Task 3 - Maintain competence and professional growth by staying current with scientifically based research, theories, and practices to provide safe and effective services for clients, the public, and other health professionals.

Knowledge of:

1. Available and credible continuing education programs (e.g., conferences, workshops, college/university courses, teleseminars, online courses, in-home study courses) and providers
2. Appropriate and relevant scientifically based consumer and professional publications (e.g., journals, books, texts, videos, DVDs, CDs, online publications and resources)
3. Appropriate agencies and organizations that establish and publish scientifically based lifestyle-modification standards and guidelines for the general public and special populations (e.g., ACSM, ACOG, USDA, OSHA, NIH, ADA, NSCA, CDC)
4. American Council on Exercise continuing education requirements and procedures

Skill in:

1. Recognizing credible resources

Task 4 - Exercise leadership by providing direction, motivation, and education and by modeling exemplary behavior to establish an environment for client success and to promote wellness in the community.

Knowledge of:

1. General professional and business practices (e.g., time management, organizational skills, appropriate attire, integrity)
2. Educational strategies to promote client safety, program success, and wellness in the community

Skill in:

1. Demonstrating professional business practices
2. Using appropriate educational strategies to promote client safety, program success, and wellness within the community.

Task 5 - Maintain an environment of continual safety by upholding industry standards to reduce the risk of injury and liability.

Knowledge of:

1. Cardiopulmonary resuscitation (CPR) and automated external defibrillator (AED) procedures
2. Worksite emergency plan
3. Appropriate emergency medical service system (EMS) activation
4. Basic first aid
5. Occupational Health and Safety Administration guidelines regarding bloodborne pathogens

6. Procedures for safe equipment operation (e.g., sizing, usage, inspection)
7. Industry standards for reducing risk of injury
8. Factors that affect liability
9. How to communicate a sense of security and safety to clients

Skill in:

1. Identifying and responding to emergency situations
2. Identifying and responding to hazards in training situations
3. Implementing the emergency plan in a professional manner
4. Communicating the rationale for various techniques that limit the risk of injury
5. Using equipment properly and safely

Task 6 - Develop risk-management strategies in accordance with recognized guidelines (e.g., IHRSA, ACE, ACSM, OSHA, NSCA, state laws) to protect the client, personal trainer, and other relevant parties.

Knowledge of:

1. Negligence (comparative and contributory) and liability laws as they pertain to personal trainers
2. Intellectual property laws as they apply to video, DVD, written materials, Internet, music, copyright, and trademark
3. Sources for and limitations of waivers and informed consents
4. Appropriate professional and general liability insurance
5. Sexual harassment and discrimination laws
6. Components of a comprehensive risk-management program
7. Credible resources for risk-management strategies (e.g., McGraw, Wong, ACSM, NSCA, OSHA, IHRSA, ACE, IDEA, Fitness Management, Athletic Business)

Skill in:

1. Complying with business laws and regulations
2. Completing appropriate reports (e.g., incident reports, accident reports, equipment and facility inspection forms, waivers, informed consents)
3. Developing and maintaining an appropriate risk-management program for a facility or business
4. Monitoring the client when exercise or fitness assessments have been terminated due to abnormal physiological responses

Task 7 - Document client-related data, communications, and progress using a secure record-keeping system in accordance with legal requirements (e.g., HIPAA, FERPA) to maintain continuity of care and to minimize liability.

Knowledge of:

1. Effective and confidential record keeping
2. Confidentiality guidelines
3. Importance of maintaining and implications of breaching client confidentiality
4. All required paperwork and documentation (e.g., waivers, informed consent, medical history, health-risk appraisal, client contracts)

Skill in:

1. Maintaining confidentiality
2. Differentiating between confidential and non-confidential documents and information

Task 8 - Participate as a member of a referral network by identifying professional contacts and community resources to ensure the highest quality of service for clients.

Knowledge of:

1. Appropriate health and allied health professions for outside referral
2. Appropriate forms and documents required when communicating with other health professionals in order to maintain continuity of client care

Skill in:

1. Identifying and networking with appropriate health and allied health professionals
2. Establishing a method for referrals
3. Creating a means of ongoing communication and follow-up with appropriate professionals

APPENDIX C

ACE Position Statement on Nutritional Supplements

It is the position of the American Council on Exercise (ACE) that it is outside the defined scope of practice of a fitness professional to recommend, prescribe, sell, or supply nutritional supplements to clients. Recommending supplements without possessing the requisite qualifications (e.g., R.D.) can place the client's health at risk and possibly expose the fitness professional to disciplinary action and litigation. If a client wants to take supplements, a fitness professional should work in conjunction with a qualified registered dietitian or medical doctor to provide safe and effective nutritional education and recommendations.

ACE recognizes that some fitness and health clubs encourage or require their employees to sell nutritional supplements. If this is a condition of employment, fitness professionals should protect themselves by ensuring their employers possess adequate insurance coverage for them should a problem arise. Furthermore, ACE strongly encourages continuing education on diet and nutrition for all fitness professionals.

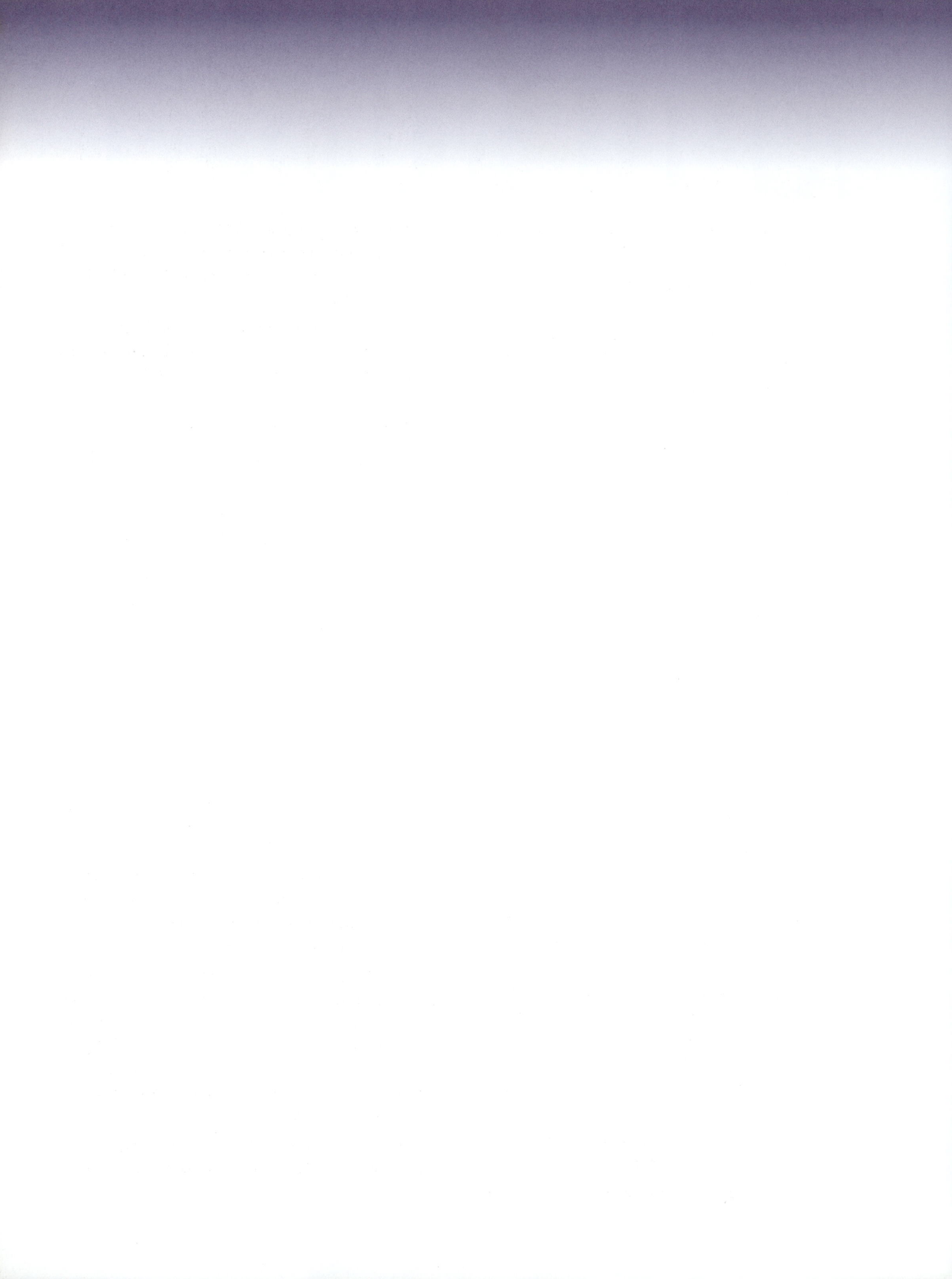

GLOSSARY

Abduction Movement away from the midline of the body.

Abrasion A scraping away of a portion of the skin or mucous membrane.

Absolute contraindication A situation that makes a particular treatment or procedure absolutely inadvisable.

Absolute strength The maximal amount of weight an individual can lift one time.

Absorption The uptake of nutrients across a tissue or membrane by the gastrointestinal tract.

Acclimatize To physiologically adapt to an unfamiliar environment and achieve a new steady state. For example, the body can adjust to a high altitude or a hot climate and gain an increased capacity to work in those conditions.

Acquired immunodeficiency syndrome (AIDS) A syndrome of the immune system caused by the human immunodeficiency virus (type HIV-1 or HIV-2) and characterized by opportunistic infection and disease.

Act of God An unforeseeable and uncontrollable occurrence, such as an earthquake or flash flood, that may cause injury.

Actin Thin contractile protein in a myofibril.

Action The stage of the transtheoretical model of behavioral change during which the individual started a new behavior less than six months ago.

Active isolated stretching (AIS) A stretching technique modeled after traditional strength-training workouts. Stretches are held very briefly in sets of a specified number of repetitions, with a goal of isolating an individual muscle in each set.

Activities of daily living (ADL) Activities normally performed for hygiene, bathing, household chores, walking, shopping, and similar activities.

Acute Descriptive of a condition that usually has a rapid onset and a relatively short and severe course; opposite of chronic.

Acute coronary syndrome A sudden, severe coronary event that mimics a heart attack, such as unstable angina.

Adduction Movement toward the midline of the body.

Adenosine trisphosphate (ATP) A high-energy phosphate molecule required to provide energy for cellular function. Produced both aerobically and anaerobically and stored in the body.

Adherence The extent to which people stick to their plans or treatment recommendations. Exercise adherence is the extent to which people follow, or stick to, an exercise program.

Adipose Fat cells stored in adipose tissue.

Adipose tissue Fatty tissue; connective tissue made up of fat cells.

Adrenocorticotropin hormone (ACTH) A hormone released by the pituitary gland that affects various important bodily functions; controls the secretion in the adrenal gland of hormones that influence the metabolism of carbohydrates, sodium, and potassium; also controls the rate at which substances are exchanged between the blood and tissues.

Aerobic In the presence of oxygen.

Aerobic capacity *See* $\dot{V}O_2$max.

Agonist The muscle directly responsible for observed movement; also called the prime mover.

Agreement to participate Signed document that indicates that the client is aware of inherent risks and potential injuries that can occur from participation.

Air displacement plethysmography (ADP) A body-composition assessment technique based on the same body volume measurement principle as hydrostatic weighing; uses air instead of water.

Alexander Technique Teaches the transformation of neuromuscular habits by helping an individual focus on sensory experiences. It is a simple and practical method for improving ease and freedom of movement, balance, support, and coordination, and corrects unconscious habits of posture and movement, which may be precursors to injuries.

Allergen A substance that can cause an allergic reaction by stimulating type-1 hypersensitivity in atopic individuals.

Alveoli Spherical extensions of the respiratory bronchioles and the primary sites of gas exchange with the blood.

Alzheimer's disease An age-related, progressive disease characterized by death of nerve cells in the brain leading to a loss of cognitive function; the cause of the nerve cell death is unknown.

Ambient temperature The temperature of the surrounding air; room temperature.

American Society of Composers, Artists and Publishers (ASCAP) One of two performing rights societies in the United States that represent music publishers in negotiating and collecting fees for the non-dramatic performance of music.

Amortization phase The transition period between the eccentric and concentric actions during plyometrics; a crucial part of the stretch-shortening cycle that contributes to power development.

Anabolic Muscle-building effects.

Anabolic-androgenic steroids (AAS) Synthetic derivatives of the male sex hormone testosterone; used for their muscle-building characteristics.

Anaerobic Without the presence of oxygen.

Anaerobic capacity The ability of an individual to perform high-intensity, anaerobic activity.

Anaerobic glycolysis The metabolic pathway that uses glucose for energy production without requiring oxygen. Sometimes referred to as the lactic acid system or anaerobic glucose system, it produces lactic acid as a by-product.

Anaerobic threshold The point during high-intensity activity when the body can no longer meet its demand for oxygen and anaerobic metabolism predominates. Also called lactate threshold.

Android Adipose tissue or body fat distributed in the abdominal area (apple-shaped individuals).

Androstenedione A steroid produced by the adrenal glands that is a precursor to testosterone and other androgens; has been used as a supplement to increase muscle strength.

Anemia A reduction in the number of red blood cells and/or quantity of hemoglobin per volume of blood below normal values.

Anemic *See* Anemia.

Aneurysm A localized abnormal dilation of a blood vessel; associated with a stroke when the aneurysm bursts.

Angina A common symptom of coronary artery disease characterized by chest pain, tightness, or radiating pain resulting from a lack of blood flow to the heart muscle.

Angina pectoris Chest pain caused by an inadequate supply of oxygen and decreased blood flow to the heart muscle; an early sign of coronary artery disease. Symptoms may include pain or discomfort, heaviness, tightness, pressure or burning, numbness, aching, and tingling in the chest, back, neck, throat, jaw, or arms; also called angina.

Angioplasty A surgical procedure that involves inserting a catheter into a blocked coronary artery. A narrow balloon is then inflated inside the artery, to widen the artery. Also called percutaneous transluminal coronary angioplasty (PTCA).

Ankylosing spondylitis Inflammatory arthritis of the spine, resembling rheumatoid arthritis, that may progress to bony ankylosis with slipping of vertebral margins; the disease is more common in males.

Anorexia *See* Anorexia nervosa.

Anorexia nervosa An eating disorder characterized by refusal to maintain body weight of at least 85% of expected weight; intense fear of gaining weight or becoming fat; body-image disturbances, including a disproportionate influence of body weight on self-evaluation; and, in women, the absence of at least three consecutive menstrual periods.

Antagonist The muscle that acts in opposition to the contraction produced by an agonist (prime mover) muscle.

Antecedents Variables or factors that precede and influence a client's exercise participation, including the decision to not exercise as planned.

Anterior Anatomical term meaning toward the front. Same as ventral; opposite of posterior.

Anterior cruciate ligament (ACL) A primary stabilizing ligament of the knee that travels from the medial border of the lateral femoral condyle to its point of insertion anterolaterally to the medial tibial spine.

Anterior shin splints Pain in the anterior compartment muscles of the lower leg, fascia, and periosteal lining. Often induced by exertional or sudden changes in activity.

Anteversion Pelvic position characterized by the ASIS (anterior superior iliac spine) being forward of the pubic symphysis.

Anxiety A state of uneasiness and apprehension; occurs in some mental disorders.

Apnea A temporary absence or cessation of breathing; when this condition occurs during sleep it is called sleep apnea.

Apneic *See* Apnea.

Arrhythmia A disturbance in the rate or rhythm of the heartbeat. Some can be symptoms of serious heart disease; may not be of medical significance until symptoms appear.

Arthritis Inflammation of a joint; a state characterized by the inflammation of joints.

Arthrokinematics The general term for the specific movements of joint surfaces, such as rolling or gliding.

Asana A posture or manner of sitting, as in the practice of yoga.

Assisted training The act of a partner offering assistance during resistance training to allow the exerciser to complete repetitions with correct form even though the exerciser may be fatigued.

Associative stage of learning The second stage of learning a motor skill, when performers have mastered the fundamentals and can concentrate on skill refinement.

Asthma A chronic inflammatory disorder of the airways that affects genetically susceptible individuals in response to various environmental triggers such as allergens, viral infection, exercise, cold, and stress.

Ataxia Failure of muscular coordination; irregularity of muscular action.

Atherogenesis Formation of atheromatous deposits, especially on the innermost layer of arterial walls.

Atherogenic dyslipidemia Formation of atheromatous deposits, especially on the innermost layer of arterial walls due to an abnormal concentration of lipids or lipoproteins in the blood.

Atherosclerosis A specific form of arteriosclerosis characterized by the accumulation of fatty material on the inner walls of the arteries, causing them to harden, thicken, and lose elasticity.

Atherosclerotic heart disease The end result of the accumulation of atherosclerotic plaques within the coronary arteries that supply the muscle of the heart with oxygen and nutrients.

Athletic trainer A healthcare professional who collaborates with physicians and specializes in providing immediate intervention when injuries occur and helping athletes and clients in the prevention, assessment, treatment, and rehabilitation of emergency, acute, and chronic medical conditions involving injury, impairment, functional limitations, and disabilities.

Atrophy A reduction in muscle size (muscle wasting) due to inactivity or immobilization.

Auscultation The technical term for listening to the internal sounds of the body (such as the heartbeat), usually using a stethoscope.

Automated external defibrillator (AED) A portable electronic device used to restore normal heart rhythms in victims of sudden cardiac arrest.

Autonomic neuropathy A disease of the non-voluntary, non-sensory nervous system (i.e., the autonomic nervous system) affecting mostly the internal organs such as the bladder muscles, the cardiovascular system, the digestive tract, and the genital organs.

Autonomous stage of learning The third stage of learning a motor skill, when the skill has become habitual or automatic for the performer.

Avulsion A wound involving forcible separation or tearing of tissue from the body.

Axial skeleton The bones of the head, neck, and trunk.

Axis of rotation The imaginary line or point about which an object, such as a joint, rotates.

Balance The ability to maintain the body's position over its base of support within stability limits, both statically and dynamically.

Ballistic stretching Dynamic stretching characterized by rhythmic bobbing or bouncing motions representing relatively high-force, short-duration movements.

Basal metabolic rate (BMR) The energy required to complete the sum total of life-sustaining processes, including ion transport (40% BMR), protein synthesis (20% BMR), and daily functioning such as breathing, circulation, and nutrient processing (40% BMR).

Base of support (BOS) The areas of contact between the feet and their supporting surface and the area between the feet.

Basic activities of daily living Any daily activity performed for self-care, including personal hygiene, dressing and undressing, eating, transferring from bed to chair and back, voluntarily controlling urinary and fecal discharge, elimination, and moving around (as opposed to being bedridden).

Behavior chain A sequence of events in which variables both preceding and following a target behavior help to explain and reinforce the target behavior, such as participation in an exercise session.

Benign A non-cancerous growth or tumor; mild disease or condition that is not life threatening.

ß-alanine A naturally occurring amino acid formed within the body.

Beta blockers Medications that "block" or limit sympathetic nervous system stimulation. They act to slow the heart rate and decrease maximum heart rate and are used for cardiovascular and other medical conditions.

Beta cell Endocrine cells in the islets of Langerhans of the pancreas responsible for synthesizing and secreting the hormone insulin, which lowers the glucose levels in the blood.

Binge eating disorder An eating disorder characterized by frequent binge eating (without purging) and feelings of being out of control when eating.

Bioelectrical impedance analysis (BIA) A body-composition assessment technique that measures the amount of impedance, or resistance, to electric current flow as it passes through the body. Impedance is greatest in fat tissue, while fat-free mass, which contains 70–75% water, allows the electrical current to pass much more easily.

Biomechanics The mechanics of biological and muscular activity.

Blood pressure (BP) The pressure exerted by the blood on the walls of the arteries; measured in millimeters of mercury (mmHg) with a sphygmomanometer.

Body composition The makeup of the body in terms of the relative percentage of fat-free mass and body fat.

Body fat A component of the body, the primary role of which is to store energy for later use.

Body mass index (BMI) A relative measure of body height to body weight used to determine levels of weight, from underweight to extreme obesity.

Bone formation The processes resulting in the formation of normal, healthy bone tissue, including remodeling and resorption.

Bone mineral density (BMD) A measure of the amount of minerals (mainly calcium) contained in a certain volume of bone.

Bone resorption The breaking down of bone by osteoclasts.

Branched-chain amino acids (BCAAs) Essential amino acids that inhibit muscle protein breakdown and aid in muscle glycogen storage. The BCAAs are valine, leucine, and isoleucine.

Breakdown training A method of resistance training wherein the exerciser lifts as many repetitions as possible until muscle fatigue sets in, then decreases the weight load and continues to lift as many repetitions as possible of the same exercise.

Broadcast Music Inc. (BMI) One of two performing rights societies in the U.S. that represent music publishers in negotiating and collecting fees for the nondramatic performance of music.

Bronchitis Acute or chronic inflammation of the bronchial tubes. *See* Chronic obstructive pulmonary disease (COPD).

Bronchodilators Medications inhaled to dilate (enlarge) and relax the constricted bronchial smooth muscle (e.g., Proventil).

Bronchospasm Abnormal contraction of the smooth muscle of the bronchi, resulting in an acute narrowing and obstruction of the respiratory airway.

Bulimia *See* Bulimia nervosa.

Bulimia nervosa An eating disorder characterized by recurrent episodes of uncontrolled binge eating; recurrent inappropriate compensatory behavior such as self-induced vomiting, laxative misuse, diuretics, or enemas (purging type), or fasting and/or excessive exercise (non-purging type); episodes of binge eating and compensatory behaviors occur at least twice per week for three months; self-evaluation is heavily influenced by body shape and weight; and the episodes do not occur exclusively with episodes of anorexia.

Bursa A sac of fluid that is present in areas of the body that are potential sites of friction.

Bursitis Swelling and inflammation in the bursa that results from overuse.

C-corporation A corporation that is designed to operate in multiple countries and with various types of investors.

Calcium channel blockers A class of blood pressure medications that relax and widen the blood vessels.

Capillaries The smallest blood vessels that supply blood to the tissues, and the site of all gas and nutrient exchange in the cardiovascular system. They connect the arterial and venous systems.

Carbohydrate The body's preferred energy source. Dietary sources include sugars (simple) and grains, rice, potatoes, and beans (complex). Carbohydrate is stored as glycogen in the muscles and liver and is transported in the blood as glucose.

Cardiac arrest The abrupt cessation of normal circulation of the blood due to failure of the heart to contract effectively.

Cardiac output The amount of blood pumped by the heart per minute; usually expressed in liters of blood per minute.

Cardiac reserve The work that the heart is able to perform beyond that required of it under ordinary circumstances.

Cardiometabolic disease A condition that puts an individual at increased risk for heart disease and diabetes and includes the following factors: elevated blood pressure, triglycerides, fasting plasma glucose, and C-reactive protein, and decreased levels of high-density lipoprotein.

Cardiopulmonary resuscitation (CPR) A procedure to support and maintain breathing and circulation for a person who has stopped breathing (respiratory arrest) and/or whose heart has stopped (cardiac arrest).

Cardiorespiratory endurance The capacity of the heart, blood vessels, and lungs to deliver oxygen and nutrients to the working muscles and tissues during sustained exercise and to remove metabolic waste products that would result in fatigue.

Cardiorespiratory fitness (CRF) The ability to perform large muscle movement over a sustained period; related to the capacity of the heart-lung system to deliver oxygen for sustained energy production. Also called cardiorespiratory endurance or aerobic fitness.

Cardiovascular disease (CVD) A general term for any disease of the heart, blood vessels, or circulation.

Cardiovascular drift Changes in observed cardiovascular variables that occur during prolonged, submaximal exercise without a change in workload.

Carnosine A substance made up of amino acids that is highly concentrated in the brain and muscle tissue; may have many beneficial antioxidant properties.

Carpal tunnel syndrome A pathology of the wrist and hand that occurs when the median nerve, which extends from the forearm into the hand, becomes compressed at the wrist.

Cartilage A smooth, semi-opaque material that absorbs shock and reduces friction between the bones of a joint.

Casein The main protein found in milk and other dairy products.

Catabolic Pertaining to the breaking down of tissue, or catabolism. Catabolism generally refers to a decrease in lean tissue, particularly muscle.

Catecholamine Hormone (e.g., epinephrine and norepinephrine) released as part of the sympathetic response to exercise.

Center of gravity (COG) *See* Center of mass (COM).

Center of mass (COM) The point around which all weight is evenly distributed; also called center of gravity.

Central nervous system (CNS) The brain and spinal cord.

Cerebrovascular accident (CVA) Damage to the brain, often resulting in a loss of function, from impaired blood supply to part of the brain; more commonly known as a stroke.

Certification A credential attesting that an individual or organization has met a specific set of standards.

Cholesterol A fatlike substance found in the blood and body tissues and in certain foods. Can accumulate in the arteries and lead to a narrowing of the vessels (atherosclerosis).

Chondromalacia A gradual softening and degeneration of the articular cartilage, usually involving the back surface of the patella (kneecap). This condition may produce pain and swelling or a grinding sound or sensation when the knee is flexed and extended.

Chronic Descriptive of a condition that persists over a long period of time; opposite of acute.

Chronic disease Any disease state that persists over an extended period of time.

Chronic fatigue syndrome (CFS) A medical condition with symptoms including fatigue, extremely low stamina, weakness, muscle pain, swelling of the lymph nodes, depression, and hypersensitivity.

Chronic obstructive pulmonary disease (COPD) A condition, such as asthma, bronchitis, or emphysema, in which there is chronic obstruction of air flow. *See* Asthma, Bronchitis, *and* Emphysema.

Circuit training A form of training that takes the participant through a series of exercise stations, sometimes with brief rest intervals in between; can emphasize muscular endurance, aerobic conditioning, muscular strength, or a combination of all three.

Claudication Cramp-like pains in the calves caused by poor circulation of blood to the leg muscles; frequently associated with peripheral vascular disease.

Closing ratio The success rate of a salesperson in making a presentation to a prospective customer and actually having the customer make a purchase to complete the sale; it is a measure of the number of sales made divided by the number of presentations given.

Co-contraction The mutual coordination of antagonist muscles (such as flexors and extensors) to maintain a position.

Cognitions Current thoughts or feelings that can function as antecedents or consequences for overt behaviors.

Cognitive domain One of the three domains of learning; describes intellectual activities and involves the learning of knowledge.

Cognitive stage of learning The first stage of learning a motor skill when performers make many gross errors and have extremely variable performances.

Collagen The main constituent of connective tissue, such as ligaments, tendons, and muscles.

Comorbidities Disorders (or diseases) in addition to a primary disease or disorder.

Comparative negligence A system used in legal defenses to distribute fault between an injured party and any defendant.

Complex carbohydrate A long chain of sugar that takes more time to digest than a simple carbohydrate.

Concentric A type of isotonic muscle contraction in which the muscle develops tension and shortens when stimulated.

Congestive heart failure (CHF) Inability of the heart to pump blood at a sufficient rate to meet the metabolic demand or the ability to do so only when the cardiac filling pressures are abnormally high, frequently resulting in lung congestion.

Connective tissue The tissue that binds together and supports various structures of the body. Ligaments and tendons are connective tissues.

Consequences Variables that occur following a target behavior, such as exercise, that influence a person's future behavior-change decisions and efforts.

Contemplation The stage of the transtheoretical model of behavioral change during which the individual is weighing the pros and cons of behavior change.

Contract A binding agreement between two or more persons that is enforceable by law composed of an offer, acceptance, and consideration (or what each party puts forth to make the agreement worthwhile).

Contractile proteins The protein myofilaments that are essential for muscle contraction.

Contracture An abnormal and usually permanent contraction of a muscle characterized by a high resistance to passive stretching.

Contraindication Any condition that renders some particular movement, activity, or treatment improper or undesirable.

Contralateral The opposite side of the body; the other limb.

Contributory negligence A legal defense used in claims or suits when the plaintiff's negligence contributed to the act in dispute.

Contusion A wound, such as a bruise, in which the skin is not broken; often resulting in broken blood vessels and discoloration.

Coronary artery disease (CAD) *See* Coronary heart disease (CHD).

Coronary atherosclerotic disease The end result of the accumulation of atherosclerotic plaques within the coronary arteries that supply the muscle of the heart with oxygen and nutrients. Also call atherosclerotic heart disease.

Coronary heart disease (CHD) The major form of cardiovascular disease; results when the coronary arteries are narrowed or occluded, most commonly by atherosclerotic deposits of fibrous and fatty tissue; also called coronary artery disease (CAD).

Corporate veil Shields individual investors in a corporation from financial or legal liability beyond their initial investment.

Corporation A legal entity, independent of its owners and regulated by state laws; any number of people may own a corporation through shares issued by the business.

Corticosteroid One of two main hormones released by the adrenal cortex; plays a major role in maintaining blood glucose during prolonged exercise by promoting protein and triglyceride breakdown.

Corticotropin releasing hormone (CRH) A hormone and neurotransmitter released by the hypothalamus in response to stress.

Cortisol A hormone that is often referred to as the "stress hormone," as it is involved in the response to stress. It increases blood pressure and blood glucose levels and has an immunosuppressive action.

Creatine A non-prescription dietary supplement that is promoted for its ability to enhance muscle strength and physical endurance.

Creatine phosphate (CP) A storage form of high-energy phosphate in muscle cells that can be used to immediately resynthesize adenosine triphosphate (ATP).

Crepitus A crackling sound produced by air moving in the joint space; also called crepitation.

Cross-training A method of physical training in which a variety of exercises and changes in body positions or modes of exercise are utilized to positively affect compliance and motivation, and also stimulate additional strength gains or reduce injury risk.

Cultural competence The ability to communicate and work effectively with people from different cultures.

Cyanosis A bluish discoloration, especially of the skin and mucous membranes, due to reduced hemoglobin in the blood.

Decisional balance One of the four components of the transtheoretical model; refers to the numbers of pros and cons an individual perceives regarding adopting and/or maintaining an activity program.

Deep Anatomical term meaning internal; that is, located further beneath the body surface than the superficial structures.

Degenerative disc disease (DDD) A condition of advancing age, and/or the result of the development of post-traumatic arthritis.

Dehydration The process of losing body water; when severe can cause serious, life-threatening consequences.

Dehydroepiandrosterone (DHEA) A steroid hormone secreted by the adrenal cortex with a wide range of biological effects.

Delayed onset muscle soreness (DOMS) Soreness that occurs 24 to 48 hours after strenuous exercise, the exact cause of which is unknown.

Dementia A deteriorative mental state characterized by absence of, or reduction in, intellectual faculties; may be caused by disease or trauma.

Deoxyribonucleic acid (DNA) A large, double-stranded, helical molecule that is the carrier of genetic information.

Depression 1. The action of lowering a muscle or bone or movement in an inferior or downward direction. 2. A condition of general emotional dejection and withdrawal; sadness greater and more prolonged than that warranted by any objective reason.

Diabetes *See* Diabetes mellitus.

Diabetes mellitus A disease of carbohydrate metabolism in which an absolute or relative deficiency of insulin results in an inability to metabolize carbohydrates normally.

Diastolic blood pressure (DBP) The pressure in the arteries during the relaxation phase (diastole) of the cardiac cycle; indicative of total peripheral resistance.

Digestion The process of breaking down food into small enough units for absorption.

Diminishing returns Principle stating that after a certain level of performance has been achieved, there will be a decline in the effectiveness of training at furthering a person's performance level.

Distal Farthest from the midline of the body, or from the point of origin of a muscle.

Diuretic Medication that produces an increase in urine volume and sodium excretion.

Dorsiflexion Movement of the foot up toward the shin.

Double taxation The imposition of taxation on corporate earnings at both the corporate level and again as a stockholder dividend.

Dual-energy x-ray absorptiometry (DEXA) An imaging technique that uses a very low dose of radiation to measure bone density. Also can be used to measure overall body fat and regional differences in body fat.

Dynamic balance The act of maintaining postural control while moving.

Dynamic stretching Type of stretching that involves taking the joints through their ranges of motion while continuously moving. Often beneficial in warming up for a particular sport or activity that involves the same joint movements.

Dysarthria A group of speech disorders caused by disturbances in the strength or coordination of the muscles of speech as a result of damage to the brain or nerves.

Dyslipidemia A condition characterized by abnormal blood lipid profiles; may include elevated cholesterol, triglyceride, or low-density lipoprotein (LDL) levels and/or low high-density lipoprotein (HDL) levels.

Dyspnea Shortness of breath; a subjective difficulty or distress in breathing.

Eating disorders Disturbed eating behaviors that jeopardize a person's physical or psychological health.

Eccentric A type of isotonic muscle contraction in which the muscle lengthens against a resistance when it is stimulated; sometimes called "negative work" or "negative reps."

Ecchymosis The escape of blood into the tissues from ruptured blood vessels marked by black-and-blue or purple discolored area.

Edema Swelling resulting from an excessive accumulation of fluid in the tissues of the body.

Effusion The escape of a fluid from anatomical vessels by rupture or exudation.

Ejection fraction The percentage of the total volume of blood that is pumped out of the left ventricle during the systolic contraction of the heart.

Elasticity Temporary or recoverable elongation of connective tissue.

Electrocardiogram (ECG or EKG) A recording of the electrical activity of the heart.

Electrolyte A mineral that exists as a charged ion in the body and that is extremely important for normal cellular function.

Emergency medical services (EMS) A local system for obtaining emergency assistance from the police, fire department, or ambulance. In the United States, most cities have a 911 telephone number that will automatically set the EMS system in motion.

Empathy Understanding what another person is experiencing from his or her perspective.

Emphysema An obstructive pulmonary disease characterized by the gradual destruction of lung alveoli and the surrounding connective tissue, in addition to airway inflammation, leading to reduced ability to effectively inhale and exhale.

Employee A person who works for another person in exchange for financial compensation. An employee complies with the instructions and directions of his or her employer and reports to them on a regular basis.

End-diastolic volume The volume of blood in a ventricle at the end of the cardiac filling cycle (diastole).

Endorphin Natural opiates produced in the brain that function to reduce pain and improve mood.

Enzyme A protein that speeds up a specific chemical reaction.

Epinephrine A hormone released as part of the sympathetic response to exercise; also called adrenaline.

Eschars Dry scabs formed on the skin following a burn or cauterization of the skin.

Essential amino acids Eight to 10 of the 23 different amino acids needed to make proteins. Called essential because the body cannot manufacture them; they must be obtained from the diet.

Essential body fat Fat thought to be necessary for maintenance of life and reproductive function.

Estrogen Generic term for estrus-producing steroid compounds produced primarily in the ovaries; the female sex hormones.

Etiology The cause of a medical condition.

Eversion Rotation of the foot to direct the plantar surface outward.

Exculpatory clause A clause within a waiver that bars the potential plaintiff from recovery.

Exercise-induced asthma (EIA) *See* Exercise-induced bronchospasm (EIB).

Exercise-induced bronchospasm (EIB) Transient and reversible airway narrowing triggered by vigorous exercise; also called exercise-induced asthma (EIA).

Expiration The act of expelling air from the lungs; exhalation.

Express partnership A partnership created through formal paperwork.

Extension The act of straightening or extending a joint, usually applied to the muscular movement of a limb.

External rotation Outward turning about the vertical axis of bone.

Extinction The removal of a positive stimulus that has in the past followed a behavior.

Extrinsic motivation Motivation that comes from external (outside of the self) rewards, such as material or social rewards.

Fartlek training A form of training during which the exerciser randomly changes the aerobic intensity based on how he or she is feeling. Also called speed play.

Fascia Strong connective tissues that perform a number of functions, including developing and isolating the muscles of the body and providing structural support and protection. Plural = fasciae.

Fasciae *See* Fascia.

Fasciitis An inflammation of the fascia.

Fast glycolytic system Anaerobic process of metabolism that breaks down glucose and glycogen into ATP during high-intensity physical activity; also called the lactate system.

Fast-twitch muscle fiber One of several types of muscle fibers found in skeletal muscle tissue; also called type II fibers and characterized as having a low oxidative capacity but a high gylcolytic capacity; recruited for rapid, powerful movements such as jumping, throwing, and sprinting.

Fat An essential nutrient that provides energy, energy storage, insulation, and contour to the body. 1 gram of fat equals 9 kcal.

Fat-free mass (FFM) That part of the body composition that represents everything but fat—blood, bones, connective tissue, organs, and muscle; also called lean body mass.

Fatty acids Long hydrocarbon chains with an even number of carbons and varying degrees of saturation with hydrogen.

Feedback An internal response within a learner; during information processing, it is the correctness or incorrectness of a response that is stored in memory to be used for future reference. Also, verbal or nonverbal information about current behavior that can be used to improve future performance.

Feldenkrais Method Consists of two interrelated, somatically based educational methods. The first, awareness through movement (ATM), is a verbally directed technique designed for group work. The second, functional integration (FI), is a nonverbal manual contact technique designed for people desiring more individualized attention.

Fetal hypoxia Brain injury occurring during and/or shortly after birth wherein the infant suffers a lack of oxygen to the brain.

FEV1 The volume of air that a person can exhale in the first second during a forced expiration test. FEV1 stands for "forced expiratory volume in one second."

Fibromyalgia Diffuse pain in the muscles and surrounding connective tissues, usually accompanied by malaise.

First ventilatory threshold (VT1) Intensity of aerobic exercise at which ventilation starts to increase in a non-linear fashion in response to an accumulation of metabolic by-products in the blood.

Flexibility The ability to move joints through their normal full ranges of motion.

Flexion The act of moving a joint so that the two bones forming it are brought closer together.

Flow-through taxation Financial profits and losses flow from the business directly to the investors. The business does not pay any taxes; rather, business profits are taxed on the investors' individual tax return and losses can be utilized by the investors to offset other personal income.

Foramina Holes or openings in a bone or between body cavities.

Frailty The condition of being frail, fragile, easily damaged; the predisposition toward increased risk of injury, illness, disability, and/or death.

Frontal plane A longitudinal section that runs at a right angle to the sagittal plane, dividing the body into anterior and posterior portions.

Functional capacity The maximum physical performance represented by maximal oxygen consumption.

Gait The manner or style of walking.

Gastrointestinal tract A long hollow tube from mouth to anus where digestion and absorption occur.

General partnership A type of business arrangement in which each partner assumes management responsibility and unlimited liability and must have at least a 1% interest in profit and loss.

General supervision A method of supervision where the worker (or trainee) does not require the constant attendance of the supervisor (or trainer).

Gestational diabetes An inability to maintain normal glucose, or any degree of glucose intolerance, during pregnancy, despite being treated with either diet or insulin.

Glucose A simple sugar; the form in which all carbohydrates are used as the body's principal energy source.

Glutamine A non-essential amino acid found in large amounts in the muscles of the body.

Glycogen The chief carbohydrate storage material; formed by the liver and stored in the liver and muscle.

Graded exercise test A test that evaluates an individual's physiological response to exercise, the intensity of which is increased in stages.

Grand mal seizure A major motor seizure characterized by violent and uncontrollable muscle contractions.

Gravity-based forces Forces that act on an object (such as the body) related to the gravitational pull of the earth.

Greater trochanteric bursitis An inflammation of the bursa sac that lies over the greater trochater of the femur. Often due to acute trauma, repetitive stress, muscle imbalance, or muscle tightness.

Gross negligence A form of negligence that is worse than normal negligence. Generally, a waiver clause cannot prevent a suit for gross negligence or for wanton or recklessness or intentional misconduct in any state or jurisdiction.

Group waiver Waiver that includes lines for multiple signatures.

Growth hormone A hormone secreted by the pituitary gland that facilitates protein synthesis in the body.

Gynoid Adipose tissue or body fat distributed on the hips and in the lower body (pear-shaped individuals).

Hatha yoga A form of yogic exercise that combines difficult postures (which force the mind to withdraw from the outside world) with controlled breathing.

Health belief model A model to explain health-related behaviors that suggests that an individual's decision to adopt healthy behaviors is based largely upon his or her perception of susceptibility to an illness and the probable severity of the illness. The person's view of the benefits and costs of the change also are considered.

Health Insurance Portability and Accountability Act (HIPAA) Enacted by the U.S. Congress in 1996, HIPAA requires the U.S. Department of Health and Human Services (HHS) to establish national standards for electronic health care information to facilitate efficient and secure exchange of private health data. The Standards for Privacy of Individually Identifiable Health Information ("Privacy Rule"), issued by the HHS, addresses the use and disclosure of individuals' health information—called "protected health information"—by providing federal protections and giving patients an array of rights with respect to personal health information while permitting the disclosure of information needed for patient care and other important purposes.

Health psychology A field of psychology that examines the causes of illnesses and studies ways to promote and maintain health, prevent and treat illnesses, and improve the healthcare system.

Heart disease A structural or functional abnormality of the heart or of the blood vessels supplying the heart that impairs its normal functioning.

Heart rate (HR) The number of heart beats per minute.

Heart-rate reserve (HRR) The reserve capacity of the heart; the difference between maximal heart rate and resting heart rate. It reflects the heart's ability to increase the rate of beating and cardiac output above resting level to maximal intensity.

Heat cramps A mild form of heat-related illness that generally occurs during or after strenuous physical activity and is characterized by painful muscle spasms.

Heat exhaustion The most common heat-related illness; usually the result of intense exercise in a hot, humid environment and characterized by profuse sweating, which results in fluid and electrolyte loss, a drop in blood pressure, lightheadedness, nausea, vomiting, decreased coordination, and often syncope (fainting).

Heat stroke A medical emergency that is the most serious form of heat illness due to heat overload and/or impairment of the body's ability to dissipate heat; characterized by high body temperature (>105° F or 40.5° C), dry, red skin, altered level of consciousness, seizures, coma, and possibly death.

Heat syncope A sudden dizziness experienced after exercising in the heat.

Heimlich maneuver First aid for choking, involving the application of sudden, upward pressure on the upper abdomen to force a foreign object from the windpipe.

Hematoma A large bruise or collection of blood under the skin, producing discoloration and swelling in the area; usually caused by trauma.

Hemodynamic Pertaining to the forces involved in the circulation of blood (e.g., heart rate, stroke volume, cardiac output).

Hemoglobin The protein molecule in red blood cells specifically adapted to carry oxygen molecules (by bonding with them).

Hemorrhagic stroke Disruption of blood flow to the brain caused by the presence of a blood clot or hematoma.

Hepatitis Inflammation of the liver, often due to viral infection.

Hepatitis B A potentially life-threatening bloodborne disease of the liver, which is transmitted primarily by sexual activity or exposure to blood.

Hernia A protrusion of the abdominal contents into the groin (inguinal hernia) or through the abdominal wall (abdominal hernia).

Herniated disc Rupture of the outer layers of fibers that surround the gelatinous portion of the disc.

High-density lipoprotein (HDL) A lipoprotein that carries excess cholesterol from the arteries to the liver.

Homeostasis An internal state of physiological balance.

Hormones A chemical substance produced and released by an endocrine gland and transported through the blood to a target organ.

HR turnpoint (HRTP) The point during incremental aerobic exercise at which the heart rate no longer increases linearly, but rather shows a curvilinear response; also called the heart rate deflection point and is related to the onset of blood lactate accumulation.

Human immunodeficiency virus (HIV) A retrovirus (family Retroviridae, subfamily Lentvirinae) that is about 100 nm in diameter and is the etiologic agent of AIDS.

Hydrolysates A product of hydrolysis, in which water reacts with a compound to produce other compounds.

Hydrostatic weighing Weighing a person fully submerged in water. The difference between the person's mass in air and in water is used to calculate body density, which can be used to estimate the proportion of fat in the body.

Hypercholesterolemia An excess of cholesterol in the blood.

Hyperextension Extension of an articulation beyond anatomical position.

Hyperglycemia An abnormally high content of glucose (sugar) in the blood (above 100 mg/dL).

Hyperlipidemia An excess of lipids in the blood that could be primary, as in disorders of lipid metabolism, or secondary, as in uncontrolled diabetes.

Hypertension High blood pressure, or the elevation of resting blood pressure above 140/90 mmHg.

Hypertension fibrinolysis Elevated blood pressure related to fibrinolysis, or increased blood platelet activity.

Hyperthermia Abnormally high body temperature.

Hypertonic Having extreme muscular tension.

Hypertonicity *See* Hypertonic.

Hypertrophy An increase in the cross-sectional size of a muscle in response to progressive resistance training.

Hypoglycemia A deficiency of glucose in the blood commonly caused by too much insulin, too little glucose, or too much exercise. Most commonly found in the insulin-dependent diabetic and characterized by symptoms such as fatigue, dizziness, confusion, headache, nausea, or anxiety.

Hyponatremia Abnormally low levels of sodium ions circulating in the blood; severe hyponatremia can lead to brain swelling and death.

Hypoperfusion A diminished blood supply to the tissues.

Hypotension Low blood pressure.

Hypothermia Abnormally low body temperature.

Hypoxia A condition in which there is an inadequate supply of oxygen to tissues.

Hypoxic *See* Hypoxia.

Iliotibial (IT) band A band of connective tissue that extends from the iliac crest to the knee and links the gluteus maximus to the tibia.

Iliotibial band syndrome (ITBS) A repetitive overuse condition that occurs when the distal portion of the iliotibial band rubs against the lateral femoral epicondyle.

Implied partnership A partnership lacking a written agreement, but in which the parties involved conduct business like a partnership.

Incision A cut in the skin, frequently from a sharp object.

Independent activities of daily living Activities often performed by a person who is living independently in a community setting during the course of a normal day, such as managing money, shopping, telephone use, traveling within the community, housekeeping, preparing meals, and taking medications correctly.

Independent contractor A person who conducts business on his or her own on a contract basis and is not an employee of an organization.

Inferior Located below.

Informed consent A written statement signed by a client prior to testing that informs him or her of testing purposes, processes, and all potential risks and discomforts.

Infrapatellar tendinitis Inflammation of the patellar tendon at the insertion into the proximal tibia.

Inherent risk Risks that can occur through normal participation in the stated activity. Inherent risks can only be avoided by declining to participate.

Insertion The point of attachment of a muscle to a relatively more movable or distal bone.

Inspiration The drawing of air into the lungs; inhalation.

Instants An event in the gait cycle that designates a component of locomotion such as the heel strike of the right foot.

Insulin A hormone released from the pancreas that allows cells to take up glucose.

Insulin-dependent diabetes mellitus (IDDM) *See* Type 1 diabetes.

Insulin resistance An inability of muscle tissue to effectively use insulin, where the action of insulin is "resisted" by insulin-sensitive tissues.

Intermediate-density lipoprotein (IDL) Formed from the degradation of very low-density lipoproteins; enables fats and cholesterol to move within the bloodstream.

Interval training Short, high-intensity exercise periods alternated with periods of rest (e.g., 100-yard run, one-minute rest, repeated eight times).

Intrinsic motivation Motivation that comes from internal states, such as enjoyment or personal satisfaction.

Inversion Rotation of the foot to direct the plantar surface inward.

Ischemia A decrease in the blood supply to a bodily organ, tissue, or part caused by constriction or obstruction of the blood vessels.

Ischemic stroke A sudden disruption of cerebral circulation in which blood supply to the brain is either interrupted or diminished.

Isokinetic A type of muscular contraction where tension developed within the muscle changes throughout the range of motion; performed with the use of special equipment; also referred to as "variable resistance" exercise.

Isometric A type of muscular contraction in which the muscle is stimulated to generate tension but little or no joint movement occurs.

Isotonic A type of muscular contraction where the muscle is stimulated to develop tension and joint movement occurs.

Ketoacidosis Occurs when a high level of ketones (beta hydroxybutyrate, acetoacetate) are produced as a by-product of fatty-acid metabolism.

Ketone An organic compound (e.g., acetone) with a carbonyl group attached to two carbon atoms. *See also* Ketosis.

Ketosis An abnormal increase of ketone bodies in the body; usually the result of a low-carbohydrate diet, fasting, or starvation.

Keyman insurance Insurance that compensates a company for the loss of a representative of the company who was performing unique and valuable functions.

Kinematics The study of the form, pattern, or sequence of movement without regard for the forces that may produce that motion.

Kinesthesis Awareness of movement.

Knowledge of results The motivational impact of feedback provided to a person learning a new task or behavior indicating the outcomes of performance.

Korotkoff sounds Five different sounds created by the pulsing of the blood through the brachial artery; proper distinction of the sounds is necessary to determine blood pressure.

Kyphosis Excessive posterior curvature of the spine, typically seen in the thoracic region.

Kyphotic *See* Kyphosis.

Laceration A jagged, irregular cut or tear in the soft tissues, usually caused by a blow. Because of extensive tissue destruction, there is a great potential for contamination and infection.

Lactate A chemical derivative of lactic acid,

which is formed when sugars are broken down for energy without the presence of oxygen.

Lactate threshold (LT) The point during exercise of increasing intensity at which blood lactate begins to accumulate above resting levels, where lactate clearance is no longer able to keep up with lactate production.

Lactic acid A metabolic by-product of anaerobic glycolysis; when it accumulates it increases blood pH, which slows down enzyme activity and ultimately causes fatigue.

Lapses The expected slips or mistakes that are usually discreet events and are a normal part of the behavior-change process.

Lateral Away from the midline of the body, or the outside.

Lateral epicondylitis An injury resulting from the repetitive tension overloading of the wrist and finger extensors that originate at the lateral epicondyle; often referred to as "tennis elbow."

Laxity Lacking in strength, firmness, or resilience; joints that have been injured or overstretched may exhibit laxity.

Lean body mass The components of the body (apart from fat), including muscles, bones, nervous tissue, skin, blood, and organs.

Lever A rigid bar that rotates around a fixed support (fulcrum) in response to an applied force.

Liability Legal responsibility.

Ligament A strong, fibrous tissue that connects one bone to another.

Limited liability corporation (LLC) A corporation that limits investors' personal financial and legal liabilities but provides flow-through taxation for investors. It is not limited to a certain number of shareholders and owners do not have to be U.S. citizens.

Limited liability partnership (LLP) A partnership in which some or all partners (depending on the jurisdiction) have limited liability; exhibits elements of both partnerships and corporations.

Limited partner An individual who retains no legal liability beyond his or her initial investment and does not have any formal input regarding partnership operations.

Limits of stability (LOS) The degree of allowable sway from the line of gravity without a need to change the base of support.

Line of gravity (LOG) A theoretical vertical line passing through the center of gravity, dissecting the body into two hemispheres.

Linear periodization A form of periodization used in resistance training that provides a consistent training protocol within each microcycle and changes the training variables after each microcycle.

Lipid The name for fats used in the body and bloodstream.

Lipoprotein An assembly of a lipid and protein that serves as a transport vehicle for fatty acids and cholesterol in the blood and lymph.

Locus of control The degree to which people attribute outcomes to internal factors, such as effort and ability, as opposed to external factors, such as luck or the actions of others. People who tend to attribute events and outcomes to internal factors are said to have an internal locus of control, while those who generally attribute outcomes to external factors are said to have an external locus of control.

Lordosis Excessive anterior curvature of the spine that typically occurs at the low back (may also occur at the neck).

Lordotic *See* Lordosis.

Low-density lipoprotein (LDL) A lipoprotein that transports cholesterol and triglycerides from the liver and small intestine to cells and tissues; high levels may cause atherosclerosis.

Macrocyle The longest timeframe in a periodized training program, usually a period of six months to one year. The goals of a macrocycle are long-term and require multiple steps to be achieved.

Magnetic resonance imaging (MRI) A diagnostic modality in which the patient is placed within a strong magnetic field and the effect of high-frequency radio waves on water molecules within the tissues is recorded. High-speed computers are used to analyze the absorption of radio waves and create a cross-sectional image based upon the variation in tissue signal.

Maintenance The stage of the transtheoretical model of behavioral change during which the individual is incorporating the new behavior into his or her lifestyle.

Malignant A cancerous tumor characterized by progressive and uncontrolled growth.

Maximal graded exercise test A physician-supervised diagnostic examination to assess a participant's physiological response to exercise in a controlled environment.

Maximal oxygen uptake ($\dot{V}O_2$max) *See* $\dot{V}O_2$max.

Maximum heart rate (MHR) The highest heart rate a person can attain. Sometimes abbreviated as HRmax.

Medial Toward the midline of the body, or the inside.

Medial collateral ligament (MCL) One of four ligaments that are critical to the stability of the knee joint; spans the distance from the medial end of the femur to the top of the medial tibia.

Medial epicondylitis An injury that results from an overload of the wrist flexors and forearm pronators.

Medial tibial stress syndrome (MTSS) Inflammation of the periosteum (connective tissue covering of the bone). Often induced by a sudden change in activity and has been associated with pes planus.

Meninges The three-layer system of membranes that envelops the brain and spinal cord.

Mesocycle The mid-length timeframe of a periodized training program, usually two weeks to a few months long. The goals of a mesocycle are designed to be steps on the way to the overall goal of the macrocycle.

MET *See* Metabolic equivalents (METs).

Metabolic equivalents (METs) A simplified system for classifying physical activities where one MET is equal to the resting oxygen consumption, which is approximately 3.5 milliliters of oxygen per kilogram of body weight per minute (3.5 mL/kg/min).

Metabolic syndrome (MetS) A cluster of factors associated with increased risk for coronary heart disease and diabetes—abdominal obesity indicated by a waist circumference ≥40 inches (102 cm) in men and ≥35 inches (88 cm) in women; levels of triglyceride ≥150 mg/dL (1.7 mmol/L); HDL levels <40 and 50 mg/dL (1.0 and 1.3 mmol/L) in men and women, respectively; blood-pressure levels ≥130/85 mmHg; and fasting blood glucose levels ≥110 mg/dL (6.1 mmol/L).

Metastasis The spreading of a disease (especially cancer) to another part of the body.

Micelles Aggregates of lipid- and water-soluble compounds in which the hydrophobic portions are oriented toward the center and the hydrophilic portions are oriented outwardly.

Microcycle The shortest timeframe in a periodized training program, usually one to four weeks long. The goals of a microcycle are short-term and are designed to be steps on the way to the overall goal of the mesocycle.

Mineral Inorganic substances needed in the diet in small amounts to help regulate bodily functions.

Minority partner A partner holding less than 50% of the company's ownership shares.

Minute ventilation ($\dot{V}_E$) A measure of the amount of air that passes through the lungs in one minute; calculated as the tidal volume multiplied by the ventilatory rate.

Mitochondria The "power plant" of the cells where aerobic metabolism occurs.

Mobility The degree to which an articulation is allowed to move before being restricted by surrounding tissues.

Morbidity The disease rate; the ratio of sick to well persons in a community.

Mortality The death rate; the ratio of deaths that take place to expected deaths.

Motivation The psychological drive that gives purpose and direction to behavior.

Motivational interviewing A method of questioning clients in a way that encourages them to honestly examine their beliefs and behaviors, and that motivates clients to make a decision to change a particular behavior.

Motor learning The process of acquiring and improving motor skills.

Motor unit A motor nerve and all of the muscle fibers it stimulates.

Muscle afferents Neurons that conduct impulses from sensory receptors into the central nervous system.

Muscle spindle The sensory organ within a muscle that is sensitive to stretch and thus protects the muscle against too much stretch.

Muscular endurance The ability of a muscle or muscle group to exert force against a resistance over a sustained period of time.

Muscular power The product of muscular force and speed of movement.

Muscular strength The maximal force a muscle or muscle group can exert during contraction.

Myocardial infarction (MI) An episode in which some of the heart's blood supply is severely cut off or restricted, causing the heart muscle to suffer and die from lack of oxygen. Commonly known as a heart attack.

Myofascial release A manual massage technique used to eliminate general fascial restrictions; typically performed with a device such as a foam roller.

Myofascial sling A continuous line of action formed by muscles, tendons, ligaments, fascia, joint capsules, and bones that lie in series or in parallel to actively moving joints or muscles.

Myofibril The portion of the muscle containing the thick (myosin) and thin (actin) contractile filaments; a series of sarcomeres where the repeating pattern of the contractile proteins gives the striated appearance to skeletal muscle.

Myofibrillar hypertrophy The increase in the size of muscle cells (myofibrils).

Myoglobin A compound similar to hemoglobin, which aids in the storage and transport of oxygen in the muscle cells.

Myosin Thick contractile protein in a myofibril.

Negative reinforcement The removal or absence of aversive stimuli following an undesired behavior. This increases the likelihood that the behavior will occur again.

Negligence Failure of a person to perform as a reasonable and prudent professional would perform under similar circumstances.

Neuromuscular efficiency The ability of the neuromuscular system to allow muscles that produce movement and muscles that provide stability to work together synergistically as an integrated functional unit.

Neuromuscular integrative action (Nia) An expressive fitness and awareness movement program and a holistic approach to health that combines movements from tai chi, yoga, martial arts, and modern ethnic dances.

Neuropathy Any disease affecting a peripheral nerve. It may manifest as loss of nerve function, burning pain, or numbness and tingling.

Neurotransmitter A chemical substance such as acetylcholine or dopamine that transmits nerve impulses across synapses.

Nia *See* Neuromuscular integrative action (Nia).

Non-insulin dependent diabetes mellitus (NIDDM) *See* Type 2 diabetes.

Nonsteroidal anti-inflammatory drug (NSAID) A drug with analgesic, antipyretic and anti-inflammatory effects. The term "nonsteroidal" is used to distinguish these drugs from steroids, which have similar actions.

Norepinephrine A hormone released as part of the sympathetic response to exercise.

Obesity An excessive accumulation of body

fat. Usually defined as more than 20% above ideal weight, or over 25% body fat for men and over 32% body fat for women; also can be defined as a body mass index of >30 kg/m^2 or a waist girth of ≥40 inches (102 cm) in men and ≥35 inches (89 cm) in women.

Occupational therapist A rehabilitation expert specializing in treatments that help people who suffer from mentally, physically, developmentally, or emotionally disabling conditions to develop, recover, or maintain daily living and work skills that include improving basic motor functions and reasoning abilities.

One-repetition maximum (1 RM) The amount of resistance that can be moved through the range of motion one time before the muscle is temporarily fatigued.

Onset of blood lactate accumulation (OBLA) The point in time during high-intensity exercise at which the production of lactic acid exceeds the body's capacity to eliminate it; after this point, oxygen is insufficient at meeting the body's demands for energy.

Operant conditioning A learning approach that considers the manner in which behaviors are influenced by their consequences.

Orthopnea Form of dyspnea in which the person can breathe comfortably only when standing or sitting erect; associated with asthma, emphysema, and angina.

Orthostatic hypotension A drop in blood pressure associated with rising to an upright position.

Osteoarthritis A degenerative disease involving a wearing away of joint cartilage. This degenerative joint disease occurs chiefly in older persons.

Osteopenia Bone density that is below average, classified as 1.5 to 2.5 standard deviations below peak bone density.

Osteoporosis A disorder, primarily affecting postmenopausal women, in which bone density decreases and susceptibility to fractures increases.

Overload The principle that a physiological system subjected to above-normal stress will respond by increasing in strength or function accordingly.

Overtraining syndrome The result of constant intense training that does not provide adequate time for recovery; symptoms include increased resting heart rate, impaired physical performance, reduced enthusiasm and desire for training, increased incidence of injuries and illness, altered appetite, disturbed sleep patterns, and irritability.

Overuse injury An injury caused by activity that places too much stress on one area of the body over an extended period.

Overweight A term to describe an excessive amount of weight for a given height, using height-to-weight ratios.

Oxygen uptake ($\dot{V}O_2$) The process by which oxygen is used to produce energy for cellular work; also called oxygen consumption.

Palpation The use of hands and/or fingers to detect anatomical structures or an arterial pulse (e.g., carotid pulse).

Palpitation A rapid and irregular heart beat.

Parasthesia An abnormal sensation such as numbness, prickling, or tingling.

Parasthesis *See* Paresthesia.

Part-to-whole teaching strategy A teaching strategy involving breaking a skill down into its component parts and practicing each skill in its simplest form before placing several skills in a sequence.

Partnership A business entity in which two or more people agree to operate a business and share profits and losses.

Patellofemoral pain syndrome (PFPS) A degenerative condition of the posterior surface of the patella, which may result from acute injury to the patella or from chronic friction between the patella and the groove in the femur through which it passes during motion of the knee.

Pathogen Any virus, microorganism or other substance capable of causing disease.

Perfusion The passage of fluid through a

tissue, such as the transport of blood through vessels from the heart to internal organs and other tissues.

Periodization The systematic application of overload through the pre-planned variation of program components to optimize gains in strength (or any specific component of fitness), while preventing overuse, staleness, overtraining, and plateaus.

Periosteum A double-layered connective tissue sheath surrounding the outer surface of the diaphysis of a long bone; serves to cover and nourish the bone.

Periostitis Inflammation of the membrane of connective tissue that closely surrounds a bone.

Peripheral artery occlusive disease (PAOD) Disease caused by the obstruction of large arteries in the arms and legs.

Peripheral neuropathy Damage to nerves of the peripheral nervous system, which may be caused either by diseases of the nerve or from the side effects of systemic illness.

Peripheral vascular disease A painful and often debilitating condition, characterized by muscular pain caused by ischemia to the working muscles. The ischemic pain is usually due to atherosclerotic blockages or arterial spasms, referred to as claudication. Also called peripheral vascular occlusive disease (PVOD).

Peripheral vascular occlusive disease (PVOD) *See* Peripheral vascular disease.

Pes cavus High arches of the feet.

Pes planus Flat feet.

Phosphagen High-energy phosphate compounds found in muscle tissue, including adenosine triphosphate (ATP) and creatine phosphate (CP), that can be broken down for immediate use by the cells.

Phosphagen system A system of transfer of chemical energy from the breakdown of creatine phosphate to regenerate adenosine triphosphate (ATP).

Physical Activity Readiness Questionnaire (PAR-Q) A brief, self-administered medical questionnaire recognized as a safe pre-exercise screening measure for low-to-moderate (but not vigorous) exercise training.

Physical therapist A rehabilitation expert specializing in treatments that help restore function, improve mobility, relieve pain, and prevent or limit permanent physical disabilities in patients of all ages suffering from medical problems, injuries, diseases, disabilities, or other health-related conditions.

Pilates A method of mind-body conditioning that combines stretching and strengthening exercises; developed by Joseph Pilates in the 1920s.

Plantarflexion Distal movement of the plantar surface of the foot; opposite of dorsiflexion.

Plasma The liquid portion of the blood.

Plyometrics High-intensity movements, such as jumping, involving high-force loading of body weight during the landing phase of the movement.

Positive reinforcement The presentation of a positive stimulus following a desired behavior. This increases the likelihood that the behavior will occur again.

Posterior Toward the back or dorsal side.

Post-exercise hypotension (PEH) Acute post-exercise reduction in both systolic and diastolic blood pressure.

Postictal state The altered state of consciousness that a person enters after experiencing an epileptic seizure.

Posture The arrangement of the body and its limbs.

Precontemplation The stage of the transtheoretical model of behavioral change during which the individual is not yet thinking about changing.

Prehypertension A systolic pressure of 120 to 139 mmHg and/or a diastolic pressure of 80 to 89 mmHg. Having this condition puts an individual at higher risk for developing hypertension.

Prehypertensive *See* Prehypertension.

Preparation The stage of the transtheoretical model during which the individual is getting ready to make a change.

Prime mover A muscle responsible for a specific movement. Also called an agonist.

Process goal A goal a person achieves by doing something, such as completing an exercise session or attending a talk on stress management.

Product goal A goal that represents change in a measurable variable, such as increases in strength scores, reductions in resting heart rate, or weight loss.

Product liability insurance Insurance that covers damages occurring due to product failure.

Professional liability insurance Insurance to protect a trainer/instructor against professional negligence or failure to perform as a competent and prudent professional would under similar circumstances.

Pronation Internal rotation of the forearm causing the radius to cross diagonally over the ulna and the palm to face posteriorly.

Proprioception Sensation and awareness of body position and movements.

Proprioceptive neuromuscular facilitation (PNF) A method of promoting the response of neuromuscular mechanisms through the stimulation of proprioceptors in an attempt to gain more stretch in a muscle; often referred to as a contract/relax method of stretching.

Protein A compound composed of a combination 20 amino acids that is the major structural component of all body tissue.

Proximal Nearest to the midline of the body or point of origin of a muscle.

Puncture A piercing wound from a sharp object that makes a small hole in the skin.

Punishment The presentation of aversive stimuli following an undesired behavior. Decreases the likelihood that the behavior will occur again.

Q-angle The angle formed by lines drawn from the anterior superior iliac spine (ASIS) to the central patella and from the central patella to the tibial tubercle; an estimate of the effective angle at which the quadriceps group pulls on the patella.

Qigong A wide variety of traditional cultivation practices that involve methods of accumulating, circulating, and working with *qi*, breathing or energy within the body. Qigong is practiced for health maintenance purposes, as a therapeutic intervention, as a medical profession, as a spiritual path, and/or as a component of Chinese martial arts.

Radiculopathy Dysfunction of a nerve root that can cause numbness or tingling, muscle weakness, or loss of reflex associated with that nerve.

Range of motion (ROM) The number of degrees that an articulation will allow one of its segments to move.

Rapport A relationship marked by mutual understanding and trust.

Rate coding The frequency of impulses sent to a muscle. Increased force can be generated through increase in either the number of muscle fibers recruited or the rate at which the impulses are sent.

Ratings of perceived exertion (RPE) A scale, originally developed by noted Swedish psychologist Gunnar Borg, that provides a standard means for evaluating a participant's perception of exercise effort. The original scale ranged from 6 to 20; a revised category ratio scale ranges from 0 to 10.

Reactive ability The ability of an individual to perform reactive movements, such as plyometrics and agility drills.

Reactive forces Forces that oppose an initial active force. For example, ground reaction forces occur at the foot when it comes in contact with the ground during running.

Reciprocal inhibition The reflex inhibition of the motor neurons of antagonists when the agonists are contracted.

Registered dietitian A food and nutrition expert that has met the following criteria: completed a minimum of a bachelor's degree at a U.S. accredited university, or other college coursework approved by the Commission on Accreditation for Dietetics Education (CADE); completed a CADE-accredited supervised practice program; passed a national examination; and completed continuing education requirements to maintain registration.

Relapse In behavior change, the return of an original problem after many lapses (slips, mistakes) have occurred.

Relative contraindication A condition that makes a particular treatment or procedure somewhat inadvisable but does not completely rule it out.

Relative strength The ratio of the amount of weight lifted to the total body weight of the person. It can be used to compare the strength of different individuals.

Relaxin A hormone of pregnancy that relaxes the pelvic ligaments and other connective tissue in the body.

Rescue medication Quick-relief or fast-acting inhaled medications taken by individuals with asthma to quickly stop symptoms.

Residual volume The volume of air remaining in the lungs following a maximal expiration.

Respiratory exchange ratio (RER) A ratio of the amount of carbon dioxide produced relative to the amount of oxygen consumed.

Respondeat superior A legal doctrine wherein the actions of an employee can subject the employer to liability; Latin for "Let the master answer."

Resting heart rate (RHR) The number of heartbeats per minute when the body is at complete rest; usually counted first thing in the morning before any physical activity.

Resting metabolic rate (RMR) The number of calories expended per unit time at rest; measured early in the morning after an overnight fast and at least eight hours of sleep; approximated with various formulas.

Return on investment (ROI) The ratio of the net income (profit minus depreciation) to the average money spent by the company overall or on a specific project. Usually expressed as a percentage, a measure of profitability that indicates whether or not a company is using its resources in an efficient manner.

Reversibility The principle of exercise training that suggests that any improvement in physical fitness due to physical activity is entirely reversible with the discontinuation of the training program.

Rheumatoid arthritis An autoimmune disease that causes inflammation of connective tissues and joints.

Rider Specific additions to a standard insurance policy.

Risk factor A characteristic, inherited trait, or behavior related to the presence or development of a condition or disease.

Risk management Minimizing the risks of potential legal liability.

Rotation Movement in the transverse plane about a longitudinal axis; can be "internal" or "external."

Royalty A payment made to the owner of a copyright, patent, or trademark in exchange for use of the protected intellectual property; typically a percentage of each sale.

Sagittal plane The longitudinal plane that divides the body into right and left portions.

Sarcomere The basic functional unit of the myofibril containing the contractile proteins that generate skeletal muscle movements.

Sarcopenia Decreased muscle mass; often used to refer specifically to an age-related decline in muscle mass or lean-body tissue.

Sarcoplasm A gelatin-like tissue surrounding the sarcomere.

Sarcoplasmic hypertrophy An increase in muscle size due to an increase in the volume of sarcoplasmic fluid as a result of high-repetition weight-lifting sets. Also called transient hypertrophy.

Sciatica Pain radiating down the leg caused by compression of the sciatic nerve; frequently the result of lumbar disc herniation.

Scoliosis Excessive lateral curvature of the spine.

Scope of practice The range and limit of responsibilities normally associated with a specific job or profession.

Secondary assessment After immediate life- or limb-threatening injuries/illnesses have been identified, this more thorough evaluation is performed to identify more subtle, yet still important, injuries.

Second ventilatory threshold (VT2) A metabolic marker that represents the point at which high-intensity exercise can no longer be sustained due to an accumulation of lactate.

Sedentary Doing or requiring much sitting; minimal activity.

Selective serotonin reuptake inhibitors (SSRI) A group of medications used to treat depression that cause an increase in the amount of the neurotransmitter serotonin in the brain.

Self-efficacy One's perception of his or her ability to change or to perform specific behaviors (e.g., exercise).

Serotonin A neurotransmitter; acts as a synaptic messenger in the brain and as an inhibitor of pain pathways; plays a role in mood and sleep.

Shaping Designing a new behavior chain, including antecedents and rewards, to encourage a certain behavior, such as regular physical activity.

Shear force Any force that causes slippage between a pair of contiguous joints or tissues in a direction that parallels the plane in which they contact.

Shin splints A general term for any pain or discomfort on the front or side of the lower leg in the region of the shin bone (tibia).

Sinoatrial node (SA node) A group of specialized myocardial cells, located in the wall of the right atrium, that control the heart's rate of contraction; the "pacemaker" of the heart.

Slow-twitch muscle fiber A muscle fiber type designed for use of aerobic glycolysis and fatty acid oxidation, recruited for low-intensity, longer-duration activities such as walking and swimming.

SMART goals A properly designed goal; SMART stands for specific, measurable, attainable, relevant, and time-bound.

SOAP note A communication tool used among healthcare professionals; SOAP stands for subjective, objective, assessment, plan.

Social support The perceived comfort, caring, esteem, or help an individual receives from other people.

Sodium bicarbonate A salt that neutralizes acids by increasing the blood's alkalinity and buffering capacity so that more lactic acid can be neutralized during physical activity.

Sole proprietorship A business owned and operated by one person.

Somatosensory system The physiological system relating to the perception of sensory stimuli from the skin and internal organs.

Specific supervision A method of supervision where the worker (or trainee) requires direct involvement of the supervisor (or trainer).

Specificity Exercise training principle explaining that specific exercise demands made on the body produce specific responses by the body; also called exercise specificity.

Sphygmomanometer An instrument for measuring blood pressure in the arteries.

Spinal stenosis A medical condition in which the spinal canal narrows and compresses the spinal cord and nerves.

Sprain A traumatic joint twist that results in stretching or tearing of the stabilizing connective tissues; mainly involves ligaments or joint capsules, and causes discoloration, swelling, and pain.

Stability Characteristic of the body's joints or posture that represents resistance to change of position.

Stages-of-change model A lifestyle-modification model that suggests that people go through distinct, predictable stages when making lifestyle changes: precontemplation,

contemplation, preparation, action, and maintenance. The process is not always linear.

Standard of care Appropriateness of an exercise professional's actions in light of current professional standards and based on the age, condition, and knowledge of the participant.

Static balance The ability to maintain the body's center of mass (COM) within its base of support (BOS).

Static stretching Holding a nonmoving (static) position to immobilize a joint in a position that places the desired muscles and connective tissues passively at their greatest possible length.

Statute of frauds A contract that must be in writing in order to be enforceable.

Statute of limitations A formal regulation limiting the period within which a specific legal action may be taken.

Steady state (HRss) Constant submaximal exercise below the lactate threshold where the oxygen consumption is meeting the energy requirements of the activity.

Stimulus control A means to break the connection between events or other stimuli and a behavior; in behavioral science, sometimes called "cue extinction."

Strain A stretch, tear, or rip in the muscle or adjacent tissue such as the fascia or tendon.

Stress fracture An incomplete fracture caused by excessive stress (overuse) to a bone. Most common in the foot (metatarsal bones) and lower leg (tibia).

Stretch reflex An involuntary motor response that, when stimulated, causes a suddenly stretched muscle to respond with a corresponding contraction.

Stretch-shortening cycle An active stretch (eccentric action) of a muscle followed by an immediate shortening (concentric action) of that same muscle. A component of plyometrics.

Stroke A sudden and often severe attack due to blockage of an artery into the brain.

Stroke volume (SV) The amount of blood pumped from the left ventricle of the heart with each beat.

Subchapter S-corporations A corporation that does not pay any income taxes. Instead, the corporation's income or losses are divided among and passed through to its shareholders.

Subcutaneous body fat *See* Subcutaneous fat.

Subcutaneous fat Fatty deposits or pads of storage fat found under the skin.

Superior Located above.

Supination External rotation of the forearm (radioulnar joint) that causes the palm to face anteriorly.

Supine Lying face up (on the back).

SWOT analysis Situation analysis in which internal strengths and weaknesses of an organization (such as a business) or individual, and external opportunities and threats are closely examined to chart a strategy.

Sympathetic nervous system A branch of the autonomic nervous system responsible for mobilizing the body's energy and resources during times of stress and arousal (i.e., the fight or flight response). Opposes the physiological effects of the parasympathetic nervous system (e.g., reduces digestive secretions, speeds the heart, contracts blood vessels)

Syncope A transient state of unconsciousness during which a person collapses to the floor as a result of lack of oxygen to the brain; commonly known as fainting.

Syndrome A collection of symptoms and signs indicating a particular disease or condition.

Synergistic dominance A condition in which the synergists carry out the primary function of a weakened or inhibited prime mover.

Systolic blood pressure (SBP) The pressure exerted by the blood on the vessel walls during ventricular contraction.

Tachycardia Elevated heart rate over 100 beats per minute.

Tai chi A Chinese system of slow meditative physical exercise designed for relaxation, balance, and health.

Tai chi chih A series of 19 movements and

1 pose that together make up a meditative form of exercise to which practitioners attribute physical and spiritual health benefits; a specific form of tai chi.

Talk test A method for measuring exercise intensity using observation of respiration effort and the ability to talk while exercising.

Target heart rate (THR) Number of heartbeats per minute that indicate appropriate exercise intensity levels for each individual; also called training heart rate.

Target heart-rate range (THRR) Exercise intensity that represents the minimum and maximum intensity for safe and effective exercise; also referred to as training zone.

Telemetry The process by which measured quantities from a remote site are transmitted to a data collection point for recording and processing, such as what occurs during an electrocardiogram.

Temporomandibular joint syndrome (TMJ) A misalignment of the joint connecting the upper and lower jaw, resulting in chronic muscle and joint pain in the jaw area.

Tendinitis Inflammation of a tendon.

Tendon A band of fibrous tissue forming the termination of a muscle and attaching the muscle to a bone.

Testosterone In males, the steroid hormone produced in the testes; involved in growth and development of reproductive tissues, sperm, and secondary male sex characteristics.

Thermoregulation Regulation of the body's temperature.

Thrombocytopenia Abnormal decrease in blood platelet number, which can result in spontaneous bruising and prolonged bleeding after injury.

Thrombotic Pertaining to thrombosis, which is blood clotting within blood vessels.

Tidal volume The volume of air inspired per breath.

Tinnitus The perception of noise, such as a ringing or beating sound, which has no external source.

Tissue plasminogen activator (tPA) A protein involved in the breakdown of blood clots.

Tonic clonic seizure The classic type of epileptic seizure consisting of two phases: the tonic phase, in which the body becomes rigid, and the clonic phase, in which there is uncontrolled jerking. Also known as a grand mal seizure.

Tonicity The elastic tension of living tissues, such as muscles and arteries.

Torsion The rotation or twisting of a joint by the exertion of a lateral force tending to turn it about a longitudinal axis.

Transient hypertrophy The "pumping" up of muscle that happens during a single exercise bout, resulting mainly from fluid accumulation in the interstitial and intracellular spaces of the muscle.

Transient ischemic attack (TIA) Momentary dizziness, loss of consciousness, or forgetfulness caused by a short-lived lack of oxygen (blood) to the brain; usually due to a partial blockage of an artery, it is a warning sign for a stroke.

Transtheoretical model of behavioral change (TTM) A theory of behavior that examines one's readiness to change and identifies five stages: precontemplation, contemplation, preparation, action, and maintenance. Also called stages-of-change model.

Transverse plane Anatomical term for the imaginary line that divides the body, or any of its parts, into upper (superior) and lower (inferior) parts. Also called the horizontal plane.

Trendelenburg gait A drop of the pelvis on the side opposite of the stance leg, indicating weakness of the hip abductors and gluteus medius and minimus on the side of the stance leg.

Triglyceride Three fatty acids joined to a glycerol (carbon and hydrogen structure) backbone; how fat is stored in the body.

Type 1 diabetes Form of diabetes caused by the destruction of the insulin-producing beta cells in the pancreas, which leads to little or no insulin secretion; generally develops in childhood and requires regular insulin injections; formerly known as insulin-dependent diabetes mellitus (IDDM) and childhood-onset diabetes.

Type 2 diabetes Most common form of diabetes; typically develops in adulthood and is characterized by a reduced sensitivity of the insulin target cells to available insulin; usually associated with obesity; formerly known as non-insulin-dependent diabetes mellitus (NIDDM) and adult-onset diabetes.

Type I muscle fibers *See* Slow-twitch muscle fibers.

Type II muscle fibers *See* Fast-twitch muscle fibers.

Umbrella liability policy Insurance that provides additional coverage beyond other insurance such as professional liability, home, automobile, etc.

Undulating periodization A form of periodization used in resistance training that provides different training protocols during the microcycles in addition to changing the training variables after each microcycle.

Valgus Characterized by an abnormal outward turning of a bone, especially of the hip, knee, or foot.

Valsalva maneuver A strong exhaling effort against a closed glottis, which builds pressure in the chest cavity that interferes with the return of the blood to the heart; may deprive the brain of blood and cause lightheadedness or fainting.

Vascular disease Any disease of the blood vessels.

Vasoconstriction Narrowing of the opening of blood vessels (notably the smaller arterioles) caused by contraction of the smooth muscle lining the vessels.

Vasodilation Increase in diameter of the blood vessels, especially dilation of arterioles leading to increased blood flow to a part of the body.

Ventilatory threshold Point of transition between predominately aerobic energy production to anaerobic energy production; involves recruitment of fast-twitch muscle fibers and identified via gas exchange during exercise testing.

Ventricular fibrillation (VF) An irregular heartbeat characterized by uncoordinated contractions of the ventricle.

Vestibular system Part of the central nervous system that coordinates reflexes of the eyes, neck, and body to maintain equilibrium in accordance with posture and movement of the head.

Vicarious liability States that employers are responsible for the workplace conduct of their employees.

Viscera The collective internal organs of the abdominal cavity.

Visceral Pertaining to the internal organs.

Visual system The series of structures by which visual sensations are received from the environment and conveyed as signals to the central nervous system.

Vital capacity The volume of air that can be maximally inhaled and exhaled in one breath.

Vitamin An organic micronutrient that is essential for normal physiologic function.

$\dot{V}O_2$max Considered the best indicator of cardiovascular endurance, it is the maximum amount of oxygen (mL) that a person can use in one minute per kilogram of body weight. Also called maximal oxygen uptake and maximal aerobic capacity.

$\dot{V}O_2$reserve ($\dot{V}O_2$R) The difference between $\dot{V}O_2$max and $\dot{V}O_2$ at rest; used for programming aerobic exercise intensity.

Waist-to-hip ratio (WHR) A useful measure for determining health risk due to the site of fat storage. Calculated by dividing the ratio of abdominal girth (waist measurement) by the hip measurement.

Waiver Voluntary abandonment of a right to file suit; not always legally binding.

Wet bulb globe temperature A composite temperature used to estimate the effect of temperature, humidity, and solar radiation on humans.

Whey The liquid remaining after milk has been curdled and strained; high in protein and carbohydrates.

Yoga Indian word for "union." A combination of breathing exercises, physical postures, and meditation that has been practiced for more than 5,000 years.

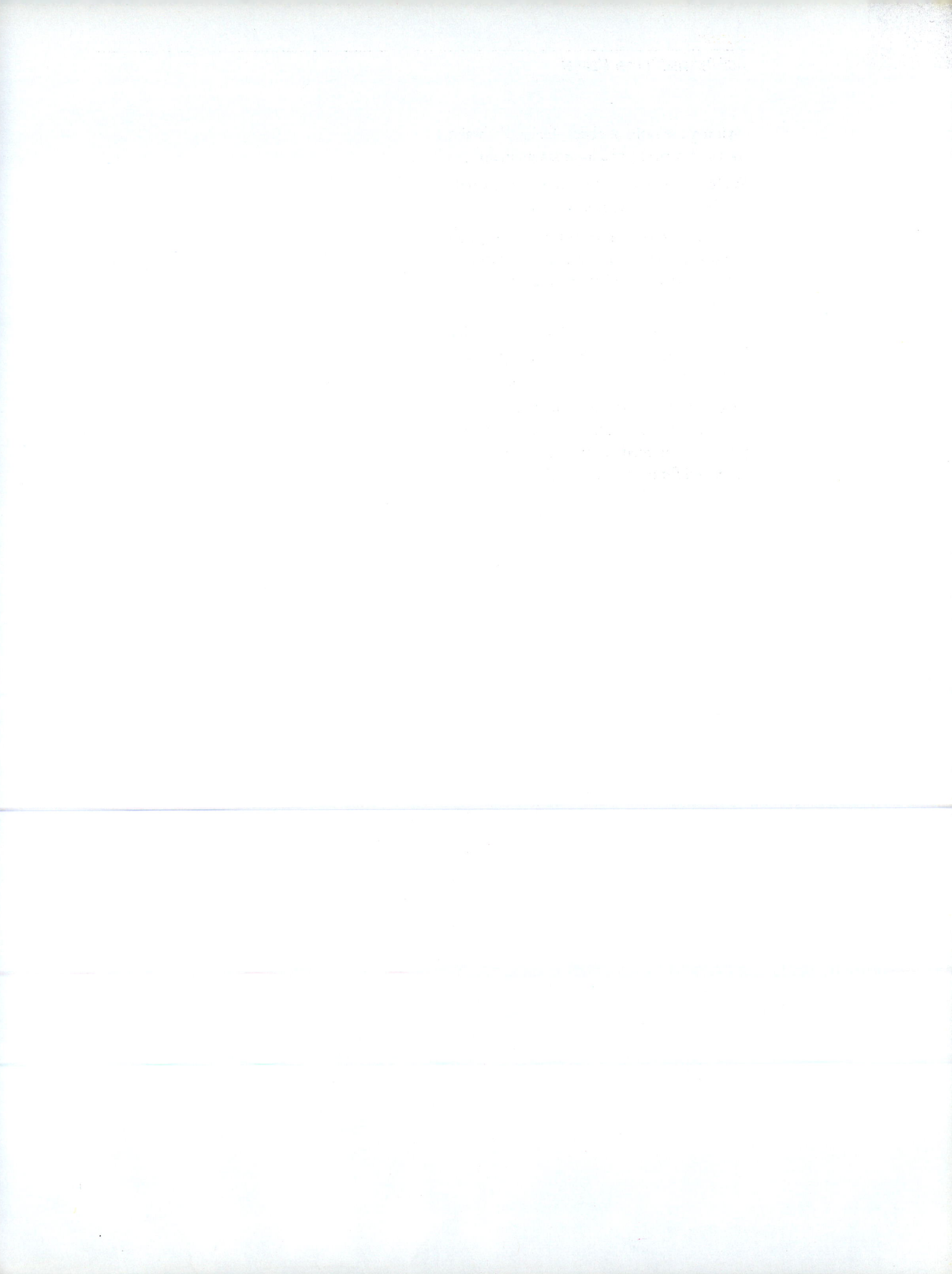

INDEX

A

ABC drills, 351t
  butt kicks, 351t, 352f
  high knees, 351t, 352f
  high marches, 351t, 352f

ABCs, 562

Abdominal circumference measurement, 187f, 187t

Abdominal skinfold measurement, 178, 179f

Abdominal strength assessments. *See also* specific tests
  contraindications to, 215
  curl-up test, 215, 215f, 216t

Abdominal thrusts, 568

Abrasion, 578

Absolute strength, 221

Access to exercise facilities, 28

Acclimatization, heat, 576

Accountant, 643

Accreditation, 15–17. *See also* Certification

ACE certification, 7–15, 604. *See also* Certification, ACE Personal Trainer

ACE Code of Ethics, 11, 659–665

ACE Educational Partnership Program, 16–17

ACE Integrated Fitness Training Model, 81–446. *See also specific topics*
  cardiorespiratory training, 369–407
  case studies, 411–446
  definition and overview, 85
  exercise program design, 81–82
  foundation, 84
  functional assessments, 84, 135–169
  functional programming for stability-mobility and movement, 245–307
  health—fitness—performance continuum, 83–84, 83f
  health-history information, 84
  initial investigational phase in, 99–132
  physiological assessments, 84, 173–240
  physiological parameters, traditional vs. new, 82, 82t
  positive experience, 86–87
  rapport in, 84
    behavioral strategies and, 86–87
    building of, 99–132
  rationale, 82–83
  resistance training, 311–364
  sequential approach, 84, 85f
  special population clientele, 95 *(See also specific populations)*
  training components and phases, 85–95, 86t
    cardiorespiratory, 92–95
    functional movement and resistance, 88–92
    overview, 87–88

ACE logo, 620

ACE name, 620

ACE Personal Trainer Certification Exam handbook, 11

ACE Personal Trainer Exam Content Outline, 10, 666–684

ACE Position Statement on Nutritional Supplements, 687

ACE professional practices and disciplinary procedures, 11–12

Achievements, major, 631

Achilles tendinitis, 551–552, 552f

ACSM's Health/Fitness Facility Standards and Guidelines, 16

Action
  cues to, 65
  in transtheoretical model of behavioral change, 68, 69t, 71

Action phase, 641

Action stage, of client–trainer relationship, 51–56, 100, 100f
  behavior contracts in, 55–56, 74
  definition of, 51–52
  effective modeling in, 54–55
  feedback in, 54
  individualized teaching in, 52, 53t
  self-monitoring systems in, 52
  "tell, show, do" in, 53–54

Active isolated stretching (AIS), 253, 253f

Activities of daily living (ADL)
  aerobic-base training for, 93
  primary movements in, 146, 150
  static balance in, 281

Activity history, 27–28

Acts of God, 611

Acute coronary syndromes, 470

Adduction, in right hip, 286, 287f

Adherence, 25–59. *See also* Motivation
- building of, trainer role in, 32–33
- definition of, 26
- empathy and rapport on, 57
- factors in, 27–29
  - categories, 27
  - environmental, 28
  - overview, 26–27
  - personal attributes, 27–28
  - physical-activity, 29
- feedback in, 31
- goal setting for, 33, 48, 50t
- leadership qualities in, 31–32

Adherence program, 638

Adoption, exercise, 26. *See also* Adherence; Motivation

Adrenocorticotropin hormone (ACTH), 453, 453f

Advanced Health & Fitness Specialist (AHFS) Certification, 19

Aerobic-base training, 92–93, 391–396
- overview of, 394t
- program design for, 395–396, 396t
- sample of, 396, 396t
- training focus of, 391, 393–395, 394t

Aerobic capacity, time for increases in, 371–372, 371f

Aerobic efficiency training, 93–94
- overview of, 394t
- program design for, 397–398
- sample of, 398, 399t
- training focus of, 396–397

Aerobic fitness. *See* $\dot{V}O_2$max

Aerobic interval training, 373

Age. *See also* Elderly
- on muscular strength and hypertrophy, 316
- on participation and adherence, 27

Agility, 174, 342

Agility drills
- cone/marker, 353t
- ladder/hurdle, 352t, 353f
- pro agility drill, 353t
- tips for, 350

Agility training, 346, 350

Agreement and release of liability waiver, 110, 602, 603f, 604–605, 610

Agreements
- to participate, 606, 607f
- written, 33, 74

Air displacement plethysmography, 177t

Airway management, emergency, 560, 560f

Alaskan spiritual dancing, 468–469

Alexander Technique, 467–468

Alignment, proper postural, 136. *See also* Posture

Allergens, asthma from, 568

Allied healthcare continuum, 5–7, 6f
- athletic trainers, 6
- nurses and physician's assistants, 5
- personal trainers, 6–7, 6f
- physical and occupational therapists, 5
- physicians, 5
- registered dietitians, 6

Alternating push-off, 347t

Alveoli, cardiorespiratory training on, 370

Ambulatory exercise, 387

Amino-acid supplements, 358

Amortization phase, 343

Anabolic-androgenic steroids (AAS), 359–360

Anaerobic capacity, 174, 316

Anaerobic capacity tests
- 300-yard shuttle run, 235–236, 236t
- Margaria–Kalamen stair climb test, 234–235, 234f, 234t

Anaerobic-endurance training, 94–95
- overview of, 394t
- program design for, 400–402, 402f
- sample of, 402, 403t
- training focus of, 398–400, 401f

Anaerobic power, 174, 231

Anaerobic-power tests
- kneeling overhead toss, 233–234, 233f
- standing long jump test, 231–232, 232t
- vertical jump test, 232–233, 232f, 233t

Anaerobic-power training, 95
- overview of, 394t
- program design for, 404
- training focus of, 403–404

Anaerobic threshold, 384. *See also* Lactate threshold (LT)

Androstenedione, 360

Aneurysm, 570

Angina, 107

Angina pectoris, 122, 569

Angiotensin-converting enzyme (ACE) inhibitors, 119, 120t

Angiotensin-II receptor antagonists, 119, 120t

Ankle edema, 107

Ankle mobilization, standing, 281, 282f

Ankle pronation
- on kinematic chain, 285–286, 285f
- on kinetic chain, 140, 141f, 141t
- in postural assessment, 139–140, 140f, 141f, 141t

Ankle splinting, 581, 581f

Ankle sprains, 549–551
- epidemiology of, 549
- exercise programming for, 550–551, 551f
- management of, 539t, 550
- signs and symptoms of, 535t, 550
- types of, 549–550, 550f

Ankle supination
- on kinematic chain, 285, 285f
- on kinetic chain, 140, 141f, 141t
- in postural assessment, 139–140, 140f, 141f, 141t

Antecedents, 72

Anterior capsule (pectoralis) stretch, 273, 273f

Anterior cruciate ligament (ACL) injuries, 534–535, 534f

Anterior cruciate ligament (ACL) rotation, 285, 285f

Anterior shin splints, 548–549, 549f

Anterior superior iliac spine (ASIS), in pelvic tilt, 143, 143f

Anthropometric measurements and body composition, 174–189. *See also* specific measurements
- air displacement plethysmography, 177t
- appropriate use/clientele, 176
- bioelectrical impedance analysis, 177t
- body composition evaluation, 183–184, 184t
- body size measurement, 185–189
  - body mass index, 185–186, 185t, 186t
  - circumference sites and procedures, 187t
  - girth measurements, 186–187, 187f, 187t
  - waist circumference, 187f, 187t, 188–189, 188t
  - waist-to-hip ratio, 188, 188t
- contraindications, 176
- correlations, 175
- dual energy x-ray absorptiometry, 177t
- goal weight calculation, 184
- hydrostatic weighing, 176–178, 177t
- lean and fat tissue measurement, 176
- magnetic resonance imaging, 177t
- near-infrared interactance, 177t
- overview, 175–176, 175t
- programming considerations, 184
- skinfold measurements, 175, 177t, 178–182
- total body electrical conductivity, 177t

Anthropometry, 174

Antihistamines, 120t, 121

Antihypertensives, 119, 120t

Anusara yoga, 462

Apley's scratch test for shoulder mobility, 162, 165–166, 165f, 166f, 166t

Apneic client, 568

Appreciation, 32

Arachnoid mater, 582

Archimedes principles, 176–178

Arm abduction, rotator cuff muscles in, 272, 272f

Arm circumference measurement, 187t

Arm lifts, prone, 278f

Arm roll, 280f

Arm squeeze and forward drive, 351f, 351t

Arm squeeze and full cycles, 351t

Arm squeeze and rear drive, 351f, 351t

Arthritis
- classification of, 503t
- exercise and, 503
- exercise guidelines for, 504, 504t
- overview of, 502–503
- sample exercise recommendation for, 504–505

Arthrokinematics, 246, 247f

Articulation, 102

Ashtanga yoga, 462

ASIS-PSIS angle, 143

Assertiveness, for relapse prevention, 34

Assessments. *See also* specific assessments
- abdominal strength
  - contraindications to, 215
  - curl-up test, 215, 215f, 216t
- balance and core, 166–169 (*See also* Balance and core assessment)
- body composition
  - body fat in, 175–176
  - contraindications to, 176

hydrostatic weighing in, 176–178, 177t
lean and fat tissue measurement in, 176
measurement techniques for, 175, 175t
choice of, 123–124
essential, conducting, 125–129
blood pressure, 126–129, 127f, 128t
heart rate, 125–126
functional, 135–169 (*See also* Functional assessments)
goals of, 123
health-related physiological, 174
needs, in resistance training, 318
physiological, 173–240 (*See also* Physiological assessments)
sequencing of, 121–123
shoulder mobility, 162–166 (*See also* Shoulder mobility assessments)
sport-skill, 230–239 (*See also* Sport-skill assessments)
static postural, 136–146 (*See also* Static postural assessment)
tools for, 124–125, 124t

Assisted exercises, 319

Associative stage of learning, 58

Asthma, 568–569
dyspnea in, 567–568
exercise and, 496–497
exercise guidelines for, 497
exercise-induced, 569
overview of, 496
sample exercise recommendation for, 496

Asthma medications, 121

Astrand-Ryhming (A-R) cycle ergometer test, 200–201, 201f, 201t

Astrand-Ryhming (A-R) nomogram, 201, 201f

Atherosclerosis, 116, 481, 569

Atherosclerotic heart disease. *See* Coronary artery disease (CAD)

Athletic shoes, 544

Athletic trainers, 6

Atrophy, disuse, 117, 312

Attitude
on behavior change, 72
on participation and adherence, 28
trainer modeling of, 55

Attitude questionnaire, 110, 113f–114f

Attorney, 642–643

Automated external defibrillator (AED)
emergency use of, 560, 566–567
legal responsibilities for, 612–613

Autonomous stage of learning, 58

Avulsion, 578

B

Back alignment, pelvic tilts and, 289f

Back injuries, 583–584, 583f, 584f

Back, low, hyperextension of, 584

Back pain
chronic, 510
low-back, 509–513, 584
exercise and, 510
exercise guidelines for, 510–512, 512f
lifting and, 584
from musculoskeletal injuries, 542–543
overview of, 509–510
sample exercise recommendation for, 513
transverse abdominis with, 256

Backpedal, 352t

Balance
in SMART goal setting, 49t
training for
static balance in, 282–284, 283t, 284f

Balance and core assessment, 166–169
blood pressure cuff test, 167–168, 168f
sharpened Romberg test, 166–167, 167f
stork-stand balance test, 167–168, 167f
worksheet for, 166, 167t

Balance, static
integrated (standing), 283–284, 284f
segmental, 281–283, 282f, 283t
training in, 282–284, 283t, 284f

Balke & Ware treadmill exercise test, 194–195, 195t

Ballistic stretches, 253, 253f

Barriers, perceived, 65, 76

Base of support (BOS), 256
controlling center of mass within, for balance training, 256
static, dynamic movement patterns over, 293–295, 293t, 294f
wide, 281, 282f

Behavioral interventions, 76

Behavioral theory models, 64–72
health belief model, 64–66
self-efficacy, 66–67
transtheoretical model of behavioral change, 26, 67–72, 103 (*See also*

Transtheoretical model of behavioral change)
understanding health behavior and, 64

Behavior change, 63–76
behavioral theory models of, 64–72 (*See also* Behavioral theory models)
cognitions and behavior in, 73
cognitive behavioral techniques in, 74–75
history of, 64
implementing strategies of, 75–76
interventions for, 76
observational learning in, 73
operant conditioning in, 72–73
personal trainer role in, 64
rapport and, 86–87
shaping in, 73
stimulus control in, 74
strategies for, 73–75
transtheoretical model of, 26, 67–72, 103 (*See also* Transtheoretical model of behavioral change)
written agreements and behavioral contracting in, 74

Behavior-change contracts, 55–56, 74

Behavior, cognitions and, 73

Behavior contracts, 33, 55–56, 74

Beliefs
on behavior change, 72
on participation and adherence, 28

Bench-press test, 1-RM, 222–225, 223f, 223t–225t. *See also* 1-RM bench-press test

Bend-and-lift movements, 89, 286, 330

Bend-and-lift patterns, 287–291
exercises for, 288
hip hinge, 287, 288f
lower-extremity alignment, 289f–290f
pelvic tilts and back alignment, 289f
squat variations, 291f
gluteals in, 286
quadriceps in, 286
in squat, 286, 287–288

Bend and lift screen, 151, 152t

Benefits, exercise
communication of, 635–638
duration and, 385–386
on health, 26
perceived, 65
of regular exercise, 82

Bent-knee marches
reverse, modified dead bug with, 262f–263f
supine, 262f

β-alanine, 358–359

Biarticulate muscle, 259

Biarticulate muscle stretching, 259

Bicycling, $\dot{V}O_2$ and energy cost of, 199, 199f

Bike test, YMCA, 197–199, 198f, 199f

Bikram yoga, 462

Bilateral presses, 299, 300f

Bilateral pull-downs, 303–304, 303f

Bioelectrical impedance analysis, 177t

Biomedical status, 27

Biopsychosocial approach, 64

Birddog, 512f

Blisters, 578

Blog, fitness, 637

Bloodborne pathogen protection, 585

Blood pressure
application of, 128–129
classification of, 128t
conducting assessment of, 126–129, 127f
in exercise, 128
exercise testing on, 122
in graded exercise tests, 191
high (*See* Hypertension)
on physical activity, 116
in SMART goal setting, 49t
strength training on, 362–363

Blood pressure cuff test, 167–168, 168f

Blood sugar, in SMART goal setting, 49t

Bodybuilding. *See* Muscle hypertrophy

Body composition, 174. *See also* Anthropometric measurements and body composition; specific measurements
aging on, 313
definition of, 175
evaluation of, 183–184, 184t
goal weight calculation in, 184
power training on, 92
programming with, 184
resistance training on, 312
skinfold measurements of, 177t, 178–182 (*See also* Skinfold measurements)
in SMART goal setting, 49t

Body composition assessment
body fat, 175–176
contraindications, 176
hydrostatic weighing, 176–178, 177t

lean and fat tissue measurement, 176
measurement techniques, 175, 175t

Body fat. *See* Fat, body

Body mass. *See also* Body size
lean, 175, 513
in SMART goal setting, 49t

Body mass index (BMI)
calculation of, 513
chart for, 185t
equations for, 185
health risks and, 186, 186t
predicted body-fat percentage from, 186, 186t
reference chart on, 186t
value of, 185–186, 185t, 186t

Body position, 42, 101

Body size. *See also* Body mass index (BMI); Weight, body
measurement of, 185–189
body mass index, 185–186, 185t, 186t
circumference sites and procedures, 187t
girth measurements, 186–187, 187f, 187t
waist circumference, 188–189, 188t
waist-to-hip ratio, 188, 188t
in SMART goal setting, 49t

Bodyweight squat test, 220–221, 221f, 221t

Bodyweight training, 357

Bone fractures, 536–537, 536f

Bone mineral density (BMD), resistance training on, 312, 313

Borg scale, 129, 129t

Boundaries, professional, 57–58

Bracing, teaching, 283

Branched-chain amino acids (BCAAs), 358

Brand, creation of, 634–635

Breathing
with warm-up and cool-down exercises, 471
yogic (pranayama), 463

Breathwork exercise, 472

Broker, insurance, 643

Bronchodilators, 121

Bronchospasm, exercise-induced, 569

Bruce protocol, for treadmill exercise testing, 192–193

Bruce submaximal treadmill exercise test
equipment in, 193
pre-test procedure for, 193
protocol and administration of, 193–194, 193t
use of, 192–193

Bruises, 578

Bursitis, 535

Bursitis, greater trochanteric, 539t, 543–544

Business concept, 631

Business description, 631–632

Business fundamentals, 625–653
accountant in, 643
attorney in, 642–643
business planning in, 630–633 (*See also* Business planning)
business structure choice in, 642
communicating benefits in, 635–638
contractors in, 643
creating a brand in, 634–635
direct-employee model in, 626–629
financial plan in, 643–646, 644f, 645f
honesty and integrity in, 626
independent-contractor model in, 600–602, 629–630
insurance broker in, 643
marketing in
for client retention, 640–641
general communication in, 641–642
professional services for starting a business in, 642–643
selling personal training in, 648–653 (*See also* Selling personal training)
service businesses in, 626
small-group training in, 638–640
starting a career in, 630
time management in, 646–648
web developer/graphic designer in, 643

Business loans, 621

Business planning, 630–633
business description in, 631–632
decision-making criteria in, 633
executive summary in, 631
financial self-assessment in, 630–631
marketing plan in, 632
operational plan in, 632
risk analysis in, 632–633, 633f
value of, 631

Business position, current, 631

Business structure, 593–600
advantages and disadvantages of, 599, 599t
choice of, 642
corporations, 597–599
franchise operations, 599–600
partnerships, 595–596
selection of, 594

sole proprietorships, 594–595, 599t
Butt kicks, 351t, 352f
Buttocks circumference measurement, 187t

C

Cables, 356–357
Caffeine, as supplement, 359
Calcium channel blockers, 119, 120t, 359
Calf circumference measurement, 187t
Calf stretches
modifications of, 552, 552f
standing, 552, 552f
Caliper, skinfold, 178
Caloric expenditure, in cardiorespiratory training, 380–382, 381t
Cancer
exercise and, 498–499
exercise guidelines for, 499–500
overview of, 498
precautions with, 500
sample exercise recommendation for, 500
Capillaries, cardiorespiratory exercise on, 370
Capsule stretches
posterior, 273, 273f
superior, 273, 273f
Carbohydrates, for hypoglycemia in diabetics, 572
Cardiac arrest
CPR for, 565–566
overview of, 565
Cardiac output, cardiorespiratory exercise on, 370
Cardiogenic shock, 585
Cardiopulmonary resuscitation (CPR), 561, 565–566
"cough," 570
legal responsibilities for, 612
Cardiorespiratory fitness (CRF), 174, 212
Cardiorespiratory fitness (CRF) testing, 189–212
cycle ergometer, 196–201 (*See also* Cycle ergometer testing)
definition of, 189
factors in, 189
field, 205–208 (*See also* Field testing, cardiorespiratory fitness)
lab or fitness center, 190–192
graded exercise tests (GXT), 190–192, 191t
treadmill exercise testing, 192–196 (*See also* Treadmill exercise testing)
maximum heart rate in, prediction equation for, 190
step, 208–212 (*See also* Step tests)
submaximal assessments, 189–190
treadmill exercise, 192–196 (*See also* Treadmill exercise testing)
use of, 189
ventilatory threshold, 202–205 (*See also* Ventilatory threshold testing)
$\dot{V}O_2$max in, 189
Cardiorespiratory training, 92–95, 369–407
in ACE IFT Model, phases of, 390–404
concept of program design, 390–391
overview, 391
phase 1: aerobic-base training, 391–396
overview, 394t
program design, 395–396, 396t
sample, 396, 396t
training focus of, 391, 393–395, 394t
phase 2: aerobic-efficiency training
overview, 394t
program design, 397–398
sample, 398, 399t
training focus, 396–397
phase 3: anaerobic-endurance training
overview, 394t
program design, 400–402, 402f
sample, 402, 403t
training focus, 398–400, 401f
phase 4: anaerobic-power training
overview, 394t
program design, 404
training focus, 403–404
three-zone training model, 385f, 391, 392t–393t
in elderly, 406–407
exercise components for, 83t
for health, fitness, and weight loss, 374–387
2008 Physical Activity Guidelines for Americans, 374
cardiovascular programming, 374–375
duration, 385–386, 386t
exercise progression, 386–387
frequency, 375, 375t
intensity, 375–385
blood lactate and VT2, 383–385, 383f–385f
caloric expenditure, 380–382, 381t
first ventilatory threshold, 380
heart rate, 375–379, 376f, 377f, 377t [*See also* Maximum heart rate (MHR)]
importance, 385
ratings of perceived exertion, 378–379

[*See also* Ratings of perceived exertion (RPE)]
talk test, 382–383
$\dot{V}O_2$ or metabolic equivalents, 378–382, 381t
length, 374
overview, 92
phase 1: aerobic-base training, 92–93
phase 2: aerobic-efficiency training, 93–94
phase 3: anaerobic-endurance training, 94–95
phase 4: anaerobic-power training, 95
physiological adaptations to exercise
cardiovascular system, 370
muscular system, 370
respiratory system, 370–371
with steady-state and interval-based exercise, 372
time for increases in aerobic capacity, 371–372, 371f
workout session
conditioning phase, 373
cool-down, 374
overview, 372
warm-up, 372–373
zones, 94
modes or types of, 387–390
ambulatory, 387
circuit training, 389
equipment-based, 388
group exercise, 388–389
lifestyle exercise, 390
mind-body exercise, 390
outdoor exercise, 389
overview, 387–388
physical activities, 387–388, 388t
seasonal exercise, 389
water-based exercise, 390
recovery and regeneration in, 404–405
in youth, 405–406

Cardiovascular disease (CVD), 481–483, 569–570
assessment of risk for, 615
exercise and coronary artery disease in, 481–482
exercise guidelines for, 482–483
risk stratification for, 107, 108t, 615
sample recommendation for, 483
types and importance of, 481

Cardiovascular disorders. *See also specific disorders*
exercise and, 481–483
on physical activity, 116

Cardiovascular drift, 373

Cardiovascular programming, 374–375

Cardiovascular risk, graded exercise test of, 191

Cardiovascular system, cardiorespiratory training on, 370

Career development, 17–19, 630

Caring, 32

Carioca, 551, 551f

Carnosine, 358

Carotid artery, 125

Carpal tunnel syndrome, 539t, 541–542, 542f

Cartilage damage, 534f, 536

Casein, 358

Case studies, of ACE IFT Model, 411–446
David (57-year-old executive, fit and active), 418–424
cardiorespiratory training
aerobic-efficiency, 421–422, 422t
anaerobic-endurance, 423–424, 425t
conclusion, 424
functional movement and resistance training, 423, 423t
goals, 418–419
history and health-risk appraisal, 418–419, 419t
trainer's assessment notes, 420t
Jan (17-year-old female athlete), 425–432
conclusion, 432
functional movement and resistance training
load, 429–431, 430t
movement, 428–429, 429t
performance, 431, 431t
goals, 426
history and health-risk appraisal, 424–426
trainer's assessment notes, 426–428, 427t–428t
Kelly (30-year-old, wedding preparation), 443–446
conclusion, 446
functional movement and resistance training
load, 445–446, 446t
movement, 444–445, 445t
trainer's assessment notes, 444, 444t
Meredith (64-year-old, active), 437–443
cardiorespiratory training
aerobic-efficiency, 440
aerobic-efficiency (progression), 442–443
anaerobic-endurance (progression), 440–441
performance, 441–442, 442t

conclusion, 443
functional movement and resistance training
load, 440
movement, 439, 439t
history and health-risk appraisal, 437–438, 437t
trainer's assessment notes, 438, 438t
Sharon (33-year-old female, fit pre-pregnancy), 412–418
cardiorespiratory training
aerobic-base, 414, 414t
aerobic-efficiency, 416, 417t
aerobic-efficiency (progression), 417–418, 418t
conclusion, 418
functional movement and resistance training
load, 416–417, 417t
movement, 415–416, 416t
goals and goal-setting, 412–413
health history and health-risk appraisal, 412, 412t
motivation, 412–413
trainer's assessment notes, 413, 414t
Stanley (28-year-old male, sedentary), 432–437
cardiorespiratory training
aerobic-base, 434–435
aerobic-base (progression), 435–436
conclusion, 437
functional movement and resistance training, 435–436, 436t
history and health-risk appraisal, 432–433, 432t

Case study, of health belief model, 65–66

Cat-camel, 261f, 512f

Catecholamines, beta blockers on, 119

C-corporations, 598–599, 599t

Center of gravity (COG)
definition of, 281
location of, 281, 282f
movement on, 281
in movement training, 89–90

Center of mass (COM), 251, 256
definition of, 281
movement on, 281

Certification. *See also* Accreditation
additional fitness, 19
continuing education for, 12
period of, 12
renewal of, 12

Certification, ACE Personal Trainer, 7–15, 604
education and experience in, 10
handbook on, 11
minimum competency in, 7
preparation and testing in, 10–11
professional responsibilities and ethics in, 11–15, 15t (*See also* Responsibilities and ethics)
ACE Code of Ethics, 11, 659–665
ACE professional practices and disciplinary procedures, 11–12
appropriate scope of practice, 15, 15t
certification period and renewal, 12
client privacy, 12–13
offering services outside scope of practice, 14–15
referral, 13
safety, 14
supplements, 14
purpose of, 7, 10
scope of practice, 7–10, 8t
updating of, 10

Cervical spine, clearing test for, 150

Cervical sprain, 583

Cervical strain, 583

Chair forward bend, 459f

Change
behavior (*See* Behavior change)
facilitating, 103–104, 104f

Chang style tai chi, 466

Chen style tai chi, original, 466

Chest pain, 569–570

Chest pass, horizontal, 348t, 349f

Chest skinfold measurements, 178, 179f

Chest toss, supine vertical, 348t, 349f

ChiRunning, 471

Choking, 568

Cholesterol. *See also* Dyslipidemia
classification of, 489, 489t
in coronary artery disease, 481
levels of, in SMART goal setting, 49t

Chondromalacia, 536

Chronic disease management, mind-body exercise for, 470

Chronic fatigue syndrome (CFS)
diagnosis of, 507, 508t
exercise and, 508
exercise guidelines for, 508–509
management of, 508

overview of, 507
sample exercise recommendation for, 509

Chronic obstructive pulmonary disease (COPD), 117

Circuit strength training, 334–335

Circuit training, 389

Circumference, 187t. *See also specific sites*

Clarifying, 103

Clarity, role, 33

Claudication
from exercise testing, 122
intermittent, 107

Clearing tests, 150, 150f

Client privacy, 12–13

Clients
developing, 636
difficult, communication with, 57
diverse population of, 5
marketing for retention of, 640–641

Client–trainer relationship
learning stages and, 58
legal aspects of, 616 (*See also* Legal responsibilities)
positive experiences in, 41, 41t
rapport in (*See* Rapport)
stages of, 39–56, 100, 100f *(See also specific stages)*
action, 51–56
investigation, 45–47
overview, 39, 39f
planning, 47–51
rapport, 40–45
trust in, 32

Closed kinetic chain (CKC) movements, 274

Closed kinetic chain (CKC) weight shifts, 279f

Closing ratio, 645

Coach, trainer as, 31–32

Code of Ethics, ACE, 11, 659–665

Cognitions, behavior and, 73

Cognitive behavioral techniques, 74–75

Cognitive stage of learning, 58

Cold illness, 576–577

Cold medications, 120t, 121

Cold pack, 579

Collaborators, 43f, 43t, 45t

Collagen
in tendons and ligaments, 579
in wound healing, 537

Commission on Accreditation of Allied Health Education Programs (CAAHEP), 17

Communication
for behavior change, 76–77
of benefits, 635–638
effective, 56–58
on adherence, 57
for behavior change, 76–77
cultural competence in, 56–57
in daily teaching interactions, 58–59
with difficult clients, 57
in investigation stage, 101
professional boundaries in, 57–58
effective listening in, 46–47
for marketing, 641–642
nonverbal, 42
verbal, 41

Communication and teaching techniques, 39–59
client–trainer relationship stages in, 39–56 (*See also* Client–trainer relationship, stages of)
effective communication in, 56–58
learning stages and client–trainer relationship in, 58

Comparative negligence, 605

Competency, minimum, 7

Complimentary session, 636

Composition, body. *See* Body composition

Compression, for musculoskeletal injuries, 538

Concentric actions, of muscle, 311

Concept, business, 631

Concussion, 581

Conditioning, operant, 72–73

Conditioning phase, 373

Cone/marker drills, 353t

Confidentiality, incident, 562

Confronting, 103

Consent, informed, 110, 606, 608, 608f–609f

Consequences, 72–73

Contemplation, 68, 69t, 71

Continuing education, 12, 17–18

Contractors, 643
independent, 600–602, 629–630

Contracts
behavioral, 33, 55–56, 74

behavior-change, 55–56
legal, 602–604, 603f

Contraindications, to exercise, 14

Contributory negligence, 605

Contusion, 578

Conversation, in motivational interviewing, 51

Cool-down, 374

Cooling, for heat illness, 575

Coordination, 174

Core
activation and conditioning of, 254–257, 255f–257f
deep (innermost) layer of, 254, 255f
definition of, 254
middle layer of, 254–255, 255f
outermost layer of, 255
in proximal stability exercises, 254–255, 255f
spine and, 255, 255f
transverse abdominis in, 255–256, 255f, 256f

Core function, 257–258, 257f, 257t, 258f
exercise progression for activation, 257, 257t
exercise progression for stabilization, 258, 259f
quadruped drawing-in (centering) with extremity movement, 257–258, 258f, 259t
supine drawing-in (centering), 257, 257f

Coronary artery disease (CAD), 569
exercise and, 481–482
on physical activity, 116
risk factors for, 107, 108t

Corporate veil, 594

Corporations, 597–599
C-corporations, 598–599, 599t
formation and maintenance of, 597
limited liability, 598, 599t
purpose and regulation of, 597
subchapter S-corporation, 597–598, 599t

Correspondence, 554

Corticotropin releasing hormone (CRH), 453, 453f

"Cough" CPR, 570

Counseling style, 103

Cramps, heat, 573

Creatine, 359

Credential, ACE, value of, 11

Crepitus, 580

Cross-training, 117, 387

Cues to action, 65

Cultural competence, in effective communication, 56–57

Curl-up, modified, 512f

Curl-up test, 215, 215f, 216t

Current business position, 631

Curved drills, cone/marker, 353t

Cutting drills, cone/marker, 353t

Cyanosis, 568

Cycle ergometer testing, 196–201
advantages of, 196–197
Astrand-Ryhming (A-R) cycle ergometer test, 200–201, 201f, 201t
contraindications to, 197
disadvantages of, 197
use of, 196
YMCA bike test, 197–199, 198f, 199f

Cycling, $\dot{V}O_2$ and energy cost of, 199, 199f

D

Dancing, Native American and Alaskan spiritual, 468–469

Dead-lift technique, 288

Decisional balance, in transtheoretical model of behavioral change, 69–70, 70f

Decision-making criteria, 633

Deconditioned individuals, muscle strengthening for, 253f, 254

Defibrillator, automated external
emergency use of, 560, 566–567
legal responsibilities for, 612–613

Deflecting, 103

Degenerative disc disease (DDD), 543

Degrees, 18–19

Dehydration, severe, 574

Dehydroepiandrosterone (DHEA), 360

Delayed-onset muscle soreness (DOMS), 87
in resistance training, 323–324
training intensity on, 322

Deliberators, 43f, 43t, 45t

Demographic variables, 27

Diabetes, 118, 490–494, 571–573, 572f
control of, 491–492
exercise guidelines for, 492
gestational, 491

overview of, 490–491
precautions with, 493, 494t
sample exercise recommendations for, 493
type 1, 491
benefits of exercise with, 492
exercise training with, 492–493
type 2, 491
benefits of exercise with, 492
exercise training with, 493

Diagonal cone jumps, 347t

Diagonals, 276f

Diaphragm, 370

Diastolic blood pressure (DBP), 116, 126
classification of, 128t
Korotkoff sound for, 127, 127f
measurement of, 128

Dietitians, registered, 6

Difficult clients, 57

Diminishing returns, in resistance training, 326

Direct-employee model, 626–629

Directing style, 103

Directors, 43f, 43t, 45t

Disciplinary procedures, 11–12

Disclosures, difficult, 47

Disease prevention, 313–314. *See also specific diseases*

Distance, for communication, 101

Distributive shock, 585

Disuse atrophy, 117, 312

Diuretics, 120t, 121

Dizziness, 107

Dominance scale, 42, 43f, 43t, 44f

Dominance, synergistic, 250

Double-progressive strength-training protocol, 324

Double taxation, 598

Drop-out. *See also* Adherence; Motivation
from exercise programs, 26–27
rate of, in vigorous-intensity exercise programs, 29

Dual energy x-ray absorptiometry, 177t

Duration, exercise
ACSM guidelines on, 385–386, 386t
for cardiorespiratory training, 385–386, 386t
definition of, 385

Dynamic and ballistic stretches, 253, 253f

Dynamic movement patterns, over static base of support, 293–295, 293t, 294f

Dynamic strengthening exercises, for good posture, 254

Dynamic stretches, 253, 253f

Dysarthria, 576

Dysfunctional fitness, 247, 284

Dyslipidemia, 488–490
classification of, 489, 489t
exercise and, 489–490
exercise guidelines for, 490
overview of, 488–489
sample exercise recommendation for, 490

Dyspnea, 107, 567–568

Dyspnea scale, 567

E

Ebbeling single-stage treadmill test, 195–196, 196f

Eccentric actions, of muscle, 311

Ecchymosis, 578

Edema, heat, 573

Educating style, 103

Education
continuing, 12, 17–18
in motivational interviewing, 51

Educational Partnership Program, 16–17

Education programs, 638

Effective communication, 56–58
on adherence, 57
for behavior change, 76–77
cultural competence in, 56–57
in daily teaching interactions, 58–59
in investigation stage, 101
professional boundaries in, 57–58

Effective listening
in communication, 46–47, 102
in motivational interviewing, 51

Effective modeling, 54–55

Ejection fraction, cardiorespiratory exercise on, 370

Elbow tendinitis, 539t, 540–541, 541f

Elderly. *See also* Age
cardiorespiratory training in, 406–407
exercise and
on cardiovascular system, 515–516

on mental health, 516
on musculoskeletal system, 516
overview of, 515
on sensory systems, 516
exercise guidelines for, 516–517
muscular strength and hypertrophy in, 316
participation and adherence in, 27
sample exercise recommendations for, 517

Elevation, for musculoskeletal injuries, 538

Emergencies and injuries, common medical, 567–586
asthma, 568–569
bloodborne pathogen protection, 585
cardiovascular disease, chest pain, and heart attack, 569–570
choking, 568
cold illness, 576–577
diabetes and insulin reaction, 571–573, 572f
dyspnea, 567–568
fractures, 580–581, 581f
head injuries, 581–583
heat illness, 573–576, 574t–576t *(See also specific types)*
HIV infection, 585–586
neck and back injuries, 583–584, 583f, 584f
seizures, 577–578
shock, 585
soft-tissue injuries, 578–580, 579f
stroke, 570–571
syncope, 570
universal precautions, 585

Emergency procedures, 559–586
assessment in, 562–564
primary, 562–563, 563f
secondary, 563–564
EMS activation in
emergency call centers, 564–565
land lines vs. cell phones, 564
when to call 9-1-1, 564, 565
first-aid kit for, 560, 560f
initial response in
automated external defibrillator, 566–567
cardiopulmonary resuscitation, 565–566
medical emergencies and injuries, 567–586 (*See also* Emergencies and injuries, common medical)
personal protective equipment for, 560
policies and procedures for, 561–562
record keeping and confidentiality in, 562
scene safety in, 560

Emotional health indicators, 49t

Emotional state appraisals, 66

Empathy, 100
on adherence, 57
cultural competence for, 56–57
in investigation stage, 102
in motivational interviewing, 51
vs. personal involvement, 57–58

Employees
direct-employee model for, 626–629
vs. independent contractors, 600–602

Empowerment, client, 30

EMS activation
emergency call centers, 564–565
land lines vs. cell phones, 564
when to call 9-1-1, 564, 565

Encouragement, 46

End-diastolic volume, cardiorespiratory exercise on, 370

Environment
in adherence, 28
for exercise testing, 124
in investigation stage, 101

Epicondylitis
lateral, 117, 540–541, 541f
medial, 540–541, 541f

Epileptic seizures, 578

Equipment
legal responsibilities for, 612–613
for resistance training
bodyweight training, 357
cables, 356–357
free weights, 357
medicine balls, 357
selectorized equipment, 356
tubing, 357

Equipment-based training, 388

Ergogenic aids and supplements
anabolic-androgenic steroids and related compounds, 359–360
β-alanine, 358–359
caffeine, 359
carnosine, 358
creatine, 359
protein and amino-acid supplements, 358
sodium bicarbonate, 358–359
vitamins and minerals, 359

Eschars, frostbite, 577

Essential body fat, 175

Ethics, 11–15, 15t. *See also* Responsibilities and ethics, professional; Scope of practice

Evaluation forms, 110–115

agreement and release of liability waiver, 110, 602, 603f, 604–605, 610
exercise history and attitude questionnaire, 110, 113f–114f
informed consent, 110, 608
medical release form, 110, 115f
testing forms, 110

Exam Content Outline, 666–684

Exculpatory clause, 503f, 604

Executive summary, 631

Exercise

in cardiovascular disease prevention, 570

Exercise adoption, 26. *See also* Adherence; Motivation

Exercise history questionnaire, 110, 113f–114f

Exercise-induced asthma (EIA), 569

Exercise-induced bronchospasm (EIB), 569

Exercise-induced feeling inventory (EFI), 130–131, 130f, 131f

Exercise program design, 81–82
2008 Physical Activity Guidelines for Americans on, 82
general recommendations in, 82, 83t

Exercise programs. *See also* specific types and indications
evaluation of, 50
formulation of, 50
healthcare professional training on, 4
personal trainer role in, 4–5

Exercise recommendations. *See also* specific indications
general, 82, 83t
for specific groups, 82

Exercise record, 554

Exercise selection and order, in resistance training, 319–320, 321f

Exercise testing. *See also* specific tests and indications
components of, 123
graded, 190–192, 191t
professionalism in, 122–123
risk stratification for, 109f–110f
termination signs or symptoms in, 107, 109f–110f, 122, 174
treadmill, 192–196 (*See also* Treadmill exercise testing)

Expenses, monthly, 644, 644f

Expense worksheet, 644, 644f

Expiration, muscles in, 370

Expression, facial, 42

Expressors, 43f, 43t, 45t

Express partnership, 595

Extinction, 73

Extremities, distal, 251

Extrinsic motivation, 30, 55

Eye contact, 42
in effective communication, 102
in effective listening, 46

Eye injuries, 582

F

Facial expression, 42, 102

Facilities, legal responsibilities for, 610–612

Fartlek training, 387

Fascia, 535

Fasciitis, 535–536

Fast glycolytic system, anaerobic-power training on, 95

Fast-twitch muscle fibers. *See* Type II muscle fibers

Fat, body, 174, 175
density of, 183
essential, 175
excess, 175–176
measurement of, 176
muscle turning to, 362
norms for, 183–184, 184t
percent
aging on, 312
equations of, 183
targeting specific deposits of, 360

Fatigue, severe, from exercise testing, 122

Feedback
in action stage, of client–trainer relationship, 54
in cognitive behavioral techniques, 75
on motivation, 30
as operant conditioning, 73
verbal persuasion as, 66

Feldenkrais Method, 468

Fibroblastic/proliferation phase, 537

Fibromyalgia
diagnosis of, 505–506, 506t
exercise and, 506
exercise guidelines for, 506

overview of, 505
sample exercise recommendation for, 507
treatment of, 506

Field testing
cardiorespiratory fitness, 205–208
1.5-mile run test, 207–208, 209t
contraindications to, 206
overview of, 205–206
Rockport fitness walking test (1 mile), 206–207, 207t
power, 230–236
anaerobic capacity
300-yard shuttle run, 235–236, 236t
Margaria–Kalamen stair climb test, 234–235, 234f, 234t
anaerobic power
kneeling overhead toss, 233–234, 233f
standing long jump test, 231–232, 232t
vertical jump test, 232–233, 232f, 233t
clients for, 231
contraindications for, 231
principles of, 230–231

Financial information, key, 631

Financial plan, 643–646, 644f, 645f

Financing, business, 621

First-aid kit, 560, 560f

First ventilatory threshold (VT1)
in aerobic-base training, 93
in aerobic-efficiency training, 93
in anaerobic-endurance training, 94
in anaerobic-power training, 95
blood lactate and, 383–385, 383f, 384f
in cardiorespiratory training, 380
on exercise intensity, 380
submaximal talk test for, 202–205
in talk test, 382
for training zones, 385, 385f
in ventilatory threshold resting, 202

Fitness
aerobic (*See* $\dot{V}O_2$max)
cardiorespiratory training for (*See under* Cardiorespiratory training)
dysfunctional, 247, 284
load training for, 333–335
new-member assessment for, 636

Fitness blog, 637

Fitness testing, 240, 240t. *See also specific types*

F.I.T.T., 374

F.I.T.T.E., 374

Flexibility, 174
exercise components for, 83t
musculoskeletal injuries and, 538
in SMART goal setting, 49t

Flexibility and muscle-length testing, 158–162
passive straight-leg raise, 161–162, 161f, 162t
range of motion by joint in, 158–159, 158t
Thomas test for hip flexion/quadriceps length, 160, 160f, 161t
worksheet for, 159, 159f

Flexibility exercises, planes for, 259–260

Flow-through taxation, 596

Fluid intake, in exercise, 576, 576t

Focused practice, 54

Foot. *See also* Ankle
stability and mobility of, 246

Footwear, proper, 544

Foramina, 543

Force, 91

Force-couple relationships, 250, 250f

Force-couples
glenohumeral joint, 250
pelvic, 250, 250f

Forearm
circumference measurement of, 187t
extensor muscles of, 541, 541f
splinting of, 581, 581f

40-yard dash, 238–239, 239f, 239t

Forward agility ladder/hurdle drills, 352t, 353f

Forward-head position, 146, 146f, 146t

Forward hops, 352t

Forward jumps, 352t

Fractures, 580–581, 581f
bone, 536–537, 536f
stress, 536, 536f, 580

Franchise operations, 599–600

Frauds, statute of, 602

Free weights, 357
vs. machines, 361–362
for strength training, 357

Frequency, exercise/training, 26
in cardiorespiratory training, 375, 375t
in resistance training, 318–319, 319t, 332, 333
in speed, agility, and reactivity training, 350

Front/lateral cone jumps, 347t

Frostbite, 577

Functional assessments, 135–169. *See also specific assessments*

in ACE IFT Model, 84
balance and core, 166–169
flexibility and muscle-length testing, 158–162
movement screens, 146–158
shoulder mobility, 162–166
static postural, 136–146

Functional movement and resistance training, 88–92
case studies of
David (57-year-old executive, fit and active)
movement, 423, 423t
stability and mobility, 421, 422t
Jan (17-year-old female athlete)
load, 429–431, 430t
movement, 428–429, 429t
performance, 431, 431t
Kelly (30-year-old, wedding preparation)
load, 445–446, 446t
movement, 444–445, 445t
Meredith (64-year-old, active)
load, 440
movement, 439, 439t
Sharon (33-year-old female, fit pre-pregnancy)
load, 416–417, 417t
movement, 415–416, 416t
stability and mobility, 413–414, 415t
Stanley (28-year-old male, sedentary)
movement, 435–436, 436t
stability and mobility, 433–434, 434t
overview of, 88
phase 1: stability and mobility training, 88–89
phase 2: movement training, 89–90
phase 3: load training, 90–91
phase 4: performance training, 91–92
principles of, 88

Functional programming, for stability-mobility and movement, 245–307. *See also specific phases*
movement in, 246–251 (*See also* Movement)
phase 1: stability and mobility training, 251–284
phase 2: movement training, 284–307 (*See also* Movement training)

G

Gait, weight transference onto stance-leg in, 286–287, 287f

Gastrocnemius stretch, 552, 552f

Gellish et al. formula, for maximum heart rate, 376

Gender
on muscular strength and hypertrophy, 314
on participation and adherence, 27

General partnerships, 595

Genuineness, 100

Gestational diabetes, 491

Gestures, 101–102

Girth measurements, 186–187, 187f, 187t

Glenohumeral joint, 272
distal mobility of, 272–280
proximal mobility of, 272

Glenohumeral joint force-couples, 250, 272

Glutamine supplement, 358

Gluteals, in bend-and-lift movements, 286

Glute bridge, 266f

Glute dominance, 286

Goals. *See also specific disorders*
process, 48
product, 48
SMART, 48, 49t

Goal setting
for adherence, 33, 48, 50t
on behavior change, 72
in cognitive behavioral techniques, 75
feedback on, 31
in planning stage of client–trainer relationship, 48–50, 49t, 50t

Goal weight calculation, 184

Golfer's elbow, 540–541, 541f

Graded exercise tests (GXT), 190–192, 191t

Grand mal seizure, 577–578

Graphic designer, 643

Greater trochanteric bursitis, 539t, 543–544

Gross negligence, 605

Group exercise, 388–389

Group Fitness Instructors, 637–638

Group waivers, 610

Growth hormone, on muscular strength and hypertrophy, 315

Guidelines, safety, 614

H

Half-kneeling lunge rise, 295, 295f

Half-kneeling triplanar stretch, 264f

Half-wall hang, 459f
Hamstrings stretch, lying, 265f
Hand gestures, 42
Hatha yoga, 458–466. *See also* Yoga, hatha
Hay-bailer patterns, 304, 306f, 307
Head immobilization, 583, 584f
Head injuries, 581–583
Head position, in postural assessment, 145–146, 146f, 146t
Head tilt–chin lift maneuver, 563f
Healing, tissue reaction to, 537
Health
  cardiorespiratory training for (*See* under Cardiorespiratory training)
  load training for, 333–335
Health behavior, 64. *See also* Behavioral theory models
Health belief model, 64–66
Health benefits. *See* Benefits, exercise
Health club membership sales, 648–653. *See also* Selling personal training
Health conditions, 116–118. *See also specific conditions*
  cardiovascular, 116
  hernia, 118
  illness or infection, 118
  metabolic, 118
  musculoskeletal, 117
  pregnancy, 118
  respiratory, 116–117
Health/Fitness Facility Standards and Guidelines, 16
Health—fitness—performance continuum, 83–84, 83f
Health history, in ACE IFT Model, 84
Health Insurance Portability and Accountability Act (HIPAA), 13, 562
Health psychology, 64, 75–76. *See also* Behavior change
Health-related physiological assessments, 174
Health-risk appraisal, 105–115
  case study example of, 111
  components of, 105–107
  evaluation forms in, 110–115
    agreement and release of liability waiver, 110, 602, 603f, 604–605, 610
    exercise history and attitude questionnaire, 110, 113f–114f
    health-history questionnaire, 110, 112f
    informed consent, 110, 608
    medical release form, 110, 115f
    testing forms, 110
  Physical Activity Readiness Questionnaire in, 105, 106f
  purposes and value of, 105
  risk stratification in, 105–107, 108t, 109f–110f (*See also* Risk stratification)
  for self-directed vs. supervised exercise, 105
Healthy lifestyle, of trainer, 54
Heart attack, 569–570
Heart rate (HR)
  assessment of, 125–126
  in cardiorespiratory training, 375–379, 376f, 377f, 377t [*See also* Maximum heart rate (MHR)]
  in exercise, 125–126
  in graded exercise tests, 191
  maximum [*See* Maximum heart rate (MHR)]
  measurement of, 126
  resting, 49t, 125
  steady state, 192
  in submaximal workload, 49t
  target exercise, Tanaka, Monahan, and Seal formula for, 197
  target heart-rate range for, 201
Heart-rate reserve (HRR) method, for exercise intensity, 375–378, 376f, 377f, 377t
Heart-rate reserve (HRR), on participation and adherence, 29
Heart-rate response to cycling, $\dot{V}O_2$ and, 199, 199f
Heat acclimatization, 576
Heat cramps, 573
Heat edema, 573
Heat exhaustion, 573–574, 574t
Heat illness, 573–576, 574t–576t. *See also specific types*
Heat index, 575–576, 575t
Heat stroke, 573–576, 574t
Heat syncope, 573
Heavy weights, vs. light weights for muscle tone vs. mass, 360–361
Heimlich maneuver, 568
Hematoma, 578
Hemorrhage control, 578–579, 579f
Hemorrhagic stroke, 570

Hepatitis, 560

Hepatitis B, 585

Hepatitis C, 585

Hernia, 118

Hexagon drill, 347t

High blood pressure. *See* Hypertension

High-density lipoprotein (HDL), 107, 108t, 109f

High knees, 351t, 352f

High marches, 351t, 352f

High-risk situations, 34–35

Hip adduction
  fundamentals of, 286, 287f
  in postural assessment, 141, 141f, 142t

Hip and thoracic spine mobility exercises, proximal, 260–271
  cat-camel, 261f
  hamstrings mobility: lying hamstrings stretch, 265f
  hip flexor mobility: lying hip flexor stretch, 263f
  hip flexor mobility progression: half-kneeling triplanar stretch, 264f
  hip mobilization
    with glute activation: shoulder bridge (glute bridge), 266f
    supine 90-90 hip rotator stretch, 267f
  monoarticulate (uniarticulate) and biarticulate muscles in, 259
  overview, 260
  pelvic tilts, 261f
  pelvic tilts progressions
    modified dead bug with reverse bent-knee marches, 262f–263f
    supine bent-knee marches, 262f
  planes for flexibility exercises in, 259–260
  posterior mobilization
    rocking quadrupeds, 271f
    table-top kneeling lat stretch, 268f
  programming principles for, 258–259
  supine 90-90 neutral back, 260f
  supportive surfaces for, 259
  thoracic (T-)spine mobilization
    prisoner rotations, 270f
    spinal extensions, 268f–269f
    spinal twists, 269f

Hip circumference measurement, 187f, 187t

Hip flexion, Thomas test for, 160, 160f, 161t

Hip flexor mobility
  half-kneeling triplanar stretch for, 264f
  lying hip flexor stretch for, 263f

Hip flexor stretch, lying, 263f

Hip-hinge exercise, 287, 288f

Hip mobilization
  with glute activation: shoulder bridge (glute bridge), 266f
  supine 90-90 hip rotator stretch, 267f

Hip rotator stretch, supine 90-90, 267f

Hips, in stability and mobility training, 251

Hip tilting, in postural assessment, 142–143, 142f, 142t, 143f

History. *See also specific disorders*
  health, 84
  medical, record keeping on, 554

HIV infection, 560
  exercise and, 585–586
  protection against, 585

Hopping, tips on, 345

Hops
  forward, 352t
  lateral, 352t

Horizontal chest pass, 348t, 349f

HR turnpoint (HRTP), 384, 384f

Human immunodeficiency virus (HIV). *See* HIV infection

Humeral rotation
  internal, 145
  internal and external, 275f
  internal and external, at shoulder, 164, 164f, 165t, 255f

Hurdle step screen, 153–155, 154f, 154t

Hurdle step test, trunk stability in, 252

Hydrolysates, 358

Hydrostatic weighing, 176–178, 177t

Hyperglycemia, 571

Hypertension, 483–485
  exercise and, 483–484
  exercise guidelines for, 484
  overview of, 483
  on physical activity, 116
  sample exercise recommendation for, 484–485
  yoga and tai chi for, 484–485

Hypoglycemia
  in diabetics, 571–572
  general points on, 571–573, 572f

Hypoperfusion. *See* Shock

Hypotension, orthostatic, with hypothermia, 577

Hypothermia, 575, 576–577
Hypovolemic shock, 585
Hypoxia
  from dyspnea, 568
  in seizure, 578

I

Ice, 538, 579
Ice massage, 579
Iliotibial (IT) band complex, 543
Iliotibial band stretch, 545, 545f
Iliotibial band syndrome (ITBS), 117, 545, 545f
Imaginal experiences, 67
Implied partnership, 595–596
Inactivity
  muscle shortening from, 248
  muscle turning to fat and, 362
Incident report, 554
Incision, 578
Independent contractors, 600–602, 629–630
Individualized teaching, 52, 53t
Individualized training programs, 76–77
Infection, 118. *See also specific types*
Inflammation, 537
Inflammatory phase, 537
Information gathering, 45–46
Informed consent, 110, 561, 606, 608, 608f–609f
Informing, 103
Infrapatellar tendinitis, 547–548
Inherent risks, 607, 610
Initial session, 636
Injury. *See also specific types*
  on participation and adherence, 29
  resistance training on risk of, 313–314
Injury analysis, 318
Inspiration
  muscles in, 370
  in ventilatory threshold resting, 202
Institute for Credentialing Excellence (ICE), 16
Instruction, legal responsibilities for, 613–614
Insulin, 571
Insulin reaction, 571–573, 572f
Insulin therapy, 118
Insurance broker, 643
Insurance, liability, 616–619. *See also* Liability insurance
Integral yoga, 462
Integrated Fitness Training Model, ACE. *See* ACE Integrated Fitness Training Model
Intellectual property, 620
Intensity, exercise/training, 375–385
  on blood lactate and VT2, 383–385, 383f–385f
  caloric expenditure in, 380–382, 381t
  on delayed-onset muscle soreness, 322
  first ventilatory threshold in, 380
  heart rate in, 375–379, 376f, 377f, 377t [*See also* Maximum heart rate (MHR)]
  importance of, 385
  %MHR and, 376, 377t
  moderate, 26
  on participation and adherence, 29
  ratings of perceived exertion in, 378, 378t, 379, 379t [*See also* Ratings of perceived exertion (RPE)]
  in resistance training, 321–322, 332, 333
  in speed, agility, and reactivity training, 350, 350t
  talk test for, 382–383
  vigorous, drop-out rate with, 29
  $\dot{V}O_2$ or metabolic equivalents in, 378–382, 381t
International Health, Racquet, and Sportsclub Association (IHRSA), 16
Internet, 637
Interval training
  aerobic, 373
  physiological adaptations to, 372
  on $\dot{V}O_2$max, 372
Interventions, behavioral, 76
Interviewing techniques
  in investigation stage, 102–103
  motivational, 50–51, 104
Intrinsic motivation, 29–30
  in motivational interviewing, 104
  via behavior-change contracts, 56
Investigation stage, of client–trainer relationship, 45–47, 99–132, 100, 100f
  assessments in
    choice of, 123–124
    conducting essential, 125–129, 127f, 128t
    goals of, 123

sequencing of, 121–123
tools for, 124–125, 124t
communication in, 101–102
definition of, 45
difficult disclosures in, 47
empathy in, 102
environment in, 101
exercise-induced feeling inventory in, 130–131, 130f, 131f
facilitating change in, 103–104, 104f
health conditions in, 116–118
health-risk appraisal in, 105–115 (*See also* Health-risk appraisal)
information gathering in, 45–46
interviewing techniques in, 102–103
listening in, 46–47
medications in, 118–121, 120t
motivational interviewing in, 104
personality style in, 101
rapport building in, 100–101 (*See also* Rapport)
ratings of perceived exertion in, 129, 129t

Iron, 359

Ischemia, 107

Ischemic stroke, 570

Isokinetic training, momentum in, 322

Isolated stretch, active, 253, 253f

Isometric actions, muscle, 311

Isometric contractions, low-grade, 253

Isotonic training, momentum in, 322

Iyengar yoga, 462

J

Jackson and Pollock formula for skinfold measurements
in men, 181t
in women, 182t

Jaw thrust method, 563f

Joint mobility, 246

Joint movement. *See* Movement; specific types

Joint stability, 246

Jumping jacks, 347t

Jumping, tips on, 345

Jumps
diagonal cone, 347t
forward, 352t
front/lateral cone, 347t
lateral, 352t, 353f
multidirectional, 347t
multiple, 347t
in place, 347t
single front/lateral box, 347t
single linear, 347t
standing long/vertical, 347t

Jump tests
standing long jump, 231–232, 232t
vertical, 232–233, 232f, 233t

K

Karvonen formula, for maximum heart rate, 376–378, 377f, 377t

Ketoacidosis, 571

Ketones, 572

Keyman insurance, 618

Kinematics, 285

Kinetic chain, ankle pronation/supination on, 140, 141f, 141t

Kneeling overhead toss, 233–234, 233f

Knees, high, 351t, 352f

Knee tucks, 347t

Knowledge
advanced, 18
in motivational interviewing, 51
on participation and adherence, 28
of results, 31

Korotkoff sounds, 126–127, 127f

Kripalu yoga, 462

Kundalini yoga, 462–463

Kyphosis, 145, 247, 584

L

Laceration, 578

Lactate acid, in ventilatory threshold resting, 202

Lactate, blood, in cardiorespiratory training, 383–385, 383f–385f

Lactate threshold (LT)
in cardiorespiratory training, 92
definition of, 384
interval training on, 372
prediction of, 371
programming exercise for, 383–385, 383f–385f
training on, 205, 205f
in ventilatory threshold resting, 202

Lactic acid, from resistance training, 314–315

Ladder/hurdle drills, agility, 352t, 353f
Lateral agility ladder/hurdle drills, 352t, 353f
Lateral epicondylitis, 117, 540–541, 541f
Lateral jumps/hops, 352t, 353f
Lateral shuffles, cone/marker, 353t
Lat stretch, table-top kneeling, 268f
Leadership qualities, 31–32
Lean body mass, 175, 513
Lean tissue measurement, 176
Lean weight, 313
Learning. *See also* Teaching
  motor, 53
  observational, 73
Learning stages, 58
Learning styles, 52, 53t
Legal guidelines, 602–610
  agreements to participate, 606, 607f
  contracts, 602–604, 603f
  exculpatory clause, 603f, 604
  informed consent, 606, 608f–609f
  inherent risks, 607, 610
  negligence, 604
  procedures, 610
  vicarious liability, 604–605
  waivers, 110, 602, 603f, 604–605, 610
Legal responsibilities, 610–614
  equipment, 612–613
  facilities, 610–612
  instruction, 613–614
  paperwork, 610
  safety guidelines, 614
  supervision, 613
Leg cramping, from exercise testing, 122
Leg-press test, 1-RM, 225–226, 225f, 227t
Legs-up-the-wall pose, 459f
Length, of cardiorespiratory training, 374
Length-tension relationships, 248–249, 248f, 249f
Liability
  personal, 596
  vicarious, 604–605
Liability insurance, 616–619
  components of, 617
  for employees and independent contractors, 618–619
  need for, 616–617
  product, 618
  professional, 617–618
  umbrella, 618
Liability waiver, 110, 602, 603f, 604–605, 610
Lifestyle exercise, 390
Lifting, proper techniques for, 584
Ligaments, collagen in, 579
Ligament strains, 534–535, 534f, 535t
Light weights vs. heavy weights, for muscle tone vs. mass, 360–361
Limb length
  discrepancy of, on hip adduction, 141, 141f
  on muscular strength and hypertrophy, 316–317
Limitations, statute of, 610
Limited liability corporation (LLC), 598, 599t
Limited liability partnership (LLP), 598, 599t
Limited partners, 596
Limits of stability (LOS), 281–282
Linear periodization, 90, 326, 327f, 328t
Line of gravity (LOG), 137, 137f, 281
Lipoprotein (lipid). *See also* Cholesterol
  classification of, 489, 489t
  levels of, in SMART goal setting, 49t
  low-density, in coronary artery disease, 481
Listening
  in client–trainer relationship, 32
  effective
    in communication, 46–47, 102
    in motivational interviewing, 51
Load training, 90–91
  goal of, 91
  for health, 333–335,
  in resistance training, 333–341
    assessment, 333
    circuit, 334–335
    objectives, 333
    for prerequisite muscular strength before performance training, 340–341
    program design, 333–340
      for muscle hypertrophy, 337–340
      for muscular endurance, fitness, and health, 333–335
      for muscular strength, 335–337
  studies on, 399
Load-volume calculation, 320
Loans, business, 621
Logo, ACE, 620
Long jump test, standing, 231–232, 232t

Lordosis
hip tilt in, 142–143, 142f, 143f
in lumbar spine, 142–143, 142f

Low back, 583f, 584. *See also* Lumbar spine
clearing test for, 150, 150f
hyperextension of, 584

Low-back pain (LBP), 509–513, 584
exercise and, 510
exercise guidelines for, 510–512, 512f
lifting and, 584
from musculoskeletal injuries, 542–543
overview of, 509–510
sample exercise recommendation for, 513

Low-density lipoprotein (LDL), in coronary artery disease, 481

Lower-cross syndrome, 142–143

Lower-extremity alignment, 289f–290f

Lower-extremity musculoskeletal injuries, 543–553
Achilles tendinitis, 551–552, 552f
ankle sprains, 535f, 549–551 (*See also* Ankle sprains)
greater trochanteric bursitis, 539t, 543–544
iliotibial band syndrome, 545, 545f
infrapatellar tendinitis, 547–548
patellofemoral pain syndrome, 546–547, 547f
plantar fasciitis, 553, 553f
shin splints, 548–549, 549f

Lumbar spine, 583f, 584. *See also* Low back
stability and mobility of, 246
in stability and mobility training, 251

Lunge matrix, 296, 297f–298f

Lunge rise, half-kneeling, 295, 295f

Lunges, 295–296, 295f–296f
directional movements for, 298f
progressions of, 296

Lunge, with resistance, 331

Lying hamstrings stretch, 265f

Lying hip flexor stretch, 263f

M

Macrocycles, 326, 327f

Magnetic resonance imaging, of body composition, 177t

Maintenance, in transtheoretical model of behavioral change, 68, 69t, 71–72

Major achievements, 631

Marches, high, 351t, 352f

Margaria–Kalamen stair climb test, 234–235, 234f, 234t

Marketing
for client retention, 640–641
general communication in, 641–642

Marketing activities, 619–620

Marketing plan, 632

Maturation/remodeling phase, 537

Maximum heart rate (MHR)
ACSM guidelines for use of, 376, 377t
calculation of
220 – age formula, 376
Gellish et al. formula, 376
Karvonen formula, 376–378, 377f, 377t
%MHR vs. 220 – age formula, 376
overestimation, 376
standard deviation, 376, 376f
Tanaka, Monahan, and Seals formula, 376
cardiorespiratory exercise on, 370
exercise intensity on, 375, 376, 377t
graded exercise tests for, 190–192, 191t
%MHR, 376, 377t
performance and, 376
prediction equation for, 190

Maximum oxygen uptake. *See* $\dot{V}O_2$max

McArdle step test, 211

McGill's torso muscular endurance test battery, 217–220
evaluation and application of, 219–220
overview and history of, 217
trunk extensor endurance test, 218–219, 219f
trunk flexor endurance test, 217–218, 217f
trunk lateral endurance test, 218, 219f

Medial collateral ligament (MCL) injuries, 534f, 535

Medial collateral ligament (MCL) rotation, 285–286, 285f

Medial epicondylitis, 540–541, 541f

Medial tibial stress syndrome (MTSS), 548–549, 549f

Medical Fitness Association (MFA), 16

Medical history, record keeping on, 554

Medical indicators, in SMART goal setting, 49t

Medical release form, 110, 115f

Medications, 118–121, 120t. *See also* specific types and agents

Medicine ball power push-up, 348f, 348t

Medicine balls, 357

Meditation, 471

Meninges, 581–582

Meniscal injuries, 534f, 536

Mesocycles, 326, 327f, 328t–329t

Metabolic conditions, 118. *See also specific conditions*

Metabolic equivalents (METs)
in cardiorespiratory training, 378–382, 381t
for training programming, 380, 381t, 382

Metabolic function, resistance training on, 313

Metabolic markers, individualized, 202

Metabolic syndrome
exercise and, 495
exercise guidelines for, 495
overview of, 494–495

Microcycles, 326, 327f, 328t–329t

Midthigh circumference measurement, 187t

Mind-body exercise, 390, 451–477
for acute coronary syndromes, 470
for chronic disease management, 470
contemporary programs of, 466–469
Alexander Technique, 467–468
Feldenkrais Method, 468
history and overview, 466
Native American and Alaskan spiritual dancing, 468–469
Nia, 468
Pilates, 466–467, 467f
differentiating characteristics of, 454
indications for, 469–470
modalities and programs of, 458–466 *(See also specific modalities and programs)*
original Chen style, 466
qigong, 464, 465f
tai chi, 464–466
yoga, 458–466
neurobiological foundations of, 452–453, 453f
outcomes and benefits of, assessing, 469
outcomes and benefits of, research-supported, 454–458
common components, 456
meta-analytic review, 454
overview, 454
qigong and tai chi, 455t, 457–458
yoga, 455t, 456–457
patterns of, 452
personal trainers and, 470–472
roots of, 453–454
taxonomy of, 452, 452t

Mind-body responses, neuroendocrine basis for, 453, 453f

Minerals, 359

Minimal encouragers, 102

Minimum competency, 7

Minority partner, 595

Minute ventilation ($\dot{V}_E$)
cardiorespiratory exercise on, 371
exercise on, 383, 383f

Mirroring, 101–102

Mitochondria, cardiorespiratory exercise on, 370

Mobility. *See also specific types*
distal, 280, 281f
joint, 246
of kinetic chain, 246, 247f
lack of, 247

Mobility exercises, distal, of glenohumeral joint, 272–280. *See also* Stability exercises, proximal, for scapulothoracic region

Mobility exercises, proximal, 258–271
hips and thoracic spine, 260–271
cat-camel, 261f
hamstrings mobility: lying hamstrings stretch, 265f
hip flexor mobility: lying hip flexor stretch, 263f
hip flexor mobility progression: half-kneeling triplanar stretch, 264f
hip mobilization
with glute activation: shoulder bridge (glute bridge), 266f
supine 90-90 hip rotator stretch, 267f
monoarticulate (uniarticulate) and biarticulate muscles in, 259
overview, 260
pelvic tilts, 261f
pelvic tilts progressions, modified dead bug with reverse bent-knee marches, 262f–263f
pelvic tilts progressions, supine bent-knee marches, 262f
planes for flexibility exercises, 259–260
posterior mobilization
rocking quadrupeds, 271f
table-top kneeling lat stretch, 268f
programming principles for, 258–259
supine 90-90 neutral back, 260f
supportive surfaces for, 259
thoracic (T-)spine
prisoner rotations, 270f
spinal extensions, 268f–269f
spinal twists, 269f
purpose of, 251
scapulothoracic region in, 251

stretching techniques in
active isolated stretch, 253, 253f
dynamic and ballistic stretches, 253, 253f
myofascial release, 253, 253f
by phase of workout session, 252–253, 253f
proprioceptive neuromuscular facilitation, 253, 253f
static stretches, 253, 253f
type I muscle fibers in, 251
type II muscle fibers in, 252

Mobility training, 88–89. *See also* Stability and mobility training

Modeling, effective, 54–55

Moderate-intensity exercise program, 26

Modified curl-up, 512f

Modified dead bug with reverse bent-knee marches, 262f–263f

Monoarticulate muscles, 259

Monotony, training, 400, 401f

Monthly expenses, 644, 644f

Mood appraisals, 66–67

Motivation, 29–31. *See also* Adherence
client empowerment in, 30
contextual, 30
definition of, 26, 29
extrinsic, 30, 55
factors in, 26
feedback in, 31
intrinsic, 29–30, 56, 104
leadership qualities in, 31–32
relapse prevention in, 34–35
self-efficacy in, 30–31
situational, 30

Motivational interviewing, 50–51, 104

Motor learning, 53, 314

Motor skills, 53

Movement, 246–251. *See also specific types*
ankle pronation/supination on kinematic chain in, 285, 285f
efficiency of, 246, 247f
five primary, 146, 284
abilities and skills in, 285
training of, 284
force-couple relationships in, 250, 250f
joint mobility in, 246
joint range of motion and, 247
joint stability in, 246
kinematics in, 285
length-tension relationships in, 248–249, 248f, 249f
mobility and stability of kinetic chain in, 246, 247f
mobility vs. stability in specific joints in, 246–247
muscle force in, 246
muscle imbalance on, 247, 248f
neural control in, 250–251, 251f
pain-compensation cycle in, 251, 251f
posture on mobility and stability in, 246–247
reciprocal inhibition in, 250
rotational, 89, 331
synergistic dominance in, 250

Movement analysis, 318

Movement compensations, 247–248

Movement efficiency pattern, 136–137, 137f

Movement screens, 146–158
bend and lift, 151, 152t
clearing tests, 150, 150f
hurdle step, 153–155, 154f, 154t
movement in, 146, 150
shoulder pull stabilization, 156–157, 156f, 156t
shoulder push stabilization, 155, 155f, 156t
thoracic spine mobility, 157–158, 157f, 157t
value of, 150

Movement training, 89–90, 284–307, 330
bend-and-lift patterns in, 287–291, 330
exercises for, 288
hip hinge, 287, 288f
lower-extremity alignment, 289f–290f
pelvic tilts and back alignment, 289f
squat variations, 291f
gluteals in, 286
quadriceps in, 286
in squat, 286, 287–288
dysfunctional fitness and, 284
pulling, 303–304, 303f, 330
pushing, 299–302, 330
exercises for
bilateral and unilateral presses, 299, 300f
overhead press, 302, 302f
thoracic matrix, 299, 301f
mechanics and muscles of, 299, 299f
resistance
five primary movements, 330–332, 331
program design, 332
rates of progression, 332
rotational (spiral), 304–307, 305f–306f, 330–331
single-leg stand patterns in, 292–298, 330
dynamic movement patterns over static base of support, 293–295, 293t, 294f

half-kneeling lunge rise, 295, 295f
lunge matrix in, 296, 297f–298f
lunge progressions in, 296
lunges, 296f
lunging effectively in, 295–296, 295f–296f
overview, 292, 292f
progression for, 295
static balance on a single leg, 293–295, 293t, 294f

Multidirectional cone/marker drill, 353t

Multidirectional jumps, 347t

Multidirectional ladder/hurdle drills, 352t, 353f

Multiple jumps, 347t

Muscle
concentric actions of, 311
eccentric actions of, 311
fat from, without exercise, 362
isometric actions of, 311

Muscle balance, importance of, 136–137, 137f

Muscle fiber type. *See* Type II muscle fibers; Type I muscle fibers

Muscle hypertrophy
age on, 316
cardiorespiratory exercise in, 370
definition of, 337
facilitation of, 337–338
gender on, 314
growth hormone and testosterone in, 315
limb length on, 316–317
load training for, 337–339
cable exercises, 339
competitive level, 339–340
FIRST recommendations, 338
post-fatigue repetitions, 340
rates of progression, 340
resting days, 339
supersets, 340
muscle fiber type on, 316
muscle length on, 316
from resistance training, 314
tendon insertion point in, 317

Muscle imbalance
assessment of, 230
causes of, 230
dysfunctional movement from, 247, 248f
factors in, 136
preventing, in resistance training, 313

Muscle isolation, for posture, 254

Muscle length
on muscular strength and hypertrophy, 316
testing of, 158–162 (*See also* Flexibility and muscle-length testing)

Muscle-mind responses, muscle-brain pathways in, 453, 453f

Muscle pump, 315

Muscle reversibility, 326

Muscle shortening
development of, 249
from inactivity, 248

Muscle spindles, in plyometric exercise, 343

Muscle strains, 533–534, 533t

Muscle-strengthening activities, frequency of, 26. *See also* Frequency, exercise/training

Muscular endurance, 174, 317
definition of, 212
load training for, 333–335
in SMART goal setting, 49t

Muscular-endurance testing, 212–221
bodyweight squat test, 220–221, 221f, 221t
considerations prior to, 213
curl-up test, 215, 215f, 216t
McGill's torso muscular endurance test battery, 217–220
evaluation and application of, 219–220
overview and history of, 217
trunk extensor endurance test, 218–219, 219f
trunk flexor endurance test, 217–218, 217f
trunk lateral endurance test, 218, 219f
push-up test, 213–214, 213f, 214t
relevance and appropriateness of, 212–213
use of, 212

Muscular fitness. *See also* Muscular endurance; Muscular strength
definition of, 212
health-related benefits of, 212

Muscular-fitness testing, 212–230. *See also specific types*
muscular endurance, 212–221 (*See also* Muscular-endurance testing)
muscular strength, 221–230

Muscular power, 317, 317f, 342

Muscular strength, 174, 221, 317
age on, 315
gender on, 314
growth hormone and testosterone in, 315
limb length on, 316–317
load training for, 335–337
muscle fiber type on, 316
muscle length on, 316

in muscular fitness, 212
in SMART goal setting, 49t
tendon insertion point, 317
Muscular strength/power/endurance relationship, 317, 317f
Muscular-strength (1-RM) testing, 221–230
1-RM bench-press test, 222–225, 223f, 223t–225t
1 RM calculation in, 229, 229t
1-RM leg-press test, 225–226, 225f, 227t
1-RM maximum prediction coefficients in, 229, 229t
1-RM squat test, 227–229, 228f
absolute vs. relative strength in, 221
considerations and contraindications for, 222
definition and use of, 221
goals of, 222
repetition table for, 224, 224t
special considerations for, 229, 229f
strength ratios in, 230, 230t
submaximal strength, 229–230, 230t
variety of, 222
Muscular system, cardiorespiratory training on, 370
Musculoskeletal conditions, on physical activity, 117
Musculoskeletal injuries, 533–554
bone fractures, 536–537, 536f
cartilage damage, 534f, 536
flexibility and, 538
footwear and, proper, 544
inflammation signs and symptoms in, 537
ligament strains, 534–535, 534f, 535t
low-back pain, 542–543 [*See also* Low-back pain (LBP)]
lower-extremity, 543–553
Achilles tendinitis, 551–552, 552f
ankle sprains, 535f, 549–551 (*See also* Ankle sprains)
greater trochanteric bursitis, 539t, 543–544
iliotibial band syndrome, 545, 545f
infrapatellar tendinitis, 547–548
patellofemoral pain syndrome, 546–547, 547f
plantar fasciitis, 553, 553f
shin splints, 548–549, 549f
management of
acute injury management in, 538
with pre-existing injuries, 537
program modification in, 537–538
muscle strains and tendinitis, 533–534, 533t
overuse conditions, 535–536
record keeping on, 554
tissue reaction to healing in, 537
upper-extremity, 538–542
carpal tunnel syndrome, 539t, 541–542, 542f
conservative management of, 539, 539t
elbow tendinitis, 540–541, 541f
rotator cuff injuries, 540, 541f
shoulder strain/sprain, 538–539, 539f, 539t
Music broadcasts, 620
Music recordings, 620
Myocardial infarction, triggering event for, 406
Myofascial release, 253, 253f
Myofibrillar hypertrophy. *See also* Muscle hypertrophy
from resistance training, 315

N

Nasal injuries, 583
National Commission for Health Certifying Agencies (NCHCA), 16
National Organization for Competency Assurance (NOCA), 16
Native American spiritual dancing, 468–469
NCCA, 16
accreditation of allied healthcare credentials through, 15–17
Department of Labor recognition of, 17
education community recognition of, 16–17
fitness and health industry recognition of, 16
Near-infrared interactance, 177t
Neck immobilization, 583, 584f
Neck injuries, 583–584, 583f, 584f
Needs assessment. *See also specific disorders*
in resistance training, 318
Negative reasons, for exercise, 55
Negative reinforcement, 72–73
Negligence, 604
comparative, 605
contributory, 605
gross, 605
Nerve radiculopathy, 543
Neural control, in movement, 250–251, 251f
Neuroendocrinology, of mind-body responses, 453, 453f
Neuromuscular efficiency, movement screens for, 136
Neuromuscular facilitation, proprioceptive, 253,

253f
Neuropathy, peripheral, in diabetic, 573
Nia, 468
9-1-1, 564, 565
Nonsteroidal anti-inflammatory drugs (NSAIDSs), for soft-tissue injuries, 579–580
Nonverbal communication, 42
Nurses, 5
Nutrition, advice on, 616
Nutritional Supplements, ACE Position Statement on, 687

O

Observational learning, 73
Obstructive shock, 585
Occupational therapists, 5
1.5-mile run test, 207–208, 209t
1-RM bench-press test, 222–225
  1 RM repetition table for, 224–225, 224t
  equipment for, 222
  pre-test procedure in, 222–223, 223f
  test protocol and administration in, 223–225, 223t
  upper-body strength from, 224, 225t
1-RM leg-press test, 225–226, 225f, 227t
1-RM maximum, 221, 317
1-RM maximum prediction coefficients in, 229, 229t
1-RM repetition table, 224–225, 224t
1-RM squat test, 227–229, 228f
1-RM testing. *See* Muscular-strength testing
Onset of blood lactate accumulation (OBLA), 204–205, 205f, 382
Open kinetic chain (OKC) movements, 274
Operant conditioning, 72–73
Operational plan, 632
Opinions, on behavior change, 72
Orientation
  in effective communication, 101
  for new members, 638
Orthopnea, 107
Orthostatic hypotension, with hypothermia, 577
Osteoporosis
  exercise and, 501
  exercise guidelines for, 501–502
  overview of, 501
  sample exercise recommendation for, 502
Outdoor exercise, 389
Overexposure, to cold, 577
Overfat, definition of, 176
Overhead presses, 299, 301f, 302
Overhead shoulder press, 302, 302f
Overhead toss, kneeling, 233–234, 233f
Overhead triceps stretch, 273, 273f
Overload, 88, 325, 386
Overtraining
  cardiorespiratory, 94
  on injury risk, 376
  signs of, 94
Overtraining syndrome, 400
Overuse conditions, musculoskeletal, 535–536
Overuse injury, 117
Overweight, 176, 513
Oxygen uptake, maximum. *See* $\dot{V}O_2$max

P

Pain-compensation cycle, 251, 251f
Paraphrasing, 46–47, 102
Participation, agreements on, 606, 607f
Partner, minority, 595
Partnership, 599t
  express, 595
  implied, 595–596
  limited liability, 598, 599t
Partnerships, 595–596
Part-to-whole teaching strategy, 288
Passion, personal, 54
Passive straight-leg (PSL) raise, 161–162, 161f, 162t
Past activity experience, behavior change and, 72
Past performance experience, 66
Patellofemoral pain syndrome (PFPS), 546–547, 547f
Patterns, single-leg stand, 292–298. *See also* Single-leg stand pattern movement training
Pectoralis stretch, 273, 273f

Pelvic force-couples, 250, 250f

Pelvic tilts, 142–143, 142f, 142t, 143f, 261f
  back alignment and, 289f
  progressions for
    modified dead bug with reverse bent-knee marches, 262f–263f
    supine bent-knee marches, 262f

Perceived barriers, 65, 76

Perceived benefits, 65

Perceived seriousness, 64–65

Perceived susceptibility, 65

Perceived threat, 64

Performance training, 91–92
  resistance training in, 341–354
    client prerequisites for, 342
    emphasis, 341
    in mid-life adults, 341
    power lifting vs. Olympic lifting in, 342–343
    power, speed, agility, and reactivity assessments, 343
    power training in, 341
    prerequisite muscular strength prior to, 340–341
    program design in
      for power, 343–346 (*See also* Plyometric exercise)
      for speed, agility, and reactivity, 346, 350–354 (*See also* Speed, agility, and reactivity training)
    resistance-training focus in, 317f, 342
    on velocity of force production, 341
    warm-up for, 342
    for weight loss, 341

Periodization
  linear, 90
  in long-term plan, 640
  for peak performance in key competitions, 350, 354t
  undulating, 90

Periodization models
  for resistance training, 326–329
    linear, 326, 327f, 328t
    sample protocols, 327, 328t–329t
    time segments of, 326, 327f
    undulating, 326–327, 327f, 329t
  for strength training, 321–322

Periosteum, 548

Periostitis, 548

Peripheral artery occlusive disease (PAOD), 487

Peripheral neuropathy, in diabetic, 573

Peripheral vascular disease (PVD), 486–488
  exercise and, 487
  exercise guidelines for, 487–488
  overview of, 486
  peripheral artery occlusive disease, 487
  peripheral vascular occlusive disease, 487, 487t
  sample exercise recommendation for, 488

Peripheral vascular occlusive disease (PVOD), 487, 487t

Personal expense worksheet, 644, 644f

Personal involvement, vs. empathy, 57–58

Personality styles, 42–45, 101
  dominance scale of, 42, 43f, 43t, 44f
  general traits in, 43t
  identifying and working with, 43, 45t
  self-assessment of, 42–43, 44f
  sociability scale of, 42, 43f, 43t, 44f

Personality traits, for personal trainers, 18

Personal liability, 596

Personal protective equipment (PPE), 560

Personal trainers. *See also specific topics*
  ACE certification of, 7–15 (*See also* Certification, ACE Personal Trainer)
  in allied healthcare continuum, 5–7, 6–7, 6f
  future of, 5
  role and scope of practice of, 3–19 (*See also* Role and scope of practice)

Persuasion, verbal, 66

Phosphagen system
  anaerobic power and, 231
  anaerobic-power training on, 95

Physical activity, 387–388, 388t. *See also* Exercise; specific activities
  for cardiorespiratory fitness, 212
  in cardiovascular disease prevention, 570
  guidelines for, 4
  health benefits of, 3–4, 4t
  illness on, 118
  recommendations for, 212
  U.S. government guidelines on, 64

Physical Activity Guidelines for Americans, 2008, 82

Physical Activity Readiness Questionnaire (PAR-Q), 105, 106f, 561

Physical appearance, resistance training on, 312

Physical capacity, resistance training on, 312

Physical therapists, 5

Physician guidelines, 10

Physician's assistants, 5

Physiological adaptations
  to cardiorespiratory training
    cardiovascular system, 370
    muscular system, 370
    respiratory system, 370–371
    with steady-state and interval-based exercise, 372
    time for increases in aerobic capacity, 371–372, 371f
  to resistance training, 314–317
    acute, 314
    long-term, 314
    motor learning, 314
    muscle hypertrophy, 314–315
    muscle remodeling, 315

Physiological analysis, 318

Physiological assessments, 173–240. *See also specific types*
  accuracy of, 240, 240t
  in ACE IFT Model, 84
  anthropometric measurements and body composition, 174–189
  cardiorespiratory fitness testing, 189–212
  health-related, 174
  muscular-fitness testing, 212–230
    muscular endurance, 212–221
    muscular strength, 221–230
  skill-related, 174
  sport-skill, 230–239
  testing and measurement in, 174
  test termination signs and symptoms in, 107, 109f–110f, 122, 174

Physiological parameters, traditional vs. new, 82, 82t

Physiological state appraisals, 66

Pilates, 466–467, 467f

Planes, for flexibility exercises, 259–260

Planning stage, of client–trainer relationship, 47–51, 100, 100f
  alternatives in, 48–50
  definition of, 47–48
  evaluation of exercise program in, 50
  motivational interviewing in, 50–51
  plan formulation in, 50
  setting goals in, 48–50, 49t, 50t

Plantar fasciitis, 553, 553f

Plaque, 569

Plumb line positions, 137f, 138–139

Plyometric exercise, 343–346
  amortization phase in, 343
  drills in, 346, 346f
    lower body, 347t
    speed, training tips for, 349
    upper body, 348f, 348t, 349f
  elements of, 343
  frequency of, 345
  intensity of, 345, 345t, 346f
  jumping and hopping tips in, 345
  for lower and upper body, 344, 344f, 344t
  precautionary guidelines in, 344–345
  repetitions and sets in, 346, 346t
  stretch-shortening cycle in, 343–344
  timing in, 343–344

Position Statement on Nutritional Supplements, ACE, 687

Positive benefits, of regular exercise, 82

Positive experience, with exercise, 86–87

Positive reinforcement, 72

Posterior capsule stretches, 273, 273f

Posterior mobilization
  rocking quadrupeds for, 271f
  table-top kneeling lat stretch for, 268f

Posterior shin splints, 548–549, 549f

Posterior superior iliac spine (PSIS), in pelvic tilt, 143, 143f

Postictal state, 578

Postnatal exercise
  exercise guidelines for, 523
  overview of, 521–522

Postural alignment, proper, 136

Postural deviations, factors in, 136

Posture
  dynamic strengthening exercises for, 254
  in effective communication, 101
  muscle isolation in, 254
  muscles in, 136
  muscle strengthening for, 253
  on stability and mobility, 246–247
  stability and mobility restoration for, 137, 137f

Power, 91
  anaerobic, 231
  calculation of, in Margaria–Kalamen stair climb test, 235
  definition of, 230–231
  equation for, 231
  muscular, definition of, 317f, 342
  in sports, 92
  strength and, 231

Power equations, 341

Power push-up, 348f, 348t

Power testing: field tests, 230–236
- anaerobic capacity
  - 300-yard shuttle run, 235–236, 236t
  - Margaria–Kalamen stair climb test, 234–235, 234f, 234t
- anaerobic power
  - kneeling overhead toss, 233–234, 233f
  - standing long jump test, 231–232, 232t
  - vertical jump test, 232–233, 232f, 233t
- clients for, 231
- contraindications for, 231
- principles of, 230–231

Power training
- for body composition, 92
- goal of, 91–92

Practice, focused, 54

Practices, professional, 11–12

Pranayama, 463

Preaching style, 103

Precautions, universal, 585

Precontemplation, in transtheoretical model of behavioral change, 68, 69t, 71

Pregnancy
- exercise guidelines for, 522–523
- exercise in, 521–522
- on physical activity, 118
- sample exercise recommendation for, 523

Prehypertension, 129

Prenatal exercise
- exercise guidelines for, 522–523
- overview of, 521–522
- sample exercise recommendation for, 523

Preparation, in transtheoretical model of behavioral change, 68, 69t, 71

Pre-participation screening. *See* Health-risk appraisal

Presses
- bilateral and unilateral, 299, 300f
- overhead, 299, 301f, 302
- overhead shoulder, 302, 302f

Prevention
- of cardiovascular disease, exercise in, 570
- disease, 313–314
- of muscle imbalance, 313
- of musculoskeletal injuries, 538
- of relapse, 34–35

PRICE, 538

PRICES, 579

Primary exercises, 319

Prisoner rotations, 270f

Privacy, client, 12–13

Pro agility test, 237, 237f, 237t

Probing, 102–103

Procedures, 610

Process goals, 48

Product liability insurance, 618

Professional boundaries, 57–58

Professionalism, 31–32

Professional liability insurance, 617–618

Professional practices, 11–12

Professional responsibilities
- business structure in, 593–600 (*See also* Business structure)
- independent contractors vs. employees, 600–602

Program design, for adherence, 32–33

Progression, exercise, 88. *See also specific exercises and sites*
- in cardiorespiratory training, 386–387
- in resistance training, 324–325

Pronation, ankle
- on kinetic chain, 140, 141f, 141t
- in postural assessment, 139–140, 140f, 141f, 141t

Prone arm lifts, 278f

Proprioceptive neuromuscular facilitation (PNF), 253, 253f

Protection. *See also* Prevention
- bloodborne pathogen, 585
- for musculoskeletal injuries, 538
- personal protective equipment for, 560

Protein supplements, 358

Proximal stability exercises, 254–258. *See also* Stability exercises, proximal

Psychological traits, on participation and adherence, 28

Psychology, health. *See* Health psychology

Pubic bone, ASIS alignment of, 143, 143f

Public Safety Answering Points (PSAPs), 564–565

Pull-downs, bilateral and unilateral, 303–304, 303f

Pulling movements, 89, 331

Pulling movement training, 303–304, 303f, 330–331

Puncture, 578

Punishment, 73

Pushing movements, 89, 331

Pushing movement training, 299–302, 330–331
exercises for
bilateral and unilateral presses, 299, 300f
overhead press, 302, 302f
thoracic matrix, 299, 301f
mechanics and muscles of, 299, 299f

Pushing the wave, 464, 465f

Push-off, alternating, 347t

Push-up
medicine ball power, 348f, 348t
power, 348f, 348t

Push-up test, 213–214, 213f, 214t

Q

Q-angle, 286

Qigong, 457–458, 464, 465f

Quad dominance, 286

Quadriceps length, Thomas test for, 160, 160f, 161t

Quadruped drawing-in (centering) with extremity movement, 257–258, 258f, 259t

Quadrupeds, rocking, 271f

Qualifications, personality traits in, 18

Questioning, 103
in effective listening, 47
in motivational interviewing, 51

R

Radial artery, 125

Radiculopathy, nerve, 543

Range of motion (ROM), 174
full, performing exercises through, 322
by joint, 158–159, 158t
plane of movement in, 247

Rapport
in ACE IFT Model, 84
on adherence, 57
attributes of, 100
behavioral strategies and, in ACE IFT Model, 86–87
building of, 99–100 (*See also* Investigation stage, of client–trainer relationship)
in investigation stage, 100–101
stages of, 100, 100f
value of, 100
components of, 100
cultural competence for, 56–57

Rapport stage, of client–trainer relationship, 40–45
first impressions in, 40–41, 41t
negative experiences in, 41
nonverbal communication in, 42
overview of, 40
personality styles in, 42–45
dominance scale of, 42, 43f, 43t, 44f
general traits in, 43t
identifying and working with, 43, 45t
self-assessment of, 42–43, 44f
sociability scale of, 42, 43f, 43t, 44f
positive experiences in, 41, 41t
verbal communication in, 41

Rate coding, power training for, 91

Ratings of perceived exertion (RPE), 129, 129t, 191t, 378–379, 378t, 379t
in aerobic-base training, 93
in aerobic-efficiency training, 93
in anaerobic-endurance training, 94
in anaerobic-power training, 95
in cardiorespiratory training, 378, 378t, 379, 379t [*See also* Ratings of perceived exertion (RPE)]
classical vs. contemporary scales of, 378, 378t
in elderly, strength training and, 356
in graded exercise tests, 191, 191t
on participation and adherence, 29
session, 379
training progression and option using, 378, 379t

Reactive ability, 346

Reactivity, 174

Reciprocal inhibition, 250

Record keeping, 554, 562

Recovery
in cardiorespiratory training, 404–405
overtraining syndrome and, 400
role of, 94–95

Referrals, 13, 47

Reflecting, 47, 103

Refreezing, after frostbite, 577

Regeneration, in cardiorespiratory training, 404–405

Registered dietitians, 6

Reinforcement
negative, 72–73
positive, 72

Relapse
prevention of, 34–35
in transtheoretical model of behavioral change, 70

Relationships, building, 636

Relative strength, 221

Repetitions
in resistance training, 320–321, 321t, 332–334
in speed, agility, and reactivity training, 350, 350t

Repetition-volume calculation, 320

Report, incident, 554

Resistance, exercise components for, 83t

Resistance training, 311–364. *See also* Functional movement and resistance training
benefits of, 312–314
body composition, 312
bone mineral density, 312, 313
injury risk and disease prevention, 313–314
metabolic function, 313
other, 313–314
physical appearance, 312
physical capacity, 312
equipment options for
bodyweight training, 357
cables, 356–357
free weights, 357
medicine balls, 357
selectorized equipment, 356
tubing, 357
ergogenic aids and supplements for
anabolic-androgenic steroids and related compounds,359–360
β-alanine, 358–359
caffeine, 359
carnosine, 358
creatine, 359
protein and amino-acid supplements, 358
sodium bicarbonate, 358–359
vitamins and minerals, 359
growth hormone and testosterone in, 315
in movement-training phase, 90
muscular strength/power/endurance relationship in, 317, 317f
myths and mistakes in, 360–363
free weights vs. machines, 361–362
light vs. heavy weights for muscle tone vs. mass, 360–361
muscle turning to fat, 362
regional fat deposit targeting, 360
strength training on blood pressure, 362–363
weightlifting in children, 361
weightlifting in elderly, 361
weight training for bulky muscles in women, 360
periodization models of, 326–329
linear, 326, 327f, 328t
sample protocols, 327, 328t–329t
time segments, 326, 327f
undulating, 326–327, 327f, 329t
physiological adaptations to, 314–317
acute, 314
long-term, 314
motor learning, 314
muscle hypertrophy, 314–315
muscle remodeling, 315
program design in, ACE IFT Model, 330–354 (*See also* specific phases)
phase 1: stability and mobility training, 330
phase 2: movement training, 330–332
phase 3: load training, 333–341
phase 3: performance training, 341–354
program progressions in, 320, 321f
traditional, 90
training principles in, 323–326
delayed-onset muscle soreness, 323–324
diminishing returns, 326
overload, 325
progression, 324–325
reversibility, 325–326
specificity, 325
training stress and microtrauma, 323
training variables in, 318–323
exercise selection and order, 319–320, 321f
needs assessment, 318
rest intervals, 322–323, 323t
training frequency, 318–319, 319t
training intensity, 321–322
training tempo, 322
training volume, 320–321, 321t
for youth, 355

Respiratory conditions, on physical activity, 116–117

Respiratory exchange ratio (RER), in ventilatory threshold resting, 202

Respiratory system, cardiorespiratory training on, 370–371

Respondeat superior, 604–605

Responsibilities and ethics, 11–15, 15t. *See also* Scope of practice

Responsibilities and ethics, professional, 11–15,

15t. *See also* Responsibilities and ethics
ACE Code of Ethics in, 11, 659–665
ACE professional practices and disciplinary procedures in, 11–12
appropriate scope of practice in, 15, 15t
certification period and renewal in, 12
client privacy in, 12–13
offering services outside scope of practice and, 14–15
referral in, 13
safety in, 14
supplements in, 14

Rest, for musculoskeletal injuries, 538

Resting heart rate (RHR), 49t
body position on, 378
in elderly, strength training and, 356
key notes on, 125
measurement of, 125–126

Resting metabolic rate (RMR), resistance training on, 312, 318

Rest intervals, in resistance training, 322–323, 323t

Restricted activity, for musculoskeletal injuries, 538

Retention, client, marketing for, 640–641

Return on investment (ROI), 631

Reverse flys with supine 90-90, 277f

Reversibility
muscle, 326
in resistance training, 325–326

Riboflavin, 359

RICE, 579

Right-angle rule, 137, 137f

Risk analysis, in business plan, 633, 633f

Risk appraisal. *See* Health-risk appraisal

Risk management, 621–622, 621t

Risk stratification, 105–107
for cardiovascular disease, 107, 108t
exercise testing and testing supervision based on, 107, 109f–110f

Rocking quadrupeds, 271f

Rockport fitness walking test (1 mile), 206–207, 207t

Role and scope of practice, 3–19
ACE Personal Trainer certification in, 7–15 (*See also* Certification, ACE Personal Trainer)
in allied healthcare continuum, 5–7, 6f
benefits of physical activity and, 3–4, 4t
career development in, 17–19
client population in, 5
in exercise program design, 4–5
scope of practice in, 7–10

Role clarity, 33

Role models, trainers as, 54–55

Romberg test, sharpened, 166–167, 167f

Rotational movements, 89, 331

Rotational movement training, 304–307, 305f–306f, 330–331
hay-bailer patterns, 304, 306f, 307
wood chops
full, 304, 306f
spiral patterns, 304, 305f

Rotator cuff injuries, 540, 541f

Rotator cuff muscles, in arm abduction, 272, 272f

Royalty, 620

Rule of threes, 401–402, 402f

Running surfaces, softer, 546

S

Safety, client, 14

Safety guidelines, 614

SAID principle, 386–387

Sarcomere length-tension relationship, 248–249, 248f, 249f

Sarcopenia, 406

Sarcoplasmic hypertrophy, 315

Scapula, normal position of, 144, 144f

Scapular protraction, 145, 145f

Scapulothoracic joint, 144, 144f, 246

Scapulothoracic proximal stability exercises
anterior capsule stretch, 273, 273f
arm roll, 280f
closed kinetic chain movements, 274
closed kinetic chain weight shifts, 279f
diagonals, 276f
fundamentals of, 272–273, 272f
humeral rotation, internal and external, 275f
open kinetic chain movements, 274
overhead triceps stretch, 273, 273f
posterior capsule stretches, 273, 273f
prone arm lifts, 278f
reverse flys with supine 90-90, 277f
shoulder packing, 274, 274f

superior capsule stretch, 273, 273f
for tissue extensibility, 273, 273f

Scapulothoracic region
in proximal mobility exercises, 251
proximal stability of, 272–280
in stability and mobility training, 251

Scar, 537

Scene safety, emergency, 560

Sciatica, 543

Scope of practice, 7–10, 8t, 614–616
for ACE-certified Personal Trainers, 8–10, 9f
appropriate, 15, 15t
definition and principles of, 7–8, 8t
dietary recommendations and, 9
laws on, 7, 10
new medical conditions and, 47
offering services outside of, 14–15
physician guidelines and, 10
signs and symptoms and, 107, 109f–110f
supplements and, 14

Seasonal exercise, 389

Second ventilatory threshold (VT2)
in anaerobic-endurance training, 94
in anaerobic-power training, 95
blood lactate and, 383f, 384–385, 384f
in cardiorespiratory training, 383–385, 383f–385f
definition of, 204
in talk test, 382
for training zones, 385, 385f
VT2 threshold test for, 204–205, 205f

Sedentary clients, initial conditioning stage for, 84

Seizures, 577–578

Selectorized equipment, 356

Self-acceptance, 55

Self-directed exercise, pre-screening for, 105, 106f

Self-discipline, 55

Self-disclosure, 47

Self-efficacy, 30–31, 66–68

Self-esteem, 67. *See also* Self-efficacy

Self-monitoring, 75

Self-monitoring systems, 52

Self-regulation, 34

Selling personal training, 648–653
changing lives in, 652
client motivation in, 650
closing the sale in, 651
earning respect and trust in, 650
emotional needs identification in, 650
empathy in, 650
first meeting in, 651
leadership in, 649
learning about client in, 652
marketing in, 649
play time in, 649–650
questions in, 651–652
sales in, 648–649
salesperson in, 649
sensitivity in, 650
seven basic rules of, 649–650
training programs in, 652–653
training session commitment in, 648
transtheoretical model of behavior change in, 652
value of professional trainer in, 651

Seriousness, perceived, 64–65

Sets
in resistance training, 332
in speed, agility, and reactivity training, 350, 350t

Shaping, 73

Sharpened Romberg test, 166–167, 167f

Shear force, 578

Shin splints, 117
fundamentals of, 548–549, 549f
vs. stress fractures, 536, 536f

Shivering, 576

Shock, 585

Shock, diabetic, 572, 572f

Shoes, athletic, 544

Shoulder bridge, 266f

Shoulder flexion and extension test, 162–163, 163f, 163t

Shoulder impingement, clearing test for, 150

Shoulder mobility assessments, 162–166
Apley's scratch test for shoulder mobility, 162, 165–166, 165f, 166f, 166t
internal and external rotation of humerus at shoulder, 164, 164f, 165t, 255f
shoulder flexion and extension test, 162–163, 163f, 163t

Shoulder packing, 274, 274f

Shoulder position, in postural assessment, 143–145, 144f, 145t

Shoulder pull stabilization screen, 156–157, 156f, 156t

Shoulder push stabilization screen, 155, 155f, 156t

Shoulder strain/sprain, 538–539, 539f, 539t

Shuffles, lateral, 353t

Side bridge, 512f

Side position, for unconscious victim, 572

Signs and symptoms. *See also specific disorders and tests*
  in graded exercise tests, 191
  of test termination, 107, 109f–110f, 122, 174

Single front/lateral box jumps, 347t

Single-leg movements, 89, 330

Single-leg stand pattern movement training, 292–298
  dynamic movement patterns over static base of support, 293–295, 293t, 294f
  half-kneeling lunge rise, 295, 295f
  lunge matrix, 296, 297f–298f
  lunge progressions, 296
  lunges, 296f
  lunges, effective, 295–296, 295f–296f
  overview, 292, 292f
  progression, 295
  static balance on a single leg, 293–295, 293t, 294f

Single leg, static balance on, 293–295, 293t, 294f

Single linear jumps, 347t

Situational motivation, 30

Sivananda yoga, 459, 460f–461f

Size, body. *See also* Body mass index (BMI); Weight, body
  measurement of, 185–189
    body mass index, 185–186, 185t, 186t
    circumference sites and procedures, 187t
    girth measurements, 186–187, 187f, 187t
    waist circumference, 188–189, 188t
  in SMART goal setting, 49t

Skill level, 49t

Skill-related physiological assessments, 174

Skills, 53–54. *See also specific skill tests*

Skinfold caliper, 178

Skinfold formulas, 178

Skinfold measurements, 175, 177, 178–182
  abdominal, 178, 179f
  chest, 178, 179f
  Jackson and Pollock formula for
    in men, 181t
    in women, 182t
  overview of, 177t
  protocol for, 183, 184t
  skinfold caliper in, 178
  skinfold formulas for, 178
  suprailium, 178, 180f
  thigh
    in men, 178, 179f
    in women, 178, 180f
  triceps, 178, 180f

Skull, 581

Slow-twitch muscle fibers. *See* Type I muscle fibers

Small-group training, 638–640

SMART goals
  for business operation, 644–646
  in cognitive behavioral techniques, 75
  for fitness, 48, 49t

SMART guidelines, 33

SOAP note, 480

Sociability scale, 42, 43f, 43t, 44f

Social networking, 637

Social support
  on behavior change, 72
  on participation and adherence, 28
  for relapse prevention, 34
  via behavior-change contracts, 55

Sodium bicarbonate, as supplement, 358–359

Softer running surfaces, 546

Soft-tissue injuries, 578–580, 579f

Sole proprietorships, 594–595, 599t

Soleus stretch, 552, 552f

Somatic yoga, 463

Specialization, 18

Special populations, 95, 480–481. *See also specific populations*

Specificity, 88, 325, 386–387

Speed, 174, 342

Speed, agility, and quickness testing, 237–240
  40-yard dash, 238–239, 239f, 239t
  pro agility test, 237, 237f, 237t
  T-test, 238, 238f, 238t
  use of, 236
  warm-up before, 236

Speed, agility, and reactivity training, 346, 350–354
  agility ladder/hurdle drills, 352t, 353f
  cone/marker drills, 353t
  definitions and components, 346, 350
  frequency, 350

intensity, 350, 350t
periodization for peak performance in key competitions, 350, 354t
repetitions and sets, 350, 350t
speed drills, 351f–352f, 351t
training tips, 350

Speed drills, 349, 351t
in plyometric exercise, 349
in speed, agility, and reactivity training, 351f–352f, 351t

Speed-endurance, 346

Speed-strength, 346

Speed training, 346, 350

Spinal column, 583–584, 584f

Spinal extensions, 268f–269f

Spinal twists, 269f

Spine, core and, 255, 255f

Spine injuries, 583–584, 584f

Spiral (rotational) movements, 89, 331

Spiral (rotational) movement training, 304–307, 305f–306f, 330–331

Spiritual dancing, Native American and Alaskan, 468–469

Splinting
of ankle, 581, 581f
of forearm, 581, 581f

Sport-skill assessments, 230–239
power testing: field tests, 230–236
anaerobic capacity
300-yard shuttle run, 235–236, 236t
Margaria–Kalamen stair climb test, 234–235, 234f, 234t
anaerobic power
kneeling overhead toss, 233–234, 233f
standing long jump test, 231–232, 232t
vertical jump test, 232–233, 232f, 233t
clients for, 231
contraindications for, 231
principles of, 230–231
speed, agility, and quickness testing, 237–240
40-yard dash, 238–239, 239f, 239t
pro agility test, 237, 237f, 237t
T-test, 238, 238f, 238t
use of, 236
warm-up before, 236
use and content of, 230

Sprain
ankle, 535f, 549–551 (*See also* Ankle sprains)
cervical, 583
shoulder, 538–539, 539f, 539t

Squat
bend-and-lift patterns, 286, 287–288
with resistance, 331
variations of, 291f

Squat test
1-RM, 227–229, 228f
bodyweight, 220–221, 221f, 221t

Stability
joint, 246
of kinetic chain, 246, 247f

Stability and mobility training, 251–284
case studies of
David (57-year-old executive, fit and active), 421, 422t
Sharon (33-year-old female, fit pre-pregnancy), 413–414, 415t
Stanley (28-year-old male, sedentary), 433–434, 434t
for deconditioned, 253f, 254
distal extremities in, 251
distal mobility in, 280, 281f
distal mobility of glenohumeral joint in, 272–280
hips and thoracic spine in, 251
lumbar spine in, 251
programming sequence for, 252, 252f
proximal mobility exercises in, for hips and thoracic spine, 258–271 (*See also* Mobility exercises, proximal)
proximal stability exercises in, 254–258 (*See also* Stability exercises, proximal)
proximal stability of scapulothoracic region in, 272–280
resistance training in, 330
static balance in
integrated (standing), 283–284
segmental, 281–283, 282f, 283t

Stability exercises, proximal, 254–258
activating the core in, 254–257, 255f–257f
core function in, 257–258, 257f, 257t, 258f
exercise progression for core activation, 257, 257t
exercise progression for core stabilization, 258, 259f
quadruped drawing-in (centering) with extremity movement, 257–258, 258f, 259t
supine drawing-in (centering), 257, 257f
core in, 254–255, 255f
for scapulothoracic region
anterior capsule stretch, 273, 273f
arm roll, 280f

closed kinetic chain movements, 274
closed kinetic chain weight shifts, 279f
diagonals, 276f
fundamentals of, 272–273, 272f
humeral rotation, 275f
open kinetic chain movements, 274
overhead triceps stretch, 273, 273f
posterior capsule stretches, 273, 273f
prone arm lifts, 278f
reverse flys with supine 90-90, 277f
shoulder packing, 274, 274f
superior capsule stretch, 273, 273f
for tissue extensibility, 273, 273f

Stability of scapulothoracic region, proximal
key factors in, 273
theory of, 272–273, 272f

Stability training, 88–89

Stages-of-change model. *See* Transtheoretical model of behavioral change

Stages of learning, 58

Stair climb test, Margaria–Kalamen, 234–235, 234f, 234t

Stance-position progressions, 283–284, 284f

Standard of care, 604

Standing ankle mobilization, 281, 282f

Standing calf stretches, 552, 552f

Standing long jump test, 231–232, 232t

Standing long/vertical jumps, 347t

Static balance
integrated (standing), 283–284, 283t, 284f
segmental, 281–283, 282f, 283t
on single leg, 293–295, 293t, 294f

Static-balance training, 282–283, 283t

Static postural assessment, 136–146
checklist for, 147f
deviation 1 in: ankle pronation/supination, 139–140, 140f, 141f, 141t
deviation 2 in: hip adduction, 141, 141f, 142t
deviation 3 in: hip tilting, 142–143, 142f, 142t, 143f
deviation 4 in: shoulder position and thoracic spine, 143–145, 144f, 145t
deviation 5 in: head position, 145–146, 146f, 146t
factors in, 136
insights from, 136
movement efficiency pattern in, 136–137, 137f
muscle balance in, 136–137, 137f
overview of, 136
plumb line positions in, 137f, 138–139
right-angle rule in, 137, 137f
stability and mobility restoration in, 137
worksheets for
anterior/posterior, 148f
sagittal, 149f

Static stretches, 253, 253f

Statute of frauds, 602

Statute of limitations, 610

Steady state, 372

Steady-state exercise, adaptations to, 372

Steady-state heart rate (HRss), 192

Step tests, 208–212
for cardiorespiratory fitness testing, 211–212
contraindications to, 208
McArdle, 211
use and principles of, 208
YMCA submaximal, 208–209, 209f, 210t

Steroids, anabolic-androgenic, 359–360

Stimulus control, 72, 74

"Stinger," 583

Stork-stand balance test, 167–168, 167f

Straight-leg raise
passive, 161–162, 161f, 162t
in supine position, 547, 547f

Strain, 579
cervical, 583
ligament, 534–535, 534f, 535t
muscle, 533–534, 533t
shoulder, 538–539, 539f, 539t

Strength. *See also specific types*
absolute, 221
muscular (*See* Muscular strength)
power and, 231
relative, 221

Strength ratios, 230, 230t

Strength testing, submaximal, 229–230, 230t

Strength training. *See also* Resistance training
on blood pressure, 362–363
for elderly, 355–356
goal of, 91
teaching exercises for, 54
for youth, 355

Stress fracture, 536, 536f, 580

Stress injuries, 580

Stress, training
in resistance training, 323
on tissue microtrauma, 323

Stretches. *See also specific types*
ballistic, 253, 253f
dynamic, 253, 253f
myofascial release in, 253, 253f
by phase of workout session, 252–253, 253f
proprioceptive neuromuscular facilitation in, 253, 253f
static, 253, 253f

Stretching
on elasticity, 373
in warm-up, 373

Stretch reflex, load training for, 91–92

Stretch-shortening cycle, 343–344. *See also* Plyometric exercise

Stroke, 570–571
exercise and, 485–486
exercise guidelines and sample recommendation with, 486
overview of, 485

Stroke volume, 125, 370

Subchapter S-corporation, 597–598, 599t

Submaximal talk test, 202–204

Submaximal talk test for VT1, 391

Submaximal workload, heart rate with, 49t

Sudden cardiac arrest
CPR for, 565–566
fundamentals of, 565

Sudden cardiac death
CPR for, 565–566
fundamentals of, 565

Sugar, blood, in SMART goal setting, 49t

Summarizing, 47

Sun salutation, 459, 460f–461f

Sunscreen, 576

Sun style tai chi, 466

Superior capsule stretch, 273, 273f

Supervision, legal responsibilities for, 613

Supination, ankle
on kinetic chain, 140, 141f, 141t
in postural assessment, 139–140, 140f, 141f, 141t

Supine 90-90 hip rotator stretch, 267f

Supine 90-90 neutral back, 260f

Supine bent-knee marches, 262f

Supine drawing-in (centering), 257, 257f

Supine vertical chest toss, 348t, 349f

Supplements. *See also specific supplements*
advice on, 616
protein and amino-acid, 358
scope of practice and, 14

Supported half-dog pose, 459f

Suprailium skinfold measurements, 178, 180f

Susceptibility, perceived, 65

"Swimmer's back," 584

SWOT analysis, 633, 633f

Syncope, 107, 570

Syncope, heat, 573

Synergistic dominance, 250

Systolic blood pressure (SBP), 116, 126
classification of, 128t
Korotkoff sound for, 127, 127f
measurement of, 128

T

Table-top kneeling lat stretch, 268f

Tachycardia, 107

Tai chi
for high blood pressure, 484–485
research-supported outcomes and benefits of, 455t, 457–458

Talk test, 93
in cardiorespiratory training, 382–383
submaximal, 202–204

Tanaka, Monahan, and Seals formula, for maximum heart rate, 376

Target exercise heart rate, Tanaka, Monahan, and Seal formula for, 197

Target heart rate, for heat acclimatization, 576

Target heart-rate range (THRR), 201

Teaching. *See also* Learning
effective communication in, 58–59
individualized, 52, 53t
techniques of, 39–59 (*See also* Communication and teaching techniques)

Television broadcasts, 620

"Tell, show, do," 53–54

Tempo, training, in resistance training, 322

Tendinitis, 533–534, 533t, 535
elbow, 539t, 540–541, 541f
infrapatellar, 547–548

Tendon
collagen in, 579

insertion point of, on muscular strength and hypertrophy, 317

Tennis elbow, 540–541, 541f

Testimonial book, 636–637

Testing forms, 110. *See also specific forms*

Testing supervision, risk stratification for, 109f–110f

Testosterone
- on muscle, in elderly, 406
- on muscular strength and hypertrophy, 315

Test termination signs and symptoms, 107, 109f–110f, 122, 174. *See also specific disorders and tests*

Thigh circumference measurement
- midthigh, 187t
- upper thigh, 187t

Thigh skinfold measurements
- in men, 178, 179f
- in women, 178, 180f

Thomas test for hip flexion/quadriceps length, 160, 160f, 161t

Thoracic spine
- in functional stability and mobility training, 251
- in postural assessment, 143–145, 144f
- stability and mobility of, 246

Thoracic spine mobility screen, 157–158, 157f, 157t

Thoracic (T-)spine mobilization exercises
- prisoner rotations, 270f
- spinal extensions, 268f–269f
- spinal twists, 269f

Threat, perceived, 64

300-yard shuttle run, 235–236, 236t

Three-zone training model, 385, 385f, 391, 392t–393t

Three-zone training model intensity markers, 391, 392t–393t

Tidal volume
- cardiorespiratory exercise on, 371
- in ventilatory threshold resting, 202

Time, exercise, 28

Time management, 646–648

Tissue plasminogen activator (tPA), 571

Tonality (voice), 102

Tonic clonic seizure, 577–578

Tools, assessment, 124–125, 124t. *See also specific tools*

Tooth injuries, 583

Torso lean, 144

Total body electrical conductivity, 177t

Training. *See specific types*

Training components and phases, 85–95, 86t
- cardiorespiratory training in, 92–95
- functional movement and resistance training in, 88–92
- overview of, 85–86, 86t, 87–88
- purpose of, 87–88

Training effect, 393–395

Training frequency. *See* Frequency, exercise/training

Training intensity. *See* Intensity, exercise/training

Training monotony, 400, 401f

Training programs. *See specific types*
- selling (*See* Selling personal training)

Training stress
- in resistance training, 323
- in tissue microtrauma, 323

Training tempo, 322

Training volume, 320–321, 321t, 332–334

Transient ischemic attack (TIA), 571

Transportation, 621

Transtheoretical model of behavioral change, 26, 67–72, 103. *See also* Adherence; Motivation
- action phase of, 641
- decisional balance in, 69–70, 70f
- examples of, 71–72
- overview of, 67
- process of change in, 68, 69t
- self-efficacy in, 68
- in selling personal training, 652
- stages of change in, 67–68

Transverse abdominis
- activation of, 256
- with back pain, 256
- in core, 255–256, 255f, 256f

Transverse plane, motion in, 89

Treadmill exercise testing, 192–196
- Balke & Ware, 194–195, 195t
- Bruce submaximal treadmill exercise test
  - equipment in, 193
  - pre-test procedure for, 193
  - protocol and administration of, 193–194,

193t
use of, 192–193
contraindications to, 193
Ebbeling single-stage, 195–196, 196f
protocols for, 192–193
use of, 192

Tree pose, 471–472, 472

Trendelenburg gait, 543

Triceps skinfold measurements, 178, 180f

Triceps stretch, overhead, 273, 273f

Triglycerides, 489, 489t

Triplanar stretch, half-kneeling, 264f

Trunk extensor endurance test, 218–219, 219f

Trunk flexor endurance test, 217–218, 217f

Trunk lateral endurance test, 218, 219f

Trust, 32

T-shirts, 637

T-test, 238, 238f, 238t

Tubing, 357

Tucks, knee, 347t

2008 Physical Activity Guidelines for Americans, 82, 374

Type I muscle fibers
in functional stability and mobility training, 251–252
in low-intensity endurance exercise, 370
on muscular strength and hypertrophy, 316
in proximal mobility exercises, 251

Type II muscle fibers
in functional stability and mobility training, 252
in higher intensity exercise, 370
on muscular strength and hypertrophy, 316
power training on, 92
in proximal mobility exercises, 252

U

Umbrella liability insurance, 618

Unconscious victim, side position for, 572

Undulating periodization, 90, 326–327, 327f, 329t

Uniarticulate muscles, 259

Unilateral presses, 299, 300f

Unilateral pull-downs, 303–304, 303f

Universal precautions, 585

Upper-body endurance tests, push-up, 213–214, 213f, 214t

Upper-body strength, from 1-RM bench-press test, 224, 225t. *See also* 1-RM bench-press test

Upper-extremity musculoskeletal injuries
carpal tunnel syndrome, 539t, 541–542, 542f
conservative management of, 539, 539t
elbow tendinitis, 539t, 540–541, 541f
rotator cuff injuries, 540, 541f
shoulder strain/sprain, 538–539, 539f, 539t

V

Valgus stress, 285, 285f

Valsalva maneuver, 118

Vasoconstriction, 121

Velocity, 91

Velocity training, movement-pattern progressions for, 344, 344f

Ventilation, minute ($\dot{V}_E$)
cardiorespiratory exercise on, 371
exercise on, 383, 383f

Ventilatory response, to exercise, 383, 383f

Ventilatory threshold 1 (VT1). *See* First ventilatory threshold (VT1)

Ventilatory threshold 2 (VT2). *See* Second ventilatory threshold (VT1)

Ventilatory threshold (VT), cardiorespiratory training on, 371

Ventilatory threshold testing, 202–205
contraindications to, 202
individualized metabolic markers in, 202
principles of, 202
submaximal talk test for VT1, 202–204

Ventricular fibrillation (VF), 566

Verbal communication, 41

Verbal persuasion, 66

Vertical jump test, 232–233, 232f, 233t

Vicarious experience, 66

Vicarious liability, 604–605

Vigorous-intensity exercise programs, drop-out rate in, 29

Viniyoga yoga, 462

Vitamin B12, 359

Vitamin D, 359

Vitamins, 359

$\dot{V}O_2$
age correction factors for, 201, 201t
in cardiorespiratory training, 378–382, 381t
energy cost of cycling and, 199, 199f

$\dot{V}O_2$max, 189, 371
cardiorespiratory training on, 371, 371f
conversion of, 199, 199f
equation for, 196
estimated, accuracy of, 189
from heart-rate response, 189
norms for, 191, 191t
relative percent concept in, 380
training based on percentages of, 378–380

$\dot{V}O_2$ reserve ($\dot{V}O_2$R), training based on, 378–380

Voice quality, 42, 102

Volume, in resistance training, 320–321, 321t, 332–334

VT1. *See* First ventilatory threshold (VT1)

VT2. *See* Second ventilatory threshold (VT1)

VT2 threshold test, 391

W

Waist circumference, 188–189
measurement of, 187f, 187t, 188–189
risk categories for, 188, 188t

Waist-to-hip ratio, 188, 188t

Waivers, 110, 602, 603f, 604–605, 610

Waivers, group, 610

Walking test
Rockport fitness (1 mile), 206–207, 207t
in SMART goal setting, 49t

Warmth, 100

Warm-up, 372–373

Water-based exercise, 390

Water depletion, 574

Web developer, 643

Website, 637

Weighing, hydrostatic, 176–178, 177t

Weight, body
calculation of goals for, 184
lean, 313
in SMART goal setting, 49t

Weightlifting
in children, 361
in elderly, 361

Weight loss, cardiorespiratory training for. *See* under Cardiorespiratory training

Weight management. *See also* Overweight
exercise and, 514
exercise guidelines for, 514
fitness membership for, 176
overview of, 513–514
sample exercise recommendation for, 515

Weights
free vs. machines, 361–362
light vs. heavy, for muscle tone vs. mass, 360–361

Weight training, for bulky muscles in women, 360

Wet bulb globe temperature (WBGT), 575

Whey, 358

Whole-body movement patterns, with gravity for resistance, 90

Winged scapulae, 145

Wood chops
full, 304, 306f
spiral patterns, 304, 305f

Work, 91

Workload, submaximal, heart rate in, 49t

Workout session, in cardiorespiratory training
conditioning phase, 373
cool-down, 374
overview, 372
warm-up, 372–373

Wrist nerves, 541, 542f

Written agreements, 33, 74

Wu style tai chi, 466

Y

Yang style tai chi, 466

YMCA bike test, 197–199, 198f, 199f

YMCA submaximal step test, 208–209, 209f, 210t

Yoga, hatha, 458–466
anusara, 462
ashtanga, 462
Bikram, 462
branches of, 458
breathing training (pranayama), 463
general precautions with, 463–464
hatha, 458–459
for high blood pressure, 484–485
history of, 458
integral, 462
Iyengar, 462

kripalu, 462
kundalini, 462–463
personal trainer use of, 471
research-supported outcomes and benefits of, 455t, 456–457
restorative, 459, 459f
Sivananda, 459, 460f–461f
somatic, 463
viniyoga, 462

Yogic breathing
pranayama, 463
with warm-up and cool-down exercises, 471

Youth
cardiorespiratory training in, 405–406
exercise and, 518
exercise guidelines for, 518–520, 519t
sample exercise recommendations for, 520–521

Z

Zinc, 359

Zone 1, 94

Zone 2, 94

Zone 3, 94

Zones, training
cardiorespiratory training, 94
VT1 and VT2 in, 385, 385f